PeriAnesthesia Nursing Core Curriculum

PREOPERATIVE, PHASE I and
PHASE II PACU NURSING

AMERICAN SOCIETY OF PERIANESTHESIA NURSES

PeriAnesthesia Nursing Core Curriculum

PREOPERATIVE, PHASE I and PHASE II PACU NURSING

Donna M. DeFazio Quinn, BSN, MBA, RN, CPAN, CAPA
Director
Orthopaedic Surgery Center
Concord, New Hampshire

Lois Schick, MN, MBA, RN, CPAN, CAPA
Per Diem Staff Nurse
Exempla Lutheran Medical Center
Wheatridge, Colorado
Per Diem Staff Nurse
Littleton Adventist Hospital
Littleton, Colorado

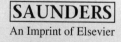
An Imprint of Elsevier

SAUNDERS
An Imprint of Elsevier

11830 Westline Industrial Drive
St. Louis, Missouri 63146

PERIANESTHESIA NURSING CORE CURRICULUM:
PREOPERATIVE, PHASE I AND PHASE II PACU NURSING

NOTICE

ISBN-13:   978-0-7216-0365-0
ISBN-10:   0-7216-0365-3

Executive Editor: Michael S. Ledbetter
Developmental Editor: Amanda Sunderman Politte
Publishing Services Manager: Melissa Lastarria
Design Manager: Bill Drone

Printed in the United States of America

Last digit is the print number: 9   8   7   6   5   4

To Gia and Tian, the sunshine of my life.
Donna M. DeFazio Quinn

To my mother, who was always there for me until her death and who was instrumental in my becoming a nurse. I also dedicate this book to my 11 older brothers and sisters for all their love, support, and guidance through the years.
Lois Schick

CONTRIBUTORS

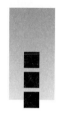

MEG BETURNE, BSN, RN, CPAN
Perioperative QI Consultant
Level III RN, Ambulatory Center
Springfield, MA

LINDA BOYUM, RN, BSN, CPAN, LHRM
Director of Nursing
Atlantic Surgery Center
Daytona Beach, FL

NANCY BURDEN, RN, MS, CPAN, CAPA
Director of Outpatient Services
Morton Plant Mease Health Care
New Port Richey, FL

KATHLYN CARLSON, MA, RN, CPAN
Staff RN, Surgical Services
Abbott Northwestern Hospital
Minneapolis, MN

THERESA L. CLIFFORD, RN, MSN, CPAN
Clinical Nurse III in Phase I PACU
Mercy Hospital;
Per Diem Staff Nurse
Western Avenue Day Surgery Center
Portland, ME

PAMELA M. DARK, RN, MSN, CAPA
Intermountain Health Care
Urban Central Region Hospitals
Surgical Services Education Coordinator
Salt Lake City, UT

JANE C. DIERENFIELD, BSN, RN, CAPA, CPAN
Kailua-Kona, HI

ROSE FERRARA-LOVE, MSN, RN, CPAN, CAPA, CNAA, BC
Nursing Instructor
Citizens School of Nursing
Alle-Kiske Medical Center
West Pennsylvania Allegheny Health System
New Kensington, PA

SUSAN JANE FETZER, RN, BA, BSN, PHD, MSN, MBA
Associate Professor
University of New Hampshire
Durham, NH
Staff Nurse
Elliot Hospital
Manchester, NH

KATY FLANAGAN, RN, CAPA
Grady Memorial Hospital
Delaware, OH

SUSAN A. GOODWIN, MS, RN, CNS, CPAN
Nurse Manager/Compliance Coordinator
Surgery Center of Edmond
Edmond, OK

VALLIRE D. HOOPER, MSN, RN, CPAN
Co-Editor, Journal of PeriAnesthesia
Nursing
Clinical Nurse Specialist, Surgical Services
St. Joseph Hospital
Assistant Clinical Professor
School of Nursing
Medical College of Georgia
Augusta, GA

LORI HOWARD, BSN, RN, CPAN
Staff Nurse, PACU
Surgery Center of Edmond
Edmond, OK

LISA P. JERAN, BSN, RN, CPAN
Clinical Supervisor
North Shore University Hospital
Long Island Jewish Healthcare System
Plainview, NY

MICHAEL KOST, CRNA, MS, MSN
Program Director
Montgomery Hospital Anesthesia Program
Morristown, PA

DINA A. KRENZISCHEK, RN, MAS, CPAN
Nurse Manager
Johns Hopkins Hospital
Baltimore, MD

MAUREEN E. LISBERGER, RN, BS, CCRN, CPAN
Aurora, CO

REX A. MARLEY, MS, CRNA, RRT
Chief Nurse Anesthetist
Northern Colorado Anesthesia Professional
Consultants
Fort Collins, CO

DONNA R. MCEWEN, RN, BSN, CNOR, CRCST
Staff Nurse
United Health Care
San Antonio, TX

LAURA F. MONETTE, RN, MS
Perioperative Clinical Nurse Specialist
Baystate Medical Center
Springfield, MA

GRATIA M. NAGLE, BA, CRNFA, CRLS, CURN
Paoli, PA

BONNIE S. NIEBUHR, MS, RN, CAE
Executive Director
American Board of Perianesthesia Nursing
Certification, Inc.
New York, NY

DEBBY NIEHAUS, BS, RN, CPAN
Clinical Nurse III
Bethesda North Ambulatory Surgery Center
Cincinnati, OH

DENISE O'BRIEN, MSN, RN, CPAN, CAPA
Clinical Nurse Specialist, Perianesthesia
Care Area
Department of Operating Rooms/PACU
University of Michigan Health System
Ann Arbor, MI

JAN ODOM-FORREN, MS, RN, CPAN, FAAN
Nursing Consultant
Louisville, KY

JUDITH E. ONTIVEROS, MSN, RN, CPAN, CAPA
Faculty
Skills Lab Coordinator
Health Sciences Division
Pasadena City College
Pasadena, CA

MARY C. REDMOND, BSN, RN, CAPA
Staff Nurse
Alegent Health Bergan Mercy Medical
Center
Omaha, NE

CAROLE A. RIES, BSN, RN, CPAN
Clinical Coordinator—SAC/PACU/ODSC
Poudre Valley Hospital Systems
Fort Collins, CO

NANCY M. SAUFL, MS, RN, CPAN, CAPA
ASPAN President 2000-2001
Coordinator, Preadmission Testing
Florida Hospital
Ormond Beach, FL

SHERRIE L. SMARTT, RN, BSN, CCRN
Critical Care Clinical Educator
Cox Health
Springfield, MO

JUDY STEVENSON, RN, BSN, CCRN
RN Educator, PACU and Same Day Surgery
Cox Health Systems
Springfield, MO
Staff Nurse
Trauma Emergency Center
Tulsa, OK

PAMELA E. WINDLE, RN, MS, CNA, CPAN, CAPA
Nurse Manager, Day Surgery Center
Post Anesthesia Care Unit
Surgical Observation Unit
St. Luke's Episcopal Hospital
Houston, TX

FOREWORD

The American Society of PeriAnesthesia Nurses (ASPAN) is committed to providing quality publications and resources for perianesthesia nurses that are current and cutting edge. Based on a variety of factors, ASPAN has determined that it is more efficacious to combine the content from the current separate cores into one core curriculum publication. This single resource provides the general information needed by nurses caring for perianesthesia patients in all settings where anesthesia or sedation/analgesia is administered.

The decision to combine the information previously contained in two separate core curriculum publications came in part as a result of the findings of a Study of Perianesthesia Nursing Practice, conducted by the American Board of Perianesthesia Nursing Certification, Inc. (ABPANC) from 1998 to 2000. This study found that all perianesthesia patients, regardless of the setting in which they receive care, have specific needs falling into four domains: physiological needs, behavioral and cognitive needs, safety needs, and advocacy needs. The knowledge needed by perianesthesia nurses to meet these needs was subsequently defined.

ASPAN remains uniquely responsible for providing the resources that meet the educational needs of perianesthesia nurses. Because the core curriculum is meant to serve a broader purpose than just certification examination preparation, the reader will find that the core curriculum includes more information that may be found on the CPAN and CAPA certification examinations. This approach ensures that ASPAN, as an education provider, can consistently meet the requests of *all* stakeholders.

To this end, ASPAN presents the first combined core curriculum. It will serve as an excellent guide to assist in the orientation of new staff, provide the framework for teaching perianesthesia nursing-related information, as well as provide an additional resource for studying in preparation for the CPAN and/or CAPA certification examinations.

Sandra Barnes, MS, RN, CPAN
President, American Society of PeriAnesthesia Nurses

PREFACE

The specialty of perianesthesia nursing is performed in a variety of settings. Once practiced only in the "recovery room," nurses now care for perioperative and post-procedure patients in an array of surroundings—hospital-based and freestanding. Perianesthesia nursing encompasses caring for patients during the preanesthesia phase (preadmission and day of surgery/procedure), in PACUs (phase I and II), ambulatory care settings, phase III settings, and special procedure areas (endoscopy, radiology, cardiovascular, oncology, etc.), labor and delivery suites, pain management services, and physician and dental offices. Nurses caring for perianesthesia patients need to possess a variety of skills and expertise. Patients undergoing operative and invasive procedures come to the facility either as a planned event or an emergency. Being able to assess the patient, develop an individualized plan of care, implement the plan, and evaluate the results requires proficiency in perianesthesia nursing.

This review text is designed to be a resource for nurses working in the perianesthesia setting. It is intended to cover perianesthesia knowledge essential to practice in both the hospital-based or freestanding setting. Regardless in which practice setting the perianesthesia nurse works, there is a group of core competencies essential to providing good nursing care. To include the wide span of knowledge perianesthesia nurses must possess, the text is divided into seven sections:

- Professional Competencies
- Environment of Care
- Life Span Considerations
- Competency of Perioperative Assessment
- Core Competencies of PACU Nursing
- Surgical Specialties
- Ambulatory Surgical Nursing Competencies

This text is also a resource for nurses preparing to take either the CPAN or CAPA certification examination. Certification in one's specialty is a way to promote quality of care to the general public, the nursing profession, and the individual nurse. When a nurse achieves certification in his or her specialty, this demonstrates commitment to his or her nursing career, provides tremendous personal satisfaction, and provides opportunities for career advancement.

The text uses an outline format to delineate areas of perianesthesia nursing practice. The text is not designed to be a complete study guide. The nurse must identify his or her own areas of strengths and weaknesses, seek out additional resources, and develop an individualized study plan that will meet one's needs.

Although designed to assist nurses in preparation of the CPAN or CAPA examination, this book can be used for other purposes such as:

- A study guide for nurses new to the perianesthesia setting
- Development of an orientation plan for the PACU
- Development of perianesthesia nursing competencies
- A reference guide for student nurses rotating through the PACU

The chapter authors are experts in their fields of practice and many of them are certified in their specialties. The information presented in this text is as accurate and current as possible. Each chapter has been reviewed numerous times to ensure accuracy.

The development of this core curriculum was sponsored by and supported by the American Society of PeriAnesthesia Nurses (ASPAN).

Donna M. DeFazio Quinn, Coeditor
Lois Schick, Coeditor

ACKNOWLEDGMENTS

This Core Curriculum brings together the specialty of perianesthesia nursing by combining the original ASPAN *Core Curriculum for Perianesthesia Nursing Practice* and the *Ambulatory Surgical Nursing Core Curriculum* into one text. From its inception to its final reality, we encountered numerous challenges, but none so monumental that it could not be overcome. We wish to thank the authors who contributed chapters to this book. The time, energy, and dedication that each exhibited is a reflection of their devotion to their profession.

We wish to thank Melissa Lastarria from the production department at Elsevier for her expertise in coordinating this project and Cindy Geiss and Beth Callaway of Graphic World for their expertise in bringing this material to a finished product. We also wish to thank Dr. Jeffrey Rosenblum for his assistance and review of Chapter 44: Renal/Genitourinary Surgery, and Lisa Jeran for her assistance and review of Chapter 28: Thermoregulation.

Our sincere appreciation goes to Mary Parker at Elsevier who worked diligently behind the scenes handling any challenge presented and resolving it without delay.

Words cannot describe our gratitude to Amanda Politte, Developmental Editor at Elsevier. Amanda kept this task on track from the start. Her assistance in organizing this enormous project is greatly appreciated. During crunch times she was always there with support, encouragement, and words of kindness to get us through the darkest days.

As Executive Editor at Elsevier, Michael Ledbetter had the forethought to believe we could combine the two core curriculums and still make a book that would meet the needs of perianesthesia nurses everywhere. Thanks for all your support in bringing this project to fruition.

A special thank you goes to my husband, Stephen Quinn, for his patience and understanding when my laptop became a permanent fixture on the kitchen table. In addition, I owe a world of gratitude to my daughters, Gia Elizabeth and Tian Xing, for their ability to make me laugh when I need it most. Their smiles and hugs were the biggest comfort of all.

Donna M. DeFazio Quinn

A special thank you goes to my sister Jean Newton who has always been there to encourage and support me. Thank you Donna for sharing your hints and expertise as a coeditor. I could not have done this without you.

Lois Schick

Contents

PeriAnesthesia Nursing Core Curriculum

PREOPERATIVE, PHASE I and PHASE II PACU NURSING

PROFESSIONAL COMPETENCIES

1 Evolution of Perianesthesia Care

JAN ODOM-FORREN

OBJECTIVES
At the conclusion of this chapter, the reader will be able to:

1. Describe three of the earliest recovery rooms.
2. Name the decade when recovery rooms became commonplace.
3. Name the one historical event that contributed most to the advent of recovery rooms.
4. Name three advances in medical technology that led to an increase in ambulatory surgeries.
5. List three reasons for consumer acceptance of ambulatory surgery.
6. Describe the development of the American Society of PeriAnesthesia Nurses (ASPAN).
7. Describe three benefits brought to perianesthesia nursing by ASPAN.

■■ Knowledge of our collective history and the evolution of postanesthesia nursing have equipped us with the tools needed to define our specialty. This knowledge is essential to developing a certification program and also guides us in resolving issues and setting goals and priorities for the specialty.

EARLY BEGINNINGS

I. Early beginnings of recovery room and ambulatory surgery
  A. Trephining of the skull and amputations identified in the year 3500 B.C. as evidenced by cave drawings
  B. New Castle Infirmary, New Castle, England (1751): rooms reserved for dangerously ill or major surgery patients
  C. Florence Nightingale, London, England (1863): separate rooms for patients to recover from immediate effects of anesthesia
  D. Ambulatory surgeries performed at Glasgow Royal Hospital for Sick Children in Scotland from 1898 to 1908
    1. Surgeries performed on 8988 children
    2. Surgeries included orthopedic problems, cleft lip and cleft palate, spina bifida, skull fracture, hernias, and others.
    3. None of the children required hospital admission.
  E. Information from Glasgow Hospital presented at a meeting of the British Medical Association in 1909
  F. Twentieth century
    1. First general anesthesia in ambulatory surgery reported in Sioux City, Iowa, in 1918
    2. 1920s-1930s: complexity of surgeries increased
    3. 1923: Johns Hopkins Hospital, Baltimore, Maryland: three-bed neurosurgical recovery unit opened by Dandy and Firor
    4. World War II: recovery units created to provide adequate level of nursing care during nursing shortage
    5. 1942: Mayo Clinic, Rochester, Minnesota

   6. 1944: New York Hospital
   7. 1945: Ochsner Clinic, New Orleans, Louisiana
   8. 1940s and 1950s: early ambulation after surgery came into acceptance.
II. Value of recovery room demonstrated in improving surgical care
   A. Anesthesia Study Commission of the Philadelphia County Medical Society report (1947): one third of preventable postsurgical deaths during an 11-year period could have been prevented by improved postoperative nursing care.
   B. Operating Room Committee for New York Hospital (1949) stated that adequate recovery room service was necessary for any hospital that provided surgical services.

ACCEPTANCE AND DECLINE OF RECOVERY ROOMS

I. Impact of changing technology on patient care
   A. 1950s: more knowledge of common postanesthesia complications
   B. 1950s-1960s: growth of surgical intensive care and postoperative respiratory support
   C. Expanding complex surgical procedures
   D. Expanding technology led to outpatient complex surgeries.
      1. Microscopic surgeries abounded.
      2. New lasers were developed (yttrium argon gas, argon, carbon dioxide).
      3. New laparoscopic instruments facilitated shorter, less invasive laparoscopic procedures.
      4. More endoscopic procedures were being performed as outpatient procedures.
      5. Video equipment and computer-assisted surgeries were now being performed.
      6. Fiber optics led to advances in ophthalmic surgeries, most of which are performed in outpatient settings.
   E. Change in anesthesia techniques and medications
   F. 1970s: recovery rooms managed routine postanesthesia patients including ambulatory, routine, and critically ill patients receiving respiratory and circulatory support
   G. Many diagnostic procedures done in ambulatory settings.
      1. X-ray procedures
      2. Laboratory tests
      3. Physical therapy
      4. Cardiopulmonary tests
      5. Pain blocks
II. Recovery rooms lose viability and identity.
   A. Staffing: shortage of skilled personnel
   B. No organized body of knowledge pertinent to postanesthesia
      1. Staff performance evaluated on the basis of trial and error
      2. No territorial restrictions: in some places considered to be extension of operating room
      3. No established standards of care

AMBULATORY SURGERY FOCUS

I. Ambulatory surgery programs established
   A. The nation's first ambulatory surgery program opened at Butterworth Hospital in Grand Rapids, Michigan, in 1961, and staff performed 879 ambulatory surgeries between 1963 and 1964.
   B. A formal ambulatory surgery program was begun at UCLA in 1962.
   C. In 1968, the Dudley Street Ambulatory Surgery Center opened in Providence, Rhode Island.
   D. The nation's first freestanding surgery facility was opened in 1970 by Dr. Wallace Reed and Dr. John Ford in Phoenix, Arizona.
      1. In 1971, the American Medical Association endorsed the use of surgicenters.

    2. In 1974, the Society for the Advancement of Freestanding Ambulatory Surgery (FASC) was formed, which was the precursor for the current Federated Ambulatory Surgery Association (FASA).

  E. The American Society for Outpatient Surgeons (ASOS; now known as American Association of Ambulatory Surgery Centers) was formed in 1978, paving the way for surgery being performed in doctors' offices.

    1. The 1980s brought a shortage of inpatient hospital beds.

    2. In 1980, the Omnibus Budget Reconciliation Act (OBRA) authorized reimbursement for outpatient surgery.

    3. In 1981, the American College of Surgeons (ACS) approved the concept of ambulatory surgery units as preadmission units for scheduled inpatients.

    4. In 1983, Porterfield and Franklin advocated for office outpatient surgery.

    5. The Society for Ambulatory Anesthesia (SAMBA) was formed in 1984.

II. The ambulatory surgery concept proliferated in the 1980s.

  A. Hospital-affiliated ambulatory surgery accounted for 9.8 million operations (45%) performed within hospital settings by 1987.

  B. By 1988, 984 freestanding outpatient surgery centers performed over 1.5 million surgical operations.

  C. By 1989, there were 984 Medicare-participating freestanding ambulatory surgery centers in the United States.

  D. The list of approved procedures that can be conducted in surgery centers was expanded in 1987 by the Health Care Financing Administration (HCFA—now known as CMS, the Centers for Medicare and Medicaid Services).

  E. In 1989, HCFA revised the payment schedule for outpatient surgeries performed on Medicare patients.

III. Freestanding recovery sites

  A. In 1979, the first freestanding recovery center opened in Phoenix, Arizona.

    1. Patients were transported directly to the recovery center from hospital postanesthesia care units (PACUs), from ambulatory surgery units (ASUs), and from physicians' offices.

    2. Some patients were transferred there from hospitals on their second or third postoperative day.

  B. In California, patients may stay in recovery centers up to three days after their surgical procedures.

  C. In the 1980s, the concept of 23-hour units led to guest services being developed for patients living more than one hour away from the site where the surgery was to be performed (hospital hotels; medical motels).

    1. Freestanding medical motels are considered a comfortable, affordable, convenient place to recuperate.

    2. Patients are cared for by family members.

    3. Home health nurses make visits.

  D. Most recent figures from the National Center for Health Statistics (NCHS) Data Center

    1. An estimated 31.5 million surgical and nonsurgical procedures were performed during 20.8 million ambulatory visits in 1996.

    2. An estimated 17.5 million (84%) of the ambulatory surgery visits were in hospitals and 3.3 million (16%) were in freestanding centers in 1996.

    3. In 2000, 63% of all surgeries were performed in outpatient settings.

IV. Economics of ambulatory surgery

  A. Cost control a primary force in the development of ambulatory surgery

    1. In 1988, 58% of surgery centers contracted with health maintenance organizations (HMOs) and 52% with preferred provider organizations (PPOs).

    2. In 1990, the American Hospital Association (AHA) reported that greater than 50% of all hospital-based surgical procedures were done on an outpatient basis.

    3. In the 1990s, 23 home observation units (recovery centers) were established in the United States.

      4. Percent of outpatient procedures approved for payment under Medicare increased.
        a. In 1982, 450 procedures approved
        b. By the early 1990s, 2500 approved procedures
        c. On July 1, 2003, 282 additional procedures added
      5. Third-party payers require many surgeries to be performed in an ambulatory setting to avoid the cost of hospitalization.
      6. Many freestanding centers have contractual arrangements with managed care plans, rehabilitation centers, and nursing homes.
      7. Outpatient facilities eliminate the costs of cafeteria, laundry, and the need for 24-hour staffing.
      8. Outpatient procedures eliminate unnecessary lab, x-ray, and electrocardiogram services.
      9. Patients recovering in 23-hour units are considered not hospitalized for purposes of reimbursement by Medicare and third-party payers.
  V. Legislation encouraged growth of ambulatory centers.
    A. Relaxation of legislation began to occur in the 1980s.
    B. By 1987, the Omnibus Budget Reconciliation Act provided for less reimbursement to hospitals, providing rates equal to those for ambulatory surgery centers.
    C. The Omnibus Budget Reconciliation Act of 1989 again increased the reimbursement rates for assigned surgical procedures in ambulatory centers.
    D. Ambulatory centers became certified.
  VI. Consumer acceptance of ambulatory surgery
    A. Awareness
      1. Increased marketing led to increased consumer awareness.
      2. Greater awareness led to greater demand for surgery in ambulatory settings.
      3. Consumers saw more physician involvement in ambulatory settings.
      4. Patient consumers felt more involved and took part in decisions.
      5. Few problems were seen with quality of care.
    B. Convenience
      1. Flexible hours
      2. Early admission and same-day discharge
      3. Less time lost from work
      4. Units easily accessible
    C. Wellness philosophy well accepted
      1. Patients could walk to the operating room.
      2. Patients could recover on stretchers or in recliners.
      3. Parents could remain with children during induction; parents and sometimes families could be present postoperatively.
      4. Patients were able to keep dentures, eyeglasses, and hearing aids with them.
      5. Patients felt more self-responsibility for their care.
    D. Reimbursement
      1. Reimbursement provided by Medicare for outpatient procedures for the elderly made ambulatory surgery a viable alternative.
      2. Employers were paying less, and consumers found ambulatory settings less expensive, making outpatient surgery an attractive option.

EMERGENCE OF ORGANIZED RECOVERY ROOM GROUPS

  I. Need to identify a special body of knowledge and skills required for practice
    A. Groups form to develop educational opportunities.
      1. Nineteen groups organized in United States
      2. Florida Society of Anesthesiologists (FSA) initiated yearly seminar in 1969.
        a. Attended by nurses from United States and Canada
        b. Dr. Frank McKechnie: very supportive of recovery room nurses

    B. Series of seminars sponsored by American Society of Anesthesiologists (ASA)—1970s

      1. Supported by solid attendance and strong interest

      2. Interest shown in development of recovery room nursing organization

II. Local and state organizations form national group

    A. Regional nursing representatives met with ASA Care Team to organize national postanesthesia nurses' association.

    B. Goals established

      1. Education for postanesthesia nurses

      2. Recognition of postanesthesia nursing as a specialty

    C. Steering committee formed, 1979

      1. Selection of name: American Society of Post Anesthesia Nurses (ASPAN)

      2. Preparation of bylaws

      3. Incorporation

      4. First ASPAN president: Ina Pipkin, RN, from Seattle, Washington

    D. First meeting of board of directors held October 1980, in Orlando, Florida

    E. Charter for component status granted to Alabama and Florida, April 1982

FIRST YEARS (OCTOBER 1980-APRIL 1982)

I. Financial development

    A. ASA grant for legal expenses

    B. Membership dues

II. Internal organization developed

    A. Committees appointed

    B. Newsletter, *Breathline,* begun in 1981

    C. Membership increased.

      1. First national conference planned

      2. Regional educational meetings held

ASPAN DEVELOPMENTS

I. Publications

    A. 1983: *Guidelines for Standards of Care*

    B. 1986: *Standards of Nursing Practice*

    C. 1986: *Journal of Post Anesthesia Nursing*

    D. 1986: *Post Anesthesia Nursing Review for Certification*

    E. 1990: *Fifty Years of Progress in Post Anesthesia Nursing 1940 -1990*

    F. 1991: *Standards of Post Anesthesia Nursing Practice*

    G. 1991: *Core Curriculum for Post Anesthesia Nursing Practice,* ed 2

    H. 1992: *Standards of Post Anesthesia Nursing Practice*

    I. 1992: *ASPAN Resource Manual*

    J. 1993: *Postanesthesia and Ambulatory Surgery Nursing Update* (WB Saunders, publisher)

    K. 1994: pediatrics added to *Redi-Ref*

    L. 1994: *ASPAN Resource Manual* published in collaboration with American Board of Post Anesthesia Nursing (ABPANC)

    M. 1994: *Ambulatory Post Anesthesia Nursing Outline: Content for Certification*

    N. 1995: *Core Curriculum for Post Anesthesia Nursing Practice,* ed 3

    O. 1995: *Standards of Perianesthesia Nursing Practice*

    P. 1996: *Certification Review for Perianesthesia Nursing* (WB Saunders, publisher)

    Q. 1996: *Research Primer*

    R. 1997: Competency-based orientation credentialing program

    S. 1998: *Revised Redi-Ref* available

    T. 1998: *Standards of Perianesthesia Nursing Practice 1998.* New additions include:

      1. Guidelines for preadmission phase

        a. Preadmission

        b. Day of surgery/procedure

  2. Guidelines for phase III (addresses ongoing care for those patients requiring extended observations/interventions after transfer/discharge from phase I or phase II)

  3. 1998 position statements

   a. Minimum staffing in phase I PACU

   b. Registered nurse use of unlicensed assistive personnel (UAP)

   c. Intensive care unit (ICU) overflow patients

 U. 1999: *Core Curriculum for Ambulatory Perianesthesia Nursing Practice* (WB Saunders, publisher)

 V. 1999: *Core Curriculum for Perianesthesia Nursing Practice,* ed 4 (WB Saunders, publisher)

 W. 1999 Position statements

  1. "Fast Tracking"

  2. "Pain Management"

  3. "On Call/Work Schedule"

 X. *2000 Standards* included a joint position statement developed by ASPAN, American Association of Critical Care Nurses (AACN), and ASA's Anesthesia Care Team Committee and Committee on "Critical Care Medicine and Trauma Medicine on ICU Overflow Patients."

 Y. *2002 Standards* included position statement on the "Nursing Shortage."

 Z. *Competency Based Orientation Manual,* ed 2, published in 2003

 AA. *Thermoregulation Guidelines* published in 2003

 BB. *Pain and Comfort Clinical Practice Guidelines and Resource Manual* published in 2003

 CC. 2003 Position Statements approved included:

  1. "Medical/Surgical Overflow Patients in the PACU and Ambulatory Care Unit"

  2. "Visitation in phase I Level of Care"

  3. "Smallpox Vaccination Programs"

II. Certification (See Appendix A on ABPANC)

 A. 1985: American Board of Post Anesthesia Nursing Certification (ABPANC) established

 B. Certification examination developed to recognize knowledge and skill of practitioners

 C. November 1986: certification examination first administered

 D. Annual certified postanesthesia nurse recognition day at national conference

 E. 1991: certification examination expanded to include ambulatory surgery nurses who work in preoperative and phase II areas

 F. 1993-1994: separate certification examinations under development for phase I PACU nurses and ambulatory postanesthesia nurses: certified postanesthesia nurse (CPAN) and certified ambulatory postanesthesia (nurse) (CAPA) designations

 G. November 1994: CAPA examination first administered

 H. 1996: Name changed to American Board of PeriAnesthesia Nursing Certification (ABPANC)

 I. 1998: 4191 CPANs, 1183 CAPAs, and 100 CPANs-CAPAs

 J. 2003: 3921 CPANs, 1730 CAPAs, and 202 CPANs -CAPAs

III. Education

 A. National conference and annual educational program

 B. Regional core curriculum workshops (2-day program available)

 C. Regional ambulatory surgery workshops

 D. Regional interpersonal and leadership skills workshops

 E. ASPAN videotapes: overviews of postanesthesia nursing

 F. National ASPAN Lecture Series established 1993

 G. Joint ASPAN/AORN (Association of Operating Room Nurses) Ambulatory Surgery Symposium, 1993

 H. Cosponsored Governmental Affairs Workshop with American Association of Nurse Anesthetists, AORN, and the American Veterans Association of Nurse Anesthetists, 1994

     I. Sponsored first Volunteer Leadership Institute (VLI) in Richmond, Virginia, September 1994, now held every 2 years

     J. Patient education videos on general anesthesia, conscious sedation, and regional anesthesia developed, 1997

     K. Continuing education articles available in *Journal of PeriAnesthesia Nursing*

     L. Consensus Conference for Perioperative Normothermia held in Bethesda, Maryland, in 1998

     M. Consensus Conference for Pain and Comfort held in Nashville, Tennessee, in 2001

IV. Specialty representation

     A. Member of National Federation for Specialty Nursing Organizations (NFSNO) since June 1983

     B. Member of National Organization Liaison Forum (NOLF)

     C. Established official liaison with ASA

     D. Official liaisons with following organizations

          1. Society of Gastroenterology Nurses and Associates (SGNA)

          2. Society of Critical Care Medicine (SCCM)

          3. FASA

     E. Increased networking with the following

          1. American Association of Nurse Anesthetists (AANA)

          2. Association of periOperative Registered Nurses (AORN)

          3. AACN

     F. Organizational affiliate of American Nurses' Association (ANA), 1992

     G. ASPAN elected to NFSNO Executive Board, 1994-1996

     H. ASPAN elected to NOLF Board, 1994

     I. ASPAN represented at AORN Perioperative World Conference in Adelaide, Australia, 1994

     J. Nursing Summit held in Chicago—a coalition of all nursing leadership to discuss Nursing's Agenda for Healthcare Reform

     K. NOLF and NFSNO combine to form new organization, Nurses Organizations Alliance (The Alliance).

     L. 2002-2003: ASPAN president represented the organization at the 10th Congress of the Cuban Nursing Society and the First Colloquium on Natural and Traditional Medicine in Havana, Cuba.

V. Other highlights

     A. 1983: members encouraged to change name of workplace from recovery room to PACU

     B. 1989: postanesthesia nurse awareness week established

     C. 1989: definition of immediate postanesthesia nursing expanded to include preoperative and phase II areas to incorporate ambulatory nurses working only in those areas

     D. 1989: presidential award established

     E. 1989: AACN formally recognized postanesthesia nursing as a critical care specialty

     F. 1991: clinical excellence and outstanding achievement awards established

     G. 1991: ASPAN becomes an ANA approver and provider of continuing education

     H. 1992-1993: research committee offers grants and conducts Delphi study to establish postanesthesia and ambulatory surgery nursing priorities.

     I. 1993: American Society of Post Anesthesia Nursing Foundation established with first board of trustees

     J. 1993: organizational task force appointed to look at size and structure of ASPAN Board, dues structure, and membership voting

     K. 1994: approved concept of specialty practice groups (SPGs)

     L. 1994: Ontario, Canada, becomes ASPAN's first affiliate member.

     M. 1994: organizational task force conducts first planning meeting.

     N. 1994: online communication by means of Internet between officers and national office

O. 1995: ASPAN name changed to American Society of PeriAnesthesia Nurses approved, change took effect July 1, 1996
P. 1995: funds for first scholarship awards donated by the ASPAN Foundation
Q. 1996: One dues structure initiated (one payment includes membership in state and national organization)
R. 1996: ASPAN website created (http://www.aspan.org)
S. 1996: *Journal of Post Anesthesia* name changed to *Journal of PeriAnesthesia Nursing*
T. 1996: preadmission testing SPG formed by ASPAN members
U. 1997: newly structured board of directors met for first time April 10 in Denver, Colorado, after the ASPAN conference
V. 1997: ASPAN Foundation receives seat and ASPAN member attends AANA Foundation Research Scholars Program
W. 1998: first meeting of the Representative Assembly on April 21 at National Conference in Philadelphia
X. 1998: ASPAN membership is more than 10,000 with 40 components
Y. Management SPG formed by ASPAN members
Z. *Competency Based Orientation Manual*, ed 2, in 2002
AA. Pain Management SPG formed by ASPAN members
BB. Publications SPG formed by ASPAN Members
CC. Geriatric SPG formed by ASPAN Members
DD. 2003: ASPAN membership is 9638 (June 2003)

BIBLIOGRAPHY

1. American Board of PeriAnesthesia Nursing Certification: Unpublished data, 1998.
2. American Society of PeriAnesthesia Nurses: Personal communication. Unpublished data, 1998.
3. Aquavella JV: Ambulatory surgery in the 1990s. *J Ambul Care Manage* 13(1):21-24, 1990.
4. DeFazio-Quinn D, editor: *Ambulatory surgical nursing core curriculum.* Philadelphia: WB Saunders, 1999.
5. American Society of Post Anesthesia Nurses: *ASPAN resource manual.* Richmond, VA: The Society, 1992.
6. American Society of Post Anesthesia Nurses: *Fifty years of progress in post anesthesia nursing 1940-1990.* Richmond, VA: The Society, 1990.
7. Bendixen H, Kinney J: History of intensive care: American College of Surgeons. In Kinney JM, Bendixen HH, Powers SR Jr, editors: *Manual of surgical intensive care.* Philadelphia: WB Saunders, 1977.
8. Burden N: PACU nursing: Our today, our tomorrows. *J Post Anesth Nurs* 3(4):222-228, 1988.
9. Burden N, Quinn D, O'Brien D, et al: *Ambulatory surgical nursing,* ed 2: Philadelphia: WB Saunders, 2000.
10. Drain CB: *Perianesthesia Nursing: A Critical Care Approach,* ed 4. Philadelphia: WB Saunders, 2003.
11. Dunn F, Shupp M: The recovery room: A wartime economy. *Am J Nurs* 43(3):279-281, 1943.
12. Feeley T: The recovery room. In Miller R, editor: *Anesthesia,* vol 3, ed 2. New York: Churchill Livingstone, 1986.
13. Fetzer SJ: Practice characteristics of the dual certificant: CPAN/CAPA. *J Perianesth Nurs* 12(4):240-244, 1997.
14. Frost E, editor: *Post anesthesia care unit: current practices,* ed 2. St Louis: Mosby, 1990.
15. Kozak LJ, Hall RP, Lawrence L: Ambulatory surgery in the United States, 1994. In *Advance Data.* Hyattsville, Md: Centers for Disease Control and Prevention, National Center of Health Care Statistics, March 14, 1997.
16. Litwack K: *Post anesthesia care nursing,* ed 2. St Louis: Mosby–Year Book, 1995.
17. Luczun ME: Postanesthesia nursing: Past, present, and future. *J Post Anesth Nurs* 5(4):282-285, 1990.
18. Ruth H, Haugen F, Grove DD: Anesthesia study commission. *JAMA* 135(14):881-884, 1945.
19. Schneider M: Trends in postanesthesia nursing. *J Post Anesth Nurs* 2(3):183-188, 1987.
20. Wetchler BV: *Anesthesia for ambulatory surgery,* ed 2. Philadelphia: Lippincott, 1990.
21. White PF: *Outpatient anesthesia.* New York: Churchill Livingstone, 1990.

2 Standards for Ethical Practice

NANCY M. SAUFL

OBJECTIVES

At the conclusion of this chapter, the reader will be able to:

1. Describe the importance of standards as they relate to perianesthesia nursing practice.

2. Identify important ethical principles.

3. List the steps for ethical decision making.

4. Define competency-based practice.

I. Definition of standard
   A. Established by authority, custom, or general consent as a model or example for measuring quality or quantity
   B. Must be the same for all persons
   C. Standard of care is determined by what a reasonably prudent nurse acting under the same circumstance would do.
   D. Authoritative statement by which the nursing profession describes the responsibilities for which practitioners are accountable
   E. Provides direction for professional nursing practice and a framework for the evaluation of practice

II. Evolution of nursing standards
   A. Prior to 1950
      1. Florence Nightingale
      2. Reports of court cases
   B. Code of Ethics published by the American Nurses Association (ANA) in 1950—nurses offer care without prejudice and in a confidential and safe manner.
   C. Standards of professional nursing practice may pertain to general or specialty practice.
      1. First generic standards for the profession established in 1973 by the ANA Congress for Nursing Practice
      2. Specialty standards followed beginning in 1974.

III. Sources of standards
   A. Accrediting organizations
      1. Joint Commission on Accreditation of Healthcare Organizations (JCAHO)
      2. Accreditation Association for Ambulatory Healthcare (AAAHC)
      3. American Association for the Accreditation of Ambulatory Surgical Facilities (AAAASF)
   B. ANA
   C. Hospital policies and procedures
   D. Specialty organizations
   E. Nursing texts and articles
   F. Common practice

IV. Standard criteria
   A. Standard—authoritative statement enunciated and promulgated by the profession by which the quality of practice, service, or education can be judged

   B. Rationale—delineates the importance to perianesthesia practice
   C. Outcome—designed to measure the results of activity (i.e., "care meets the same standards of practice wherever the care is provided in the healthcare organization")
   D. Criteria—describes the principles to be used in implementing practices to meet the standard; reflects the actual activities that take place to ensure the standard is met (i.e., the phase II professional nurse ensures the availability of appropriate transportation for the patient from the facility)
V. *ANA Standards of Clinical Nursing Practice,* ed 2 (generic in nature; originally published by the ANA in 1991; apply to all registered nurses engaged in clinical practice, regardless of setting)
   A. Standards of care—describe a competent level of nursing care as demonstrated by the nursing process; delineate care that is provided to all patients
      1. Assessment—the nurse collects patient health data.
      2. Diagnosis—the nurse analyzes the assessment data in determining diagnoses.
      3. Outcome identification—the nurse identifies expected outcomes individualized to the patient.
      4. Planning—the nurse develops a plan of care that prescribes interventions to attain expected outcomes.
      5. Implementation—the nurse implements the interventions identified in the plan of care.
      6. Evaluation—the nurse evaluates the patient's progress toward attainment of outcomes.
   B. Standards of professional performance—describe a competent level of behavior in the professional role; all nurses are expected to engage in professional role activities appropriate to their education and position.
      1. Quality of care—the nurse systematically evaluates the quality and effectiveness of nursing practice.
      2. Performance appraisal—the nurse evaluates own nursing practice in relation to professional practice standards and relevant statutes and regulations.
      3. Education—the nurse acquires and maintains current knowledge and competency in nursing practice.
      4. Collegiality—the nurse interacts with, and contributes to the professional development of, peers and other health care providers as colleagues.
      5. Ethics—the nurse's decisions and actions on behalf of patients are determined in an ethical manner.
      6. Collaboration—the nurse collaborates with the patient, family, and other health care providers in providing patient care.
      7. Research—the nurse uses research findings in practice.
      8. Resource utilization—the nurse considers factors related to safety, effectiveness, and cost in planning and delivering patient care.
VI. Agency for Healthcare Research and Quality (AHRQ), formerly the Agency for Healthcare Policy and Research (AHCPR) (officially changed to AHRQ in 1999)
   A. Established in 1989 to enhance the quality, appropriateness, and effectiveness of health care services and access to those services
   B. Standard of practice—implies that patients will receive care according to standard
   C. Guideline—designed to guide practitioners, patients, and consumers in decisions regarding health care
   D. In 1992, released the first of a series of clinical practice guidelines: *Acute Pain Management: Operative or Medical Procedures and Trauma* (four major goals):
      1. Reduce the incidence and severity of patients' acute postoperative or posttraumatic pain
      2. Educate patients about the need to communicate unrelieved pain
      3. Enhance patient comfort and satisfaction
      4. Contribute to fewer postoperative complications, and in some cases, shorter stays after surgical procedures

  E. For more information, write or call: AHRQ, 2101 E. Jefferson St. # 501, Rockville, Maryland 20852l; 301-594-1364; e-mail: http://www.ahrq.org/info/customer.htm; Web site: http://www.ahrq.org

VII. *Standards of Perianesthesia Nursing Practice*—2002

  A. ASPAN history of standards

   1. 1983: *Guidelines for Standards of Care* published

   2. 1986: *Standards of Nursing Practice* published

   3. 1989: Definition of immediate postanesthesia nursing expanded to include preoperative and phase II areas to incorporate ambulatory nurses working only in those areas

   4. 1991: *Standards of Post Anesthesia Nursing Practice* published; included data for initial, ongoing, and discharge assessment (phase I and phase II)

   5. 1992: *Standards of Post Anesthesia Nursing Practice* published

   6. 1995: *Standards of Perianesthesia Nursing Practice* published; included preanesthesia and postanesthesia information (preanesthesia or preprocedural, phase I, and phase II)

   7. 1998: *Standards of Perianesthesia Nursing Practice* revised; included the addition of postanesthesia phase III, focusing on the provision of care for patients requiring extended observation/intervention after transfer/discharge from phase I and phase II

   8. 2000: *Standards of Perianesthesia Nursing Practice* revised

   9. 2002: *Standards of Perianesthesia Nursing Practice* revised

  B. Perianesthesia nursing scope of practice—ASPAN describes the perianesthesia nursing scope of practice as the assessment for, diagnosis of, intervention for, and evaluation of physical or psychosocial problems or risks for problems that may result from the administration of sedation and analgesia or anesthetic agents and techniques. Perianesthesia nursing practice is systematic in nature and includes the nursing process, decision making, analytical and scientific thinking, and inquiry. The environment includes, but is not limited to:

   1. Preanesthesia phase

    a. Preadmission

    b. Day of surgery or procedure

    c. Postanesthesia care units (PACUs)

    d. Phase I

    e. Phase II

    f. Ambulatory care settings

    g. Phase III settings

    h. Special procedures areas (i.e., cardioversion, electroconvulsive therapy, endoscopy, radiology, oncology, etc.)

    i. Labor and delivery suites

    j. Pain management services

    k. Physician and dental offices

  C. Specialty of perianesthesia nursing encompasses the care of the patient and family or significant other along the perianesthesia continuum of care:

   1. Preanesthesia phase

    a. Preadmission—the nursing roles in this phase focus on preparing the patient and family or significant other physically, psychologically, socioculturally, and spiritually for their experiences; interviewing and assessment techniques are used to identify potential or actual problems that may result.

    b. Day of surgery or procedure—the nursing roles in this phase focus on validation of existing information and completion of preparation of the patient and family or significant other physically and emotionally for their experiences.

   2. Postanesthesia phase I—the nursing roles in this phase focus on providing postanesthesia nursing care to the patients in the immediate postanesthesia period, transitioning them to phase II, the inpatient setting, or to an intensive care setting for continued care. Basic life-sustaining needs are of the highest priority and constant vigilance is required during this phase as the needs of the patients are neither minimal nor episodic.

3. Postanesthesia phase II—the nursing roles in this phase focus on preparing the patient and family or significant other for care in the home, phase III, or an extended care environment.

4. Postanesthesia phase III—the nursing roles in this phase focus on providing ongoing care for those patients requiring extended observation or intervention after discharge from phase I or phase II. Interventions are directed toward preparing the patient for self-care and/or the family or significant other for care in the home.

D. The scope of perianesthesia nursing practice is also regulated by:
1. Hospital or facility policies and procedures
2. State and federal regulatory agencies
3. National accreditation bodies
4. Professional nursing organizations

E. Perianesthesia nursing interacts with other professional groups to advance the delivery of quality care. These groups include but may not be limited to:
1. American Association of Critical Care Nurses (AACN)
2. American Association of Nurse Anesthetists (AANA)
3. American Board of Perianesthesia Nursing Certification (ABPANC)
4. ANA
5. American Society of Anesthesiologists (ASA)
6. Anesthesia Patient Safety Foundation (APSF)
7. Association of periOperative Registered Nurses (AORN)
8. Federated Ambulatory Surgery Association (FASA)
9. National League for Nursing (NLN)
10. National Student Nurses Association (NSNA)
11. Nursing Organizations Alliance (NOA)
12. Society for Ambulatory Anesthesia (SAMBA)
13. Society for Office-Based Anesthesia (SOBA)

F. Standards
1. Standard I: Patient Rights—"Perianesthesia nursing practice is based on philosophic and ethical concepts that recognize and maintain the autonomy, confidentiality, dignity and worth of individuals."
2. Standard II: Environment of Care—"Perianesthesia nursing practice promotes and maintains a safe, comfortable and therapeutic environment for patients, staff and visitors."
3. Standard III: Staffing and Personnel Management—"An appropriate number of professional nursing staff with demonstrated competence are available to meet the individual needs of patients and families in each level of perianesthesia care based on patient acuity, census, and physical facility."
4. Standard IV: Performance Improvement—"The professional perianesthesia nurse monitors and evaluates perianesthesia care on an ongoing basis. Identified problems are resolved through a collaborative multidisciplinary approach to assure the quality and appropriateness of patient care."
5. Standard V: Research—"Perianesthesia nurses participate in research by reviewing literature, designing studies, conducting studies, analyzing results, and/or incorporating findings into practice."
6. Standard VI: Assessment—"The professional perianesthesia nurse performs a systematic and continuous assessment of the patient and assures that all data are collected, documented, and communicated."
7. Standard VII: Planning and Implementation—"The professional perianesthesia nurse develops and coordinates the implementation of a dynamic plan of care based on analysis of the individual patient assessment."
8. Standard VIII: Evaluation—"The professional perianesthesia nurse continuously evaluates the patient's progress toward the desired outcomes and revises the plan of care and interventions as necessary."

G. Resources
   1. American Hospital Association (AHA) *A Patient's Bill of Rights*
   2. Nine provisions of the ANA's *Code of Ethics for Nurses with Interpretive Statements* (approved June 30, 2001)
   3. Patient classification and recommended staffing guidelines
      a. Staffing is based on patient acuity, census, and physical facility.
      b. The professional nurse uses prudent judgment in determining nurse-to-patient ratios and staffing mix to reflect patient acuity and nursing intensity.
   4. Criteria for initial, ongoing, and discharge assessment and management
      a. Preadmission
      b. Day of surgery or procedure
      c. Operative or procedure report
      d. Initial assessment: phase I
      e. Ongoing assessment and management: phase I
      f. Discharge assessment: phase I
      g. Initial assessment: phase II
      h. Ongoing assessment and management: phase II
      i. Discharge assessment: phase II
      j. Initial and ongoing assessment and management: phase III
   5. Recommended equipment for preanesthesia phase, PACU phase I, phase II, and phase III
   6. Emergency drugs and equipment
   7. ASA standards
      a. "Statement on Routine Preoperative Laboratory and Diagnostic Screening"
      b. ASA "Basic Standards for Preanesthesia Care"
      c. ASA "Standards for Postanesthesia Care"
   8. Agency for Health Care Research and Quality: *Abbreviated Acute Pain Management Flowchart* (Note: no longer available.)
   9. Competent support staff
   10. "Use of Support Personnel in the Postanesthesia Care Units and Ambulatory Care Units": Joint Statement of American Society of Post Anesthesia Nurses (ASPAN) and ASA, October 1990
   11. ANA Position Statement: "Role of the Registered Nurse in the Management of Analgesia by Catheter Techniques (Epidural, Intrathecal, Intrapleural, or Peripheral Nerve Catheters)"
   12. Association of Women's Health, Obstetrics and Neonatal Nurses (AWHONN) Position Statement: "Role of the Registered Nurse (RN) in the Care of the Pregnant Woman Receiving Analgesia/Anesthesia by Catheter Techniques (Epidural, Intrathecal, Spinal, PCEA Catheters)"
   13. ANA Position Statement: "Role of the Registered Nurse in the Management of Patients Undergoing Sedation for Short-Term, Therapeutic, Diagnostic or Surgical Procedures"
   14. Safe transfer of care
   15. American Society of PeriAnesthesia Nurses: "Clinical Guideline for the Prevention of Unplanned Perioperative Hypothermia"
      a. Define normothermia.
      b. Define hypothermia.
      c. Alert healthcare providers of the importance of maintaining perioperative normothermia.
      d. Provide ways to address the management of unplanned perioperative hypothermia.
      e. Improve patient outcomes.
   16. American Society of PeriAnesthesia Nurses Internet resources
H. ASPAN position statements
   1. "A Position Statement on Entry into Nursing Practice"
   2. "A Position Statement on Air Safety in the Perianesthesia Environment"

3. "A Position Statement on the Perianesthesia Patient with a Do-Not-Resuscitate Advance Directive"
   a. ASPAN recommends that, at the time of surgery and prior to receiving any anesthetic medication, a patient with an active do-not-resuscitate (DNR) advance directive must reconsider this designation and reclarify wishes about resuscitation during the perianesthesia period.
   b. To limit potential for ethical dilemmas, the patient's informed consent will include discussion of the advance directive, living will, or physician order that specifies DNR or do-not-intubate (DNI) during a candid and well-documented conversation with physicians and appropriate significant other(s).
   c. Each facility establishes and communicates a policy that identifies resources and procedures that detail the management of a patient's DNR or DNI status during the perianesthesia period.
4. "A Position Statement on Perianesthesia Advanced Practice Nursing"
5. "A Position Statement on Minimum Staffing in Phase I PACU"
   a. It is the position of ASPAN that two licensed nurses, one of whom is a registered nurse competent in postanesthesia nursing, will be present in the phase I PACU whenever a patient is recovering from anesthesia.
6. "A Position Statement on Registered Nurse Utilization of Unlicensed Assistive Personnel"
7. "A Position Statement on Fast Tracking"
   a. It is the position of ASPAN that wherever fast tracking is practiced a collaborative plan of care be developed between the anesthesiology department and perianesthesia services. The plan should address the following:
      (1) Appropriate patient selection
      (2) Preoperative education of the patient and family
      (3) Appropriate selection and management of anesthetic agents
      (4) Assessment criteria used to evaluate patient readiness in bypassing phase I at the end of the surgical procedure
      (5) Discharge criteria
      (6) Monitoring and reporting patient outcomes
8. "A Position Statement on Pain Management"
9. "A Position Statement on On Call/Work Schedule"
10. "A Joint Position Statement on ICU Overflow Patients" developed by ASPAN, AACN, and ASA's Anesthesia Care Team Committee and Committee on Critical Care Medicine and Trauma Medicine, September 1999
11. "A Position Statement on the Nursing Shortage"
12. "A Position Statement on Medical-Surgical Overflow Patients in the Postanesthesia Care Unit"
13. "A Position Statement on Visitation in Phase I Level of Care"
14. "Position Statement on Smallpox Vaccination Programs"
VIII. "Perianesthesia Standards for Ethical Practice"—The perianesthesia nurse provides care that encompasses compassion, collaboration, and trust. The principles of the "Perianesthesia Standards for Ethical Practice" include a moral obligation to promote the welfare, health, and safety of the patients we serve, and to advocate on the patient's behalf whenever necessary.
   A. Competency
      1. Maintains personal accountability
      2. Participates in professional continuing education
      3. Adheres to ASPAN's Standards
      4. Complies with institutional policies and procedures
      5. Accepts responsibility
      6. Participates in performance improvement
      7. Utilizes competency-based orientation
      8. Remains current on new products
      9. Practices with compassion

   B. Responsibility to patients
- **1.** Provides quality care
- **2.** Confirms informed consent
- **3.** Explains procedures
- **4.** Maintains confidentiality
- **5.** Participates in patient teaching
- **6.** Answers questions accurately
- **7.** Communicates pertinent information
- **8.** Provides communication aides
- **9.** Advocates for spiritual comfort
- **10.** Respects patient's decisions
- **11.** Protects patients from harm
- **12.** Advocates for patients
- **13.** Delegates tasks appropriately
- **14.** Aggressively provides pain control
- **15.** Includes the patient's family and/or support system
- **16.** Evaluates the patient's environment for safety
- **17.** Ensures that all patients are cared for by a professional nurse

   C. Professional responsibility
- **1.** Adheres to policies, procedures, and standards
- **2.** Provides comparable level of care regardless of physical setting
- **3.** Discusses patient information appropriately
- **4.** Maintains accurate patient records
- **5.** Safeguards patient confidentiality
- **6.** Participates in activities that contribute to professional development
- **7.** Promotes certification
- **8.** Acts as a mentor
- **9.** Demonstrates fair management of resources
- **10.** Maintains an awareness of changing practice issues
- **11.** Recognizes a need to care for one's self
- **12.** Follows policies, procedures, and laws

   D. Collegiality
- **1.** Collaborates with peers and colleagues
- **2.** Promotes respectful relationships

   E. Research
- **1.** Obtains appropriate Institutional Review Board (IRB) approvals
- **2.** Protects the rights of research participants
- **3.** Protects confidentiality
- **4.** Uses findings to support clinical practice
- **5.** Identifies problems to be considered for research

IX. Competency-based practice

   A. Comprehensive guide to competency and skill development for perianesthesia nurses

   B. May be used to orient new perianesthesia nurses

   C. May be used for annual skills renewal and annual updates for the perianesthesia nursing staff

   D. Provides the perianesthesia nurse a framework of essential performance criteria, thus establishing basic competencies needed to practice in diverse perianesthesia settings

   E. Competencies
- **1.** Preanesthesia
  - **a.** Preanesthesia testing
  - **b.** Preoperative teaching
  - **c.** Preoperative history and assessment
  - **d.** Day of surgery preparation
- **2.** Airway management
- **3.** Circulation
- **4.** Neurological

    5. Renal
    6. Moderate sedation and analgesia
    7. Anesthesia agents and adjuncts
        a. General inhalation agents
        b. Muscle relaxants
        c. Regional anesthesia
        d. Intravenous agents
    8. Perianesthesia fluid management and resuscitation
    9. Patient comfort
        a. Pain and comfort management
        b. Nausea and vomiting
    10. Thermoregulation
        a. Malignant hyperthermia
        b. Hypothermia
    11. Age-specific competencies
        a. Pediatric
        b. Adolescent
        c. Adult
        d. Elderly
    12. Postoperative education and teaching
    13. Medical imaging and interventional radiology
    14. Legal and documentation
    15. Transcultural nursing
    16. Mentoring
X. Unlicensed assistive personnel in the perianesthesia setting
    A. Value of utilizing competent unlicensed assistive personnel (UAP) in perianesthesia settings
    B. Foremost concern is to promote safe environment for the perianesthesia patient.
    C. Guidelines to be utilized
        1. Perianesthesia nursing profession defines and supervises the education, training, and utilization for UAPs involved in direct patient care.
        2. Perianesthesia RN is responsible for and accountable for the provision of nursing practice.
        3. Perianesthesia RN supervises and determines appropriate utilization of any UAP involved in direct patient care.
        4. Purpose of the UAP is to enable the professional perianesthesia nurse to provide nursing care for the patient.
    D. Competency-based orientation and credentialing for the UAP
        1. Basic life support
        2. Airway management
        3. Care of the patient with emesis
        4. Care of the patient requiring oral intake
        5. Care of the patient with hypothermia
        6. Care of the patient with malignant hyperthermia
        7. Care of the patient requiring monitoring
        8. Care of the patient with seizure disorder
        9. Care of the patient with catheters and drains
        10. Care of the patient requiring comfort measures
        11. Care of the patient receiving intravenous fluids
        12. Care of the patient requiring oral or nasal suctioning
        13. Safe transport of the perianesthesia patient

To obtain a copy of *Standards of Perianesthesia Nursing Practice 2002; Competency Based Orientation and Credentialing Program 2002;* and/or *Competency Based Orientation and Credentialing Program for Unlicensed Assistive Personnel in the Perianesthesia Setting 2001;* contact ASPAN at 10 Melrose Avenue, Suite 110, Cherry Hill, NJ 08003; at 1-877-737-9696 (toll-free); or at http://www.aspan.org.

XI. Ethical issues
  A. Ethics
    1. The science relating to moral action and moral values
    2. Concerned with motives and attitudes and their relation to the good of the individual
  B. Professional responsibilities and duties
    1. Duty of veracity: a duty to tell the truth
    2. Rule of confidentiality: a duty to control disclosure of personal information about patients to others
    3. HIPAA—Health Insurance Portability and Accountability Act
      a. Requires health care organizations to comply with federal regulations for privacy and electronic transactions
      b. Portability standards
      c. Accountability standards
      d. Privacy standards
    4. Duty of advocacy: nurse supports the best interests of the individual patient.
    5. Accountability: answerable to others for one's actions
    6. Duty of fidelity: obligation to be faithful to commitments to self and others
  C. Ethical theories
    1. Utilitarianism: defines "good" as happiness or pleasure
      a. Greatest good for the greatest number of people
      b. The end justifies the means.
    2. Deontology: system of ethical decision making based on moral obligation or commitment to others
      a. Emphasis on the dignity of human beings
    3. Principalism: incorporates various existing ethical principles and attempts to resolve conflicts by applying one or more of them
  D. Ethical principles
    1. Beneficence: views the primary goal of health care as doing good for patients
    2. Nonmaleficence: requirement that health care providers prevent or do no harm to their patients
    3. Autonomy: freedom of action as chosen by an individual
    4. Justice: duty to be fair to all people
  E. Ethical decision making: goal is to determine right from wrong in certain situations in which the lines are unclear.
    1. Decision making process
      a. Obtain as much information as possible.
      b. State the problem or dilemma as clearly as possible.
      c. List all possible choices of action.
      d. Evaluate the consequences of each choice.
      e. Make a decision.
    2. Moral model
      a. Massage the dilemma.
      b. Outline the options.
      c. Resolve the dilemma.
      d. Act by applying chosen option.
      e. Look back and evaluate entire process.
  F. Relationship of law and ethics
    1. Legal system is founded on rules and regulations that are formal and binding; ethical values are subject to philosophical, moral, and individual interpretation.
    2. Legal right may or may not be ethical
    3. Moral right may or may not be a legal right.
    4. Law influences ethical decision making and ethics can influence legal decision making.

    G. "Perianesthesia Standards for Ethical Practice"
      1. Included in ASPAN's *Standards of Perianesthesia Nursing 2002*
    H. American Nurses Association, *Code of Ethics for Nurses with Interpretive Statements* (nine provisions approved July 2001)
      1. The nurse practices with compassion and respect.
      2. The nurse's primary commitment is to the patient.
      3. The nurse advocates for the health, safety, and rights of the patient.
      4. The nurse is accountable for individual nursing practice.
      5. The nurse owes the same duties to self as to others.
      6. The nurse participates in maintaining and improving health care environments and conditions.
      7. The nurse participates in the advancement of the profession.
      8. The nurse collaborates with other health professionals.
      9. The profession of nursing is responsible for articulating nursing values, for maintaining the integrity of the profession, and for shaping social policy.
    I. The nursing shortage
      1. The American Nurses Association, the National Council of State Boards of Nursing, and the National Federation of Licensed Practical Nursing, Inc: "Joint Statement on Maintaining Professional and Legal Standards During a Shortage of Nursing Personnel"
      2. American Society of PeriAnesthesia Nurses: *A Position Statement on the Nursing Shortage*

BIBLIOGRAPHY

1. Agency for Healthcare Research and Quality: *Clinical practice guideline: Acute pain management: Operative or medical procedures and trauma.* AHCPR Pub 92-00322. Rockville, MD: US Dept of Health and Human Services, 1992. (Note: no longer available. Archived at the National Library of Medicine at http://www.ncbi.nlm.nih.gov/books/bv.fcgi?rid+hstat6.chapter.8991)
2. American Hospital Association: *A patient's bill of rights.* First adopted by the AHA in 1973; revision approved October 1992. Available at http://www.hospitalconnect.com/aha/about/pbillofrights.html. Accessed January 2003.
3. American Nurses Association: *Code for nurses with interpretive statements.* Washington, DC: American Nurses Publishing, 2001.
4. American Nurses Association: The role of the registered nurse in management of analgesia by catheter techniques (spinal, intrathecal, intrapleural, or peripheral nerve catheters), 1991. Available at http://www.nursingworld. org. Accessed January 2003.
5. American Nurses Association: The role of the registered nurse in the management of patients receiving IV conscious sedation for short-term therapeutic, diagnostic or surgical procedures, 2001. Available at http://www.nursingworld.org. Accessed January 2003.
6. American Nurses Association: *Nursing's social policy statement.* ANA Publication No. NP-107. Washington, DC: American Nurses Publishing, 1995.
7. American Nurses Association: *Standards of clinical nursing practice,* ed 2. Washington, DC: American Nurses Publishing, 1998.
8. American Nurses Association: *Joint statement on maintaining professional and legal standards during a shortage of nursing personnel,* 1992. Available at http://www.nursingworld.org. Accessed January 2003.
9. American Society of PeriAnesthesia Nurses: *2002 standards of perianesthesia nursing.* Cherry Hill, NJ: American Society of PeriAnesthesia Nurses, 2002.
10. American Society of PeriAnesthesia Nurses: *Position statements.* Available at http://www.aspan.org. Accessed May 2003.
11. American Society of PeriAnesthesia Nurses: *Competency based orientation and credentialing program.* Cherry Hill, NJ: American Society of PeriAnesthesia Nurses, 2002.
12. American Society of PeriAnesthesia Nurses: *A competency based orientation and credentialing program for unlicensed assistive personnel in the perianesthesia setting.* Cherry Hill, NJ: American Society of PeriAnesthesia Nurses, 2000.
13. Association of periOperative Registered Nurses: *Standards, recommended practices, guidelines.* Denver, Colo: Association of periOperative Registered Nurses, 2002.
14. Association of Women's Health, Obstetric and Neonatal Nurses: The role of the registered nurse in care of pregnant women receiving analgesia/anesthesia by catheter techniques (epidural, intrathecal, spinal, PCEA catheters), 2001. Available at http://www.awhonn.org. Accessed January 2003.

15. Brent NJ: *Nurses and the law: A guide to principles and applications.* Philadelphia: WB Saunders, 1997.

16. Brunsen CD, Eichhorn JH: Risk management: Avoiding complications and litigation. In White PF, editor: *Ambulatory anesthesia and surgery.* Philadelphia: WB Saunders, 1997, pp 691-699.

17. Burden N, DeFazio Quinn D, O'Brien D, et al: *Ambulatory surgical nursing.* Philadelphia: WB Saunders, 2000.

18. Connelly J: Emotions, ethics and decision making in primary care. *J Clin Ethics* 9(3):225-234, 1998.

19. Faden R: Managed care and informed consent. *Kennedy Inst Ethics J* 7(4):377-379, 1997.

20. Gastmans G: Challenges to nursing values in a changing nursing environment. *Nurs Ethics* 5(3):236-245, 1998.

21. Gray C: Understanding and complying with HIPAA. *J Perianesth Nurs* 18(3):182-185, 2003.

22. Green C: Ethical issues in perianesthesia nursing. *J Perianesth Nurs* 15(4):229-236, 2000.

23. Gue DG, Fox S: Guide to medical privacy and HIPAA. Washington, DC: Thompson Publications Group, 2002.

24. Guido GW: *Legal issues in nursing,* ed 2. Stamford, CT: Appleton & Lange, 1997.

25. HIPAA Advisory: The HIPAA privacy, security, transaction, and code sets, and national resources, 1996. Available at http://www.hipaadvisory.com. Accessed January 2003.

26. Jeran L: Patient temperature: An introduction to the clinical guideline for the prevention of unplanned hypothermia. *J Perianesth Nurs* 16(5):303-304, 2001.

27. Joint Commission on Accreditation of Healthcare Organizations: Sentinel event alert: A follow-up review of wrong site surgery, 2002. Available at http://www.jcaho.org/about+us/news+ Accessed December 2001.

28. Joint Commission on Accreditation of Healthcare Organizations: *Comprehensive accreditation manual for hospitals.* Overbrook, Ill: Joint Commission on Accreditation of Healthcare Organizations, 2001.

29. Kolcaba K, Wilson L: Comfort care: A framework for perianesthesia nursing. *J Perianesth Nurs* 17(2):102-113, 2002.

30. Mamaril M: Fast-tracking the postanesthesia patient: The pros and cons. *J Perianesth Nurs* 15(2):89-93, 2000.

31. Odom J:. Implementation of nursing standards. In Quinn D, editor: *Ambulatory surgical nursing core curriculum.* Philadelphia: WB Saunders, 1999, pp 10-15.

32. Odom J: Legal and ethical issues. In Quinn D, editor: *Ambulatory surgical nursing core curriculum.* Philadelphia: WB Saunders, 1999, pp 27-35.

33. Redman BK, Fry ST: Nurses' ethical conflicts: What is really known about them? *Nurs Ethics* 7(4):360-365, 2000.

34. United States Congress. Health insurance portability and accountability act. *104th Congress, Public Record,* 104-191, 1996.

35. White G: The code of ethics for nurses. *Am J Nurs* 101:73-75, 2001.

36. Wood J: Ethical decision-making. *J Perianesth Nurs:*16(1):6-10, 2001.

37. Zickuhr MT: Nursing practice, nursing standards, and nursing practice. In Litwack K, editor: *Core curriculum for perianesthesia nursing practice,* ed 4. Philadelphia: WB Saunders, 1999.

3 The Nursing Process

SUSAN JANE FETZER

OBJECTIVES

At the conclusion of this chapter the reader will be able to:

1. Describe the application of the nursing process to each phase of perianesthesia care.

2. List the resources used for data collection during the preadmission assessment.

3. Identify the frequently applied North American Nursing Diagnosis Association (NANDA) diagnostic labels for actual and possible nursing diagnosis during the perianesthesia period.

4. Describe methods used to evaluate perianesthesia nursing care patient outcomes.

I. Overview of nursing process
   A. Nursing process is a systematic, rational method of providing individualized nursing care.
   B. A cyclic process that follows a logical sequence of interrelated phases
   C. Derived from the scientific method of problem solving and decision making
   D. Five phases compose the nursing process: assessment, diagnosis, planning, implementation, outcome evaluation.
   E. Goals of nursing process
      1. Establish a patient database.
      2. Identify health care needs.
      3. Determine goals of care, priorities of care, and expected patient outcomes.
      4. Direct nursing interventions necessary to meet patient needs.
      5. Evaluate effectiveness of nursing systems in achieving expected patient outcomes.
II. Nursing process: assessment
   A. Information-gathering phase of nursing process
   B. Types of data included in assessment
      1. Subjective data
         a. Primary sources include data obtained from patient reports, descriptions, and perceptions:
            (1) Health history completed by the patient
            (2) Focused data obtained during preadmission interview
               (a) Contact person in case of emergency
               (b) Patient telephone number for discharge follow up
               (c) Allergies to foods (especially milk products, shellfish)
               (d) Allergies to medications
               (e) Sensitivities to medications
               (f) Contact allergies (especially latex, tape, iodine products)
               (g) Presence of implants or prostheses (e.g., pacemakers, contact lenses, hearing aids)
               (h) Anesthetic intolerance (e.g., drug intolerance, risk factors for malignant hyperthermia, risk factors for pseudocholinesterase deficiency)
               (i) Current prescription medications
               (j) Personal habits including frequency and last use of tobacco, alcohol, street drugs, over-the-counter medications, herbal supplements
               (k) Type, amount, and time of last oral intake

        (3) Patient's report of the perianesthesia experience

        (4) Information obtained during postdischarge follow up interview

   b. Secondary sources include data obtained from family and significant others.

        (1) Parental reports of child behavior

        (2) Spouse, caretaker report of adult behavior

2. Objective data

   a. Includes data obtained from nursing observation

        (1) Physical appearance during preadmission interview, during surgery, and the perianesthesia period

        (2) Patient behavior during preoperative and discharge teaching

        (3) Patient behavior during preadmission interview, when experiencing local or regional anesthesia, and during the postanesthesia period

   b. Includes data obtained through nursing examination

        (1) Preanesthetic physical assessment

           (a) Vital sign measurements

           (b) Systems assessment: skin, respiratory, cardiovascular, musculoskeletal, neurological, psychosocial, and hematological

           (c) Assessment related to specific surgical or anesthetic procedure anticipated (e.g., visual acuity for elderly patient scheduled for cataract surgery, assessment of radial pulse of patient scheduled for carpal tunnel release)

           (d) Focused cultural or spiritual requirements

              (i) Dietary (e.g., milk products, food taboos)

              (ii) Family dynamics (e.g., patriarchal caste)

              (iii) Medical restrictions (e.g., blood transfusion, disposal of tissues)

              (iv) Spiritual rituals (e.g., removal of clothing or jewelry)

              (v) Communication (e.g., sign, non-English speaking, nonverbal)

        (2) Intraoperative physical assessment

           (a) Vital sign monitoring

           (b) Systems assessment depends on type of anesthesia and surgical procedure: respiratory, cardiovascular, neurological, skin

        (3) Postanesthesia physical assessment

           (a) Vital sign monitoring

           (b) Systems assessment: respiratory, cardiovascular, musculoskeletal, neurological, endocrine, urinary, skin are compared with preanesthetic baseline.

           (c) Appearance of surgical site

           (d) Level of pain, nausea, dizziness

           (e) Status of patient dependent equipment

              (i) Drains, tubes

              (ii) Pumps, warming devices

              (iii) Intravenous, arterial lines

              (iv) Blood collection systems

3. Tertiary sources of objective data

   a. Preanesthetic phase

        (1) Previous medical records

        (2) Current medical history and physical

        (3) Laboratory, radiology, cardiology, and diagnostic procedure reports

        (4) Information sources can include community health nurses, primary care physicians, physician consultants, physical therapists, dietitians, pharmacists, social workers.

   b. Intraoperative phase

        (1) Circulating nurse record

        (2) Anesthesia record

        (3) Operative report or progress note

        c. Postanesthesia phase

          (1) Laboratory, radiology, cardiology reports as needed

   C. Organization of assessment data

     1. Data can be organized and documented using systems or medical model approach (i.e., cardiac, respiratory, neurological, etc.).

     2. Data can be organized and documented using functional health patterns.

        a. Health perception–health management pattern

        b. Nutritional–metabolic pattern

        c. Elimination pattern

        d. Activity–exercise pattern

        e. Sleep–rest pattern

        f. Cognitive–perceptual pattern

        g. Self-perception–self-concept pattern

        h. Role–relationship pattern

        i. Sexuality–reproductive pattern

        j. Coping–stress tolerance pattern

        k. Value–belief pattern

     3. Data can be organized and documented using a nursing model (e.g., Orem's Self-Care Deficit Theory).

   D. Nursing data is analyzed.

     1. Data from multiple sources is compared.

     2. Data is compared with standards and norms.

     3. Data is examined for gaps and inconsistencies.

     4. Patterns are identified.

   E. Data is organized and documented so that findings are communicated to health care providers.

   F. All assessment data is considered confidential and communicated only to health care providers who have a work-related right to know.

III. Nursing process: diagnosis

   A. Definition: A nursing diagnosis is a clinical judgment about the patient's response to actual or potential health problems.

   B. Nursing diagnosis is derived from an analysis of assessment data.

   C. Purpose

     1. Communicate nursing judgment

     2. Provide universally understood judgment across settings and specialties

     3. Clearly identify the domain of nursing

     4. Promotes accountability and professional autonomy

   D. Components of a nursing diagnosis

     1. Nursing diagnosis includes diagnostic label, defining characteristics, and related factors.

     2. Diagnostic label

        a. Also referred to as a problem

        b. Directs the nurse-sensitive patient outcome

        c. NANDA identifies over 150 diagnostic labels.

        d. Examples of frequently occurring perianesthesia diagnostic labels

          (1) Preoperative diagnostic labels

            (a) Anxiety: uneasiness, the source of which is often nonspecific or unknown to the individual

            (b) Fear: a feeling of dread with an ability to identify its sources

            (c) Knowledge deficit: state in which a person lacks the skills or information to successfully manage his or her own health care (e.g., knowledge deficit related to postoperative pain management)

            (d) Fluid volume deficit: decreased intravascular, extracellular, or intracellular fluid

          (2) Intraoperative

            (a) Perioperative positioning injury, risk for: state in which the patient is at risk for injury as a result of the environmental conditions found in the perioperative setting

      (b) Body temperature, risk for altered: state in which the patient is at risk for failure to maintain body temperature within normal range

      (c) Gas exchange, impaired: excess or deficit in oxygenation or carbon dioxide elimination at the alveolar-capillary membrane

      (d) Decreased cardiac output: a state in which the heart is unable to pump blood with enough force to meet the body's metabolic demands

      (e) Ineffective peripheral tissue perfusion: a decrease in oxygen resulting in the failure to nourish tissues at the capillary level

      (f) Infection, risk for: state in which a patient is at increased risk for being invaded by pathogenic organisms

      (g) Hypothermia: state in which a patient's core body temperature is reduced below 96.8° F (36° C)

  (3) Phase I

      (a) Airway clearance, ineffective: inability to clear secretions or obstructions from the respiratory tract to maintain a clear airway

      (b) Breathing pattern, ineffective: state in which a patient's inhalation or exhalation pattern does not promote adequate ventilation

      (c) Gas exchange, impaired: excess or deficit in oxygenation or carbon dioxide elimination at the alveolar-capillary membrane

      (d) Decreased cardiac output: state in which the heart is unable to pump blood with enough force to meet the body's metabolic demands

      (e) Thought process, altered: disruption in such mental activities as conscious thought, reality orientation, problem solving, judgment, and comprehension

      (f) Acute pain: state in which patient experiences and reports the presence of severe discomfort or an uncomfortable sensation

      (g) Nausea: state in which patient experiences an unpleasant, wavelike sensation in the back of the throat, epigastrium, or abdomen; may be associated with vomiting

      (h) Hypothermia: state in which a patient's core body temperature is reduced below 96.8° F (36° C)

      (i) Anxiety: uneasiness, the source of which is often nonspecific or unknown to the individual

      (j) Fear: feeling of dread with an ability to identify its sources

      (k) Ineffective peripheral tissue perfusion: decrease in oxygen resulting in the failure to nourish tissues at the capillary level

      (l) Fluid volume excess: increased isotonic fluid retention

     (m) Fluid volume deficit: decreased intravascular, extracellular, or intracellular fluid

      (n) Impaired urinary elimination: disturbance in urine elimination

      (o) Impaired physical mobility: state in which a patient experiences a limitation of ability for independent movement

      (p) Impaired skin integrity: state in which a patient's skin is impaired

      (q) Impaired tissue integrity: state in which a patient experiences damage to mucous membrane, corneal, integumentary, or subcutaneous tissue

  (4) Phase II

      (a) Acute pain: state in which patient experiences and reports the presence of severe discomfort or an uncomfortable sensation

      (b) Nausea: state in which patient experiences an unpleasant, wavelike sensation in the back of the throat, epigastrium, or abdomen; may be associated with vomiting

      (c) Impaired urinary elimination: disturbance in urine elimination

      (d) Self-care deficit (dressing, bathing, toileting): state in which a patient experiences an impaired ability to perform an activity of daily living

      (e) Knowledge deficit: state in which a patient lacks the skills or information to successfully manage his or her own health care (e.g., postdischarge care)

      (f) Impaired physical mobility: state in which a patient experiences a limitation of ability for independent movement (e.g., post-closed reduction for extremity fracture)

3. Risk nursing diagnosis (previously labeled potential nursing diagnosis)

    a. Represents nursing judgment that patient is more vulnerable to develop an actual problem than others in the same situation

    b. Patient database contains evidence of risk factors for the actual diagnosis, but no defining characteristics are evident.

    c. Examples of perianesthesia risk nursing diagnoses

      (1) Risk for impaired skin integrity (e.g., risk may be due to poor health status, chronic steroid use)

      (2) Risk for aspiration (e.g., risk may be due to history of stroke with residual weakness)

      (3) Risk for imbalanced body temperature (e.g., hypothermia risk may be due to age, type of surgical procedure)

E. Determining nursing diagnosis

  1. Defining characteristics

    a. Cues that describe the behavior

      (1) Subjective data

      (2) Objective data

      (3) Data organized into patterns

      (4) Two to three defining characteristics verify the nursing diagnosis.

      (5) Examples of perianesthesia defining characteristics

    b. Preoperative

      (1) Defining characteristics: increased tension, withdrawal, increased heart rate

      (2) Nursing diagnosis: fear—feeling of dread with an ability to identify its sources (e.g., intravenous insertion)

    c. Phase I

      (1) Defining characteristics: decreased vital capacity, dyspnea, decreased respiratory rate

      (2) Nursing diagnosis: ineffective breathing pattern—state in which a patient's inhalation or exhalation pattern does not promote adequate ventilation

    d. Phase II

      (1) Defining characteristics: urgency, retention

      (2) Nursing diagnosis: impaired urinary elimination—disturbance in urine elimination

  2. Related factors

    a. Definition: conditions or circumstances that cause or contribute to the problem

    b. Indicate what should change in order to return patient to improved state

    c. Assist in identifying nursing interventions

    d. Examples of perianesthesia-related factors

      (1) Preoperative

        (a) Nursing diagnosis: fluid volume deficit—state of decreased intravascular, interstitial, and/or intracellular fluid

        (b) Defining characteristics: thirst, decreased blood pressure, increased pulse rate, dry mucous membranes

        (c) Related factors: inadequate fluid intake secondary to nothing by mouth (NPO) requirements for surgery

        (2) Phase I

           (a) Nursing diagnosis: ineffective airway clearance—inability to clear secretions or obstructions from the respiratory tract to maintain clear airway

           (b) Defining characteristics: dyspnea, crackles, increased respiratory rate, restlessness, wide-eyed

           (c) Related factors: postextubation laryngospasm

        (3) Phase II

           (a) Nursing diagnosis: nausea—an unpleasant, wavelike sensation in the back of the throat, epigastrium, or abdomen

           (b) Defining characteristics: sick to stomach, increased salivation

           (c) Related factors: surgical anesthetics, movement from surgical suite

  3. Risk factors

    a. Similar to related factors and defining characteristics

    b. Describe events that put patient at risk

    c. Only found in risk for (potential) nursing diagnoses

    d. Examples of perianesthesia risk factors

      (1) Age—elderly have higher risk for impaired skin integrity.

      (2) Nutritional status—diabetic patients have higher risk for impaired skin integrity.

      (3) Personal habits—smokers have higher risk for ineffective airway.

      (4) Co-morbid diseases—dialysis patients have higher risk for fluid excess.

IV. Nursing process: planning

  A. Planning includes setting goals and expected outcomes of care.

    1. Goals (i.e., long-term goals) are broad statements of patient and family behaviors that are measurable or observable and realistic.

    2. Goals reflect the effect of nursing care.

    3. Goals may be achieved after discharge from perianesthesia care.

    4. Goals are patient centered and focused on what patient is expected to achieve.

    5. Examples of perianesthesia goals

      a. Preoperative

        (1) Patient will state maintenance of NPO status preoperatively.

        (2) Patient will be knowledgeable about postoperative pain assessment.

        (3) Patient will have heart rate within acceptable limits and not demonstrate pacing behaviors preoperatively.

      b. Phase I

        (1) Patient's temperature will be within normal range within 30 minutes of arrival.

        (2) Patient will report a pain score under 3 on 1-10 scale.

        (3) Patient's vital signs will be within 20% of preoperative levels.

      c. Phase II

        (1) Patient will be free of postoperative infection.

        (2) Patient will be knowledgeable about postoperative wound care.

        (3) Patient will resume self-care activities of daily living without pain.

  B. Nursing Outcomes Classification (NOC) system classifies standardized nurse-sensitive outcomes.

    1. Components of NOC

      a. Patient outcomes are nurse-sensitive.

        (1) A nursing intervention will be used to produce or influence the outcome.

        (2) A nursing intervention occurred before the observation of the outcome.

        (3) Interventions that produced or influenced the outcome are within the nurse's scope of practice.

      b. Outcome includes a label with definition.

        (1) Describes the complete meaning of outcome concept

        (2) Clear and simple

        (3) Describes a state, behavior, or perception that is inherently variable and can be measured and quantified

(4) Describe in nonevaluative terms (e.g., words such as *decreased, improved* not appropriate)
  c. Outcome includes indicators.
    (1) Defined: an observable patient outcome that is sensitive to nursing intervention
    (2) Indicators serve to characterize a patient's state.
      (a) In expected range (IER)
      (b) Within normal limits (WNL)
  d. Outcomes are assessed on a measurement scale.
    (1) Seventeen scales from NOC classification
    (2) Each Likert scale includes five points.
2. Examples of perianesthesia nurse-sensitive outcomes
  a. Preoperative
    (1) Outcome: fear control—personal actions to eliminate or reduce disabling feelings of alarm aroused by an identifiable source
    (2) Indicators: uses effective coping strategies, maintains concentration, uses relaxation techniques to reduce fear
    (3) Measurement scale: 1-5
      (a) 1 = never demonstrated
      (b) 2 = rarely demonstrated
      (c) 3 = sometimes demonstrated
      (d) 4 = often demonstrated
      (e) 5 = consistently demonstrated
  b. Perioperative
    (1) Outcome: thermoregulation—balance among heat production, heat gain, and heat loss
    (2) Indicators: body temperature WNL, shivering when cold
    (3) Measurement scale: 1-5
      (a) 1 = extremely compromised
      (b) 2 = substantially compromised
      (c) 3 = moderately compromised
      (d) 4 = mildly compromised
      (e) 5 = not compromised
  c. Phase I
    (1) Outcome: circulation status—extent to which blood flows unobstructed, unidirectionally, and at an appropriate pressure through large vessels of the systemic and pulmonary circuits
    (2) Indicators: systolic blood pressure (BP) (IER), heart rate (IER), peripheral pulses strong, peripheral pulses symmetrical
    (3) Measurement scale: 1-5
      (a) 1 = extremely compromised
      (b) 2 = substantially compromised
      (c) 3 = moderately compromised
      (d) 4 = mildly compromised
      (e) 5 = not compromised
  d. Phase II
    (1) Outcome: ambulation, walking—ability to walk from place to place
    (2) Indicators: walks at slow pace, bears weight
    (3) Measurement scale: 1-5
      (a) 1 = does not participate
      (b) 2 = requires assistive person and device
      (c) 3 = requires assistive person
      (d) 4 = independent with assistive device
      (e) 5 = completely independent
C. Planning is documented in writing to inform all health care providers.
  1. Preprinted, standardized care plans or critical paths are guides adapted to each patient.

2. Individualized care plans include assessments and diagnoses that are specific to the patient.
3. Care plan usually consists of preprinted document, which is individualized.

V. Nursing process: implementation
   A. Nursing implementation consists of those activities or interventions performed by the nurse or delegated to unlicensed health personnel.
   B. Purpose of interventions
      1. Reduce risks (e.g., preop: determine preoperative NPO status during interview)
      2. Monitor health status (e.g., phase I: record BP every 10 minutes)
      3. Resolve, prevent, or manage problem (e.g., phase I, II: assess respiratory status, encourage deep breathing)
      4. Facilitate independence and assist with self-care (e.g., phase II: educate about urinary catheter care prior to discharge)
      5. Promote wellness (e.g. phase II: educate on lifestyle and dietary changes following removal of urinary tract stone)
   C. Types of interventions
      1. Direct care: actions performed through direct interaction with patient (e.g., obtaining vital signs)
      2. Indirect care: actions performed away from the client but on behalf of the client (e.g., monitoring laboratory values)
      3. Independent: activities initiated by the registered nurse on the basis of knowledge and skill (e.g., teaching patient about wound care for discharge)
      4. Dependent: activities carried out under the physician's order (e.g., administering ketorolac for pain)
      5. Collaborative: activities carried out in conjunction with other health team members (e.g., reinforcing crutch walking initiated by physical therapy)
      6. Interventions for high-risk nursing diagnoses
         a. Reduce or eliminate risk factors.
         b. Prevent occurrence of problem.
         c. Monitor onset of problem.
      7. Interventions for possible nursing diagnoses: collect additional data to confirm or rule out diagnoses.
      8. Interventions for collaborative problems
         a. Monitor for change in status.
         b. Manage problem with physician-prescribed therapy.
         c. Evaluate response of prescribed therapy.
   D. Nursing interventions may be selected from the Nursing Interventions Classification (NIC) system
      1. NIC classifies nursing activities using standardized language.
      2. Priority interventions are research based.
      3. Characteristics of interventions
         a. Consistent with the nursing diagnosis
         b. Implemented safely or delegated appropriately
         c. Documented
      4. Interventions include the following actions:
         a. Directly performing an activity
         b. Assisting the patient to perform the activity
         c. Supervising the performance of the activity by patient or caregiver
         d. Delegating the activity to unlicensed assistive personnel
         e. Teaching patients
         f. Counseling patients about health care alternatives
         g. Monitoring for potential complications
      5. Examples of interventions by perianesthesia nurses
         a. Preoperative
            (1) Obtain baseline vital signs.
            (2) Reinforce preoperative teaching.

            (3) Initiate intravenous access for antibiotic prophylaxis.

            (4) Measure patient for antiembolism stockings.

      b. Intraoperative

            (1) Monitor vital signs.

            (2) Position patient to maintain skin integrity.

            (3) Provide emotional support during local anesthetic.

            (4) Administer conscious sedation.

      c. Phase I

            (1) Monitor vital signs.

            (2) Encourage deep breathing.

            (3) Administer pain medication.

            (4) Reposition.

      d. Phase II

            (1) Reinforce preoperative teaching prior to discharge.

            (2) Encourage fluid intake.

            (3) Identify environmental factors that may create risk for falls at home.

            (4) Administer oral pain medication.

VI. Nursing process: evaluation

   A. Evaluation of the nursing process requires a determination of the achievement of nurse-sensitive patient outcomes.

   B. Steps in patient outcome evaluation

     1. Perform assessment to determine patient status.

     2. Compare assessment findings to expected outcomes.

     3. Determine extent of expected outcome achievement.

       a. Completely met

       b. Partially met

       c. Not met

     4. Identify variables that have affected achievement of expected outcomes (e.g., unexpected anesthetic technique, development of postoperative nausea, inability to contact adult caregiver).

     5. Decide whether to continue, modify, or terminate the plan of care.

       a. Continue plan if outcome not achieved but variables impeding care are not identified.

       b. Modify plan if outcome not achieved but variables impeding care have been identified and can be resolved.

       c. Terminate plan if outcome met.

VII. Communicating the nursing process

   A. Communicating nursing process includes written documentation and oral reporting to health care providers.

   B. All phases of nursing process are communicated.

   C. Purpose of communicating nursing process

     1. Informs other health care providers of patient status

     2. Assists in identifying common response patterns

     3. Provides foundation for evaluation of services (e.g., quality improvement, research)

     4. Creates a legal document

     5. Validates service rendered for reimbursement

   D. Written documentation by perianesthesia nurse includes:

     1. Patient history

     2. Standardized care plan or critical path flow sheet

     3. Flow sheet for assessment findings and vital signs

     4. Nurses' progress notes for variations from norm

     5. Discharge teaching instructions

   E. Oral communication

     1. Used when providing change of shift report, or providing report to other health care providers (e.g., anesthetist, unlicensed caregiver)

     2. Delivered in private environment to ensure patient confidentiality

     3. Should stress unusual or abnormal findings

VIII. Nursing process specific to perianesthesia nursing

   A. The steps of the nursing process in the perianesthesia environment are accomplished almost simultaneously due to the quick procedural time.

   B. Assessment of the patient from the preadmission interview to the postdischarge follow up is an ongoing process.

   C. A strong emphasis is placed on identifying priority nursing diagnoses.

   1. Airway related

   2. Breathing related

   3. Circulation related

   4. Disturbing symptoms: pain, nausea, urinary retention

   5. Knowledge deficits

   D. Evaluations of expected patient outcomes may occur after discharge during follow up telephone contact.

   E. Documentation of instructions for aftercare and the patient's understanding are crucial following anesthesia.

   F. Documentation of care must comply with predetermined standards established by third-party payers for reimbursement purposes.

BIBLIOGRAPHY

1. Alfaro-LeFevre R: *Applying nursing process: A step by step guide,* ed 5. Philadelphia: Lippincott, 2002.

2. Johnson M, Maas M, Moorehead S: *Nursing outcomes classification,* ed 2. St Louis: Mosby, 2000.

3. Johnson M, Bulechek G, McCloskey Dochterman J, et al. *Nursing diagnoses, outcomes and interventions: NANDA, MIC, NOC linkages.* St Louis: Mosby, 2001.

4. McCloskey JC, Bulecek GM. *Iowa intervention project: Nursing intervention classification (NIC),* ed 3. St Louis: Mosby, 2000.

5. North American Nursing Diagnosis Association: *Nursing diagnoses: Definitions and classification 2001-2002.* Philadelphia: North American Nursing Diagnosis Association, 2001.

6. Wilkinson J: *Nursing diagnosis handbook,* ed 7. Upper Saddle River, NJ: Prentice Hall, 2000.

4 Patient and Family Education

PAMELA M. DARK

OBJECTIVES

At the conclusion of this chapter the reader will be able to:

1. Utilize the nursing process to provide patient and family education (assessment, nursing diagnosis, planning, implementation, and outcome evaluation).
2. Define Joint Commission on Accreditation of Health Care Organizations (JCAHO) standards for patient and family education.
3. Identify elements of a needs assessment.
4. Identify barriers to learning.
5. Design a patient education plan based on information obtained in the needs assessment.
6. Develop patient education that addresses the five teaching domains.
7. Develop components of patient teaching utilizing the three domains of learning.
8. Develop teaching strategies that meet the needs of patients with different learning styles.
9. Develop methods for evaluation of patient education.
10. Utilize information obtained from evaluations to improve the education process.

I. Define JCAHO standards for patient and family education.
   A. JCAHO's goal of the patient and family education function is to improve patient health outcomes by promoting healthy behavior and involving the patient in care and care decisions.[10]
   B. Expectations:
      1. Provide information that will enhance knowledge and skills necessary to promote recovery and improve function.
      2. The patient receives education and training specific to the patient's assessed needs, abilities, learning preferences, and readiness to learn as appropriate to the care and services provided by the hospital or facility (JCAHO PF.3).
      3. Consider barriers in education assessment.
         a. Cultural
         b. Religious
         c. Physical limitations
         d. Cognitive limitations
         e. Language
         f. Financial barriers
      4. Educate patients about safe and effective use of medications according to their needs.
      5. Educate patients about safe and effective use of equipment and supplies and means of obtaining them.
      6. Counsel patients.
         a. To foods and diets appropriate to illness
         b. To possible food–drug interactions

7. Provide patients leaving a facility with information on obtaining follow-up care and accessing community resources.[4]
8. Provide patients with education about pain and pain management as part of treatment.
9. Provide patients with information about their responsibilities in their care including self-care activities.
   a. Patients have been identified as having responsibilities as well as rights.
10. Provide discharge instructions that contain information about
    a. Diet
    b. Activity
    c. Medications
    d. Follow-up care
    e. Plan of care
    f. Contact number if the patient has questions
11. Provide documentation of education to patient and family.
    a. Verbally
    b. Written form
12. Provide patients with information about available resources that will facilitate habilitation or rehabilitation.
13. Promote the patient education process among appropriate staff and disciplines that are providing care or services.
14. Care is planned for and coordinated by the facility providing the patient services.

II. Assessment
   A. Identify elements of a "needs assessment."
      1. "Needs assessment: The process of determining through data collection what a person, group, organization, or community must learn and/or wants to learn to provide appropriate education programs to meet the required or desired needs of the learners"[1]
      2. Ascertain learning needs.[1]
         a. Readiness to learn (willingness or ability to accept information)
         b. Emotional intelligence (chemical changes that facilitate the process of receiving and interpreting information)[3]
         c. Knowledge of disease or care management
            (1) Where do you obtain your health information (e.g., physician, nurse, magazines, books, pharmacist, etc.)?
         d. Functional barriers (reading ability, language, means of learning, sensory problems)
            (1) Reading level—most individuals are at five grade levels below last completed year of school.
            (2) Ask patient to read something simple (e.g., something posted in patient room).
            (3) Assess comprehension—reading tests do not determine what was learned or understood, only that the person can read the material.
         e. Cultural or spiritual beliefs (see Chapter 22)
      3. Learning needs are identified deficits in knowledge that exist between a desired level of performance and the actual level of performance.
         a. Exist due to a lack of knowledge, attitude, or skills[1]
      4. Consider options for obtaining information.
         a. Informal conversations
         b. Questionnaires
         c. Observations
         d. Structured interviews
            (1) Telephone
            (2) Face to face
         e. Focus groups
         f. Patient charts

  g. Risk management reports

  h. Committee requests

  i. Professional society standards or requirements

  j. Changes in patient populations

  k. Patterns of care delivery

  l. Regulatory requirements

 5. Motivation for learning

  a. Internal is more lasting and more self-directive.

  b. Need for learning is recognized.

   (1) Patients who are ill do not absorb information well—this improves as health returns.

  c. Encourage motivation.

   (1) Provide nonthreatening environment.

   (2) Encourage self-direction and independence.

   (3) Demonstrate a positive attitude about patient's ability to learn.

   (4) Offer continuing support and encouragement as attempts are made to learn.

   (5) Create learning situations in which patient is likely to succeed.

B. Consider the patient as an individual with specific needs, abilities, values, knowledge, and skills.

 1. Start with what the learner knows.

  a. Determine what the patient, family, or significant other feels that they need to know.

   (1) Collect data from patient, family, or significant other.

   (2) Determine what the patients consider needs and problems and what motivates them.

 2. Determine learning style (way that individual processes information).

  a. Adults often use more than one method of learning, but have a primary learning preference.

  b. Children have a more defined preference for one of the learning styles.

  c. May need to use more than one method to provide information

  d. Learning styles

   (1) Visual: Learn through seeing. Like to see the big picture or diagrams. Like demonstrations, or watching videos, will prefer to have written material to coincide with the verbal instructions.

   (2) Auditory: Learn through hearing. Like to listen to audio tapes, lectures, debates, discussion, and verbal instructions.

   (3) Kinesthetic: Learn through physical activities and through direct involvement. Like to be "hands-on," moving, touching, experiencing, will respond well to hands-on learning with equipment and return demonstration of skills.

 3. Prioritize needs

  a. Maslow's hierarchy of needs provides a guideline for determining patient needs.

   (1) Physiological needs

   (2) Safety and security needs

   (3) Belonging and love needs

   (4) Esteem needs

   (5) Self-actualization needs

  b. Involve patient and family in determining what they consider important to learn.

 4. Determine availability of resources.

  a. Focus on what is available and what information can be provided to patient and family for the present and/or future use.

 5. Consider time-management issues.

  a. What can be provided in the time frame available?

  b. Minimize distractions.

      6. Assessment of readiness to learn
        a. Utilize *PEEK* method.[1]
          (1) Physical readiness (measure of ability, complexity of task, environmental effects, health status, gender)
          (2) Emotional readiness (anxiety level, support system, motivation, risk-taking behavior, frame of mind, development stage)
          (3) Experiential readiness (level of aspiration, past coping mechanisms, cultural background, locus of control, orientation)
          (4) Knowledge readiness (present knowledge base, cognitive ability, learning disabilities, learning styles)
        b. Demonstrates an interest in learning
        c. Observation
        d. Patient or chart
        e. Timing
          (1) What is occurring at the moment?
          (2) How much time is involved in teaching (brief and basic)?
        f. Health beliefs and practices
        g. Cultural factors
        h. Economic concerns and resources
        i. Support systems
    C. Sources of information:
      1. Statistics from the literature or experience, such as who is most likely to develop specific complications
      2. Patient history
      3. Consider the age of the patient
        a. Developmental needs
        b. What do patients need to learn?
          (1) Avoid providing graphic details. Provide general information and more specific information if requested by patient.
          (2) Information about process—what will happen along the way?
      4. Educational background and primary language
      5. Cultural factors
        a. "Do you seek the advice of another health practitioner?"
        b. "Do you use herbs or other medications or treatments?"
        c. "What language do you use most often when speaking and writing?"
      6. What knowledge, skills, values, and attitudes does the patient have?
III. Nursing diagnosis:
    A. Identify barriers to learning.
      1. Preoperative
        a. Knowledge deficits and information seeking behaviors, risks for developing problems
          (1) Process issues
          (2) Safety issues
          (3) Risks for injury, infection
          (4) Anxiety
          (5) Hypothermia or hyperthermia
          (6) Potential coping inability, ineffective coping
          (7) Ineffective or absent support system
          (8) Body image disturbance
          (9) Caregiver role strain
         (10) Risk for altered development
         (11) Fears
         (12) Fluid volume deficits
         (13) Latex allergy risk or problem
         (14) Impaired mobility
         (15) Pain management concerns (acute and chronic)
         (16) Nutritional deficits and concerns

    2. Postoperative
       a. Knowledge deficits and risks for developing problems
         (1) Airway management problems
         (2) Safety concerns
         (3) Hypothermia or hyperthermia
         (4) Nutritional concerns and needs
         (5) Altered mental status
         (6) Activity intolerance or inability
         (7) Aspiration risk
         (8) Body image disturbance
         (9) Caregiver role strain
         (10) Communication impaired
         (11) Risk for altered, delayed, or regressed development
         (12) Altered family processes
         (13) Fear
         (14) Fluid volume deficit or excess
         (15) Grieving
         (16) Latex allergy risk or problem
         (17) Impaired mobility
         (18) Nausea
         (19) Impaired memory
         (20) Ineffective pain management (acute and chronic)
         (21) Nutritional concerns and deficits
         (22) Impaired skin integrity
         (23) Altered sleep patterns and inadequate sleep
         (24) Impaired tissue integrity
         (25) Urinary elimination concerns
         (26) Altered sexuality
         (27) Risk for development of constipation
   3. Determine specific problems of patient and family or significant other.
   4. Nursing diagnosis may be formal or informal.
       a. May be incorporated into a care process model or map
   5. Diagnosis may be related to altered health responses or dysfunction.
       a. May be anticipated or actual problems

IV. Planning: Design a patient education plan based on information obtained in the needs assessment.
   A. Develop teaching plan based on mutually predetermined behavioral outcomes to meet individual needs.[1]
      1. Assess suitability of education materials used for patients.
        a. Reading level can be assessed using a variety of assessment tools.
         (1) Simple checks include font size and type style, color contrast between the ink and the paper, appearance (does it look hard to read?), number of components and facts in each paragraph, and the use of familiar words in an unfamiliar context.
         (2) Avoid the use of medical terminology—explain in terms the patient and family can understand.
         (3) Use words of less than three syllables. Use simple, smaller words.
         (4) Write shorter sentences.
         (5) Active voice—avoid passive voice.
         (6) Reading materials should be at a fifth grade or lower reading level.
   B. The needs of the patient are assessed first.
      1. Address immediate and emerging needs—explain rationale for what will be occurring.
        a. Physical
        b. Psychological
        c. Social

      d. Nutritional status

      e. Functional status

      f. Pain

      g. Necessary diagnostic tests based on patient diagnosis and condition—not routine testing

      h. Discharge planning

        (1) Starts at first contact with patient and progresses through each additional contact

   2. Determine teaching priorities.

   3. Develop learning objectives.

      a. Desired outcomes

        (1) State the desired client behavior or performance.

        (2) Reflect an observable, measurable activity

        (3) May add conditions or modifiers as required to clarify what, where, when, or how the behavior will be performed

        (4) Include criteria specifying the time by which learning should have occurred.

      b. Learning objectives can reflect the learners' command of simple to complex concepts.

      c. Must be specific about what behaviors and knowledge (cognitive, psychomotor, affective) the learner must have to accomplish the desired outcome

        (1) Example: Describe signs and symptoms of wound infection. Identify equipment needed for wound care. Describe appropriate actions if questions or complications arise.

   4. Select specific content to be addressed.

   5. Select teaching strategies to be utilized based on information obtained in needs assessment.[2]

      a. Explanation (cognitive)

      b. One to one discussion (affective, cognitive)

      c. Answering questions (cognitive)

      d. Demonstration (psychomotor)

      e. Discovery (cognitive, affective)

      f. Group discussions (affective, cognitive)

      g. Practice (psychomotor)

      h. Printed and audiovisual materials (cognitive)

      i. Role-playing (affective, cognitive)

      j. Modeling (affective, psychomotor)

      k. Computer-assisted learning programs (all types of learning)

   6. Teach basics before progressing to more difficult concepts.

   7. Allow time for questions and review of contents for clarification.

C. Specific patient population requirements—will have bearing on ability to learn and interact

   1. Age-specific—Infant, child, adolescent, adult, and geriatric

      a. Emotional, cognitive, communication, educational

      b. Developmental age—not just age of patient

        (1) Are there any developmental delays or injuries that may have impacted the ability to learn?

      c. Family's, significant other's, or guardian's expectations for and involvement in care

      d. Emotional or behavioral disorders

      e. Alcoholism or drug dependency

      f. Possible victims of abuse or neglect

      g. Patients with history of posttraumatic stress disorder (PTSD) or previous unpleasant experiences

      h. Cultural preferences

      i. Past and present health care practices

      j. Language barriers

        (1) New legislation requires the use of qualified interpreters for limited English proficiency (LEP) patients representing the largest minority group in the area.

        (2) The patient has the option of declining the interpreter and using a family member or friend, but this must be documented on the patient record.

        (3) Qualified interpreters must be used for all "life-threatening" information such as diagnosis, patient histories, surgical procedures, medical procedures, procedural consents, and discharge instructions (unless declined by the patient).

        (4) Information can be taken and given over the phone via an authorized interpreter if the interpreter is not available to come to the hospital or facility site.

D. Pediatric concerns when addressing educational needs

  1. Pediatric stages of growth and development

  2. Psychosocial development (Erikson)[13]

    a. Experiences can be favorable or unfavorable.

    b. Birth to one year (trust vs. mistrust)

      (1) Establishment of trust dominates.

      (2) Trust exists in relationship to someone or something.

    c. One to three years (autonomy vs. shame and doubt)

      (1) Autonomy is centered on the children's increased ability to control their bodies, themselves, and their environments.

      (2) Want to do things for themselves by using newly acquired motor skills (walking, climbing, and mental powers of selection and decision making)

      (3) Much of learning is acquired through imitation of activities and behavior.

      (4) Negative feelings arise when made to feel small and self-conscious, when consequences of behavior and choices are negative, when shamed by others, or forced to be dependent in areas where independence has been demonstrated.

    d. Three to six years (initiative vs. guilt)

      (1) Characterized by energetic and intrusive behavior and a strong imagination. Children explore the world with all of their senses and abilities.

      (2) No longer guided by outsiders; have developed a conscience that warns and protects or threatens them

      (3) A sense of guilt occurs when in conflict with others or they are made to feel that their behaviors are bad.

      (4) Must learn to maintain initiative without encroaching on the rights of others

    e. Six to twelve years (industry vs. inferiority)

      (1) Children want to engage in activities and behaviors that they can complete. Need a sense of achievement

      (2) Learn to compete and cooperate with others; learn the rules

      (3) Important stage in learning to develop relationships with others

      (4) May feel inadequate and inferior if too much is expected of them or they believe they cannot measure up to standards set for them by others

    f. Twelve to eighteen years (identity vs. role confusion)

      (1) Development characterized by rapid and marked physical changes

      (2) Adolescents' perception of their bodies changes and diminishes.

      (3) Become overly preoccupied with others' perceptions of themselves

      (4) Face difficulty in dealing with concepts that others expect of them and the values of society

  3. Cognitive development (Piaget)

    a. Cognitive development consists of age-related changes that occur in mental activities.

    b. Intelligence enables individuals to make adaptations to the environment that increase the probability of survival.[13]

    c. Three stages of reasoning
- (1) Intuitive
- (2) Concrete operational
- (3) Formal operational

    d. Concrete reasoning for children begins at about 7 years of age

    e. Birth to two years (sensorimotor)
- (1) Six substages that are governed by sensations
- (2) Progress from simple reflex activity to simple repetitive behaviors to imitative behavior
- (3) Develop a sense of cause and effect
- (4) Display a high level of curiosity, experimentation, and enjoyment of new things
- (5) Begin to develop a sense of self, become aware of a sense of permanence
- (6) Begin to use language and thought

    f. Two to seven years (preoperational)
- (1) Children interpret objects in sense of relationships or the use to themselves. Unable to see things from any perspective but their own
- (2) See things in sense of concrete and tangible; lack the ability to use deductive reasoning
- (3) Use imaginative play, questioning, and other interactions to develop the ability to make associations between ideas
- (4) Thought is dominated by what children see, hear, or experience. Have increasing use of language and symbols to represent objects in their environment

    g. Seven to eleven years (concrete operations)
- (1) Become increasingly logical and articulate
- (2) Are able to sort, classify, order, and organize information to use in problem solving
- (3) Develop a new concept of permanence
- (4) Able to deal with multiple aspects of a situation simultaneously
- (5) Do not yet have the ability to deal with abstract concepts
- (6) Problems are solved in concrete systematic methods based on what children recognize.
- (7) Become less self-centered through interactions with others; thinking becomes socialized
- (8) Can consider points of view outside their own

    h. Eleven to fifteen years (formal operations)
- (1) Able to be adaptable and flexible
- (2) Can think in abstract terms and symbols and are able to draw logical conclusions from observations
- (3) Can make hypotheses and test them
- (4) Consider abstract, theoretical, and philosophical matters
- (5) May confuse the ideal with the practical, but in most cases can deal with the contradictions and resolve issues
- (6) Nonsocial stimulating experience that starts outside the child
- (7) Attention attracted by objects in the environment: light, color, taste, odors, textures, and consistencies
- (8) Use of body senses to experience

E. Stress:
1. Can be physiologic, psychological, or emotional
2. Some individuals are more vulnerable than others.
3. Responses can be behavioral, psychological, or physiologic.
4. Children are more vulnerable when a number of stressors are present.
5. Identify behaviors indicative of stress.

      6. Must listen to children—be aware of fears and concerns

      7. Physical comforting and reassuring is beneficial to children.

  F. Coping: individual reactions to stressors

      1. Strategies are specific to the person.

      2. Styles are relatively unchanging personality characteristics or outcomes of coping.

      3. Children have a more internal center of control.

      4. Strategies that use relaxation are effective in reducing stress.

  G. Fears

      1. Vary with age of child[13]

         a. Infants

           (1) 0-6 months: Loss of support, loud noise, bright lights, sudden movement

           (2) 7-12 months: Strangers, sudden appearance of unexpected and looming objects, animals, or heights

         b. Toddlers (1-3 years): Separation from parents, the dark, loud or sudden noise, injury, strangers, certain persons (e.g., the physician), certain situations (e.g., trip to the dentist), animals, large objects or machines, change in environment

         c. Preschoolers (3-5 years): Separation from parent, supernatural beings such as monsters, or ghosts, animals, the dark, noises, "bad" people, injury, death

         d. School-age children (6-12 years): Supernatural beings, injury, storms, the dark, staying alone, separation from parent, things seen on television or in movies, injury, tests and failure in school, consequences related to unattractive physical appearance, death

         e. Adolescents: Inept social performance, social isolation, sexuality, drugs, war, divorce, crowds, gossip, public speaking, plane and car crashes, death

  H. Adult concerns when addressing educational needs

      1. Early adulthood: 20-40 (intimacy vs. isolation)

         a. Have a commitment to work and relationships

           (1) Have they planned appropriately for the impact that surgery may have on their work, social, and personal life?

         b. Concerned with emancipation from parents and in building an independent lifestyle[9]

         c. Concerned with forming an intimate bond with another and choosing a mate

           (1) Seeks love, commitment, and industry of an intense lasting relationship

           (2) Relationships include mutual trust, cooperation, acceptance, sharing of feelings and goals.

           (3) Without secure personal identity, the adult cannot form a love relationship. The result is a lonely, isolated and withdrawn person

         d. Has reached maximum potential for growth and development

         e. All body systems operate at peak efficiency.

         f. Nutritional needs depend on maintenance and repair requirements and on activity levels.

         g. Sensible nutrition is a major problem for many adults.

         h. Cognitive function has reached a new level of formal operations and the capacity for abstract thinking.

         i. Less egocentric, operates in a more realistic and objective manner

         j. Is close to the maximum ability to acquire and use knowledge

         k. Work is an important factor in the young adult and is tied closely with ego identity.

         l. Begins to self-reflect in the late twenties to early thirties: "Where am I going?" "Why am I doing these things in my life?"

         m. Thirties are characterized by settling down.

  n. Strives to establish a niche in society and to build a better life
  o. Risk for stress is increased since there are many situations that require choices to be made.
  p. Single parents often have additional stress of decreased financial resources for themselves and/or children.
2. Middle adulthood: 40-64 years (generativity vs. stagnation)[9]
  a. Realization that life is half over has occurred.
  b. Accepting and adjusting to the physical changes of middle age
    (1) Effects of aging are becoming more apparent—wrinkles, graying or thinning hair, changes in body function, redistribution of fat deposits, decreased physical stamina and abilities.
    (2) Decreased respiratory capacity and cardiac function, visual changes
    (3) Sensory function remains intact except for some visual changes (e.g., decreased accommodation for near vision or presbyopia)
    (4) Females—menopause: Decrease in estrogen and progesterone—brings attendant symptoms of atrophy of reproductive organs, hot flashes and mood swings
    (5) Men: Decrease in testosterone, which causes a decreased sperm and semen production, and less intense orgasms
  c. Adjusting to aging parents
  d. Reviewing and redirecting career goals
  e. Helping adolescent children in their search for identity
    (1) Often feel caught in a "squeeze" between simultaneously changing needs of adolescent children and aging parents
  f. Accepting and relating to the spouse as a person
  g. Coping with an empty nest at home
  h. Aware of occasional death of peers—reminder of own mortality
  i. Leading causes of death are cardiovascular disease, cancer, and stroke.
  j. Morbidity is increased.
    (1) Often related to increase in obesity
    (2) Resulting hypertension, cardiovascular disease, diabetes and mobility dysfunction, and arthritis
    (3) Chronic smoking leads to health problems at this stage.
  k. Intelligence levels remain generally constant.
    (1) Is further enhanced by knowledge that comes with life experiences, self-confidence, a sense of humor, and flexibility
    (2) Interested in how new knowledge is applied, not just in learning for learning's sake
  l. Adults have an urge to contribute to the next generation.
    (1) Needs to be needed, to leave something behind
    (2) If fulfillment does not occur, stagnation is experienced—boredom, a sense of emptiness in life which leads to being inactive, self-absorbed, self-indulgent, a chronic complainer.
  m. Role realignment occurs in relationships with aging parents.
    (1) Once parents die, middle-aged adults are more vulnerable and realize limited quantities of time are left.
  n. Be alert for depressive symptoms, suicide risk factors, abnormal bereavement, signs of physical abuse or neglect, malignant skin lesions, peripheral arterial disease, and other body dysfunction (applies to young adulthood and late adulthood as well).
3. Maturity—65 years to death (integrity vs. despair)[9]
  a. Fastest growing segment of the population
  b. Developmental tasks include
    (1) Adjusting to changes in physical strength and health
    (2) Forming a new family role as an in-law and/or a grandparent
    (3) Adjusting to retirement and reduced incomes
    (4) Developing postretirement activities that enhance self-worth and usefulness

(5) Arranging satisfactory physical living quarters
(6) Adjusting to the death of spouse, family members, and friends
(7) Conducting a life review
(8) Preparing for the inevitability of one's own death

  c. Illness affects aging people more than those in other age groups.
    (1) Incidence of chronic disease increases, resistance to illness decreases, and recuperative power decreases.
    (2) Body aches and pains increase.
    (3) Increasingly dependent on the health care system for advice, health teaching, and physical care

  d. Widely diverse response to disease and health concerns is dependent on subjective attitude, physical activity, nutrition, personal habits, and occurrence of physical illness.

  e. Intellectual function depends on factors such as motivation, interest, sensory impairment, educational level, deliberate caution, and a tendency to conserve time and emotional energy rather than acting assertively.[9]
    (1) Decreased ability to read materials printed in normal or small font size
    (2) Loses ability to read materials printed in or on backgrounds of green and blue

  f. Decreased ability for complex decision making
    (1) Do not provide information for more than one task at a time. Giving a list of steps to follow produces confusion and inability to follow-through.

  g. Decreased speed of performance—requires more time to process and to complete tasks

  h. Memory may be affected.

  i. If so, short-term memory more so than long-term memory

  j. Retirement often involves financial adjustment.
    (1) May impact ability to manage disease processes if money is not available for medications or food

  k. Options to live alone may change as ability to care for self decreases.

  l. Reminded of limited time remaining as aging continues
    (1) Life review occurs.

  m. Feels content with life or has feelings of futility, despair, resentment, hopelessness, and a fear of death

  n. Decreased ability to read materials in normal or small font size

I. Develop patient education that addresses the five teaching domains.

  1. Situational and procedural information
    a. Examples
      (1) Explain process—preoperatively, intraoperatively, postoperatively.
      (2) Who will patient come into contact with?
      (3) Family's or significant other's role in process
      (4) Children—what parental or guardian role is, when parent or guardian will leave child and when will be back with them again

  2. Sensation and discomfort information
    a. Examples:
      (1) "What will occur?" "How will you feel?"
      (2) Pain management
      (3) Anxiety
      (4) "What will you hear?" Hearing is last sense to leave, first to return—may hear things even if not completely awake.

  3. Patient role information
    a. Examples
      (1) Explain procedures, follow up, medications.
      (2) Instruct about home health follow up, ways to manage at home.

  4. Skills training
    a. Examples
      (1) Teach skills (e.g., how to do a dressing change, empty drains, management of pain)

       5. Psychosocial support
         a. Examples
            (1) Assist in decision making.
            (2) Reinforce what may already be known.
            (3) Change: provide alternative behaviors or thoughts.
            (4) Maximize current level of functioning.

J. Develop components of patient teaching utilizing the three domains of learning.
    1. Types of learning
    2. Transfer of learning—not automatic or immediate
       a. Memory
          (1) Must move from short-term to long-term memory
    3. Problem solving
    4. Affective and attitude learning
       a. Addresses attitudes, behaviors, and feelings
       b. Most difficult domain in which to effect learning
    5. Psychomotor learning
       a. Motor skills
       b. Best taught by demonstration and hands-on experiences
       c. Provide the opportunity to practice.
       d. Return demonstration (e.g., use of incentive spirometer, crutch walking demonstration and practice)
    6. Cognitive learning
       a. Addresses the patient's understanding
       b. Incorporates use of facts, details and information basic to intellectual learning[3]
       c. Multiple methods best address this learning need.
       d. People remember
          10% of what they read
          20 % of what they hear
          30 % of what they see
          50 % of what they see and hear
          90% of what they say and do[3]

V. Interventions: Develop strategies that meet the needs of patients with different learning styles.
  A. Teaching is performed using specific methods of instruction and tools.
    1. Optimal time for learning depends primarily on the learner.
    2. Pace of the teaching session affects learning.
    3. Environment selected must be conducive to learning.
       a. Avoid distractions such as noise and interruptions.
    4. Teaching aids can foster learning and help focus learner's attention.
    5. Learning is more effective when the learner discovers the content for himself or herself.
       a. Provide stimulating motivation and stimulating self-direction.
       b. Provide feedback.
    6. Repetition reinforces learning.
    7. Organize information ahead of time.
    8. Use lay person's vocabulary.
    9. Teaching strategies
  B. Utilize specific teaching strategies.
    1. Group teaching
    2. Computer-assisted instruction
    3. Discovery and problem solving
    4. Behavior modification
  C. Develop patient education that addresses the five teaching domains.
  D. Develop teaching strategies that meet the needs of patients with different learning styles.
  E. Role of play in development
    1. Play assists in development of sensorimotor skills, intellectual development, socialization, creativity, and self-awareness. Has therapeutic and moral value

   2. Content of play
      a. Social-affective play
         (1) Take pleasure in relationships with people
         (2) Starts with smiling, cooing, progresses to initiating games and activities
         (3) Varies among cultures
      b. Sense-pleasure play
      c. Skill play
         (1) Repeat actions over and over
         (2) Determination to accomplish and develop new skills may produce a sense of frustration and pain.
      d. Unoccupied behavior
         (1) Not playful, but focus attention on anything that strikes the children's interest
         (2) Daydream, fiddle with clothes or other objects, or walk aimlessly
      e. Dramatic or pretend play
         (1) Dramatic or symbolic play begins in late infancy (11 to 13 months)
         (2) Predominant form of play in preschool child
         (3) As interactions with others increase, children attribute meaning to activities.
         (4) Acting out daily events provides modeling of behaviors of family and members of society.
         (5) Interacting with the environment develops a greater understanding of the world.
      f. Games
         (1) Found in all cultures
         (2) Repetitive activities allow progression to more complicated games and activities.
         (3) Challenge development of independent skills: puzzle solving, playing solitaire, computer or video games
         (4) Different ages participate in different games—simple to more complex
         (5) Preschoolers hate to lose and will try to cheat or change the rules, or demand exceptions.
         (6) School age and adolescents enjoy competitive games—mental and physical.
F. Transcultural teaching[2]
   1. Obtain teaching materials, pamphlets, and instructions in languages used by clients in the health care setting.
      a. Utilize a translator to evaluate materials.
   2. Use visual aids, such as pictures, charts, or diagrams to communicate meaning.
      a. Audiovisual material may help portray the intent of simple information.
   3. Use concrete rather than abstract words.
      a. Use simple language—short sentences, short words.
      b. Present only one idea at a time.
   4. Allow time for questions.
   5. Avoid the use of medical terminology.
   6. If understanding another's pronunciation is a problem, validate a brief meaning in writing.
   7. Use humor cautiously.
   8. Do not use slang words or colloquialisms.
   9. Do not assume that a client who nods, uses eye contact, or smiles is indicating an understanding of what is being taught.
   10. Invite and encourage questions during teaching.
   11. When explaining procedures or functioning related to personal areas of the body, it might be appropriate to have a nurse of the same sex do the teaching.

         12. Include the family in the planning and teaching.

         13. Consider the client's time orientation.

         14. Identify cultural health practices and beliefs.

            a. Provide education to patient in preferred language.

            b. Provide written materials in preferred language.

VI. Evaluation

   A. Develop methods of evaluation for patient education materials and processes.

      1. Both an ongoing and final process

      2. Evaluate achievement of desired outcomes.

         a. Established by patient, family, significant other and nursing collaboration

         b. Learning objectives and goals of education directed by nursing diagnosis

            (1) Cognitive learning demonstrated by acquisition of knowledge that directly impacts behavior changes

            (2) Psychomotor learning is best evaluated by observing how well the client carries out a procedure.

            (3) Affective learning is more difficult to observe. May be evaluated by determining if patient has made changes to behaviors that will improve long-term health status and by patient obtaining health education that impacts long-term health

      3. Evaluation of content[6]

         a. Purpose

            (1) Is it clearly stated?

            (2) Is it clearly understood?

         b. Content topics

            (1) That which is of greatest interest will become focus of patient efforts.

         c. Scope

            (1) Limited to purpose or objectives

         d. Summary and review

            (1) Reinforces and reiterates information addressed

      4. Literacy demand

         a. Reading grade level

            (1) Utilize reading formulas.

            (2) Keep materials at fifth grade or lower.

         b. Writing style

            (1) Active voice is more easily understood.

            (2) Conversational style

         c. Vocabulary

            (1) Common, explicit words are used.

         d. Sentence construction

            (1) New facts and behaviors are learned more quickly when learner is told the context first.

         e. Learning enhancement (road signs)

            (1) Headers or captions

      5. Graphics (illustrations, lists, tables, charts, graphs)

         a. Cover graphic

            (1) Material is judged by first impression.

            (2) Friendly, attractive, and clearly portrays intent of material

         b. Type of illustration

            (1) Simple line drawings promote realism without distracting details.

            (2) Avoid medical textbook drawings or abstract art or symbols.

         c. Relevance of illustrations

            (1) Avoid nonessential details such as room background, elaborate borders, and unneeded color.

            (2) Will detract from intent of material

         d. Graphics

            (1) If used, must have clear explanations (step by step, or how- to instructions)

            (2) Easily misunderstood

    e. Captions
       (1) Can quickly tell a reader what the graphic is about and where to focus
       (2) Brief and simple
6. Layout and typography
    a. Layout
       (1) Illustrations are on the same page adjacent to the text.
       (2) Layout and sequence of information are consistent, easy to predict flow.
       (3) Visual cuing devices (shading, boxes, arrows) are used to direct attention to specific points or key content.
       (4) Adequate white space is used to reduce appearance of clutter.
       (5) Use of color supports and is not distracting from the message.
       (6) Line length is 30-50 characters and spaces.
       (7) High contrast between paper and type
       (8) Paper has non-gloss or low-gloss surface.
    b. Typography
       (1) Type size and font make test easy or difficult to read at all levels.
       (2) Test type is uppercase and lowercase serif or sans serif.
       (3) Type size is at least 12 point.
       (4) Typographic cues (boldface, size, color) emphasize key points.
       (5) No ALL CAPS for long headers or running text
    c. Subheadings or "chunking"
       (1) Less than seven independent items—more easily remembered
       (2) Three to five items for lower literacy levels
7. Learning stimulation and motivation
    a. Interaction included in text and/or graphic
       (1) Chemical changes occur when the patient responds to the questions.
       (2) Memory is enhanced and retention occurs.
       (3) Moves to long-term memory
       (4) Ask to solve problems, to make choices, or to demonstrate, and so forth.
    b. Desired behavior patterns are modeled, shown in specific terms.
       (1) People learn more readily by observation and by doing it themselves, rather than by being told.
    c. Motivation
       (1) More motivated to learn when the tasks or behaviors are doable
       (2) Divide complex tasks into small parts—will experience small successes in understanding or problem solving.
8. Cultural appropriateness
    a. Cultural match: Logic, language, experience (LLE)
       (1) Does the LLE match the intended audience?
    b. Cultural image and examples
       (1) Present cultural images and examples in a realistic and positive way.
9. Evaluate the effectiveness of the teaching that was provided by the nurse.
    a. Consider all factors of the teaching experience.
       (1) Timing
       (2) Teaching strategies
       (3) Amount of information provided
       (4) Was the teaching helpful?
       (5) Was the patient, family, or significant other overwhelmed by the amount or type of information?
       (6) Request feedback from the patient, family, and significant other.
       (7) Were the needs of the patient considered when providing the education?
       (8) Were the patient's preferences for learning considered in providing the education?

10. Documentation of teaching process is essential.
    a. Provides a legal record that the teaching occurred
    b. Provides a record for referral and review with the patient at a later date (e.g., follow-up phone contact)
    c. Did the patient respond to the education?
    d. Documentation components
       (1) Diagnosed learning needs
       (2) Learning objectives
       (3) Topics taught
       (4) Client outcomes
       (5) Need for additional teaching
       (6) Resources provided
11. Were the tools and methods utilized appropriate?
12. Were there any barriers to assessing, planning, and delivering the education?
13. Were the evaluation and analysis objective?

B. Utilize information obtained from evaluations to improve the education process.
   1. Effectiveness of education is evaluated by changes in behavior, knowledge attained, attitudes, and skills development.
   2. Methods of evaluation
      a. Concurrent and retrospective
         (1) Self-report of patient, family or significant other
         (2) Direct observation
         (3) Retain copy of materials provided to patient.
   3. Methods of measurement
      a. Defined quality indicators that determine patient outcomes
      b. Observation
      c. Interview
      d. Checklist
      e. Written or oral testing (where appropriate)
      f. Patient demonstrates comprehension of information provided in postprocedural behaviors.
      g. Patient satisfaction surveys
      h. Postprocedure contacts
         (1) Surveys
         (2) Telephone contact
         (3) Other contacts
   4. Utilize feedback to improve the process for the future.
      a. Include actual information and skills taught.
      b. Teaching strategies used
      c. Time framework and content for each class
      d. Teaching outcomes and methods of evaluation

BIBLIOGRAPHY

1. Bastable SB: *Nurse as educator: Principles of teaching and learning.* Sudbury, MA: Jones and Bartlett, 1997.
2. Berman AJ, Burke K, Erb G, et al: *Fundamentals of nursing: Concepts, process, and practice,* ed 6. Upper Saddle River, NJ: Prentice Hall Health, 2000.
3. Burden N: *Ambulatory surgical nursing,* ed 2. Philadelphia: WB Saunders, 2000.
4. Canobbio MM: *Mosby's handbook of patient teaching,* ed 2. St Louis: Mosby, 2000, p ix.
5. American Society of PeriAnesthesia Nurses, DeFazio Quinn DM, editor: *Ambulatory surgical nursing core curriculum.* Philadelphia: WB Saunders, 1999.
6. Doak CC, Doak LG, Root JH: *Teaching patients with low literacy skills,* ed 2. Philadelphia: Lippincott, 1996.
7. Engel J: *Pocket guide to pediatric assessment,* ed 4. St Louis: Mosby.
8. Intermountain Health Care, Urban Central Region Hospitals Quality Resource Department: Fact sheets: Patient education. Salt

Lake City: Intermountain Health Care, Urban Central Region Hospitals Quality Resource Department, May 2003.

9. Jarvis C: *Physical Examination and Health Assessment,* ed 2. Philadelphia: WB Saunders, 1996.

10. Joint Commission for Accreditation of Healthcare Organizations: Joint Commission Standards: *Provision of Care, Treatment, and Services.* 2003.

11. Litwack K: *Core curriculum for perianesthesia nursing practice,* ed 4. Philadelphia: WB Saunders, 1999.

12. Redman BK: *The practice of patient education.* St Louis: Mosby, 2001.

13. Wong DL, Whaley LF, Wilson D, et al: *Whaley & Wong's nursing care of infants and children,* ed 6. St Louis: Mosby, 1999.

5 Nursing Research

SUSAN JANE FETZER

OBJECTIVES
At the conclusion of this chapter the reader will be able to:

1. Define nursing research.

2. Describe the purpose of nursing research.

3. Describe the nurse's role in protection of patients from unethical or harmful research.

4. Identify the components of a research proposal.

5. Differentiate the research process from the quality assurance process.

6. Identify three topics in perianesthesia nursing practice that are in need of research.

7. Identify three methods of applying ambulatory perianesthesia research in practice.

I. Definition of nursing research
  A. Scientific method: controlled, systematic process for conducting studies in which data are collected under constant conditions to decrease error so that all data are collected in the same manner
  B. Research: process of applying the scientific method to answer questions
  C. Nursing research: process of applying the scientific method to answer questions about nursing education, nursing practice, and nursing administration
II. Goals of nursing research
  A. Maximize patient outcomes from nursing interventions
  B. Establish a unique body of knowledge that validates the impact of perianesthesia nursing
  C. Maximize effectiveness and efficiency of perianesthesia nursing care delivery
III. Objectives of nursing research
  A. Validate interventions used by perianesthesia nurses
  B. Uncover perianesthesia phenomena not previously realized
  C. Develop and test theories able to explain, predict, and control perianesthesia nursing practice and patient outcomes
  D. Substantiate the unique contribution of perianesthesia nurses as health care providers
IV. Developing and planning a research study
  A. Phases
    1. Proposal development
    2. Institutional review approval
    3. Data collection
    4. Analysis
    5. Communication of findings
  B. Proposal development
    1. Definition: A proposal is the plan the researcher intends to implement to solve the research problem by answering the research question or supporting the research hypothesis.
    2. Proposal precedes the implementation of a research study.
      a. Assists the researcher to think through all steps in a study so nothing is missed

     b. Allows the researcher to make changes before investing time and money in procedures that may not be appropriate

     c. Encourages researcher to plan study with such clarity that it can be replicated (e.g., reproduced with another group)

     d. Provides an opportunity for peer review that allows constructive criticism from others who are knowledgeable about topic and research process for purpose of improving the study

     e. Proposal will be reviewed by the human subjects committee or institutional review board (IRB) prior to data collection.

3. Components of the proposal contains

     a. Introduction and problem statement

       (1) Introduction defines problem and provides background information so reader can understand why study needs to be conducted.

       (2) One to two paragraphs at the beginning of a research proposal that introduces the topic to the reader

       (3) Problem statement is a description of a dilemma or situation.

         (a) Dilemma or situation requires resolution by scientific inquiry and the development of new knowledge.

         (b) Situation has not been satisfactorily resolved by past research studies.

         (c) Dilemma exists because of a knowledge gap in the nursing literature.

         (d) Example of perianesthesia nursing introduction and problem statement (from Shertzer and Keck,[4] pp. 90-91):

> Pain is a common problem in the PACU resulting in negative consequences for the patient. Length of stay in the PACU contributes to total cost of the surgical experience. Unrelieved pain is one of the most common causes of delayed stay in the PACU, therefore, contributing to higher cost.

> The traditional means to provide pain relief in the PACU has been through the used of medications. The effect of medications differs from person to person because of great variability in personal responses to pain. Experts have suggested that a combination of pharmaceutical and nonpharmaceutical therapies have the greatest potential for providing optimal pain relief. Music and quiet conversation by staff have the potential to provide pain relief and improve patient satisfaction with the PACU experience. The effect of music with noise control in the PACU on pain reports is not known.

         (e) Perianesthesia topics that can be developed into research problems

           (i) Preoperative

             [a] Effectiveness of take-home preoperative video on patient compliance with preoperative regimen

             [b] Completeness of data provided by patient for preoperative database

             [c] Appropriate scheduling of preadmission visits

           (ii) Phase I

             [a] Role of registered nurse during conscious sedation

             [b] Speed of patient rewarming on pain management

             [c] Competency of unlicensed personnel

           (iii) Phase II

             [a] Validity of discharge criteria for regional anesthesia patients

             [b] Effectiveness of postoperative telephone calls in measuring patient outcomes

[c] Use of bladder scanner to determine postoperative voiding necessity

b. Proposal purpose statement

(1) The purpose statement provides a direction the researcher will take to solve the research problem.

(2) Includes the extent of the research project and the clinical context in which the researcher is interested

(3) Presents one sentence that clarifies and provides the specific reason for the research

(4) Example of perianesthesia nursing purpose statement (from Shertzer and Keck,[4] p. 93)

The purpose of the study was to investigate the effect of soothing music and control of noise on patients' perceived pain in PACU.

(5) Perianesthesia purpose statements in need of research

    (i) Preoperative

      [a] The purpose of the study is to determine the effectiveness of a take-home preoperative video on patient compliance with preoperative regimen.

      [b] The purpose of the study is to describe the completeness of the data provided by the patient for the preoperative database.

      [c] The purpose of the study is to determine the most appropriate scheduling of preadmission visits.

    (ii) Phase I

      [a] The purpose of the study is to describe the role of the registered nurse during moderate sedation and analgesia.

      [b] The purpose of the study is to describe the relationship between the speed of patient rewarming and perceived pain.

      [c] The purpose of the study is to determine the relationship between the availability of unlicensed personnel and nursing satisfaction.

    (iii) Phase II

      [a] The purpose of the study is to determine the validity of discharge criteria for regional anesthesia patients.

      [b] The purpose of the study is to determine effectiveness of postoperative telephone calls in measuring patient outcomes.

      [c] The purpose of the study is to determine the relationship between bladder scan volume and postoperative voiding urgency.

c. Proposal review of literature

(1) The review of literature presents and clarifies what has been previously written or studied on the proposed topic.

(2) The researcher seeks out available solutions to the research problem in the existing literature before planning the study.

(3) Includes a written summary of previous research related to the study problem and purpose

(4) Provides the reader with a comprehensive background on the research topic

(5) Types of literature

    (a) Research-based literature—qualitative or quantitative research studies that follow steps of the scientific method found in nursing and nonnursing journals

    (b) Theoretical—opinions or empirical experience articles found in nursing and nonnursing journals

    (c) Research-based literature is preferred.

      (6) Literature breadth and depth
        (a) Breadth—wide variety of topics because area of research not well defined
        (b) Depth—focused review on single concept when area of research is extensively documented in existing literature

d. Proposal research question and/or hypotheses
  (1) Study purpose is narrowed down further to focus on one or two research questions and/or hypotheses.
  (2) Research question
    (a) Definition: an interrogative statement posed by the researcher when little is known about the topic
    (b) Used when there is insufficient past research to predict a relationship between two characteristics (variables) or an effect of one variable on another
    (c) Components include the group to be studied and the characteristics (variables) under investigation.
    (d) Examples of perianesthesia nursing research questions
      (i) Preoperative
        [a] What preoperative information do cataract patients retain?
        [b] How do parents describe the effect of pediatric preoperative tours on the child's behavior?
        [c] What are the characteristics of patients who do not comply with fasting limits (e.g., nothing by mouth [NPO]) preoperatively?
      (ii) Phase I
        [a] What are the educational characteristics of RNs administering conscious sedation?
        [b] What is the older nurse's experience of being on-call?
        [c] How long does it take an elderly patient to regain movement after spinal anesthesia?
      (iii) Phase II
        [a] What is the effect of ketorolac on discharge temperature of elderly patients?
        [b] What is the most frequent reason for inability to contact patients by phone for discharge follow-up?
        [c] What are the factors associated with the ambulatory perianesthesia nurse's proficiency with cardiopulmonary resuscitation?
  (3) Research hypothesis
    (a) Definition: a formal declaration of an expected relationship or cause and effect between two characteristics (variables) made by the researcher based on established theory and/or past research
    (b) Statement that offers a potential solution to the research problem that can be supported by the existing literature and the researcher's experience
    (c) The hypothesis is always determined prior to the study and offers a framework for the research methodology.
    (d) Components of a hypothesis
      (i) Group being studied
      (ii) Characteristics (variables) being studied
      (iii) The direction of the expected relationship (e.g., positive, negative, increased, decreased)
    (e) Examples of perianesthesia nursing research hypotheses
      (i) Preoperative
        [a] Cataract patients who are provided with face-to-face preoperative education will remember more

information than cataract patients who are given an audiovisual preoperative video.

[b] Patients scheduled for breast biopsy will report more anxiety if the time between preadmission interview and day of surgery is longer than three days.

[c] There is a positive relationship between patient educational level and compliance with NPO guidelines.

(ii) Phase I

[a] There will be a positive relationship between the postanesthesia care unit (PACU) nurse's years of experience and comfort with administering moderate sedation and analgesia.

[b] Patients who receive intravenous ketorolac preoperatively will report less postoperative pain than patients who receive intravenous ketorolac intraoperatively.

[c] Patients who receive supplemental oxygen during postoperative transport to PACU will report less nausea than patients who do not receive supplemental oxygen.

(iii) Phase II

[a] Discharge assessment phone calls placed after 5:00 P.M. will be more successful than phone calls placed before 5:00 P.M.

[b] There is a negative relationship between duration of preoperative NPO status and ability to void prior to discharge in cystoscopy patients.

[c] Pediatric patients who participate in preoperative pediatric tours will recover faster than patients who do not participate.

(4) Research variables

(a) Definition: any quality or characteristic that is likely to change and/or is observed or measured by the researcher

(b) The independent variable is a characteristic selected by the researcher and believed to affect another characteristic (i.e., dependent variable).

(c) The dependent variable is the characteristic believed by the researcher to change when the independent variable is changed.

(d) The independent variable is the cause or antecedent; the dependent variable is the effect or outcome.

(e) Demographic variables are characteristics of the group (e.g., patients) being measured (i.e., gender, age, type of anesthesia, type of surgery, height, weight).

(f) The independent, dependent, and demographic variables require definition and measurement by the researcher; other characteristics, which may impact the research study, should be controlled.

(g) The independent and dependent variables are found in the purpose statement and the research question or the hypothesis.

(h) Examples of perianesthesia nursing variables of interest

(i) Preoperative

[a] Type of preoperative teaching strategy (e.g., face to face, video)

[b] Timing of preadmission visits (e.g., two days preoperative, day of surgery)

[c] Preoperative temperature

(ii) Phase I

[a] Postoperative temperature

      [b] Report of nausea
      [c] Oxygen saturation
    (iii) Phase II
      [a] Duration of time to discharge
      [b] Bladder volume
      [c] Report of pain
    (iv) Demographic variables—patients
      [a] Age
      [b] Gender
      [c] Surgical procedure
    (v) Demographic variables—providers
      [a] Years of experience
      [b] Certification status
      [c] Educational background
(i) Examples linking independent (IV) and dependent variables (DV) of interest
    (i) Type of teaching strategy (IV) and preoperative knowledge using a posttest score (DV)
    (ii) Time of preadmission visit (IV) and anxiety behavior (DV)
    (iii) Type of health care provider (IV) and patient satisfaction (DV)
    (iv) Warming device (IV) and postoperative temperature (DV)
    (v) Intravenous fluid administration volume (IV) and time to postoperative void (DV)
    (vi) Certification of RN provider (IV) and amount of conscious sedation administered (DV)
    (vii) Use of ketorolac (IV) and postoperative pain (DV)
    (viii) Postoperative phone call (IV) and patient satisfaction (DV)
    (ix) Use of pediatric tours (IV) and child anxiety behavior upon discharge (DV)
(5) Proposal methodology
  (a) Definition: the blueprint or plan taken by the researcher to collect the data required to answer the research question or support the research hypothesis
  (b) Includes all procedures required to collect the research data: design, sample, setting, instrument, procedure, data analysis
  (c) Researcher includes rationales for decisions on how, when, where data is collected as these decisions may affect the research results.
  (d) The researcher seeks to design the methodology so that the findings will have implications for nursing in general, not just the group being studied (e.g., generalizability).
(6) Proposal research design
  (a) Definition: the approach the researcher will use to collect the data—qualitative or quantitative
  (b) Depends on the purpose of the study and the research question or hypothesis
  (c) Qualitative research design
    (i) Focuses on the perianesthesia experience from the perspective of the patient
    (ii) Emphasis is on the holistic approach to the patient.
    (iii) Seeks to examine meaning of and insight into a patient's experience
    (iv) Used when previous research on the topic is limited or absent
    (v) Data is collected using words and narratives of patients.

(vi) Examples of topics using qualitative research designs in perianesthesia nursing

    [a] Preoperative

      [1] Experience of waiting for surgery

      [2] Patient's account of preadmission screening

      [3] A narrative response to advanced directive questions prior to surgery

    [b] Phase I

      [1] Patient's account of the experience of postanesthetic shivering

      [2] One patient's account of midazolam-induced amnesia

      [3] Experience of parents during the child's surgery

    [c] Phase II

      [1] A narrative response to inquiry about satisfaction with caregivers

      [2] Patients' experience with postdischarge nausea

      [3] Parental satisfaction with discharge instructions

(d) Quantitative research design

   (i) Focuses on understanding one part of the patient's experience

   (ii) Emphasis is placed on one or two selected variables of interest to the researcher.

   (iii) Used when a variable is in need of description (e.g., descriptive research), a relationship is being examined (e.g., correlational research), or cause and effect is being tested (e.g., experimental research)

   (iv) Data collected for quantitative research can be reduced to numbers for statistical analysis.

   (v) Examples of topics using quantitative research designs in perianesthesia nursing

    [a] Preoperative

      [1] Characteristics of patients who fail to follow preoperative instructions (descriptive research)

      [2] Effect of pediatric tours on parental anxiety (experimental research)

      [3] Relationship between NPO duration and preoperative blood pressure (correlational research)

    [b] Phase I

      [1] Relationship between fluid volume replacement intraoperatively and incidence of postoperative nausea (correlational research)

      [2] Incidence of hypothermia among the elderly patient (descriptive study)

      [3] Effect of Reiki therapy on report of postoperative pain (experimental study)

    [c] Phase II

      [1] Effect of ketorolac on discharge temperature (experimental research)

      [2] Incidence of postdischarge nausea (descriptive research)

      [3] Relationship between admission temperature and discharge temperature (correlational research)

(7) Proposal research sample

  (a) Definition: the individuals (i.e., patients, nurses, and family members) who agree to participate and provide data for the research study

  (b) Individuals who provide data are referred to as participants (qualitative design) or subjects (quantitative design).

(c) Sample is selected from the population of all individuals with the characteristic of interest.

(d) Sample is selected so that the individuals are representative of all the individuals who are known to have the variable(s) of interest to the researcher.

(e) Sample size

    (i) Qualitative design: data collected from participants until data saturation is obtained

    (ii) Quantitative design

        [a] Number of variables being studied

        [b] Type of variables being studied

        [c] Statistical analysis selected

        [d] Instrument used to measure variables

        [e] Power analysis (statistical calculation) used to determine number of subjects

(f) Types of samples

    (i) Simple random sample: random selection of study subjects from population of interest using flip of a coin or random numbers table

    Example: sample randomly selected from the population of thyroidectomy patients because it would be difficult and costly to study all patients in this category

    (ii) Stratified random samples: dividing subjects into layers or strata on the basis of specific attributes

    Example: PACU nurse wishes to study implementation of PACU standards of practice; hospitals are stratified by geographic location (east, west, north, south) and bed size (<100, 100-300, >300).

    (iii) Systematic random sampling: random selection of sample from a list or membership roster

    Example: American Society of PeriAnesthesia Nurses (ASPAN) membership roster (population of PACU nurses) is used to obtain a sample of PACU nurses for a study on attitudes toward research.

    (iv) Cluster sample: selection of a cluster of institutions in a geographic area

    Example: sample of patients selected from several PACUs from several hospitals in a metropolitan area

    (v) Convenience or accidental sample: obtaining subjects within readily available location or handy population

    Example: PACU nurse studies effect of music therapy on pain in first 50 adult perianesthesia patients having orthopedic surgery who agree to participate.

        [a] Problem with convenience samples: Patients studied may not be representative of all patients admitted to all PACUs in all states.

    (vi) Purposive sample: selected intentionally on the basis of a particular attribute and frequently used in instrument development

    Example: PACU nurse testing the ability of a new questionnaire to measure attitudes of ambulatory surgical patients' families regarding family visits in PACU would purposefully ask surgical patients' family members to participate in study. (Note: Families studied may not be representative of all types of ambulatory surgical patients' families.)

    (g) Sample criteria
        (i) Researcher makes decision on demographic characteristics of participants or subjects for the study
       (ii) Inclusion criteria—demographic characteristics the researcher desires
     (iii) Exclusion criteria—demographic characteristics that will make the participant or subject ineligible for the study
     (iv) Examples of selection criteria for perianesthesia nursing research sample
          [a] Fifty male patients having regional anesthesia for herniorraphy
          [b] All cataract patients requiring conscious sedation during the month of June
          [c] Every other adult patient requiring general anesthesia who is not allergic to aspirin
          [d] Children from 3 to 7 years old who are accompanied by a parent
          [e] Registered nurses who have been members of ASPAN for at least 10 years

(8) Research setting
    (a) Definition: location or environmental condition under which the study data are collected
    (b) A description of the setting allows the reader to determine whether the research environment is similar to the reader's environment and the findings are applicable to the reader's practice.
    (c) Examples of a perianesthesia nursing research setting
        (i) Waiting area of preadmission testing department
       (ii) Phase I PACU of a rural acute care facility with four operating suites and six postanesthesia bays
     (iii) Hospital-based surgery center caring for 30 pediatric surgical cases per week
     (iv) Operating room with temperature controlled at 60° F and humidity of 75%
      (v) Waiting area of the surgeon's office
     (vi) Patient's home

(9) Research instrument
    (a) Definition: any device (e.g., monitor, questionnaire, interview) that produces or records data required by the research project
    (b) Selection of the instrument depends on the variable being studied, the availability of the instrument, the expertise of the researcher, and the subject's capabilities.
    (c) The instrument should be able to actually measure what the researcher intends (i.e., be a valid representation of the variable).
    (d) The instrument should be able to collect consistent measurements of the variable being studied (i.e., be a reliable representation of the variable).
    (e) The researcher describes the instrument clearly before the data is collected.
        (i) Reports or establishes the instrument's reliability
       (ii) Reports or establishes the instrument's validity
     (iii) Describes the nature of the instrument (e.g., number of questions, type of questions, type of device)

(iv) Provides rationale for selection of the instrument
(v) Provides source for instrument and any previous use of instrument
(f) Examples of perianesthesia nursing research instruments
(i) Visual Analog Pain Scale (VAS)
(ii) Tympanic thermometer in core mode
(iii) Speilberger's State–Trait Anxiety Questionnaire
(iv) Postanesthesia discharge criteria modified by Aldrete
(v) Written posttest on care of surgical dressing
(10) Research procedure
(a) Definition: description of the steps taken to implement research data collection, including the selection of the sample, the identification of the setting, the administration of the research instrument, and any protocols for the independent variable
(b) Procedure is provided with sufficient detail to allow the study to be replicated (repeated with a different group of participants) by other researchers.
(c) Procedure described in chronological order of implementation
(11) Data analysis methods
(a) Definition: Procedures used to analyze the data
(b) Qualitative analysis will include ways in which the researcher will determine themes.
(c) Quantitative analysis
(i) Descriptive procedures, correlational procedures, or tests of hypotheses
(ii) Based on the type of data collected and the format of hypothesis
(iii) Statistical experts are consulted to determine the appropriate statistical procedures.

V. Ethical issues in nursing research
A. The researcher is required to protect the vulnerable patient from harmful effects and to ensure that benefits to participants outweigh risks of participating in the research.
B. Ethical research behaviors include objectivity, cooperation with institutional guidelines, integrity, and honesty.
C. Any research on human subjects requires review and approval by an IRB or human subjects committee prior to collecting data.
1. Composition of the IRB includes nurses, physicians, and other health care professionals; clergy, community members, attorneys, and ethicists also participate on the IRB.
2. IRB independently determines the ethical implications of the research methodology.
D. IRB determines the requirements for participant's informed consent either in writing or verbally.

VI. Communicating the results of a research project
A. Upon completion of data collection, the researcher includes in the report findings, discussion of findings, conclusions, implications, and recommendations.
B. Findings
1. A demographic summary of the sample is provided.
2. Results of the data analysis are provided in the order of the research questions or hypotheses.
3. Tables are used to illustrate findings.
4. Statistical notations are used to describe findings (e.g., $p = .001$).
C. Discussion of findings
1. An interpretation of the findings
2. Related research that supports or refutes the study findings is discussed from the perspective of the researcher's findings.

3. Examples of perianesthesia nursing research findings
   a. Findings from this study indicated that face-to-face preoperative instructions improve posttest scores significantly more than video teaching did.
   b. Findings of this study revealed that two days prior to surgical intervention is the appropriate time for a preadmission interview.
   c. Findings from this study did not identify a difference in patient satisfaction between care delivered by unlicensed providers and licensed providers.
   d. Findings from this study indicated no difference in postoperative temperature between patients who received ketorolac and patients who received acetaminophen.
   e. Findings from this study showed that postoperative follow-up phone calls made in the afternoon were more successful than those made in the morning.
D. Conclusions
   1. Definition: one or two specific statements of new knowledge that has been revealed by the research findings
   2. The conclusion attempts to answer the research problem presented at the beginning of the study.
   3. Examples of perianesthesia nursing research conclusions
      a. The findings of the study support the conclusion that patients who receive face-to-face preoperative teaching learn better.
      b. The conclusion of this study is that the timing of preoperative visits can impact patient anxiety related to their surgical experience.
      c. The conclusion of this study is that level of patient education is a predictor of compliance with NPO guidelines.
      d. The research findings support the conclusion that pediatric preoperative tours reduce parental anxiety but have no effect on the child anxiety prior to discharge.
      e. The findings of the study support the conclusion that patients who receive preoperative analgesics have less postoperative nausea.
E. Implications and recommendations
   1. Definition: suggestions offered by the researcher as to ways the research conclusions could be utilized in nursing practice, nursing education, nursing administration, or by future researchers
   2. Implications for practice translate the research findings into usable interventions to improve patient outcomes.
   3. At least one implication is reported for each research conclusion.
   4. Examples of perianesthesia nursing research implications
      a. The study suggests that preoperative teaching be conducted by trained perianesthesia nurses during individualized face-to-face sessions.
      b. The study findings suggest that preadmission visits should be scheduled a maximum of two days before the day of surgery.
      c. The study findings recommend that NPO guidelines be explained based on the patient's educational level.
      d. The study findings suggest that parental tours may be just as effective as pediatric tours in reducing postoperative anxiety behaviors of children.
      e. The researcher recommends that the study be repeated using male and female patients of a wide range of ages.
VII. Quality improvement and the research process
   A. Quality improvement (i.e., quality assurance, total quality improvement, and total quality management) projects are designed to measure performance against preestabished criteria.
   B. Quality improvement projects do not follow all the steps of the research process (see Table 5-1).
   C. Purpose of quality improvement project is to solve an institutional problem or improve, or evaluate current practice.

■ TABLE 5-1
■ ■ **Comparison Between Research and Quality Improvement Using Key Characteristics**

Characteristic	Research	Quality Improvement
Seeks to solve a problem	Yes	Yes
Seeks to develop new knowledge	Yes	No
Requires defining the problem	Yes	Yes, but problem may be to examine current practice for improvement areas.
Requires a purpose statement	Yes	No
Requires a question or hypothesis to be answered	Yes	No
Project is supported by outside literature.	Yes	No
Sample is representative of population.	May be, if using quantitative methods	No, sample of convenience
Sample size is important.	Yes	No
Setting is described for replication.	Yes, important for future researchers	No, setting is institution specific.
Instrument has preestablished validity and reliability.	Yes, validity and reliability strengthen study.	Not needed, frequently an institution-created tool is used
Procedure is clearly described.	Yes, permits replication	Not necessary because one person is collecting data
Multiple methods used for data analysis depending on type of question or hypothesis	Yes, use of themes, descriptive, correlational, and effect statistics	No, data analyzed using descriptive statistics (mean, percentage)
Institutional review board approval required	Yes, mandatory	No, permission to survey granted by institution's administration
Findings, discussion, conclusion, recommendations follow from question or hypothesis.	Yes	No, findings are discussed in light of improvement of quality.
Publication in peer-reviewed journal	Yes, results are disseminated to encourage knowledge development.	No, results are shared with internal stakeholders.

VIII. Utilization of research findings
    A. Research findings can be located in a variety of sources.
        1. Poster displays at national and local conferences and meetings of professional organizations
        2. Oral presentations at continuing education meetings
        3. Local and national publications
            a. Specialty journals: *Journal of PeriAnesthesia Nursing (JOPAN), Breathline*
            b. Clinical journals: *AORN Journal, American Journal of Critical Care, AANA Journal*
            c. Research journals: *Nursing Research, Applied Nursing Research, Western Journal of Nursing Research*
    B. Evidence-based practice
        1. Definition: integration of clinical judgment with the most current, relevant, and defensible research evidence
        2. Philosophy introduced in early 1990s to implement most sound practice within limits of existing knowledge
        3. Shift in care based on clinical practice to care based on empirical evidence

■ TABLE 5-2
■ ■ Evidence-based Practice

Level (strength) of Evidence	Type of Evidence
I	Systematic review of all randomized control trials on the topic
II	One research study on the topic that used a randomized control trial
III.1	Controlled research trials without randomization
III.2	Cohort or case-controlled study
III.3	Dramatic results in uncontrolled experiments
IV	Descriptive studies, expert opinion, expert committees

    4. Evidence includes many sources.
      a. Research studies
      b. Knowledge from basic sciences
      c. Clinical expertise
    5. For a given practice, level of evidence varies and can be rated (Table 5-2) evidence.
  C. Communicating research to colleagues
    1. Perianesthesia nursing journal club can be used to communicate findings to colleagues.
      a. A journal club is composed of a group of nurses who meet regularly to discuss and analyze research related to their practice.
      b. Familiarizes colleagues with a wide variety of publications and research issues
    2. Policy and procedure committee utilizes research findings.
      a. Applies research conclusions to standard of care in the institution
      b. Notes procedures that are research based by including references of research studies
      c. Revises policies and procedures as new knowledge is discovered by nurse researchers
  D. Professional responsibility
    1. Nurses have a professional responsibility to maintain practice currency by reading, discussing, and participating in perianesthesia nursing research.
    2. Research utilization should be included in all professional job descriptions.
  E. Perianesthesia nurses participating in nursing research are responsible for
    1. Being aware of the research purpose and methodology
    2. Validating that the research project has undergone independent review
    3. Advocating for the participant's informed consent
    4. Supporting the research data collection procedure where possible

BIBLIOGRAPHY

1. Burns N, Grove SK: *The practice of nursing research: Conduct critique and utilization,* ed 4. Philadelphia: Saunders, 2001.
2. Fetzer SJ, Vogelsang J. *Research primer for perianesthesia nurses.* Thorofare, NJ: American Society of PeriAnesthesia Nurses, 2001.
3. Fetzer SJ, Hand MC: A profile of perianesthesia nursing patient outcome research, 1994-1999. *J PeriAnesthNurs* 16(5):315-324, 2001.
4. Shertzer KE, Keck JF: Music in the PACU environment. *J PeriAnesthNurs* 16(2):90-102, 2001.
5. Windle P: Ethical considerations in nursing research. *J PeriAnesthNurs* 17(10):49-52, 2001.

6 Legal Issues

JAN ODOM-FORREN

OBJECTIVES
At the conclusion of this chapter the reader will be able to:

1. Identify five common causes of nursing liability.

2. Discuss methods for prevention of a malpractice suit.

3. Describe the four elements of negligence.

4. Discuss phases of litigation that can occur with a malpractice suit.

LEGAL CONCEPTS

I. Sources of law
   A. Constitutional—system of laws for governance of a nation; may be federal or state
   B. Statutory—made by the legislative branch of the government
   C. Administrative—laws enacted by administrative agencies charged with implementing particular legislation
   D. Judicial—laws made by the courts that interpret legal issues that are in dispute

II. Types of law
   A. Common law—derived from principles rather than rules and regulations
   B. Civil law—based on rules and regulations
      1. Administered through courts as damages or money compensation
      2. Most important area is *tort* law which involves compensation to those wrongfully injured
   C. Criminal law—conduct that is offensive or harmful to society as a whole
   D. Substantive law—concerns the wrong, harm, or duty that caused the lawsuit
   E. Procedural law—concerns the process and rights of the individual charged with violating substantive law

III. Legal definitions
   A. See Box 6-1.

IV. Negligence law
   A. Tort law—a civil wrong that allows the injured party to seek reparation; concerns any action or omission that harms someone
      1. Negligence
      2. Malpractice
      3. Assault and battery
      4. Invasion of privacy
      5. False imprisonment
      6. Defamation
   B. Essential elements of professional negligence (malpractice)
      1. Duty—once you, as a nurse, undertake the care of a patient, you are under a duty to act in accordance with the standard of care (e.g., you establish a duty to the patient when you take report on a patient in the postanesthesia care unit and accept that patient into your care).
      2. Breach of duty—failure to act in accordance with the standard of care
         a. May be an act of omission (e.g., a failure to administer a medication that was ordered)
         b. May be an act of commission (e.g., administration of a medication to which the patient had an allergy)

■ BOX 6-1
■ **LEGAL TERMINOLOGY**

Assault
An attempt or threat that causes a person to fear physical touch or injury

Battery
The unauthorized touching of an individual's body, any extension of it, or anything attached to it in an offensive or injurious manner

Defendant
Person or entity against whom plaintiff's allegations are made

Expert Witness
A person who serves to educate the court and jury about the subject under consideration, including the appropriate standard of care

Malpractice (Professional Negligence)
A type of negligence that involves a standard of care that can be reasonably expected from professionals (e.g., attorneys, nurses, physicians, accountants); failure to act as a reasonably prudent nurse would act under similar circumstances

Negligence
Deviation from the standard of care that a reasonable person would use in a certain set of circumstances

Plaintiff
The person or party who brings the lawsuit and alleges harm

Standard of Care
The care and judgment exercised by a reasonable, prudent person (nurse) under the same or similar circumstances

3. Causation—plaintiff must prove that the breach of duty was the cause of damages (e.g., the administration of the medication to which the patient had an allergy caused an anaphylactic shock resulting the patient's death).
    a. Most difficult element to prove
4. Damages—actual loss or damages must be established (e.g., death, nerve damage, fracture).
5. Plaintiff must prove all four elements of negligence for the cause of action to succeed.
C. Employer liability
    1. Respondent superior—"let the master speak"—employer is vicariously liable for negligent acts of employee if the act occurred during an employment relationship and within part of the employee's job responsibilities.
    2. Corporate liability—health care delivery system can be sued when it breaches any direct duty to the patient.
D. *Res ipsa loquitur*—"the thing speaks for itself"; a rule of evidence that allows a supposition of negligence on the part of the defendant (e.g., permanent loss of neuromuscular control of arm after routine hysterectomy)
    1. Defendant must be solely in control at the time injury occurred, and injury would not have occurred if defendant had exercised due care.
    2. Plaintiff must have done nothing to contribute to negligence (e.g., foreign object left inside patient after surgery).
E. Intentional torts—intent is necessary, and there must be a willful action against the injured person.
    1. Assault—an action that causes apprehension or unwarranted touching (e.g., threatening a patient)

      2. Battery—unauthorized touching of one person by another (e.g., lack of consent for treatment)

      3. False imprisonment—unjustifiable detention of a person without a legal warrant (e.g., not allowing a patient to go who wants to leave against medical advice)

  F. Quasi-intentional torts

      1. Invasion of privacy—patient's right to privacy is recognized.

         a. Using a person's likeness or name without consent for commercial advantage

         b. Unreasonable intrusion into person's private affairs

         c. Public disclosure of private facts about a person

         d. Placing a person in a false light in the public's eye

      2. Defamation—wrongful injury to another's reputation

         a. Includes libel (written form) or slander (spoken form).

  G. Standards of care—minimal requirements that define an acceptable level of care

      1. May be established by

         a. State Nurse Practice Act

         b. Federal agency guidelines and regulations

         c. American Nurses Association (ANA)

         d. American Society of PeriAnesthesia Nurses (ASPAN) or other national specialty organization

         e. Joint Commission on Accreditation of Healthcare Organizations (JCAHO) or other accrediting bodies, such as Accreditation Association for Ambulatory Health Care (AAAHC)

         f. Hospital or ambulatory surgery facility rules and procedures

         g. State Board of Nursing

         h. Common practice

         i. Nursing texts and articles

      2. Determined by expert witnesses for judicial system

         a. Essential in professional negligence cases

LIABILITY ISSUES

I. Possible causes of nursing liability for the perianesthesia nurse

  A. Failure to adequately assess or monitor a patient

      1. Nurse must possess competency to assess and/or monitor patient.

      2. Assessment and monitoring of patient are actually performed.

      3. If assessment and monitoring reveal reportable condition, nurse must notify physician.

      4. Nurse must continue to assess and monitor to evaluate effectiveness of intervention.

  B. Errors in the use of equipment

  C. Errors in medication or treatment

      1. Failure to follow five rights: right drug, right dose, right patient, right route, right time

  D. Failure to communicate

      1. To another nurse

      2. Changes in patient condition to a physician

  E. Patient falls

  F. Operating room errors (e.g., sponges/instruments left inside patient)

  G. Mix-ups during patient transfers (e.g., wrong surgery on patient)

  H. Failure to report or act on deviations from accepted practice

      1. Nurses expected to exercise independent judgment and object when physician's orders are inappropriate

      2. Report facts to manager or otherwise follow chain of command

  I. Failure to follow a physician's order promptly and accurately

  J. Failure to follow institutional or facility procedures

    K. Failure to properly teach patient or caregiver accurate and appropriate discharge instructions
      1. Should receive discharge instructions before admission or surgery
      2. Use preprinted discharge instructions.
      3. Give verbal and written instructions.
    M. Premature discharge for the ambulatory surgery patient
    N. Failure to ensure the presence of an informed caregiver (responsible adult)
    O. Failure to assess the ambulatory surgery patient on admission (e.g., nothing by mouth [NPO] status, any signs or symptoms that might affect reaction to anesthesia or surgery, medication use that day)

II. Prevention of liability
    A. Documentation
      1. Accurate and comprehensive documentation essential
      2. Purposes of documentation
        a. To communicate the patient's condition to other health professionals
        b. To assess for improvements that might be needed by risk management and quality management
        c. To obtain data for research
        d. To obtain reimbursement—from the government and insurance
        e. As a legal record
        f. To use as data for quality-of-care review
      3. Nurses' notes first place an attorney will look
        a. Written with time and date and in chronological order
        b. Contains most detailed information regarding the patient
      4. Documentation guidelines
        a. Chart accurately.
          (i) It is very difficult to prove that something was done if it is not charted.
          (ii) On the other hand, deliberate inaccuracies can totally destroy defense and expose nurse to criminal charges of fraud.
        b. Chart objectively.
          (i) Describe only what you observe.
          (ii) Do not use words such as "seems," "apparently," or "appears."
        c. Write legibly, and use standard abbreviations adopted by the health care facility.
        d. Do not use the chart to criticize or complain.
          (i) Use other appropriate avenues if there is criticism of another nurse.
        e. Do not destroy or obliterate documentation.
          (i) Do not use correction fluid or any other kind of eradicator.
          (ii) Draw one line through the error, initial, and date the line.
        f. Do not leave vacant lines; sign every entry.
        g. Chart as promptly as possible after the care is given.
        h. Correct grammar, spelling, and punctuation make a difference.
        i. Do not chart for someone else or allow someone else to chart for you.
        j. Use appropriate procedure for documenting a late entry.
        k. Document patient and/or family teaching.
        l. Document disposition of any personal belongings.
        m. Document any nursing interventions and patient responses to those interventions.
        n. Document any communication with a physician or supervisor concerning a patient's condition.
    B. Electronic documentation guidelines
      1. Protect the user identification code or password given for personal use.
        a. No one else should be given access to that password or document for the user.
      2. Only access information and document in chart as authorized to do so.
        a. An attempt to access an electronic chart on a patient without authorization is a breach of confidentiality and privacy.

   3. Never ignore electronic reminders that information is coded incorrectly, important data overlooked, or flags for critical information about the patient (e.g., lab work).
      a. Systems alert nurses if a portion of the nursing process is absent.
   4. Know the facility procedure for how to handle late entries.
   5. Stay updated when changes in documentation format occur.
C. Incident reports
   1. Use has changed from punitive measure to a documentation of unusual events.
      a. Should be no fear of reprisal or other negative consequences
      b. Atmosphere of trust and cooperation essential for system to be of best value
   2. All actual and potential injuries must be reported.
      a. Should be initiated by the person who observed the event or the first to become aware of the incident
      b. Incorporate patient's description into the report by use of direct quotes.
   3. Documentation should be factual and objective.
      a. Include information regarding patient, description of the incident, any injuries sustained, and outcome of event.
   4. Allows risk manager to assess situation and decide on best corrective action
   5. Record fact about event in nurses' notes, but not fact that incident report filed.
D. Telephone calls
   1. Document any telephone calls made to report changes in patient condition.
   2. Important information to include
      a. Specific time call was made
      b. Who made the call?
      c. Who was called?
      d. To whom information was given
      e. All information given
      f. All information received
   3. When obtaining consents (and any other time appropriate), have another witness listen in.
E. Personal accountability
   1. Know your state Nurse Practice Act.
   2. Know the national standards for perianesthesia nursing practice.
   3. Continuing education is essential.
      a. Read professional journals and books.
      b. Attend pertinent seminars.
      c. Maintain membership in professional organization pertinent to specialty.
   4. Policies and procedures
      a. Will be held accountable for knowing and following hospital or ambulatory facility's policies and procedures
      b. Policies and procedures should not conflict with one another.
      c. Policies and procedures should reflect actual practice.
   5. Patient relations
      a. Important aspect of prevention of liability
      b. Old adage is true: "Happy patient rarely sues."
      c. Do not criticize other health care providers in the presence of the family or patient.
      d. Maintain good communication and rapport with the patient and family.

THE LEGAL PROCESS

I. Phases of litigation
   A. Evaluation for suit—review of medical record
   B. Pleadings

  1. Complaint—outlines alleged negligence, states the injury, and may indicate an amount of compensation demanded
      a. Notify insurer and hospital after complaint received.
  2. Answer—defendant is allowed a certain period of time to respond to allegations.
      a. Attorney prepares the answer.
  C. Prelitigation panels—required by some states
      1. Medical review panel
      2. Medical tribunal
      3. Arbitration panel
  D. If you've been sued
      1. Do not discuss the case with anyone other than the risk manager or your attorney.
      2. Do not talk to the plaintiff, the plaintiff's attorney, or anyone testifying for the plaintiff.
      3. Do not discuss with reporters.
      4. Do not alter patient's chart or hide any information from your attorney.
  E. Discovery (pretrial phase)—attempts to narrow issues for trial by gathering and clarifying facts
      1. Interrogatories—list of written questions that seeks information to support or refute the complaint
      2. Production of documents—may be requested (e.g., ambulatory surgery facility records, incident reports, anesthesia records, policies and procedures, discharge teaching forms)
      3. Deposition—oral testimony of any person thought to have information pertaining to the case
          a. Testimony given under oath
          b. Recorded by court reporter
  F. Settlement negotiations—may continue throughout process and occur at any time in the process
  G. Trial of lawsuit—may be a judge or jury trial
      1. Jury selection
      2. Opening statements by plaintiff and defendant
      3. Plaintiff presents case—uses expert witnesses.
      4. Defendant presents case—uses expert witnesses.
      5. Defense may make motion for directed verdict against plaintiff—argues that the plaintiff has not met the burden of proof.
      6. Closing statements by plaintiff and defendant
      7. Jury instructions by the judge
      8. Jury deliberations
      9. Verdict
      10. Appeal (optional)

ISSUES OF CONSENT

  I. Informed Consent
  A. Consent obtained after the patient has been fully informed by the physician or dentist about the risks and benefits of the treatment, alternatives, and consequences of no treatment
  B. Types of consent
      1. Express—given by direct words, either written or oral
      2. Implied—inferred by the patient's conduct or may be legally presumed in emergency situations
  C. If patient not legally competent adult, patient's parents, legal guardian, or—in some states—next of kin or friend can make health care decisions.
  D. Treatment without consent
      1. Assault and/or battery
      2. Negligent failure to obtain consent

 E. Exceptions to duty to disclose
  1. Some emergency situations—life or well-being of the individual is threatened and consent cannot be obtained or would result in a delay of treatment.
  2. Therapeutic privilege—physician believes information would be harmful to the patient; very restricted.
  3. Patient has waived right to consent—does not want to be informed.
  4. Lack of decision-making capacity—information must be shared with proxy decision-maker or guardian.
 F. Documentation of consents
  1. Nurses who sign as witnesses are only witnessing signature of person signing consent form.
  2. If patient has additional questions, nurse should refer questions to physician.
  3. If physician fails to discuss questions further with the patient, nurse must report that information through the appropriate chain of command.
  4. If English is not primary language of patient, an interpreter must be used.
II. Advanced directives
 A. Living will—directive from competent individual to medical personnel and family members regarding treatment he or she wishes to receive when he or she can no longer make the decisions himself or herself
 B. Natural Death Act
  1. State-legislated legally recognized living wills with statutory enforcement
  2. Protects practitioner and ensures patient's wishes are followed
 C. Durable power of attorney for health care—allows competent patients to appoint an individual to make health care decisions if they become incompetent to do so
 D. Patient Self-Determination Act (PSDA)
  1. Passed in 1990 as part of federal Omnibus Budget Reconciliation Act (OBRA)
  2. Requires hospitals and other facilities on admission to advise all patients of their rights to refuse treatments and of any relevant state laws dealing with advanced directives
 E. Do-not-resuscitate directives—require documentation that the patient's decision was made after consultation with physician and understanding of options
 F. Health Insurance Portability and Accountability Act of 1996 (HIPAA)
  1. A major goal of the Act is to ensure that individuals' health information is properly protected while allowing the flow of health information needed to provide and promote high-quality health care and to protect the public's health and well being.
  2. Major purpose is to define and limit the circumstances in which an individual's protected health information may be used or disclosed by covered entities.

BIBLIOGRAPHY

1. Aiken TD, Catalano JT: *Legal, ethical, and political issues in nursing.* Philadelphia: Davis, 1994.
2. American Society of Post Anesthesia Nurses: *Standards of perianesthesia nursing practice.* Cherry Hill, NJ: American Society of Post Anesthesia Nurses, 2002.
3. Ashley RC: How do I know if I have been sued as a nurse and what do I do? *Crit Care Nurse* 22(3):82-83, 2002.
4. Ashley RC: The anatomy of a lawsuit: Part 1. *Crit Care Nurse* 22(4):68-69, 2002.
5. Ashley RC: The anatomy of a lawsuit: Part 2. *Crit Care Nurse* 22(5):82-83, 2002.
6. Berry FA: What to do when sued. *Curr Rev Post Anesth Nurs,* 14(19):153-160, 2002.
7. Brent NJ: *Nurses and the law: A guide to principles and applications,* ed 2. Philadelphia: WB Saunders, 2001.
8. Brunson CD, Eichhorn JH: Risk management: Avoiding complications and litigation. In White PF, editor. *Ambulatory Anesthesia and Surgery.* Philadelphia: WB Saunders, 1997, pp 691-699.
9. De Kornfeld TJ: Medico-legal considerations in the recovery room. *Curr Rev Post Anesth Nurs* 14(3):17-24, 1992.
10. Feutz-Harter S: Nursing case law update. *J Nurs Law* 1(2):57-61, 1994.
11. Fiesta J: Failure to assess. *Nurs Manage* 24(9):16-17, 1993.
12. Flores JA: What if you're named in a lawsuit? *RN* 65(12):65-68, 2002.

13. Guido GW: *Legal issues in nursing,* ed 2. Stamford, CT: Appleton & Lange, 1997

14. Health and Human Services, US Department of: Summary of the HIPAA Privacy Rule, 2003. Available at http://www.hhs.gov/ocr/hipaa. Accessed April 2003.

15. Hall JK: *Nursing: Ethics and law.* Philadelphia: WB Saunders, 1996.

16. Kelly LY, Joel LA: Legal aspects of nursing practice. In *The nursing experience: Trends, challenges, and transitions.* New York: McGraw-Hill, 1996, pp 481-522.

17. Kemmy JA: OR nursing law: Legal implications of perioperative documentation. *AORN J,* 57(4):954, 956, 968, 1993.

18. Litwack K: Legal and ethical issues in PACU practice. In *Post Anesthesia Care Nursing,* ed 2. St Louis: Mosby–Yearbook, 1995, pp 42-69.

19. Odom J: Legal issues in perianesthesia nursing. *Dissector J Perioper Nurs Coll N Z Nurse Organ* 30(4):9-11, 2003.

20. O'Keefe JE: *Nursing practice and the law: Avoiding malpractice and other legal risks.* Philadelphia: Davis, 2001

21. Quan KP, Gee DC: Legal responsibilities and informed consent: United States and international perspectives. In White PF, editor: *Ambulatory anesthesia and surgery.* Philadelphia: WB Saunders, 1997, pp 682-690.

22. Springhouse Corporation: *Nurse's handbook of law and ethics.* Springhouse, PA: Springhouse, 1992.

23. Tammelleo AD: Patient sues nurse for failure to obtain consent. *Regan Rep Nurs Law* 33(10):4, 1993.

24. Zuffoletto JM: OR nursing law: Anatomy of a lawsuit. *AORN J* 56(5):933-936, 1992.

25. Zuffoletto JM: OR nursing law: Proving causation, damages in malpractice cases. *AORN J* 58(3):589-592, 1993.

ENVIRONMENT OF CARE

SECTION TWO
Specific Problems
ENVIRONMENT OF CARE

7 Practice Settings

DONNA M. DEFAZIO QUINN

OBJECTIVES

At the conclusion of this chapter the reader will be able to:

1. Define the scope of practice for perianesthesia nursing.

2. Identify three phases of perianesthesia care.

3. List the three phases of postanesthesia care.

4. Name six areas where operative or procedural care can be delivered.

I. Perianesthesia care
  A. Definition
    1. Scope of practice involves
      a. Diagnosis of,
      b. Intervention for,
      c. Evaluation of physical or psychosocial problems or risks for problems that may result from the administration of sedation/anesthesia or anesthetic agents and techniques.[1]
    2. Includes
      a. Nursing process
      b. Decision making
      c. Analytical and scientific thinking
      d. Inquiry
  B. Environment
    1. Preanesthesia phase
      a. Preadmission interview accomplished via
        (1) In-person visit to facility
        (2) Telephone
        (3) Preoperative questionnaires
        (4) Preoperative education sessions
        (5) Preadmission testing clinics
        (6) Internet-based and Web-based interactive programs
      b. Day of surgery preparation accomplished in
        (1) Holding unit
        (2) Outpatient surgery unit
        (3) AM Admit unit
        (4) Labor and delivery suites
        (5) Physician office
        (6) Dental office
        (7) Additional preoperative or preprocedural holding areas (cardiac, endoscopy, electroconvulsive therapy [ECT], oncology, etc.) as designated by the facility
      c. Resources available for patient education
        (1) One-on-one with RN
        (2) Video
        (3) Audiocassette
        (4) Pamphlets
        (5) Printed instruction
        (6) Web-based teaching modules

        (7) Preoperative tours

        (8) Group lecture

  2. Intraoperative and procedural phase

    a. Operating room

    b. Special procedures room

    c. Radiology

    d. Cardiac labs

    e. Interventional suites

    f. Physician office

    g. Pain management settings

    h. Emergency departments

    i. Other areas throughout the facility

  3. Postanesthesia phase

    a. Phase I

        (1) Nursing focus is on providing care during the immediate postanesthesia period.

        (2) Preparing patient for transfer to phase II, inpatient nursing unit, or intensive care unit.

    b. Phase II

        (1) Nursing focus on continued recovery of patient, and

        (2) Preparing patient for transfer to phase III, home, or to an extended care facility

        (3) Patient and family education

    c. Phase III

        (1) Focus is to provide ongoing care for those requiring extended observation or intervention after discharge.

        (2) Interventions are directed toward preparing the patient for self-care.

C. Practice settings for perianesthesia care

  1. Hospitals

    a. Traditional operating rooms

    b. Ambulatory surgery units within the hospital setting, hospital outpatient departments (HOPDs)

    c. Special care units

        (1) Endoscopy

        (2) Radiology

        (3) Labor and delivery Suites

        (4) ECT labs

        (5) Cardiac labs

        (6) Emergency departments

        (7) Pain management units

        (8) Burn units

        (9) Intensive care units

  2. Surgical hospitals

  3. Clinics

    a. Within the hospital setting

    b. Freestanding

  4. Ambulatory surgery centers

    a. Freestanding

        (1) On hospital campus

        (2) In community setting

  5. Physician offices

    a. Surgical specialties include, but not limited to

        (1) Plastic

        (2) Dental

        (3) Dermatology

        (4) Ophthalmology

   6. Recovery settings
   a. Main postanesthesia care unit (PACU)
      (1) Usually in close proximity to operating room suites
      (2) Phase I area for postoperative care
      (3) May incorporate phase II care
   b. Phase II PACU
      (1) May be included in phase I area,
      (2) Adjacent to phase I unit, or
      (3) Located in another area of the facility
   c. Phase III PACU
      (1) Twenty-three hour observation suites
         (i) Within the hospital or facility setting
         (ii) Outside the hospital or facility setting
      (2) Rehabilitation centers and suites
         (i) Within the hospital setting
         (ii) Outside the hospital setting
      (3) Physician office with overnight capability
      (4) Designated recovery areas for specialty services (radiology, cardiac labs, ECT labs, etc.)
      (5) Recovery care centers
         (i) On hospital campus
         (ii) Within the community
D. Special considerations
   1. Standardization of nursing care regardless of where perianesthesia care is delivered
   2. Availability of emergency resources—equipment, personnel, and predetermined processes

BIBLIOGRAPHY

1. American Society of PeriAnesthesia Nurses: *Standards of perianesthesia nursing practice.* Cherry Hill, NJ: American Society of PeriAnesthesia Nurses, 2002.
2. Barnes S: Patient preparation: The physical assessment. *J PeriAnesth Nurs* 17:16-17, 2002.
3. Burden N, DeFazio Quinn DM, O'Brien D, et al: *Ambulatory surgical nursing.* Philadelphia: WB Saunders, 2001.
4. Drain CB: *Perianesthesia nursing: A critical care approach,* ed 4. Philadelphia: WB Saunders, 2003.
5. Sullivan EE: A successful practice: Pre-admitting test center. *J PeriAnesth Nurs* 16:198-200, 2001.

8 Policies and Procedures

DONNA M. DEFAZIO QUINN

OBJECTIVES

At the conclusion of this chapter the reader will be able to:

1. List five important functions for policies and procedures.

2. Describe the proper format of the page layout of policies and procedures.

3. Identify 10 important policies and procedures related to the postanesthesia care unit (PACU).

4. Describe the process for obtaining administrative approval of policies and procedures.

5. Describe the process for revising policies and procedures

I. Policies
   A. Definition
      1. Guidelines to assist in decision making
         a. Increases likelihood of consistency in decisions and actions
         b. Means to ensure practice is in compliance with standards
      2. Defines responsibility
      3. Element of the organization that is an extension of the mission statement
      4. Provides order and stability so unit can work as a coordinated group
      5. Directs action for thinking about and solving recurring problems related to the objectives of the organization
   B. Developed by
      1. Nursing executive
      2. RNs
      3. Designated nursing staff members
      4. Input from ancillary health care team members
   C. Functions
      1. Promotes teamwork
      2. Provides clarity and uniformity
         a. Identifies what is expected in a specific manner
         b. Encourages consistency in practice
      3. Defines limits of authority and responsibility
      4. Aids in delegation
      5. Serves as a resource for accreditation and regulatory agencies
         a. Accrediting bodies
            (1) Joint Commission for Accreditation of Healthcare Organizations (JCAHO)
            (2) Accreditation Association for Ambulatory Health Care (AAAHC)
            (3) American Association for the Accreditation of Ambulatory Surgical Facilities (AAAASF)
         b. State licensing agency
         c. Regulating agencies
            (1) Centers for Medicare and Medicaid Services (CMS)

      6. Provides a basis for change
         a. If current practice is not known, it is difficult to know what needs to be changed.
      7. Establishes a mechanism for consistent treatment of staff and a framework for staff assignments
      8. Provides a safeguard for nursing personnel when legal action ensues
         a. Nurses are held accountable for practice consistent with existing policies at the time of the action.
         b. Adherence to policies provides a defense for actions taken.
      9. Establishes a consistent level of expectation of staff members
         a. Orientation clearly identifies individual's responsibility to know and adhere to policies.
     10. Process is never ending.
         a. Continually need to update polices and procedures based on
            (1) Changes in practice
            (2) Changes in regulatory requirements
            (3) Changes in standards
            (4) Changes in technology
         b. Staff members need to be involved in process.
            (1) Annual review of policies as a whole
            (2) Ongoing review of various policies throughout the year

II. Procedures
  A. Definition
      1. Instructions that detail steps necessary to complete a task
      2. Includes
         a. Necessary steps and process
         b. Supplies
         c. Equipment
         d. Personnel
         e. Documentation
  B. Functions
      1. Reminder for tasks performed infrequently
      2. Resource for orienting new staff members
      3. Facilitates cost containment
         a. Identifies necessary supplies
         b. Reduces unnecessary waste
      4. Increases productivity
         a. Decreases time lost seeking answers
      5. Provides a means to measure quality and appropriateness of care when auditing nursing practice

III. Format of policies and procedures
  A. Page layout
      1. Title
      2. Number
      3. Authorizing signatures and approving body
      4. Review date
      5. Revision date
  B. Common divisions
      1. Administration
      2. Anesthesia
      3. Environment of care
      4. Employee health
      5. Infection control
      6. Materials management
      7. Medical records
      8. Patient care
      9. Personnel
    10. Pharmacy

        11. Quality management
        12. Registration
        13. Risk management
        14. Safety
  IV. Overview of policies and procedures needed

    The following content outline suggests general required policies and procedures. It is not the intent of this chapter to provide an all-inclusive list of possible policies and procedures.

    A. Table of contents
    B. Facility and unit philosophy and objectives
    C. Scope of service
    D. Mission, vision, values statements
    E. Administrative organizational chart
        1. Chain of command
            a. Governing body
            b. Job descriptions
            c. Staffing patterns
            d. Standards of care
        2. Medical staff
            a. Physician privileges
            b. Physician credentialing procedure
            c. Medical advisory committee
    F. Patient rights
        1. Rights and responsibility statement
        2. Ethical treatment
        3. Patient grievance process
        4. Advance directives
        5. Health Insurance Portability and Accountability Act (HIPAA) Privacy Notice
    G. Admission
        1. Criteria
        2. Approved procedure list
        3. Appropriateness of patients based on American Society of Anesthesiologists (ASA) classification
        4. Population served
        5. Preoperative assessment
    H. Discharge
        1. Criteria and scoring system
        2. Patient instructions
        3. Responsible adult escort
    I. Anesthesia requirements
        1. Anesthesia consent
        2. Monitoring of patients receiving anesthesia
        3. Fast-tracking guidelines
    J. Patient charges
        1. Self-pay patients
        2. Discounts
        3. Turnover of accounts to collection agency
    K. Business office
        1. Precertification guidelines
        2. Co-pay collections
        3. Scheduling process
    L. Consents
        1. Informed consent
        2. Minors
        3. Power of attorney
        4. Sterilization
        5. Administration of blood products

      6. "Do Not Resuscitate" (DNR) orders
      7. Experimental treatment
      8. Procurement of forensic evidence
      9. Electroconvulsive therapy
    10. Cardioversion
    11. Hepatitis B immunization
    12. Release of medical information

M. Emergency procedures
    1. Emergency transfers
    2. Emergency eye wash station
    3. Cardiopulmonary resuscitation (CPR), basic cardiac life support (BCLS), advanced cardiac life support (ACLS) standards, pediatric advanced life support (PALS)
    4. Malignant hyperthermia crisis
    5. Cardiac arrest

N. Equipment
    1. Operative
    2. Emergency
    3. Preventative maintenance program
    4. Repairs
    5. Medical device reporting
    6. Biomedical engineering requests

O. Facilities management
    1. Emergency generator
    2. Maintenance of fire warning system
    3. Preventative maintenance program
    4. Occupational Safety and Health Administration (OSHA) regulations

P. Environment of care plans
    1. Safety management
    2. Utilities management
    3. Life safety management
    4. Medical equipment management
    5. Employee safety
    6. Security management
    7. Hazardous materials management
    8. Emergency preparedness

Q. Infection control
    1. Universal precautions
    2. Personal protective equipment
    3. Disposal of contaminated needles, sharps
    4. Transmission-based precautions
    5. Hepatitis B vaccine
    6. Hand washing
    7. Housekeeping procedures
    8. Operating room (OR) attire
    9. Traffic patterns
    10. Visitors
    11. Restricted areas

R. Information systems
    1. Description and use of systems
    2. Confidentiality and security agreements
    3. Systems backup and retention policy
    4. System access and password policy

S. Employee health
    1. Annual requirements
    2. Immunizations including hepatitis B
    3. Tuberculosis testing requirements
    4. Sick leave
    5. Worker's compensation

   T. Patient care
   1. OR standards of care
   2. PACU standards of care
   3. National, state, and facility standards of care
   4. Nurse-to-patient ratios
   5. Preoperative testing requirements
   6. Intraoperative monitoring procedures
   7. Moderate sedation and analgesia guidelines
   8. Postoperative monitoring procedures
   9. Patient education requirements
   U. Physician orders
   1. Standing preoperative orders
   2. Standing anesthesia orders
   3. Standing orders for ophthalmology; total joint, and so forth
   V. Quality management
   1. Overview of quality management program
   2. Goals of quality management program
   3. Description of indicators and benchmarks
   W. Patient records
   1. Consents
   2. Confidentiality and HIPAA requirements
   3. Order of medical record
   4. Medical record retention
   5. Release of information
   X. Safety
   1. Latex allergy
   2. Fire safety
   3. Electrical safety
   4. Hazardous material training
   5. Emergency preparedness training
   6. Glutaraldehyde exposure monitoring
   7. Waste gas monitoring
   8. Exposure control plan
   9. Postexposure follow-up
   10. Bomb threat
   11. Violence in the workplace
   12. Body mechanics
   13. Radiation safety
   14. Control of radioactive materials
   Y. Staff member rules and responsibilities
   1. Orientation
   2. Confidentiality
   3. Security
   4. Competency requirements
   5. Performance appraisals
   6. Required education and certifications
   7. Conflict of interest statement
   Z. Supplies
   1. Procurement, ordering
   2. Sterilization
   3. Storage
   4. Annual inventory
V. Approval process for policies and procedures
   A. Varies according to individual institution
   B. May be approved by one or a combination of the following
   1. Individual department
   2. Director of nursing
   3. Nursing leadership committee

       4. Surgical committee
       5. Anesthesia department
       6. Medical executive committee
       7. Chief executive officer
       8. Governing board of directors
VI. Use of manuals
    A. Readily available to staff members
       1. Staff members familiar with contents of manual
       2. Manuals available on information network
       3. Staff members identify needed policies and procedures.
       4. Staff members identify needed revisions to established policies and procedures.
    B. Used as reference
VII. Revision of manuals
    A. Annual reviews to update and revise
    B. Annual review with staff
    C. Process to review revisions with staff
    D. Legal issues
       1. Maintain accurate file, noting revisions.
       2. Include reason for revision.
       3. Date
       4. Potential exists to provide specific policy in place on specific past date for litigation purposes.
       5. Old policies kept on hand for 7 years
       6. Old policies should be clearly marked with beginning and end dates.

BIBLIOGRAPHY

1. Burden N, Quinn DMD, O'Brien D, et al: *Ambulatory surgical nursing*. Philadelphia: WB Saunders, 2000.
2. Drain CB: *Perianesthesia nursing: A critical care approach*. Philadelphia: Elsevier Science, 2003.
3. Joint Commission for Accreditation of Healthcare Organizations: *2003 Comprehensive Accreditation Manual for Hospitals (CAMH)*. Oakbrook Terrace, IL: Joint Commission for Accreditation of Healthcare Organizations, 2003.

9 Regulatory Agencies and Accreditation

NANCY BURDEN

OBJECTIVES

At the conclusion of this chapter the reader will be able to:

1. List three levels of government that regulate health care.

2. Give three examples of activities addressed by state nurse practice acts.

3. Name at least three agencies within the U.S. Department of Health and Human Services.

4. Describe the major components of Health Insurance Portability and Accountability Act (HIPAA) regulations.

5. Give five examples of issues administered or regulated by state or local agencies.

REGULATORY AND ACCREDITATION ISSUES

Standards are the foundation from which the nurse develops and expands an individual and collective level of service. Standards related to the care of the patient are created and promulgated primarily by professional societies and educational institutions. Professional nursing and medical standards, however, must function within a larger collection of regulations, laws, and requirements.

Most laws and regulations exist to protect the public, patients, and health care workers. Some address financial and economic issues. All levels of government—federal, state, and local—exert control over various areas of practice. Participation in Medicare, Medicaid, and other federally funded programs is dependent on meeting numerous requirements. An example is the requirement of the Civil Rights Act to provide translation service for non-English–speaking patients.

Accreditation is a voluntary decision; however, both federal and private payers look for accreditation and expect that providers will be accredited by a national accrediting body. Three such organizations exist that affect perianesthesia settings.

This chapter provides an overview of important regulatory bodies and laws but is, by no means, a comprehensive list. It is essential that nurses, nurse managers, and administrators understand the implications of regulatory compliance and know the entities that affect their specific areas of practice.

I. Professional regulation[4,7]
   A. Nursing boards
   B. State nurse practice acts
      1. Regulate professional nursing practice
      2. Identify scope of practice
      3. Protect autonomy of the professional nurse
      4. Protect public from unlicensed personnel practicing nursing
      5. Require that ethical and professional conduct standards be met such as American Nurses Association's Code for Nurses
      6. Disciplinary actions
   C. Certification boards
      1. Specialty specific
      2. Promote high level of education, experience, and application

    D. Other health care providers with professional regulation
- 1. Physicians
- 2. Nurse anesthetists
- 3. Advanced registered nurse practitioners
- 4. Physician assistants
- 5. Radiology technologists
- 6. Pharmacists

II. Facility-specific regulation
- A. Policies and procedures for human resources, clinical, and professionals
- B. Employment requirements
- C. Drug free workplace regulations
- D. Remember that policies are a promise to perform in a specific manner.
- E. Ensure actual practice and policies conform

III. County and local regulation
- A. Business licensing
- B. Fire and disaster plans
- C. Emergency management plans
- D. Building codes
- E. Impact fees
- F. Environmental regulations

IV. State regulations
- A. Vary by state
- B. Often define and/or enforce federal mandates
- C. Examples of state regulations
  - 1. Facility licensing—hospitals, ambulatory surgery centers, pharmacies
  - 2. Professional licensing
  - 3. Risk management
  - 4. Biohazardous waste handling
  - 5. Pharmacy licensing and regulation
  - 6. Public health laws
  - 7. Radiation control
  - 8. Health statistics reporting
  - 9. Child, adult, elder abuse reporting

V. Federal regulations, standards, and guidelines[10]
- A. Americans with Disabilities Act (ADA)
  - 1. Administered by Department of Justice, Civil Rights Division
  - 2. Prevention of discrimination based on disabilities
  - 3. Remove barriers to access—physical, process, and attitude
  - 4. Reasonable modification of policies, practices, and procedures to accommodate
  - 5. Auxiliary aids such as qualified interpreters, telecommunications devices for the deaf (TDDs), large print materials
  - 6. Applies to prospective employees
  - 7. Sets hiring and interviewing guidelines
  - 8. Expects reasonable accommodation for otherwise qualified candidates
- B. Centers for Disease Control and Prevention (CDC)[2]
  - 1. Conducts research
  - 2. Recommends disease prevention strategies affecting health care workers
    - a. Hand washing standards
    - b. Tuberculosis screening for health care workers
    - c. Immunization against hepatitis
  - 3. Provides accurate health care information
  - 4. Investigates disease outbreaks
- C. Civil Rights Acts of 1957, 1960, 1964, 1968[3,9]
  - 1. Administered by Department of Justice, Civil Rights Division
  - 2. Antidiscrimination statutes
  - 3. Prohibit discrimination on basis of national origin, race, age, gender, and other factors

    4. Develop comprehensive language assistance program
      a. Assess facility's language needs
      b. Develop formal written policy
      c. Train staff
      d. Monitor program continually
  D. Clinical Laboratory Improvement Amendments (CLIA) Program
    1. The Centers for Medicare and Medicaid Services (CMS) regulates all laboratory testing to ensure quality.
    2. Labs must be certified to receive Medicare or Medicaid reimbursement.
    3. CLIA waivers for specific point of care testing apparatus
  E. CMS (formerly Health Care Financing Administration [HCFA])
    1. Medicare and Medicaid
      a. Payment and coordination of health care benefits
      b. Fraud and abuse prevention and reporting
      c. False Claims Act (protects and rewards whistleblowers who report fraudulent claims against federal government)
      d. Antikickback statutes
    2. State Children's Health Insurance Program (SCHIP)
    3. HIPAA of 1997
    4. CLIA
  F. Consolidated Omnibus Budget Reconciliation Act (COBRA) of 1986
    1. Applies to certain former employees, spouses, dependent children, retirees
    2. Right to temporary continuation of health insurance coverage at group rates
  G. Drug Enforcement Administration (U.S. DEA)[11]
    1. Controlled Substances Act (CSA), Title II of the Comprehensive Drug Abuse Prevention and Control Act of 1970
      a. Categorizes drugs regulated under federal laws into five schedules based upon the substance's medicinal value, harmfulness, and potential for abuse or addiction
        (i) Schedule I—highest (heroin, lysergic acid diethylamide [LSD], hashish, etc.)
        (ii) Schedule II—high (morphine, phencyclidine (PCP), codeine, cocaine, methadone, Demerol®, Benzedrine, etc.)
        (iii) Schedule III—medium (codeine with aspirin or Tylenol®, anabolic steroids, etc.)
        (iv) Low (Darvon®, Talwin®, phenobarbital, Equanil®, Librium®, diazepam, etc.)
        (v) Lowest (over the counter or prescription compounds with codeine, Lomotil®, Robitussin-AC®, etc.)
      b. System of distribution for those authorized to handle controlled substances
      c. Registration of those authorized to handle controlled substances
      d. Documentation and inventory control requirements
      e. Storage security regulations
    2. Works in conjunction with U.S. Department of Health and Human Services (HHS)
  H. Emergency Medical Treatment and Active Labor Act (EMTALA)[5]
    1. Part of COBRA of 1986
    2. Regulations passed in 1998
    3. Part of Code that governs Medicare
    4. Primary purpose is to prevent hospitals from rejecting patients, refusing to treat them, or transferring them because of patient's inability to pay.
  I. Employee Retirement Income Security Act (ERISA)
    1. To ensure pension and other promised benefits
    2. Connected to Internal Revenue Code
  J. Fair Labor Standards Act (FLSA)
    1. Also known as Wage and Hour Regulations
    2. Defines exempt and nonexempt requirements for overtime

3. Clarifies how pay issues are to be communicated
4. Sets guidelines for age appropriate work and hours

K. U.S. Department of HHS
   1. Far reaching regulatory control—umbrella department for many agencies
   2. CMS
   3. Fraud prevention and reporting
   4. Freedom of Information Act
   5. Biologicals—blood, organs, tissues
   6. Poverty Guidelines
   7. National Practitioner Data Bank (NPDB)
   8. Agency for Healthcare Research and Quality (AHRQ)
   9. Food and Drug Administration (FDA)
   10. CDC

L. HIPAA of 1997
   1. Title I—protects health insurance for workers who change or lose their jobs
   2. Title II—requires Department of HHS to establish national standards for
      a. Electronic health care transactions
      b. Addressing security of health care information
      c. Protecting privacy of health care information
   3. Congress added Administrative Simplification section to standardize code sets, formats, and identifiers to save money.
   4. Protected health information (PHI)
   5. Privacy Rule—empowers patients and gives them more control over their PHI, how it is used, where it is shared
   6. T, P, O—treatment, payment and operations—these are the three areas where PHI can be shared freely, albeit confidentially

M. Medical device reporting[1]
   1. U.S. FDA
   2. Safe Medical Devices Act of 1990
   3. Objective to provide mechanism to identify and monitor significant adverse events related to medical devices
   4. Responsibilities by manufacturers and device users (medical facilities)
   5. MedWatch Program is mandatory reporting mechanism.
   6. Deaths or serious injuries must be reported within 10 workdays.

N. National Fire Protection Association (NFPA)[6]
   1. Develops, publishes, and disseminates timely consensus codes and standards intended to minimize the possibility and effects of fire and other risks
   2. Standards referenced by agencies and regulator bodies for compliance

O. Occupational Safety and Health Administration (OSHA)[8]
   1. Division of the U.S. Department of Labor
   2. Williams-Steiger Occupational Safety and Health Act of 1970
   3. Protection of workers—examples
      a. Environmental Safety Standards (e.g., fire safety, escape routes)
      b. Ergonomic controls
      c. Hazard Communication Standard (e.g., Material Safety Data Sheets)
      d. Materials Handling and Storage Hazards and Controls
      e. Needlestick Safety and Prevention Act
   4. Exposure Control Plan
      a. Occupational Exposure to Bloodborne Pathogens—Standard 29 CFR 1010.1030
      b. Determine employee exposure risk
      c. Outline methods to control exposure
      d. Use engineering controls and work safety practices to improve safety (e.g., needleless systems, one hand techniques)
      e. Provide personal protective equipment
      f. Housekeeping, laundry practices
      g. Hepatitis B vaccination program

        h. Evaluation of exposures

        i. Documentation

    P. Patient Self-Determination Act

        1. Advance directives

           a. Living will

           b. Durable power of attorney

        2. Facility must have written polices and procedures that meet requirements for advance directives.

        3. Written information for patients—requirements vary by type of medical facility

        4. Educate staff on advance directive policies and requirements

VI. Accrediting agencies

    A. Joint Commission on Accreditation of Healthcare Organizations (JCAHO) (http://www.jcaho.org)

        1. Voluntary program

        2. Acute care, ambulatory, long-term care, other types of facilities

        3. Recognized by third-party payers and government agencies

        4. Surveys will be totally unannounced by 2006.

        5. Strong emphasis on safety initiatives

    B. Accreditation Association for Ambulatory Health Care, Inc. (AAAHC) (http://www.aaahc.org)

        1. Surveys many types of ambulatory health care providers

        2. Emphasizes constructive consultation and education

        3. Recognized by third-party payers and government agencies

    C. American Association for Accreditation of Ambulatory Surgery Facilities (AAAASF) (http://www.aaaasf.org)

        1. To ensure high standards in office-based surgery

        2. Single specialty and multispecialty facilities owned and operated by surgeons who are certified by a board recognized by the American Board of Medical Specialties (ABMS)

        3. Requires peer review and quality and process improvement programs to be in place

■ ■■ The Internet has become an excellent resource for all levels of regulation—state, federal, accrediting, and in some cases, local and county. Accessing such sites will provide a wealth of information to be applied to the work setting. Generic search engines can assist in that search, but using more specific sites can improve the search for health and regulatory related information. Here are a few that are specific to regulatory issues in health care.

- http://www.firstgov.gov is an excellent starting point for federal searches, but also has the added benefit of links to every state.
- http://www.hippo.findlaw.com is the address for Health Hippo, a collection of health care policy and regulatory materials from advance directives to productive rights, the FDA to fraud and abuse, and more.
- http://www.allsearchengines.com then allows a link into health and medicine search engines.
- http://www.nlm.nih.gov is the portal into the National Library of Medicine, another significant link.

BIBLIOGRAPHY

1. Centers for Devices and Radiological Health, Office of Surveillance and Biometrics: *Medical device reporting: An overview.* Rockville, MD: Department of Health and Human Services, 1996.
2. Centers for Disease Control and Prevention: Available at http://www.cdc.gov. Accessed on April 7, 2003.
3. Federated Ambulatory Surgery Association: ASC's struggle to provide language translation. *Fed Ambul Surg Assoc Update* 19:5, 2002.
4. Flook D: The professional nurse and regulation. *J PeriAnesth Nurs* 18(3):160-167, 2003.
5. Garan, Lucow, Miller, PC: Available at http://www.emtala.com. Accessed on April 7, 2003.

6. National Fire Protection Association: Available at http://www.nfpa.org. Accessed April 18, 2003.

7. New York State Nurses Association: Talking points: Protecting the Nurse Practice Act. Available at http://www.nysna.org. Accessed April 7, 2003.

8. Occupational Safety and Health Administration: Available at http://www.osha.gov. Accessed on April 17, 2003.

9. US Department of Justice, Civil Rights Division: *Civil rights division activities and programs.* Washington, DC: US Department of Justice, 2002.

10. US Department of Justice: Title III highlights. Available at http://www.usdoj.gov/crt/ada. Accessed on April 18, 2003.

11. US Drug Enforcement Administration: Available at http://www.dea.gov. Accessed on April 18, 2003.

10 Safety

DEBBY NIEHAUS

OBJECTIVES

At the conclusion of this chapter the reader will be able to:

1. Identify the physical structure of the perioperative environment.

2. Identify components of a safe environment in which to deliver competent care to all perianesthesia patients.

3. Discuss the minimum required policies and procedures for safety in the perianesthesia setting.

4. List special considerations for caring for latex-sensitive and allergy patients.

5. Discuss five staff expectations for a safe environment.

I. Joint Commission on Accreditation of Healthcare Organizations (JCAHO) 2004 National Patient Safety Goals
   A. Focus
      1. Help accredited organizations address specific areas of concern in regard to patient safety
      2. Each goal includes no more than two recommendations
      3. Usually no more than six goals established each year
      4. Goals are reevaluated each year
      5. New goals announced in July each year and become effective on January 1 the following year
   B. 2004 Goals
      1. Improve accuracy of patient identification
         a. Use at least two patient identifiers before blood draws or administration of medications.
         b. Before the start of any surgical or invasive procedure, conduct a final verification process (time out) to confirm correct patient, procedure, and site.
      2. Improve the effectiveness of communication among caregivers.
         a. Process to verify verbal or telephone orders.
         b. Standardization of abbreviations, acronyms, and symbols
      3. Improve safety of using high-alert medications.
         a. Remove concentrated electrolytes from patient care units.
         b. Standardize and limit the number of drug concentrations available.
      4. Eliminate wrong site, wrong patient, wrong procedure surgery.
         a. Create preoperative verification process.
         b. Implement process to mark surgical site; involve patient.
      5. Improve safety of using infusion pumps.
         a. Ensure free-flow protection.
      6. Improve effectiveness of clinical alarm systems.
         a. Implement regular preventative maintenance and testing.
         b. Ensure alarms are activated with appropriate settings and sufficiently audible.
      7. Reduce the risk of health care–acquired infections.
         a. Comply with current Centers for Disease Control (CDC) hand-hygiene guidelines.
         b. Manage as sentinal events all identified cases of unanticipated death or major permanent loss of function associated with a health care–acquired infection.

II. Physical structure—safe environment
  A. American Society of PeriAnesthesia Nurses (ASPAN) standard on environment of care
    1. Nursing practice promotes a safe, comfortable, and therapeutic environment for patients, staff, and visitors (ASPAN 2002 Standards).
  B. Patient safety provided through dynamic assessment and care management along with having emergency equipment and medications readily available
    1. ASPAN 2002 Standards, Resource 4: Criteria for initial, ongoing, and discharge assessment and management
    2. ASPAN 2002 Standards, Resource 5: Equipment for preanesthesia phase, PACU phase I, phase II, phase III
    3. ASPAN 2002 Standards, Resource 6: Emergency drugs and equipment
  C. Lobby and reception area
    1. Exterior signs clearly marked to direct to entrance or route to follow written in large letters that are easily read
    2. Wide entrance door, clear path for the handicapped and elderly; facility complies with regulations of the American with Disabilities Act (ADA)
    3. Reception desk in sight of entrance door
    4. Knowledgeable receptionist or clerk to direct or answer questions
    5. Positive first impression of personnel who are identified (name badge per facility policy)
    6. Area conveys sense of cleanliness, comfort, and professionalism.
    7. Waiting area relaxing with sturdy furniture, well-positioned lighting, nearby telephone, and handicapped accessible rest rooms
    8. Diversion—TV, music, magazines, vending (separate from waiting patients); separate, enclosed play area for families with children or an area with least traffic (books and safe toys that do not create a hazard)
    9. Separate, enclosed area for physician to speak with waiting family members and significant others
    10. No loose carpets or slick finishes on wood or solid surface floors
    11. Staff or volunteer in waiting room to assist and keep family informed
  D. Business and administrative area
    1. Office space as needed for admitting, scheduling, billing, executive director, nurse manager, anesthesia personnel, doctor dictation and consult room, and conference room and staff education area
    2. Promotion of safety, health, and emotional well-being of business staff
      a. Appropriate lighting, ventilation, and temperature control
      b. Furnishings for good body mechanics
      c. Standard office equipment with noise reduction measures
      d. Telephone answering machine or voice mail
      e. Computerized management information system, ergonomic seating, and work area
  E. Consultation and diagnostic area
    1. Located close to reception for easy accessibility
    2. Two-way communication system for summoning assistance
    3. Consultation room
      a. Table and chairs for interview and/or family consultation with doorways that are handicapped and wheelchair accessible
      b. Provision for privacy
  F. Diagnostic area
    1. Lab area for obtaining patient specimens, appropriate supplies, gloves, eye protection, and access for hand washing
    2. Bathroom handicapped accessible with emergency call light
    3. Stretcher for electrocardiogram or lab work equipped with safety rails, straps and steps or lifts in area to assist in patient transfer
    4. Safety measures if radiology services provided (i.e., lead aprons and dose badges for staff; lead protection for patient as appropriate)

G. Preoperative admitting
   1. Patients to be admitted after surgery may be taken to assigned room in AM admitted through AM Admit Unit, or to assigned nursing floor for hospital admission or preoperative regimen, then transferred to preoperative area.
   2. Outpatients and office surgery patients admitted to preoperative area for admission
       a. May be open area with minimal separation with curtains or glassed walls and doors and audio and visual separation
       b. In some facilities, postanesthesia care unit (PACU) area doubles as preadmission unit.
   3. Preanesthesia areas with a relaxing décor in calming colors and quiet surroundings with restricted traffic; may provide soft music
   4. Toys provided for young children are appropriate to age and have no safety issues such as sharp edges, loose parts, or pieces that can be swallowed.
       a. Facility policy outlines inspection and cleaning regime for toys.
   5. Preoperative area distinctly separate from the postoperative area
   6. Bathroom is handicapped accessible with a call light.
   7. Lockers are provided for storage and safekeeping of personal belongings.
   8. Patient admitted to bed, recliner, or stretcher (depends on facility practice); check for recommended weight limits if a bariatric patient
   9. Documentation forms for physician, nurse, anesthesia, and other health care providers
       a. Documentation in patient medical record as required by policy and mandated standards
   10. Intravenous poles and solutions, oxygen delivery system, and suction equipment easily accessible in admission area and wherever moderate sedation and analgesia is administered
   11. Patient monitoring devices and emergency equipment in working order; alarms on and audible whenever in patient use
   12. All medications readily available
   13. All medications routinely checked for outdates
   14. Easy access to emergency call system
   15. Emergency access plan posted by all telephones
   16. Plan in place for computer and telephone downtime
H. Operating rooms (all surgical facilities)
   1. Follow recommended standards and practice of the Association of periOperative Registered Nurses (AORN), AORN Standards, Recommended Practice and Guidelines, 2002.
   2. Follow established Center for Medicare and Medicaid Services (CMS) guidelines.
   3. Follow National Fire Protection Association (NFPA) Life Safety Code.
   4. Emergency equipment and supplies readily accessible
       a. Emergency crash carts
       b. Emergency medications
       c. Defibrillator—checked daily on battery
       d. Malignant hyperthermia (MH) cart
       e. Access to emergency personnel and paramedic units
   5. ASPAN 2002 Standards, Resource 5: Equipment for preanesthesia, PACU phase I, phase II, phase III (includes Malignant Hyperthermia Association of the United States [MHAUS] emergency recommendations)
   6. ASPAN 2002 Standards, Resource 6: Emergency drugs and equipment
   7. Emergency power generator and emergency light fixtures with recommended scheduled battery check
   8. Emergency backup oxygen supply readily available
   9. Battery-powered monitors readily available

10. Battery-powered vacuum (suction) unit readily available
11. Anesthesia equipment, supplies, and drugs readily accessed
    a. Process in place to ensure all anesthesia supplies and equipment checked daily
12. Two-way communication for summoning help to the operating room (OR) from the preoperative and postoperative areas
13. All ORs provide for separate and proper safe storage of supplies, sterile instruments, cleaning supplies, and sterilization of equipment.
14. Safety of patients, staff, physicians, and ancillary personnel is ensured through implementation of safe practices and infection control guidelines.
15. Emergency spill kits and material safety data sheets (MSDS) information readily available
16. Staff members review program for hazardous material handling and disposal on an annual basis.
17. Ongoing routine inspection of equipment by staff and clinical engineering
    a. Routine inspection of electrical devices and wall plugs
    b. Grounding devices inspection tagged and dated
    c. Pillows and padding for positioning and restraints
    d. Ensure properly functioning OR tables brakes, accessory pieces, and lifts.
    e. Anesthesia waste gas scavenging functioning properly
18. ASPAN 2002 Standards, Position Statement: Air safety in the perianesthesia environment
19. Strict adherence to principles of asepsis
20. Infection control program in place as specified by JCAHO or other accrediting organization based on patient population served (i.e., children, women, adults, and elderly)
21. ORs in close proximity to PACU for reduced patient transfer time
    a. Ideal if adjacent
    b. System for OR to communicate directly with PACU
22. Follow manufacturer's recommendations for weight limits for OR tables or stretchers for bariatric patient and staff safety
    a. Have proper transfer system (i.e., bariatric lift or adequate personnel)
    b. Employees educated on proper body mechanics

I. Phase I: PACU
    1. Maintain adequate respect for patients' physical and psychological needs and privacy but not to exclusion of safety.
    2. Adequate space to allow nursing care from either side of stretcher or bed or from the head and foot of patient
    3. Adequate competent staffing and ongoing nursing assessment for a safe environment
    4. ASPAN 2002 Standards, Resource 3: Patient classification/ recommended staffing guidelines
    5. ASPAN 2002 Standards, Resource 4: Criteria for initial, ongoing, and discharge assessment and management
    6. Patient care supplies readily accessible and within reach at bedside
    7. Each station includes
        a. Oxygen delivery system, vacuum station, suction
        b. Monitoring devices—cardiac monitor, pulse oximeter, noninvasive blood pressure monitor, and thermometer
    8. Ice machine for patient ice chips or if needed in MH crisis
    9. Patient warming devices
        a. Hot air warming devices
        b. Thermal blanket warming device
    10. Open room design for optimal visualization

11. Distinct separation of postoperative patients and those patients having other procedures in the phase I PACU
    a. Chronic pain procedures
       (1) Check state laws—facility may not be eligible for reimbursement if procedure done in PACU and not a licensed "bed" with state license.
    b. Preoperative administration of regional block
    c. Special procedures
12. Private recovery area (separate room within confines of PACU)
    a. Serves to provide care to patients requiring isolation
    b. Can be used for recovery of crying child
    c. Can serve as a private area for special circumstances
       (1) Trauma patients who are not expected to recover—allows visitation by family
       (2) Overnight stays in PACU
       (3) Any patients needing privacy because of other special circumstances
13. Desks or bedside units ergonomic in comfort and easy view of patients
14. Adjoins phase II with easy access for bed or stretchers through doorways
15. Hospital-based PACU
    a. Assign ambulatory patients to an area separated from sicker inpatients along with separation of children from adults if possible to reduce patient emotional discomfort, chance of infection, reduced attention paid to healthier outpatient
16. Freestanding center
    a. Favor liberal visiting policy, close proximity to waiting room, and provide patients with space for family members to sit with them
    b. Easy chairs, handicapped accessible rest rooms, and changing areas equipped with safety rails, emergency call systems, and so forth are made available to patients in many combined phase I and II units.
    c. A need for unobstructed safe access and assisted transfer in the immediate postoperative period
    d. Outside access to allow for ease and safety for discharge and ambulance transfer of patients to acute care hospital if required
17. ASPAN 2002 Standards, Resource 4: Criteria for Initial, ongoing, and discharge assessment and management
18. ASPAN 2002 Standards, Resource 5: Equipment for preanesthesia phase, PACU phase I, phase II, phase III

J. Phase II PACU
    1. May be private room on a nursing unit where patient transferred after sufficiently recovered and discharged from phase I perianesthesia unit
    2. Postoperative room that serves to provide for protective patient isolation because of poor immune system, contaminated wound drainage, or contagious disease
    3. Private rooms may be provided on return to same day surgery unit.
    4. Freestanding phase II
       a. Casual, homelike atmosphere with sturdy easy chairs for patients
       b. Provides continued nursing care and observation
       c. Provides setting for education and home care instructions for patients along with family or significant other
       d. Encourages self-care, ambulation, and a return to a level of function as close to the preoperative state as the procedure allows
    5. Open design ambulatory phase II
       a. Provision necessary for privacy related to care (i.e., partial walls, curtains, screens with safety in mind and nurse visualization)
       b. Stretchers or recliners depending on surgery and type and duration of anesthesia (should be in safe working order, patient's weight needs)
       c. Discharge area large enough to accommodate at least one family member or significant other

> **d.** Separate area for pediatric patients and family, if possible
> **e.** Cabinets or furniture for patient care items, equipment storage, and discharge supplies (i.e., crutches, sling, sitz bath, emesis basins)
> **f.** Basic emergency equipment and supplies available although usually in cabinet or in chair side stand.
> > (1) Ambu bags, oxygen mask, portable oxygen, portable suction
> > (2) Emesis basin, tissues, waterproof pads
> **g.** Ready access to emergency carts, equipment, and personnel
> **h.** Bathroom(s) in close proximity and handicapped accessible

6. Accessibility to waiting area and exit for efficient patient discharge
   a. Separate exit door for convenience, privacy, and handicapped access
   b. Short route for those patients who are discharged ambulating
   c. Wheelchair ramp available and protected from weather
7. Telephone or intercom access to hospital or other emergency care personnel if needed and emergency plan with phone numbers posted by all phones
8. Adequate competent staffing to provide for safe patient environment
9. ASPAN 2002 Standards, Resource 4: Criteria for initial, ongoing, and discharge assessment and management
10. ASPAN 2002 Standards, Resource 3: Patient classification/recommended staffing guidelines
11. ASPAN 2002 Standards, Resource 5: Equipment for preanesthesia phase, PACU phase I, phase II, phase III
12. Patients may be "fast tracked" and bypass phase I and be admitted directly to phase II if meet criteria for phase II admission.
13. ASPAN sets forth a position statement "to safeguard the delivery of postanesthesia care in a safe, appropriate and cost effective manner."
14. ASPAN 2002 Standards, Position Statement: Fast tracking

III. Support services and safety
  A. Supplies and equipment
     1. Proper storage for equipment
     2. Supplies readily available
     3. Outside shipments unboxed in receiving area—separate from sterile supplies to decrease potential of introducing contaminants and vermin to restricted areas
     4. Inventory system in place for rapid location and retrieval of specific items
     5. Equipment stored adjacent to or near area of intended use
     6. Delicate instruments and equipment stored in a protected area (e.g., microscopes, c-arms)
     7. ASPAN 2002 Standards, Resource 5: Equipment for preanesthesia phase, PACU phase I, phase II, and phase III
  B. Housekeeping and linen
     1. Cleaning supplies and equipment stored out of sight of patients and visitors
     2. General housekeeping duties performed during downtimes
     3. Cleaning solutions and chemicals properly labeled and stored safely with adequate ventilation (e.g., anesthetic gases, formaldehyde, ethylene oxide)
     4. MSDS available in central location for all hazardous chemicals on unit
     5. Appropriate supplies available for cleaning
     6. Personnel assigned to clean operating rooms are properly trained and provided with appropriate personnel protective equipment (PPE).
     7. Mop heads are changed after each use.[19]
     8. Separation of soiled and clean linen is maintained at all times.
     9. Scrub clothing stored within confines of changing rooms
     10. Linen carts are stored to avoid contamination.
  C. Mechanical and electrical
     1. New equipment is evaluated and tested prior to use.
        a. Clinical engineering is responsible for servicing and safety.
        b. Inspected for safety; proper function prior to use

        c. Labeled with inspection sticker according to facility policy

        d. Routinely rechecked periodically according to facility policy

    2. Hospital-integrated unit

        a. Clinical engineering responsible for servicing and safety of equipment

    3. Freestanding facility

        a. Individual(s) may be assigned or contracted for mechanical work.

        b. Manager and clinical staff members should have basic knowledge and written instructions regarding proper use of facility systems.

           (1) Electrical breaker switches

           (2) Water shut-off valves

           (3) Backup oxygen source

           (4) Piped-in gas shut-off valves

           (5) Emergency generator

           (6) Security system

           (7) Heating, ventilation, air conditioning (HVAC) units

           (8) Humidifier controls

        c. Emergency contact number of service technicians readily available

D. Staff support services

    1. Comfort and safe working environment provided for all staff members and physicians

    2. Lounge for staff and physician use separate from clinical area

    3. Area for education, staff meeting, completion of projects

    4. Reference library, medical reading material, Internet access

    5. Parking area for staff and physicians

        a. Adequate parking spaces for employees and patients

        b. Separate entrance from patient entrance

        c. Well lighted for security purpose

    6. Dictation area

        a. Private area to ensure confidentiality

        b. Quiet area without distractions

        c. Easy access to medical records

        d. Provisions to maintain privacy of medical records

IV. General safety considerations

A. Overview

    1. Dependent on physical conditions of facility and safety plan

    2. Policies and procedures in place to ensure safe practices

    3. Safety-minded attitude and practice of staff members

    4. Practice habits of employees and physicians

    5. Administrative support reflective of compliance with safety standards

B. JCAHO Standards related to safety

    1. Approximately 50% directly related to safety

    2. Additional standards indirectly related to safety

    3. JCAHO accreditation means quality care and safety to public.

C. Other accrediting organizations

    1. CMS

    2. Accreditation Association for Ambulatory Health Care (AAAHC)

    3. American Association for Accreditation of Ambulatory Surgery Facilities (AAAASF)

    4. State agencies

        a. Refer to specific standards published by each

D. Safety management program

    1. Safety committee

        a. Discuss issues needing attention

           (1) Issues identified following inspections, drills, or other events

        b. Determine corrective action needed

    2. Safety plans
       a. Safety management
         (1) Process to review, as frequently as necessary, but not less than every two years, all applicable service safety policies and procedures
         (2) Promotion of hazard surveillance program, including response to product safety recalls
         (3) Reporting of all accidents involving patients, visitors, or staff; including evaluation, conclusion, recommendations, and action taken
         (4) Use of safety-related information in the orientation of new employees and continuing education of all employees
         (5) Annual evaluation of the effectiveness of the safety program
       b. Life safety (fire) management
       c. Utilities
       d. Medical equipment management
       e. Employee (worker) safety management
       f. Security management
       g. Hazardous materials management
       h. Emergency preparedness management
E. Patient safety (see Box 10-1)
    1. Care is delivered by competent health care providers.
    2. Standards of perianesthesia and perioperative nursing care (ASPAN/AORN) are adhered to.
    3. Support staff and unlicensed assistive personnel (UAP) function under the direction of perianesthesia or perioperative nurse
    4. Clinical staff demonstrate competency for required duties
       a. Assessed annually
       b. Documented in personnel file
    5. Professional nurse demonstrates knowledge of
       a. Standards
       b. Policies
       c. Procedures
       d. Nurse practice act
F. Visitor safety
    1. Well-marked signage
    2. Uncluttered and well-lighted hallways
    3. Dry, nonskid floors in waiting areas
    4. No loose carpet, rugs, tiles
    5. Toys and books for children
       a. Properly stored to reduce clutter
       b. Should be age appropriate
       c. No small loose pieces—choking hazard for small child
       d. Large toys and blocks pose a danger of tripping
       e. Toys with many parts may be thrown around waiting area, posing a hazard.
       f. Toys need to be disinfected on a routine basis.
    6. Visitors providing hands-on care
       a. Not routinely allowed except in special circumstances where visitor is caregiver with special knowledge on moving and caring for patient
    7. Document and report any visitor incidents per facility policy
       a. Injuries
       b. Falls
       c. Medical occurrences
G. Employee safety (see Box 10-2)
    1. Security of personnel is maintained.
    2. Infection control practices
       a. Personnel follow established policies and procedures.
       b. Universal precautions are maintained.

■ BOX 10-1
■ **PATIENT EXPECTATIONS FOR A SAFE ENVIRONMENT**

1. The competence of all health providers is ensured.
   - All professional health care providers are currently licensed.
   - All nonprofessional health care providers are appropriately trained and supervised.
   - Providers are currently certified in basic cardiac life support (BLS/CPR) and, in the PACU, in ACLS.
   - Providers are knowledgeable of specific perianesthesia health care needs.
   - Providers continually update and demonstrate necessary competencies.
   - Emergency drills are practiced by all providers as required by local, state, federal, and/or regulatory recommendations.
   - All employees are knowledgeable of the policies and practices of the facility.
2. The patient is appropriately attended.
   - Patients have a method for summoning assistance within reach at all times.
   - Heavily sedated or anesthetized patients and children are attended at all times.
   - Patients at high risk for falls are identified, and interventions employed.
   - An anesthesia provider or other physician who is appropriately qualified in resuscitative techniques is present or immediately available until all patients operated on that day have been evaluated and discharged.
3. Safety practices are in place to protect the patient during times of dependence.
   - An identification bracelet is provided and visually checked before administration of medications or start of a procedure along with another patient identifier that shall not be the patient's room number.
   - The name of the patient's primary physician is documented on the medical record for reference in case of an emergency situation.
   - Safety devices are used (e.g., nonskid slippers or flooring, side rails and safety straps, wheel locks on stretchers, recliners, and wheelchairs).
   - Providers protect the patient from pressure and injury through knowledge of proper body mechanics, positioning, and padding of pressure points.
   - The patient is asked for verbal identification and the type and site of surgery before transfer to the OR.
   - Prior to the start of any invasive procedure or surgery, a final verification process is performed (time out) to confirm the correct patient, procedure, and site.
   - Sharp objects and unprotected needles are not placed in contact with or near the patient at any time.
   - Sponges, needles, and instruments are accounted for before closing of body cavities.
   - Radiopaque sponges are used whenever a body cavity is entered.
   - The patient is appropriately protected from radiation, electrical, or laser injuries.
   - Intubated patients in the PACU will have endotracheal cuffs inflated until the time of extubation unless specific contraindications exist.
   - Patients with artificial airways in place are constantly attended and are positioned to prevent aspiration.
   - Suction is immediately available for unconscious patients.
   - Two licensed providers, one of whom is a registered nurse competent in phase I postanesthesia nursing, are present at all times when a postoperative patient is in the building or department.
   - Two providers are available to help with the initial ambulation of patients who are at high risk for falling—the very elderly or physically weak, postspinal or postepidural patients, those unable or not allowed to bear weight on one leg, and those with a history of fainting or difficulty in ambulating.
   - Discharge of the patient who has received anesthesia or sedation is allowed only when that patient is accompanied by a responsible adult.
4. Appropriate and safe equipment is available.
   - All technical and electronic equipment is tested for safety by the clinical engineer or equivalent before initial use and in an ongoing manner.

■ BOX 10-1 *Cont'd*
■ **PATIENT EXPECTATIONS FOR A SAFE ENVIRONMENT**

- Unsafe or questionable equipment is taken out of service and labeled immediately.
- Monitoring devices are calibrated and serviced periodically as designated by the manufacturer.
- Directions for use are readily available for all equipment.
- Emergency equipment is checked periodically for function and staff familiarity.
- Stretchers, wheelchairs, and recliners are periodically inspected.
- There is emergency access to replacement equipment in the event of a failure.
- Portable emergency equipment allows for safe transport to another unit or facility.
- An internal and external communication system is available throughout the facility.

5. Medications are stored and administered safely.
   - An adequate stock of medications is maintained.
   - Security of medication from tampering, theft, and unauthorized use is ensured.
   - All medications remain in their original wrapping. If they are transferred to another container, they are conspicuously labeled by the pharmacist who transfers them.
   - Expiration dates, color, and clarity are checked before use.
   - Outdated medications are removed from the storage area of medications in use.
   - Emergency drugs are checked for expiration dates at least monthly and are replaced immediately if used or outdated.
   - Storage of medication is temperature and humidity controlled as indicated for individual drugs.
   - Oral, injectable, and topical drugs are stored separately.
   - Allergies are identified and consistently documented in a prominent and consistent location on all patient records. This may include having the patient wear a bracelet noting any allergies.
   - Nurses follow safe standards of practice by identifying the drug, dose, route, time, patient's name, one additional demographic patient identifier other than room number, and allergies before administering any medication.
   - All patients are observed for untoward or allergic effects of medications administered.

6. The principles of asepsis are maintained.
   - All providers are knowledgeable of and practice proper techniques to prevent the spread of disease and germs.
   - Strict aseptic technique is followed in the OR and for invasive procedures such as catheter insertion or irrigation, venipunctures, dressing changes, and injections.
   - All personnel are truthful and ethical about any break in sterile technique. They immediately report such an occurrence and take necessary steps to correct or address any resulting problems and to avoid future occurrences.
   - Sterility of supplies is ascertained through ongoing monitoring of autoclave function, checking of expiration dates, rotating of stock, and monitoring of individual techniques of packaging for sterilization.
   - Providers with highly contagious diseases will not be involved in the care of surgical patients.

7. Decisions about health care are made thoughtfully and with regard to the individual.
   - A physician knowledgeable of the patient directs the patient care, including discharge.
   - All pertinent data and diagnostic test results are available and are assessed before administration of anesthesia or the onset of the procedure.

PACU, postanesthesia care unit; *BLS,* basic life support; *CPR,* cardiopulmonary resuscitation; *ACLS,* advanced cardiac life support; *OR,* operating room.
From Burden N, DeFazio Quinn DM, O'Brien D, et al: *Ambulatory surgical nursing.* Philadelphia: WB Saunders, 2000, p 100-101.

■ BOX 10-2
■ **STAFF EXPECTATIONS FOR A SAFE ENVIRONMENT**

1. Personal security is addressed.
   - Alarm systems, security devices, and locks are maintained as appropriate to the risks inherent to the geographic location of the facility
   - Entrances and parking lots are well lighted.
   - A security guard is provided in high-risk areas.
   - One person is not left alone in the facility.
   - Narcotics, needles, syringes, and prescription pads are appropriately locked and/or kept out of sight when not in use.
2. Policies and practices are in place to prevent the spread of disease.
   - Universal precautions approved by the CDC (Centers for Disease Control and Prevention) are practiced.
   - The facility provides sufficient protective clothing, gloves, goggles, and storage containers for wastes, antiseptics, and sinks for hand washing.
   - Needles are discarded in appropriate containers without recapping or breaking.
   - Personnel and patients with highly communicable diseases (measles, mumps, chickenpox, and influenza) are not allowed in the facility.
   - Aseptic technique is maintained.
3. Policies and practices are in place to prevent exposure to, or injury from, radiation, laser equipment, electrical, and other equipment.
   - Defibrillators are stored in the "disarmed" mode.
   - Appropriate gear (goggles, lead aprons) is available for protection against injury from potentially dangerous equipment.
   - Warning signs are posted conspicuously when laser equipment or radiation is in use.
   - Radiology technicians announce their intentions before taking an exposure to allow staff members to put on protective apparel or to leave the immediate area.
   - Adequate instruction regarding equipment usage is provided for all staff members.
   - Equipment is safety checked before its use and periodically thereafter.
   - Equipment that is faulty or suspected to be faulty is removed from service immediately and is labeled for repair immediately.
4. Individual health practices are encouraged.
   - The facility provides or requires a periodic physical examination of all employees. This includes appropriate diagnostic testing.
   - The facility supports and provides immunization against hepatitis B for high-risk personnel.
   - The facility requires appropriate skin testing for tuberculosis.
   - Vacation and personal leave time is supported administratively for the emotional and physical well-being of employees.
   - Appropriate stress reduction practices are encouraged.
5. Ongoing educational programs and information sessions are provided to instruct personnel on safety habits.
   - Information is available regarding body mechanics, use of electrical equipment, storage, and disposal of toxic wastes, and so forth.
   - Information is available in the native language of employees who are unable to understand English.
   - Periodic fire and disaster drills are held to increase employees' awareness of personal responsibilities and ways to protect themselves and patients from danger during an emergency.
6. Storage of chemicals and toxic or dangerous materials protects personnel.
   - Unit-specific material safety data sheets (MSDS) for all toxic materials stored in the building or department are available and are easily accessible to all employees.
   - Adequate ventilation and sturdy storage shelves are provided.
   - No smoking is allowed near volatile materials or other combustibles.
   - Policies for handling dangerous materials are available and are communicated to all employees.

■ BOX 10-2 *Cont'd*
■ **STAFF EXPECTATIONS FOR A SAFE ENVIRONMENT**

> - Emergency eye wash stations are readily available wherever there is potential for exposure and eye wash stations are tested periodically to ensure proper function.
> 7. Employees in high-risk areas are protected from anesthesia waste gases.
>   - A scavenging system is in place for retrieval and elimination of anesthetic waste gases from the operating room.
>   - Anesthesia equipment is maintained and inspected for leaks and cracks. Damaged equipment is discarded or repaired.
>   - Ventilation systems are cleaned regularly.
>   - Anesthetic gases are not turned on before actual induction of the anesthesia.
>   - Female employees of childbearing age receive appropriate medical care and counseling.
>   - Employees in high-risk areas receive annual physical examination; these may include liver and kidney function tests if deemed appropriate by the employee's physician.
> 8. A policy is in place regarding employee incidents, injury, or exposure to a biologic hazard.
>   - Access to emergency care is immediately available should an employee be injured.
>   - A mechanism is in place for reporting any incident involving staff safety.
>   - Follow-up of injuries or incidents includes a plan to prevent similar future occurrences.
> 9. A mechanism exists that allows staff participation in establishment of a safe and pleasant working environment.
>   - All staff members will be educated regarding possible health and safety hazards in the workplace. Education will occur during initial orientation and will be reviewed on an annual basis.
>   - Facility personnel are involved in the safety management program.
>   - A mechanism is in place for employees to express suggestions or concerns regarding workplace safety.

From Burden N, DeFazio Quinn DM, O'Brien D, et al: *Ambulatory surgical nursing.* Philadelphia: WB Saunders, 2000, p 102.

      c. Aseptic technique is maintained.
      d. Tuberculosis screenings
      e. Hepatitis B vaccine offered and provided
  V. Policies and procedures
    A. Fire and disaster
      1. Basic fire prevention methods and codes per National Fire Protection Association (NFPA)
      2. A written plan for fire safety and evacuation
        a. Posted throughout facility
        b. Staff demonstrate proper techniques for patient evacuation.
      3. Periodic, regular mock drills involving staff members recommended
        a. Nearest fire extinguisher
        b. Fire alarm pull boxes
        c. Location of fire exit(s) and door(s)
        d. Types of fire extinguishers available and appropriate use of each
        e. At least quarterly, check licensure requirements.
      4. Department manager responsible for ensuring all employees properly trained in fire safety
      5. Emergency telephone numbers posted by phone
      6. Fire drills performed at least quarterly
      7. Disaster drills performed twice a year; one drill needs to include influx of patients
        a. Staff participate in annual fire safety training
    B. Safety
      1. Establish standards for education and training.

2. Equipment inspected and maintained on a routine basis (preventative maintenance program)
3. Staff members instructed in
   a. Proper body mechanics
   b. Hazardous chemicals, biohazards, and MSDS
   c. Electrical and fire safety
   d. Workplace violence
   e. Bomb threats
      (1) Procedure for notifying authorities
      (2) Procedures for maintaining calmness during evacuations
   f. Handling threatening phone calls
      (1) Techniques to diffuse the situation
      (2) Procedure to track the caller
      (3) Need to plan for evacuation
   g. Natural disasters
      (1) Tornado
      (2) Lightning
      (3) Earthquake
      (4) Mass casualty
      (5) Explosions
   h. Chemical spills
4. Evacuation plan and egress routes reviewed and practiced at least annually
   a. Mock drills with play actors beneficial
C. Infection control practices
   1. Follow CDC guidelines
   2. Hand washing to prevent spread of or acquiring nosocomial contaminates
   3. JCAHO or other agency standards for infection control program
      a. Surveillance
      b. Identification
      c. Prevention
      d. Control of infection
      e. Reporting of infections
   4. Isolation procedure
      a. Procedure details how patients requiring isolation are cared for.
      b. Body substance isolation protects against contact of
         (1) Blood, saliva, semen
         (2) Urine feces, vaginal secretion, amniotic fluid
         (3) Wound drainage, cerebrospinal fluid, synovial fluid
      c. Protective barriers
         (1) Gloves, mask
         (2) Goggles, hoods, safety glasses
         (3) Hair and shoe coverings
         (4) Waterproof gowns
      d. Respiratory isolation for airborne disease (tuberculosis, childhood disease exposure)
         (1) Measles, pertussis, chickenpox, colds
         (2) Recent cough, fever, congestion, croup, sore throat
         (3) Policy details highly susceptible or pregnant staff members' role in avoiding patient contact.
         (4) When alternative care area is utilized because of absence of isolation room
            (a) PACU care is delivered by PACU nurse
            (b) PACU nurse competent in isolation procedures
            (c) Same level of care is administered regardless of where recovery takes place
      e. Standard precaution guidelines
      f. Personal protective equipment (PPE) readily available
      g. Staff receives annual training in infection control policies and procedures.

D. Cardiopulmonary resuscitation (CPR), advanced cardiac life support (ACLS), pediatric advanced life support (PALS)
    1. Annual review of CPR by qualified trainer
    2. Demonstrated competency of all staff in CPR every two years
    3. PACU phase I staff nurses maintain current ACLS and/or PALS as appropriate to patient population served.
    4. ASPAN 2002 Standards, Standard III: Staffing and Personnel Management

E. Dress code
    1. Determined by proximity and frequency of access to ORs (AORN and ASPAN)
        a. Unrestricted area
            (1) Traffic not limited
            (2) Street clothes may be worn.
        b. Semirestricted
            (1) Processing and storage areas for instruments and supplies
            (2) Corridors leading to the restricted areas of the surgical suite
                (a) Staff wear surgical attire.
                (b) Patients wear gowns, hair, and foot coverings.
        c. Restricted
            (1) Operating rooms, clean center core and scrub sink
            (2) Surgical attire and masks required

F. Waste gas levels
    1. Monitoring in operating rooms and PACU phase I per Occupational Safety and Health Administration (OSHA)
    2. Positive-pressure ventilation; 15 air exchanges per hour in OR; 6 air exchanges in PACU
    3. Smoke evacuator used to remove surgical plume
    4. Policy and procedure on maintenance of OR air handling system
    5. ASPAN 2002 Standards, Position Statement on air safety in the perianesthesia environment

G. Unscheduled admissions and cancellations
    1. Patients requiring postoperative admission to an acute care setting should not be scheduled in a freestanding facility.
    2. Unforeseen circumstances requiring admission postoperatively include
        a. Uncontrolled pain
        b. Prolonged nausea and/or vomiting
        c. Extensive surgery beyond what was scheduled
        d. Need for postoperative monitoring
            (1) Rule out myocardial infarction
            (2) Stroke
            (3) Ventilator support
        e. Unable to meet discharge criteria
            (1) Unstable vital signs
            (2) Diabetes
            (3) Hypertension
            (4) Cardiac abnormalities
            (5) Respiratory status
    3. Cancellations
        a. Patient did not meet nothing by mouth (NPO) requirements
        b. Uncontrolled diabetes, hypertension, cardiac condition
        c. Acute illness
        d. Abnormal lab work
        e. Unable to rule out possible pregnancy
        f. Insurance or financial coverage
        g. Patient consent issues (e.g., guardianship, power of attorney, minors)
        h. Patient unable to fulfill obligation for required transportation home
        i. ASPAN 2002 Standards, Resource 13: Safe transfer of care
        j. Patient lacking competent home care support

  VI. Emergency drugs and equipment
    A. Based on American Heart Association ACLS and PALS guidelines
    B. Provide drugs and equipment according to population served.
    C. Refer to ASPAN 2002 Standards, Resource 6: Emergency Drugs and Equipment.
 VII. Latex allergy or sensitivity
    A. Identification of known patient allergy or sensitivity when case scheduled
      1. Schedule as first case of the day when possible or have operating room vacant for one hour prior to start of case.
        a. Case order not an issue where facilities have adopted a latex-free environment
      2. Procedure in place to identify latex allergy patients to all staff members involved in care of the patient
      3. Document and communicate latex allergy patient care needs to
        a. Preadmission testing unit
        b. Radiology (if applicable)
        c. Laboratory
        d. Pharmacy
        e. Nursing care unit
        f. Central Supply for latex-free supplies if not readily available on unit
        g. All health care team members involved in patient's care
    B. Preanesthesia care
      1. Obtain history including any latex allergy testing and results.
      2. Identify patients not previously identified but at high risk for being latex sensitive.
        a. History of rash, pruritis, edema, or burning after tape removal, reaction to Band-Aids, rubber gloves, blowing up balloons, or latex condom use
        b. Skin eruption at examination site when gloves used in dental, medical, or obstetrical exams
        c. Patient with multiple drug and food allergies
        d. Allergy to tropical fruits, kiwi, banana, tomatoes, potatoes, avocado, strawberry
        e. Multiple gastrointestinal or genitourinary procedures (i.e., spina bifida)
        f. Patients with occupational exposure to latex (health care or food workers)
      3. Document and communicate patient information.
      4. Follow established policy and procedure.
      5. Latex-free supply cart readily available
        a. Includes drugs and supplies needed to treat anaphylactic reaction
      6. Support patient and family.
    C. Intraoperative care
      1. Communicate and document
        a. Operating room personnel and ancillary personnel aware of patient's allergy and sensitivity
        b. Latex-free supplies available
        c. Surgical suite properly prepared
          (1) Ideally surgical suite located at end of corridor or last suite
          (2) Outside traffic limited
          (3) Closed room maintained while patient is in area
          (4) Open packs and supplies in hall or substerile room adjoining suite
          (5) OR table covered
          (6) All monitoring equipment latex free or covered per guidelines
      2. Notify anesthesia personnel that latex-free supplies needed in surgical suite.
      3. Emergency medications readily available
    D. Postanesthesia care
      1. Utilize latex-free supplies.
      2. Provide care in a separate location.

3. Follow established policy and procedure guidelines to provide a latex-free environment.
4. Provide support to patient and family.
5. Provide patient/family education.
6. Provide home care instructions.
7. Provide resources for patient to obtain additional information regarding
   a. Latex-containing and latex-free products
   b. Medic-Alert band
   c. Emergency medications and use (epinephrine autoinjectable and/or diphenhydramine) *Benadryl*
8. Notification to primary care physician (if new reaction)
9. Procedure on reporting reactions to manufacturer or government agency if reaction to a medical device
10. Essential that all health care workers follow established policies on communication and documentation

VIII. Staff orientation and continuing education programs
  A. Preparation of the orientee for the expected scope of practice
     1. ASPAN standards
     2. AORN standards
     3. The Society of Gastroenterology Nurses and Associates (SGNA) standards
     4. State Nurse Practice Act
  B. Formulation of skills and knowledge required to function effectively
     1. Competency-based practice

■ BOX 10-3
■ **EMPLOYEE OWNERSHIP IN THE ENVIRONMENT**

Own your space—it is part of you.
- Neatness counts—and helps you work more efficiently.
- Personalize your work area—you spend one third of your day there.
- Watch for and correct safety concerns.
- Separate food and medications, and date each when opened

Consider the patient's point of view.
- You are the most important part of the environment.
- Smiles, genuine concern, and neat appearance matter.
- Do not bring food or beverages into the clinical area where patients can see or smell them.
- Avoid loud noises and private conversations in the patient care area.
- Provide privacy for the patient and honor confidential information.
- Childproof the area to keep children safe.

Conserve resources.
- Use supplies wisely.
- Label supply locations and maintain appropriate stock levels.
- Do not hoard supplies and linens.
- Log out and turn off computers at the end of the day.
- Turn electricity off when a room or piece of equipment is not being used.
- Set room temperature for comfort, and do not continually change settings.

Know your environment.
- Learn and remember security systems and locking mechanisms.
- Know procedure for summoning help for any kind of emergency.
- Ask if you are unsure of how to use a piece of equipment.
- Take responsibility to learn about all the departments and processes in the facility so that you can answer any patient's question.
- Be prepared to give accurate directions to patients for both inside and outside the facility.

From Burden N, DeFazio Quinn DM, O'Brien D, et al: *Ambulatory surgical nursing.* Philadelphia: WB Saunders, 2000, p 119.

    C. Staff members educated in
1. General safety management issues
2. Departmental safety plans
3. Special hazards related to assigned duties
4. Safety practices related to the population served (pediatrics, geriatrics)

    D. ASPAN, Competency based orientation credentialing program: 2002 edition

    E. Use of unlicensed assistive and support personnel in the perianesthesia setting
1. ASPAN 2002 Standards, Position Statement: Registered nurse utilization of unlicensed assistive personnel
2. ASPAN 2002 Standards, Resource 9: Competent support staff

IX. Special considerations for bariatric surgery patients

    A. Special equipment to meet bariatric patient needs
1. Wheelchair
2. Stretcher
3. OR table
4. Bedside commode
5. Bariatric hover mat to transport from stretcher to postoperative bed
6. Lifts that meet bariatric weight limits or adequate personnel present to assist with moving, lifting, or transporting patient
   a. Lifts provide for staff and patient safety when moving and transporting patient
   b. Perianesthesia nurse determines the mode, number, and competency level of personnel required for transport

X. Employee responsibilities

    A. Take ownership in the workplace environment (see Box 10-3).
1. Take pride in the way the environment looks.
2. Assess the environment from the patient's perspective.
3. Conserve resources.
4. Be aware of your environment.

BIBLIOGRAPHY

1. Aker J: Safety of ambulatory surgery. *J Post Anesth Nurs* 16(6):353-358, 2001.
2. American Society of PeriAnesthesia Nurses: *ASPAN competency based orientation and credentialing program.* Cherry Hill, NJ: American Society of PeriAnesthesia Nurses, 2002.
3. American Society of PeriAnesthesia Nurses: *ASPAN standards of nursing practice.* Cherry Hill, NJ: American Society of PeriAnesthesia Nurses, 2002.
4. Association of periOperative Registered Nurses: *AORN standards: Recommended practice and guidelines.* Denver, CO: Association of Operating Room Nurses, 2002.
5. Barnes S: Considering bypass of phase I PACU? *J Post Anesth Nurs* 17(3):193-195, 2002.
6. Brown B, Riippa M, Shaneberger K: Promoting patient safety through preoperative patient verification. *AORN J* 74(5):690-698, 2001.
7. Burden N, Quinn DD, O'Brien D, et al: *Ambulatory surgical nursing,* ed 2. Philadelphia: WB Saunders, 2000.
8. Cope KA, Merritt WT, Krenzischek D, et al: Phase II collaborative pilot study: Waste anesthetic gas levels in the PACU. *J Post Anesth Nurs* 17(4):240-250, 2002.
9. Floyd PT: Latex allergy updates. *J Post Anesth Nurs* 15(1):26-30, 2000.
10. Fortunato NH: *Berry & Kohn's operating room technique,* ed 9. St. Louis: Mosby, 2000.
11. Joint Commission for Accreditation of Healthcare Organizations: Joint Commission Standards. Available at http://www.jcaho.org. Accessed December 2002.
12. Krenzischek D, Schafer J, Nolan M, et al: Phase I collaborative pilot study: Waste anesthetic gas levels in the PACU. *J Post Anesth Nurs* 17(4):227-239, 2002.
13. Litwack K: *Core curriculum for post anesthesia nursing practice,* ed 4. Philadelphia: WB Saunders, 1999.
14. Marley R: Patient care after discharge from the ambulatory surgical center, *J Post Anesth Nurs* 16(6):399-419, 2001.
15. Mecca RS: Safety in the post anesthesia care unit, part I: Clinical safety, *Curr Rev PeriAnesth Nurse* 23(21):247-259, 2001.
16. Mecca RS: Safety in the post anesthesia care unit, part II: Clinical safety, *Curr Rev PeriAnesth-Nurse* 23(22):263-274, 2002.
17. Meeker MH, Rothrock JC: *Alexander's care of the patient in surgery,* ed 11. St Louis: Mosby, 1999.

18. Michel LL, Myrick C: Current and future trends in ambulatory surgery and their impact on nursing practice. *J Post Anesth Nurs* 3(3):347-349, 1990.

19. Phippen ML, Wells MP: Patient care during operative and invasive procedures. Philadelphia: WB Saunders, 2000, pp 160.

20. Redmond M: Malignant hyperthermia: Perianesthesia recognition, treatment, and care. *J Post Anesth Nurs* 16(4):259-270, 2001.

21. Saufl N: JCAHO's patient safety standards. *J Post Anesth Nurs* 17(4):265-269, 2002.

22. Sullivan E: Life safety in the perianesthesia care environment: Planning for internal disasters. *J Post Anesth Nurs* 15(3):177-179, 2000.

23. Watkins AC: Fast-tracking after ambulatory surgery. *J Post Anesth Nurs* 16(6):379-387, 2001.

11 Continuous Quality Improvement

MEG BETURNE

OBJECTIVES

At the conclusion of this chapter the reader will be able to:

1. Describe important functions of total quality management in the perianesthesia setting.

2. Recognize major changes that have occurred in health care and their impact on quality improvement.

3. Identify personnel and levels of an organization responsible for quality.

4. Identify different dimensions of quality.

5. Recognize the different types of customers in the health care market.

6. List useful sources of data collection.

7. List useful tools for identifying patterns or trends.

8. Describe how the focus of outcome studies is changing in the perianesthesia setting

    I. Total quality management (TQM)
        A. A philosophy that quality is a responsibility shared by all and applicable to all levels of the organization
        B. Works to enhance the performance of important processes involved in the delivery of health care, having as much to do with achieving greater organizational efficiency and cost savings as improving quality of care
        C. Continuous improvement focusing on the customer, within and external to the institution, to identify root causes of problems and opportunities for improvement to achieve greater quality and efficiency
        D. Focuses on practices, nonclinical as well as clinical aspects of care
        E. Views quality as an entity subject to measurement, the scientific method and data-driven problem solving
        F. Joint Commission on Accreditation of Healthcare Organizations (JCAHO) views quality quantitatively measurable with a result focus.
    II. Dimensions of quality
        A. Effectiveness: The power of a particular procedure or treatment to improve health status improvement
        B. Efficiency
            1. The delivery of a maximum number of comparable units of health care for a given unit of health resources used
            2. Organization and supervision to combat variation in patient care
        C. Accessibility
            1. The ease and convenience with which health care can be reached in the face of financial, organizational, cultural, and emotional barriers
        D. Acceptability
            1. The degree to which health care satisfies patients'
              a. Sensitivity to timing issues
              b. Logical flow of activities

      c. Tactful, clear communication, including patient feedback

      d. Accommodation of special needs

  E. Provider competence

    1. The provider's ability (including technical and interpersonal skills) to use the best available knowledge and judgment to produce the health and satisfaction of customers

      a. Ability to convey trust and confidence

      b. Ability to perform the promised service dependably and accurately

      c. Ability for tactful problem solving

      d. Willingness to help patients and provide prompt service

      e. Empathetic caring and individualized attention to patients and families

  F. Tangibles

    1. The appearance of physical facilities, equipment, personnel, and communication materials (brochures, educational handouts)

    2. Clear directions—easily readable signage

III. TQM history

  A. Evolved from Japanese industry after World War II by Edward Deming

    1. Dr. Deming developed sampling and data quality improvement strategies and assisted the Japanese in developing high-quality merchandise.

    2. His philosophy for quality improvement was adapted by U.S. automakers in the 1980s.

  B. Joseph Juran delineated the fundamental components of a comprehensive approach to the management of quality.

    1. He identified the elements of a system to measure, improve, and lead to optimal outcomes.

    2. His principles were adopted by health care organizations in the late 1980s.

    3. Efficiency (resource use) and quality (performance) viewed as aspects of the whole

  C. TQM has become

    1. A cornerstone and guiding force in businesses, public agencies, and health care industry in 1990s

    2. Essential in today's changing health care marketplace and resultant need for health care providers to deliver more cost-effective care so that they may survive an increasing competitive environment

IV. Measuring quality

  A. Traditional ways of measuring quality

    1. Chart audit

      a. Peer review process used in hospitals until the 1970s

      b. Involved review of small sample of patient records by medical staff with judgment made as to quality of care provided

    2. Structure standards

      a. Qualifications of the providers, the physical facility, equipment, and other resources and the characteristics of the organization and its financing

    3. Process

      a. What occurs during the encounters between patients and providers

        (1) Clinical process deficiency is an avoidable error or unnecessary step in the prevention, diagnosis, and treatment of a health problem.

    4. Outcomes

      a. Things that do or do not happen as a result of medical intervention, including complication rates, functional capacity and performance, cost effectiveness, and patient satisfaction

        (1) Is the number one competitive factor next to cost in health care

        (2) Survey target areas for JCAHO and Accreditation Association for Ambulatory Health Care (AAAHC)

        (3) One of the most crucial expectations of managed care and third-party payers

(4) The endpoint of outcomes research are clinical practice guidelines intended to assist practitioners and patients in choosing appropriate health care for specific conditions.

V. Changes in the health care marketplace
  A. Since 1990, insurers have been directing patients to providers within managed care entities, such as health maintenance organizations (HMOs) and preferred provider organizations (PPOs).
  B. Insurers seek low-cost providers, based on prenegotiated payment for entire sets of services.
  C. To support their decision making, insurers rely on claims databases that facilitate identification of quality of care and cost-effective providers.
  D. In point-of-service plans (POSs), members use providers outside managed care approved networks; they are charged co-payments and deductibles higher than those charged for in-network services.
  E. Insurers are now adopting prospective payment, a bundling of the physician, ancillary, and institutional fees into a highly competitive price along with capitation—a financing mechanism in which an annual payment is made to a set of providers who contract to provide specified benefits package for each insured individual during the contract year
  F. Vertical integration is driving reimbursement reform; it refers to services provided across the spectrum of settings and institutions.

VI. Outcomes
  A. Objective measurement
    1. Patient satisfaction
    2. Efficiency
    3. Cost reduction and effectiveness
    4. Results of service
  B. Need to measure to stay competitive in health care industry
  C. The most important concerns are
    1. Positive patient outcomes
    2. Cost effective delivery of care
    3. Provide return on investment
  D. Measure against established standards and guidelines
    1. Benchmarking—defining competitors' best features from both internal and external customers' perspectives and then adopting the best practices of these organizations to operations and subsequently exceeding the benchmark performance
  E. Focus on results of performance or nonperformance of a function or process

VII. Customers
  A. Managing quality requires improving the capability and reliability of processes to meet the needs of the customers who depend on those processes; quality improvement is "customer centered."
    1. In health care, the patient is the most important customer.
    2. External customers include patients and their family members, payers and purchasers such as insurance companies, employers, government agencies, and regulatory agencies such as JCAHO, physician offices, nursing homes, and the community.
    3. Internal customers include health care providers, nursing staff, medical assistants, specialty services, customer relations managers, frontline personnel and management.

VIII. Gathering data and analysis
  A. Define current practice.
  B. Define customer needs and expectations.
    1. What complaints and dissatisfaction are most likely to drive away existing or new customers?
    2. What level of quality does the competition deliver and how does it compare with ours?

   3. What are our most costly deficiencies?
   4. What deficiencies in our internal processes have the most adverse effect on our customers?
C. Select a team.
   1. Verify team has representation from identified problem area.
   2. Evaluate team for personal knowledge, flexibility for meetings and assignments, and ability to work with departments to implement remedy.
D. The initial step in improving a process is the adoption of operational definitions and the identification of the key measures that should be tracked.
E. Clearly define the problem statement so all team members are thinking about the same problem; identify changes needed in process or area to be improved.
   1. Differentiate between sporadic versus chronic problems.
   2. Define boundaries (beginning and end points) of process to be improved.
   3. Generate and organize theories.
   4. Determine manageable time frame (usually 6-12 months).
F. Design data collection and train data collectors.
G. Collect and analyze specific, objective data in a uniform fashion.
H. Patterns or trends can be identified with
   1. Checklist—identifies how often certain events are happening, simple tool to assist in data collection
   2. Flowchart—pictorial representation showing all of the steps of a process (a graphic sequence of events)
   3. Histogram—data-gathering tool used to show the frequency of events, distribution showing patterns
   4. Control chart—a "run chart" with statistically determined upper control limit and lower control limits (determines how much variation can be expected)
   5. Pareto chart—special form of vertical bar graph to help determine which problems to solve in what order (highest to lowest)
   6. Cause and effect diagram—represents relationship between some effect and all the possible causes influencing it, organizes the potential causes of a problem to help find the root cause
   7. Scatter diagram—clarifies the relationship that exists between two factors
   8. Benefit/cost analysis
   9. Control spreadsheet
   10. Run chart—tool for displaying the variation in data over time
   11. Cost of poor quality—identifies forces that oppose or support options selected, identifies driving and restraining forces
   12. Force field analysis—technique that displays the driving (positive) and restraining (negative) forces surrounding any change
   13. Brainstorming followed by affinity diagramming—generating as many ideas, concerns, problems, or options as possible in a short time, then diagramming these ideas
   14. Databases—compilation of related information systematically organized
I. Evaluate data and validate current practice or identify opportunities for improvement using the following criteria:
   1. Total cost
   2. Impact
   3. Benefit/cost relationship
   4. Cultural impact, resistance to change
   5. Risk
   6. Health, safety, and the environment
J. Determine required resources (people, money, time, and materials).
K. Implement changes with pilot program.
L. Change process as indicated by deficiencies.
M. Evaluate effectiveness using in-process and end-result measures.

   IX. Sources of data collection

      A. Objective surveys and questionnaires

         1. Should be consumer oriented

         2. Solicit both consumer complaints and opinions.

      B. Phone call or written survey

         1. Postoperative phone call is an important tool for evaluating patient's postoperative condition, reinforcing teaching, and obtaining performance feedback.

         2. Mail-back questionnaires tend to generate low response (20-40%).

         3. Sources of gathering data

            a. Health care providers (MDs, DOs, DPMs, NPs, PAs)

            b. Third-party payers

            c. Patients

            d. Family members and friends

            e. Nursing staff (RNs, LPNs)

            f. Management

            g. Specialty and support services

            h. Medical assistants, technical associates, unlicensed assisted personnel (UAP)

         4. Patient records

         5. Satisfaction gap analysis

         6. Observation

         7. Variance reports (occurrence reports)

         8. Infection control reports

         9. Issues uncovered during a JCAHO visit

         10. Reviews and audits

            a. Data on cost of poor quality

            b. Records of quality department

            c. Internal audit

            d. Management engineering

         11. Long-term strategic goals

         12. Other quality improvement projects

      C. Computer-based patient input through available websites or dedicated computer terminals in hospitals

      D. Patient focus groups

      E. Open-ended interviews, either structured or informal

   X. Indicators

      A. Monitor and improve the quality of all aspects of care

      B. May include clinical criteria, clinical standards, practice guidelines, protocols, and a performance database

      C. Stated in objective terms

      D. Are measurable

         1. Accuracy, risk adjustment, and cost are measured through control of information technology.

         2. Based on current knowledge or structure and projected needs, standards, or industry changes

      E. Classified as outcome, process, or structure

  XI. Collecting data

      A. Numerator identification

         1. Number of times the behavior or condition is met

      B. Denominator identification

         1. Total number of patients, cases, medical records, or other variables surveyed or studied

      C. Compliance rate

         1. Calculated by dividing the numerator by the denominator

      D. Frequency of data collection

         1. Related to frequency of activity monitored

            a. Significance of event or activity monitored

  b. Common cause variation
   (1) Inevitable, inherent variation in the system or process
   (2) Can be reduced through clinical pathways, care maps, practice analysis, and feedback regarding best practices
  c. Special cause variable
   (1) Variation resulting from sources outside the system, unplanned events, freak occurrences, human error
  d. Essential consideration to decide which episode of the process is the most important to address
  e. Designated time or length of study

XII. Unique issues for ambulatory care
  A. Low incidence of severe adverse events
  B. Transient but disturbing side effects such as postoperative pain, nausea and vomiting, dysphagia, and extended somnolence may influence a patient-based assessment for quality of care.
   1. Delayed recovery may prevent discharge home and require need for continued care and observation overnight.
  C. Short length of stay
   1. Brief window to obtain desired outcomes
   2. Families or significant others share responsibility for postoperative care of patient at home.
   3. Emphasis is on active patient involvement in provision of care with wellness as the focus.
   4. Cross-training of nurses and support personnel reduces number of different persons treating a patient as well as enhances continuity of care.
   5. Simplified paperwork and documentation leaves more time for direct care.
  D. Free-standing center must have predetermined plan and agreement with hospital for emergency admission of patients to continuity of quality care.
  E. Age no longer a barrier; well-controlled systemic disease does not disqualify patient from receiving care in an ambulatory setting
   1. With elderly patient, it minimizes separation from family and environment.
   2. Must consider risks of anesthetic, surgery, home care
   3. With young patient: premature infant or ex-preemies that need postoperative apnea monitoring not appropriate candidates
  F. Payment structure
   1. Fixed or "packaged" fees for standard surgical procedures (PPO/HMO)
   2. Complications or unplanned admissions to the hospital may incur more expenses.
    a. Overnight observation and pain control at a 23-hour unit in the ambulatory surgery or designated hospital unit after an outpatient procedure is less costly than at the acute care hospital setting and allows more complicated and extensive list of procedures to be done in a lower-cost outpatient setting.
    b. Recovery care centers provide low-cost alternative to hospitalization for patients having outpatient surgery who may need observation or care for 24 to 72 hours after surgery but not care in a more costly hospital setting.
   3. Timeliness of care
   4. Convenience
  G. Teaching
   1. Encompasses all ages of patient
   2. Thorough postoperative instructions to patient and family member or significant other
   3. Use of collaborative approach with patient, including patient empowerment
   4. Nurses must consider
    a. Educational background of patient, family member, or significant other

        b. Literacy; knowledge, skills, values, and attitudes of patient

        c. Determine readiness to learn, learning style, and timeliness of instructions

        d. Language barriers

        e. Physical impairments (deaf patient requiring signer to interpret verbal instructions) and mental or physical handicaps

        f. When and where to obtain follow-up care documented

        g. What to do in case of emergency documented

        h. Patient and family compliance

        i. Patient safety

        j. Traditional outcomes

          (1) Have historically been assessed in terms of surgical and anesthesia-related complications

            (a) Unplanned hospital admissions

            (b) Prolonged recovery time after anesthesia

            (c) Unscheduled postoperative physician or emergency room visit

            (d) Mortality

            (e) Major morbidity

          (2) More recent outcomes focus on patient experience

            (a) Incidence of postoperative nausea and vomiting

            (b) Pain or surgical discomfort

            (c) Dizziness

            (d) Sore throat

            (e) Shivering

            (f) Return to usual activities

            (g) Patient satisfaction

XIII. Issues for postanesthesia care unit (PACU), phase I

    A. Severe adverse events

       1. Return of patient to the operating room because of loss of peripheral pulses, large blood loss, hematoma formation, wound dehiscence

       2. Patient reintubation

       3. Inability to extubate patient (delayed awakening and/or return of muscular strength and function)

       4. Issues of respiratory compromise: Laryngospasm/bronchospasm, croup, stridor, wheezing, retractions

       5. Spontaneous pneumothorax

       6. Emergence delirium

       7. Malignant hyperthermia

       8. New onset of ST depression or elevation

       9. New onset of life-threatening dysrhythmia

     10. Patient with chest pain, changes in electrocardiogram, rise in level of cardiac enzymes, nausea and sweating (rule out myocardial infarction)

     11. Marked hypotension, hypertension, tachycardia, or bradycardia

     12. Pulmonary embolism, pulmonary edema

     13. Inability to maintain adequate oxygen saturation, greater than 90%, in patients with a baseline saturation of 90% or greater preoperatively

     14. Marked fluid imbalance noted from assessing output, skin turgor, and blood pressure

     15. Tissue injury, burn, and skin breakdown

     16. Severe hypothermia

    B. Disturbing side effects that may influence a patient-based assessment for quality of care

       1. Surgical pain and referred pain

       2. Nausea and vomiting

       3. Shivering

       4. Mild hypothermia

       5. Full bladder

       6. Pruritis

       7. Delay in moving extremities after regional and local anesthesia
       8. Headache, muscle aches
       9. Pins and needle sensation, numbness in extremities
     10. Drug reaction (nonanaphylactic)
     11. Somnolence

  C. Other patient care issues
       1. High level of noise and increased use of lights may cause overstimulation.
       2. Lack of privacy with only curtains separating patients
       3. Delay in reaching PACU from the operating room
       4. Prolonged stay in PACU because of unavailability of nursing unit beds
       5. Inadequate supply of beds for the morbidly obese patients
       6. Close proximity of preoperative and postoperative patients
       7. Close proximity of adult and pediatric patient populations
       8. Close proximity of PACU patients and intensive care unit overflow patients
       9. Less chance for visitation because of overcrowded conditions
     10. Lack of appropriate isolation rooms for the increased number of methicillin-resistant *Staphylococcus aureus* (MRSA) and vancomycin-resistant *Enterococcus* (VRE) cases
     11. Acute pain issues in a chronic pain patient
     12. Presence of phase I and phase II patients in the same recovery area, requiring a different focus and approach to care
     13. Cross-training of operating room nurses, pediatric PACU nurses, preoperative holding unit staff and support personnel reduces the number of persons treating the patient.

  D. Staff satisfaction issues
       1. Presence of Pyxis machines for dispensing medications and medical supplies reduces time spent in ordering and stocking; keeps adequate supply in close proximity to patient care areas.
       2. Proper use of UAPs enables the PACU nurse to provide nursing care for the patient.
       3. Simplified nursing flow sheets, checklists, and computer documentation allows more time for direct care.
       4. Practice guidelines, established protocols, policies, and standards guide the PACU nurse from admission to discharge of patients.

EXAMPLES OF QUALITY IMPROVEMENT PROJECTS IN PHASE I AND II PACU

1. Hypothermia in total joint patients can be studied through a collaborative approach with the operating room staff and the nurses on the orthopedic floor. Begin with data collection to determine if there is a problem and how widespread it is. Use a standardized collection tool. Review what techniques are currently in place to prevent or control hypothermia in this at-risk population. Try a new strategy and evaluate its use with another data collection. It may take several interventions (strategies) before one or more are found that really impact this problem. It is a good idea to brainstorm this and other issues with your colleagues across the country or post it on the American Society of PeriAnesthesia Nurses (ASPAN) website (http://www.aspan.org). It is very important to continue to monitor the effect of interventions on a regular basis until the problem no longer exists. If it resurfaces in the future, then another data collection can be done and the process can begin again. The use of warming blankets and space blankets in the operating room, the maintenance of an appropriate ambient room temperature, and the proper covering of exposed body parts not involved in the surgical procedure are important interventions. In the PACU, the use of heated oxygen, warming blanket and warmed intravenous fluids will help to restore the patient to a normothermic state.

2. Use of oxygen for transport of patients from the operating room to the PACU: If you have noticed that your PACU patients have a low oxygen (O_2) saturation on arrival when they have not received O_2 support on transport, get a multidisciplinary team together and investigate the problem. Keep meticulous, consistent records. Review the literature for references on the topic. After the data collection is completed, write up a proposal to include the purchase of x number of oxygen tanks and holders. Then educate the operating room and PACU staffs. Implement the strategy and evaluate the results. If there is a positive correlation, (between patients on oxygen during transfer having a good O_2 saturation versus those that arrive in PACU without oxygen), then you will have proved your case. Continue to monitor at regular intervals to ensure consistent results and to check on compliance with this strategy.

3. Patient education project for the ambulatory setting: If you notice that a patient population (elderly patients having abdominal aortic aneuryism surgery) is experiencing a learning deficit (they are unaware of the medication that is being dispensed to them from the physician's office to take the morning of surgery prior to arrival), then it is good to follow up with data collection. If a high percentage, of these patients do not know the name, dose, purpose, side effects or possible allergic reactions, then the strategy to implement would be to deliver a stack of preprinted medication sheets (appropriate for drug being dispensed) to the physician office. Bring a stack of facility brochures and/or promotional articles, and request the medication sheet be placed in each brochure and handed out to patients at their preoperative visits. Not only is it a great opportunity to educate this patient population, but it also helps with safety and informs future patients about you and your facility. Once again, after the strategy has been implemented, data should be collected at regular intervals to check on positive outcomes and compliance with strategy.

BIBLIOGRAPHY

1. Berk J, Berk S: *A total quality management overview, everyone has a customer: Total quality management, implementing continuous improvement.* New York: Sterling, 1993.

2. Crosby PB: *Quality without tears: The art of hassle-free management.* New York: McGraw-Hill, 1995.

3. Gaucher E, Coffey R: *Total quality in healthcare: From theory to practice.* San Francisco: Jossey-Bass, 1993.

4. Goonan K: *The Juran prescription: Clinical quality management.* San Francisco: Jossey-Bass, 1995.

5. Iacono M: Performance assessment and improvement. J PeriAnesth Nurs 16(3): 195-197, 2001.

6. Iacono M: Conflict, communication, and collaboration: Improving interactions between nurses and physicians. *J PeriAnesth Nurs* 18(1):42-46, 2003.

7. *Juran quality improvement pocket guide.* Wilton, CT: Juran Institute, 1993.

8. Kildea-Pahl D, Baltimore J, Kosiara B: Outpatient surgery care unit work process redesign. *J PeriAnesth Nurs* 16(2):70-81, 2001.

9. Kitowski T: Evaluation of an acute pain service. *J PeriAnesth Nurs* 17(1):21-29, 2002.

10. Kleinbeck SVM: Is meta-analysis clinically useful for perianesthesia nurses? *J PeriAnesth Nurs* 16(3):151-157, 2001.

11. Litwak K: *Core curriculum for perianesthesia practice.* Philadelphia: WB Saunders, 1999.

12. McGoldrick KE: *Ambulatory anesthesia: A problem-oriented approach.* Baltimore: Williams & Wilkins, 1995.

13. Shelton P: *Measuring and improving patient satisfaction.* Gaithersburg, MD: Aspen, 2000.

14. Sultz H, Young K: *Health care USA: Understanding its organization and delivery.* Gaithersburg, MD: Aspen, 2001.

15. *2002 Standards of Perianesthesia Nursing Practice.* Cherry Hill, NJ: American Society of PeriAnesthesia Nurses, 2002.

16. Vogelsang J: Quantitative research versus quality assurance, quality improvement, total quality management, and continuous quality improvement. *J PeriAnesth Nurs* 14(2): 78-81, 1999.

LIFE SPAN CONSIDERATIONS

12 Human Growth and Development

DONNA M. DEFAZIO QUINN

OBJECTIVES
At the conclusion of this chapter the reader will be able to:

1. Define growth and development.

2. Identify the stages of growth and development.

3. Compare Freud's theory of psychosocial development with Erikson's theory.

4. List the four stages of cognitive development.

5. Explain the five stages of language development.

6. Relate the effects of positive influence on the development of self-esteem.

7. Identify eight factors that could influence growth and development.

   I. Overview of growth and development
     A. Definition
       1. Growth and development
         a. Often used interchangeably
         b. Each has distinct definition
       2. Growth
         a. Implies a change in quantity (quantitative change)
           (1) An increase in physical size of a whole or any of its parts
           (2) Can be measured in
             (a) Inches, centimeters (height)
             (b) Kilograms or pounds (increased organ mass, weight)
             (c) Numbers (increased vocabulary, increased number of relationships with others, increased number of physical skills that can be performed)
         b. Increase in number and size of cells
           (1) Reflected in an increase in the size and weight of the whole or any of its parts
       3. Development
         a. A complex concept not easily measured or studied
         b. Gradual growth and expansion; viewed as a qualitative change
           (1) Increased function (skill) and complexity (capacity)
           (2) Occurs through growth, maturation, and learning
         c. Move from lower case to a more advanced stage of complexity
           (1) Continuous orderly series of conditions
           (2) Leads to activities, new motives for activities, and eventual patterns of behavior
           (3) Expansion of capabilities to provide greater facility in functioning
         d. Developmental process
           (1) Continuous, complex, and irreversible
           (2) Involves aging
             (a) Most rapid during fetal stage
             (b) Is a lifelong process

      e. Progression of development

        (1) Simple to complex

          (a) Infant's vocalizations before speech refinement

        (2) General to specific

          (a) Infant's palmar grasp prior to acquiring finer control of pincer grasp

        (3) From head to toe (cephalocaudally)

          (a) Infant gains head and neck control prior to gaining control of trunk and limbs.

        (4) From inner to outer (proximodistally)

          (a) Control of near structures before control of structures farther away from the body center

          (b) Infant coordinates arms to reach before gaining hand and finger coordination.

    f. Predictability of development

      (1) Sequence of development is invariable.

      (2) Precise age will vary.

      (3) Wide normal range allows for individual variances.

    g. Uniqueness of development

      (1) Each child has own genetic potential for growth and development.

      (2) May be deterred or modified at any stage

II. Stages of growth and development

  A. Prenatal

    1. Period of life from conception to birth

      a. Crucial period in developmental process

      b. Health and well-being of the infant directly related to adequate prenatal care

      c. Direct relationship between maternal health and certain manifestations in the newborn

  B. Newborn or neonatal

    1. From birth through the first month of life

    2. Major physical adjustment to extrauterine existence

  C. Infancy

    1. Begins at end of first month of life and ends at one year of age

    2. Period of rapid motor, cognitive, and social development

    3. Establishes basic trust

      a. Foundation for future relationships

  D. Early childhood (see Box 12-1)

    1. Toddler

      a. From 1 to 3 years

    2. Preschool

      a. From 3 to 6 years

    3. Characteristics of early childhood

      a. Characterized by intense activity and discovery

      b. Marked physical and personality development

      c. Motor development advances steadily

      d. Acquire language skills

      e. Expand social relationships

      f. Learn role standards

      g. Gain self-control and mastery

      h. Develop increasing awareness of dependence and independence

      i. Begin to develop self-concept

  E. Middle childhood or school-age years

    1. From age 6 to 11 or 12 years

    2. Child is directed away from family group and centered around peer relationships.

    3. Steady advancement in physical, mental, and social development

■ BOX 12-1
■ **EMERGING PATTERNS OF BEHAVIOR FROM 1 TO 5 YEARS OF AGE***

15 Months
Motor: Walks alone; crawls up stairs
Adaptive: Makes a tower of three cubes; makes a line with crayon; inserts pellet in bottle
Language: Jargon; follows simple commands; may name a familiar object (ball)
Social: Indicates some desire or needs by pointing; hugs parents

18 Months
Motor: Runs stiffly; sits on small chair; walks up stairs with one hand held; explores drawers
 and wastebaskets
Adaptive: Makes a tower of four cubes; imitates scribbling; imitates vertical stroke; dumps
 pellet from bottle
Language: 10 words average; names pictures; identifies one or more parts of body
Social: Feeds self, seeks help when in trouble; may complain when wet or soiled; kisses
 parents with pucker

24 Months
Motor: Runs well; walks up and down stairs, one step at a time; opens doors; climbs on
 furniture; jumps
Adaptive: Tower of seven cubes (six at 21 months); circular scribbling; imitates horizontal
 stroke; folds paper once imitatively
Language: Puts three words together (subject, verb, object)
Social: Handles spoon well; often tells immediate experiences; helps to undress; listens to
 stories with pictures

30 Months
Motor: Goes up stairs alternating feet
Adaptive: Tower of nine cubes; makes vertical and horizontal strokes, but generally will not
 join them to make a cross; imitates circular stroke, forming closed figure
Language: Refers to self by pronoun "I"; knows full name
Social: Helps put things away; pretends in play

36 Months
Motor: Rides tricycle; stands momentarily on one foot
Adaptive: Tower of 10 cubes; imitates construction of "bridge" of three cubes; copies a circle;
 imitates a cross
Language: Knows age and sex; counts three objects correctly; repeats three numbers or a
 sentence of six syllables
Social: Plays simple games (in "parallel" with other children); helps in dressing (unbuttons
 clothing and puts on shoes); washes hands

48 Months
Motor: Hops on one foot; throws ball overhand; uses scissors to cut out pictures; climbs well
Adaptive: Copies bridge from model; imitates construction of "gate" of five cubes; copies cross
 and square; draws a man with two to five parts besides head; names longer of two lines
Language: Counts four pennies accurately; tells a story
Social: Plays with several children with beginning of social interaction and role-playing; goes
 to toilet alone

60 Months
Motor: Skips
Adaptive: Draws triangle from copy; names heavier of two weights
Language: Names four colors; repeats sentence of 10 syllables; counts 10 pennies correctly
Social: Dresses and undresses; asks questions about meaning of words; domestic role-playing

*Data are derived from those of Gesell (as revised by Knobloch), Shirley, Provence, Wolf, Bailey, and others. After 5 years
the Stanford-Binet, Wechsler-Bellevue, and other scales offer the most precise estimates of developmental level. In order to
have their greatest value, they should be administered only by an experienced and qualified person. From Behrman RE,
Kliegman RM, Jenson HB: *Nelson Textbook of Pediatrics,* ed 17. Philadelphia: WB Saunders, 2004, p 39.

■ TABLE 12-1
■ ■ Summary of Personality, Cognitive, and Moral Development Theories

Stage/age	Psychosexual Stages (Freud)	Psychosocial Stages (Erikson)	Cognitive Stages (Piaget)	Moral Judgment Stages (Kohlberg)
I Infancy Birth to 1 year	Oral-sensory	Trust vs. mistrust	Sensorimotor (birth to 2 years)	
II Toddlerhood 1 to 3 years	Anal-urethral	Autonomy vs. shame and doubt	Preoperational thought, preconceptual phase (transductive reasoning, e.g., specific to specific) (2-4 years)	Preconventional (premoral) level Punishment and obedience orientation
III Early childhood 3 to 6 years	Phallic-locomotion	Initiative vs. guilt	Preoperational thought, intuitive phase (transductive reasoning) (4-7 years)	Preconventional (premoral) level Naïve instrumental orientation
IV Middle childhood 6 to 12 years	Latency	Industry vs. inferiority	Concrete operations (inductive reasoning and beginning logic) (7-11 years)	Conventional level Good-boy, nice-girl orientation Law-and-order orientation
V Adolescence 12 to 18 years	Genitality	Identity and repudiation vs. identity confusion	Formal operations (deductive and abstract reasoning) (11-15 years)	Postconventional or principled level Social-contract orientation Universal ethical principle orientation (no longer included in revised theory)

From Wong D, editor, Wilson D, Hockenberry-Eaton M, et al: *Wong's essentials of pediatric nursing,* ed 6. St Louis: Mosby, 2001, p 102.

   4. Emphasis is on developing skill competencies.
   5. Social cooperation and moral development take on importance.
      a. Relevant for later life stages
   6. Critical period in the development of self-concept
 F. Later childhood or adolescence and young adulthood
   1. From the beginning of the twelfth year to the end of the twenty-first year
   2. Period of rapid maturation and change
   3. Considered to be a transition that begins with the onset of puberty and extends to the point of entry into the adult world
   4. Biologic and personality maturation are accompanied by physical and emotional turmoil.
   5. Self-concept is redefined.
   6. In late adolescence the child begins to internalize all previously learned values and focus on an individual rather than a group identify.
 III. Theories of development—overview (see Table 12-1)
   A. Freudian
      1. Psychosocial
      2. Emphasis on development of personality

      B. Erikson
          1. Psychosocial development
      C. Sullivan
          1. Interpersonal development
      D. Piaget
          1. Cognitive development
      E. Kohlberg
          1. Moral development
      F. Skinner, Watson
          1. Learning theory; behaviorism
          2. Focus entirely on behavior
          3. Internalize processes such as thoughts and feelings
      G. Maslow
          1. Humanistic
          2. Focus on characteristics that contribute to healthy personality development
IV. Freudian
      A. Three components of personality
          1. Id
              a. Develops during birth
              b. The unconscious mind
              c. Inborn component that drives instincts
              d. Obeys pleasure principle of immediate gratification of needs
                  (1) Raw libido seeking pleasure
          2. Ego
              a. Develops during toddler years
              b. Represents the conscious mind
                  (1) Reality component
                  (2) Mediates conflict
              c. Functions as conscious or controlling self
              d. Finds realistic means of gratifying instincts
              e. Blocks irrational thinking of the id
          3. Superego
              a. Develops during preschool years
              b. Conscience
              c. Functions as moral arbitrator
                  (1) Puts good or bad labels on behavior
              d. Represents the ideal
              e. Prevents individual from expressing undesirable instincts that could threaten social order
      B. Psychosexual development (See Table 12-2)
          1. Stages of development
              a. Oral
              b. Anal
              c. Phallic
              d. Latency
              e. Genital
          2. Sexual instincts significant in development of personality
          3. Psychosexual used to describe any sensual pleasure
          4. Theory focuses on desire to satisfy biological needs.
              a. Theory difficult to verify
              b. Of little value when attempting to predict future behaviors
              c. Psychosexual development usually complete by 6 years of age
      C. Oral stage
          1. Birth to 1 year of age
          2. Sources of pleasure
              a. Sucking
              b. Biting

■ TABLE 12-2
■ ■ **Personality Traits Associated with Freud's First Three Stages of Psychosexual Development**

Stage	Age	Source of Pleasure	Personality Traits
Oral	Birth to 1 year	Oral activities —sucking —biting —chewing —vocalizing	Pessimism or optimism Determination or submission Gullibility or suspiciousness Admiration or envy Cockiness or self-belittlement
Anal	1 to 3 years	Anal region —withhold or expel feces	Stinginess or overgenerosity Constrictedness or expansiveness Rigid punctuality or tardiness Stubbornness or acquiescence Orderliness or messiness
Phallic	3 to 6 years	Genitals	Brashness or bashfulness Stylishness or plainness Gaiety or sadness Blind courage or timidness Gregariousness or isolationism

From Quinn DMD: *Ambulatory surgical nursing core curriculum.* Philadelphia: WB Saunders, 1999, p 236.

      c. Chewing
      d. Vocalizing
   3. Oral personality traits
      a. Pessimism or optimism
      b. Determination or submission
      c. Gullibility or suspiciousness
      d. Admiration or envy
      e. Cockiness or self-belittlement
  D. Anal stage
    1. One to 3 years of age
    2. Focus on anal region
    3. Child develops ability to withhold or expel feces at will.
    4. Toilet training can have lasting effects on personality development.
    5. Anal personality traits
      a. Stinginess or overgenerosity
      b. Constrictedness or expansiveness
      c. Rigid punctuality or tardiness
      d. Stubbornness or acquiescence
      e. Orderliness or messiness
  E. Phallic stage ·
    1. Three to 6 years of age
    2. Focus on genitals
    3. Recognition of difference between sexes
    4. Phallic personality traits
      a. Brashness or bashfulness
      b. Stylishness or plainness
      c. Gaiety or sadness
      d. Blind courage or timidness
      e. Gregariousness or isolationism
  F. Latency period
    1. Six to 12 years of age
    2. Elaboration of previous learned traits and skills
    3. Physical and psychic energies funneled into acquiring knowledge of vigorous play

G. Genital stage
   1. Twelve years and over
   2. Begins at puberty
   3. Genital organs become major source of sexual tensions and pleasures.
   4. Energy used to form friendships and prepare for marriage
H. Nursing implications of Freud's theory
   1. Children and parents may have many questions concerning
      a. Normal sexual development
      b. Sex education
   2. Nurses must understand normal sexual growth and development.
      a. Assist children and parents to form healthy attitudes about sex

V. Erikson
   A. Theory of psychosocial development most widely used
   B. Emphasis on healthy personality rather than pathologic approach
      1. Stresses rational and adaptive natures of individual
      2. Explains child's behaviors in mastering developmental tasks
   C. Eight stages of development
      1. Each stage has two components—favorable and unfavorable aspect of conflict
      2. Progression to next stage depends on resolution of conflict
      3. Conflict never mastered completely—remains a recurrent problem throughout life
   D. Trust versus mistrust stage (stage I)
      1. Birth to 1 year of age
      2. "Getting" and "taking in" from all the senses
      3. Exists only in relation to something or someone
      4. Consistent, loving care by mother essential to development of trust
      5. Mistrust develops when
         a. Trust-promoting activities absent
         b. Basic needs inconsistently or inadequately met
      6. Individual develops quality of hope and belief that one can attain deep and essential wishes.
         a. Results in faith and optimism
   E. Autonomy versus shame and doubt (stage II)
      1. One to 3 years of age
      2. Development centered on child's ability to control his or her body, himself or herself, and the environment
      3. Uses his or her power to do things independently
         a. Walking
         b. Climbing
         c. Selection and decision making
      4. Learns to conform to social rules
      5. Doubt and shame arise when
         a. Child made to feel unimportant or self-conscious
         b. Choices are disastrous.
         c. Shamed by others
         d. Forced to be dependent when he or she is capable of assuming control
      6. Achieves autonomy through imitation
         a. Parents are key socializing intermediaries.
         b. Results in self-control and willpower
   F. Initiative versus guilt stage (stage III)
      1. Three to 6 years of age
      2. Characterized by vigorous, intrusive behavior and a strong imagination
      3. Explores physical world with all senses
      4. Develops a conscience
      5. Responds to an inner voice that warns and threats

    6. Guilt arises when
      a. Child undertakes goals or activities that are in conflict with those of parent
      b. Made to feel activities are bad
    7. Achieves initiative through identification
      a. Family is key socializing agent.
      b. Results in direction and purpose; ability to imagine and pursue

G. Industry versus inferiority stage (stage IV)
    1. Six to 12 years of age
    2. Carries tasks and activities through to completion
    3. Learns to complete and cooperate with others
    4. Learns rules
    5. Successful child develops a sense of mastery and self-assurance.
    6. Inferiority develops when
      a. Too much is expected of child
      b. Child believes he or she cannot meet standards set for him or her by others
    7. Achieves industry through education
      a. Teachers and peers are socializing agents.
      b. Develops competence, skill, and intelligence to complete task

H. Identity versus role confusion stage (stage V)
    1. Twelve to 18 years of age
    2. Characterized by marked physical changes
    3. Engrossed in how he or she appears to others as compared with his or her own self-concept
    4. Struggle with
      a. Ability to maintain current role and future role as defined by peers
      b. Integrating concepts and values with those of society
      c. Decision for an occupation
    5. Role confusion develops when unable to resolve core conflicts.
    6. Mastering identity results in devotion and fidelity.
    7. Achieves identity through peer pressure and role experimentation

I. Intimacy versus isolation stage (stage VI)
    1. Occurs in early adulthood
    2. Intimacy established on a sense of identity
    3. Capacity to develop
      a. An intimate love relationship
      b. Intimate interpersonal relationships with friends, partners, and significant others
    4. Isolation develops when intimacy not present.
    5. Intimacy develops when there is mutuality among peers.
    6. Key socializing agents
      a. Lovers
      b. Spouses
      c. Close friends
    7. Develops affiliation and love

J. Generativity versus stagnation stage (stage VII)
    1. Young and middle adulthood
    2. Creation and care of next generation
    3. Essential element is to nourish and nurture.
    4. Failure results in self-absorption and stagnation.
    5. Key socializing agents are spouse, children, and cultural norms.
      a. Results in production and care; commitment and concern for what has been generated

K. Ego integrity versus despair stage (stage VIII)
    1. Old age
    2. Results from satisfaction with life and acceptance of what has been
    3. Despair is a result of remorse for what might have been.

        4. Ego integrity results in renunciation and wisdom and concern with life in the face of death.

        5. Process achieved through introspection

VI. Sullivan

    A. Interpersonal development

        1. Recognizes importance of environment in development

        2. Has some predictive value

        3. Does not recognize biologic maturation process

    B. Emphasis on interpersonal relationships and importance of social approval or disapproval in developing a self-concept

        1. Unfavorable reactions result in tension and anxiety.

        2. Favorable reactions result in comfort and security.

    C. Infants

        1. Mother gratifies and comforts child.

        2. Relationship gradually extends to other family members.

    D. Toddler

        1. Becomes more outgoing

        2. Directs social gestures to wider audience

            a. Relatives

            b. Neighborhood children

        3. Engages in aspects of social learning

            a. Peer play

            b. Family events

    E. School age

        1. Wider range of relationships

            a. Authority figures at school and in community

        2. Develops peer relationships

        3. Shares intimacy and common interests with peers

    F. Adolescent

        1. Personal identity

            a. Friends of same sex

            b. Friends of opposite sex

VII. Piaget: Cognitive development

    A. Cognition

        1. Process by which developing individuals become acquainted with the world and objects it contains

        2. Cognitive development allows child ability to

            a. Reason abstractly

            b. Think in a logical manner

            c. Organize intellectual functions into higher structures

    B. Sequence of four stages (sensorimotor, preoperational, concrete operational, formal operational)

        1. Prior practice or teaching has little effect on development of new cognitive skills.

        2. Suitable cognitive maturity or readiness necessary to progress to next stage

    C. Sensorimotor stage of intellectual development

        1. Birth to 2 years of age

        2. Consists of substages that are governed by sensations through which simple learning takes place

        3. Progresses from simple reflex activities to simple repetitive behaviors that imitate behaviors

        4. Develops sense of cause and effect

            a. Directs behavior toward object

            b. Solves problems through trial and error

            c. High level of curiosity

            d. Develops sense of self through interactions with environment

                (1) Able to differentiate self from environment

5. Awareness that object has permanence
   a. Important prerequisite for all other mental activity
D. Preoperational period of intellectual development
   1. Two to 7 years of age
   2. Egocentricity is predominant characteristic.
      a. Defined as inability to put oneself in place of another
   3. Interprets objects and events in terms of their relationship or use of them
   4. Sees only his or her perspective
      a. Cannot see another's point of view
   5. Preoperational thinking is concrete and tangible.
   6. Lacks ability to make deductions or generalizations
   7. Thoughts dominated by what he or she sees, hears, and experiences
   8. Increasing ability to use language to represent objects in his or her environment
   9. Increasing ability to elaborate on concepts and make simple associations between ideas
   10. Cannot understand that, for every action or operation, there is an action or operation that cancels it
   11. Develops intuitive reasoning later in stage
   12. Begins to understand weight, length, size, and time
E. Concrete operational stage
   1. Seven to 11 years of age
   2. Thoughts become more logical and coherent.
   3. Able to problem solve
   4. Classifies, sorts, orders, and organizes facts
   5. Able to deal with a number of different aspects of a situation simultaneously
   6. Unable to deal with abstract
   7. Problem solves in concrete, systematic fashion, based on what he or she can perceive
   8. Thoughts become less self-centered.
   9. Can consider points of view other than his or her own
   10. Develops socialized thinking
F. Formal operational stage
   1. Twelve to 15 years of age
   2. Characterized by adaptability and flexibility
   3. Can think in terms of the abstract
   4. Able to draw conclusions from a set of observations
   5. Can make and test hypotheses
   6. May confuse the ideal with the practice
VIII. Kohlberg: Moral development (see Table 12-3)
A. Based on cognitive development theory
B. Proceeds in an invariant sequence of stages
C. Cannot acquire higher levels of moral reasoning until appropriate cognitive development has occurred
D. Preconventional level of morality
   1. Morality is external.
      a. Children conform to rules imposed by adults.
   2. Stage 1: The punishment and obedience orientation
      a. Child determines if action is good or bad based on consequences
      b. Obeys those in power
      c. Avoids punishment
      d. Possesses no concept of the underlying moral order
   3. Stage 2: The instrumental relativist orientation
      a. The right behavior is that which satisfies the child's own needs.
      b. Possesses elements of fairness, reciprocity, and equal sharing
      c. Do not possess elements of loyalty, gratitude, or justice

    E. Conventional level
       1. Child concerned with
         a. Conformity and loyalty
         b. Maintaining, supporting, and justifying the social order
         c. Personal expectations of those significant to him or her
       2. Child values maintenance of family regardless of consequences
       3. Stage 3: The interpersonal concordance or "good boy—nice girl" orientation
         a. Behavior that meets approval of others is viewed as good.
         b. Conformity to the norm is the "natural" behavior.
         c. Earn approval by being "nice"
       4. Stage 4: The "law and order" orientation
         a. Correct behavior is
           (1) Obeying rules
           (2) Doing one's duty
           (3) Showing respect for authority
           (4) Maintaining social order
         b. Rules and authority can be social or religious.
    F. Postconventional, autonomous, or principled level
       1. Child reaches cognitive formal operational stage.
       2. Attempts to define moral values and principles
       3. Stage 5: The social contract, legalistic orientation
         a. Correct behavior defined in terms of general individual rights and standards agreed to by society
         b. Emphasis on
           (1) Legal point of view
           (2) Possibility of changing law in terms of societal needs and rational considerations

IX. Skinner, Watson: Learning theory
    A. Learning occurs when behavior changes as a result of experience.
    B. Child
       1. Acquires new behaviors
       2. Produces alterations in existing behavior through
         a. Forming associations through conditioning
         b. Observing models
       3. Behavior is determined (conditioned) by
         a. Environmental events
         b. Experiences
         c. Consequences
       4. Rewarded behaviors are repeated.
       5. Punished behaviors are not repeated.
    C. Conditioning
       1. Learning through association
         a. Establishing a connection between a stimulus and a response
       2. Operant or instrumental conditioning
         a. Involves rewards or reinforcements to encourage specific behaviors
         b. Applicable to toddler and preschooler learning
       3. Avoidance conditioning
         a. Discourages undesirable behaviors through punishment
         b. Success depends on child's subjective assessment of reward or punishment.

X. Maslow: Humanistic theory
    A. Focuses on attributes or characteristics that contribute to healthy personality development
    B. Concerned with uniqueness and potential of individuals
       1. Humans motivated by two need systems
         a. Basic
           (1) Food, water, and shelter

TABLE 12-3
Theories of Growth and Development

	Piaget's Periods of Cognitive Development	Freud's Stages of Psychosexual Development	Erikson's Stages of Psychosocial Development	Kohlberg' Development
Infancy	Period 1 (birth-2 yr): Sensorimotor period. Reflexive behavior is used to adapt to the environment; egocentric view of the world; development of object performance	Oral stage. Mouth is a sensory organ; infant takes in and explores during oral passive substage (first half of infancy); infant strikes out with teeth during oral aggressive substage (latter half of infancy)	Trust vs. mistrust. Development of a sense that the self is good and the world is good when consistent, predictable, reliable care is received; characterized by hope	Stage 0 (0-2 yr): Naivete and egocentrism. No moral sensitivity; de basis of what pleases the child; infants like love what helps them and disl them; no awareness of the effect of thei actions on others "Good is what I like and want."
Toddlerhood	Period 2 (2-7 yr): Preoperational Thought. Thinking remains egocentric, becomes magical, and is dominated by perception.	Anal stage. Major focus of sexual interest is anus; control of body functions is major feature.	Autonomy vs. shame and doubt. Development of sense of control over the self and body functions; exerts self; characterized by will	Stage 1 (2-3 yr): Punishment-obedience orientation. Right or wrong is determine consequences: "If I get caught and for doing it, it is wrong. If I am not caught or punished, then it must be right." Premorality or preconventional morality
Preschool Age		Phallic or Oedipal/Electra stage. Genitals become focus of sexual curiosity; superego (conscience) develops; feelings of guilt emerge.	Initiative vs. guilt. Development of a can-do attitude about the self; behavior becomes goal-directed, competitive, and imaginative; initiation into gender role; characterized by purpose.	Child conforms to rules out of self-interest: "I'll do this for you if you do this for me"; behavior is guided by an "eye for an eye" orientation. "If you do something bad to me, then it' if I do something bad to you."
School age	Period 3 (7-11 yr): Concrete operations. Thinking becomes more systematic and logical, but concrete objects and activities are needed.	Latency stage. Sexual feelings are firmly repressed by the superego; period of relative calm.	Industry vs. inferiority. Mastering of useful skills and tools of the culture; learning how to play and work with peers; characterized by competence	Morality of conventional role conformity (7-10 yr): Good boy or girl orientation. Morality is based on avoiding disappro disturbing the conscience; child i socially sensitive.

	Cognitive (Piaget)	Psychosexual (Freud)	Psychosocial (Erikson)	Moral (Kohlberg)
Adolescence	Period 4 (11 yr–adulthood): Formal operations New ideas can be created; situations can be analyzed; use of abstract thinking	Puberty or genital Stage Stimulated by increasing hormone levels; sexual energy wells up in full force, resulting in personal and family turmoil.	Identity vs. role confusion Begins to develop a sense of "I"; this process is lifelong; peers become of paramount importance; child gains independence from parents; characterized by faith in self.	Stage 4 (begins at about 10-12 yr): Law and order orientation Right takes on a religious or metaphysical quality for authority rules for their own sake. Morality of self-accepted moral princ stage 5: Social contract orientation Right is determined by what is best f majority; exceptions to rules c person' longer justifies the means; laws are for mutual good and mutual cooperation.
Adulthood			Intimacy vs. isolation Development of the ability to lose the self in genuine mutuality with another; characterized by love Generativity vs. stagnation Production of ideas and materials through work; creation of children; characterized by care Ego integrity vs. despair Realization that there is order and purpose to life; characterized by wisdom	Stage 6: Personal principle orientation Achieved only by the morally mature individual; few people reach this level; these people do what they think is right, regardless of others' opinions, legal sanctions, or personal sacrifice; actions are guided by internal standards; integrity is of utmost importance; may be willing to die for their beliefs. Stage 7: Universal principle orientation This stage is achieved by only a rare few; Mother Teresa; Gandhi, and Socrates are examples; these individuals transcend the teachings of organized religion and per as part of the cosmic order the reason for their existence, and live for their beliefs.

From James SR, Ashwill JW, Droske SC: *Nursing care of children*. Philadelphia: WB Saunders, 2002, pp 70-71.

        b. Growth needs-internally motivated and reinforced
          (1) Beauty
          (2) Self-fulfillment
     2. Needs arranged in a hierarchy
        a. Lower-level needs assume dominance.
        b. When one level need is satisfied, the next becomes predominant.
  C. Theory does not address developmental stages or shaping of human behaviors.

XI. Biologic growth
  A. During childhood, variations in growth of tissues and organs produce changes in body proportions.
  B. First year
     1. Period of rapid growth
     2. Lengthening of trunk
     3. Accumulation of subcutaneous fat
  C. First year to puberty
     1. Legs grow more rapidly.
     2. Body becomes slender and elongated.
  D. Puberty
     1. Feet and hand sizes increase.
        a. Appear large in relation to rest of body
        b. Source of embarrassment
     2. Trunk growth increases.
     3. Onset of puberty approximately 2 ½ years earlier for girls than boys
     4. Rapid linear growth followed by lateral growth
     5. Child "fills out" during later stages of adolescent growth.
  E. Height
     1. Occurs as a result of skeletal growth
     2. Considered a stable measurement of general growth
     3. When maturation of skeleton is complete, linear growth ceases.
  F. Weight
     1. Weight gain considered indication of satisfactory growth progress in child
     2. Variable
     3. Subject to numerous intrinsic and extrinsic factors
  G. Neurologic growth
     1. Rapid brain cell growth from 30 weeks to 1 year of age
     2. Growth consists of
        a. Increase in cytoplasm around nuclei of existing cells
        b. Increase in number and intricacy of communication with other cells
        c. Advancing peripheral axions in relation to expanding body dimensions
     3. Brain growth
        a. Measured by head circumference
        b. Increases six times during first year
     4. Lymph tissue
        a. Lymph nodes, thymus, spleen, tonsils, adenoids, blood lymphocytes
          (1) Increase rapidly
          (2) Reach adult dimensions by age 6
          (3) Tissue reaches size approximately twice that of adult by age 12.
            (a) Rapid decline to stable adult dimension by adolescence

XII. Language development
  A. Child born with mechanism and capacity to develop speech and language skills
     1. Requires intact physiologic function of
        a. Respiratory system
        b. Speech control center in cerebral cortex
        c. Articulation and resonance structures of the mouth and nasal cavity

    2. Child also requires
        a. Intact and discriminating auditory apparatus
        b. Intelligence
        c. A need to communicate
        d. Stimulation
B. Components of language
    1. Phrenology learned first
        a. Basic units of sound that are combined to produce words
    2. Semantics of language learned next
        a. Words and sentences convey an expressed meaning.
    3. Gain knowledge of syntax
        a. The form or structure of language (rules)
    4. Pragmatics
        a. Principles specifying how language is used in different contexts and situations
C. Stages of language development
    1. Prelinguistic stage
        a. Period before child speaks first meaningful word
        b. Develops systematically over first 10 to 12 months
        c. Involves crying, cooing, and babbling
    2. Holophrastic stage
        a. Speech consists of one- or two-word statements.
        b. Includes holophrases
            (1) Single words with meaning of entire sentence
    3. Telegraphic stage
        a. Speech includes content words only.
        b. From 18 to 24 months
    4. Preschool period
        a. Produce lengthy sentences
        b. Speech increases in complexity.
        c. From 30 months to 5 years
    5. Middle childhood period
        a. Refines language skill
        b. Increases linguistic competence
        c. From 6 to 14 years
        d. Uses bigger words
        e. Understands complex syntactic structures of language
D. Theories of language development
    1. Learning theory
        a. Language is acquired as child hears and responds to speech.
        b. How child learns to speak (two theories)
            (1) Operant conditioning—adults reinforce child's attempt to produce grammatical speech
            (2) Acquires language by listening to and imitating speech of adults
    2. Nativists theory
        a. Inborn linguistic processor specialized for language learning
        b. Critical period for language development exists
        c. Most proficient at learning language between 2 years of age and puberty
    3. Interactional proponents
        a. Child is biologically prepared to acquire language.
        b. Recognizes crucial role of environment in language learning
E. Factors affecting language development
    1. Delayed, lack of, or impaired speech can result from
        a. Congenital structural defects of mouth and nasopharynx
        b. Hearing deficit
        c. Neurologic dysfunction
        d. Maternal deprivation
        e. Emotional factors

■ BOX 12-2
■ **GUIDELINES FOR COMMUNICATING WITH CHILDREN**

- Allow children time to feel comfortable.
- Avoid sudden or rapid advances, broad smiles, extended eye contact, or other gestures that may be seen as threatening.
- Talk to the parent if the child is initially shy.
- Communicate through transition objects such as dolls, puppets, stuffed animals before questioning a young child directly.
- Give older children the opportunity to talk without the parents present.
- Assume a position that is at eye level with child.
- Speak in a quiet, unhurried, and confident voice.
- Speak clearly, be specific, use simple words, and use short sentences.
- State directions and suggestions *positively.*
- Offer a choice only when one exists.
- Be honest with children.
- Allow them to express their concerns and fears.
- Use a variety of communication techniques.

From James SR, Ashwill JW, Droske SC: *Nursing care of children.* Philadelphia: WB Saunders, 2002.

  F. Guidelines for communicating with children (see Box 12-2)
    1. Do not exclude child in interactions.
    2. Be aware that nonverbal communication conveys the most significant message.
XIII. Self-concept and self-esteem
  A. Self-concept
    1. Perception of whole self
    2. Not present at birth
      a. Develops gradually as a result of unique experiences
      b. Learned during childhood
      c. Is a product of socialization
    3. Is subjective; may not reflect reality
    4. Answers the question "Who am I?" and "What am I?"
    5. Formed by
      a. Self-selected mental images
      b. Attitudes
      c. How he or she thinks others see him or her
  B. Self-esteem (see Box 12-3)
    1. Personal, subjective judgment of one's worthiness
      a. Derived from and influenced by social groups
      b. Individual's perception of how he or she is valued by others
    2. Factors affecting child's development of self-esteem[13]
      a. Temperament
      b. Personality
      c. Ability and opportunity to accomplish age-appropriate developmental tasks
      d. Significant others
      e. Social roles undertaken
      f. Expectations of social roles
    3. Methods to develop and preserve self-esteem
      a. Needs to feel worthwhile
      b. Needs recognition for achievements
      c. Needs approval of parents and peers
      d. For inappropriate behavior, stress "behavior" is unacceptable, not the child.

■ BOX 12-3
■ **SELF-ESTEEM IN CHILDREN: COMMUNICATION PRACTICES**

Techniques to Enhance Self-Esteem	Practices that Harm Self-Esteem
■ Praise efforts and accomplishments.	■ Criticize efforts and accomplishments.
■ Use active listening skills.	■ Be too busy to listen.
■ Encourage expression of feelings.	■ Tell children how they should feel.
■ Acknowledge feelings.	■ Give no support for dealing with feelings.
■ Use developmentally based discipline.	■ Use physical punishment.
■ Use "I" statements.	■ Use "you" statements.
■ Be nonjudgmental.	■ Judge the child.
■ Set clearly defined limits and reinforce them	■ Set no known limits or boundaries.
■ Share quality time together.	■ Give time grudgingly.
■ Be honest.	■ Be dishonest.
■ Describe behaviors observed when praising and disciplining.	■ Use coercion and power as discipline.
■ Compliment the child.	■ Belittle, blame, or shame the child.
■ Smile.	■ Use sarcastic, caustic, or cruel "humor."
■ Touch and hug the child.	■ Avoid coming near child even when the child is open to touching, holding, or hugging. Touch only when performing a task.
■ Rock the child.	■ Avoid comforting through rocking.

From James SR, Ashwill JW, Droske SC: *Nursing care of children.* Philadelphia: WB Saunders, 2002, p 62.

     e. Needs constructive communication
       (1) Use of "I" messages
       (2) Conveys feelings and needs
       (3) Does not destroy child's self-esteem
   4. Positive experiences during developmental phases
     a. Child is successful in early motor and verbal experiences.
     b. Develops positive self-concept and high self-esteem
     c. Receives encouragement and positive recognition form others
     d. Exposed to appropriate role models
     e. Permitted to experience fear, disappointment, and frustration
     f. Encouraged to finish tasks and reach goals
     g. Results in an individual with sturdy identity and high level of self-actualizing behavior
   5. Negative experiences during developmental phases
     a. Leads to negative self-concept and low self-esteem
     b. Child receives insufficient or negative recognition from others.
     c. Child exposed to inappropriate role models
     d. Child is prevented from finishing tasks and reaching goals.
     e. Results in an individual with frail identity and self-destructive behavior
XIV. Factors influencing growth and development
  A. Heredity
   1. Inherent characteristics influence development
     a. Sex of child directs pattern of growth and behavior of others toward child
     b. Physical characteristics are inherited.
       (1) Can influence how child grows and interacts with environment
  B. Gender
   1. Sex differences that influence behaviors in childhood
     a. Boys
       (1) More aggressive physically
       (2) Engage in rough and tumble play
       (3) Aggressive fantasies

(4) Competitive behavior more common
(5) Difficulty sitting still
(6) Engage in more exploratory behavior
(7) High activity level in presence of other boys
(8) Greater impulsiveness
(9) Subject to distraction
(10) More extensive sphere of relationships
(11) Highly oriented toward peer groups
(12) Congregate in large groups
(13) View themselves as more powerful and with more control over events
(14) Respond to a challenge, especially when it appeals to their ego or competitive feelings
   b. Girls
     (1) More aggressive verbally
     (2) More likely to associate in pairs or small groups
     (3) Involved in more intense relationships with a few close friends
     (4) More concerned with the welfare of the group
     (5) More apt to compromise in situations involving conflict
     (6) May be superior regarding motivation to achieve
     (7) More likely to comply to adult commands
     (8) More nurturant or helping behavior
C. Culture
  1. Ethnicity, demographic setting, socioeconomic class, parental occupation, and family structure
  2. Attitude and expectations differ with respect to the sex of the child.
D. Lifestyle
  1. Different family structures
    a. Two parent
    b. One parent
    c. Extended family
    d. Other variations
E. Play
  1. Activity with meaning and purpose
  2. May be directly related to expanding
    a. Social development
    b. Intellectual development
    c. Motor development
    d. Language development
  3. Play used to accomplish developmental tasks and master the environment
F. School
  1. Contributes to development in the form of
    a. Skill training
    b. Cultural transmission
    c. Self-actualization
G. Neighborhood
  1. Offers child opportunity to experience world outside the home
    a. Accepting
    b. Supportive of child's physical and psychosocial needs
    c. Reinforcing of child's self-confidence and safety
H. Disease
  1. Disorders
    a. Skeletal (dwarfism)
    b. Chromosome anomalies (Turner syndrome)
    c. Disorders of metabolism
     (1) Vitamin D-resistant rickets
     (2) Mucopolysaccharidoses
     (3) Endocrine disorders

      d. Klinefelter syndrome and Marfan syndrome

      e. Chronic illness

      f. Congenital cardiac anomalies

      g. Respiratory disorders

        (1) Cystic fibrosis

      h. Malabsorption syndromes

      i. Defects in digestive enzyme systems

I. Neuroendocrine

   1. Possible relationship exists between hypothalamus and endocrine system that influences growth.

   2. Peripheral nervous system may influence growth.

      a. Muscles deprived of nerve supply degenerate.

   3. All hormones affect growth in some manner.

      a. Growth hormone, thyroid hormone, and androgens given to a person deficient in these hormones

        (1) Stimulates protein anabolism

        (2) Produces retention of elements essential for building protoplasm and bony tissue

J. Prenatal factors

   1. Smoking may produce smaller infant.

   2. Fetal alcohol syndrome infants

      a. Exhibit prenatal and postnatal growth deficiencies in height and weight

      b. May produce significant central nervous system alterations that may not be evident until the child is older

   3. Fetal exposure to drugs such as marijuana, cocaine, and heroin

      a. Associated with intrauterine growth retardation and prematurity

   4. Nutritional needs

      a. Poor nutrition may have negative influence on development from time of implantation of ovum until birth.

      b. Severe maternal malnutrition associated with permanent reduction in total number of fetal brain cells

        (1) Has critical effect on child's intellectual functioning

K. Season, climate, and oxygen concentration

   1. Some evidence that

      a. Growth in height faster in spring and summer months

      b. Growth in weight more rapid in autumn and winter

   2. Effects of hypoxia on growth

      a. Children with disorders that produce chronic hypoxia characteristically smaller than children of same chronological age

      b. Children native to high altitudes smaller than children of lower altitudes

L. Nutrition

   1. Single most important influence on growth

   2. Satisfactory nutrition closely related to good health throughout lifetime

   3. Malnutrition

      a. Defined as undernutrition, primarily resulting from insufficient calorie intake

      b. May result from

        (1) Inadequate dietary intake

          (a) Quality

          (b) Quantity

        (2) Disease that interferes with

          (a) Appetite

          (b) Digestion

          (c) Absorption

        (3) Excessive physical activity

        (4) Inadequate rest

        (5) Disturbed interpersonal relationships

        (6) Other environmental or psychological factors

    M. Stress

        1. Abnormal conditions that tend to disrupt normal functions of the body or mind

        2. Imbalance between environmental demands and coping resources

        3. Some children more vulnerable than others

            a. Affected by age, temperament, life situation, and state of health

            b. Response can be behavioral, physiologic, or psychologic.

        4. Methods of coping

            a. Respond by trying to change the circumstance (primary control coping)

                (1) Tantrums

                (2) Aggressive behavior

            b. Trying to adjust to circumstances (secondary control coping)[1]

                (1) Withdrawal

                (2) Submission

        5. Fear

            a. Emotional reaction to a specific real or unreal threat or danger

                (1) Child perceives threat.

                    (a) Person

                    (b) Animal

                    (c) Situation

                (2) Perceives threat to be stronger than himself or herself and capable of harm

            b. Alleviate fear by

                (1) Presence of adult who will offer protection

                (2) Becoming familiar with source of threat (animal)

    N. Media

        1. Television

            a. Pervasive force

            b. Primary source of socialization in children

            c. Major source of information

                (1) Unhealthy messages regarding sex and violence

                (2) Alcohol consumption synonymous with having a good time

                (3) Food products promoting unhealthy nutritional practices

        2. Reading materials

            a. Books, newspapers, magazines

                (1) Provide enjoyment

                (2) Increase child's knowledge

        3. Movies

            a. Not closely associated with reality

            b. Usually provide opportunity for desirable social learning

            c. Child may be unable to distinguish between reality and fantasy.

                (1) Results in fears

BIBLIOGRAPHY

1. Band EB, Weisz JR: How to feel better when it feels bad: children's perspectives on coping with everyday stress. *Dev Psychol* 24:247-253, 1988.

2. Bantz DL, Siktberg L: Teaching families to evaluate age-appropriate toys. *J Pediatr Health Care* 7(3):111-114, 1993.

3. Behrman RE, Kliegman RM, Jenson HB: *Nelson textbook of pediatrics,* ed 16. Philadelphia: WB Saunders, 2000.

4. Burden N, DeFazio Quinn DM, O'Brien D, et al: *Ambulatory surgical nursing,* ed 2. Philadelphia: WB Saunders, 2000.

5. Hall C, Reet M: Enhancing the state of play in children's nursing. *J Child Health Care* 4(2):49-54, 2000.

6. James SR, Ashwill JW, Droske SC: *Nursing care of children: Principles and practice,* ed 2. Philadelphia: WB Saunders, 2002.

7. Johanson LS: Teaching using G.R.O.W.T.H. *Nurse Educ* 25(1):7, 2000.

8. Koenig JM, Zorn CR: Using storytelling as an approach to teaching and learning with diverse students. *J Nurs Educ* 41(9):393-399, 2002.

9. Matteson-Kane M: Teddy bear teachers. *Nurse Educ* 26(5):214,220, 2001.

10. McDowell BM: Using toy critiques to teach growth and development. *Nurse Educ* 27(5):199-200, 2002.
11. Overbay JD: Comics and childhood development. *Nurse Educ* 26(6):262-263, 2001.
12. Phippen ML, Wells MP: Patient care during operative and invasive procedures. Philadelphia: WB Saunders, 2000.
13. Savedra MC, Tesler MD, Holzemer WL, et al: *Adolescent pediatric pain tool (APPT): Preliminary user's Manual*. San Francisco: University of California, 1989.
14. Sieving R, Zirbel-Donish S: Development and enhancement of self-esteem in children. *J Pedia HealthCare* 4(6):290-296, 1990.
15. Wong, D, editor, Wilson D, Hockenberry-Eaton M, et al: *Wong's essentials of pediatric nursing*, ed 6. St Louis: Mosby, 2001.

13 The Pediatric Patient

DONNA M. DEFAZIO QUINN

OBJECTIVES

At the conclusion of this chapter the reader will be able to:

1. Name the stressors associated with hospitalization in the infant, toddler, preschooler, and school-age child.
2. Identify four nursing goals for performing the preoperative assessment.
3. Identify the three degrees of dehydration in the pediatric patient.
4. Categorize the causes, signs and symptoms, and treatment of respiratory acidosis, respiratory alkalosis, metabolic acidosis, and metabolic alkalosis.
5. Identify four potential causes of hypothermia in the pediatric patient.
6. Describe four precautionary measures for prevention of hypothermia in the pediatric patient.
7. State the causes, signs and symptoms, and nursing interventions for stridor, croup, laryngospasm, bronchospasm, and airway obstruction in the pediatric patient.

I. Preparation for hospitalization
   A. Elective surgery
      1. Outpatient
         a. Child arrives at facility morning of procedure.
         b. Undergoes procedure
         c. Recovers from procedure
         d. Is discharged home same day
      2. Inpatient
         a. Usually admitted day of surgery through AM admissions unit
         b. Undergoes procedure
         c. Recovers from procedure
         d. Transferred to nursing unit for continued recovery
      3. Advantages of outpatient surgery
         a. Minimal separation from parents
         b. Decreased risk of infection because of decreased exposure to hospital environment
         c. Reduced psychological trauma to child and parents
         d. Decreased cost
      4. Advantages of postoperative admission
         a. Provision of skilled nursing care that parents may not be able to provide
         b. Ability to administer potent analgesics
         c. Ability to administer required postoperative treatments
      5. Disadvantages—outpatient
         a. Facility may be freestanding.
         b. Not connected to hospital
         c. May require transport to hospital if child requires overnight admission
         d. Does not allow for follow-up care and continued observation
         e. Care can be a burden to family.
         f. Less continuity of care
         g. Increased difficulty in managing pain

6. Disadvantages—inpatient
   a. Increased anxiety because of unfamiliar environment
   b. Potential for acquired hospital infection
B. Emergency surgery (see Box 13-1)
   1. Child usually not prepared for admission
   2. Child and parents emotionally distraught
C. Response to hospitalization
   1. Response varies according to
      a. Developmental age
      b. Presence of support system
      c. Consistency of care providers
      d. Past exposure to hospital
D. Factors affecting response (see Box 13-2)
   1. Age
      a. Preparation for hospitalization varies by age
      b. Based on child's growth and development
   2. Cognitive development
   3. Family member's response
      a. Child knows when parent is upset.
         (1) Anxiety transferred to child
         (2) Child's anxiety level increases.
            (a) Parent does not answer child's questions.
            (b) Parent talks in whispers so child does not hear.
      b. Reaction of family members depends on
         (1) Coping strategies
         (2) Sociocultural environment
         (3) Availability of support systems
         (4) Prior experiences with hospitalization
      c. Nursing interventions to assist family members
         (1) See Box 13-3.
II. Stressors associated with hospitalization
   A. Infant and toddler
      1. Separation anxiety (major stressor)
         a. Stages
            (1) Protest: child is agitated, resists caregivers, screams, cries, actively searches for parent, clings to parent, is inconsolable.
            (2) Despair: child becomes quiet, withdrawn, sad and apathetic, experiences hopelessness, refuses to play, acts disinterested.
            (3) Detachment: child becomes interested in environment, appears content, plays quietly, does not search for parent, seems to form relationship with caregivers, may ignore parents if they return.
      2. Fear of injury and pain
         a. Child may perceive reaction from parents.
         b. Reaction affected by previous experiences
         c. Child reacts by crying, avoiding painful stimuli, pushing painful stimuli away.
         d. Reaction may be result of intrusion on self, whether painful or not.
      3. Loss of control
         a. Disruption of normal daily routines and rituals
         b. Offer choices to return some control to child
         c. May regress in behaviors associated with feeding, toileting, and so forth.
   B. Preschooler (early childhood)
      1. Separation anxiety
         a. Reaction less intense than infant and toddler
         b. Reactions include tantrums, regression, anger, uncooperativeness.
         c. May repeatedly ask when parents will return or why they cannot be there

■ BOX 13-1
■ **WORKING WITH CHILDREN IN EMERGENCIES: DEVELOPMENTAL GUIDELINES**

Infants
- Allow the use of pacifier.
- Use a quiet, soothing voice.
- Touch, rock, or cuddle the infant. Holding the infant securely or swaddling a young infant can also be comforting.
- Keep the infant warm; if the infant must be undressed, use warming lights to ensure a comfortable temperature.
- As much as possible, allay parents' fears so they will not be communicated to the infant.
- Remember that infants experience pain.

Toddlers
- Give treatments and perform procedures with the toddler sitting up on the stretcher or examining table or on the parent's lap.
- Perform the most distressing or intrusive parts of the examination last.
- Reassure family members as much as possible—the child will benefit from their confidence.
- Allow the child to have familiar objects (transitional objects) such as a blanket, doll, or toy to help feel safe.
- Keep frightening objects out of the child's line of vision. Also try to keep machines that make loud noises away.
- Praise ("you are so brave") and distraction (bubbles, puzzles) will decrease anxiety and increase cooperation.

Preschoolers
- Explain a procedure or treatment a few seconds rather than minutes beforehand, because allowing the child time to think about it may result in frightening fantasies or exaggerations.
- Talk to preschool children throughout procedures, describing the sensations they are feeling or will feel and telling them how they can help.
- Distract the child with noises or bright objects. Counting with some preschool children might help to calm them during procedures.
- Avoid criticizing the preschool child for crying, struggling, or fighting during a procedure.
- Reassuring a child that the child did try his or her best to cooperate will help to build a positive self-image.
- Encourage the preschool child to talk about how the illness or injury occurred. If the child is inappropriately taking responsibility for the illness or injury, try to reassure that the child is not to blame for the situation.
- Remember that preschool children can seem to understand more than they actually do. Health care providers often overestimate understanding in a child of this age, so be sure to explain things in words the child understands.
- Use positive terms, such as "make better" and "help," and avoid more frightening terms, such as "shot" and "cut."
- Use adhesive bandages over small wounds and injection sites. Preschool children might imagine their blood leaking out through puncture wounds.

School-Age Children
- Offer simple choices whenever possible to help the child feel more in control. The school-age child is capable of deciding in which arm to have an injection or in which hand to hold a nebulizer. Talk directly to the child, explaining procedures in simple terms. When explaining treatments or care options to the parent, include the child.
- Ask the child about the level of understanding, and allow time for questions.
- Address the child's fears or concerns directly, rather than treating them as foolish or inconsequential.
- Give rewards, such as a sticker or inexpensive toy, after a procedure, regardless of the child's behavior. Think of this gesture as a reward for undergoing the procedure, not as a judgment of "good" or "bad" behavior.

From James SR, Ashwill JW, Droske SC: *Nursing care of children,* ed 2. Philadelphia: WB Saunders, 2002, p 275.

■ BOX 13-2
■ DEVELOPMENTAL APPROACHES TO THE HOSPITALIZED CHILD

Neonate
- Anticipate needs, and fulfill them in a timely manner.
- Provide opportunities for nonnutritive (comfort) sucking and oral stimulation, using a pacifier.
- Provide swaddling, with the infant's hands drawn to the midline and close to the face. Use facilitated tucking and soft talking to soothe.
- If the infant is very ill, provide a quiet, soothing environment. Pay close attention to light and sound stimulation.
- When stimulation is appropriate, provide stimulation for each sense (e.g., mobiles, music, smell, soft stuffed animals). Use contrasting colors and textures.
- Watch for cues of overstimulation, such as eye avoidance, extension of arms, splaying of fingers, and "zoning-out" behavior.
- Before painful procedures, provide comforting touch and nonnutritive sucking. Follow painful procedures with tucking, holding, and cuddling.
- Model and share appropriate behaviors with family members regarding stimulation, touch, verbalization, and feeding.
- Provide consistent caregivers when parents are not available.
- Collaborate with parents on ways to provide them care.
- Involve the parents in the care of their infant as much as possible.
- Encourage parents to room-in if possible.

Infant
- For the younger infant, provide the same care given for neonate.
- The older infant will begin to anticipate painful procedures and fight. Use sheets and blankets to provide swaddling if necessary. Allow nonnutritive sucking for comfort.
- Expect regressive behavior, and inform parents to expect it and why.
- Limit the number of caregivers to whom the infant must adjust.
- Request that parents bring the infant's security object (e.g., blanket, stuffed animal).
- Encourage parents to be present during procedures.

Toddler
- Expect regression, and inform parents about behaviors.
- Follow home routines and rituals.
- Involve parents in the care of the toddler.
- Provide for rooming-in if possible.
- Allow opportunities for mobility when it can be done safely.
- Employ all possible methods of pain control when the child must have a painful procedure.
- Anticipate temper tantrums when the child's frustration level is high.
- Maintain a safe environment for toddler's physical acting out and temper tantrums.
- Encourage the child to be independent (e.g., feed self, use potty chair, put on socks).
- Provide support when the toddler needs to be dependent (e.g., hold after a procedure, comfort if parents leave).
- Approach with a positive attitude ("I am going to give you your medicine").

Preschooler
- Provide safe ways to act out aggression (e.g., with punching bags, painting, clay).
- Take time for communication. Answer questions with simple, concrete explanations. Explain all procedures honestly. Allow for choices whenever possible.
- Expect egocentric behavior.
- Provide for a safe and secure environment (e.g., with a night light, view of others, objects from home).
- Be consistent.
- Ask the parents how the child usually copes in new situations.
- Tell the child that he or she did not cause the illness.
- Involve the parents in care, and follow home routines.

Continued

■ BOX 13-2 *Cont'd*
■ **DEVELOPMENTAL APPROACHES TO THE HOSPITALIZED CHILD**

- Place the child with other children of the same age if possible.
- Provide for play activities in the playroom and in the room.
- Accept regression if it occurs, and explain it to parents.
- Encourage the child to be independent (e.g., feeding, dressing, toileting).

School-Age Child
- Inform the child of limits, and enforce them (e.g., no water fights, wheelchair races, leaving the unit).
- Involve the child in planning and implementing care (e.g., allow child to choose from menu and assist with some procedures).
- Explain all procedures, and allow the child time for questions and answers. Use medical and scientific terminology and diagrams, body outlines, or anatomically correct dolls to explain the procedure.
- Accept regression, but encourage independence.
- Provide privacy.
- Encourage the child to assist in keeping the room and belongings in order.
- Assist the child in contacting friends. Encourage parents to contact the teacher and have school friends send cards and letters.
- If the child's condition supports visits and calls from friends, encourage this contact.
- Provide for the educational needs of the child by encouraging parents to bring in work and by scheduling study times. If the child will have a prolonged period of hospital or home care, arrange for a teacher to work with the child. Some hospitals have a hospital-based teacher.

Adolescent
- Provide privacy for care and visiting.
- Encourage the adolescent to wear street clothes and perform normal grooming.
- Encourage questions about appearance and the effects of illness on the adolescent's future.
- Use scientific and medical terminology to prepare the adolescent for procedures.
- Use body outlines and diagrams, and give the rationale for the procedure.
- When possible, provide for a special activity area that is limited to adolescent use. Introduce the child to other adolescents on the unit.
- Encourage peers to call and visit if the adolescents can tolerate this action.
- Assist parents in communicating, supporting, and guiding their adolescents by providing them with information about growth and development.
- Allow favorite foods to be brought in if the adolescent does not need a special diet.
- Approach the adolescent with caring, understanding, and acceptance.
- Provide for educational needs, as for a school-age child.

From James SR, Ashwill JW, Droske SC: *Nursing care of children,* ed 2. Philadelphia: WB Saunders, 2002, p 315.

2. Fear of injury and pain
   a. Fear of mutilation
   b. Lack of understanding causes child to imagine that things are worse than they actually are.
   c. Reacts to strangers, loud noises, machines, and equipment
   d. Reacts to intrusive procedures that cause bleeding
   e. Reaction based on previous experiences
   f. Child may cling to parent.
   g. May fear illness caused by something they did wrong
   h. Pain
      (1) Reaction to pain includes
         (a) Crying
         (b) Restlessness
         (c) Whimpering

■ BOX 13-3
■ **NURSING CARE: THE FAMILY WITH A HOSPITALIZED CHILD**

Focused Assessment
- Assess factors that affect a family's adjustment to illness and hospitalization.
- Compare assessment with concerns expressed on the child's admission history.
- Was the admission an emergency?
- Were there previous admissions? If yes, how did the parents perceive those hospitalizations?
- How serious is the illness or trauma?
- Are some factors unknown, such as the cause of the disease, illness, or injury, or the child's prognosis?
- Special attention should be given to any information obtained in the admission interview.
- Determine if the parents and siblings are experiencing stress and how they are coping with the hospitalization.
- Encourage communication using open-ended statements such as "this must be difficult for you" to encourage communication in the crisis.

Identify the parents' needs for sleep, nutrition, and information.

Nursing Diagnosis: Interrupted family process related to the child's hospitalization and illness.

Expected Outcome: The parents will participate in the child's care, meet the needs of other family members, use appropriate support systems, identify ways to cope, and assist the child to move from a sick role to a well role.

Intervention	Rationale
1. Orient the parents to the hospital, and provide information related to their physical needs (e.g., food, sleep, bathing).	1. The parent's physical needs must be met for them to meet the child's needs and their own emotional needs. Meeting their needs indicates support by the caregiver.
2. Encourage family members (parents, siblings) to express their feelings and to ask questions about the child's illness, procedure, or surgery.	2. Expression decreases anxiety and clarifies misconceptions.
3. Provide the family with information about the child's condition, treatment, and support systems. Begin to prepare them for the child's discharge.	3. Information gives parents a sense of control and decreases their anxiety.
4. Identify with the family the ways in which they are coping; support their parenting skills.	4. Individuals are not always aware of their coping mechanisms, and the nurse should help the family evaluate the effectiveness of theirs.
5. Refer the family to other professionals (e.g., social worker, clinical psychologist, clinical specialist, psychiatrist, clergy) when their problems are not within the scope of nursing.	5. Early identification of family problems can decrease the possibility of escalation of the problems. Collaboration with other health professionals can bring a holistic approach to the care of the child and family.

Evaluation
- Are the parents able to participate in their child's care while meeting the needs of other family members?
- Do family members support each other and seek other resources when necessary?
- Are family members able to describe and use positive coping skills?
- Are the parents able to assist the child to move from a sick to a well role?

From James SR, Ashwill JW, Droske SC: *Nursing care of children,* ed 2. Philadelphia: WB Saunders, 2002, p 326.

           (d) Active resistance to caregiver

           (e) Screaming

        (2) May be able to verbally express pain

        (3) Can respond to pain assessment tools

        (4) Nursing assessment may not be truly accurate.

  3. Loss of control

    a. Reacts to loss of control and disruption of routine

    b. May regress

      (1) Temper tantrums, toileting, and so forth

      (2) Exhibits negative behavior

C. School age

  1. Separation anxiety

    a. Less affected because child is accustomed to periods of separation

    b. Reacts with inappropriate behavior

  2. Fear of injury and pain

    a. Fears

      (1) Death

      (2) Disfigurement

      (3) Mutilation

      (4) Procedures involving the genitals

    b. Child understands cause and effect.

    c. May express guilt about illness

    d. Pain

      (1) Able to express concern regarding pain

      (2) Methods to control reaction to pain

        (a) May want to watch procedure being performed

        (b) May request nurse to talk to them during procedure

  3. Loss of control

    a. Illness causes child to feel helpless and dependent.

    b. Expresses anger at loss of independence

    c. Reactions include boredom, frustration, anger at caregivers, disinterest, refusing to cooperate.

    d. Offer opportunities to promote independence

      (1) Assist in own care

      (2) Assist with treatments

      (3) Make choices regarding fluid and food intake

D. Reaction of siblings to hospitalization

  1. Siblings may experience

    a. Jealousy

    b. Insecurity

    c. Resentment

    d. Confusion

    e. Anxiety

  2. Have difficulty understanding why ill sibling is getting all the attention

    a. Amount of stress experienced by well child varies according to

      (1) Well child's age and developmental level

      (2) Closeness to ill sibling

      (3) Who is caring for well child while sibling is hospitalized?

      (4) How often can well child visit ill sibling?

      (5) Changes in parental behavior

  3. May worry they will be ill like sibling

  4. Strategies to meet needs of siblings

    a. Encourage ill child to retell experience to siblings

      (1) May be uncomfortable for parents but helps put the illness, accident, or injury in perspective

      (2) If sibling expresses guilt, address concerns directly.

      (3) Provide parents with educational materials they can use with siblings.

(4) Schedule for siblings to visit.

(5) If unable to visit, send photographs.

(6) Encourage telephone communication between siblings.

III. Communicating with the pediatric patient (see Table 13-1)

    A. Types of communication

        1. Verbal

            a. Uses the spoken word

            b. May be hampered by language barriers

            c. May be misunderstood

        2. Nonverbal

            a. Most reliable

            b. Not so easily controlled

            c. Child's natural method of expression

    B. Communication skills

        1. Listening

            a. Nurse needs to understand level of language development and cognitive level of child.

            b. Need to provide child with explanations

                (1) Assists in establishing trust between child and nurse

        2. Observation

            a. Provides cues about child

            b. Observe

                (1) Eyes

                    (a) Happy

                    (b) Sad

                (2) Quality of voice

                (3) Facial expression

                    (a) Smiling or crying

                    (b) Relaxed or tense

                    (c) Makes eye contact or avoids eye contact

                (4) Body posture

                    (a) Relaxed or stiff

                    (b) Open or closed body posture (arms crossed in front of body versus arms loosely at sides)

                    (c) Facing nurse or turned away from nurse

                (5) Movement

                    (a) Holds still or resists touch by nurse

                    (b) Moving around room or staying still near parent

                    (c) Cooperative versus kicking and flailing

                    (d) Nodding head with understanding

                    (e) Biting, shaking, twitching, banging fist

                (6) Vocal clues

                    (a) Crying

                    (b) Whining

                    (c) Silence

                    (d) Tone of voice (shaky versus loud and confident)

                (7) Interaction between parent and child

                    (a) How parent responds to child overall

                    (b) How parent responds to child's behavior

                        (i) Good behavior rewarded

                        (ii) Unacceptable behavior receives attention.

                    (c) How parent physically handles child

                    (d) How parent answers child's questions

                    (e) How parent enlists the cooperation of the child

        3. Silence

            a. Child may be quiet because he or she is

                (1) Afraid

                (2) Shy

TABLE 13-1

Developmental Milestones and Their Relationship to Communication Approaches

Development	Language Development	Emotional Development	Cognitive Development	Suggested Communication Approach
INFANTS (0-12 MO) Infants' experience the world through the senses of hearing, seeing, smelling, tasting, and touching.	Crying, babbling, cooing Single-word production Able to name some simple objects	Dependent on others; high need for cuddling and security Responsive to environment (sounds, visual stimuli, etc.) Distinguish between happy and angry voices as well as between familiar and strange voices Beginning to experience separation anxiety	Interactions largely reflexive Beginning to see repetition of activities and movements Beginning to initiate interactions intentionally Short attention span (1-2 min)	Use calm, soft, soothing voice. Be responsive to cries. Engage in turn-taking vocalizations (adult imitates baby sounds). Talk and read regularly to infants. Prepare infant as you are about to perform care. Talk to infant about what you are about to do. Use a slow approach and allow child time to get to know you.
TODDLERS (1-2 YR) Toddlers experience the world through the senses of hearing, seeing, smelling, tasting, and touching.	Two-word combinations emerge Participate in turn-taking in communication (speaker/listener) "No" becomes a favorite word. Able to use gestures and verbalize simple wants and needs.	Strong need for security objects Separation/stranger anxiety heightened Participate in parallel play Thrive on routines Beginning development of independence: "Want to do by self" Still very dependent on significant adults	Experiment with objects Participate in active exploration Begin to experiment with variations on activities Begin to identify cause-and-effect relationships Short attention span (3-5 min)	Learn the toddler's words for common items, and use them in conversations. Describe activities and procedures as they are about to be done. Use picture books. Use play for demonstrations. Be responsive to child's receptivity toward you, and approach cautiously. Preparation should occur immediately before the event.
PRESCHOOL CHILDREN (3-5 YR) Preschool children use words they do not fully understand, nor do they accurately	Further development and expansion of word combination (able to speak in full sentences) Growth in correct grammatical	Like to imitate activities and make choices Strive for independence but need adult support and encouragement Demonstrate purposeful	Begin developing concepts of time, space, and quantity Magical thinking prominent World seen only from child's perspective	Seek opportunities to offer choices. Use play to explain procedures and activities. Speak in simple sentences, and explore using relative concepts. Use picture and story books, puppets.

Language/Communication	Social/Psychosocial	Cognitive	Nursing Implications
understand many words used by others. Use pronouns. Clearer articulation of sounds. Vocabulary rapidly expanding; may know words without understanding meaning	attention-seeking behaviors. Learn cooperation and turn-taking in game playing. Need clearly set limits and boundaries	Short attention span (5-10 min)	Describe activities and procedures as they are about to be done. Be concise; limit length of explanations (<5 min). Engage in preparatory activities 1-3 hr before the event.

SCHOOL-AGE CHILDREN (6-11 YR)

Language/Communication	Social/Psychosocial	Cognitive	Nursing Implications
School-age children communicate thoughts and appreciate viewpoints of others. Words with multiple meanings and words describing things they have not experienced are not thoroughly understood. Expanding vocabulary enables child to describe concepts, thoughts and feelings. Development of conversational skills	Interact well with others. Understand rules to games. Very interested in learning. Build close friendships. Beginning to accept responsibility for own actions. Competition emerges. Still dependent on adults to meet needs	Able to grasp concepts of classification, conversation. Concrete thinking emerges. Become very oriented to "rules". Able to process information in serial format. Lengthened attention span (10-30 min)	Use photographs, books, diagrams, charts, videos to explain. Make explanations sequential. Engage in conversations that encourage critical thinking. Establish limits and set consequences. Use medical play techniques. Introduce preparatory materials 1-5 days in advance of the event.

ADOLESCENTS (12 YR AND OLDER)

Language/Communication	Social/Psychosocial	Cognitive	Nursing Implications
Adolescents are able to create theories and generate many explanations for situations. They are beginning to communicate like adults. Able to verbalize and comprehend most adult concepts	Beginning to accept responsibility for own actions. Perception of "imaginary audiences". Need independence. Competitive drive. Strong need for group identification. Frequently have small group of very close friends. Question authority. Strong need for privacy	Able to think logically and abstractly. Attention span up to 60 min.	Engage in conversations about adolescent's interests. Use photographs, books, diagrams, charts, and videos to explain. Use collaborative approach and foster and support independence. Introduce preparatory materials up to 1 wk in advance of the event. Respect privacy needs.

From James SR, Ashwill JW, Droske SC: *Nursing care of children*, ed 2. Philadelphia: WB Saunders, 2002, pp 58-59.

                    (3) Angry
                    (4) Busy
            b. Need to assess environment to determine cause of silence
            c. May be used by child to block communication
            d. May be used to promote positive communication
                    (1) Allows child to process thoughts and feelings
                    (2) Seek to understand what has been communicated.
        C. Communicating at the child's level of understanding
            1. See Table 13-2
    IV. Educational strategies
        A. Infant (0-12 months)
            1. Developmental characteristics
                a. Unable to understand explanations
                b. Is sensitive to gentle voice, touch, and movement
                c. Stranger anxiety occurs at 6-8 months
            2. Teaching strategies
                a. Main focus is to teach parents.
                b. Use soft voice and gentle tone in communicating.

■ TABLE 13-2
■ ■ Communication with the Child in the Perioperative Setting

Don't Say	Do Say	Child's Perspective
We are going to put you on a stretcher.	A special bed with wheels	Child may interpret as "stretch her"—"Why are they going to stretch me?"
The doctor will give you some gas.	The doctor will give you a special medicine that you will breathe through a mask like this (show mask).	"Why are they going to give me gasoline?"
The doctor will put you to sleep for your operation.	We will give you some medicine that will put you in a very deep sleep so that the doctor can do the operation and you won't feel anything. When it's all over, you will wake up.	"They put my kitty to sleep and he never woke up."
The doctor will cut you open—make an incision.	Make a tiny opening.	"He is going to cut me with a knife?"
Take your vital signs	Check your temperature to see how warm you are and how fast your heart is beating	Taking can be misinterpreted; do not "take" anything from the child.
Put some electrodes on your chest	Put some sticky Band-Aids (stickers) on you so we can get a picture of your heart.	Involve child in process; supply child with printout of ECG that he/she will be able to take home and show his/her friends (great for show and tell).
Put a dressing on	You will have a bandage on.	"Why will they dress me?"
Give you a shot—a little stick—just like a bee sting	Give you a little medicine under your skin	"When you get shot, you get hurt real bad." "Are you going to shoot me with a gun?"
Hook you up to a monitor	Attach some wires so you can see your heart beat on a TV screen	"Are you going to hook me like I hook the fish when I go fishing?"
Hurt	Boo-boo, owie, uncomfortable, discomfort	Communicate at child's developmental level with words he/she is familiar with.

From Quinn DMD: *Ambulatory surgical nursing core curriculum.* Philadelphia: WB Saunders, 1999, p 262.

    c. Talk to and touch infant prior to procedure.
    d. Provide favorite security object before beginning procedure.
    e. Spend time with child before procedure.
    f. Involve parents in care.
B. Toddler (1-3 years)
    1. Developmental characteristics
      a. Perceives separation from parents as a threat
      b. Limited coping skills
      c. Limited ability to express emotions and feelings
      d. Fantasizes about what happens and why
      e. Short attention span
      f. Limited vocabulary
      g. No concept of time
    2. Teaching strategies
      a. Encourage parental presence.
      b. Describe machines and equipment.
      c. Use play as a method of expression.
      d. Tell child it is OK to cry.
      e. Communicate in simple words child can understand (see Table 13-2).
      f. Limit teaching to 5-10 minutes.
      g. Allow hands on of demonstration of equipment.
      h. Provide explanations as close to the procedure time as possible.
C. Preschooler (3-6 years)
    1. Developmental characteristics
      a. Magical thinking
      b. Limited coping behaviors
      c. Fear of body mutilation
      d. Increased verbal skills
      e. Understands concrete explanations
    2. Teaching strategies
      a. Explain why to eliminate children thinking they caused the situation.
      b. Ask children to repeat back to assess their understanding.
      c. Avoid threatening words.
      d. Encourage parental presence for stressful interventions.
      e. Give clear explanations of which body part will or will not be affected.
      f. Use visual aids, books, models, and so forth to explain procedures.
      g. Limit teaching sessions to 10-15 minutes.
      h. Involve child in teaching session—allow handling of equipment, supplies, models, and so forth.
        (i) Allow child opportunity to ask questions.
      j. Explain what child will feel, hear, and so forth.
D. School-age child (6-12 years)
    1. Developmental characteristics
      a. Eager to learn and accomplish new skills
      b. Concept of time has improved.
      c. Cannot apply logic to abstract problems
      d. Increased attention span
      e. Looks to peers for support
      f. Increased neuromuscular development
      g. Becoming more independent
      h. Views hospitalization as a punishment
        (i) Exhibits competitive behavior
    2. Teaching strategies
      a. Use books in teaching.
      b. Focus on concrete aspects of the procedure.
      c. Provide information 1-2 days in advance.
      d. Teaching sessions can last 30-45 minutes.
      e. Provide education in a group setting.

        f. May still request parents for support

        g. Offer continued reassurance.

        h. Provide explanations to alleviate children thinking they caused the situation.

    E. Preoperative education

        1. Include child in preparation.

        2. Communicate with child in language appropriate for age and developmental level.

        3. See Table 13-2.

V. Preoperative assessment

    A. Goals

        1. Decrease anxiety level for child and parents

        2. Establish a trusting relationship with child

        3. Assist parents and family to

            a. Design and implement a plan of care.

                (1) Process (what's going to happen)

                (2) Expectations (time frames for preoperative, intraoperative, and postoperative)

                (3) Potential complications associated with procedure (pain, bleeding, nausea and vomiting, etc.)

            b. Plan preoperative preparation of child based on developmental level.

        4. Prevent postoperative complications.

            a. Awareness of preoperative health status

                (1) Cardiac

                    (a) Congenital problems

                (2) Respiratory

                    (a) Recent colds, congestion, asthma

                (3) Report any abnormal findings to anesthesiologist.

    B. Decision to perform procedure on an outpatient basis based on

        1. Type of procedure to be performed

        2. Parental readiness and acceptance of procedure

        3. Patient status

            a. Child in good health

            b. Generally Anesthesiologists Society of America (ASA) class I or II, occasionally class III

            c. If chronic illness, should be optimally prepared

    C. Laboratory requirements

        1. Vary according to hospital or facility policy

        2. Current trend is towards no requirements for healthy children.

        3. Generally only hematocrit for child less than 1 year of age

    D. Nothing by mouth (NPO) guidelines

        1. Vary according to hospital or facility policy

        2. Stomach should be free of solids prior to anesthesia.

        3. Clear liquids up to 2-4 hours preoperatively.

    E. Physical exam

        1. Use play therapy.

            a. Perform procedure on teddy bear or doll first.

            b. Have child hold stethoscope.

            c. Have parent hold infant and approach from behind.

        2. Listen to what the child has to say.

        3. Give simple, easy-to-understand instructions; give one at a time.

        4. Be honest with child.

        5. Do painful procedures last.

        6. Note birthmarks, bruises, loose teeth (document on record).

VI. Preanesthesia evaluation (see Box 13-4)

    A. Performed by anesthesia provider and/or RN

        1. Evaluate for conditions requiring special treatment (e.g., anemia, asthma).

■ BOX 13-4
■ **THE PREANESTHETIC HISTORY**

Child's Previous Anesthetic and Surgical Procedures
Review anesthetic record for information about mask and endotracheal tube size, type and size of laryngoscope used, difficulties with mask ventilation or intubation; history of hyperthermia or acidosis.

Perinatal Problems (Especially for Infants)
Need for prolonged hospitalization
Need for supplemental oxygen or intubation
History of apnea and bradycardia

Other Major Illnesses and Hospitalizations

Family History of Anesthetic Complications, Malignant Hyperthermia, or Pseudocholinesterase Deficiency

Respiratory Problems
Chronic exposure to environmental tobacco smoke
Obstructive apnea, breathing irregularities, or cyanosis (especially in infants younger than age 6 mo)
History of snoring or obstructive breathing pattern
Recent upper respiratory tract infection
Recurrent respiratory infections
Previous laryngotracheitis (croup)
Asthma or wheezing during respiratory infections

Cardiac Problems
Murmurs
Dysrhythmia
Exercise intolerance
Syncope
Cyanosis

Gastrointestinal Problems
Reflux and vomiting
Feeding difficulties
Failure to thrive
Liver disease

Exposure to Exanthems or Potentially Infectious Pathogens

Neurologic Problems
Seizures
Developmental delay
Neuromuscular diseases
Increased intracranial pressure

Hematologic Problems
Anemia
Bleeding diathesis
Tumor
Immunocompromise
Prior blood transfusions and reactions

Renal Problems
Renal insufficiency, oliguria, anuria
Fluid and electrolyte abnormalities

Continued

■ BOX 13-4 *Cont'd*
■ **THE PREANESTHETIC HISTORY**

Psychosocial Considerations
Posttraumatic stress
Drug abuse, use of cigarettes or alcohol
Physical or sexual abuse
Family dysfunction
Previous traumatic medical and surgical experiences
Psychosis, anxiety, depression

Gynecologic Considerations
Sexual history (sexually transmitted diseases)
Possibility of pregnancy

Current Medications
Prior administration of corticosteroids

Allergies
Drugs
Iodine
Latex products
Surgical tapes
Food allergies (especially soy and egg albumin)

Dental Condition (Loose or Cracked Teeth)

When and What the Child Last Ate (especially in emergency procedures)

From Behrman RE, Kliegman RM, Jenson HB: *Nelson textbook of pediatrics,* ed 17. Philadelphia: WB Saunders, 2004, p 343.

      2. Evaluate for recent exposure to communicable and infectious diseases (e.g., chickenpox, human immunodeficiency virus, hepatitis).
      3. Counsel patient and parents regarding anesthesia and surgery.
   B. Physical examination
      1. General observation of the patient
      2. Vital signs
      3. Assess airway for potential difficulty with mask induction or intubation.
      4. Assess respiratory status (presence of wheezing, coughing, etc.).
      5. Assess ability to perform venous access after induction.
      6. Assess behavior to determine need for premedication.
   C. Implications of anesthesia to preexisting diseases (see Table 13-3)
      1. Chronically ill child may present for outpatient surgery
         a. Diagnostic or therapeutic procedure (e.g., insertion of venous access device)
   D. Premedication
      1. Decreases fear and anxiety
      2. Allows easier transition of child from parents to anesthesia provider
      3. Techniques to assist in preparation of the child preoperatively (based on child's cognitive development)
         a. Explain purpose of procedure.
            (1) Use pictures, diagrams, dolls, video, and so forth.
            (2) Use words child can understand.
         b. Describe sequence of events.
         c. Describe potential discomfort.
         d. Allow time for ample discussion.
      4. Premedication should not be substituted for lack of preprocedure education.

■ TABLE 13-3
■ ■ Specific Pediatric Diseases and Their Anesthetic Implications

Disease	Implications
RESPIRATORY SYSTEM	
Asthma	Intraoperative bronchospasm that may be severe
	Pneumothorax
	Optimal preoperative medical management essential; may require preoperative steroids
Difficult airway	May require special equipment and personnel
	Should be anticipated in children with dysmorphic features or acute airway obstruction as in epiglottitis or laryngotracheobronchitis or with airway foreign body
	Patients with Down syndrome may require evaluation of atlanto-occipital joint
	Patients with storage diseases may be at high risk.
Bronchopulmonary dysplasia	Barotrauma with positive pressure ventilation
	Oxygen toxicity, pneumothorax a risk
Cystic fibrosis	Airway reactivity, bronchorrhea
	Risk of pneumothorax, pulmonary hemorrhage
	Atelectasis
	Assess for cor pulmonale.
Sleep apnea	Must rule out pulmonary hypertension and cor pulmonale
	Requires careful postoperative observation for obstruction
Cardiac	Need for antibiotic prophylaxis for subacute bacterial endocarditis
	Use of air filters; careful purging of air from intravenous equipment
	Need to understand effects of various anesthetics on the hemodynamics of specific lesions
	Preload optimization and avoidance of hyperviscous states in cyanotic patients
	Possible need for preoperative evaluation of myocardial function and pulmonary vascular resistance
	Provide information about pacemaker function and ventricular device function.
HEMATOLOGIC	
Sickle cell	Possible need for simple or exchange transfusion based on preoperative Hgb and percent Hgb S
Oncology	Pulmonary evaluation of patients who have received bleomycin, *bis*-chloroethyl-nitrosourea, chloroethyl-cyclohexyl-nitrosourea, methotrexate, or radiation to the chest
Rheumatologic	Limited mobility of temporomandibular joint, cervical spine, arytenoids cartilages
	Requires careful preoperative evaluation
	May be difficult airway
GASTROINTESTINAL	
Esophageal, gastric	Potential for reflux and aspiration
Liver	High overall morbidity and mortality in patients with hepatic dysfunction
	Altered metabolism of some drugs
	Potential for coagulopathy
Renal	Altered electrolyte and acid–base status
	Altered clearance of some drugs
	Need for preoperative dialysis with selected cases
	Succinylcholine to be used with extreme caution and only when serum potassium level is recently shown to be normal

Continued

■ TABLE 13-3 *Cont'd*
■ ■ **Specific Pediatric Diseases and Their Anesthetic Implications**

NEUROLOGIC

Seizure disorder	Avoid anesthetics that may lower threshold.
	Ensure optimal control preoperatively.
	Preoperative anticonvulsant levels.
Increased intracranial pressure	Avoid agents that increase cerebral blood flow.
	Avoid hypercarbia.
Neuromuscular disease	Avoid depolarizing relaxants; at risk for hyperkalemia.
	May be at risk for malignant hyperthermia
Developmental delay	May be uncooperative at induction
Psychiatric	Monoamine oxidase inhibitor (or cocaine) may interact with meperidine, resulting in hyperthermia and seizures.
	Selective serotonin reuptake inhibitors may induce or inhibit various hepatic enzymes that may alter anesthetic drug clearance.
	Illicit drugs may have adverse effects on cardiorespiratory homeostasis and may potentiate the action of anesthetics.

ENDOCRINE

Diabetes	Greatest risk is unrecognized intraoperative hypoglycemia; if insulin is administered, monitor blood glucose level intraoperatively; must provide glucose and insulin with adjustment for fasting condition and surgical stress.

SKIN

Burns	Difficult airway
	Risk of rhabdomyolysis and hyperkalemia from succinylcholine
	Fluid shifts
	Bleeding coagulopathy
Immunologic	Retroviral drugs may inhibit benzodiazepine clearance.
	Immunodeficiency requires careful infection control practices.
	May require cytomegalovirus-negative blood products, irradiation, or leukofiltration
Metabolic	Careful assessment of glucose homeostasis in infants

From Behrman RE, Kliegman RM, Jenson HB: *Nelson textbook of pediatrics,* ed 17. Philadelphia: WB Saunders, 2004, p 344.

5. Options for premedication
   a. Oral
      (1) Midazolam
         (a) 0.5 mg/kg orally (PO)
         (b) Nursing considerations
            (i) May cause respiratory depression
      (2) Diazepam
         (a) 0.1 to 0.5 mg/kg PO
         (b) Nursing considerations
            (i) Slow onset
            (ii) Prolonged action
            (iii) Insufficient dose may cause disinhibition and decreased patient cooperation.
      (3) Oral transmucosal fentanyl
         (a) Lollipop may be viewed by child as candy.
         (b) 10 to 15 µg/kg oral transmucosal
         (c) Nursing considerations
            (i) High incidence of itchy nose
            (ii) May cause respiratory depression, nausea, vomiting

    b. Nasal

       (1) Midazolam (not Food and Drug Administration [FDA] approved)

          (a) 0.2 to 0.3 mg/kg intranasal

       (2) Ketamine

          (a) 3 mg/kg intranasal

    c. Intramuscular (IM)

       (1) Midazolam, ketamine

          (a) Painful

          (b) Reserved for sedation of highly distressed or uncooperative child

             (i) Midazolam: 0.08 to 0.5 mg/kg IM

             (ii) Ketamine: 2 to 5 mg/kg IM

          (c) Nursing considerations

             (i) Increases heart rate and blood pressure

             (ii) Accumulation of pharyngeal secretions may cause laryngospasm.

             (iii) Contraindicated with increased intracranial pressure

    d. Rectal

       (1) Barbiturates

          (a) Methohexital

             (i) 1% to 10% solution to 20-30 mg/kg per rectum

             (ii) Nursing considerations

               [a] Unpredictable systemic bioavailability

               [b] May cause rectal irritation or defecation

               [c] Contraindicated in temporal lobe epilepsy or porphyria

          (b) Pentobarbital or secobarbital: 2-4 mg/kg per rectum

             (i) Nursing considerations

               [a] May cause paradoxical reaction

               [b] Contraindicated in porphyria

       (2) Benzodiazepines

          (a) Midazolam: 0.4-1 mg/kg per rectum

          (b) Diazepam: 0.1-0.5 mg/kg per rectum

       (3) Ketamine: 8 to 10 mg/kg per rectum

    e. Anticholinergics

       (1) Current trend to limit use

          (a) Drying of secretions is unpleasant in awake child.

          (b) Need for drying secretions diminished because of current available anesthetics

       (2) Used when

          (a) Prolonged surgery in prone position

          (b) Airway surgery

          (c) Ophthalmic surgery to block the oculocardiac reflex

       (3) Nursing considerations

          (a) Atropine can cause fever, extremely dry mouth, flushing, tachycardia.

          (b) Glycopyrrolate

             (i) No central nervous system (CNS) effects

             (ii) Long duration

          (c) Scopolamine

             (i) May cause confusion

             (ii) Long duration

6. Nursing interventions

    a. If premedication is administered

       (1) Continuous observation of child necessary

          (a) Prevent from falling or becoming injured

          (b) Resuscitation equipment immediately available

       (2) Nursing staff skilled in airway management

VII. Intraoperative anesthetic considerations

Although the nurse is not involved in the administration of anesthetic agents, an understanding of anesthetic agents and techniques will assist the nurse in providing answers to both patients' and parents' questions as well as ensuring a safe postoperative recovery from the anesthetic agents.

A. Placement of intravenous (IV) catheter

    1. May be inserted prior to induction with older or cooperative child

        a. May use eutectic mixture of local anesthetics (EMLA)

        b. Requires application to site 1 to 2 hours in advance of venipuncture

    2. Usually inserted after mask induction on young child

B. Emotional responses to anesthetic induction (see Table 13-4)

    1. Decrease by allowing parent in operating room.

    2. Hospital or facility policy dictates acceptance of this practice.

C. Induction of anesthesia

    1. Induction technique dependent on

        a. Specific patient risks

        b. Disease status

        c. Preoperative medical condition

        d. Presence or absence of IV line

        e. Child's or parent's choice

    2. Selected technique discussed with parents and child during preoperative interview

    3. Allowing child to practice beforehand with selected equipment (inhalation mask) helpful

        a. Use play therapy.

        b. Assist in decreasing child's anxiety level caused by new and unfamiliar procedure.

        c. Involve parents as appropriate.

    4. Ideal method is one that causes the child the least distress.

    5. IV induction

        a. Medically indicated if child is coming in for emergency surgery

            (1) Child is at increased risk for aspiration of gastric contents.

    6. Rapid sequence induction

        a. Patient inhales 100% oxygen prior to induction.

            (1) Prolongs the time to arterial desaturation with apnea

---

■ TABLE 13-4
■ ■ **Emotional Responses to Anesthetic Induction**

Age	Typical Responses and Implications
0-8 mo	Fewer anticipatory responses Generally calm with strangers Mask induction well tolerated
8 mo-2 yr	Separation anxiety is high. Most difficult for mask induction Premedication, preinduction useful
3-7 yr	Separation anxiety still present Mask induction aided by parental presence
7-11 yr	Generally calm with mask induction Fear of needles Fear of loss of control
12-18 yr	Generally prefers intravenous to mask induction

From Behrman RE, Kliegman RM, Jenson HB: *Nelson textbook of pediatrics,* ed 16. Philadelphia: WB Saunders, p 301, 2000.

  b. Anesthesia induced with rapid acting hypnotic and a muscle relaxant

  c. Cricoid pressure is applied to occlude the esophagus.

   (1) Prevents reflux of gastric contents into the pharynx

 7. Risks associated with rapid sequence induction

  a. Unknown if muscle paralysis will cause inability to intubate the trachea or ability to ventilate by mask

  b. The fixed dose of hypnotic may cause hypertension or hypotension.

  c. The younger the infant, the shorter the time before child becomes hypoxic after preoxygenation induction

  d. Cricoid pressure does not protect against aspiration.

 D. Inhalation induction technique

  1. Medically indicated in situations where spontaneous breathing needs to be preserved

   a. Foreign body in the airway

  2. Most widely accepted technique of induction in the United States

  3. Well accepted for children 4 to 10 years of age

  4. Technique

   a. Proceed in quiet surroundings.

   b. Avoid delays once in operating room.

   c. Use flavored aromas on mask.

   d. Administer nitrous oxide (odorless) in conjunction with oxygen first.

   e. Introduce more aromatic vapor anesthetics.

VIII. Anesthetic agents

 For complete information regarding anesthetic agents, see Chapter 26.

 IX. Perianesthesia considerations

  A. Metabolism

   1. Infants have greater nutritional requirements to minimize loss of body protein.

    a. Develop disturbances more rapidly than adults

    b. Complications increase proportionately with increase in time of fluid restriction.

   2. Infants and small children should have priority on surgery schedule in order to limit food and fluid deprivation to as short a time as possible.

   3. Intake (may vary according to hospital or facility policy)

    a. Infants

     (1) Regular formula or diet up to 6 hours before anesthesia

     (2) Clear liquids up to 2 to 4 hours before

     (3) Should not miss more than two feedings

     (4) Oral intake resumes promptly after recovery from anesthesia.

    b. Toddler and preschool children

     (1) Usually permitted clear liquids up to 6 hours preoperatively

    c. Children over 5 years of age

     (1) NPO after midnight or 8 hours prior to induction of anesthesia

     (2) Exceptions necessary for children with diabetes or other special problems

     (3) Postoperative oral intake resumed as tolerated

  B. Fluid and electrolyte balance

   1. Infants and young children more vulnerable to changes (see Box 13-5)

   2. Dehydration

    a. Dehydration causes disturbances in acid–base balance.

     (1) Caused by decrease in fluid intake or fluid loss

     (2) Causes rapid extracellular fluid loss

     (3) Results in electrolyte imbalance

     (4) Results in intracellular fluid loss

     (5) Causes cellular dysfunction

     (6) Can result in hypovolemic shock and death

■ BOX 13-5
■ **PEDIATRIC DIFFERENCES RELATED TO FLUID AND ELECTROLYTE BALANCE**

Infants
- Because of the higher percentage of water in the extracellular fluid (ECF), infants can lose fluids equal to their ECF within 2 to 3 days.
- Infants are less able to concentrate urine because of immature renal function.
- Infants have a higher rate of peristalsis than older children.
- Infants have an immature lower esophageal sphincter, making them more prone to gastroesophageal reflux, which can lead to dehydration and electrolyte disturbances.
- Infants have a harder time compensating for acidosis because of their decreased ability to acidify urine.

Infants and Young Children
- Infants and young children have a higher metabolic turnover of water relative to adults because of a higher metabolic rate. (If losses are not replaced rapidly, imbalance occurs.)
- Infants and young children are unable to verbalize or communicate thirst.

Infants and Children
- In comparison with adults, infants and children have a proportionately greater body surface area in relation to body mass, resulting in a greater potential for fluid loss via the skin and gastrointestinal tract.
- Infants and children have a higher proportionate water content (premature infants have 90%, full-term infants 75% to 80%, preschool children 60% to 65%, and adolescents and adults approximately 55% to 60%), with a larger proportion of fluid in the extracellular space.
- The immune system of infants and children is not as robust as an adult's immune system, rendering young children more susceptible to infectious diseases, fever, gastroenteritis, and respiratory infections, all of which can result in fluid and electrolyte disturbances and fluid-volume deficit.
- Infants and children are at higher risk because of increased exposure to infections in a day care or nursery setting.

From James SR, Ashwill JW, Droske SC: *Nursing care of children*, ed 2. Philadelphia: WB Saunders, 2002, p 508.

    b. Degrees of dehydration[14]
        (1) Mild
            (a) 3% to 5% loss of body weight
            (b) Fluid volume loss less than 50 ml/kg
        (2) Moderate
            (a) 6% to 9% loss of body weight
            (b) Fluid volume loss less than 50-90 ml/kg
        (3) Severe
            (a) 10% or more loss of body weight
            (b) Fluid volume loss 100 ml/kg or greater
    c. Nursing assessment
        (1) Measure intake and output.
        (2) Assess skin color, temperature, and turgor.
        (3) Assess perfusion.
            (a) Vital signs
                (i) Rapid, weak, thready pulse
                (ii) Increased respiratory rate
                (iii) Decreased blood pressure
        (4) May be irritable, lethargic, confused; infant cry may be high pitched and weak
    d. Treatment (see Box 13-6)
        (1) Correct imbalance.
        (2) Treat underlying cause.

■ BOX 13-6
■ **MAINTENANCE FLUID REQUIREMENTS AND MINIMUM URINE OUTPUT**

Daily Fluid Requirements by Body Weight
≤10 kg:	100 ml/kg
10-20 kg:	1000 ml + 50 ml/kg for each additional kilogram between 10 and 20 kg
20+ kg:	1500 ml + 20 ml/kg for each additional kilogram over 20 kg

Minimum Urine Output by Age/Group
Infants and toddlers:	>2-3 ml/kg/hr
Preschoolers and young school-age children:	> 1-2 ml/kg/hr
School-age children and adolescents:	0.5-1 ml/kg/hr

From James SR, Ashwill JW, Droske SC: *Nursing care of children,* ed 2. Philadelphia: WB Saunders, 2002, p 516.

C. Hypervolemia
  1. Infants and toddlers at increased risk
    a. Excessive IV fluid administration
    b. Increase in antidiuretic hormone and aldosterone being produced in response to stress of surgery
  2. Signs and symptoms
    a. Restlessness
    b. Increased activity
    c. Periorbital edema
      (1) Occurs before alterations in vital signs
      (2) May be more prominent on dependent side (side child is lying on)
    d. Tachycardia
    e. Dyspnea
      (1) Accompanied with grunting respirations and
      (2) Adventitious lung sounds
  3. Interventions
    a. Administer IV fluids using graduated fluid chamber (Soluset) or infusion pump
    b. Monitor intake and output
    c. If periorbital edema noted, decrease IV fluid rate.
    d. Notify physician.
D. Disturbances in acid–base balance
  1. Need to maintain pH between 7.35 and 7.45 (see Chapter 25)
    a. Crucial in order to maintain
      (1) Cellular function
      (2) Enzyme activity
      (3) Neuromuscular membrane potentials
    b. Respiratory system and kidney work to maintain pH within normal limits
    c. Respiratory system works rapidly
    d. Renal system works slower; 1 to 2 days
  2. To correct acidosis (pH below normal)
    a. Lungs will
      (1) Increase respiratory rate and depth
      (2) Remove carbon dioxide (CO_2)
      (3) Increase pH
    b. Kidneys will
      (1) Excrete hydrogen ions
      (2) Conserve bicarbonate
      (3) Increase pH
  3. To correct alkalosis (pH above normal)
    a. Lungs will
      (1) Decrease respiratory rate and depth
      (2) Decrease pH

      b. Kidneys will

        (1) Conserve hydrogen ions

        (2) Decrease pH

  4. Imbalance involving respiratory or metabolic mechanism

     a. Types of imbalances

       (1) Respiratory acidosis

         (a) Causes

           (i) Pulmonary disease

           (ii) Airway obstruction

           (iii) Respiratory failure

           (iv) CNS depression from sedation or anesthesia

         (b) Signs and symptoms

           (i) Increased heart rate

           (ii) Dysrhythmias

           (iii) Increased respiratory rate and depth

         (c) Treatment

           (i) Aimed at correcting ventilation defect

             [a] Oxygen

             [b] Intubation

             [c] Mechanical ventilation

             [d] Administration of sodium bicarbonate

       (2) Respiratory alkalosis

         (a) Causes

           (i) Hyperventilation

           (ii) Hypoxia

           (iii) Compensation from metabolic acidosis

           (iv) Sepsis

         (b) Signs and symptoms

           (i) Increased respiratory rate and depth

           (ii) Dysrhythmias

         (c) Treatment

           (i) Oxygen

           (ii) Rebreathing mask

           (iii) Mechanical ventilation

           (iv) Sedatives

       (3) Metabolic acidosis

         (a) Causes

           (i) Increased metabolic rates

             [a] Fever

             [b] Respiratory distress syndrome

             [c] Seizures

           (ii) Ketoacidosis

           (iii) Interference with normal metabolism

           (iv) Loss of bicarbonate

           (v) Acute and chronic renal failure

         (b) Signs and symptoms

           (i) Increased heart rate

           (ii) Dysrhythmias

           (iii) Cold, clammy skin (mild to moderate acidosis)

           (iv) Warm, dry skin (severe acidosis)

           (v) Changes in level of consciousness (from confusion to stupor to coma)

         (c) Treatment

           (i) Treat underlying cause.

           (ii) Sodium bicarbonate replacement

           (iii) Potassium replacement

           (iv) Mechanical ventilation

(4) Metabolic alkalosis
    (a) Causes
        (i) Volume depletion
    (b) Signs and symptoms
        (i) Dysrhythmias
        (ii) Increased heart rate
        (iii) Changes in level of consciousness (confusion to stupor)
        (iv) Muscular weakness
    (c) Treatment
        (i) Treat underlying cause.
        (ii) Administer fluids with sodium chloride and potassium.
        (iii) Isotonic saline
        (iv) Histamine H2 receptor antagonist (cimetidine) *Tagamet*

E. Body temperature
  1. Infants and children
    a. Heat loss occurs by
      (1) Evaporation—skin becomes wet; evaporative heat loss can occur.
      (2) Radiation—heat transfers from body surface to surfaces in room not in direct contact with body.
      (3) Conduction—air currents pass over skin.
        (a) Can be caused by cold diapers and blankets
      (4) Convection—heat loss at a surface caused by fluid flowing across at a lower temperature.
  2. Assessment of infants
    a. May exhibit mottling
      (1) Caused by immature temperature-regulating mechanism
  3. Measurement of temperature
    a. Methods
      (1) Axillary
        (a) For infants and children <4 to 6 years of age
        (b) For uncooperative, immunosuppressed, neurologically impaired
        (c) For patient who has undergone oral surgery
        (d) Reading is approximately 1 degree lower than the body's core temperature
      (2) Oral
        (a) For children >6 years of age
        (b) Avoid liquids 30 minutes prior to oral temperature assessment.
        (c) Inaccurate readings may be caused by oral intake, oxygen administration, nebulizer treatments, and crying
      (3) Rectal
        (a) Taken only when no other route is feasible
      (4) Digital
        (a) May be used for oral, axillary, or rectal readings
        (b) Disposable covers over probe prevent cross-contamination
      (5) Tympanic
        (a) Frequently used for pediatric patients
        (b) Provides quick measurement
        (c) Temperature correlates with oral and rectal readings.
        (d) Placing traction on pinna to expose tympanic membrane increases accuracy of reading.
    b. Documentation
      (1) Important to document method used to obtain reading
      (2) Provides health care professional with consistent measurement when evaluating fluctuations in temperature
  4. Hypothermia (a core temperature less than 36° C [96.8° F])
    a. Child has difficulty maintaining temperature.
      (1) Result of body being stressed from illness or injury

      b. Occurs rapidly in child because of
        (1) Increased body surface area
        (2) Decreased mass
        (3) Lack of insulating subcutaneous fat
        (4) Infants less than 6 months lack involuntary shivering mechanism
      c. Potential causes of hypothermia
        (1) Vasodilating anesthetic agents (halothane, isoflurane, enflurane)
        (2) Muscle relaxants
        (3) Environmental causes (cool environment of operating room)
        (4) Administration of cool IV fluids
      d. Danger to small child
        (1) Increased oxygen consumption
        (2) Increased vasoconstriction
          (a) Results in hypoxemia, hypoglycemia and metabolic acidosis
          (b) Depletes metabolic energy stores
          (c) Causes fluid and electrolyte imbalance
      e. Must be kept warm to minimize heat loss and prevent hypothermia
        (1) Body temperature decreases in operating room because of cooler temperatures
        (2) Room temperature should be maintained as warm as 85° F (29° C)
        (3) Continuous monitoring during anesthesia period
        (4) Other precautionary measures
          (a) Warm blankets
          (b) Warm air devices
          (c) Radiant heat lamps
          (d) Wrapping head
          (e) Heated humidification of inspired gases
          (f) Drapes must permit some evaporative heat loss to maintain equalization of body temperature.
          (g) Solutions should be warmed.
            (i) Skin preparations
            (ii) Irrigation solutions
   5. Hyperthermia (a core temperature greater than 38° C [100.4° F])
      a. Can see cases where core temperature greater than 104° F (40° C)
      b. Causes
        (1) Fever
        (2) Dehydration
        (3) Infection
        (4) Decrease in sweating from atropine administration
        (5) Environmental causes (warm operating room)
        (6) Excessive drapes
        (7) Medications that disturb temperature regulation such as general anesthetics (malignant hyperthermia [MH])
          (a) Refer to Chapter 28 for complete information on MH.
  F. Respiratory assessment
   1. High priority because of impact of ineffective ventilation on cardiac function
   2. Majority of cardiac arrhythmias and arrests related to respiratory failure
   3. Airway problems most common on emergence and immediate postoperative period
   4. Anatomic differences
      a. Large tongue in proportion to mouth size; potential for airway obstruction
      b. Shorter neck; potential for compromised airway and difficult intubation
      c. Normal narrowing of trachea at cricoid cartilage ring
        (1) Provides an anatomic cuff when tracheal intubation is used

(2) Cuffed endotracheal tubes not used for children under 9 years of age because of anatomic cuff

(3) Smaller endotracheal tube used to eliminate risk of stenosis

  d. Smaller airway opening

(1) Reduction in airway radius causes potential increase in airflow resistance.

(2) Small amount of mucous, edema, or foreign body may cause airway obstruction significant to compromise gas exchange.

  e. Infant is obligatory nose breather; difficult breathing through mouth.

  f. Infants and young children use abdominal muscles to inhale.

  g. Cartilage of larynx easily compressed

(1) Can cause narrowing of airway

(2) Occurs when neck is flexed or extended

(3) More susceptible to spasm

  h. Epiglottis is short, stiff, U-shaped.

(1) Difficult intubation

(2) Swelling narrows opening; potential for airway obstruction

  i. Tonsillar tissue normally enlarged until early school-age

  j. Rib cage

(1) Intercostal musculature poorly developed

(2) Accessory muscles do not contribute to inspiration.

(3) Child more dependent on effective movement of diaphragm for ventilation

5. Assessment

  a. Evaluation of skin color

  b. Respiratory rate (normally higher than adult)

  c. Pattern of breathing

  d. Depth of respirations

  e. Quality of breath sounds

6. Measurement—respirations

  a. Inform child of procedure; avoid excitement

  b. Observe respiratory rate and effort for one full minute.

  c. Evaluate quality and symmetry of chest movement.

  d. Allow infant or toddler to cry prior to performing comfort measures.

(1) Ensures deep breathing in child who cannot follow commands

(2) May initiate coughing if secretions are present

  e. Observe for signs of respiratory distress.

(1) Increased heart rate one of first signs

(2) Grunting

(3) Stridor

(4) Wheezing

    (a) Inspiratory

    (b) Expiratory

(5) Croupy cough

(6) Flared nostrils

(7) Sternal retractions

(8) Increased work of breathing

(9) Cyanosis

(10) Apneic periods

  f. Increased respiratory rate

(1) Response to respiratory distress is an increase in respiratory rate.

(2) Potential causes include

    (a) Respiratory distress

    (b) Excess fluid volume

    (c) Pain

    (d) Hypothermia

    (e) Elevated temperature

    g. Decreased respiratory rate

        (1) Potential causes include

            (a) Administration of anesthetic agents

            (b) Administration of opioids—decreased respiratory rate may be compensated by increased depth of respirations.

            (c) Pain

7. Abnormal respiratory findings

    a. Depressed respiratory rate

        (1) Causes

            (a) Anesthesia

            (b) Narcotic, barbiturate, sedative administration

            (c) Hypothermia

        (2) Signs and symptoms

            (a) Shallow, slow, or absent respirations

        (3) Nursing interventions

            (a) Stimulate patient.

            (b) Oxygen administration

            (c) Chin lift

            (d) Insertion of oral airway

            (e) Suction

            (f) Notify anesthesiologist, surgeon.

    b. Stridor

        (1) Definition

            (a) Shrill, harsh sound

            (b) Heard during inspiration, expiration, or both

            (c) Produced by air flowing through a narrowed segment of the respiratory tract

        (2) Causes

            (a) Tracheal irritation

            (b) Edema

        (3) Signs and symptoms

            (a) Crowing respirations

        (4) Nursing interventions

            (a) Administer humidified oxygen.

            (b) Elevate head of bed.

            (c) Notify anesthesiologist, surgeon.

            (d) Physician may order racemic epinephrine.

    c. Croup

        (1) Definition

            (a) Term used to describe a group of conditions

            (b) Characterized by inspiratory stridor, croupy cough, hoarseness, and varying degrees of respiratory distress

        (2) Causes

            (a) Irritation caused by intubation

            (b) Endotracheal tube too large

            (c) Traumatic or repeated intubations

            (d) Coughing with endotracheal tube in place

            (e) Change of patient position while intubated

            (f) Surgical procedure greater than 1 hour in duration

            (g) Surgical trauma

        (3) Signs and symptoms

            (a) Usually occur soon after extubation—usually within 1 hour

            (b) May intensify within 4 hours

            (c) Completely resolved in 24 hours

            (d) Signs

                (i) Stridor

                (ii) Thoracic retractions

                (iii) Hoarseness

     (iv) Crouplike cough

     (v) Varying degrees of obstruction cause varying degrees of distress

   (4) Nursing interventions

    (a) Humidified oxygen

    (b) Elevate head of bed.

    (c) Notify anesthesiologist, surgeon.

    (d) Physician may order racemic epinephrine; dexamethasone; reintubation if airway severely compromised; hydration.

    (e) Calm child.

     (i) Judicious use of narcotics

     (ii) Parental presence

    (f) Consider overnight admission; edema may rebound after administration of racemic epinephrine.

 d. Laryngospasm

  (1) Definition

   (a) Approximation of true vocal cords or both true vocal cords and false cords

  (2) Cause

   (a) Inadequate depth of anesthesia with sensory stimulation

    (i) Secretions

    (ii) Manipulation of airway

    (iii) Surgical stimulation

   (b) Irritant trigger

  (3) Signs and symptoms

   (a) Use of accessory muscles

    (i) Always auscultate lungs since "rocking motion of chest" may be misinterpreted.

   (b) Partial to complete obstruction

  (4) Nursing interventions

   (a) Administer 100% oxygen.

   (b) Continuous positive pressure by mask.

   (c) Notify anesthesiologist, surgeon; may administer muscle relaxants.

   (d) Remove stimulus.

   (e) Jaw thrust

 e. Bronchospasm

  (1) Causes

   (a) Preexisting airway disease (asthma)

   (b) Allergy, anaphylaxis

   (c) Histamine release

   (d) Aspiration

   (e) Mucous plug

   (f) Foreign body

   (g) Pulmonary edema

  (2) Signs and symptoms

   (a) Increased respiratory rate

   (b) May have mild, moderate, or severe dyspnea

   (c) Intercostal retractions

   (d) Inspiratory and expiratory wheezing

  (3) Nursing interventions

   (a) Administer oxygen.

   (b) Suction secretions; remove foreign body.

   (c) Notify anesthesiologist, surgeon.

   (d) Physician may order

    (i) Inhaled bronchodilators (nebulized albuterol or metaproterenol)

    (ii) Terbutaline

■ TABLE 13-5
■ ■ Normal Vital Signs by Age

Age	Temperature*		Pulse rate (beats/min)	Respiratory Rate (breaths/min)	Blood Pressure (mm Hg)
	Degrees Fahrenheit	Degrees Celsius			
Newborn	96.8-99 (axillary)	36-37.2 (axillary)	120-160	30-60	Systolic: 46-92 Diastolic: 38-71
3 yr	97.5-98.6 (axillary)	36.4-37 (axillary)	80-125	20-30	Systolic: 72-110 Diastolic: 40-73
10 yr	97.5-98.6 (oral)	36.4-37 (oral)	70-110**	16-22	Systolic: 83-121 Diastolic: 45-79
16 yr	97.5-98.6 (oral)	36.4-37 (oral)	55-90	15-20	Systolic: 93-131† Diastolic: 49-85

*The normal range of the child's temperature will depend on the method used. Temperatures exhibit circadian rhythms at all ages.
**After age 12 yr, a boy's pulse is 5 beats/min slower than a girl's.
†After age 14 yr, blood pressure in boys is higher than in girls.
From James SR, Ashwill JW, Droske SC: *Nursing care of children*, ed 2. Philadelphia: WB Saunders, 2002, p 235.

          (iii) Epinephrine
          (iv) Antihistamine
           (v) Dexamethasone
          (vi) Support ventilation; reintubation
       (e) Consider overnight admission
    f. Airway obstruction
      (1) Causes
        (a) Tongue
        (b) Soft tissue edema
        (c) Retained packs, sponges
      (2) Signs and symptoms
        (a) Use of accessory muscles
        (b) Nasal flaring
        (c) Abdominal, diaphragmatic contractions
        (d) Decrease in inhaled air
      (3) Nursing interventions
        (a) Administer oxygen.
        (b) Chin lift
        (c) Suction.
        (d) Notify anesthesiologist, surgeon.
G. Cardiovascular assessment
  1. Vital signs
    a. Measure vital body functions
    b. Provide basis for decisions concerning overall health of child
    c. Vary depending on state of the child (see Table 13-5)
      (1) Resting vital signs (sleeping)
      (2) Awake vital signs (crying)
  2. Anatomy
    a. Chest wall thin in infants and young children
      (1) Less subcutaneous fat and muscle tissue than older child
      (2) Potential to auscultate innocent murmurs
  3. Heart rate
    a. Regulated by autonomic nervous system
    b. Increased heart rate results in increase in cardiac output.
    c. Decreased heart rate results in decreased cardiac output.

4. Electrocardiogram (ECG) monitoring
   a. T waves in infants much larger because electrodes are situated much closer to the heart
   b. May be same size as QRS complex
   c. Accurate assessment necessary to avoid erroneous or double counting
   d. Monitor in lead II for best P wave configuration
   e. Lead placement
      (1) Place on extremities to decrease artifact from breathing.
      (2) Do not place leads on bony prominence.
      (3) To decrease potential of trauma on fragile ribs, snap leads to electrodes before placing on child.
5. Measurement of pulse
   a. Apical pulse rate recommended for infants and children <2 years of age
   b. Assess prior to administering medications.
   c. Inform child of procedure.
   d. Allow child to play with stethoscope.
   e. Radial pulse may be used for children >2 years of age.
6. Measurement of blood pressure
   a. Choose appropriate cuff size.
      (1) Based on midpoint limb circumference
      (2) Inappropriate size will cause blood pressure to be artificially elevated or decreased.
   b. Measure in same extremity with patient in same position for increased consistency.
   c. Inform child of procedure.
7. Assessment findings
   a. Cyanosis, tachypnea
      (1) Sign of impending respiratory failure
      (2) Indication of cardiovascular compromise and possible hemodynamic instability
   b. Tachycardia
      (1) Normal method of increasing cardiac output
      (2) Possible causes include
         (a) Decreased perfusion caused by impending shock
         (b) Elevated temperature
         (c) Pain
         (d) Early respiratory distress
         (e) Administration of medications (atropine, morphine, epinephrine)
   c. Bradycardia
      (1) Of great concern in pediatric patient
      (2) Possible causes include
         (a) Respiratory distress (late sign)
         (b) Hypoxia
         (c) Vagal response
         (d) Increased intracranial pressure
         (e) Administration of Prostigmin *(neostigmine)*
   d. Hypertension
      (1) Possible causes include
         (a) Excess intravascular fluid
         (b) Carbon dioxide retention
         (c) Pain
         (d) Increased intracranial pressure
         (e) Administration of medications such as ketamine, epinephrine
   e. Hypotension
      (1) Possible causes include
         (a) Anesthetic agents such as halothane, isoflurane, enflurane

(b) Administration of opioids

(c) Late sign of shock

H. Postoperative assessment

1. Airway (refer to respiratory assessment section in this chapter for in-depth discussion)

   a. Respiratory rate

      (1) Pattern, depth, and quality of breath sounds

   b. Assess breath sounds.

   c. Assess respiratory effort.

      (1) Observe for dyspnea, tachypnea, wheezing, use of accessory muscles of ventilation, persistent coughing accompanied by frothy secretions.

      (2) Tachypnea is often the first sign of respiratory distress in infant.

      (3) Support airway.

      (4) Increase oxygen delivery (humidified).

      (5) Bag-valve mask

      (6) Prepare for possible endotracheal intubation.

2. Breathing

   a. Monitor oxygen saturation level.

   b. Listen

      (1) Snoring indicates possible obstruction from the tongue.

         (a) Chin lift or jaw thrust maneuver

         (b) Place on side.

         (c) Position sitting up with tongue falling forward.

      (2) Gurgling indicates possible secretions.

         (a) Suction.

3. Circulation, perfusion

   a. Evaluate heart rate.

      (1) Assess ECG rate and rhythm.

   b. Assess distal perfusion (palpation of peripheral pulses).

   c. Evaluate blood pressure.

   d. Assess skin color.

4. Check dressing if present.

   a. Note and record amount of drainage if present.

   b. Reinforce if necessary.

   c. Inspect areas underneath bed linens to identify potential bleeding sites.

5. Assess for bleeding in areas without dressing.

   a. Throat following tonsillectomy, oral, dental procedures

   b. Genitourinary area

6. Inspect IV site.

   a. Secure IV by wrapping area with gauze to prevent removal by infant, toddler, or small child.

   b. Assess and regulate infusion rate.

7. Assess skin color and integrity.

   a. Observe for any abnormalities that may not have been present preoperatively (e.g., scratches, bruises).

   b. Wash antiseptic from skin (e.g., Betadine).

8. Assess level of consciousness.

   a. Reactive, unreactive, restless, responsive, combative, cooperative, and so forth

   b. Restrain if necessary.

   c. Pad side rails to prevent injury.

9. Pain

   a. Myths

      (1) Children do not feel pain.

      (2) Children will not remember having pain.

      (3) A child is not in pain if he or she can be distracted or is sleeping.

      (4) A child can tolerate pain better than an adult can.

      (5) Medication should not be given to a child unless he or she exhibits obvious signs of pain.

      (6) A child cannot tell you where it hurts.

      (7) It is best to medicate children using the intramuscular route.

      (8) Addiction is a dangerous side effect of pain management in the pediatric patient.

b. Physiologic changes

    (1) Observe for

      (a) Increased heart rate

      (b) Increased blood pressure

      (c) Increased respiratory rate

      (d) Decreased oxygen saturation

      (e) Flushed skin

      (f) Restlessness

      (g) Sweating

      (h) Dilated pupils

    (2) Above physiologic changes are mimicked when child exhibits fear and anxiety.

    (3) Assess further to determine cause of physiologic changes.

c. Assessment

    (1) Assess according to developmental level (see Box 13-7).

    (2) Consider child's previous pain experiences.

      (a) Obtain history from parent, child.

      (b) Identify child's normal response to pain.

      (c) Identify child's normal words to communicate pain.

    (3) Assessment tools

      (a) Used to obtain more objective data related to pain assessment

      (b) Types

        (i) Self-report

        (ii) Behavioral instruments

      (c) Benefits

        (i) Gives child an effective means to communicate the pain he or she is feeling.

        (ii) Allows consistent means for child to express pain level

      (d) Examples

        (i) Oucher or Faces pain-rating scale

          [a] Consists of drawings or pictures of faces ranging from smiling to crying

        (ii) Numeric scale

          [a] Usually a line with numbers (0 to 10) with 0 meaning no pain and 10 meaning the worst possible pain

        (iii) Poker chip tool

          [a] Uses four poker chips, with each chip representing a little bit of pain; child is asked to take as many chips as he or she has pain

        (iv) Word Graphic Rating Scale

      (a) Uses descriptive words on a scale; child is asked to identify the degree of pain

d. Postoperative pain (see Box 13-8)

    (1) Treatment plans begin preoperatively.

      (a) Age-appropriate education prior to procedure

      (b) Discussion of proposed plan

      (c) Hands-on play with medical equipment

    (2) Intraoperative treatment

      (a) Regional blocks

      (b) Analgesics administered intraoperatively

■ BOX 13-7
■ **PAIN ASSESSMENT ACCORDING TO DEVELOPMENTAL LEVEL**

Neonate and Infant
- Changes in facial expression, including frowns, grimaces, wrinkled brow, expression of surprise, and facial flinching
- Increases in blood pressure and heart rate and decrease in arterial saturation
- High-pitched, tense, harsh crying
- Generalized or total-body response in neonate and young infant that becomes more purposeful as the infant matures
- May thrash extremities; may exhibit tremors
- Older infants: rub painful area, pull away, or guard the involved part

Toddler
- Loud crying
- Verbalizes words that indicate discomfort ("ouch," "hurt," "boo-boo")
- Attempts to delay procedures perceived as painful
- Generalized restlessness
- Guards the site
- Touches painful areas
- May run from the nurse

Preschooler
- May think the pain is punishment for some deed or thought
- Crying, kicking
- Describe the location and intensity of pain (e.g., "ear hurts bad")
- Regression to earlier behaviors (loss of bladder and bowel control)
- Withdrawal
- Denies pain to avoid a possible injection
- May have been told to "be brave" and deny pain even though it is present

School-age Child
- Able to describe pain and quantify pain intensity
- Fears body harm
- Has an awareness of death
- Stiff body posture
- Withdrawal
- Procrastinates or bargains to delay procedure

Adolescent
- Perceives pain at a physical, emotional, and mental level
- Understands cause and effect
- Describes pain and quantifies pain intensity
- Increased muscle tension
- Withdrawal and decreased motor activity
- Uses words such as "sore," "ache," or "pounding" to describe pain

From James SR, Ashwill JW, Droske SC: *Nursing care of children*, ed 2. Philadelphia: WB Saunders, 2002, p 422.

    (3) Postanesthesia care unit (PACU)
        (a) Analgesics, opioid administration
           (i) Orally
          (ii) Intravenously, through existing line—intermittent or continuous infusion
         (iii) Combination therapy
             [a] Opioids, with acetaminophen or nonsteroidal antiinflammatory drugs
         (iv) As needed dosing not recommended—results in inadequate pain relief

■ BOX 13-8
■ **NURSING CARE OF THE CHILD IN PAIN**

Focused Assessment
Regardless of setting (in-patient, clinic, home), the nursing assessment for the child in pain begins in the same way if the child is verbal. The child is questioned to determine what word or words are used for pain. Then the parents are questioned as to cultural or spiritual beliefs or practices that might impact pain issues. The nurse should remember that parents are to be used as the first resource to help assess the child and the child's response to intervention. Then a pain history is taken from child and parent, including physical, emotional, or psychosocial factors that might affect the child in regard to pain.

The current pain is assessed as to onset, duration, location, intensity, and quality. An age-appropriate pain tool is used to assess the intensity of pain. The same tool is used consistently, and it becomes a part of the child's chart as a future reference. Behavioral and physiologic changes are noted also. If the child is preverbal or nonverbal, a behavioral assessment is completed along with use of an assessment tool designed for nonverbal children. Response to the interventions, pharmacologic and nonpharmacologic, is assessed again using pain tools, parents' input, and observation of behavioral and physiologic data.

Nursing Diagnosis: Acute pain related to physical or biologic factors: edema, disease process, infection, invasive procedure, surgery, trauma

Expected Outcomes: The child will experience a decrease in pain to an acceptable level, as evidenced by reduced pain level on an assessment tool, as well as demonstrate a relaxed body posture, decreased crying, fussiness, restlessness, and facial grimacing.
The child will return to the activity level experienced before the onset of pain.

Intervention	Rationale
1. Observe and document behavioral and physiologic signs of pain in the child. Note both verbal and nonverbal responses. Assess vital signs.	1. Assessment of pain in children is based on behavioral and physiologic changes. Children may have difficulty verbalizing pain. The nurse will have to depend on behavioral changes alone to assess infants and other children who are nonverbal or unable to communicate clearly. Physiologic changes vary in response to pain and should be evaluated together with a behavioral assessment.
2. Assess for other factors that might be affecting the child: separation, fear, anxiety, loss of control, as well as spiritual or cultural beliefs regarding pain.	2. The child's perception of pain and ultimate reaction to pain may be influenced by other factors.
3. Monitor pain based on the child's developmental stage.	3. Infants and children at each developmental level have their own unique way of reacting to and coping with pain.
4. Use a developmentally appropriate pain assessment tool. The tool should be a part of the child's chart for easy reference.	4. Infants and children may have difficulty communicating about their pain. Assessment tools provide more consistent, objective, and quantitative information.
5. Question the child if possible to assess the onset, duration, location, and type of pain and what type of pain relief measures works best.	5. Such factors will influence the choice of analgesic.
6. Note if the child's pain level is different when at rest, ambulating, playing, or during procedures.	6. Pain relief measures can be improved by a thorough understanding of cause and effect.

Continued

■ BOX 13-8 *Cont'd*
■ **NURSING CARE OF THE CHILD IN PAIN**

7. Implement nonpharmacologic pain reduction strategies:	7. Nonpharmacologic pain management strategies can enhance pharmacologic measures and should be implemented before administering analgesics.
a. Distraction	**a.** Distraction interrupts the transmission of pain.
b. Relaxation techniques	**b.** Relaxation is also thought to interrupt pain.
c. Cutaneous stimulation, such as massage or warm or cold compresses	**c.** Cutaneous stimulation blocks pain transmission.
d. Quiet, calm environment	**d.** A quiet, calm environment is more conducive to rest and sleep, which enhance the effects of analgesia.
e. Repositioning	**e.** A change in position may relieve pressure or provide for a more relaxed, comfortable body.
f. Decreased environmental noise and light	**f.** A quiet, comfortable environment can have a soothing, relaxing effect on the child and parent.

From James SR, Ashwill JW, Droske SC: *Nursing care of children*, ed 2. Philadelphia: WB Saunders, 2002, pp 434-435.

(v) Patient-controlled analgesia (PCA)
   [a] Allows for timely administration of medication, improving analgesic efficacy
   [b] Allows for the patient to participate in self-care
   [c] Patients individually selected for PCA based on manual dexterity and conceptual understanding
   (b) Assess at regular intervals.
   (c) Assess during vital sign checks.
   (d) Whenever possible, administer medications through a noninvasive route, orally, or an existing IV line.
(4) Nursing considerations
   (a) Administer analgesics as prescribed.
   (b) Avoid waiting until child experiences severe pain before medicating.
   (c) Avoid palpating surgical site unless necessary.
   (d) Medicate prior to performing nursing activities that could be painful (dressing change, deep breathing, ambulation).
   (e) Involve parents in process.
(5) Nonpharmacologic interventions for pain management
   (a) Provide distraction (playing, singing, taking a deep breath, blowing bubbles, watching television, reading).
   (b) Provide relaxation opportunities (hold baby in comfortable position, rock, assist child to get into a comfortable position, ask child to take a deep breath and hold it-then to go "limp as a rag doll" while exhaling slowly).
   (c) Behavioral contracting
      (i) Set up a reward system using stars or tokens (for younger children).
      (ii) Use a written contract (for older children) that includes measurable goals and identified rewards.
   (d) Guided imagery (child describes the details of a pleasurable experience; concentrates on pleasurable experience during painful procedure)
   e. Medications (see Chapter 29)

10. Thermoregulation
   a. Assess temperature on admission, every hour, and at discharge (may vary according to facility policy).
      (1) Hypothermia
         (a) Implement warming measures.
      (2) Hyperthermia
         (a) Potential for malignant hyperthermia
I. Discharge (see Box 13-9)
   1. Process
      a. Planning usually begins before admission.
      b. Encourage parental participation in child's care
      c. Encourage child to participate in own care based on physical and developmental abilities.
         (1) Involvement helps maintain and improve coordination, muscle tone, and circulation.
         (2) Fosters positive self-esteem and self-control
         (3) Assists child to view hospitalization in a more positive manner
      d. Seek child's input when developing plan of care.
   2. Criteria
      a. Facility-specific criteria
   3. Instructions
      a. Procedure-specific
      b. Anesthesia
         (1) Written instruction on how to contact anesthesia department should questions arise regarding anesthesia-related concerns or complications.
         (2) Two adults to accompany child on discharge; one to drive and one to attend to needs of the child
         (3) Child safely secured in restraint device appropriate for age
   4. Nurse's role (see Table 13-6)
      a. Clarify misconceptions for both parent and child.
      b. Encourage child to talk about experience.

■ BOX 13-9
■ **INFORMATION FOR DISCHARGE**

After assessing the family's knowledge, provide the information families need to know to help the child's transition from hospital to home:
- Information about the illness or trauma and expected outcomes. Tell the parents when they should consult the primary care physician or nurse.
- Medications or treatments to be given at home and information about times, route, side effects, and any special care to be taken when giving the medication. Providing written information is valuable.
- Information about any special nutritional needs
- Specific activities the child may, may not, and sometimes should participate in
- The date when the child may return to school
- The date to bring the child back to the hospital, clinic, or office for follow-up care
- Information about any referral agency needed for the child or family
- The unit phone number and primary nurse's name

Explain, demonstrate, and request a return demonstration of any treatments or procedures that will be done at home. This teaching should be an ongoing process and not left until the time of discharge, because learning takes place at different rates.

From James SR, Ashwill JW, Droske SC: *Nursing care of children*, ed 2. Philadelphia: WB Saunders, 2002, p 325.

■ TABLE 13-6
■ ■ Common Nursing Diagnoses for Pediatric Patients Undergoing Operative or Invasive Procedures

Diagnosis	Risk Factors, Defining Characteristics, and Related Factors	Expected Outcome
Risk for infection	Risk factors —immature immune response —poor nutritional state —thin epidermis —small surface area —immature ability to handle respiratory secretions —inability to control bowels and bladder functions —surgical incision —anesthesia —invasive monitoring —central catheters —total parenteral nutrition infusion —ostomies —open wounds —blood sampling —traumatic delivery —trauma or accident	The child does not experience a wound infection.
Risk for impaired skin integrity	Risk factors —thin epidermis —decrease in normal skin lubricants —decrease in subcutaneous fat —surgical incision —infection —poor nutritional state —drainage in contact with the skin —open wounds —ostomies —invasive monitoring —application of extraneous objects such as electrosurgical dispersive electrode pneumatic tourniquet, tape, casting material, adhesive drapes —application of chemical agents such as prepping solutions	The child's skin integrity is maintained.
Risk for fluid volume deficit	Risk factors —Large body surface area in relation to size —immature kidney function —increased fluid needs due to increased percentage of body weight in water (infant's body weight 80% water compared with adult 50% to 60% of body weight in water) —inability to concentrate urine —increased volume of gastrointestinal secretions —surgery —anesthesia —exposed epidermis leading to increased evaporative water losses —poor intravenous access —narrow margin between adequate hydration and fluid overload	Adequate fluid volume is maintained. —The kidneys remain perfused and output is 1 ml/kg/hour. —Blood pressure is maintained. —Vital signs remain stable. —Blood urea nitrogen and creatinine values are within normal limits. —The child maintains body temperature.

■ TABLE 13-6 *Cont'd*
■ ■ **Common Nursing Diagnoses for Pediatric Patients Undergoing Operative or Invasive Procedures**

Diagnosis	Risk Factors, Defining Characteristics, and Related Factors	Expected Outcome
	—increased losses from the gastrointestinal tract due to nasogastric tubes and ostomies —increased fluid losses from seizures, fever, crying, time spent undergoing ventilation, suctioning and nothing-by-mouth (NPO) status	
Risk for hypothermia during the procedure period	Risk factors —thin epidermis —large body surface in relation to size —thin layer of subcutaneous fat —chemical thermogenesis in brown adipose tissue —exposure of the epidermis to the outside environment —increased evaporative water loss —exposure of internal organs —exposure to cold intravenous fluids and skin preparation solutions —age (neonate) —low body weight	The child's body temperature is maintained within normal limits throughout the procedure period.
Risk for ineffective breathing patterns	Risk factors —age (neonate or infant) —chest and abdominal operative procedures —decreased ability to handle oral secretions —large size of infant head compared with the adult head (attaining a good "stiff" position for alignment of the airway axes is more difficult) —large tongue size of the infant compared with the adult tongue (laryngoscopy and visualization of the larynx are more difficult) —position of the vocal cords in the infant (makes the airway seem anterior, resulting in difficulty when trying to visualize the larynx with laryngoscopy) —difference in metabolic requirements and oxygen consumption in neonates and infants (a neonate may require 6 ml/kg/minutes of oxygen compared with 3 ml/kg/minute in an adult) —presence of fetal hemoglobin during the first 6 months of life (fetal hemoglobin has more affinity for oxygen, thus allowing more oxygen to be carried to the tissues but less to be released at the tissue level) —Nonshivering thermogenesis to produce body heat (can be detrimental because oxygen consumption and carbon dioxide production increase) —alveolar minute ventilation in the neonate, which is twice that of an adult, requires an increased ventilatory rate to meet metabolic demands for oxygen consumption	The child's respirations are adequate to maintain sufficient oxygen to meet cellular requirements.
Risk for injury (tissue burn) related to electrosurgery	Risk factors —use of electrosurgery generator not equipped with contact quality monitoring —use of dry adhesive return electrode	The patient is free from injury (tissue burns) related to the use of electrosurgery.

Continued

■ TABLE 13-6 *Cont'd*
■ ■ Common Nursing Diagnoses for Pediatric Patients Undergoing Operative or Invasive Procedures

Diagnosis	Risk Factors, Defining Characteristics, and Related Factors	Expected Outcome
	—use of noncontact quality monitoring return patient electrode —use of high power settings —coiling of active and return electrodes —contact of active and return electrodes with metal that is attached to the patient or patient drapes	
Risk for injury (ignition incident) secondary to the use of electrosurgery, laser, or other heat source	Risk factors —oxygen-enriched environment —use of noncuffed endotracheal tube —high power settings of the electrosurgical generator —accumulation of smoke plume at the operative site	The patient is free from injury (ignition incident) related to the use of electrosurgery, laser, and other heat sources.
Alteration in comfort: pain	Defining characteristics —verbal or nonverbal communication of pain —guarding or protective behavior —self-focusing —narrowed focus as evidenced by an altered perception of time, withdrawal from social contact, and impaired thought processes —moaning and crying —facial mask of pain as evidenced by a lack of luster in the eyes, a "beaten" appearance, fixed or scattered movement, and facial grimace —alteration in muscle tone, which may range from listless to rigid —autonomic response (diaphoresis, increased blood pressure and pulse, pupillary dilation, and increased or decreased respiratory rate) Related factors —procedure —lack of knowledge concerning pain management techniques	The child's comfort level is sufficient throughout the procedure period.
Fear	Defining characteristics —describes or acts out the focus of perceived threat or danger —describes or acts out feelings of dread, nervousness, or concern about impending surgery, hospitalization, and intrusive procedures —verbalizes an expectation of danger to the self —increased questioning or information seeking —restless behavior —narrowed focus of attention that progresses to fixed attention on the impending event —diaphoresis —increased heart rate —increased respiratory rate —crying —clinging to a parent or other significant person	The child exhibits signs of control and expresses feelings (verbal or nonverbal) of security during the operative or invasive procedure period.

Continued

■ TABLE 13-6 *Cont'd*
■ ■ **Common Nursing Diagnoses for Pediatric Patients Undergoing Operative or Invasive Procedures**

Diagnosis	Risk Factors, Defining Characteristics, and Related Factors	Expected Outcome
	—combative behavior toward caregiver	
	—decreased ability to express concerns and describe sensations	
	Related factors—lack of cognitive understanding concerning hospitalization, surgery, and intrusive procedures	
	—fantasy thoughts	
	—active imagination	
	—sensed parental fear or anxiety	
	—perceived inability to control event	

From Phippen ML, Wells MP: *Patient care during operative and invasive procedures.* Philadelphia, WB Saunders, 2000, pp 663-665.

    c. Review necessary information, including, but not limited to
       (1) Necessary physical care
          (a) Encourage child and/or parent participation.
          (b) Return demonstration assists in verifying child and/or parental understanding.
       (2) Necessary equipment and/or supplies needed to care for child (crutches, dressings, etc.)
       (3) Instructions on activities of daily living (play activities, sports, return to school)
       (4) Diet
       (5) Medication administration
       (6) Potential complications
          (a) Expected
          (b) Unexpected
       (7) Emergency contact information
       (8) Follow-up appointment with physician
       (9) Necessary home health agency referrals
       (10) Assessment of parental capability to meet child's needs
    d. Reinforce physician's instructions.
    e. Allow time for questions and answers.
    f. Provide written instructions.
  5. Postoperative telephone evaluation
    a. Usually performed the day after surgery
    b. Assess patient's progress.
    c. Identify postoperative complications.
    d. Evaluate need for referral to physician.
    e. Answer questions or concerns.
    f. Reinforce discharge instructions.

BIBLIOGRAPHY

1. Anthony D, Jasinski DM: Postoperative nausea and vomiting in children. *J PeriAnesth Nurs* 15(6):401-407, 2000.
2. Asher ME: Evidence-based practice, part 2: Reliability and validity of selected acute pain instruments. *J PeriAnesth Nurs* 16(1):35-40, 2001.
3. Barnes S: Perioperative considerations for the child with an upper respiratory tract infection. *J PeriAnesth Nurs* 15(6):392-396, 2000.
4. Behrman RE, Kliegman RM, Jenson HB: *Nelson textbook of pediatrics,* ed 16. Philadelphia: WB Saunders, 2000.

5. Burden N, DeFazio Quinn DM, O'Brien D, et al: *Ambulatory surgical nursing,* ed 2. Philadelphia: WB Saunders.

6. Carpenter KH: Developing a pediatric patient/parent hospital preparation program. *AORN J* 67(5):1042, 1045-1046, 1998.

7. Cassady JF, Wysocki TT, Miller KM, et al: Use of a preanesthetic video for facilitation of parental education and anxiolysis before pediatric ambulatory surgery. *Anesth Analg* 88(2):246-250, 1999.

8. Collett L, D'Errico DO: Suggestions on meeting ASPAN standards in a pediatric setting. *J PeriAnesth Nurs* 15(6):386-391, 2000.

9. Fina DK, Lopas LJ, Stagnone JH, et al: Preparing for surgery: Providing the details. *J PeriAnesth Nurs* 16(1):31-32, 2001.

10. Fortner PA: Preoperative patient preparation: Psychological and educational aspects. *Semin Perioper Nurs* 7(1):3-9, 1998.

11. Goldstein NA, Fatima M, Campbell TF, et al: Child behavior and quality of life before and after tonsillectomy and adenoidectomy. *Arch Otolaryngol Head Neck Surg* 128(7): 770-775, 2002.

12. Hamers JPH, Abu-Saad HH, Geisler FEA, et al: Sedation/analgesia for diagnostic and therapeutic procedures in children. *J PeriAnesth Nurs* 15(6):415-422, 2000.

13. Hollinger I: Current trends in pediatric anesthesia. *Mt Sinai J Med* 69(1,2):51-54, 2002.

14. James SR, Ashwill JW, Droske SC: *Nursing care of children: Principles and practice.* ed 2. Philadelphia: WB Saunders, 2002.

15. Kain ZN, Caldwell-Andrews AA, Wang SM, et al: Parental intervention choices for children undergoing repeated surgeries. *Anesth Analg* 96(4):970-975, 2003.

16. Kain ZN, Caldwell-Andrews A, Wang SM: Psychological preparation of the parent and pediatric surgical patient. *Anesthesiol Clin North America* 20(1):29-44, 2002.

17. Kain ZN, Mayes LC, Wang SM, et al: Parental presence and a sedative premedicant for children undergoing surgery: A hierarchical study. *Anesthesiology* 92(4): 925-927, 2000.

18. Kristensson-Hallstrom I: Parental participation in pediatric surgical care. *AORN J* 71(5):1021-1024, 2000.

19. Lamontagne LL, Hepwoth JT, Salisbury MH: Anxiety and postoperative pain in children who undergo major orthopedic surgery. *Appl Nurs Res* 14(3):119-124, 2001.

20. Lamontagne LL: Children's coping with surgery: A process-oriented perspective. *J Pediatr Nurs* 15(5):307-312, 2000.

21. Lesperance MM, D'Errico C: Efficiency of the operating room vs the short procedure room: squeezing the balloon. *Arch Otolaryngol Head Neck Surg* 129(4):427-428, 2003.

22. Lucier MM, Brisson D: Extubation of pediatric patients by PACU nurses. *J PeriAnesth Nurs* 18(2):91-95, 2003.

23. Lucier MM, Brisson D: The effect of paracetamol, fentanyl, and systematic assessments on children's pain after tonsillectomy and adenoidectomy. *J PeriAnesth Nurs* 14(6):357-366, 1999.

24. Mazurek Melnyk B: Intervention studies involving parents of hospitalized young children: An analysis of the past and future recommendations. *J Pediatr Nurs* 15(1):4-13, 2000.

25. Merkel S, Malviya S: Postoperative pain management: Morphine versus ketorolac. *J PeriAnesth Nurs* 17(1):30-42, 2002.

26. Mills MD: Tonsillectomy and adenoidectomy pathway plan of care for the pediatric patient in day surgery. *J PeriAnesth Nurs* 12(6):387-395, 1997.

27. Moline BM: Separation and induction behaviors in children: Are parents good predictors? *J PeriAnesth Nurs* 15(1):6-11, 2000.

28. Munro H: Postoperative nausea and vomiting in children. *J PeriAnesth Nurs* 15(6): 401-407, 2000.

29. Odegard KC, Modest SA, Laussen PC: A survey of parental satisfaction during parent present induction of anaesthesia for children undergoing cardiovascular surgery. *Paediatr Anesth* 12(3):261-266, 2002.

30. Oldfield SJ: Parent-child patterns of coping. *J Child Health Care* 5(1):11-18, 2001.

31. Patel RI, Verghese ST, Hannallah RS, et al: Fast-tracking children after ambulatory surgery. *Anesth Analg* 93(5):918-922, 2001.

32. Phippen ML, Wells MP: Patient care during operative and invasive procedures. Philadelphia: WB Saunders, 2000.

33. Sandlin D: Pediatric pain, tools and assessment. *J PeriAnesth Nurs* 15(6):408-414, 2000.

34. Savedra MC, Tesler MD, Holzemer WL, et al: *Adolescent pediatric pain tool (APPT): Preliminary user's manual.* San Francisco: University of California, 1989.

35. Stephens BK, Barkey ME, Hall HR: Techniques to comfort children during stressful procedures. *Adv Mind Body Med* 15(1):49-60, 1999.

36. Summers S: Extubation of pediatric patients by PACU nurses. *J PeriAnesth Nurs* 18(2):91-95, 2003.

37. Tait AR, Voepel-Lewis T, Malviya S: Perianesthesia care of adult and pediatric strabismus surgery patients. *J PeriAnesth Nurs* 13(1):16-23, 1998.

38. Tweddell JS, Hoffman GM: Postoperative management in patients with complex congenital heart disease. *Semin Thorac Cardiovasc Surg Pediatr Card Surg Annu* 5(1):187-205, 2002.

39. VanDijk M, Peters JW, Bouwmeester NJ, et al: Are postoperative pain instruments use-

ful for specific groups of vulnerable infants? *Clin Perinatol* 29(3):469-491, 2002.

40. Voepel-Lewis T, Tait AR, Malviya S: Another option for pediatric preanesthesia education. *J PeriAnesth Nurs* 16(4):278-278, 2001.

41. Voepel-Lewis T, Malviya S: Nurses' attitudes toward parental visitation on the postanesthesia care unit. *J PeriAnesth Nurs* 12(1):2-6, 1997.

42. Wong D, editor, Wilson D, Hockenberry-Eaton M, et al: *Wong's essentials of pediatric nursing,* ed 6. St Louis: Mosby, 2001.

43. Zuwala R, Barber KR: Reducing anxiety in parents before and during pediatric anesthesia induction. *AANA J* 69(1):21-25, 2001.

14 The Adolescent Patient

DONNA M. DEFAZIO QUINN

OBJECTIVES

At the conclusion of this chapter the reader will be able to:

1. Identify three stressors associated with hospitalization.

2. List five nursing interventions used to approach the hospitalized adolescent.

3. Name five nursing interventions to communicate effectively with an adolescent.

4. Identify five educational strategies used to educate the adolescent.

5. Describe four signs that the nurse might observe that may indicate the adolescent is in pain.

I. Growth and development
  A. Definition
    1. Eleven to 21 years of age
    2. Transition from childhood to adulthood
      a. Biologic changes
      b. Psychosocial changes
    3. Three stages
      a. Early adolescence
      b. Middle adolescence
      c. Late adolescence
  B. Early adolescence
    1. Ten to 13 years of age
    2. Period of growth acceleration
      a. Increase in appetite in response to rapid growth
    3. Biologic development
      a. Girls
        (1) Development of breast tissue
        (2) Begin to put on fat
        (3) Slightly taller and heavier than boys
        (4) Beginning of hair growth
          (a) Pubic
          (b) Axillary
        (5) Menarche
      b. Boys
        (1) Enlargement of testes
        (2) Gynecomastia
        (3) Spermatogenesis
    4. Motor development
      a. Increase in gross muscle mass
      b. Increase in fine motor coordination
      c. Prone to ligament tears
      d. Awkward, gangly period

5. Psychosocial development
   a. Erikson
      (1) Stage of identity versus role confusion (12 to 18 years of age)
         (a) Corresponds to Freud's genital stage
         (b) Characterized by rapid physical changes
         (c) Adolescents become preoccupied with appearance (how they look to others).
   b. Freud
      (1) Genital stage (age 12 and older)
         (a) Begins with puberty
         (b) Reproductive system and sex hormones mature
         (c) Genital organs become major source of sexual tensions and pleasures.
         (d) Also period of forming relationships and preparing for marriage
   c. Other characteristics
      (1) Shy, awkward
      (2) Adjusting to middle school
      (3) Move from operational thinking to formal, logical operations
         (a) Ability to manipulate abstractions
         (b) Able to reason from principles
         (c) Able to weigh multiple points of view according to varying criteria
         (d) Able to think about the process of thinking
      (4) More at ease with same sex
         (a) Tend to move away from family
         (b) Increased activity with peers
         (c) Conformity
         (d) Cliques
      (5) Increase in self-consciousness
         (a) Adolescents meticulous about their appearance
         (b) Feel everyone is looking at them
      (6) Low self-esteem
      (7) Increase in rebellious behavior
      (8) Increase in independence
      (9) Increase in sexual interest
         (a) Interest is greater than sexual activity.
         (b) Often have questions about sexual changes they are experiencing
C. Middle adolescence
   1. Fourteen to 16 years of age
   2. Biologic development
      a. Girls
         (1) Increase in height
         (2) Increase in breast size
         (3) Increase in growth of pubic hair
         (4) Sexual maturation occurs.
         (5) Develop hips
         (6) Growth acceleration declines.
         (7) Appetite decreases.
      b. Boys
         (1) Change in voice
         (2) Larynx enlarges.
         (3) Muscle mass enlarges followed by increase in strength.
         (4) Widening of shoulders
         (5) Growth of facial hair
         (6) Rapid increase in height
         (7) Increase in appetite

        (8) Increase in size of genitalia

        (9) Gynecomastia decreases.

    c. Both sexes

       (1) Increase in acne

       (2) Development of sweat glands (increase in body odor)

       (3) Completion of dentition

       (4) Sensory and language development complete

       (5) Capacity of cardiovascular pump increases

          (a) Heart size doubles.

          (b) Blood pressure, blood volume, and hematocrit increase.

       (6) Lung capacity doubles.

       (7) Physiologic increase in sleepiness

  3. Motor development

    a. Increase in physical endurance

    b. Increased skill in sports

    c. Increase in fine and gross muscle coordination

    d. Increase in fine motor skill activities

  4. Psychosocial development

    a. Increased conflicts with parents

    b. Mood swings

       (1) Impulsive

       (2) Impatient

       (3) Narcissistic

       (4) Moody

    c. Tests established limits

    d. Privacy very important

    e. Peer group very important

    f. Abstract thoughts increase.

       (1) Tend to question and analyze everything

       (2) Become more self-centered

  5. Sexual development

    a. Sexual experimentation begins.

    b. Degree of sexual activity varies.

    c. Begin to sort out sexual identity

       (1) Beliefs regarding love, honesty, and propriety

    d. Choose either celibacy, monogamy. or polygamous experimentation

    e. Knowledgeable regarding risk of pregnancy, AIDS, and other sexually transmitted diseases

       (1) Knowledge does not necessarily control behavior.

  6. Development of self-concept

    a. Period of experimentation

       (1) Peers less important

       (2) Change style of dress

       (3) May change group of friends

    b. Deal with inner turmoil

  7. Development of relationships

    a. Parental relationship strained

       (1) May become distant

       (2) Dating may become source of conflicts.

    b. Physical attractiveness still important

    c. Popularity is critical for peer relationships and self-esteem.

    d. Begin to identify career path

       (1) Life skills

       (2) Opportunities

    e. Positive role models crucial at this stage of development

D. Late adolescence

  1. Seventeen to 20 years of age or beyond

    2. Biologic development

      a. Growth slows.

      b. Physically mature

      c. Structure and reproductive growth almost complete

      d. No neurologic developmental changes apparent

      e. Cardiopulmonary capacity relatively mature

    3. Psychosocial development

      a. Aware of own strength and limitations

      b. Establishes own value system

      c. Cognition tends to be less self-centered

      d. Ability to think abstractly

      e. Able to express thoughts and feelings about various aspects of life

        (1) Justice, patriotism, history

      f. Idealistic about love, social issues, ethics, and lifestyles

      g. Conformity less important

      h. More consistency of emotions

      i. Able to control anger

      j. Turbulence with parents decreases.

      k. Prepares to leave home

      l. Social relationships more mature

    4. Sexual development

      a. More commitment to intimate relationships

      b. Form stable relationships and attachments

      c. More realistic concept of partner's role

    5. Self-concept

      a. More secure body image and gender-role definition

      b. Sexual identity secured

      c. Self-esteem increases.

        (1) More stable body image

        (2) Comfortable with physical growth

      d. Social roles defined and articulated

        (1) Career decisions become pressing.

        (2) Self-concept increasingly tied to role in society (students, workers, parents)

    6. Relationships

      a. Separation from parents complete (emotional and physical)

      b. Gained independence from family

      c. Peer group not so important as individual friendships

      d. Relationships are characterized by giving and sharing.

      e. Testing possibility of permanent male–female relationship

II. Stressors associated with hospitalization

  A. Separation anxiety

    1. May or may not want parents involved

    2. May become more dependent on parents

    3. Separation from friends increases anxiety.

  B. Fear of injury or pain

    1. Fear how illness is viewed by peers

      a. Activity limitations

      b. Appearance

    2. May refuse to cooperate if treatment does not fit into lifestyle

    3. May project image of "calm and cool" even though they are terrified

    4. May question everything or appear confident in that they know it all

    5. Able to describe degree of pain

  C. Loss of control

    1. May resist dependence

    2. Want to be in control

    3. May react to loss of control with anger, withdrawal, uncooperativeness, and refusal to follow rules

■ BOX 14-1
■ **DEVELOPMENTAL GUIDELINES FOR WORKING WITH ADOLESCENTS IN EMERGENCIES**

- Preserve the adolescent's modesty; offer adolescents a choice as to whether they want their parents present when obtaining history and during the examination.
- Consider the legal issues regarding the right to privacy for pregnant adolescents and adolescents with sexually transmissible diseases.
- Provide an opportunity for questions.
- Listen to the adolescent's concerns nonjudgmentally and without belittling the young person.
- Developing a teasing relationship with an adolescent is often a temptation, but this has potential for harm—the adolescent is easily embarrassed.
- Explain procedures or treatments carefully and allow choices. Adolescents are capable of complex abstract thinking and can make intelligent and reasoned decisions about their own care.

From James SR, Ashwill JW, Droske SC: *Nursing care of children.* Philadelphia: WB Saunders, 2002, p 275.

    4. A planned procedure (scheduled surgery) allows a greater sense of control than an unplanned (emergency) procedure.
    5. Often feel isolated and unable to obtain adequate support
  D. Emergency admissions (see Box 14-1)
III. Interventions to minimize stress
  A. Preparation
    1. Give information about proposed procedure.
      a. Adolescent very anxious regarding self-image and identity
      b. Information will help to reduce psychological stress and elicit more cooperation.
        (1) Explain tests and procedures.
        (2) Provide information on how the adolescent will feel during certain tests and procedures.
        (3) Provide information regarding when results of tests will be known.
        (4) Discuss approximate length of time in each phase of hospitalization (preadmission, operating room, postanesthesia care unit [PACU], etc.)
        (5) Discuss impact of procedure on daily living (expected return to school, driving, etc.).
        (6) Adolescent more accepting of information provided by health care professional rather than parent
      c. May be concerned regarding cause of illness (need for surgery); provide necessary information
    2. Allow choices when possible.
      a. Induction of anesthesia
      b. Parental presence
    3. Intraoperative
      a. Monitoring devices that will be applied (electrocardiogram [ECG], pulse oximeter, blood pressure [BP])
      b. Sensations from anesthetics administered
      c. Endotracheal intubation after "asleep" or loss of consciousness obtained
      d. Only surgical area exposed; respect adolescent's privacy
        (1) Sterile drapes applied
        (2) Only area exposed to staff view is operative area.
      e. Will remain unconscious throughout procedure; will not talk or do anything to cause them embarrassment

IV. Developmental approach to the hospitalized adolescent
  A. Nursing interventions
      1. Provide privacy.
      2. Avoid stereotyping adolescent as difficult and unmanageable.
      3. Adolescent reacts to not only information given, but also manner in which it is delivered.
      4. Encourage wear of normal street clothes when possible.
      5. Encourage questions regarding appearance and the effects of the current illness and surgery on the adolescent's future.
      6. Incorporate scientific and medical terminology into explanations and preparations for procedures.
      7. Provide adolescent with body outlines, diagrams, or other graphics when explaining procedures; include rationale.
      8. If possible, utilize special area on unit reserved for adolescents.
      9. Introduce adolescent to other adolescents on unit.
      10. Encourage peer communication if length of stay is prolonged.
          a. Telephone
          b. Visitation by peers
      11. Assist parents with communicating to adolescent (see Box 14-2).
          a. Offer support.
          b. Provide with growth and development information.
      12. Approach adolescent with caring, understanding, and acceptance.
  B. Cause and effect
      1. Puts into perspective why adolescents think and act the way they do
      2. Adolescent uses formal rules of logic and evidence to assess cause and effect.
      3. Understands why something happens the way it does
  C. Handling emotion
      1. Uses a range of modalities from sophisticated verbal or written expression to motoric activity

---

■ BOX 14-2
■ **GUIDELINES FOR COMMUNICATING WITH ADOLESCENTS**

Build a Foundation
- Spend time together.
- Encourage expression of ideas and feelings.
- Respect their views.
- Tolerate differences.
- Praise good points.
- Respect their privacy.
- Set a good example.

Communicate Effectively
- Give undivided attention.
- Listen, listen, listen.
- Be courteous, calm, and open-minded.
- Try not to overreact. If you do, take a break.
- Avoid judging and criticizing.
- Avoid the "third degree" of continuous questioning.
- Choose important issues when taking a stand.
- After taking a stand:
    - Think through all options.
    - Make expectations clear.

From James SR, Ashwill JW, Droske SC: *Nursing care of children*. Philadelphia: WB Saunders, 2002, p 130.

        2. May regress in behavior

        3. Thoughts, feelings, fears may be shared with friends, especially peers.

    D. Major fears and worries

        1. Uncertainty about self as a person

        2. Concerned about whether or not body, thought, and feelings are normal

        3. Nursing interventions

            a. Involve in decision making

            b. Give information sensitively.

            c. Explore tactfully what is known or unknown.

                (1) Fearful that nurse may think they are "dumb"

  V. Legal issues

    A. Consent of minors

        1. Governed by state laws

        2. Exemptions to parental consent for medical treatment

            a. Emancipated minors

                (1) Live away from home

                (2) No longer subject to parental control

                (3) Economically self-supporting

                (4) Married

                (5) Member of military service

            b. Emergencies

                (1) May be treated without parental consent during medical emergency

                    (a) Physician judgment

                    (b) Delay would jeopardize health or life of minor.

            c. Mature minor rule

                (1) Emerging trend in law

                (2) Recognizes minor is mature enough to understand nature of illness and risks and benefits of therapy

                (3) Should receive treatment at their own request

  VI. Guidelines for communicating with the adolescent (see Box 14-2 and Table 14-1)

    A. Build a foundation.

        1. Spend time together.

        2. Encourage expression of ideas and feelings.

            a. May talk quite freely when given opportunity

            b. Adolescents have language and culture all their own.

            c. More willing to discuss concerns with an outsider

            d. Occasionally will answer in monosyllables

                (1) Opposed to contact with nurse

                (2) Adolescents may not feel safe enough to reveal themselves.

                (3) May not want to communicate in front of parents

        3. Respect adolescent's views.

        4. Tolerate differences.

        5. Praise good points.

        6. Respect adolescent's privacy.

            a. Maintain confidentiality of information provided.

            b. Issues regarding pregnancy, sexual activity, substance abuse

        7. Set a good example.

    B. Communicate effectively.

        1. Give undivided attention.

        2. Be alert for signals indicating readiness to talk.

        3. Listen, listen, listen.

        4. Be courteous, calm, and open-minded.

        5. Try not to overreact to anything the adolescent says or does.

        6. Avoid passing judgment or criticizing.

 VII. Physical assessment of the adolescent

    A. Approach

        1. Best to use straightforward approach

■ TABLE 14-1
■ ■ **Developmental Milestones and Their Relationship to Communication Approaches**

Development	Language Development	Emotional Development	Cognitive Development	Suggested Communication Approach
Adolescent (12 years and older) Adolescents are able to create theories and generate many explanations for situations. They are beginning to communicate like adults.	Able to verbalize and comprehend most adult concepts	Beginning to accept responsibility for own actions Perception of "imaginary audiences" Need independence Competitive drive Strong need for group identification Frequently have small group of very close friends Question authority Strong need for privacy	Able to think logically and abstractly Attention span up to 60 min	Engage in conversations about adolescent's interests. Use photographs, books diagrams, charts, and videos to explain. Use collaborative approach and foster and support independence. Introduce preparatory materials up to 1 week in advance of the event. Respect privacy needs.

From James SR, Ashwill JW, Droske SC: *Nursing care of children.* Philadelphia: WB Saunders, 2002, p 59.

  2. Avoid being condescending.
  3. Involve in decision of who should be present for exam
 B. Technique
  1. Move from head to toe.
  2. Perform genital exam in the middle of exam.
   a. Allow ample time for questions and answers.
  3. Assure adolescent regarding normal growth and development.
  4. Answer questions or concerns regarding what is happening to their bodies.
  5. Drape appropriately to preserve dignity.
 C. Nursing considerations
  1. Admission to hospital or ambulatory surgery center (ASC) may be viewed as a threat to adolescent's independence; results in loss of control.
  2. May react by not cooperating or withdrawing
  3. May resent dependency on others and have difficulty accepting restrictions
   a. Identify nothing by mouth (NPO) status.
   b. Explain consequences of not telling the truth regarding NPO status.
  4. Involve in decision making and planning.
  5. Accept childish methods of coping.
  6. Provide support.
  7. Give explanations and consequences.
VIII. Preoperative, intraoperative, and postoperative considerations
 A. Preoperative interview
  1. Role of family
   a. Identify importance of family to adolescent.
   b. Ascertain if adolescent wants parent(s) present.
   c. Questions might not be answered in presence of parents.
   d. Allow parents to accompany adolescent to holding area if requested.
   e. Inform parents of necessity to remain at facility.
  2. Employ communication techniques to ensure a full understanding of procedure by adolescent.
  3. Answer all questions truthfully and honestly.

       4. Provide for privacy.

          a. Conduct procedures that violate privacy only after induction of anesthesia (hair removal, skin prep, insertion of urinary catheters, etc.).

       5. Allow choices when possible.

          a. Type of anesthesia induction

          b. Site of intravenous

  B. Guidelines for preoperative preparation

       1. Adolescent capable of abstract thought and reasoning

          a. Supplement explanations with reasons

          b. Explain long-term consequences of procedure.

          c. May fear death and disability

          d. Encourage questions regarding fears, options, and alternatives.

       2. Conscious of appearance

          a. Provide privacy.

          b. Discuss how procedure may affect appearance (visible scar, correction of deformity).

          c. Emphasize physical benefits of procedure.

       3. Adolescent very concerned with present

          a. Immediate effects of procedure more important than future benefits.

       4. Adolescent striving for independence

          a. Involve in decision making.

          b. Impose few restrictions.

          c. Suggest methods for maintaining control.

          d. Accept regression to more childish ways of coping.

          e. May have trouble accepting new authority figures and may resist complying with procedures (NPO guidelines)

       5. Need for support

          a. May show false bravery to nurse

          b. Very anxious but may not be able to verbalize concerns

  C. Emergency situations (see Box 14-1)

       1. Parents experience stress.

          a. Fear and anxiety most common emotion

          b. Parental fears

             (1) Child may die.

             (2) Child may experience pain.

             (3) Child's body may be permanently altered.

       2. Cause of stress is unique to circumstance.

       3. Parents may experience guilt.

          a. Feel responsible for injury

          b. They are submitting child to a painful experience.

          c. They do not have the knowledge to make educated decisions concerning the child's care.

       4. Include family members in child's care to reduce feelings of helplessness.

  D. Admission assessment

       1. Necessary to anticipate postoperative complications

          a. Assess cardiac, respiratory, and neurologic functions.

          b. Recent or current cold, chest sounds

       2. Observe verbal and nonverbal behavior prior to surgery.

       3. Vital signs, including temperature

       4. Allergies and sensitivities, including latex

       5. Use of alcohol, tobacco, recreational drugs

       6. Sexual assessment

          a. Use of birth control

          b. Possible pregnancy

       7. Educate (refer to Chapter 4 for complete information)

          a. What is going to happen?

          b. Time frames

       c. Postoperative routine in PACU
          (1) Oxygen
          (2) Position
          (3) Dressing checks
          (4) Intravenous
          (5) Pain assessment and treatment

  8. Educational strategies
       a. Developmental characteristics
          (1) Struggling with identity role
          (2) Concerned with body image
          (3) Peer relations extremely important
          (4) Struggling with independence versus dependence
          (5) Thinks abstractly
          (6) Understands complex language
          (7) Verbalizes fears
          (8) Seeks privacy
          (9) Able to cope with situations
       b. Teaching strategies
          (1) Clearly explain how the body is affected by surgery or procedure.
          (2) Expect feelings of anger and grief as a result of change to body image.
          (3) Educate in group sessions with peers.
          (4) Give control over teaching session.
             (a) Where held
             (b) When held
             (c) Preferred methods of learning
             (d) Collaborative decision making
          (5) Use scientific names with explanations.
          (6) Use diagrams, printed materials.
          (7) Encourage verbalization of fears.
          (8) Ascertain if adolescent wants parents involved.
          (9) Provide opportunities for adolescent to express anxieties.
          (10) Provide information openly and honestly.
          (11) Expect regression during periods of stress.

E. Intraoperative
  1. Provide reassurance prior to induction.
       a. Hold hand.
       b. Offer support.
       c. Assure preservation of privacy and dignity.
       d. Provide for patient safety.

F. Postoperative
  1. Respiratory assessment
       a. Monitor rate and depth of ventilation.
       b. Monitor oxygen saturation.
       c. Observe for tongue obstruction.
       d. Observe for respiratory depression from narcotics and muscle relaxants.
  2. Cardiovascular assessment
       a. Assess vital signs and perfusion.
       b. Heart rate: 60-90 beats per minute (BPM) (awake); 50-90 BPM (sleeping)
       c. Blood pressure: 112-128 mm Hg systolic; 66-80 mm Hg diastolic
  3. Thermoregulation
       a. Respond to cold environment by increasing metabolism.
          (1) Leads to increase in oxygen consumption
       b. Hypothermia
          (1) Monitor vital signs including core temperature, pulse, respiratory rate, degree of emergence from anesthesia, continuous ECG

(dysrhythmias and cardiovascular depression associated with hypothermia).
  c. Hyperthermia
      (1) Malignant hyperthermia
4. Emergence delirium
  a. Description
      (1) Dissociative state
      (2) No response to verbal commands
      (3) Appears confused and disoriented
      (4) Generalized purposeless movements
      (5) Lasts 30 seconds to 5 minutes
  b. Nursing interventions
      (1) Protect from injury
      (2) Generally will fall back to sleep and reawaken without recollection
      (3) Avoid stimulation—provide quiet environment.
  c. Causative factors
      (1) Preoperative anxiety
      (2) Postoperative pain
      (3) Hypoxia
      (4) Hypotension
      (5) Urinary distention
5. Assessment of pain (see Box 14-3)
  a. Perceive pain on three levels
      (1) Physical
      (2) Emotional
      (3) Mental
  b. Able to understand cause and effect of pain
      (1) Can describe pain
      (2) Can describe their feeling regarding pain
      (3) Can describe strategies that have helped with past experiences of pain
  c. Not unusual for adolescents to deal with pain through regressive behavior
      (1) Increased dependence on parent
      (2) Expects the nurse to know they are in pain—should not have to ask for pain medication
  d. Observed signs include
      (1) Increased muscle tension
          (a) Facial grimacing
          (b) Muscle rigidity
      (2) Withdrawal
          (a) Decreased interest in environment and usual activities
      (3) Decreased motor activity
          (a) Reluctant to move

■ BOX 14-3
■ **PAIN ASSESSMENT OF THE ADOLESCENT**

- Perceives pain at a physical, emotional, and mental level
- Understands cause and effect
- Describes pain and quantifies pain intensity
- Increased muscle tension
- Withdrawal and decreased motor activity
- Uses words such as "sore," "ache," or "pounding" to describe pain

From James SR, Ashwill JW, Droske SC: *Nursing care of children.* Philadelphia: WB Saunders, 2002, p 422.

(4) Verbalizes with words such as "ache," "sore," "pounding," and so forth to describe pain
    (a) May grunt, groan, or sigh
    (b) Rarely cries or screams
        (i) Physical resistance and aggression are unusual unless the adolescent is totally unprepared for the procedure.
        (ii) Very concerned with maintaining composure and are embarrassed and ashamed if he or she loses control
    (c) Describes pain intensity and quality
    (d) May hesitate to disclose pain unless he or she is sure nurse is willing to listen
  e. Assessment tools
    (1) Self-report
        (a) Visual analog scale (VAS)
            (i) Mark on a line (no pain to worst pain) a point that corresponds to adolescents' pain levels.
        (b) Verbal numerical score
            (i) Choose a number from 0 to 10 (0 = no pain, 10 = worst pain imaginable) that corresponds to their pain levels.
    (2) Adolescent pediatric pain tool (APPT)
        (a) Patient draws on front and back of body outlines to locate pain.
        (b) Indicates pain intensity on a Word Graphic Rating Scale
        (c) Circles words that describe the quality of pain
  f. Pharmacologic interventions
    (1) Nonsteroidal antiinflammatory drugs (NSAIDs)
        (a) Oral
            (i) For mild to moderate pain
            (ii) Can be administered preoperatively
            (iii) Contraindicated in patients with renal disease and those at risk of or with actual coagulopathy
            (iv) May mask fever
            (v) Can be given in conjunction with opioid
        (b) Parenteral
            (i) Ketorolac
                [a] For moderate to severe pain
                [b] May be useful when opioids contraindicated
    (2) Opioids-for moderate to severe pain
        (a) Oral
            (i) May be as effective as parenteral in appropriate doses
            (ii) Administer as soon as oral intake tolerated
            (iii) Route of choice
        (b) Intramuscular (IM)
            (i) Painful
            (ii) Absorption unreliable
            (iii) Avoid IM route if possible.
        (c) Subcutaneous (SC)
            (i) Preferred route to IM
            (ii) Painful
            (iii) Absorption unreliable
            (iv) Avoid SC route if possible.
        (d) Intravenous
            (i) Preferred route after major surgery
            (ii) Can be administered continuous or intermittently
            (iii) Used for patient-controlled analgesia (PCA)
            (iv) Increased risk for respiratory depression
        (e) PCA
            (i) Provides steady level of analgesia
            (ii) Not routinely used in outpatient setting

(f) Epidural, intrathecal
  (i) Provides good analgesia
  (ii) Increased risk of respiratory depression
  (iii) May have delayed onset
  (iv) Requires careful monitoring
  (v) Not routinely used in outpatient setting
(3) Local anesthetics
  (a) Limited indications
  (b) Provides effective regional analgesia
  (c) Limited duration of action
  (d) May be used for orthopedic procedures
    (i) Arthroscopy
    (ii) Anterior cruciate ligament repairs
    (iii) Other joint procedures
      [a] Shoulder
      [b] Elbow
      [c] Wrist
      [d] Foot
      [e] Ankle
    (iv) General surgery
      [a] Injected into incisional area
g. Dosage
(1) Acetaminophen (Tylenol)
  (a) Dose
    (i) 10-15 mg/kg orally, every 4 hours
  (b) Comments
    (i) Can be given rectally
    (ii) Lacks peripheral antiinflammatory activity of NSAIDs
    (iii) Does not inhibit platelet function
    (iv) Maximum of 60 mg/kg per day
(2) Aspirin
  (a) Dose
    (i) 10-15 mg/kg orally, every 4 hours
  (b) Comments
    (i) Contraindicated in presence of fever or other viral diseases
    (ii) Inhibits platelet aggregation
    (iii) May cause postoperative bleeding
    (iv) Associated with Reye syndrome
(3) NSAIDs
  (a) Ketorolac
    (i) Dose
      [a] 0.75-1.0 mg/kg intravenous route—administer slowly, every 6 hours as needed (PRN)
      [b] 1.0 mg/kg intramuscularly, every 6 hours PRN
    (ii) Comments
      [a] Only NSAID approved for parenteral analgesia
    (iii) Limit use to 48-72 hours
  (b) Ibuprofen
    (i) Dose
      [a] 10 mg/kg orally, every 6-8 hours
    (ii) Comments
      [a] Available as oral suspension
      [b] Available as several brand names and generic
  (c) Naprosyn
    (i) Dose
      [a] 5 mg/kg orally, every 12 hours
    (ii) Comments
      [a] Longer half-life than other NSAIDs

(4) Opioids
    (a) Fentanyl
        (i) Dose
            [a] 1.0 µg/kg, intravenous bolus every one half hour
            [b] 1-2 µg/hour, intravenous infusion
        (ii) Comments
            [a] Rapid onset
            [b] Short duration
            [c] Useful for painful procedures
            [d] Potential for respiratory depression; monitor closely
    (b) Morphine
        (i) Dose
            [a] 0.2-0.4 mg/kg orally, every 4-6 hours
            [b] 0.1 mg/kg intravenously, every 2 hours
        (ii) Comments
            [a] Observe for respiratory depression.
            [b] Common side effects include nausea and vomiting and histamine release.
    (c) Meperidine
        (i) Dose
            [a] 1-5 mg/kg intramuscularly, every 3-5 hours
            [b] 1.0 mg/kg intravenous bolus, every 2 hours
        (ii) Comments
            [a] Observe for respiratory depression.
            [b] Dizziness, nausea, and vomiting common in ambulatory patient
            [c] Used for the treatment of shivering in the postoperative patient
    (d) Codeine
        (i) Dose
            [a] 1.0 mg/kg orally, every 3 hours
        (ii) Comments
            [a] Monitor for respiratory depression.
            [b] Dizziness, nausea, vomiting, and hypotension more frequent in ambulatory patient
            [c] Dose may be limited because of nausea and vomiting.
    (e) Oxycodone (Percocet, Percodan, Tylox)
        (i) Dose
            [a] 0.2 mg/kg orally, every 3-4 hours
        (ii) Comments
            [a] Suppresses respirations
            [b] Dizziness, nausea, vomiting, and hypotension more common in ambulatory patient
    (f) Hydrocodone (Lortab, Lorcet, Vicodin)
        (i) Dose
            [a] 0.2 mg/kg orally, every 3-4 hours
        (ii) Comments
            [a] Suppresses respirations
            [b] Dizziness, nausea, vomiting, and hypotension more common in ambulatory patient
6. PACU phase I considerations
  a. Safety
    (1) Side rails up
    (2) When adolescent wakes up out of control
        (a) Speak in strong voice.
        (b) Orient to place.
        (c) Explain foul language is unacceptable in PACU environment.
  b. Prevent complications.

    c. Transport from operating room to PACU.
      (1) Safely
      (2) Position on side.
      (3) Safety strap in place
      (4) Oxygen administered
    d. Length of stay
      (1) No general rule
      (2) Institutional policy
      (3) Utilize discharge criteria rather than time.
    e. Replacing fluid deficits
      (1) Properly hydrated
    f. Equipment
      (1) Generally same as adult
7. PACU phase II considerations
    a. Pain management
    b. Patient and family anxiety
      (1) Maintain calm, reassuring manner.
      (2) Provide privacy.
      (3) Encourage expression of feelings.
      (4) Give encouragement and positive feedback.
      (5) Encourage parental presence if approved by patient.
    c. Discharge criteria
      (1) Individual criteria established by facility
      (2) Comply with standards (ASPAN, state, and regulatory agencies).
    d. Discharge instructions
      (1) Follow-up visit with surgeon
      (2) Provide information regarding procedure findings.
      (3) Provide instructions regarding home care.
        (a) Activity
        (b) Diet
        (c) Procedure-specific instructions
        (d) Drug and food interaction sheet
      (4) Enforce importance of compliance with postoperative instructions.
      (5) Parental involvement as requested by adolescent
        (a) If not involved, be sure to review information with parents separately to ensure their understanding of postoperative instructions.

BIBLIOGRAPHY

1. Behrman RE, Kliegman RM, Jenson HB: *Nelson textbook of pediatrics.* ed 16. Philadelphia: WB Saunders, 2000.
2. Burden N, DeFazio Quinn DM, O'Brien D, Gregory Dawes BS: *Ambulatory surgical nursing,* ed 2. Philadelphia: WB Saunders, 2000.
3. Gillies ML, Smith LN, Parry-Jones WL: Postoperative pain assessment and management in adolescents. *Pain* 79(2-3): 207-215, 1999.
4. James SR, Ashwill JW, Droske SC: *Nursing care of children: Principles and practice,* ed 2. Philadelphia: WB Saunders, 2002.
5. Malviya S, D'Errico C, Reynolds P, et al: Should pregnancy testing be routine in adolescent patients prior to surgery? *Anesth Analg* 83(4):854-858, 1996.
6. McGrath MH, Mukerji S: Plastic surgery and the teenage patient. *J Pediatr Adolesc Gynocol* 13(3):105-118, 2000.
7. Savedra MC, Tesler MD, Holzemer WL, et al: *Adolescent pediatric pain tool (APPT): Preliminary user's manual.* San Francisco: University of California, 1989.
8. Vetter TR, Heiner EJ: Discordance between patient self-reported visual analog scale pain scores and observed pain-related behavior in older children after surgery. *J Clin Anesth* 8(5):371-375, 1996.
9. Wong D, editor, Wilson D, Hockenberry-Eaton M, et al: *Wong's essentials of pediatric nursing,* ed 6. St Louis: Mosby, 2001.

15 The Adult Patient

VALLIRE D. HOOPER

OBJECTIVES

At the conclusion of this chapter the reader will be able to:

1. Identify developmental issues associated with each stage of adulthood.

2. Define health, wellness, and illness.

3. List three types of health and illness behaviors.

4. Identify the effects of the stress response on the body's adaptation to surgery.

5. List three characteristics unique to the adult learner.

I. Definitions
   A. Growth
      1. Increase in body size
      2. Change in structure, function, or complexity of body cell content and metabolic and biochemical processes
      3. Occurs up to some point of optimum maturity
   B. Development
      1. Growth responsibility arising at a certain time in the course of development
         a. Successful achievement
            (1) Satisfaction
            (2) Continued success in future tasks
         b. Failure
            (1) Unhappiness
            (2) Disapproval by society
            (3) Difficulty with later developmental tasks and functions
   C. Maturation and learning
      1. Maturation: emergence of genetic potential for changes in form, structure, complexity, integration, organization, and function
      2. Learning
         a. The process of gaining specific knowledge or skill
         b. Acquiring habits and attitude
         c. Results from experience, training, and behavioral changes
      3. Adequate maturation must be present for learning to occur
II. Stages of adulthood
   A. Young adulthood
      1. Definitions
         a. Age
            (1) Young-young adult: 25-30 years of age
            (2) Old-young adult: 30-45 years of age
         b. Birthdate and generation
            (1) Generation X: Born between 1964 and 1980
               (a) The most educated group of individuals in the United States
               (b) Come from families with the highest divorce rate in the country
               (c) The largest group of latchkey children ever known
                  (i) Adept at self-management
                  (ii) Adept at managing their environments
                  (iii) Comfortable with independent decision making

(d) Less optimistic about the future

(e) Never feel financially secure

(f) Abhor vagueness

(g) Are extremely protective of their time

(h) Communicate directly, sometimes almost abruptly

(i) Many late Generation X-ers have a different perspective on world history.

    (i) Have no recollection of the Reagan era

    (ii) Have only known one Germany

    (iii) The Vietnam War is as ancient as World War II.

    (iv) They don't remember the Challenger blowing up.

    (v) They have always had acquired immunodeficiency syndrome (AIDS) in their world.

(2) Baby Boomers: Born between 1946 and 1964

    (a) Most were raised in a two-parent home

        (i) Mother's responsibilities were caring for the children and the home.

        (ii) Father was the breadwinner, authority figure, and rarely questioned.

    (b) Experienced many social reforms in our country

        (i) Civil rights movement

        (ii) Antiwar protests

    (c) Experienced a lot of gains from a thriving economy

    (d) Embrace the attitude of "only the best"

    (e) Classified as workaholics

        (i) Take great interest in material rewards

        (ii) Value promotion and recognition

        (iii) Committed to making the world a better place

2. Developmental issues

  a. Settling down

  b. Developing a more conservative, traditional viewpoint

  c. Must enter and successfully manage multiple new roles simultaneously

    (1) Work

    (2) School

    (3) Marriage

    (4) Home

    (5) Child rearing

  d. Primary tasks

    (1) Finding an occupation

    (2) Staying in one place

    (3) Establishing a new family

3. Sociocultural issues

  a. Consistent positive influences

    (1) Continuous economic growth

    (2) Abundance of material goods and technology

    (3) Rapid social changes

    (4) Sophisticated medical care

  b. Constant threats

    (1) Terrorist attacks

    (2) Pollution

    (3) Overpopulation

    (4) Loss of natural resources

  c. Instant media coverage and Internet access make the world small and outer space a not-so-distant place.

    (1) All information is easily accessible and readily available.

    (2) Instant, up close, and continuous coverage of traumatic events may cause psychologic stress.

        (a) Depression

(b) Panic and anxiety disorders
(c) Posttraumatic stress disorder
   d. Other influences
      (1) Changes in women's roles
      (2) Decreasing birth rates
      (3) Increasing longevity
   4. Issues affecting response to ambulatory surgery (see Box 15-1)
 B. Middle age
   1. Definition
      a. Covers ages 45 to 65
         (1) Consider the physiologic age and condition of the body
         (2) Also consider psychologic age: how old the person acts and feels
      b. Age divisions
         (1) Early middle age: 40-55
         (2) Late middle age: 56-64
      c. Social class will affect age assignment.
         (1) Poorer person will perceive prime or midpoint as occurring at an earlier age.
   2. Developmental and sociocultural issues
      a. Becoming one of the largest segments of the population
         (1) Earn the most money
         (2) Pay a major portion of the bills and taxes
      b. Yield much power in
         (1) Government
         (2) Politics
         (3) Education
         (4) Religion
         (5) Science
         (6) Business
         (7) Communication
      c. Common experiences
         (1) Good physical and mental health
         (2) Personal freedom
         (3) Good command of self and the environment
   3. Issues affecting response to ambulatory surgery (see Box 15-1)
III. Health, wellness, and illness
 A. Definitions
   1. Health
      a. Defined by the World Health Organization (WHO), 1947, as a state of complete physical, social, and mental well-being; not merely the absence of disease
      b. Is often described on a continuum of wellness and illness

■ BOX 15-1
■ **DEVELOPMENTAL ISSUES AS RELATED TO AMBULATORY SURGERY**

Young Adulthood
Little or no insurance coverage
Needs to return to work or school as soon as possible
May need help with care of home, children, or parents
May expect sophisticated medical technology to be able to fix anything with very little "down" time

Middle Age
Physical condition often better indicator of surgical/anesthesia response than chronological age
More financially stable
Better insurance coverage
May be balancing many professional, civic, and family responsibilities

2. Wellness
   a. The ability to adapt, relate effectively, and to function at near maximum capacity
   b. Need to examine functioning in four areas
      (1) Physiologic factors: structures and functions of the body
      (2) Psychologic factors: self-concept as affected by various demographic variables
         (a) Age
         (b) Sex
         (c) Race
         (d) Education
         (e) Economic status
         (f) Other
      (3) Sociocultural factors
         (a) Interrelationships with others
         (b) Environmental factors
         (c) Lifestyle
      (4) Developmental factors: related to completion of developmental tasks
3. Disease and illness
   a. Disease
      (1) A state of nonhealth
      (2) Biological dysfunction is present
      (3) Major focus of the medical model
      (4) Can be legitimized by the health care provider
   b. Illness
      (1) The patient's personal perspective of the disease state
      (2) Related to the psychosocial impact of the disease on the individual
      (3) Individual influences on perception of illness severity
         (a) Personality
         (b) Demographic characteristics
         (c) Presence of support systems
B. Health care and prevention
   1. Levels of health care
      a. Health promotion: activities to improve or maintain optimum health
      b. Disease prevention: actions to prevent disease or disability
      c. Diagnosis and treatment: emphasizes early recognition and treatment of health problems
      d. Rehabilitation: designed to limit incapacity caused by health problems as well as to prevent recurrences
   2. Levels of prevention
      a. Primary prevention: ways to prevent illness
      b. Secondary prevention: early identification and treatment of health problems
      c. Tertiary prevention: activities designed to return the physically or emotionally compromised person to the highest possible level of health
   3. The ambulatory arena is now involved in all levels of health care and prevention.
IV. Health and illness behavior
   A. Health behavior
      1. Activities undertaken by those believing themselves to be healthy
      2. Purpose is to prevent disease or detect it in an asymptomatic stage.
      3. Examples
         a. Breast self-exam (BSE)
         b. Regular exercise
         c. Prudent heart living

      d. Routine checkups

      e. Ambulatory procedures

         (1) Routine screening colonoscopy

         (2) Follow-up cardiac catheterization in nonsymptomatic patient

B. Illness behavior

   1. Activities carried out in response to a set of symptoms by those who feel ill

   2. Allows the individual to determine his or her state of health and need for treatment

   3. Limited to health-seeking behavior to identify and/or assess the changes occurring or to search for a solution

   4. Influences affecting illness behavior

      a. Recurrence of symptoms

         (1) The more frequent or severe the symptoms, the more likely that outside help will be sought

      b. Visibility and consequences

         (1) The more apparent the symptoms, the more illness behavior exhibited

         (2) If the disorder is attached to stigma, the individual will be less likely to seek help.

         (3) Help will usually be sought for life-threatening symptoms.

      c. Perceived seriousness or severity

         (1) Disorders perceived as serious lead to earlier illness behavior.

         (2) Influences on perception of symptom severity

            (a) Social class

            (b) Health belief system

            (c) Hierarchy of other needs and desires

      d. Availability of treatment and the medical care system

         (1) Distance, costs, convenience, time, effort, and fear of outcome affect willingness to seek help.

         (2) Individual subordination by the health care system also affects willingness to seek treatment.

      e. Knowledge and significance of symptoms

         (1) Lack of knowledge of symptom significance often influences the individual to seek help.

      f. Cultural and social expectations

         (1) Cultural and ethnic backgrounds affect symptom interpretation and notion of when it is acceptable to seek health care.

         (2) Lower classes are more influenced by symptoms interfering with important roles.

         (3) The elderly use more health care services.

         (4) Women seek medical attention more frequently than men.

C. Sick role behavior

   1. Activities undertaken by individuals who consider themselves ill for the purpose of getting well

   2. Is learned and influenced by evaluation and legitimization from others

   3. Is assumed when one accepts being ill, initiates some form of action, and demonstrates a desire to be well again

   4. Four major role components, divided into rights and obligations

      a. Rights

         (1) Exemption from normal responsibilities

            (a) Dependent on the nature and severity of the illness

            (b) Requires validation or legitimization by others and the physician

            (c) Once legitimized, person is obligated to avoid responsibilities.

         (2) Right to be cared for

            (a) Person is not expected to recover by an act of will or decision.

            (b) Is not responsible for becoming sick and therefore has a right to be cared for

        (c) Physical dependency and the need for emotional support are acceptable.

    b. Obligations

        (1) Obligation to want to become well

            (a) Being ill is seen as undesirable.

            (b) The sick role can result in secondary gains.

            (c) Motivation to recover is of primary importance.

        (2) Obligation to seek and cooperate with technically competent help

            (a) The individual needs the technical expertise that health care professionals can provide.

            (b) Cooperation with these professionals for the goal of getting well is mandatory.

  5. Ambulatory implications

    a. Patient may need to be educated that sick role behavior is acceptable and often expected following ambulatory procedures.

    b. Ambulatory procedures often reduce the amount of time spent in the sick role.

V. Stress response syndrome

  A. Definitions

    1. Stress

      a. A socio-psychophysiologic phenomenon

      b. A composite of intellectual, behavioral, metabolic, and other physiologic responses to a stressor or stressors of internal or external origin

      c. Influenced by environmental, psychologic, and social factors

      d. Uniquely perceived by the individual

    2. Stressors (stress agents)

      a. May be internal or external

      b. Examples

        (1) Cold

        (2) Heat

        (3) Infectious organisms

        (4) Disease processes

        (5) Fever

        (6) Pain

        (7) Imagined events

        (8) Intense emotional involvement

    3. Stress response

      a. Initiated in response to a stressor

      b. Is protective and adaptive by nature

      c. Regulated by the nervous and endocrine systems

        (1) Sympathetic nervous system (SNS)

        (2) Pituitary gland

        (3) Adrenal gland

      d. The magnitude of the response depends on the perceived severity of the threat.

    4. Survival depends on one's ability to balance between stressors and adaptive capacities.

  B. General adaptation syndrome (GAS)

    1. Developed by Hans Selye

    2. Most widely accepted and frequently used physiologic theory of stress and adaptation

    3. Three stages

      a. Alarm stage

        (1) Begins with the first exposure to the stressor

        (2) Fight or flight mechanism (SNS) is activated.

            (a) Heart rate increases.

            (b) Cardiac output (CO) increases.

            (c) Stroke volume increases.

    (d) Peripheral vasoconstriction
    (e) Increased perspiration
    (f) Gastrointestinal upset
   (3) In most situations, the body's defensive forces are mobilized to deal with the stressor.
   (4) Death can occur in this stage if the stressor is strong enough to result in exhaustion of the body's adaptive mechanisms and energy supply.
  b. Stage of resistance or adaptation
   (1) Reflects "adaptation" as the body fights back
   (2) Psychologic mobilization occurs
   (3) Influences on ability to adapt
    (a) Physical functioning
    (b) Coping skills
    (c) Total number of stressors experienced
  c. Stage of exhaustion
   (1) A progressive breakdown of compensatory mechanisms and homeostasis
   (2) Occurs only if the stress becomes overwhelming, is not removed, or if the individual is ineffective in coping with it
   (3) All energy for adaptation is exhausted.
   (4) Physiologic and psychologic collapse will ensue.
C. Physiologic responses to stress
 1. The initial response is stimulated by the central nervous system (CNS).
 2. Information is then forwarded to the hypothalamus, which integrates and coordinates the homeostatic adjustments
 3. Hypothalamus stimulates the autonomic nervous system (ANS) and the anterior and posterior pituitary
 4. The physiologic responses to hypothalamic stimulation and their effects on the surgical patient are listed in Table 15-1
D. Psychosocial responses to stress
 1. Primary theory is the stress-appraised event theory by Lazarus.
  a. Looks at stress and adaptation from the viewpoint of cognition, perception, and transaction
   (1) The way the individual interprets the situation will determine if he or she perceives it as stressful.
  b. Positive and negative events can result in stress.
  c. Emphasis is on the process or dynamics of what is happening.
 2. Cognitive appraisal
  a. The mental process used by the person to assess an event in relation to his or her well-being and available coping resources and options.
  b. Evaluative forms
   (1) Irrelevant appraisal
    (a) Occurs if the event is considered to be of no concern or impact on the current level of well-being
   (2) Benign–positive appraisal
    (a) Occurs if the event is considered as indicative of a positive state of affairs
    (b) The event shows that all is well.
   (3) Stressful appraisal
    (a) Occurs with a negative evaluation of the present or future state of well-being
    (b) Occurs in three forms
     (i) Harm–loss: damage or injury has already taken place.
     (ii) Threat: harm or loss has not yet occurred but is expected.
     (iii) Challenge
      [a] The possibility for growth or mastery is perceived.
      [b] The opportunity for gain outweighs the possible risk of harm.

■ TABLE 15-1
■ ■ Physiologic Responses to Hypothalamic Stimulation

Responding Organ/ System	Organ/system Action	Physiologic Response	Surgical Adaptation	Surgical Maladaptation
Autonomic Nervous system (ANS)	Simulates the sympathetic nervous system (SNS) to stimulate:			
	Exocrine glands Epinephrine and norepinephrine release	Sweating Decreases insulin and increases glucagon releases: See net increase in blood glucose and protein and fat catabolism	No impact Increased amino acids for wound healing Increased wound healing Increased energy available Increased blood sugar Increased energy available for adaptation	No impact Negative nitrogen balance that may negatively impact tissue repair unless reversed Development of excessive scar tissue and adhesions Increased blood sugar is detrimental to diabetics. Increased heat loss may result in hypothermia, shivering, and increased oxygen demand.
		Constriction of vascular smooth muscle: Increase in blood pressure (BP)	Shifts blood away from periphery to the vital organs Decreases blood loss by increasing clotting	May decrease renal perfusion Increased thrombus formation
		Cardiopulmonary responses: Increased heart rate and contractility Bronchodilatation	Increased myocardial perfusion Increased oxygen and perfusion to vital organs Increased oxygen exchange Improved ventilation	Increased workload for heart: May lead to heart failure Hypertension No maladaptation as a result of bronchodilatation
		Kidneys are stimulated to release renin: Converted to aldosterone by angiotensin II		
		Aldosterone results in sodium and	Increased blood volume helps to reduce	Hypervolemia Hypertension Circulatory overload

■ TABLE 15-1
■ ■ Physiologic Responses to Hypothalamic Stimulation

Responding Organ/ System	Organ/system Action	Physiologic Response	Surgical Adaptation	Surgical Maladaptation
		water retention at the renal tubules. See increased blood volume.	hypovolemia: Maintenance of blood pressure and cardiac output	Heart failure
Anterior pituitary	Releases adrenocorticotropin hormone (ACTH): Stimulates the adrenal cortex to release aldosterone and cortisol	Aldosterone results in increased blood volume. Cortisol results in an increase in blood glucose and protein and fat catabolism.	Increased blood sugar Increased wound healing Increased energy Increased antiinflammatory response	Prolonged antiinflammatory response may lead to infection. See above for other maladaptive responses.
Posterior pituitary	Stimulates the release of vasopressin/ antidiuretic hormone (ADH)	Causes sodium and water retention at the renal tubules: Results in increased blood volume	See above.	See above.

3. Coping modes
   a. Defined as those efforts used to manage the environmental and internal demands exceeding personal resources; mobilized in response to an event perceived as stressful
   b. Accomplished by eight coping modes
      (1) Escape–avoidance
         (a) Wishful thinking and other behavioral efforts to escape or avoid the problem
      (2) Confrontive
         (a) Aggressive efforts to alter the situation
         (b) Involves some degree of hostility and risk taking
      (3) Distancing
         (a) Attempt to detach from the situation and thus minimize the significance
      (4) Self-control
         (a) Strive to regulate one's feelings and actions
      (5) Seeking social support
         (a) Seek information, tangible and emotional support
      (6) Accepting responsibility
         (a) Acknowledge one's own role in the problem
         (b) Attempt to rectify the situation
      (7) Planful problem solving
         (a) Deliberate and analytical approach to altering the situation
      (8) Positive reappraisal
         (a) An effort to focus on the positive side or opportunity for personal growth

    E. Behavioral responses to stress

        1. Anger, hostility, antagonism, noncompliance

        2. Depression, apathy, crying, inability to concentrate, depression

        3. Grief, shock, denial, withdrawal

        4. Acceptance, information seeking, planning, decision making

    F. Factors affecting response to stressors

        1. Nature of specific stressors encountered

        2. What the stressors mean to the patient

            a. May differ based on past experience and development

            b. Ill patients may become less mature, less discriminating, and less reality oriented.

        3. Patient's characteristic mode of coping with stress

            a. Depends on personality

            b. Threat of hospitalization or surgery may be responded to by

                (1) An aggressive manner

                (2) Resignation

                (3) Seeking constant information

        4. Patient's current psychologic resources

            a. Determines the person's resiliency and ability to endure the stress without decompensation

            b. Affected by

                (1) Level of self-esteem and social support

                (2) Presence or absence of any underlying depression or chronic anxiety

        5. Hardiness factor

            a. A personality characteristic

                (1) A sense of control over one's life

                (2) Involvement and commitment to productive activities

                (3) Anticipation of change as an exciting positive challenge

            b. Acts as a buffer between stress and illness

VI. Stress management

    A. Assessment of current level of stress

    B. Intervention

        1. Physical relaxation and stress management

            a. Progressive relaxation

            b. Acupuncture and acupressure

            c. Biofeedback

            d. Massage

            e. Therapeutic touch

        2. Cognitive methods of relaxation and stress management

            a. Thought stopping

            b. Positive self-talk

            c. Assertive communication training

            d. Laughter, humor, play, tears

            e. Guided imagery

        3. Time and resource management

        4. Other nursing interventions

            a. Acknowledge individual feelings and behaviors.

            b. Develop trusting relationship.

            c. Involve family and significant others.

VII. Health promotion and prevention

    A. Activities designed to improve or maintain optimum health

    B. Likelihood to participate in such behaviors is influenced by internal and external cues.

        1. Internal cues include bodily states such as feeling good or energetic.

        2. External cues

            a. Interactions with significant others

        b. Impact of media communication

        c. Visual stimuli from the environment

  C. Strategies include

    1. Physical, physiologic

        a. Proper nutrition

        b. Balance of exercise and rest

        c. Cessation of destructive health habits (smoking, alcohol, or drug abuse)

        d. Health screening

    2. Emotional

        a. Effective communication

        b. Promotion of self-esteem, self-confidence, security

        c. Anxiety reduction measures

        d. Crisis resolution

    3. Cognitive

        a. Coping methods

        b. Visualization and imagery

        c. Health education

    4. Social

        a. Family, friend, peer relations

        b. Group associations and processes

        c. Maintenance of cultural ties

    5. Spiritual and moral

        a. Values clarification

        b. Acknowledgment of meaning and purpose of life

        c. Establishment of belief system

        d. Establishment of moral and ethical behaviors

VIII. Preoperative health history interview

  A. Should focus on age-specific issues in addition to general preoperative assessment and preparation

  B. Young adulthood

    1. Generally a healthy population

    2. Pertinent health problems include

        a. Upper respiratory infection

        b. Influenza

        c. Essential hypertension

        d. Mitral valve prolapse

        e. Iron deficiency anemia

        f. Simple diarrhea

        g. Cystitis

        h. Acute pyelonephritis

        i. Chronic fatigue syndrome

        j. AIDS

        k. Hepatitis B

        l. Cervical, breast, and testicular cancer

  C. Middle age

    1. Variety of health problems may begin to develop.

    2. Pertinent health problems include

        a. Sinusitis

        b. Hiatal hernia

        c. Duodenal peptic ulcer disease

        d. Angina pectoris

        e. Secondary hypertension

        f. Hyperthyroidism

        g. Hyperuricemia or gout

        h. Diabetes type II

        i. Acute and chronic prostatitis

        j. Lumbosacral strain

IX. Health teaching–learning
- **A.** Teaching is a critical nursing intervention that is crucial to successful outcomes in the ambulatory setting.
  - **1.** Teaching and learning processes are related.
  - **2.** Teaching–learning process is easily integrated into the nursing process.
- **B.** Definitions
  - **1.** Learning
    - **a.** Process of acquiring wisdom, knowledge, or skill
    - **b.** Overt changes in behavior may be observed.
  - **2.** Teaching
    - **a.** Process of sharing knowledge and insight
    - **b.** Facilitating another to learn knowledge, insight, and skills
  - **3.** Health education
    - **a.** Transmits information, motivates, and helps people adopt and maintain healthful practices and lifestyles
    - **b.** Is concerned with the environment, professional training, and research to maintain and evaluate the process
    - **c.** Traditionally focuses on what the professional thinks is good or needed by the patient
    - **d.** Positive approaches are generally more effective than fear
- **C.** Phases of the teaching–learning process
  - **1.** Assessment
    - **a.** Begins with an assessment of the nurse's teaching abilities
    - **b.** Gather information about the patient, his or her learning needs, and his or her readiness to learn
      - (1) Patient's level of understanding, ability to comprehend, and any obstacles to learning (sensory losses, language barriers) should be identified during the general psychosocial assessment.
      - (2) Assessment should also include patient's interest level, attentiveness, and current understanding about upcoming procedure.
    - **c.** A realistic teaching plan should be established based on
      - (1) Patient's current level of knowledge
      - (2) Nurse's ability to provide the new information needed by the patient
      - (3) A plan to identify and dispel patient misconceptions should also be included.
  - **2.** Diagnosis
    - **a.** Diagnose the patient's learning needs.
    - **b.** Set teaching priorities.
  - **3.** Planning
    - **a.** Set goals with the patient.
    - **b.** Determine behavioral objectives.
    - **c.** Select teaching and evaluation methods.
      - (1) Content and type of information
      - (2) Type of media used
      - (3) Who will be involved?
      - (4) The environment and time frame in which it will be provided
  - **4.** Intervention
    - **a.** Use appropriate strategies for instruction.
  - **5.** Evaluation
    - **a.** Evaluate patient outcomes.
    - **b.** Revise and reevaluate as needed.
- **D.** Characteristics of the adult learner
  - **1.** Readiness to learn is determined by life tasks, roles, and immediate problems.
  - **2.** Application of learning is related to the relevancy of the problems.
  - **3.** Orientation to learning is independent and self-directed.

      4. Value of experiences
         a. Experiences are internalized.
         b. Experiences provide a foundation for further learning.
         c. May contribute to resistance to change
      5. Rate of learning
         a. Resistant to learning nonrelevant material
         b. Aging process increases time needed to complete some learning tasks.
      6. Barriers to learning
         a. Family, work, or community responsibilities may compete with learning time and energy.
         b. Anxieties about self-image may also threaten ability to learn.
      7. Cultural differences
         a. Unique beliefs should be respected.
         b. Use interpreters and/or audiovisual aids for persons who do not speak English.
         c. Be knowledgeable of cultures, ethnic groups, and religions commonly encountered in your environment.
      8. Educational background
         a. Identify level of formal education attained by the patient.
         b. Remember that level of formal education does not equate with one's ability to learn.
         c. Determine patient's reading level.
         d. Determine patient's health knowledge.
         e. Determine patient's feelings about education and learning.
         f. Use pictures for patients with low literacy skills.
   E. Domains of learning
      1. Cognitive: concerns the learner's knowledge and understanding
      2. Affective: concerned with the learner's attitudes, emotions, and ways of adjusting to an illness
      3. Psychomotor: concerned with motor skills
   F. Goals of teaching
      1. To forewarn or provide information
      2. To teach skills (Foley care, dressing changes, etc.)
      3. Assist in decision making and planning
      4. Family involvement in patient care
      5. Reinforcement of existing knowledge
      6. Explain procedures, follow-up, and medications
      7. Discuss future events, expectations
      8. Advice about home health follow-up, home management
      9. Encourage change, provide alternative behaviors or thoughts
   G. Maximizing teaching–learning effectiveness
      1. Allow sufficient time.
      2. Choose appropriate time and environment.
      3. Confirm patient readiness.
         a. Preoperative: admission details are taken care of.
         b. Postoperative: pain controlled, stable, awake, family present
      4. Actively involve the learner.
      5. Use creativity in approaches.
      6. Encourage learner to contribute to ideas.
      7. Use humor or novelty to help learner relax and retain the content.
      8. Organize material logically and present it in manageable amounts.
      9. Highlight or point out important information.
     10. Differentiate between similar concepts and contrasting information.
     11. Allow practice as much as possible, giving constructive feedback.
   H. Common barriers to effective teaching–learning
      1. Providing false reassurance
      2. Invading privacy
      3. Minimizing or ignoring feelings

4. Not listening
5. Giving wrong information
6. Violating trust relationship
7. Noisy environment
8. Lack of privacy
9. Physiologic distraction (pain, nausea, vomiting, etc.)

BIBLIOGRAPHY

1. Black J, Hawks J, Keene A: *Medical-surgical nursing*, ed 6. Philadelphia: WB Saunders, 2001.
2. Burden N, Quinn DMD, O'Brien D, et al: Preparing the patient. In Burden N, editor: *Ambulatory Surgical Nursing.* Philadelphia: WB Saunders, 2000, pp 346-362.
3. Burmeister WL: Hiring/developing future leaders. Presented at Southern Company training session, Birmingham, AL, 2000.
3. Burrell LO: Contemporary nursing practice. In Burrell LO, Gerlach MJM, Pless BS, editors: *Adult nursing: Acute and community care*, ed 2. Stamford, CT: Appleton & Lange, 1997, p 3.
4. Hooper VD: The next generation. *J PeriAnesth Nurs* 17:219-221, 2002.
5. Lambert VA, Lambert CE, Gugino HS: Crisis and stress. In Burrell LO, Gerlach MJM, Pless BS, editors: *Adult nursing: Acute and community care*, ed 2. Stamford, CT: Appleton & Lange, 1997, p 74.
6. Litwack K: The adult patient. In Litwack K, editor: *Core curriculum for post anesthesia nursing practice*, ed 3. Philadelphia: WB Saunders, 1995, p 47.
7. Lubkin IM, Larson PD, editors: *Chronic illness: Impact and interventions*, ed 5. Boston: Jones & Bartlett, 2002.
8. McCance KL, Huether SE, editors: *Pathophysiology*, ed 4. St Louis, Mosby, 2002.
9. Meisenhelder JB: Anniversary responses to terrorism. *Am J Nurs* 102(9):24AA-24EE, 2002.
10. Murray RB, Zentner JP, editors: *Nursing assessment and health promotion: Strategies through the life span*, ed 5. Norwalk, CT: Appleton & Lange, 1993.
11. Watson DS: Wanted: A few good nurses. *AORN J* 76:8-11, 2002.
12. Zimmerman PG: Generation X staff. *J Emerg Nurs* 26:492-495, 2000.

16 The Elderly Patient

LOIS SCHICK

OBJECTIVES

At the conclusion of this chapter the reader will be able to:

1. Using a systems approach, identify changes that occur with aging.

2. Describe the demographics of the elderly patient.

3. Identify potential problems that may occur after a surgical procedure.

4. Discuss the purpose of a preoperative assessment.

5. Identify postoperative priorities in consideration of the physiologic changes that occur with aging.

Elderly patients present a unique challenge for the perianesthesia care unit (PACU) nurse. Physiologic changes of aging combined with pathologic conditions necessitating surgical intervention mandate careful assessment, planning, and implementation of the nursing process and PACU care plan.

   I. Definition of elderly
      A. Greater than 65 years old
         1. 65 to 75 years: "young-old"
         2. 75 to 85 years: "old"
         3. >85 years: "old-old"
      B. Life expectancy[34]
         1. Men: 81 years
         2. Women: 84 years
      C. Number of elderly in United States is increasing.[34]
         1. By 2030, the older population will double to about 70 million people
         2. Members of the minority groups are projected to represent 25% of the older population in 2030.
         3. Over 2 million Americans celebrated their sixty-fifth birthday in 2000 (5574 per day).
         4. Elderly account for one third of all health care costs.
         5. There were 50,545 persons aged 100 or more in 2000 (0.02% of total population).
         6. Postoperative cognitive dysfunction in the elderly may persist at least 3 months after otherwise uncomplicated surgery.
      D. The Silent Generation (also known as the Veteran Generation) (people born before 1946)[20,36]
         1. Comprise 10% of today's work force
         2. Rely on tried and true ways of doing things
         3. Core values include
            a. Dedication and sacrifice
            b. Hard work
            c. Conformity
            d. Law and order
            e. Respect for authority
            f. Patience
            g. Duty before reward
            h. Adherence to rules
               (1) Honor

    4. Veteran Generational Personality
- **a.** Likes consistency and uniformity
- **b.** Likes things on a grand scale
- **c.** Are conformers
- **d.** Believe in "logic" not "magic"
- **e.** Are disciplined
- **f.** Are past oriented and history absorbers
- **g.** Believe in law and order

II. Proposed theories of aging
- **A.** Random mutation of DNA
- **B.** Cumulative abnormalities of DNA
- **C.** Damage to tissues by free radicals
- **D.** Biologic clock
- **E.** Genetic program of life expectancy
- **F.** Failure of growth substance
- **G.** Production of an "aging factor"

III. Physiologic changes of aging: Changes in both structure and function
- **A.** Functional age is impacted by
  - **1.** Chronic disease processes
  - **2.** Personal attitudes and outlook
  - **3.** Family and friends network
- **B.** Age-related diseases
  - **1.** Cerebral arteriosclerosis
  - **2.** Alzheimer's
  - **3.** Parkinson's
- **C.** Central nervous system (CNS)
  - **1.** Neurogenic atrophy and reduction of peripheral nerve fibers
    - **a.** Decreased blood flow and CNS activity
      - (1) Causing slower reaction times
      - (2) Reduced ability to cope with body stressors
      - (3) Diminished ability to respond to demands on cardiovascular systems
      - (4) Prolonged emergence from pharmacologic interventions (e.g., benzodiazepines) and decreased pain perception
    - **b.** Decreased cognitive function
      - (1) Loss of memory and decreased understanding
      - (2) Lengthening of learning speed
      - (3) Higher risk of confusion
      - (4) Short attention span
      - (5) Decreased sensory abilities
        - (a) Impaired hearing acuity
          - (i) Men especially lose high-frequency sounds.
          - (ii) Deafness
          - (iii) Decrease in acoustic acuity
        - (b) Vestibular changes may also alter balance and/or cause vertigo.
        - (c) Visual precision is reduced.
          - (i) Lenses fail (as in cataracts)
          - (ii) Glaucoma
        - (d) Decreased tactile perception
        - (e) Acuity of smell diminished
          - (i) May impair hygiene
    - **c.** Homeostatic mechanism slows altering sympathetic and parasympathetic responsiveness.
      - (1) Decreased sensitivity to baroreceptors
      - (2) Change in thermoregulation
        - (a) Affected by autonomic impairment
        - (b) Changes to skin and blood vessels

        (c) Impaired by many chronic medications

        (d) Elderly are vulnerable to heat stroke and hypothermia.

  d. Compromised perfusion caused by arteriosclerotic changes

    (1) Increased incidence of organic brain syndrome

    (2) Increased incidence of cerebrovascular accidents (strokes)

    (3) Increased incidence of microemboli

    (4) Decreased cerebral blood flow

    (5) Decreased cerebral metabolic oxygen consumption

    (6) Decreased CNS activity

  e. Nursing implications

    (1) Allow additional time to assimilate information and give responses.

    (2) Prepare for possible increased length of stay in ambulatory surgery.

    (3) Encourage use of sensory aids.

        (a) Hearing aids

        (b) Visual aids

        (c) Glasses

            (i) Contacts

            (ii) Magnifying glass

    (4) Include family member or responsible adult in instructions

    (5) Verbal communication

        (a) Face patient when speaking.

        (b) Raise speaking volume, not pitch.

        (c) Speak slowly and clearly.

    (6) Observe for prolonged or toxic effects of drugs.

    (7) Encourage lower doses.

    (8) Safety measures

        (a) Handrails

        (b) Other assistive devices

            (i) Canes, walkers, nonslip shower chairs

        (c) Nonskid footwear

        (d) Physical support by caretaker

        (e) Observation

D. Cardiovascular system

  1. Most changes are caused by arteriosclerotic changes.

    a. Loss of large artery elasticity

      (1) Coronary

      (2) Aorta

      (3) Carotid

      (4) Iliac

      (5) Femoral

      (6) Popliteal

      (7) Renal

    b. Decreased organ perfusion and decreased compensatory regulation from loss of elasticity

    c. Vessel fragility

    d. Increase in systolic blood pressure

  2. Loss of tissue elasticity

    a. Organ perfusion decreases

      (1) Myocardium

      (2) Decreases optimal regulation of all body systems

    b. Peripheral circulation impaired

      (1) Lowers tolerances to stress responses (heart workload increases)

      (2) Along with decreased collagen, increases difficulty of venipuncture

        (a) Aging collagen makes tough "rolling" veins.

        (b) Loss of elasticity likely to cause bleeding around site during and

              after venipuncture
- (3) Higher risk for bruising
- (4) Increases peripheral vascular resistance
  - (a) Restricts left ventricular ejection
  - (b) Promotes cardiac hypertrophy
- (5) Potential for orthostatic hypotension
- c. Increased susceptibility to clotting disorders
  - (1) Stroke
  - (2) Thrombosis
  - (3) Embolism
3. Cardiac conduction system
   - a. Decreased heart rate
     - (1) Resulting from increased parasympathetic activity
     - (2) Resulting from degenerative changes in conduction system
   - b. Dysrhythmias and blocks occur more frequently.
   - c. Can lead to CNS changes
   - d. Myocardial changes
     - (1) Left ventricular hypertrophy
     - (2) Increased myocardial irritability, leading to dysrhythmias
     - (3) Fibrosis of endocardial lining, leading to endocardial thickening and rigidity, decreased contractility
     - (4) Calcification of valves, leading to valve incompetence
4. Altered hemodynamics
   - a. Pump effectiveness diminishes because of atrophy of myocardial fibers.
   - b. Decrease in cardiac output (1% per year after 30 years of age)
   - c. Slower circulation time
   - d. Prolonged onset of action and clearing times for drugs
   - e. Increased blood pressure
   - f. Systolic blood pressure increases with aging reflecting development of poorly compliant arterial walls.
   - g. Heart rate decreases, suggesting increase in activity of parasympathetic nervous system.
   - h. Slowed circulation time, leading to slower onset of drug effects
   - i. Decreased cardiac reserve; stressors
     - (1) Fever
     - (2) Tachycardia
     - (3) Exertion
     - (4) Anxiety
     - (5) Hypoxemia
     - (6) Pain
5. Orthostatic hypotension
   - a. Decreased blood vessel tone, leading to peripheral pooling of blood, increased risk for deep vein thrombosis (DVT)
   - b. Baroreceptor failure
   - c. Medications (most common cause)
     - (1) Antihypertensives
     - (2) Diuretics
     - (3) Tricyclic antidepressants
     - (4) Phenothiazines
     - (5) Alcohol
   - d. Decreased tolerance to volume changes
6. Nursing considerations
   - a. Observe responses to medications.
     - (1) Allow adequate time for response before repeating.
     - (2) Use lower range of medication dosage and encourage team to utilize lower dosages.
   - b. Monitor for cardiac inadequacy.

(1) Lungs
  (a) Provide adequate oxygenation.
      (i) Encourage deep breathing.
      (ii) Watch for fluid overload while ensuring adequate hydration.
(2) Heart
  (a) Assess heart sounds.
  (b) Cardiac monitoring for arrhythmias
  (c) Assess lung sounds.
  (d) Avoid extremes of blood pressure.
      (i) Watch for orthostatic changes.
  (e) Encourage slow position changes.
  (f) Vascular considerations
      (i) Gentle venipunctures
  (g) Avoid tourniquets where possible.
      (i) Minimize use of automatic blood pressure devices.
      (ii) Adequate pressure on sites after venipuncture or catheter removal
  (h) Encourage early ambulation.

E. Respiratory system
  1. Airway
    a. Edentia
      (1) Impacts patency of airway
      (2) Creates difficulty in intubation
    b. Decreased bone mass of jaw
  2. Anatomic changes
    a. Increased anteroposterior (AP) diameter
    b. Progressive flattening and decreased muscle strength of diaphragm
    c. Increased chest wall rigidity
      (1) Arthritic changes in rib cage
    d. Reduction in alveolar surface
    e. Narrowing of intervertebral disks
      (1) Reduces total lung capacity by 10%
    f. Loss of skeletal muscle mass, leading to wasting of diaphragm and skeletal muscles
    g. Loss of teeth changes jaw structure, leading to difficult airway maintenance.
  3. Physiologic changes
    a. Reduction in pulmonary elasticity
    b. Decreased chest wall mobility
    c. Loss of alveolar septa, leading to air trapping
    d. Decreased pulmonary compliance
    e. Increased airway resistance
    f. Decreased cough and gag reflex, leading to risk of aspiration
    g. Ventilation and perfusion alterations develop.
      (1) Decreased tidal volume
      (2) Decreased vital capacity
      (3) Decreased inspiratory reserve
      (4) Decreased cardiac output
      (5) Decreased aerobic capacity
      (6) Increased dead space
      (7) Decreased oxygen and carbon dioxide exchange
      (8) Decreased oxygen content of blood
          (a) $PaO_2 = 100 - (0.4 \times \text{Age in years}) = \text{mm Hg}$
          (b) For example, in an 80 year old: $PaO_2 = 100 - (0.4 \times 80)$ = 68 mm Hg (vs. normal PaO_2 of 100 mm Hg)
    h. Environmental changes impact the respiratory system.

(1) Smoker
(2) Dust
    (a) Air pollution
4. Nursing considerations
  a. Airway
    (1) Assess airway constantly.
    (2) Protect unconscious airway.
      (a) Suction oropharynx as needed.
      (b) Support and position.
    (3) Provide appropriate airways and oxygen delivery supplies.
    (4) Returning dentures can help support the airway.
  b. Secretions and effective cough
    (1) Position
      (a) With head elevated when possible
      (b) To maximize chest expansion
    (2) Encourage coughing and deep breathing.
    (3) Ensure reflexes have returned prior to administering oral fluids.
  c. Oxygenation
    (1) Monitor oxygen saturation (e.g., pulse oximeter).
    (2) Support with oxygen as necessary.
  d. Pain
    (1) Alleviate pain.
    (2) Employ anxiety and stress-reduction tactics.

F. Gastrointestinal change
  1. Decreased salivation
  2. Decreased peristalsis
    a. Gastric emptying delayed
    b. Increased risk of aspiration
    c. Increased problem of constipation
  3. Decreased hepatic blood flow resulting from arteriosclerotic changes
  4. Decreased microsomal enzyme activity
    a. Delayed drug metabolism (e.g., fentanyl, vecuronium)
  5. Decreased absorption of orally administered drugs and nutrients (e.g., ferrous sulfate iron and calcium)
  6. Malnutrition possible
    a. Can increase perioperative morbidity
    b. Can compromise postoperative recovery and wound healing
    c. Most reliable indicator of malnutrition is hypoalbuminemia
  7. Nursing considerations
    a. Careful administration of oral fluids and food
      (1) Start with small amounts.
      (2) Begin when sitting up if possible.
    b. Elevate head of bed for most effective gastric emptying.
    c. Consider ulcers with complaint of chest pain.
      (1) Observe for prolonged or toxic drug effects.

G. Renal and genitourinary changes
  1. Decreased bladder capacity (200 ml)
  2. Decreased muscle tone and weakened sphincters
    a. Especially in women after multiple obstetric deliveries
    b. May result in incontinence
    c. Increased residual urine
  3. Enlarged prostate (men) may result in urinary incontinence and retention.
  4. Atrophic changes of vagina and urethral mucosa in women
  5. Decreased renal plasma flow
  6. Decreased glomerular filtration rate
    a. Resulting from decreased blood flow
    b. Decreases 1% to 1.5% per year after 30 years of age

        c. Results in decreased renal metabolism
           (1) Decreased clearance of medications and metabolites
           (2) Examples: fentanyl, vecuronium, midazolam
     7. Response time to correct fluid and electrolyte balance increased
        a. May increase risk of fluid overload
        b. Decreased ability to concentrate urine
        c. Inability to conserve sodium, leading to hyponatremia
        d. Decreased activity of renin or aldosterone, leading to hyperkalemia
     8. Nursing implications
        a. Observe for fluid imbalance.
           (1) Monitor intake and output.
           (2) Encourage oral fluids postoperatively.
        b. Observe for effects of electrolyte imbalance.
           (1) Monitor and/or observe for cardiac dysrhythmias, electrocardiogram (ECG) changes.
           (2) Consider that hyponatremia may be a cause of confusion.
        c. Observe for prolonged medication effect.
           (1) Use lower dosage range of medications, and encourage smaller medication dosage by team.
           (2) Provide support for toileting needs.
               (a) Toilet frequently (offer urinal or bedpan).
               (b) Assist to bathroom.
               (c) Facilitate genitourinary hygiene.
               (d) Provide protection for bedding and clothing.
               (e) Reassure and support emotionally.
               (f) Regard privacy to diminish embarrassment.
  H. Musculoskeletal changes
     1. Osteoporosis: inappropriately low bone mass for age, gender, and race
        a. Leads to decline in bone matrix
        b. Peak bone mass around 30-40 years of age
        c. Mineral content of bone (bone density) decreases.
           (1) After 40 years of age
           (2) For men, 0.5% per year
           (3) About 1.0% per year for women
        d. Skeletal support compromised
        e. Bone reabsorption exceeds bone formation.
        f. Increased risk of fractures, pain, skeletal deformities
           (1) Repair of hip fractures is one of top five surgeries done in elderly patients.
        g. Decrease in flexibility
        h. Risk factors
           (1) Age
           (2) Female
           (3) Low body weight
           (4) Caucasian race
           (5) Cigarette smokers
     2. Degenerative changes in vertebrae increase difficulty of spinal anesthesia and intubation.
        a. Degeneration of bone causes
           (1) Pathologic changes
               (a) Vertebral degeneration
     3. Kyphoscoliosis
        a. Limits chest expansion and capacity
        b. Limits success in establishing spinal or epidural injection
        c. Compression fractures
        d. Increased potential for pathologic fracture
        e. Higher incidence of traumatic fractures (falls especially)
     4. Osteoarthritis

      a. Specific cause unknown, but there is demonstrated relationship with

        (1) Advancing age

        (2) Wear and tear of joints throughout life span

      b. Structural changes in the joint

        (1) Probably starts in cartilage

        (2) Leads to

          (a) Reduced mobility of joint

          (b) Difficult ambulation

          (c) Potential for falls

          (d) Pain

          (e) Less flexibility

      c. May compromise intraoperative positioning

    5. Nursing considerations

      a. Careful positioning throughout perioperative experience

        (1) Support for back

        (2) Alignment

        (3) Protection of bony processes

      b. Observe for prolonged or toxic effects of regional agents.

      c. Provide for pain relief.

      d. Assist patient with physical tasks related to strength.

        (1) Moving

        (2) Ambulation

        (3) Exercise

          (a) Gentle movement

          (b) Encourage frequent activity.

      e. Safety concerns

        (1) Concerted fall prevention program

          (a) Support when walking: cane, walker, rails

          (b) Treaded (skid-resistant) footwear

          (c) Education for patient and caretakers

             (i) Potential for accidental falls: Use skid-resistant slippers, handrails and other safety measures.

I. Endocrine changes

  1. Decreased ability to metabolize glucose

    a. Results in glucose intolerance

    b. Pancreatic function declines.

      (1) Increased incidence of adult-onset diabetes mellitus

      (2) Greatest between 60 and 70 years of age

    c. Plasma renin concentrating ability decreases 30% to 50%.

  2. Decreased production of renin, aldosterone and testosterone

  3. Decreased vitamin D absorption

  4. Increased activation and increased plasma concentration of antidiuretic hormone

J. Dermatologic changes

  1. Loss of subcutaneous fat

    a. Compromises thermoregulation

    b. Increased risk of hypothermia

    c. Loss of padding for bony prominences

  2. Increase in overall body fat (especially women)

    a. Increased availability of lipid-storage sites

      (1) Reservoir for lipid-soluble (fat-soluble) drugs: diazepam, midazolam, enflurane

      (2) Prolongs drug action

  3. Loss of sweat glands

  4. Decreased skin pigmentation caused by decreased production of melanocytes; pallor does not equal anemia

   a. Provide warmed blankets and warm environment during and after operative event.

   b. Protect skin with
      (1) Proper positioning
      (2) Padding on bony prominences
      (3) Use paper or other nontearing skin tape.

   c. Remember, loss of pigmentation mimics pallor.
      (1) Do not rely on skin color to assess for anemia or cardiac distress.

   d. Provide careful positioning and safety instructions.

5. Epidural atrophy and loss of collagen

   a. Increases risk of skin breakdown and injury

   b. Decreases skin elasticity and turgor

6. Nursing considerations

   a. Provide warmed blankets and warm environment during and after operative event.

   b. Protect skin with
      (1) Proper positioning
      (2) Padding on bony prominences
      (3) Use paper or other nontearing skin tape.

   c. Remember, loss of pigmentation mimics pallor.
      (1) Do not rely on skin color to assess for anemia or cardiac distress.

K. Hematologic and immune system

   1. Decreased bone marrow production

   2. Decreased T-cell function

   3. Increased autoantibodies

   4. May see anemia and autoimmune diseases (Chapter 34)

L. Sensory changes

   1. Visual changes

      a. Decreased visual acuity

      b. Decreased peripheral vision

      c. Decreased accommodation (presbyopia)

      d. Retinal vascular changes

      e. Cataract formation

      f. Increased incidence of glaucoma

   2. Auditory changes

      a. Decreased sensitivity to sound (presbycusis)

      b. Loss of high-pitched sound perception

      c. Impairment of sound localization

   3. Tactile changes

      a. Decreased sensation

      b. Decreased response to pain

   4. Taste and smell acuity decreases.

M. Laboratory changes

   1. Decreased potassium

      a. Medications, diuretics

      b. Diet deficient in potassium

   2. Decreased sodium

      a. Dilutional

      b. True decrease

      c. Renal failure

   3. Decreased hemoglobin

      a. Blood loss (gastrointestinal and postmenstrual uterine bleeding)

      b. Malabsorption of iron

      c. Malnutrition

N. Neuropsychiatric changes

1. Acute brain syndrome
   a. Physiologic
   b. Rapid onset
   c. Reversible
   d. Possible causes—always rule out hypoxemia first!
      (1) Medication intolerance
      (2) Metabolic disturbance
      (3) Electrolyte imbalance
         (a) Hypernatremia and hyponatremia
      (4) Nutritional deficit
      (5) Depression
      (6) Stress, fear, anxiety
2. Chronic brain syndrome
   a. Associated with arteriosclerosis
   b. Degenerative changes
      (1) Alzheimer's disease
      (2) Cerebrovascular accident (CVA; stroke)
      (3) Dementia
3. Depression
   a. Causes: isolation, illness, loss, biochemical changes
   b. Symptoms: fatigue, insomnia, anorexia, somatic changes
O. Pathophysiologic conditions in elderly
   1. Of people 75 years old, 86% have one or more of the following chronic conditions.
      a. Cardiovascular: hypertension, atherosclerosis, dysrhythmias, valve disease
      b. Cerebral: cerebrovascular accident, cognitive degeneration
      c. Pulmonary: chronic obstructive pulmonary disease (COPD), asthma
      d. Endocrine: diabetes mellitus, hypothyroidism
      e. Neurologic: Parkinson's disease
      f. Musculoskeletal: arthritis
      g. Sensory: visual and hearing loss
      h. Hepatic: cirrhosis
   2. Physical status changes increase anesthetic and surgical risk.
IV. Psychosocial considerations for the elderly
   A. Maintain and promote autonomy.
      1. Independence
         a. Encourage performance of self-care.
         b. Address issues of concern.
            (1) Advance directives
            (2) Quality-of-life issues
         c. Talk with, not "around," the patient.
         d. Inquire about preferences.
            (1) Name use (e.g., "What do you prefer that I call you?")
            (2) Time schedules (eating, sleeping, etc.)
      2. Competence
         a. Reduced ability to provide self-care leads to depression and reduced self-worth.
         b. Abilities to perform may alter with time of day, health status, and life events
         c. Elders require more practice with new skills.
         d. Repetition and clarification enhance learning.
   B. Encourage self-acceptance.
      1. Maintain patient dignity.
      2. Invite expression of fears.
         a. Death and dying
         b. Change in body image and function
      3. Review coping mechanisms.

      4. Present patient with decision alternatives when possible.

  C. Time concept is altered.

    1. Employ tactics for time orientation.

      a. Time perception of elapsed time

      b. Past, present, and future

  D. Social awareness

    1. Elders are experiencing life role changes.

      a. May outlive friends and family (especially old-old)

      b. Caregivers become the patient (drastic role change when other party is already ill and debilitated).

    2. Encourage participation of significant others.

V. Elder abuse (usually related to family or other caregiver)

  A. Types

    1. Material and financial

    2. Physical

      a. Sexual

      b. Beating, slapping, kicking

      c. Neglect

        (1) Passive

        (2) Active (especially old-old)

        (3) Self

      d. Emotional

      e. Verbal

        (1) Threatening physical abuse or isolation

        (2) Humiliation

        (3) Intimidation

      f. Withholding (e.g., care, food, company)

  B. Detection

    1. Physical assessment and evidence of bodily harm

      a. Bruises

      b. Skin tears

      c. Burns

      d. Evidence of restraint

    2. Emotional abuse (difficult to assess)

      a. Fear of violence

      b. Social isolation

  C. Mandatory reporting

    1. Different laws in each state

  D. Resources

    1. Adult protection programs

    2. Domestic violence programs

    3. Services

      a. Financial advocacy

      b. Social advocacy

      c. Religious groups

VI. Pharmacologic alterations in aging

  A. Alterations in organs responsible for drug metabolism and clearance

    1. Lungs

    2. Kidneys

    3. Liver

  B. Protein binding of medications impaired

    1. Increases amount of available (free, unbound) drug

      a. Free drug is active drug, increasing drug effects.

  C. Storage of lipid-soluble medications increased

    1. Unpredictable clearance and elimination

  D. Prolonged action and elimination of medications

    1. Require decreased doses of medications

    2. Increased risk of cumulative drug effects

      3. Increased risk of adverse drug reactions

  VII. Considerations before surgery (see Box 16-1)

    A. Advantages of ambulatory surgery for the elderly

      1. Decreased risk of nosocomial infections

        a. Wound infections

        b. Respiratory infections

      2. Decreased incidence of mental confusion

        a. Environment less disruptive

        b. Decreased disruption in personal routine

      3. Minimized length of stay away from home environment

      4. Cost-effectiveness

    B. Disadvantages of ambulatory surgery for the elderly

      1. Compliance to the plan of care

        a. Diminishing abilities

          (1) Cognitive (e.g., forgetfulness)

            (a) Unable to complete care regime

            (b) Unable to cope with changes in routine

              (i) New medication protocols

              (ii) Care related to procedure

          (2) Physical

            (a) Diminished stamina and strength for self-care

            (b) Increased potential for falls

            (c) Unaware of wound contamination

        b. Lack of support system at home

          (1) Transportation issues and other logistic issues

          (2) Financial concerns (unable to obtain medications, supplies)

          (3) Lack of caregiver or significant other

          (4) Reduced or nonexistent circle of friends (especially in the old-old)

    C. Preoperative assessment

      1. To obtain precise baseline

        a. Consider physiologic not chronologic age

        b. Age alone does not determine risk.

      2. To obtain information about preexisting disease

        a. Especially with ambulatory patients

        b. Includes medications used and appropriateness of use

        c. Acute versus chronic conditions

        d. Evaluation of risk

      3. To review or obtain laboratory information

        a. Anemia common

        b. Electrolyte imbalance

          (1) Hypokalemia resulting from diuretics

          (2) Hyponatremia resulting from inability to conserve sodium

          (3) Glucose levels in diabetic patients

      4. To identify special needs

        a. Prostheses

        b. Language and communication barriers

        c. Mobility aids

■ BOX 16-1

■ **COMMON SURGICAL PROCEDURES DONE ON THE ELDERLY PATIENT**

Ophthalmic: cataract, vitrectomy
Genitourinary: cystoscopy, transurethral resection of the prostate
Orthopedic: open reduction and internal fixation—hip, joint replacement
Cardiovascular: pacemaker, carotid endarterectomy
General: herniorrhaphy

       d. Barriers to ambulatory patient returning home

         (1) Transportation

         (2) Caregiver availability, ability to care for self

         (3) Access to follow-up care

    5. To anticipate postoperative sequelae and to reduce risk factors

    6. To begin patient teaching

    7. To maximize preoperative physical status

       a. Pulmonary function

       b. Nutritional status, including hydration

       c. Medication protocol

  D. Multidisciplinary assessment

    1. PACU nurse

    2. Anesthesiologist

    3. Surgeon

    4. Medical consultation as needed

VIII. Intraoperative considerations for the elderly

  A. Sensory

    1. Avoid loud noises.

       a. Music

       b. Conversation not including the patient

    2. Allow patient to keep sensory aids if possible.

    3. Maintain voice, tactile, or visual contact with awake patient.

  B. Environment

    1. Remember thermostatic needs.

       a. Increased risk when core body temperature falls below 96.8° F (36° C)

    2. Protective measures

       a. Raise room temperature.

       b. Use warming blankets or devices.

       c. Warm anesthetic gases, solutions, IV fluids.

       d. Cover patient's head.

  C. Positioning

    1. Change slowly and gently; avoid extremes.

    2. Lift patient! Do not pull!

    3. Support back of neck (prevent discomfort from kyphosis or arthritis, for example).

    4. Pad and support to protect pressure points.

  D. Circulation: remember that hypotension and slowed circulation predispose patient to thrombus formation and emboli.

    1. Use antiembolitic stockings or sequential compression devices.

       a. Especially high-risk patient

       b. Prolonged (>2 hours) procedures

    2. Observe for points of pressure that might inhibit blood flow to extremities.

  E. Nurse-monitored local anesthesia; monitoring notes

    1. Elders do not tolerate fluid or blood loss well.

       a. When patient approaches hypovolemia, small changes can have large impact.

       b. Monitor fluid loss and output carefully.

    2. Impending crisis may be indicated by fluctuations in cardiac rate and rhythm.

IX. Anesthetic options for elderly patient

  A. General anesthesia

    1. Smooth induction and rapid recovery

    2. Inhalation requirements less

       a. Minimum alveolar concentration (MAC) decreases by 4% per year after 40 years of age.

    3. Delayed clearance or metabolism of IV anesthetic agents

       a. Decrease dose of barbiturates, benzodiazepines, opioids.

    4. Increased risk of hypothermia

     5. If edentulous, may be difficult to ventilate by mask

     6. Arthritis may limit cervicospinal mobility for intubation.

  B. Regional anesthesia

     1. Minimal physiologic alterations

     2. Decreased cardiopulmonary complications

     3. Less postoperative confusion

     4. Provides postoperative analgesia

     5. Spinal anesthesia

        a. Lower abdomen and lower extremity surgery

        b. Duration prolonged in elderly

        c. Hypotension may be pronounced.

        d. May be complicated by musculoskeletal changes

        e. Low incidence of spinal headaches

     6. Epidural anesthesia

        a. Less hypotension

        b. Greater cardiovascular stability

        c. Reduced anesthetic dose requirements

  C. Intravenous (IV) sedation and analgesia

     1. Increased sedating effects of benzodiazepines

     2. Increased respiratory depressant effects of narcotics

     3. Because of coexisting diseases, may not be appropriate for RN to administer intravenous conscious sedation

  D. Ambulatory surgery

     1. Minimizes separation from family and environment

     2. May be appropriate depending on type of surgery

        a. Must consider risks of anesthetic, surgery, home care

X. Postoperative priorities for the elderly patient in phase I (see Box 16-2)

  A. Reduction of morbidity and mortality

  B. Ventilation

     1. Promote optimal gas exchange.

        a. Provide high-humidity oxygen.

        b. Promote deep breathing and coughing.

        c. Prevent atelectasis.

        d. Elevate head of bed to facilitate lung expansion.

     2. Prevent respiratory infections.

        a. Sterile suctioning of endotracheal tube

        b. Protect patient from aspiration.

■ BOX 16-2
■ **NURSING DIAGNOSIS**

Examples of related nursing diagnostic categories include:
Impaired gas exchange
Potential for infection
Ineffective breathing pattern
Alteration in fluid volume (excess or deficiency)
Ineffective thermoregulation: hypothermia
Knowledge deficit: preoperative/postoperative information
Alteration in comfort: pain
Sensory-perceptual alteration
Ineffective airway clearance
Impaired physical mobility
Self-care deficit

       c. Promote deep breathing (prevent pneumonia).

   3. Monitor for compromised function.

       a. Observe for residual drug effects.

       b. Maintain artificial airways.

       c. Use pulse oximetry monitoring.

       d. Consider preexisting disease.

C. Fluid balance

   1. Correct preoperative dehydration.

       a. Nothing by mouth (NPO) status

       b. Diuretic therapy

       c. Poor nutritional status

       d. Presence of nausea and vomiting

   2. Prevent fluid overload.

       a. Assess preexisting cardiopulmonary disease.

       b. Monitor intake and output.

       c. Assess breath sounds.

   3. Monitor urine output.

       a. Decreased bladder capacity

       b. Urinary retention (men), incontinence (women)

       c. Perioperative diuretics

       d. Perioperative fluid intake

       e. Decreased awareness of distension

D. Activity—"stir-up" routine

   1. Promotes circulation and ventilation

   2. Permits assessment of neurologic status

       a. Deviations from preoperative status

   3. Monitor for orthostatic hypotension when mobilizing outpatients.

       a. Mobilize more slowly than younger adults.

E. Thermoregulation

   1. Rewarm patient.

   2. Document temperature.

   3. Normothermia promotes cardiovascular stability.

F. Comfort

   1. Positioning

       a. Care in turning; turn frequently

       b. Anatomic and surgical alignment

       c. Pad bony prominences

   2. Skin care

       a. Avoid excessive tape application.

       b. Remove tape and ECG leads carefully.

       c. Dry wet skin promptly.

       d. Hold venipuncture sites after removal of needle.

       e. Remove skin preparation solutions to decrease irritation.

   3. Pain management

       a. Titrate narcotics.

       b. Pain increases myocardial oxygen demand.

       c. Consider decreased sensory response to pain.

       d. Evaluate presence of residual preoperative or anesthetic drugs.

   4. Psychologic support

       a. Reorientation

       b. Avoid sensory deprivation and overload.

       c. Avoid use of restraints.

       d. Continue verbal and tactile communication.

       e. Provide hearing aids, glasses, and dentures.

       f. Provide simple, clear instructions—ascertain patient's level of understanding.

       g. Rule out hypoxemia as cause of postoperative agitation.

        h. Maintain dignity and respect.

XI. PACU phase II

  A. Physical status

     1. Ensure safety.

        a. Ambulate carefully.

          (1) Sit on edge of stretcher to gain balance.

          (2) Provide physical support for walking.

             (a) Use orthopedic and prosthetic devices as necessary.

             (b) Lower stretcher

             (c) Step stool with caution (they tip!)

          (3) Encourage, while allowing patient to find own pace of movement.

        b. Return all sensory aids prior to ambulation.

        c. Monitor neuromuscular status.

     2. Psychologic interventions

        a. Promote wellness concept.

          (1) Return clothes and belongings promptly.

          (2) Reunite with family members, responsible adult, significant others.

        b. Communicate with patient expecting:.

          (1) Slower thought processes, movements, and responses

          (2) Old does not mean stupid!

     3. Home preparation

        a. Include support persons when reviewing home instructions.

        b. Verify plans for home support.

          (1) Ascertain patient, family, or responsible adult's understanding of and ability to comply with discharge instructions.

          (2) Elderly caring for elderly may not be adequate or responsible.

          (3) Arrange time and place for postoperative contact.

             (a) Recovery issues evaluation

               (i) Consider tool easily understood by patient.

               (ii) Introducing a Likert-type scale to patient prior to surgery would be beneficial.

               (iii) Discuss possible topics of postoperative telephone contact.

        c. Instruct on return to normal preoperative medication regime.

        d. Instructions

          (1) Avoid sedating medications.

          (2) Provide clear verbal instructions.

          (3) Provide large-print written instructions.

             (a) Large simple diagrams or pictures

          (4) Ascertain understanding (patient and other care providers as necessary).

             (a) By demonstration

             (b) Return demonstration

          (5) Repeat instructions.

BIBLIOGRAPHY

1. Allen A: Caring about the elderly: Opportunities and obligations. *J Post Anesth Nurs* 8(2):131-133, 1993.
2. Bejelle A: Rheumatic diseases. In Birren JE, editor: *Encyclopedia of gerontology.* San Diego: Academic Press, 1996, p 451.
3. Burden N: *Ambulatory surgical nursing.* Philadelphia: WB Saunders, 2000.
4. Birren J, editor: *Encyclopedia of gerontology.* San Diego: Academic Press, 1996.
5. Callahan L: General considerations in planning anesthetic care for the geriatric patient. *Anesth Today* 3(1):10-14, 1991.
6. Cassel CK, Cohen HJ, Larson EB, et al, editors: *Geriatric medicine,* ed 3. New York: Springer, 1997.
7. Clyne M, Forlenza M: Consumer-focused preadmission testing: A paradigm shift. *J Nurs Care Qual* 11(3):9-15, 1997.
8. Drain C: *The Post Anesthesia Care Unit.* Philadelphia: WB Saunders, 1994.

9. Ebert Thomas: Physiology of the cardiovascular effects for general anesthesia in the elderly. *Syllabus on Geriatric Anesthesiology*. Available at http://www.asahq.org/clinical/geriatrics/phy.htm. Accessed on May 5, 2003.

10. Ferrara-Love R: Geriatric considerations for the ambulatory surgery patient. Presentation at Issues for a New Millennium. conference co-sponsored by Chesapeake Bay Society of PeriAnesthesia Nurses and American Society of PeriAnesthesia Nurses, Stevensville, MD, 1997.

11. Gibson JR Jr, Mendenhall MK, Axel NJ: Geriatric anesthesia: Minimizing the risk *Geriatr Clin North America* 1:313-321, 1985.

12. Hazen SE, Larsen PD, Martin JLH: General anesthesia and elderly surgical patients. *AORN J* 65(4):815-822, 1997.

13. Lancaster KA: Patient teaching in ambulatory surgery. *Nurs Clin North America* 32(2):417-427, 1997.

14. Lien C: Thermoregulation in the elderly. *Syllabus on Geriatric Anesthesiology*. Available at http://www.asahq.org/clinical/geriatrics/thermo.htm. Accessed on May 5, 2003.

15. Linden I, Engberg IB: Nursing discharge assessment of the patient post-inguinal herniorrhaphy in the ambulatory surgery setting. *J Post Anesth Nurs* 9(1):14-18, 1994.

16. Litwack K: *Post anesthesia care nursing*, ed 2. St Louis: Mosby, 1995.

17. Litwack K: The elderly patient in the post anesthesia care unit. *Nurs Clin North America* 28(3):507-518, 1993.

18. Litwack K: *The elderly surgical patient*. Sacramento, CA: CME Resource, 1995.

19. Lynch SH: Elder abuse: What to look for, how to intervene. *Am J Nurs* 97(1):27-33, 1997.

20. Martin C: Transcend generational timelines. *Nurs Manage* 34(4):24-28, 2003.

21. Martin-Sheridan D: Geriatrics and anesthesia practice. In Nagelhout J, Zaglaniczny K, editors: *Nurse anesthesia*. Philadelphia: WB Saunders, 1997, pp 981-987.

22. McLeskey C: Pharmacokinetic and pharmacodynamic differences in the elderly patient undergoing anesthesia. *Anesth Today* 3(1):1-9, 1991.

23. McLeskey C, Nibel D: Anesthesia for the geriatric outpatient. In White P, editor: *Outpatient anesthesia*. New York: Churchill Livingstone, 1990.

24. Muravchick S: Geriatric anesthesia: Are you ready? *Syllabus on Geriatric Anesthesiology*. Available at http://www.asahq.org/clinical/geriatrics/geron.htm. Accessed on May 5, 2003.

25. Norman J: *Gerontological nursing*. Sacramento, CA: CME Resource, 1994.

26. Oberle K, Allen M, Lynkowski P: Follow-up of same day surgery patients. *AORN J* 59(5):1016-1025, 1994.

27. Ross B: Aging and the respiratory system. *Syllabus on Geriatric Anesthesiology*. Available at http://www.asahq.org/clinical/geriatrics/aging.htm. Accessed on May 5, 2003.

28. Roy R, Price A: Geriatric patients. In McGoldrick K, editor: *Ambulatory anesthesiology: A problem-oriented approach*. Baltimore: Williams & Wilkins, 1995, pp 111-126.

29. Stiff J: Evaluation of geriatric patient. In Rogers M, Tinker J, Covino B, et al, editors: *Principles and practice of anesthesia*. St Louis: Mosby, 1993, pp 480-492.

30. Stoelting R, Miller R: *Basics of anesthesia*, ed 4. Philadelphia: Churchill Livingstone, 2000, pp 376-385.

31. Sung Y-F: Age-related diseases. *Syllabus on Geriatric Anesthesiology*. Available at http://www.asahq.org/clinical/geriatrics/age_related.htm. Accessed on May 5, 2003.

32. Tasch M: Cardiovascular and autonomic nervous system aging. *Syllabus on Geriatric Anesthesiology*. Available at http://www.asahq.org/clinical/geriatrics/cardio.htm. Accessed on May 5, 2003.

33. Thereault J: Aging and the central nervous system. *Syllabus on Geriatric Anesthesiology*. Available at www.asahq.org/clinical/geriatrics/aging_central.htm. Accessed on May 5, 2003.

34. US Department Health and Human Services: A profile of older Americans. Available at http://www.aoa.gov/prof/ Statistics/profile/2002profile.pdf. Accessed in November 2003.

35. Worfolk JB: Keep frail elders warm! *Geriatr Nurs* 18(1):7-11, 1997.

36. Zemke R, Raines C, Flipczak R: *Generations at work*. New York: AMACOM, 2000.

COMPETENCY OF PREOPERATIVE ASSESSMENT

17 Preoperative Assessment Programs

DONNA M. DEFAZIO QUINN

OBJECTIVES

At the conclusion of this chapter the reader will be able to:

1. Identify three reasons why preoperative interviews should be conducted in advance.

2. List three options available for conducting preoperative assessments and interviews.

3. Express four benefits of providing preoperative tours for patients.

4. Describe four disadvantages of using Web-based programs to obtain patient information preoperatively.

I. Purpose of preoperative programs
   A. Provide comprehensive assessment and teaching regarding the perioperative and perianesthesia experience (see Box 17-1)
   B. Timing of preoperative assessment
      1. Far enough in advance to
         a. Obtain additional diagnostic testing and/or consultation if needed
         b. Alter current medical regimen if necessary (discontinue anticoagulant therapy)
         c. Obtain equipment, supplies, and other items necessary for postoperative care
         d. Make arrangements in family schedule (home care, day care, transportation, etc.)
         e. Prepare patient physically and emotionally for surgery
      2. Not too far in advance that patient forgets preoperative instructions
   C. Benefits of a preoperative assessment program
      1. Identify issues needing further follow-up prior to admission to avoid costly delays and cancellations.
         a. Additional diagnostic screenings
         b. Postoperative care needs
            (1) Supplies, prescriptions
            (2) Equipment for home care (crutches, walker, continuous passive motion [CPM], etc.)
            (3) Arrangement for visiting nurse services (if appropriate)
            (4) Transportation home if outpatient surgery (to avoid unnecessary postoperative stay and unsafe transportation plans)
            (5) Responsible adult caregiver
      2. Preoperative diagnostic screening is based on specific clinical indicators or risk factors.
         a. Age
         b. Preexisting disease or illness
         c. Surgical procedure being performed
      3. Potential safety issues are identified.
         a. Patient and family history

■ BOX 17-1
■ **GOALS OF PREANESTHESIA ASSESSMENT FOR AMBULATORY SURGERY PATIENTS**

- To optimize patient care, satisfaction, and comfort
- To minimize perioperative morbidity and mortality by assessing factors that affect the risk of anesthesia or that might alter the planned anesthesia technique
- To minimize surgical delays or cancellations on the day of surgery
- To assess the appropriateness of the patients and the procedure for the ambulatory surgery facility
- To evaluate the patient's health status, thus determining which specific preoperative investigations and consultations are required to formulate a plan of patient care
- To communicate patient management issues effectively between care providers (e.g., anesthetist, surgeon, primary care provider)
- To ensure efficient and cost-effective patient evaluation

From Cassidy J, Marley RA: Preoperative assessment of the ambulatory patient. *J PeriAnesth Nurs* 11:334-343, 1996.

     (1) Malignant hyperthermia
     (2) Pseudocholinesterase deficiency
   b. Mobility issues
   c. Ability of patient to care for himself or herself if lives alone
   d. Quality and amount of caregiver assistance
   e. Compliance with preoperative instructions
     (1) Nothing by mouth (NPO) requirements
     (2) Procedure-related instructions for preoperative preparations (i.e., bowel prep, antiseptic shower, etc)
     (3) Preoperative medications
       (a) Medications that need to be stopped the day of surgery
       (b) Medications that need to be administered the day of surgery
       (c) Medications that need to be stopped prior to surgery
         (i) Anticoagulant therapy
         (ii) Acetaminophen
         (iii) Herbals
  4. Provide preoperative teaching.
   a. Procedure-specific instructions
   b. Compliance with preoperative instructions
   c. Review of preoperative and postoperative expectations
   d. Importance of caregiver support
  5. Patient satisfaction
   a. Convenient for the patient
   b. Informative
   c. Allows patient to get response to questions or concerns
II. Types of preoperative assessment programs
  A. Hospital-based preoperative assessment clinics
   1. Patient scheduled for preoperative appointment once surgery booked
   2. Appointment may include
    a. Diagnostic testing
     (1) Labs
     (2) Electrocardiogram (ECG), cardiac stress testing, and so forth
     (3) Radiological exams
     (4) Procedure-specific diagnostic testing
   3. Patient may be interviewed by
    a. Anesthesia provider
    b. Specially trained preanesthesia assessment nurse
    c. Nurse practitioner or physician assistant
    d. Medical students, interns, residents

     4. Advantages

        a. Allows patient the opportunity to build patient rapport and ask questions

        b. Allows interviewer to adequately assess patient's understanding of preoperative and postoperative instructions

     5. Disadvantages

        a. May not be feasible for emergent cases or add-ons

        b. Busy lifestyle may preclude patients from taking time out for in-person interview.

        c. Travel distance may preclude patient from attending scheduled interview.

        d. Elderly or handicapped may have difficulty getting to scheduled interview.

        e. Staffing costs

B. Ambulatory surgery center based

     1. Patient comes to the center or is telephoned for preadmission testing and interview.

     2. Diagnostic testing may be performed at this time or on day of procedure.

     3. Anesthesiologist may interview the patient.

     4. RN obtains patient's medical history and performs preoperative teaching.

C. Physician office based

     1. May provide patient with "preoperative teaching booklet"

     2. RN, physician assistant, or registered nurse practitioner may perform preoperative assessment and teaching.

D. Telephone interviews

     1. RN interviews patient and completes a questionnaire.

     2. Shortened interviews can be done for repeat patients who have had no change in medical condition since last visit.

E. Web-based assessment and teaching programs

     1. Facility based

        a. Specifically designed to meet needs of facility

        b. May include virtual preoperative tour

     2. Independent Web based

        a. Purchased service

     3. Process

        a. Patient accesses a designated secure Web site to complete a medical history.

        b. Questionnaire is then reviewed by an RN for accuracy and need to follow-up with patient.

        c. Program may offer preoperative teaching module (see Box 17-2).

            (1) Patient proceeds at own pace.

        d. Interactive module allows patient to ask questions and receive responses in a timely manner.

     4. Advantages

        a. Patient completes information during leisure time.

        b. Patient does not have to take time off from work.

        c. Able to proceed at own pace

■ BOX 17-2

■ **ADVANTAGES OF COMPUTER-BASED PREOPERATIVE EDUCATION**

- Consistency—quality and content is standardized.
- Individualized instruction—patients proceed at their own pace and can repeat and review information.
- Privacy—only the patient sees incorrect answers, avoiding embarrassment over incorrect or personal answers.
- Time efficiency—reduces professional time spent presenting information common to most patients
- Accessibility—it can be used at any time, for inpatients as well as outpatients.

From Burden N, Quinn DMD, O'Brien D, et al: *Ambulatory surgical nursing.* Philadelphia: WB Saunders, 2000, p 349.

     5. Disadvantages
       a. Decreased opportunity to build personal rapport with patient
       b. No person available to answer questions or provide explanations
       c. Possible lack of Internet access
       d. Potential anxiety over privacy issues
       e. Potential for actual breech of privacy

F. Questionnaire
    1. Patient completes an abbreviated questionnaire at time of scheduling or shortly thereafter.
    2. RN reviews questionnaire to determine if patient's medical history warrants an in-person interview and/or diagnostic testing.
    3. Healthy patients are contacted via telephone to review preoperative instructions.

G. Preoperative group sessions
    1. May be generalized or pertinent to specific patient population
    2. Helpful to include various team members in session
      a. Admissions
      b. Preadmission operating room and postanesthesia care unit (PACU) nurse
      c. Anesthesia
      d. Social services
      e. Case managers
      f. Financial counseling
      g. Nutritional services
      h. Rehabilitation services
      i. Visiting nurse services
    3. Patients may benefit from talking with patients who are undergoing same procedure and/or patients who have already undergone procedure (cardiac, bariatric surgery).
    4. Allows nurse to reach a multitude of patients at one time
    5. Helpful to review the clinical pathway and expectations for the specific surgical procedure
    6. Patient and family have opportunity to have any questions answered in advance.
    7. Not always convenient for patients to attend

H. Preoperative tours—Pediatric
    1. Benefits of program
      a. Provides information to patient, family, significant others
      b. Minimizes postoperative complications through proper education
      c. Decreases anxiety by reviewing preoperative process
      d. Allows opportunity to review clinical pathway and expectations of recovery
      e. Allows child to see surrounding so it will be familiar on day of surgery
      f. Allows opportunity for patient and family to get questions answered
      g. Allows opportunity for child to practice "leaving parents" to go into procedure room and then reunite—builds trust
    2. Types of pediatric programs
      a. Tour of facility with hands-on practice with common equipment child will encounter
        (1) Blood pressure cuff
        (2) Thermometer
        (3) Face mask
        (4) Casting materials, slings, crutches, and so forth
      b. Safari adventure through the perioperative area
      c. "Dress-up" programs
      d. Role-playing activities
      e. Procedure specific, (e.g., cardiac, urological, orthopedic)

I. Preoperative tours—adult
    1. Useful for patients undergoing major surgical interventions

       2. Can be done in a group or individually
       3. Review of preoperative and postoperative expectations assists in deceasing patient anxiety.
       4. Allows patient and family to see where the family will wait
    J. Additional alternatives to preoperative assessment
       1. In-home assessment program
          a. Labor intensive
          b. May be beneficial for severely handicapped or patients undergoing major procedure
       2. Community preadmission testing centers
          a. Conveniently located in the community
          b. Flexible hours
       3. Preoperative videos
          a. Can be generalized or surgery specific
          b. Can focus on pediatric population
          c. Allows viewing in own home in familiar surroundings
          d. Can be reviewed numerous times until patient is comfortable with content
       4. Educational pamphlets and brochures
          a. Distributed to patient at surgeon's office
          b. Can be as brief or detailed as necessary to meet patient needs
          c. Provides concrete information patient can look at in comfort of own home when anxiety level is decreased
          d. May explain surgical procedure in detail
          e. May help to spur questions patient would otherwise not have considered
       5. Primary care provider
          a. Performs preassessment diagnostic testing
          b. May provide medical clearance
III. Conclusion
    A. Preoperative patient education extremely important to
       1. Provide patient with necessary information to make surgical experience a positive one
       2. Assess patient's understanding of and potential compliance with preoperative and postoperative instructions
    B. Attaining goals
       1. Can achieve goals of preoperative assessment and teaching in varied ways
       2. Does not matter which method is used as long as the end result is achieved
       3. Provide patient with written materials to reinforce teachings
       4. Have different approaches available to meet varied needs of patients and families

BIBLIOGRAPHY

1. American Society of PeriAnesthesia Nurses: *ASPAN standards of nursing practice.* Cherry Hill, NJ: American Society of PeriAnesthesia Nurses, 2002.
2. Association of Operating Room Nurses: *AORN standards: Recommended practice and guidelines.* Denver, CO: Association of Operating Room Nurses, 2002.
3. Burden N, Quinn DD, O'Brien D, et al: *Ambulatory surgical nursing,* ed 2. Philadelphia: WB Saunders, 2000.
4. Fischer SP: Cost-effective preoperative evaluation and testing. *Chest* 115(5):96S-100S, 1999.
5. Gibby GL: How preoperative assessment programs can be justified financially to hospital administrators. *Int Anesthesiol Clin* 40(2):17-30, 2002.
6. Krenzischek DA, Wilson L, Poole E: Evaluation of ASPAN's preoperative patient teaching videos on general, regional, and minimum alveolar concentration/conscious sedation anesthesia. *J PeriAnesth Nurs* 16;(3):174-180, 2001.
7. Lee DS, Lee SS: Pre-operative teaching: How does a group of nurses do it? *Contemp Nurse* 9(1):80-88, 2000.
8. Lin PC, Lin LC, Lin JJ: Comparing the effectiveness of different educational programs for patients with total knee arthroplasty. *Orthop Nurs* 16(5):43-49, 1997.
9. Malkin KF: Patients' perceptions of a preadmission clinic. *J Nurs Manage* 8(2):107-113, 2000.

10. Oermann MH: Effects of educational intervention in waiting room on patient satisfaction. *J Ambul Care Manage* 26(2):150-158, 2003.

11. Oermann MH, Masserang M, Maxey M, et al: Clinic visit and waiting: Patient education and satisfaction. *Nurs Econ* 20(6):292-295, 2002.

12. Oermann MH, Webb SA, Ashare JA: Outcomes of videotape instruction in clinic waiting area. *Orthop Nurs* 22(2):102-105, 2003.

13. Pellino T, Tluczek A, Collins M, et al: Increasing self-efficacy through empowerment: Preoperative education for orthopaedic patients. *Orthop Nurs* 17(4):48-59, 1998.

14. Pollard JB, Zboray AL, Mazze RI: Economic benefits attributed to opening a preoperative evaluation clinic for outpatients. *Anesth Analg* 83(2):407-410, 1996.

15. Ryan P: The benefits of a nurse-led preoperative assessment clinic. *Nurs Times* 96(39):42-43, 2000.

16. Stephens P: Pre-anaesthesia assessment clinics. *Anaesthesia* 56(1):84, 2001.

17. Sullivan EE: A successful practice: Preadmitting test center. *J PeriAnesth Nurs* 16(3):198-200, 2001.

18. Wadsworth L, Smith A, Waterman H: The nurse practitioner's role in day case preoperative assessment. *Nurs Stand* 16(47):41-44, 2002.

19. Ziolkowski L, Strzyzewski N: Perianesthesia assessment: Foundation of care. *J PeriAnesth Nurs* 16(6):359-370, 2001.

18 History and Physical Examinations

ROSE FERRARA-LOVE

OBJECTIVES
At the conclusion of this chapter the reader will be able to:

1. State goals of preoperative history and physical exams.

2. Plan a subjective and objective patient exam.

3. Discuss the importance of completing a system review.

I. The nursing history and physical examination
   A. General health
      1. Questions and observations regarding overall health include
         a. General appearance
         b. Height
         c. Weight
            (1) Often converted to kilograms to facilitate rapid calculation of medication doses in mg/kg format
               (a) Weight in pounds (divided by 2.2 equals weight in kilograms)
               (b) Weight in kilograms (multiplied by 2.2 equals weight in pounds)
            (2) Obesity
               (a) Many freestanding surgical centers enforce weight restrictions because of increased risk of anesthesia complications.
                  (i) Usually 300 pounds (136.4 kg)
            (3) Recent unplanned weight loss
         d. Recent or current infection
            (1) Upper respiratory infections
            (2) Lower respiratory infections
         e. Allergies
            (1) Food
            (2) Drugs
            (3) Environment
         f. Nutritional habits
         g. Physical handicaps
            (1) Use of adjuncts for walking
      2. Physical examination includes observation.
         a. Skin
            (1) Color
            (2) Turgor
            (3) Elasticity
            (4) Presence of bruises
               (a) May necessitate report to authorities if abuse is suspected
            (5) Other injuries
            (6) Dryness
            (7) Lesions
               (a) Include mucous membrane

       (8) Cleanliness

       (9) Dental hygiene

  b. Abnormalities

       (1) Posture

       (2) Gait

       (3) Mobility

          (a) Use of wheelchair, walker, or cane should be noted.

       (4) Pain at rest

  c. Physical characteristics

       (1) Potential complications for intubation

          (a) Short, stocky neck

          (b) Cervical fusion or arthritis

          (c) Thick tongue

          (d) Temporal mandibular joint disease

          (e) Dental or orthopedic abnormalities

  d. Vital signs should be obtained to identify aberrancies and for baseline measurements.

       (1) Blood pressure

          (a) Dynamic measurements that change minute to minute

             (i) Response to

                [a] Environment

                [b] Physiologic demands

          (b) Average ranges

             (i) 100–135 mm Hg systolic

             (ii) 60–80 mm Hg diastolic

          (c) Orthostatic measurements with underlying cardiac or hypertensive history

       (2) Pulse

          (a) Average range 60–100 beats per minute

       (3) Respirations

          (a) Average rate

             (i) 12–20 breaths per minute

             (ii) 16-25 breaths per minute in elderly

          (b) Use of accessory muscles of respiration

          (c) Shape and symmetry

          (d) Sternal abnormalities

             (i) Pectus carinatum

                [a] Chicken breast or pigeon breast

             (ii) Pectus excavatum

                [a] Breastbone caves in resulting in sunken chest appearance

             (iii) Anterior-posterior diameter increased

                [a] May be normal with

                   [1] Age

                   [2] Hyperinflation

          (e) Abnormal breathing patterns

             (i) Küssmaul *— deep gasping / severe diabetic ketoacidosis coma —*

            (ii) Cheyne-Stokes *— apnea 10-60 seconds > increasing depth and frequency of resps.*

            (iii) Biot's *can be normal in children.*

Short breaths → long irreg periods of apnea seen in TICP

       (4) Temperature

          (a) Oral temperatures considered normal at 96.4° F (35.8° C)

          (b) Rectal temperatures average slightly less than 1° F higher.

          (c) Axillary temperatures are approximately one half to 1° F lower.

          (d) Tympanic thermometers offer comfortable, rapid, and accurate readings.

             (i) Approximately ½° F to 1° F higher than oral readings

          (e) Variances in normal ranges

             (i) Normal physiologic status

(f) Extrinsic forces
   (i) Medication
   (ii) Recent exercise
   (iii) Effort
   (iv) Anxiety and fear

B. Medication history
   1. Medication protocol affects types of medications and anesthetic agents used.
      a. Helps avoid untoward drug interactions or withdrawal episodes
   2. Include in history form
      a. Names
      b. Dosages
      c. Frequency
      d. Length of time prescribed
      e. Effects
      f. Nonprescription drugs
         (1) Aspirin
            (a) Prolongs bleeding time
      g. Herbal preparations
      h. Habit-forming drugs usage
         (1) Tobacco
            (a) Number of pack years
               (i) Number of packs per day × number of years
               (ii) Attempts to stop
         (2) Alcohol
            (a) Type
            (b) Amount
            (c) Frequency
            (d) Changes in reaction to alcohol intake
         (3) Recreational
         (4) Prescription
      i. Side effects
      j. Allergic reactions
         (1) Specific drug
            (a) May know only category of drug (i.e., antibiotic)
            (b) Identify if related categories will be used in the ambulatory surgery center (ASC).
         (2) Specific reaction
            (a) True allergy or expected side effect
         (3) Usually documented in red
            (a) Highly visible
               (i) On medical record
            (b) On patient identification band
         (4) Environmental and food allergies
            (a) Allergy to eggs may have possible cross-sensitivity with propofol.
            (b) Allergy to bananas, kiwis, peaches, water chestnuts may have link with latex allergies.
               (i) Cutaneous exposure
                  [a] Anesthesia masks, head straps, rebreathing masks, tourniquets, electrocardiogram (ECG) patches, adhesive tape, surgical gloves
                  [b] Other sources include elastic bandages, rubber positioning rings, rubber shoes, elastic clothing, balloons, Koosh balls, sporting equipment
               (ii) Mucous membrane
                  [a] Nasogastric tubes, balloons, nipples, pacifiers, products used in dentistry, urinary catheters, glove contact with vaginal mucosa, enema kits, rectal pressure catheters

(especially in patients with spina bifida and impaired bowel control)
- [b] Other sources include condoms.
  - (iii) Inhalation
    - [a] Often associated with glove powder
  - (iv) Internal tissue
    - [a] Intraoperative resulting from surgical gloves contacting the peritoneum or internal organs
  - (v) Intravascular
    - [a] Disposable syringes, medication aspirated from vials with latex stoppers, injection of medication via ports of intravenous tubing (latex can leech into solutions injected)

C. Nutrition status
  1. Weight history
     a. Typical day's diet
        (1) Salt
        (2) Saturated fats
        (3) Food habits
            [a] Ethnicity
  2. Physiologic processes dependent upon proper nutrition
     a. Wound healing
     b. Oxygen transport
     c. Enzymes synthesis
     d. Clotting factors
     e. Resistance to infection
  3. Diseases associated with poor nutrition
     a. Crohn's disease
     b. Malignancies
     c. Chronic obstructive pulmonary disease (COPD)
     d. Ulcerative colitis
  4. Indications of malnutrition
     a. Anorexia
     b. Recent weight loss
     c. Dull hair
     d. Brittle nails
     e. Diagnostic tests
        (1) Decreased lymphocytes
        (2) Decreased serum albumin and transferrin levels
  5. Obesity complicates
     a. Administration of anesthesia
        (1) Requires higher-than-normal levels of anesthetic agents
            (a) Fat-soluble agents tend to prolong effects.
        (2) Increased stress on cardiovascular system
            (a) Increased oxygen needs
            (b) Increased carbon dioxide production
                (i) Associated with increased body mass
     b. Technical aspects of performing procedure
        (1) Often difficult to intubate
            (a) Difficult to maintain airway
                (i) Increased risk of aspiration
                (ii) Increased intraabdominal pressures
            (b) Gastric contents higher in volume and more acidic
        (2) Problems with positioning
            (a) Weight of abdominal and chest contents can cause respiratory embarrassment when in Trendelenburg position.
        (3) Difficult to perform venipuncture
     c. Patient's recovery
        (1) Electrolyte and fluid balance essential for homeostasis

       (a) Regulates cardiac rhythm

       (b) Muscle strength

       (c) Distribution and metabolism of drugs

          (i) Mental alertness

       (d) Table 18-1 highlights signs and symptoms of electrolyte imbalances.

    (2) Signs of dehydration

       (a) Loss of skin turgor

       (b) Listlessness

       (c) Orthostatic hypotension

       (d) Rapid and thready pulse

       (e) Dryness of mucous membranes

       (f) Thirst

    (3) Cardiovascular

       (a) Symptoms of cardiac disease

          (i) Chest pain or tightness

       (b) Palpitations

       (c) Chronic fatigue

       (d) Loss of appetite

       (e) Angina

       (f) Swelling of the ankles

       (g) Paroxysmal nocturnal dyspnea (PND)

       (h) Exhaustion

    (4) Particular importance

       (a) Recent cardiac surgery

       (b) Myocardial infarction (MI)

          (i) Considered most important indicator of anesthesia morbidity

       (c) Generally elective, nonurgent surgery postponed for at least 6 months after an MI

       (d) Angina

       (e) Aortic stenosis

       (f) Poorly controlled dysrhythmias

       (g) Congestive heart failure

       (h) Extremes in blood pressure

          (i) Presence of pacemaker

    (5) Physical examination parameters

       (a) Apical pulse

          (i) Rate

       (b) Rhythm

       (c) Quality

       (d) At least one blood pressure reading

       (e) Palpation of peripheral pulses

       (f) Observation for edema

       (g) Clubbing of fingers

       (h) Cyanosis

       (i) Distention of neck veins

       (j) General energy level

       (k) Respiratory ease

       (l) Auscultation of heart for murmurs

          (i) Systolic murmur over right sternal border, second intercostal space may indicate presence of aortic stenosis

          (ii) Associated with unexpected dysrhythmias

       (m) Diminished stroke volume

6. Cardiac drugs

  a. Maintain normal routine preoperatively.

    (i) Do not skip doses.

       (a) Beta blockers

■ TABLE 18-1
■ ■ Signs and Symptoms of Electrolyte Imbalance

Electrolyte Normal Value	Physiologic Functions	Excess	Deficiency
Potassium (K) 3.5-5.0 mEq/L	—Nerve conduction —Muscle contraction —Enzyme action for cellular energy production —Regulates intercellular osmolality	—Generalized muscle weakness and flaccidity; can affect respiratory muscles, paresthesia —Cardiac: bradycardia, ventricular ectopy and fibrillation, 3 degree heart block, asystole (>7.0 mEq/L) —ECG changes: flat or absent P wave, wide QRS, peaked T wave, prolonged PR interval	—Muscle weakness, flaccidity, fatigue, leg cramps, ↓ deep tendon reflexes, shallow respirations, weak, thready pulse, hypotension —Cardiac: atrial dysrhythmias, premature ventricular contractions (PVCs), AV blocks, cardiac arrest (<2.5 mEq/L) —ECG changes: flat or inverted T wave, depressed ST segment, U wave present, potentates digitalis toxicity, premature atrial contractions (PACs) or PVCs
Sodium (Na) 135-145 mEq/L	—Transmission and conduction of nerve impulses —Regulates vascular osmolality —Regulates body fluids and acid/base balance —Regulates neuromuscular activity via sodium pump	—Excitement; thirst; dry, sticky tongue and mucous membranes; oliguria; flushed skin; confusion; lethargy; coma; convulsions; hypo- or hypertension; elevated temperature	—Abdominal cramping, anorexia, malaise, nausea and vomiting, muscle weakness, headache, confusion, lethargy, convulsions, coma
Calcium (Ca) 9-11 mg/dl	—Nerve and muscle activity —Myocardial contractility —Maintains cell permeability —Converts prothrombin to thrombin —Formation of teeth and bones	—Lethargy, depression, apathy, anorexia, nausea and vomiting, muscle weakness, headache, confusion, decreased attention span, slurred speech, hypertension. —Cardiac: heart block, PVCs, idioventricular rhythms, cardiac arrest —ECG changes: shortened QT interval	—Anxiety, excitement, hyperreflexia, grimacing, numbness and tingling of lips or fingers, muscle cramps and spasms, laryngospasm, convulsions, tetany, dysrhythmias including ventricular tachycardia (VT) —Positive Trousseau's sign: carpal spasm after inflation of blood pressure cuff on upper arm to 20 mm Hg over systolic for 3 minutes, shows tetany —Positive Chevostk's sign: abnormal facial spasm when facial nerve in front of ear is tapped —ECG changes: prolonged QT interval

From Quinn DMD: *Ambulatory surgical nursing core curriculum.* Philadelphia: WB Saunders, 1999, p 69.

(b) Calcium channel blockers
(c) Antihypertensives
D. Peripheral vascular disease
  1. Inspection
    a. Skin color
    b. Hair distribution
    c. Edema
    d. Varicosities
      (i) Stasis ulcers
      (ii) Capillary refill time
  2. Palpation
    a. Peripheral pulses
      (1) Characteristics
        (a) Absent = 0
        (b) Weak, thready = 1+
        (c) Normal = 2+
        (d) Full, bounding = 3+
    b. Rigidity of vessels
      (1) Palpable vibration (thrill)
  3. Auscultation
    a. Bruit
      (1) Humming sound from narrow or bulging artery
  4. Symptoms
    a. Peripheral cyanosis
    b. Pain
    c. Cold
    d. Intermittent claudication — *lameness, limping pain calf muscle during walking subsides with rest. Results from inadequate blood supply.*
    e. Central vessel involvement
      (1) Confusion
      (2) Transient blindness
      (3) Hemiparesis
  5. Nursing interventions
    a. Intraoperative passive range of motion
    b. Use of padding of bony prominences intraoperatively
      (1) Heels
      (2) Elbows
      (3) Shoulders
      (4) Hips
      (5) Coccyx
    c. Encouragement of active exercises before and after surgery
    d. Use of antiembolism stockings
    e. Explanation of symptoms of thrombophlebitis
    f. Encouragement of adequate fluid intake
    g. Have patient immediately report any of the following symptoms postoperatively.
      (1) Pain in the leg, especially increased calf pain when foot is dorsiflexed (positive Homan's sign) *bend part toward dorsum or posterior aspect of body Foot backward at ankle toes - away from sole of foot hand - bent backward, overextended*
      (2) Fever
      (3) Chills
      (4) Swelling
      (5) Redness
      (6) Heat
      (7) Tenderness in leg
E. Respiratory
  1. History
    a. Infectious or chemical influences
    b. Smoking habits
    c. Chronic cough

        d. Previous lung surgery

        e. Emphysema

           (1) Patients may not admit to emphysema as a disease.

           (2) Look for symptomatology.

              (a) Dyspnea

                 (i) Minimal exertion

              (b) Rest

              (c) Chronic cough

              (d) Barrel chest

              (e) Elevation of shoulders

              (f) Pursed lip breathing

              (g) Cyanosis

              (h) Clubbing of fingers

              (i) Tachypnea

              (j) Predisposition to respiratory infections

           (3) Shortness of breath

           (4) Current or past episodes of

              (a) Pneumonia

              (b) Tuberculosis

              (c) Bronchitis

              (d) Asthma

    2. Physical examination

        a. Auscultation of the chest

           (1) Crackles

              (a) Typically short, explosive, discontinuous sounds

              (b) May be heard in patients with

                 (i) Pulmonary emphysema

              (c) Bronchitis

              (d) Asthma

              (e) Pulmonary congestion

                 (i) Caused by congestive heart failure (CHF)

           (2) Rhonchi

              (a) Coarser, rattling sounds with lower pitch

                 (i) Generally heard over large airways

           (3) Wheezes

              (a) Continuous, musical sound

                 (i) Asthma or emphysema

              (b) Particularly expiration

        b. Baseline breath sounds

           (1) Comparison for postanesthetic findings

              (a) Aspiration

              (b) Fluid overload

              (c) Bronchospasm

        c. Baseline oximetry readings

           (1) Observation of

              (a) Rate

              (b) Depth

              (c) Ease of breathing

        d. Cyanosis

        e. Symmetry of chest movements

        f. Use of accessory muscles

        g. Production of sputum

        h. Upper airway including anatomic structures

           (1) Short, stocky neck

           (2) Excessive skin or fat on back of neck

           (3) Thick tongue

           (4) Previous cervical fusion

           (5) Temporal mandibular joint disease

(6) Down syndrome
   (a) Thick, protruding tongue
   (b) Skin folds on posterior neck
   (c) Instability of atlantalaxial joint in cervical spine
      (i) Found in approximately 10% to 20% of persons with Down syndrome
      (ii) Dislocation or subluxation of this joint can occur with hyperextension of neck.
   (d) Cervical cord compression with nerve damage and possible death in 5% to 10% of those predisposed

F. Neurologic
   1. Assessment
      a. General affect
         (1) Behavior
         (2) Speech patterns
         (3) Orientation
         (4) Gait
      b. Fine motor movements
         (1) Writing
         (2) Cough
         (3) Blink
         (4) Swallow
         (5) Pupil reflexes
      c. Motor abilities
         (1) Muscle strength
         (2) Vision
         (3) Hearing
      d. Presence of
         (1) Headache
         (2) Dizziness
         (3) Paralysis
         (4) Seizures
         (5) Loss of motor control
      e. Preexisting neurologic deficit
         (1) More complete examination
            (a) Cerebral
            (b) Motor
            (c) Cranial nerves
               (i) Table 18-2 describes abnormalities in function of the cranial nerves.
            (d) Reflex functions

G. Sensory and prosthetic
   1. Patients may not provide accurate information about sensory deficits.
      a. Embarrassment
      b. Vanity
      c. Assessment skills
         (1) Hearing loss
            (a) Patient may lean or turn toward conversation.
            (b) Answer questions inappropriately or not at all
            (c) Watch interviewer's lips
            (d) Provide interpreter in American Sign Language if patient is knowledgeable in use.
               (i) Provide information and answers to questions that patient can understand.
         (2) Visual impairment
            (a) Difficulty seeing documents
            (b) Should have instructions, consents, and other forms read to them prior to having them signed

■ TABLE 18-2
■ ■ **Abnormalities in Cranial Nerve Function**

Name	Type*	Function	Test Abnormality
I. Olfactory	S	Smell	Coffee, tobacco
II. Optic	S	Vision	Visual acuity Pupillary reaction, visual fields
III. Oculomotor	M	Eye movement	Ptosis; lateral and downward deviation of eye
IV. Trochlear	M	Eye movement	Medial and upper deviation of eye
V. Trigeminal (3 branches— opthalmic, maxillary, mandibular)	S	From skin of face and cornea	Loss of sensation on one side of face
VI. Abducens	M	Eye movement	Medial deviation of eyeball
VII. Facial	S	Taste—anterior tongue	Inability to grimace on one side of face
	M	Muscles of facial expression	
VIII. Acoustic auditory vestibulocochlear	S	Hearing	Watch ticking; whispered voice
	S	Equilibrium	Vertigo; nystagmus
IX. Glossopharyngeal	S	Taste on posterior portion of tongue	Loss of gag reflex; deviation of uvula toward the unaffected side
	M	Pharyngeal muscles	
X. Vagus	S	From thoracic and abdominal organs	As with IX plus hoarseness
	M	Pharyngeal and laryngeal muscles plus thoracic and abdominal organs	
XI. Spinal accessory	M	Sternocleidomastoid and trapezius muscles	Inability to shrug one shoulder or to move chin to one side against pressure of examiner's hand
XII. Hypoglossal	M	Tongue movement	Deviation of tongue to affected side

*S, sensory; M, motor.
From Quinn DMD: *Ambulatory surgical nursing core curriculum.* Philadelphia: WB Saunders, 1999, pp 73.

  2. Note that this occurred on patient record.
   a. Emphasis is to ensure effective communication and understanding between patient and staff throughout surgical experience.
   b. Patient must be able to understand instructions and explanations.
    (1) May need sensory aids such as
     (a) Hearing aids
     (b) Glasses or contact lenses
     (c) Electronic voice stimulator
     (d) Historically banned from operating room
      (i) Current wellness-centered care approach brings more liberal policy.
      (ii) As long as there is no threat to patient safety, potential for loss or harm to device, these devices are often allowed to remain with the patient.
      (iii) Decision usually made by anesthesiologist
     (e) Reassures patients that they may retain these devices and promotes psychological health

        (f) Same is true for dentures, wigs, prosthetic limbs, and bras.
           (i) Essential for self-image and security
           (ii) If they must be moved, reassure patients that they will be returned as soon as possible.
           (iii) Personal privacy and dignity will be maintained.
           (iv) Some ASCs are reevaluating the policy of removing dentures from all patients.
              [a] Unless having general anesthesia, usually not necessary

    c. Documentation of presence of
        (1) Loose or chipped teeth
        (2) Permanent bridgework
           (a) Avoid accidental injury during airway or tube insertion.
           (b) Identify potential complications of airway management.
           (c) Establish preexisting problems for legal reasons.

H. Musculoskeletal
  1. History
    a. Arthritis
    b. Scoliosis
    c. Osteoporosis
    d. Sciatica
    e. Vertebral disc problems
    f. Amputations
    g. Prior fractures
    h. Frequent falls
  2. Physical assessment
    a. Muscle strength
    b. Gait
    c. Mobility
    d. Range of motion
    e. Use of orthopedic appliances or prostheses
    f. Need for assistive devices
        (1) Walker
        (2) Cane
        (3) Wheelchair

I. Integumentary
  1. Assessment
    a. Observation
        (1) Color
        (2) Temperature
        (3) Texture
        (4) Dryness
        (5) Turgor
        (6) Loss of elasticity
           (a) Normal change in aging
           (b) Can also indicate dehydration
        (7) Integrity
           (a) Easy bruising or petechiae
               (i) Could indicate hematologic problems
        (8) Jaundice
           (a) Could indicate history of hepatitis
        (9) Cyanosis or mottling
           (a) May indicate serious vascular or cardiac disease

J. Communicable diseases
  1. Scabies
  2. Pediculosis (lice)
  3. Impetigo
    a. Presence of rash, especially in children

     4. Tuberculosis
        a. Making a comeback with advent of human immunodeficiency virus (HIV)
        b. Newer strains often drug resistant
     5. History of
        a. Recent fever
        b. Upper respiratory symptoms
        c. Measles (rubeola)
        d. German measles (rubella)
        e. Chickenpox (varicella)
           (1) Treatment prior to admission to ASC
           (2) Other people, including patients in contact, could contract disease or infestation.
           (3) Wound infection potential as result of self-contamination

K. Gastrointestinal
     1. History
        a. Previous surgery
           (1) Diversional surgery
           (2) Colostomy
        b. Gastrointestinal bleed
        c. Cancer
        d. Hiatal hernia
        e. Chronic diarrhea or constipation
        f. Presence of postoperative nausea and vomiting (PONV)
           (1) If predisposition known, psychological and pharmacological interventions can be initiated to prevent occurrence.
           (2) PONV unpleasant but potential for aspiration strong
        g. Aspiration risk
        h. Pyloric obstruction
        i. Intestinal obstruction
        j. Esophageal diverticula
        k. Diminished pharyngeal reflexes
        l. Obesity
        m. Advanced pregnancy
        n. Unknown compliance with nothing by mouth (NPO) requirements
     2. Assessment
        a. Mouth
        b. Pharynx
        c. Esophagus
        d. Stomach
        e. Large intestine
        f. Small intestine
        g. Pancreas
        h. Liver
        i. Gallbladder

L. Renal and hepatic
     1. Many anesthetic drugs are metabolized in the kidneys and liver.
     2. History or presence of renal or hepatic disease is of great concern.
        a. Pseudocholinesterase
           (1) Enzyme necessary for metabolism of succinylcholine and ester-type local anesthetics
     3. Kidney function
        a. Excretion of urine
        b. Influences fluid and electrolyte and acid–base balance
        c. Nitrogenous wastes from protein metabolism are excreted.
        d. Electrolytes are maintained.
           (1) Sodium, potassium, chloride
           (2) Excretion of some drugs is also dependent on kidney function.

4. Liver function
   a. Metabolism of bilirubin
   b. By-products of red blood cell breakdown
   c. Protein synthesis
      (1) Particularly albumin
      (2) Chronic liver disease patients have decreased serum protein levels.
   d. Drug biotransformation
      (1) Protein-bound drugs (thiopental and bupivacaine) have fewer sites to bind.
      (2) Unbound portions remain active in bloodstream, creating prolonged or enhanced effects.
5. Physical assessment
   a. Renal disease
      (1) May not be evident until 50% or more function is lost
   b. Liver disease
      (1) Jaundice
      (2) Spider angiomata
      (3) Ecchymosis
      (4) Ascites
      (5) Pedal edema
      (6) Scleral icterus → *covers white of the eye*
6. History   *Pigmentation with bile - jaundice*
   a. Cirrhosis
      (1) Chronic alcohol or drug abuse
   b. Hepatitis
   c. Immune disorders
   d. Extreme forms of dieting
   e. Liver or kidney insufficiency or failure
   f. Extremes in blood pressure
   g. Anemia
   h. Electrolyte imbalance
   i. Depression
M. Endocrine
   1. Diverse diseases; can affect many processes necessary for tolerance of anesthesia and surgery
   2. Hormones regulate
      a. Response to stress
      b. Rate of metabolism
      c. Blood pressure
      d. Pulse rates
      e. Blood glucose levels
      f. Urine production
      g. Electrolyte balance
      h. Table 18-3 lists principal hormones and symptoms from imbalances.
   3. Diabetes
      a. Complications secondary to diabetic condition
         (1) Delayed wound healing
         (2) Retinopathy
         (3) Kidney failure
         (4) Peripheral artery disease
         (5) Potential for
            (a) Ketoacidosis
            (b) MI
            (c) Severe hypoglycemia
      b. Requires special instructions especially with regard to insulin and diet on day of surgery
         (1) Often asked to bring own insulin to ASC

■ TABLE 18-3
■ ■ **Endocrine Imbalances**

Hormone	Hyposecretion	Hypersecretion
Thyroid hormone	Children—cretinism Adults—myxedema ↓BMR, tiredness, mentally slow, bradycardia	Hyperthyroidism, ↑ BMR*, always hungry, irritable, tachycardia, weight loss
Parathyroid hormone	Spontaneous discharge of nerves, spasms, tetany, death	Weak, brittle bones; kidney stones
Insulin	Diabetes mellitus	Hypoglycemia
Adrenocortical hormones	Addison's disease (body does not synthesize enough glucose, unable to deal with stress, sodium loss in urine may lead to shock)	Cushing's disease (edema gives full moon face, fat around trunk, ↑ blood glucose levels, depressed immune response)

*BMR, basal metabolism rate.
From Quinn DMD: *Ambulatory surgical nursing core curriculum.* Philadelphia: WB Saunders, 1999, p 77.

       (2) May be asked to bring own food if ASC does not serve food or serves only donuts or sweet rolls for postoperative nourishment

N. Hematologic
  1. Disorders of the blood may involve
    a. Red blood cells
      (1) Anemia
      (2) Sickle cell anemia
      (3) Thalassemia
      (4) Polycythemia
    b. Lymphocytes and plasma cells
      (1) Agranulocytosis
      (2) Leukemia
      (3) Multiple myeloma
    c. Lymph nodes and spleen
      (1) Lymphoma
      (2) Infectious mononucleosis
    d. Platelets and clotting factors
      (1) Hemorrhagic disorders
      (2) Purpura
      (3) Coagulation disorders
        (a) Hemophilia
        (b) Hypoprothrombinemia
  2. Physical examination
    a. Observation
      (1) Petechiae and bruising
      (2) Pallor and cyanosis
        (a) Skin and mucous membranes
      (3) Hepatomegaly
      (4) Splenomegaly
  3. History of
    a. Fatigue
    b. Lassitude
    c. Easy bruising
    d. Frequent nosebleeds
    e. Hematuria

        f. Blood in stools

        g. Excessive bleeding after minor injuries or dental extractions

    4. Leukemia and acquired immunodeficiency syndrome (AIDS)

        a. May be scheduled in ASC to avoid hospitalization and subsequent nosocomial infections

II. Psychosocial assessment

  A. Evaluation of emotional, cognitive, social, and cultural assessments occurs during physical assessment.

  B. Emotional assessment

    1. Most patients express a moderate to high degree of anxiety and fear facing surgery.

        a. Patients have a right to feel anxiety.

            (1) Placating or belittling the situation is seen as demeaning to the patient.

            (2) Credibility of staff is undermined by this approach.

    2. Anxiety and fear are similar but different.

        a. Anxiety is described as a vague, unknown, or unidentified source evoked by a threat to one's existence or personality.

        b. Fear is related to a more specific person or occurrence.

            (1) Some common fears related to surgery are

               (a) Possibility of not waking up after anesthesia

               (b) Having a mask placed on the face

               (c) Regaining consciousness during the surgery

               (d) Making a fool of oneself

               (e) Feeling the operation

               (f) Anticipated postoperative pain

               (g) Outcome of surgery

        c. Ambulatory surgery would seem to provoke less fear and anxiety, but this is not the case.

            (1) Home recuperation can add additional pressure.

               (a) Fear of facing emergencies at home without medical attention

               (b) Concern about family members who would have to care for them

               (c) Inadequate pain medication

               (d) Need to have another adult for transportation and home support

                  (i) Threat to independence

               (e) Embarrassment at having to ask for help

               (f) Problems of obtaining other person to provide support

               (g) Pressure of arriving on time

                  (i) Many people do not sleep the night before for fear of not waking in time.

               (h) May be primary caregiver for spouse

                  (i) Concern over their care while in surgery and during recuperation period

    3. Preoperative interview important

        a. Assess emotional state.

            (1) Objective observations

               (a) General appearance

               (b) Nervousness

               (c) Decreased attention span

               (d) Lack of eye contact

               (e) Increase heart rate

               (f) Lack of self-confidence

               (g) Decreased concentration

               (h) Rapid speech patterns

               (i) Diaphoresis

               (j) Dry mouth

               (k) Clammy skin

               (l) Pressure of arriving on time

               (m) Nausea

(n) Urinary frequency

(o) Hyperventilation

(p) Precordial chest pain

(2) Subjective information

(a) Patient

(b) Family

(3) Provide answers to questions.

(a) Information and support allow patient to gain understanding of upcoming surgery.

(b) Trust develops with surgical staff.

(c) By allowing patient to express feelings, staff can help patients to identify coping mechanisms to deal with rational and irrational fears.

(d) Anxiety can influence amount of teaching patients understand.

(i) Mildly anxious patients receive the most complete instructions.

(ii) Moderately anxious patients receive less information.

(iii) Give more attention to their specific areas of concern.

(iv) Severely anxious patients should receive only basic information.

(v) Need encouragement to verbalize fears

(e) Patients in state of panic are unable to learn.

(f) No instructions should be given.

(g) Physician should be notified of patient's status.

(4) Cognitive assessment

(a) Evaluate patient's understanding of procedure.

(b) Ask open-ended questions to elicit and encourage patient's response in own words.

(c) Avoid yes and no answers.

(d) Evaluate prior to having patient sign consent.

(e) Patient and/or family must be sufficiently intelligent and responsible to provide care.

(f) Understand and comply with preoperative and postoperative instructions

(g) Knowledge of hygiene

(h) Nutrition requirements

(i) Complying with NPO status

C. Illiteracy

1. Written instructions of no use to person who cannot read or understand what is read

2. Estimated more than 23 million Americans are illiterate

a. Cannot read at the level most health care information is written (fifth-grade level)

(1) Many may be able to sign name without reading form.

(a) Clear verbal instructions particularly important

b. Language barrier

(1) English as a second language

(a) Need for interpreter to provide information

(i) Preferably *not* a family member

(ii) May be protecting patient by withholding information they feel patient should not know

D. Social assessment

1. Concept of ambulatory surgery is family based and home based.

a. Patients need strong support system.

b. Equally important are those persons be responsible for aftercare.

2. Evaluation of home situation important during preoperative planning process

a. Elderly patients

(1) Surgical patient may be healthier of couple (spouse/companion).

(a) Often require outside help
(i) Neighbors
(b) Other family members
(c) Home health provider
(d) Physical environment of home
(i) Number of stairs
(e) Bathroom location
(f) May need to utilize social services to provide discharge planning
(g) Proximity of home to surgical center

  E. Cultural assessment
   1. Cultural and ethnic beliefs play role in patient's attitudes about health care.
      a. Difficult to separate beliefs from modern health care
      b. May be considered superstitions by health-care workers
         (1) Spiritual control over body
         (2) Faith healing
         (3) Being one with the environment
      c. Health care workers must respect patient's cultural beliefs.

III. Diagnostic assessment
  A. 1970s-1980s
   1. Many ambulatory surgery centers cared for essentially healthy individuals.
      a. Diagnostic practices were limited to few tests.
         (1) Fingerstick hemoglobin and hematocrit screen
         (2) Dipstick urinalysis
            (a) Provided sufficient data to safely administer anesthesia
  B. Today—sicker patients having surgery on an outpatient basis.
   1. Diagnostic requirements now include a variety of basic and complex testing.
      a. Often same requirements as hospitalized counterparts
   2. Preoperative testing is done to reduce risks associated with anesthesia and surgery.
      a. Provides information about whether the patient can tolerate surgical procedures
  C. Debate over amount and type of preoperative testing
   1. Cost-effectiveness
      a. Current trend is toward ordering only those tests specifically indicated by abnormal clinical symptoms or history.
   2. Clinical thoroughness
      a. Diagnostic testing is expensive.
         (1) Benefit thought to outweigh expense
            (a) Offers early detection of previously undiagnosed diseases
            (b) Provides information regarding general health and ability to tolerate surgery of patient

BIBLIOGRAPHY

1. Benady S: Patient's herbal habits may hinder anesthesia response. *Medical Post* 36(6), 2000. Accessed at http://search.medicalpost.com/mpcontent/article.jsp?content=/content/EXTRACT/RAUART/3624/33B.html.
2. Burden N, Quinn DMD, O'Brien D, et al: *Ambulatory surgical nursing.* Philadelphia: WB Saunders, 2000.
3. Delgan JH, Vallerand AH: *Davis's Drug Guide for Nurses*, ed 8. Philadelphia: Davis, 2003.
4. Drain C: *Perianesthesia nursing: A critical care approach*, ed 4. Philadelphia: WB Saunders, 2003.
5. Fischback F: *Manual of laboratory and diagnostic tests.* Philadelphia: Lippincott, 2000.
6. Flanagan K: Preoperative assessment: Safety considerations for patients taking herbal products. *J PeriAnes Nurs* 16(1):19-26, 2001.
7. Lewis SM, Heitkemper MM, Dirksen SR: *Medical-surgical nursing: Assessment and management of clinical problems*, ed 5. St Louis: Mosby, 2000.
8. Wertheimer L: Analysis: Recently taken herbal remedies may pose surgical complication. *All Things Considered*. Washington, DC: National Public Radio, July 10, 2001.

19 Preexisting Medical Conditions

LOIS SCHICK

OBJECTIVES

At the conclusion of this chapter the reader will be able to:

1. Identify patients with an increased perioperative risk.

2. Recognize the reasons for the increased risk.

3. State the specific perioperative nursing care priorities for the high-risk patient.

4. Describe techniques to reduce perioperative morbidity and mortality.

I. Preexisting medical conditions
   A. Increase American Society of Anesthesiologists (ASA) classification
   B. Increase perioperative risk, morbidity, and mortality
   C. May require multiple medications
      1. Increased potential for drug interactions
      2. Increased potential for laboratory test alterations
      3. Increased potential for noncompliance
   D. Level of disease control may jeopardize ambulatory status.
II. Cardiovascular diseases
   A. Hypertension
      1. Definition: systolic >140 mm Hg and/or diastolic >90 mm Hg
         a. Ideal pressure of 115/76 or less
      2. Incidence: 24% of U.S. population; greater in males than females
         a. Ideal pressure present in only 4% of adult U.S. population
      3. Significance: risk factor for coronary artery disease, cerebrovascular accidents, congestive heart failure, arterial aneurysm, and end-stage renal failure
      4. Etiology and findings
         a. Medical evaluation and clearance
            (1) Mild hypertension: within 2 months of surgery
            (2) Moderate hypertension: within 2 weeks of surgery
            (3) Severe hypertension (diastolic >110 mm Hg): immediate evaluation with surgery canceled
         b. Advise patient to take routine prescription antihypertensive medication on day of surgery with a sip of water.
         c. Ask about presence of heart disease during preoperative interview.
         d. Postoperative systemic hypertension warrants prompt assessment and treatment to minimize risks of myocardial ischemia, heart failure, stroke, and bleeding.
            (1) Pain assessment
            (2) Fluid overload assessment
   B. Coronary artery disease (CAD)
      1. Definition: accumulation of plaque within the coronary arteries
      2. Incidence: extremely common, males predominance under age 55; equal in males and females over age 55

3. Significance: increased risk for myocardial infarction (MI), diabetes, smoking, hypertension, renal disease, dysrhythmias, congestive heart failure (CHF), sudden death
4. Etiology: physiologic, environmental, aging, diet, biochemical
    a. Myocardial oxygen delivery does not meet myocardial oxygen demand, resulting in myocardial ischemia.
    b. Myocardial oxygen supply does not reach myocardium after thrombosis of coronary artery, resulting in MI.
5. Treatment: coronary vasodilators (nitrates), activity, diet, education
6. Perioperative significance
    a. If history of MI, elective surgery should wait minimum of 6 months to decrease risk of reinfarction with very high mortality.
    b. Requires evaluation and clearance from a cardiologist
    c. May increase intraoperative monitoring requirements
    d. Assess for signs of CHF; if present, surgery is canceled.
    e. Signs of CHF include
        (1) Shortness of breath
        (2) Dyspnea on exertion or nocturnal
        (3) Jugular venous distension
        (4) Crackles
        (5) Edema
    f. Assess incidence and triggers of chest pain.
        (1) If new onset (<2 months) or unstable, postpone surgery pending cardiologist evaluation.
        (2) All prescription medications to be taken on morning of surgery with sip of water
    g. Second and third postoperative days are most common time for MI in noncardiac surgical patients.
    h. Ischemia intraoperative designates patient as "high risk" in postoperative period.
C. CHF
    1. Definition
        a. Left-sided and/or right-sided heart dysfunction producing decreased systolic emptying and decreased ventricular compliance
        b. Heart is unable to meet demands of peripheral tissues.
    2. Incidence
        a. Most common inpatient diagnosis for patients over 65 years of age
        b. Greater in males than in females for ages 40-75
        c. Males equal to females for over age 75
    3. Significance: increased risk for pulmonary edema, dyspnea, peripheral edema
    4. Etiology: CAD, myocardial infarction, rheumatic heart disease, volume overload, congenital heart disease, noncompliance with medications
    5. Treatment: diuretics, inotropic therapy, oxygen, low-sodium diet, ventricular assist devices (VAD)   *influencing the force of muscle contractility*
    6. Perioperative significance
        a. If symptomatic (see section II.B), surgery is canceled.
        b. Auscultate breath sounds on arrival, on admission to postanesthesia care unit (PACU) phase I, and prior to discharge.
        c. Strict intake and output records
        d. Increased perioperative mortality (10% to 50%)
        e. Obtain cardiologist clearance prior to surgery.
        f. Opioids may be used for maintenance of anesthesia.
        g. Regional anesthesia is acceptable for peripheral operations.
D. Mitral valve prolapse (MVP)
    1. Definition: prolapse or stenosis of mitral heart valve that results in resistance to left ventricular emptying (increased afterload)
    2. Incidence: age <30 congenital; age >70 degenerative

3. Significance: increased risk of angina, syncope, fatigue, dyspnea, click or heart murmur on auscultation, pulmonary embolism, dysrhythmias
4. Etiology: congenital, rheumatic heart disease, aging
5. Treatment: prolapse often requires no treatment; stenosis requires valve replacement, digoxin, or other antidysrhythmics (including angiotensin-converting enzymes [ACE] inhibitors, beta blockers), diuretics, low-sodium diet, anticoagulation therapy, and education.
6. Perioperative significance
   a. Patients require antibiotic endocarditis prophylaxis prior to dental work or other invasive procedures regardless of age, cause, disease severity.
   b. May be anticoagulated on warfarin; if so, check prothrombin time/International Normalized Ratio (PT/INR)
      (1) Patient may be asked to stop warfarin 3 days prior to surgery.
   c. Risk of pulmonary edema is significant.
   d. Avoid hypertension and acute increases in sympathetic tone.

E. Dysrhythmias
   1. Definition: alteration in conduction system requiring pharmacologic or surgical (automatic implantable cardiac defibrillator [AICD], pacemaker) intervention
   2. Incidence: very common (dysrhythmias)
      a. Use of pacemakers and AICDs increases with age.
      b. Common outcome of coronary artery disease
   3. Significance: increased risk of myocardial infarction and progression to lethal dysrhythmias
   4. Etiology: CAD, CHF, valve disease, myocardial infarction, hypoxia, hypercarbia, electrolyte imbalance, acid–base alterations, altered activity of the autonomic nervous system, drugs (i.e., volatile anesthetics, catecholamines)
   5. Treatment: pharmacologic, education, pacemaker (heart block, asystole), cardioversion, AICD (ventricular fibrillation)
   6. Perioperative significance
      a. Patient to take antidysrhythmic medications on day of surgery
      b. Inquire about type of pacemaker and setting (patient may have pacer identification card); document in chart (may need to call cardiologist).
      c. Have external pacemaker readily available.
      d. Have cardiologist available, although not necessarily in the operating room (OR).
      e. If patient has an AICD, cautery should not be used during surgery.
         (1) If cautery must be used, AICD is turned off.
         (2) External defibrillator must be available in OR suite for immediate use if needed.

III. Pulmonary diseases
   A. Chronic obstructive pulmonary disease (COPD)
      1. Definition: term includes chronic bronchitis and emphysema.
         a. Bronchitis signs include cough, increase sputum production, dyspnea, wheezing.
         b. Emphysema signs include barrel chest, pursed lip breathing, decreased breath sounds, dyspnea.
      2. Incidence: 20% to 30% of adults less than 40 years of age; greater in males than in females
      3. Significance: hypoxia, hypercapnia ↑ amt CO_2 in blood
      4. Etiology: cigarette smoking, air pollution, occupational exposure to smoke
      5. Treatment: bronchodilators, possibly anticholinergics and corticosteroids, patient education to stop smoking   an agent that blocks para symph nerve fibers
      6. Perioperative significance
         a. Encourage patient to stop smoking 8-10 weeks prior to surgery; be aware that most patients will not comply.

b. General anesthesia may exacerbate symptoms and disease; regional anesthesia avoids intubation and use of controlled ventilation.

c. Patient's respirations controlled by hypoxic drive.
   (1) High flow, high concentration oxygen may produce apnea.
   (2) Nasal cannula <3 L oxygen preferred delivery system unless unable to maintain saturation

d. Encourage deep breathing and coughing after general anesthesia; postoperative pulmonary infections common.

e. Ask patient to bring inhalers used to the facility on day of surgery.

f. Pulmonary function tests may be ordered preoperatively.

B. Asthma
   1. Definition: tracheobronchial disorder characterized by obstruction to airflow secondary to narrowing of airways, edema, and inflammation
   2. Incidence: 10 million new cases each year; 50% patients under age 10; 7% to 19% of all children
   3. Significance: increased risk of laryngospasm and bronchospasm on induction, hypoxemia, decreased peak flow rates
   4. Etiology: allergic factors, smoke, infection, cold air, exercise
   5. Treatment: bronchodilators (beta-2 agonists), corticosteroids (acute asthma), mast cell stabilizers, education
   6. Perioperative significance
      a. Encourage patient to avoid known irritants to minimize perioperative wheezing.
      b. Auscultate breath sounds preoperatively and postoperatively
      c. Increased risk of bronchospasm on intubation and emergence
      d. Halothane, isoflurane, enflurane, and ketamine may be used because they cause bronchodilation during administration.
      e. Ask patient to bring any inhalers used to the facility on the day of surgery.
      f. If on steroids, determine last use and dose; may need steroid preoperatively.
      g. Question patient on the frequency, severity, and management of attacks.
      h. Cancel surgery if patient has an upper respiratory infection.

C. Smoking
   1. Definition: use of inhaled tobacco
   2. Incidence: extremely common; teenagers, adults, and elderly. Young female is fastest growing group.
   3. Significance: increased risk of COPD, heart disease, hypoxia, poor tissue healing, postoperative pulmonary complications six times greater than that of nonsmoker, hyperreactive airway
   4. Etiology: access to and use of product
   5. Treatment: cessation, nicotine patch, Smokers Anonymous, self-withdrawal
   6. Perioperative significance
      a. Patient has elevated carboxyhemoglobin levels.
      b. Carbon monoxide has greater affinity for hemoglobin than does oxygen.
      c. Increased risk of bronchospasm and laryngospasm on induction, intubation, emergence
      d. Encourage patient to stop smoking 8 weeks prior to surgery; be aware that most will not comply.
      e. If chronic productive cough, preoperative antibiotics may be used.
      f. Anesthesia considers deep extubation if severe reactive airway disease

IV. Renal diseases
   A. Acute renal failure (ARF)   *presence of nitrogenous bodes esp. urea in bld*
      1. Definition: rapid, increasing azotemia with or without oliguria
      2. Significance: patient will experience urinary changes, fluid volume excess, metabolic acidosis, sodium alterations, potassium excess, calcium deficit and phosphate excess, nitrogenous waste accumulation.
      3. Incidence: 5% of adult population have co-existing renal disease that could contribute to perioperative morbidity.

    4. Etiology: prerenal (i.e., hypovolemia, CHF); renal (intrinsic) (injury to the renal tubules from ischemia or nephrotoxins); and postrenal (obstructive) (urinary outflow tracts are obstructed by prostatic hypertrophy or cancer of prostate or cervix)

    5. Patient inappropriate for ambulatory surgery

  B. Chronic renal failure (CRF)

    1. Definition: progressive, irreversible disruption of the excretory and regulatory function of the nephron

    2. Incidence: common—160,000 new cases per year; more common in African-Americans; rare in children; equal in males and females

    3. Significance: patients commonly diabetic with multiple laboratory alterations, hypertension, and anemia

    4. Etiology: pyelonephritis, polycystic kidneys, autoimmune, diabetes, drug-induced nephropathy (antibiotics, nonsteroidal antiinflammatory drugs [NSAIDs]), hypertension, congenital

    5. Treatment: renal replacement therapy, hemodialysis, peritoneal dialysis, ultrafiltration, renal transplantation, diet, patient education

    6. Perioperative significance

      a. Avoid nephrotoxic drugs.

      b. Consider decreased doses of medications eliminated through kidneys.

      c. Anemia may compromise oxygenation, especially with hematocrit <18%.

      d. Monitor electrolytes and renal function preoperatively, especially potassium, blood urea nitrogen (BUN), and creatinine.

      e. Obtain preoperative glucose level in diabetic patients.

      f. Avoid same-arm venipunctures and blood pressures if patient has arteriovenous (A-V) fistula for hemodialysis.

      g. Increased risk for infection

      h. Determine date of last dialysis; if off schedule, anticipate fluid and electrolyte imbalance.

      i. Avoid potassium-containing solutions, morphine, meperidine, and pancuronium. _→ Pavulon   neuromuscular blocking agent_

      j. Obtain preoperative weight.

      k. Careful intake and output; may be on fluid restriction

      l. Poor tolerance for physiologic stress

      m. Instruct patient to take antihypertensive medications on day of surgery.

      n. Use of lactated Ringer's or dextrose in lactated Ringer's may lead to acidosis; use normal saline or dextrose 5% in one half normal saline.

V. Liver diseases

  A. Cirrhosis—liver failure

    1. Definition: hepatic fibrosis producing portal hypertension including ascites, variceal bleeding, hepatic encephalopathy

    2. Incidence: 30,000 deaths per year; greater in males than in females

    3. Significance: inappropriate for ambulatory surgery

    4. Etiology: excessive alcohol ingestion, chronic viral hepatitis

    5. Treatment: Parenteral vitamin K if prothrombin times are prolonged, monitor arterial blood gases (ABG), pH, and urine output. Monitor for hypoglycemia. Ensure adequate hydration.

  B. Hepatitis

    1. Definition

      a. Acute hepatitis is an inflammatory disease of hepatocytes most often caused by a virus although drugs and toxins can also cause it.

      b. Chronic hepatitis (active): widespread destruction of hepatocytes causing cirrhosis and hepatic failure

      c. Chronic hepatitis (persistent): nonprogressive inflammatory disease confined to portal areas

2. Incidence (varies with cause)
   a. Hepatitis A: 25% of cases; elective surgery should not be performed on patients.
   b. Hepatitis B: 200,000 young adults per year
   c. Hepatitis C: most common cause of acute viral hepatitis; greater in males than in females
3. Significance: hepatitis in presence of alcoholism increases risk of cirrhosis.
   a. Depending on extent of disease, may have alterations in coagulation, fluid and electrolytes, and wound healing
4. Etiology: viral
   a. Hepatitis A: transmitted enterically (fecal–oral via food)
   b. Hepatitis B: transmitted sexually, via contaminated blood (needle sticks) and body fluids
   c. Hepatitis C: transmitted via blood transfusions and body fluids, although in 50% of cases route of transmission unknown
5. Treatment: supportive because disease is viral
   a. Hepatitis A: immune globulin, hepatitis A vaccine, treat at home unless dehydrated
   b. Hepatitis B: prevention—vaccine Hepatitis B, Hepatitis B immune globulin for passive immunization, bed rest and orthotopic liver transplantation for liver failure
   c. Hepatitis C: type 1 interferon with or without ribavirin; orthotopic liver transplantation for liver failure
6. Perioperative significance
   a. Patients with acute hepatitis are inappropriate for ambulatory surgery.
   b. Patients with chronic persistent hepatitis should be evaluated by a gastroenterologist prior to surgery.
   c. Vigilance to universal precautions
   d. Consider obtaining preoperative liver enzymes to compare with previous levels.
      (1) Increases reflect worsening of disease.
      (2) Requires medical evaluation prior to surgery
   e. Anticipate hypoglycemia and potential fluid overload postoperatively.
   f. Be cognizant of potential for delayed awakening from prolonged drug metabolism or encephalopathy.

C. Alcohol abuse
   1. Definition: illness characterized by significant impairment associated with persistent and excessive use of alcohol
      a. Impairment may be physiologic, psychologic, or social.
   2. Incidence: 10% of men; 3.5% of women; 11% to 15% of all adults; highest incidence is between 18 and 39 years of age
   3. Significance: associated with malnutrition, poor compliance, hypertension, pulmonary disease with concomitant cigarette use, stroke, diabetes, gastrointestinal (GI) disease
   4. Etiology: biologic, psychologic, and sociocultural factors
   5. Treatment: detoxification and withdrawal of use
   6. Perioperative significance
      a. Compliance with preoperative and postoperative instructions may be poor.
      b. Determine usual consumption, time, and amount of last drink.
      c. Malnutrition may compromise wound healing.
      d. Aberrant responses to narcotics and benzodiazepines
      e. At risk for cirrhosis, alterations in coagulation, and bleeding
      f. Delirium tremens may require heavy sedation or restraints to prevent patient self-injury.
         (1) First sign of delirium tremens in patient still sedated following general anesthesia may be tachycardia.

(2) Occurrence of delirium tremens in perioperative period associated with high incidence of morbidity and mortality

g. Increased incidence of aspiration pneumonitis
   (1) Concomitant pulmonary disease will require aggressive postoperative pulmonary hygiene.

h. Long-term consumption impairs hepatic metabolism; short-term consumption inhibits drug metabolism.

i. Polyneuropathy is a relative contraindication to regional anesthesia.

j. Patients arriving intoxicated for ambulatory procedures should have surgery canceled.

VI. Neuromuscular, skeletal, connective tissue diseases
   A. Scoliosis
      1. Definition: C-shaped or S-shaped lateral curvature of the vertebral spine
         a. Kyphosis: anterior flexion of vertebral column
         b. Scoliosis: lateral curvature of vertebral column
      2. Incidence: greater in women than in men (80% women)
      3. Significance: most commonly diagnosed and treated in childhood during maximal growth period
      4. Etiology: congenital, fracture, osteomalacia
      5. Treatment
         a. In childhood and adolescence: exercises, weight reduction, bracing, casting, surgery (spinal fusion with rod placement)
         b. In adults: spinal fusion
      6. Perioperative significance
         a. Severe deviations (>50 degrees) can compromise cardiopulmonary function; obtain preoperative pulmonary function tests.
         b. Curvature can cause lower back pain.
         c. Deformity may compromise intraoperative positioning.
         d. Mitral valve prolapse present in 25% of patients; will require antibiotic prophylaxis
         e. Patients with concomitant myopathies likely to require postoperative ventilation; inappropriate as outpatients
         f. Pulmonary function may be decreased after general anesthesia, requiring aggressive pulmonary care.
   B. Arthritis: rheumatoid and osteoarthritis
      1. Definitions
         a. Rheumatoid: chronic inflammatory disease of multiple joints producing disability and disfigurement
         b. Osteoarthritis: degenerative disease of articular cartilage with minimal inflammation
      2. Incidence
         a. Rheumatoid: 1 in 1000 children; greater in females than in males; most common between ages 30 and 50
         b. Osteoarthritis: 63% to 85% of Americans over 65 years of age; 20 million patients
      3. Significance
         a. Rheumatoid: increased incidence of cardiopulmonary involvement
         b. Osteoarthritis is the most common form of joint disease.
      4. Etiology
         a. Rheumatoid: unknown, includes genetics, altered immune response, trauma
         b. Osteoarthritis: aging, genetics
      5. Treatment: goal is to maintain joint function and to minimize disability.
         a. Rheumatoid: symptomatic, NSAIDs, gold, methotrexate, corticosteroids
         b. Osteoarthritis: NSAIDs and heat
      6. Perioperative significance
         a. Rheumatoid arthritis
            (1) Joint stiffness worse in morning; consider afternoon scheduling.

(2) Pericardial effusion, thickening present in one third of adults

(3) Pleural effusion is the most common pulmonary alteration.

  b. Osteoarthritis

(1) Corticosteroids not recommended; increased risk of degenerative joint changes

  c. Arthritis (both types)

(1) Cervical spine and temporomandibular joint (TMJ) involvement may restrict neck mobility for intubation; may require use of fiberoptic bronchoscopy.

(2) Limited joint mobility may compromise intraoperative positioning.

(3) NSAIDs can alter platelet function and coagulation and cause mild anemia.

(4) Obtain preoperative coagulation studies, hemoglobin, and hematocrit.

C. Neuromuscular diseases

  1. Muscular dystrophy

  a. Definition

(1) Progressive disease of muscle resulting in painless degeneration and atrophy of skeletal muscles

(2) Caused by increased permeability of skeletal muscle membranes and decreased cardiopulmonary reserve

  b. Inappropriate for ambulatory surgery

  2. Myasthenia gravis

  a. Definition: chronic autoimmune disease of the neuromuscular junction resulting in rapid exhaustion and weakness of voluntary skeletal muscles

  b. Incidence: 1 in 20,000 adults; greater in females than in males; females ages 20-30, males >60 years of age

  c. Significance: disease classified as type I to IV based on skeletal muscle involvement and severity of symptoms

(1) Type I: involvement of only extraocular eye muscles

(2) Type IIA: slow, progressive mild skeletal muscle weakness without respiratory muscle involvement

(3) Type IIB: severe, rapidly progressive form of skeletal muscle weakness with respiratory muscle weakness

(4) Type III: acute onset, rapid deterioration of skeletal muscle strength with high mortality

(5) Type IV: severe skeletal muscle weakness that results from progression of type I or type II

  d. Etiology: unknown; thymus gland abnormality; autoimmune disease of neuromuscular junction mediated by reduction in number of acetylcholine receptors at neuromuscular junction

  e. Treatment: anticholinesterase drugs (pyridostigmine, Mestinon), corticosteroid, immunosuppressants, plasmapheresis, thymectomy

  f. Perioperative significance

(1) Not appropriate for ambulatory surgery if type IIB, III, or IV

(2) Will likely require prolonged postoperative ventilatory support

(3) Anticholinesterase drugs alter effects of nondepolarizing muscle relaxants with variable responses.

(4) Very susceptible to respiratory depression

(5) Consider epidural analgesics.

  3. Parkinson's disease (paralysis agitans)

  a. Definition: slow adult-onset, progressive disease of central nervous system degeneration characterized by the classic triad of resting tremor, rigidity, and bradykinesia *Extreme slowness of movement*

  b. Incidence: 50,000 new cases per year; greater in males than in females; onset >40 years of age

  c. Significance: do not assume presence of mental status changes.

  d. Etiology: possible genetic predisposition

     e. Treatment: no cure

        (1) Goal is to control symptoms and to slow disease course.

        (2) May include levodopa in combination with Sinemet; bromocriptine, and lergotrile; amantadine, which reduces symptoms via presumed anticholinergic and enhanced dopamine effect; anticholinergics; stereotaxic surgery; experimental treatment with fetal adrenal implantation.

     f. Perioperative significance

        (1) Physical limitations may increase need for assistive devices.

        (2) Continue levodopa on day of surgery—interruption of drug for 6-12 hours can result in loss of drug's therapeutic effect, including difficulty in maintaining ventilation.

        (3) Levodopa may produce orthostatic hypotension, dysrhythmias, hypertension.

        (4) Use of phenothiazines (Compazine) and butyrophenones (Droperidol) contraindicated—may produce extrapyramidal effects

        (5) Depression common in advanced stages of disease (if monoamine oxidase (MAO) inhibitors are being used, notify anesthesiologist)

        (6) Intravascular volume depletion and inadequate response to hypotension make blood pressure (BP) and heart rate fluctuate.

        (7) Ketamine may cause exaggerated sympathetic response.

        (8) Potential hyperkalemic response to succinylcholine

        (9) Postoperative period

           (a) Close attention to respiratory status

           (b) Close attention to central nervous system (CNS) state

           (c) Begin anti-Parkinson's therapy immediately postoperative

VII. Endocrine diseases: Characterized by an overproduction or underproduction of single or multiple hormones

  A. Diabetes mellitus (DM)

    1. Definition

     a. Chronic, systemic disease producing altered glucose metabolism and hyperglycemia

     b. Insulin dependent diabetes mellitus (IDDM, type I, ketosis prone) commonly develops in childhood and adolescents.

        (1) Patient produces no insulin.

        (2) Requires insulin to sustain life

     c. Noninsulin dependent diabetes mellitus (NIDDM, type II, Nonketosis prone) develops after age 35.

        (1) Commonly managed with diet and oral hypoglycemic agents

        (2) May require insulin

     d. Incidence: 2.4% of U.S. population (5.5 million people)

     e. Significance: increased risk of macroangiopathy (coronary artery disease, cerebrovascular disease, peripheral vascular disease), microangiopathy (retinopathy, nephropathy), and CNS disorder (autonomic nervous system neuropathy, peripheral neuropathy)

     f. Etiology

        (1) IDDM: autoimmune, viral, genetic, environmental

        (2) NIDDM: genetic, obesity

     g. Treatment: diet, oral hypoglycemic agents (not with IDDM), insulin, exercise, BP control; pancreas transplant is option if renal disease is end stage in IDDM cases.

     h. Perioperative significance

        (1) Ultimate goal is to mimic normal metabolism, avoid hypoglycemia, excessive hyperglycemia, ketoacidosis, and electrolyte disturbances.

(2) Patients will require glucose-containing intravenous (IV) solutions to prevent hypoglycemia and insulin to prevent ketosis and hyperglycemia.

    (a) Goal: blood glucose level of 120-180 mg/dl

(3) Diabetic patients ideally scheduled early in the day to avoid prolonged fasting (NPO).

(4) Continue insulin on the day of surgery (some physicians request half normal dose—check facility policy); alternative is to hold insulin on day of surgery and to monitor blood glucose levels during surgery.

(5) Oral hypoglycemic agents commonly held as hypoglycemia common without caloric intake

(6) Obtain preoperative electrocardiogram (ECG), electrolytes, glucose (may vary with facility policy)

    (a) Most common cause of perioperative morbidity in diabetic patients is ischemic heart disease.

(7) Presence of autonomic nervous system dysfunction may increase risk of aspiration and cardiovascular instability.

(8) Peripheral neuropathy may influence selection of regional anesthesia.

(9) Regional: diabetic nerves may be more prone to edema especially if epinephrine used.

(10) IV solutions commonly contain potassium.

(11) All supplemental insulin to be given IV to prevent unpredictable subcutaneous absorption

(12) Limited joint mobility and obesity may make intubation difficult.

(13) Infections and end-organ risk substantially increased with blood sugar >250 mg/dl.

  B. Adrenocortical insufficiency (Addison's disease)

    1. Definition: absence of cortisol and aldosterone owing to destruction of the adrenal cortex

    2. Incidence: 1 in 100,000, all ages, no race or gender predominance

    3. Significance: endocrine and metabolic alterations

    4. Etiology: autoimmune, tuberculosis (TB), acquired immune deficiency syndrome (AIDS), adrenal hemorrhage in anticoagulated patient

    5. Treatment: corticosteroid replacement, surgical excision of adrenal gland(s)

    6. Perioperative significance

      a. Steroid dose may be increased for patients undergoing surgical procedure because patients are unable to increase release of endogenous cortisol to meet physiologic stress; can lead to cardiovascular collapse.

      b. Most minor ambulatory procedures require no change of steroid dose.

      c. Instruct patient to take steroid medication on morning of surgery.

      d. Correct hypovolemia, hyperkalemia, hyponatremia, hypoglycemia.

      e. Benzodiazepine preoperative OK

      f. Chest x-ray for pneumothorax if adrenalectomy

      g. Increased pancreatitis seen with left adrenalectomy

      h. Perioperative steroids may

        (1) Decrease wound healing

        (2) Increase infections

        (3) Increase stress ulcers

        (4) Increase glucose intolerance

        (5) Increase BP

VIII. Hematologic diseases

  A. Anemia

    1. Definition: deficiency of erythrocytes (red blood cells)

      a. Females: hemoglobin <11.5 g/dl (hematocrit 36%)

      b. Males: hemoglobin <12.5 g/dl (hematocrit 40%)

2. Incidence: common
3. Significance: will compromise oxygen delivery to cells
4. Etiology: iron deficiency (infants and small children only); chronic disease in adults (GI bleed, menstrual loss); thalassemia (decreased synthesis of normal hemoglobin)
5. Treatment: ferrous sulfate; address source if chronic loss
6. Perioperative significance
   a. No minimally accepted standard of hemoglobin concentration required for surgery
   b. Low hemoglobin does not require transfusion.
   c. Low hemoglobin does not compromise wound healing.
   d. Low hemoglobin does not increase the risk of infection.
   e. Decision to transfuse intended only to increase the oxygen-carrying capacity.
   f. Patients with compromised oxygenation are not candidates for ambulatory surgery.
   g. Keep patient warm postoperatively, prevent shivering.
   h. Maintain high PaO_2.
   i. Avoid hyperventilation or acute alkalosis.
B. Sickle cell anemia
   1. Definition: chronic hemoglobinopathy with varying quantities of hemoglobin S (normal is hemoglobin A), resulting in vascular occlusion and compromised tissue oxygenation
   2. Incidence: sickle cell trait 8% to 10% of all African-Americans (defined as hemoglobin S concentration <50%), 0.2% of all African-Americans with sickle cell disease (hemoglobin S 70% to 98%), 1 in 500 African-Americans
      a. Also present in persons from India and Saudi Arabia
   3. Significance: characterized by chronic hemolysis (anemia) and acute vasoocclusive crisis that causes organ failure and can be life threatening
   4. Etiology: inherited, autosomal recessive
   5. Treatment: minimize factors that cause sickling, including hypoxia, acidosis, hypothermia, hemoglobin concentration <8.5 g/dl, dehydration, pain, infection
   6. Perioperative significance
      a. Patients in sickle cell crisis inappropriate for ambulatory surgery
      b. Patients with sickle cell trait not at increased risk during perioperative period
      c. Patient with sickle cell disease must be free of infection, hydrated, and hemodynamically stable preoperatively.
      d. Obtain sickle cell lab test in all African-Americans under age 15.
         (1) If, by age 15 patient has never been tested nor diagnosed, can omit.
         (2) Most commonly diagnosed in childhood
      e. Anesthetic goal: avoid acidosis secondary to hypoventilation, maintain oxygenation, prevent circulatory stasis, maintain body temperature.
      f. Postoperative goal: maintain oxygenation, maintain intravascular fluid volume, maintain body temperature, utilize analgesics.
         (1) Palliative care for painful crisis
         (2) Simple and exchange transfusions
         (3) Hydroxyurea to increase fetal hemoglobin
C. The anticoagulated patient
   1. Definition: administration of oral anticoagulant to induce alterations in coagulation to prevent thrombus formation
   2. Incidence: used in patients with synthetic heart valves, history of atrial fibrillation, sinus arrhythmia with enlarged left atrium, left ventricular dysfunction, CHF, history of thrombolic events
   3. Significance: concomitant valve disease or replacement
   4. Etiology: Coumadin therapy alone or with aspirin or dipyridamole
   5. Treatment: discontinue drug, vitamin K

      6. Perioperative significance

        a. Increased risk of surgical bleeding

        b. Coumadin ideally stopped 3 days before elective procedure

          (1) May not be possible for patients with prosthetic valves

        c. Obtain prothrombin time (PT) day of surgery.

        d. Consider bleeding time and platelet count.

        e. Inquire about the use of aspirin and NSAIDs in addition to Coumadin use.

        f. Increased risk of cerebrovascular accident (CVA) with atrial fibrillation patients off Coumadin

IX. Infectious diseases

  A. Human immunodeficiency virus (HIV) infection, AIDS

      1. Definition: destruction of lymphocytes with decline in immune function

      2. Incidence: >250,000 infectious persons; young adults 25-44; greater in males than in females

      3. Significance: increased risk of opportunistic infections in CNS, GI tract, lungs (TB)

      4. Etiology: HIV spread via sexual activity, blood transfusions, IV drug use, fetal transmission, needle stick

      5. Treatment: supportive, antiretroviral chemotherapy (combination drug therapy) some disease slowing with investigational drug therapy; prophylaxis against opportunistic infections including pneumococcal vaccine, hepatitis B vaccine, influenza vaccine, isoniazid, trimethoprim–sulfamethoxazole

      6. Perioperative significance

        a. Meticulous attention to universal precautions

        b. Chest x-ray to rule out interstitial pneumonitis

        c. Must consider extent of organ system involvement when approving ambulatory status (pneumonia, dementia, cardiomyopathy, renal dysfunction)

        d. Asymptomatic patient who is HIV positive will respond in normal manner to anesthetic agents.

  B. TB

      1. Definition: bacterial pulmonary infection characterized by asymptomatic conversion of a TB skin test or presence of fever and nonproductive cough in an "at-risk" patient

      2. Incidence: 100 in 100,000 population; greater in males than in females; increased risk with elderly in nursing homes, HIV-positive patients, homeless, prisoners, Asian and Latin America immigrants

      3. Significance: can affect bones, joints, meninges, kidney, and skin

      4. Etiology: *Mycobacterium tuberculosis* via droplet aerosol transmission (coughing and sneezing)

      5. Treatment: isoniazid, rifampin, pyrazinamide, streptomycin, and ethambutol in combination varying with severity of disease

      6. Perioperative significance

        a. Highest risk of disease is within 8-12 weeks of exposure.

        b. Rifampin colors urine, tears, and secretions orange.

        c. Isoniazid can cause peripheral neuritis and hypersensitivity—can prevent with pyridoxine.

        d. Compliance issues predominate with number of drugs and length of treatment.

        e. Not infectious after 2 weeks of therapy and negative acid fast bacilli (AFB) culture

        f. Chest x-ray will show infiltrate with or without effusion.

        g. Homeless patients will have significant discharge limitations.

        h. Patients with active TB require respiratory isolation.

        i. Limit traffic, use disposable equipment, wear protective clothing, and remove unessential equipment in the surgical suite when patients are done.

X. Substance abuse

  A. Illicit drug use

   1. Definition: self-administration of drug(s) that deviate(s) from accepted medical or social use, which, if sustained, can lead to physical and psychologic dependence

   2. Incidence: varies with drug; includes alcohol, cocaine, opioids, barbiturates, benzodiazepines, amphetamines, marijuana, hallucinogens

   3. Significance: physical withdrawal requires inpatient hospitalization—should not be attempted in perioperative period.

   4. Etiology: biologic, social, environmental, psychologic factors

   5. Treatment: medical management of withdrawal, behavioral, and supportive counseling

   6. Perioperative significance

    a. Can manifest cross-tolerance to drugs making it difficult to predict anesthetic and/or analgesic requirements; usually increased

    b. May have concomitant problems of HIV, hepatitis, TB, malnutrition

    c. Frequently has associated personality disorders

    d. Patients acutely affected by substances are not candidates for ambulatory surgery.

XI. Obesity

  A. Definition: weight >20% of ideal body weight

   1. Morbidly obese: double normal body weight

  B. Incidence: 20% to 30% of adult men, 30% to 40% of adult women; greater in females than in males; all ages

  C. Significance: may have concomitant heart disease, diabetes, pulmonary insufficiency

  D. Etiology: food intake greater than energy expenditure; genetic, endocrine, acquired disease

  E. Treatment: medically supervised weight loss with nutritional counseling, increase exercise and activity; surgical: gastric stapling or bypass or intestinal bypass

  F. Perioperative significance

   1. Increased risk of aspiration; administer metoclopramide, H2 antagonist

   2. Decreased use of positive pressure ventilation to preoxygenate to prevent distention and vomiting

   3. Increased difficulty in intubation

   4. May be chronically hypoxemic and hypercarbic; sleep apnea common

   5. Increased duration of action of lipid-soluble drugs

   6. Increased morbidity from cardiovascular disease

   7. Increased risk of deep venous thrombosis—consider antiembolism precautions.

   8. Increased risk of wound infection

   9. Respiratory insufficiency, pneumonia, and thromboembolic phenomena avoided postoperatively by

    a. Minimal sedation

    b. Appropriate pain control

    c. Early ambulation

BIBLIOGRAPHY

1. Braun: Definition of hypertension. Available at http://www.braun.com/medical/blood-pressure/infocenter/background/Accessed on June 24, 2003.
2. Burden N, Quinn D, O'Brien D, et al: *Ambulatory surgical nursing.* Philadelphia: WB Saunders, 2000.
3. Drain C: *Perianesthesia nursing: A critical care approach.* St Louis: Elsevier, 2003.
4. Fogoros R:: Doctors drop the ball on hypertension. Published March 4, 2002. Available at http://www.heartdisease.about.com/library/weekly/aa030402a.htm. Accessed on June 23, 2003.
5. Faust, R: *Anesthesiology review,* ed 3. New York: Churchill Livingstone, 2002.
6. Litwack K: *Post anesthesia care nursing,* 2nd ed. St Louis: Mosby–Yearbook, 1995.
7. Roisen M, Fleischer L: *Essence of anesthesia practice,* ed 2. Philadelphia: WB Saunders, 2002.
8. Stoelting R, Dierdorf S: *Handbook for anesthesia and co-existing disease,* ed 2. New York: Churchill Livingstone, 2002.

20 Complementary and Alternative Therapies

SUSAN A. GOODWIN and JANE C. DIERENFIELD

OBJECTIVES

At the conclusion of this chapter the reader will be able to:

1. Define the terms complementary therapies, alternative therapies, and integrative medicine.

2. Discuss the influence of Eastern medicine, including Traditional Chinese Medicine and East Indian contributions.

3. Compare and contrast 27 commonly used herbs, vitamins, and dietary supplements.

4. Summarize five complementary therapies that could be used in the perianesthetic period.

5. Briefly define additional complementary and alternative therapies.

I. Overview of complementary therapies
   A. Definitions
      1. Conventional medicine is practiced by MDs, or DOs, and other allied health professionals, such as registered nurses, psychologists, or physical therapists.
         a. Is taught at U.S. medical schools, and is generally provided at U.S. hospitals
         b. Commonly known as Western medicine and is based on biology and pathology
      2. Complementary therapies (CTs)
         a. Are a group of diverse medical and health care systems, practices, and products that are not presently considered to be a part of conventional medicine
         b. Are taken or used in conjunction with conventional medicine
         c. Are based on Eastern philosophy, which is based on balance and harmony
         d. Oriental medicine began approximately 5000 years ago.
            (1) The Yellow's Emperor's Classic of Internal Medicine was written 2000 years ago.
      3. Alternative therapies (ATs)
         a. Are the same group of diverse medical and health care systems, practices, and products that are not presently considered to be a part of conventional medicine
         b. Are used in place of conventional medicine
      4. A therapy by itself is not complementary or alternative
         a. The use or lack of use of conventional medicine is what defines a therapy as complementary or alternative.
   B. Integrative medicine is the eventual combination of complementary therapies and medicine.
      1. Reliable evidence of efficacy of complementary medicine is needed prior to its integration into clinical practice.
   C. A study of complementary medicine articles published in mainstream medical literature as retrieved from Medline from 1966 through 1996 demonstrated a significant increase.

    1. Clinical trial articles of complementary medicine increased from 1987 through 1996.

II. Current utilization of complementary and alternative therapies
- A. Terms
  1. "Complementary and alternative medicines" (CAMs) is commonly used.
     - a. In the medical literature
     - b. By the National Center for Complementary and Alternative Medicine
  2. The term CAMs will be used to correctly refer to the literature, or when referring to medical practice.
  3. In this chapter, "complementary and alternative therapies" (CATs) will be used to describe these interventions.
     - a. This term more appropriately describes nursing practice.
- B. A follow-up study of use of CAMs in the United States from 1990 through 1997 demonstrated an increase in the use of at least one CAM from 33.8% in 1990 to 42.1% in 1997.
  1. The probability of using an alternative medicine practitioner increased from 36.3% in 1990 to 46.3% in 1997.
  2. In 1997, the visits to alternative medicine practitioners exceeded the projected number of visits to primary care physicians by an estimated 243 million.[12]
- C. The National Center for Complementary and Alternative Medicine
  1. In 1992, the National Institute of Health (NIH) established for Office of Alternative Medicine (OAM) with the mission of providing the American public with reliable information about the safety and effectiveness of CAMs.
     - a. Budget for 1992 was $2 million.
  2. In 1998, Congress expanded the OAM into the National Center for Complementary and Alternative Medicine (NCCAM).
  3. In 2001, the NCCAM had an annual budget of $89.1 million.
  4. Complementary and alternative medicine is defined by the NCCAM as a group of diverse medical and health care systems, practices, and products that are not presently considered to be part of conventional medicine.
- D. A partial listing of complementary and alternative therapies
  1. Acupuncture
  2. Aromatherapy
  3. Ayurveda
  4. Chiropractic
  5. Dietary supplements
  6. Energy healing
  7. Herbal therapies
  8. High-dose vitamin or megavitamin therapies
  9. Homeopathy
  10. Magnetic therapy
  11. Massage
  12. Meditation
  13. Naturopathy
  14. Osteopathic
  15. Prayer
  16. Qigong
  17. Reiki
  18. Relaxation techniques
  19. Therapeutic touch
  20. Yoga
- E. Recent trends in CATs in the United States
  1. National surveys indicate that CATs are widely used in the United States and are increasing in popularity.
  2. Use of CATs tends to be higher among patients who are
     - a. Female
     - b. Middle aged or younger, 35-49 years of age

       c. White
       d. Married
       e. Employed
       f. More affluent
       g. Better educated, with some college education
       h. Have more insurance
       i. Live in the Western part of the United States
  3. People who use CATs also use medical doctors.
       a. The more visits a patient made to a medical doctor, the more likely he or she was to use alternative medicine.[15]
  4. CATs are used less frequently by
       a. African-Americans
       b. People 65 or older
  5. CATs are used most frequently for
       a. Chronic pain
       b. Anxiety and/or depression
       c. Urinary tract problems
       d. Back problems
       e. Headaches
       f. Allergies
       g. Arthritis
       h. Digestive problems
       i. Cancer
       j. Diabetes
       k. Acquired immune deficiency syndrome (AIDS)
       l. To prevent future illness form occurring
       m. To maintain health and vitality
  6. Unsupervised use, which is a form of expanded self-care, is the usual method of use for most CATs.
       a. In other words, there is usually no involvement of either a medical doctor or an alternative medicine practitioner.
  7. The increasing use of CATs has occurred despite the fact that the majority of costs have been paid out-of-pocket.

F. Use of CATs throughout the world
  1. In Denmark in 1987, 10% of the population used CATs.
  2. In Australia in 1993, 49% of the population used CATs.
  3. In 1996, France spent $99 million on herbal remedies and $503 million on homeopathic remedies.
  4. The United Kingdom spent $94 million of herbal remedies and $30 million on homeopathic remedies.
  5. Germany spent $541 million on herbal remedies and $528 million on homeopathic remedies.
  6. In Germany, herbal medicine is well integrated into the medical culture.
       a. Tens of millions of prescriptions are written by physicians for herbal medicines each year.

G. Reasons for use of CATs
  1. Dissatisfaction with conventional treatment
  2. A desire to try all options, especially among cancer patients
  3. Anecdotal information from friends or acquaintances
  4. A belief that CATs are less harmful than conventional therapies
  5. Many CATs are holistic and encompass a spiritual component, which is lacking in conventional medicine.

H. Implications for further study
  1. The use of traditional randomized, double-blind, placebo-controlled, clinical trials with CATs present certain challenges.
  2. It would be extremely difficult to design and implement randomized, double-blind, placebo-controlled, clinical trials of all the CATs that are in use today.

3. Many of the CATs have been in use for thousands of years, with vast anecdotal success.
4. Treatment plans with CATs are often individualized and are thus hard to replicate.
5. CATs are increasingly being integrated with conventional medicine, rather than being used alone or in the place of conventional medicine.
6. Pharmaceutical companies invest between $350 and $500 million in a 10-year period to bring a new drug to market—when the drug is marketed, the money is recouped.
7. Obtaining financial support for research on herbs is difficult, because there is no financial incentive for investment by pharmaceutical companies; the herb is readily available, cannot be patented, and is thus not financially lucrative.

I. Guidelines for CAMs in medical practice
1. In April 2002, the Federation of State Medical Associations of the United States developed guidelines for the use of CAMs in medical practice.
2. They encompass education and regulation of physicians who use CAMs in their practice.
3. Third-party payers require Current Procedural Terminology (CPT) codes for reimbursement for services rendered.
4. Currently, there are only eight CPT codes for CAMs and CATs.
   a. CPT codes are a proprietary product of the American Medical Association (AMA).[11]
   b. To date, the AMA has not created additional codes for CAMs.
5. More than 4000 Alternative Billing Codes have been created by Alternative Link (http://www.alternativelink.com).
   a. However, these have not been embraced by the AMA.
   b. Not yet formally accepted by third-party payers
6. Some third-party payers are beginning to offer reimbursement for certain CATs.

III. Preoperative assessment of perianesthetic patients
A. Lack of report of CATs
1. In one study of patients 65 or older, 57% made no mention of their use of CATs to their doctor.[15]
2. In a study of CATs from 1990 through 1997, more than 60% of patients did not disclose their usage of CATs to the medical doctor.
3. The flourishing use of herbal preparations increases the need to specifically question preoperative patients about their use of herbals.
4. Many people do not view herbals as "medicine" or may be reluctant to disclose their uses of complementary therapies to conventional practitioners, such as nurses or doctors.
5. The preoperative nurse must make specific and repeated inquires to the patient about the potential use of herbals.

B. Herbals
1. Are plant-derived products used for medicinal and health purposes (see Table 20-1)
2. Thirty percent of all modern drugs are derived from plants.
3. The use of herbals has increased significantly in the past 10 years.
4. Herbals may have many allergic reactions as well as interactions with prescription drugs.
5. Perioperative patients are exposed to a great number of pharmacological agents during their surgical experience.
   a. The potential for adverse drug interactions is much higher than during their everyday life.
   b. The potential interactions with anesthetic drugs include
      (1) Coagulation disturbances
      (2) Prolongation of anesthetic sedation
      (3) Adverse cardiovascular effects
      (4) The American Society of Anesthesiologists recommends that patients discontinue herbal medicines at least 2 weeks prior to surgery.

TABLE 20-1
■ ■ Herbs

Herb	Actions	Uses	Side Effects	Perianesthetic Implications	Preoperative Discontinuation
Aloe vera	Relieves pain, decreases inflammation and swelling. Is antiinflammatory, and may encourage wound contraction. May increase blood flow. Useful for first- and second-degree burns. May be useful in the treatment of psoriasis.	*Topical:* Emollient. Encourages healing of a wound, burn, hemorrhoids, insect bites, poison ivy or oak, skin rashes, sunburn, and yeast infections. *Oral:* Treats or prevents constipation.	Rare topical allergic reactions. Oral gel can reduce absorption of many drugs.	Oral use may cause hypokalemia due to cathartic effects.	Not necessary
Arnica	Is an immunostimulant. May increase macrophage activity and blood circulation to injured area. Has antiinflammatory and mild analgesia properties. Is frequently combined with goldenseal.	*Topical and Oral:* Relieves muscle, joint, and cartilage pain from bruises, contusions, hyperextensions, bursitis, and arthritis.	Long-term topical use can lead to toxic skin reactions. Internal use has a very narrow dosing range. The FDA classes arnica as unsafe for internal use. The German Commission E does not recommend internal use because of potentially toxic effects.	May be the source of preoperative skin irritations. May have minimal anticoagulant effects.	2 weeks
Black cohosh	Estrogenic activity. Also causes hypotensive effects via decreased vascular spasm. Also has sedative, antiinflammatory and antispasmodic effects.	Is approved by the German Commission E for the treatment of PMS, dysmenorrhea, and menopausal symptoms, including reduction in hot flashes and mood changes. May inhibit bone loss caused by menopause. Appears to increase the normal growth of vaginal cells, thereby reducing vaginal dryness and dyspareunia. Alleviates insomnia. Used as an antiinflammatory for arthritis. Remifemin, a European form of black cohosh, is available in the United States.	GI discomfort, frontal headache, nausea, heaviness in the legs, weight problems, dilated pupils, and flushed face. Avoid use during pregnancy.	May cause hypotension and bracycardia. May potentiate antihypertensive medications.	2 weeks

Continued

TABLE 20-1
■ Herbs *Cont'd*

Herb	Actions	Uses	Side Effects	Perianesthetic Implications	Preoperative Discontinuation
Chamomile	Mild sedative. Also has antispasmodic, antibacterial, antipyretic, and antiinflammatory activity.	Used as an antiemetic, for indigestion, to decrease cramping secondary to diarrhea, and as an aid for sleep. Can be used for dysmenorrhea and to treat arthritis.	Allergic reactions are common, especially in patients who are allergic to ragweed and include contact dermatitis, urticaria, bronchospasm, and pharyngeal edema.	May potentiate sedation. Anticoagulant effects due to platelet inhibition.	2 weeks
Cranberry	Prevents *E. Coli* from adhering to bladder wall and the urinary tract. Acidifies the urine.	To acidify the urine and treat urinary tract infections. Decreases the incidence of urinary stones.	None with normal doses. Very large doses may result in diarrhea.	None known	Not necessary
Echinacea	Has antiinflammatory, immunostimulating, bacteriostatic, bacteriocidal, and free-radical scavenging effects. Causes activation of cell-mediated immunity. Enhances phagocytosis. Decreases the activity of viruses.	Is used for the prophylaxis and treatment of viral, bacterial and fungal infections, especially the common cold. Begin use at the first sign of a cold to decrease cold symptoms and duration. If used for longer than 8 weeks, the effectiveness declines. Also used to treat chronic wounds, ulcers, and arthritis. Used in Germany along with chemotherapy to treat cancer.	Use longer than 8 weeks could cause immunosuppression and hepatotoxicity (some controversy exists about this). Echinacea should not be used with other hepatotoxic drugs, such as anabolic steroids, amiodarone, methotrexate, or ketoconazole. Do not give concomitantly with immunosuppressants. Can cause transplant rejection. Use with caution in patients with asthma or allergic rhinitis.	Causes inhibition of hepatic enzymes. May affect many anesthetic agents.	2 weeks
Evening primrose oil	Chemical constituents are prostaglandin precursors, which have antiinflammatory properties.	Used for PMS symptom relief, diabetic neuropathy, numerous skin conditions, and chronic autoimmune diseases such as rheumatoid arthritis, Raynaud's syndrome, and multiple sclerosis.	Lowers seizure threshold and increases anticonvulsant requirements. Nausea, softening of stools, and headache.	May interact with drugs that are anticonvulsants. Inhibits platelet aggregation.	2 weeks

Feverfew	Is a prostaglandin inhibitor. Has been shown to suppress 86-88% of prostaglandin production.	Used to treat migraines and can reduce the number as well as severity of migraines. Also used to treat fever and arthritis.	NSAIDs may negate the effects of feverfew in the treatment of migraines. May cause mouth ulcers.	Anticoagulant effects due to platelet inhibition.	2 weeks. Discontinuation after prolonged use can cause a rebound effect, resulting in symptoms of migraine, insomnia, and anxiety. A slow withdrawal may reduce these effects.
Garlic	Can lower the risk of developing artherosclerosis through its antihypertensive and anticholesterolemic effects, as well as platelet inhibition. Has antibacterial and antiviral properties. Appears to prevent some cancers.	Used to treat hypertension, hypercholesterolemia, arteriosclerosis, and infection.	Inhibits platelet function and fibrinogen. Concomitant use with aspirin, NSAIDs, or anticoagulants is not recommended. May cause nausea, hypotension, and allergy. Bad breath is a common side effect.	Anticoagulant effects due to platelet inhibition. Can cause hypotension.	2 weeks
Ginger	Has antiemetic, antispasmodic, and antiinflammatory properties. Is a potent inhibitor of thromboxane synthetase.	Is used to treat PONV, motion sickness, sea sickness, hyperemesis gravidarum, intestinal gas, and indigestion. Also used to treat arthralgias.	Inhibits platelet function. May cause GI upset when taken on an empty stomach.	Anticoagulant effects due to platelet inhibition. May cause hypotension or bradycardia.	2 weeks. However, there have been studies in which ginger was given just prior to surgery to reduce PONV, and no increased bleeding was seen.

Continued

TABLE 20-1
■ ■ Herbs *Cont'd*

Herb	Actions	Uses	Side Effects	Perianesthetic Implications	Preoperative Discontinuation
Gingko biloba	Its components act as antioxidants, alter vasoregulation, alter neurotransmitter and receptor activity, and inhibit platelet-activating factor.	Stabilizes and perhaps improves cognitive function in patients with dementia. Used for peripheral vascular disease, vertigo, tinnitus, and erectile dysfunction. Slows macular degeneration and protects the retina, especially in diabetic retinopathy.	Mild GI upset and headache. Inhibits platelet function and fibrinogen. Concomitant use with aspirin, NSAIDs, or anticoagulants is not recommended. May diminish effectiveness of anticonvulsants.	Anticoagulant effects due to platelet inhibition.	2 weeks
Ginseng	A number of ginseng products exist, whose effects vary widely. It is important to be familiar with which ginseng is used. In general, acts as an adaptogen, protecting the body against stress and restoring homeostasis. The underlying mechanism appears to be similiar to steroids. Acts as an immunostimulant. Has a hypoglycemic effect.	Used to reduce stress and improve vitality. Can also be used for mild depression, chronic fatigue syndrome, fibromyalgia, and stress-induced asthma. Improves cognitive function, attention span, psychomotor performance, and concentration.	May cause headache, tremulousness, and insomnia. Avoid in patients with bipolar syndrome and psychosis. Avoid concurrent use with estrogens and corticosteroids due to additive effects. May lower blood glucose levels; should not be used in patients with diabetes. Concomitant use with aspirin, NSAIDs, or anticoagulants is not recommended due to inhibition of platelet function.	Anticoagulant effects due to platelet inhibition. Can cause hypertension or tachycardia. May potentiate sedation. Hypoglycemia.	2 weeks
Goldenseal	Has antibacterial properties. May reduce gastric inflammation. Is frequently combined with arnica.	Is used for its antibacterial and antifungal properties to treat conjunctivitis, gastric and duodenal ulcers, thrush, and strep throat.	Excessive doses can cause jaundice and elevated liver enzymes. Is contraindicated with diarrhea, GI cramping, and nausea and vomiting.	Use cautiously with heparin. May augment or diminish effects of antihypertensives.	2 weeks

Kava-kava	Acts as a sedative-hypnotic possibly by potentiating GABA inhibitory neurotransmission. Has mild analgesic and muscle-relaxing effects. Has abuse potential.	Alleviates stress, anxiety, tension, and nervousness. Used as an anxiolytic and sedative. Relieves tension headaches and muscle spasms (restless leg syndrome, TMJ pain).	Avoid concomitant use with barbituates, alcohol, and benzodiazepines as excessive sedation can occur. Do not use with antiparkinsonian drugs. Decreases platelet function. Heavy use produces kava dermopathy, characterized by reversible, scaly, cutaneous eruptions accompanied by jaundice. The sale of kava has recently been banned in Canada and the United Kingdom due to reported liver damage with kava use.	Excessive sedation can occur with anesthetic drugs. Anticoagulant effects due to platelet inhibition. / 24 hours
Ma huang (ephedra)	Known as ephedra. Ephedrine, a sympathomemetic amine, is the predominant active compound. It increases heart rate and blood pressure, bronchodilates, has antiinflammatory properties, and inhibits prostaglandins.	Commonly used as a decongestant for allergies and hay fever. Used to promote weight loss, increase energy, and treat bronchospastic disorders such as asthma or bronchitis. Also used as an aphrodisiac.	Causes dose-dependent increases in blood pressure and heart rate. Can cause palpitations, coronary spasm, MI, and stroke. Concomitant use of ephedra and MAOIs can result in hyperpyrexia and hypertension.	May cause hypertension or arrhythmias. When given halothane, may cause ventricular arrhythmias. / 7 days
Peppermint	Relaxes the lower esophageal sphincter. Antispasmodic, smooth muscle relaxant.	Used for nausea, rhinitis, heartburn, flatulence, and nausea.	Avoid in patients with hiatal hernia and GERD, as the relaxation of the lower esophageal spincter may worsen symptoms.	None known / Not necessary
Saw palmetto	Increases urinary flow, decreases nocturia, and decreases postvoid residual volumes. Acts as a urinary antiseptic.	Relief of benign prostatic hypertrophy symptoms, such as frequent urination, difficulty in initiating urination, and high residual volume.	Mild GI distress	None known / Not necessary

Continued

TABLE 20-1
Herbs Cont'd

Herb	Actions	Uses	Side Effects	Perianesthetic Implications	Preoperative Discontinuation
St. John's Wort	Acts similarly to MAOIs or SSRIs by inhibiting serotonin, norepiniphrine, and dopamine reuptake by neurons.	Is licensed in Germany for the treatment of anxiety, depression, and sleep disorders. Use of St. John's Wort for moderate depression may be no more effective than a placebo.	Avoid concomitant use with MAOIs and SSRIs, which could result in a serotonin syndrome. May inhibit the absorption of iron. Causes photosensitivity. Through enzyme induction, increases the metabolism of many drugs, including cyclosporine, alfentanil, midazolam, lidocaine, calcium channel blockers, warfarin, and SSRIs. Avoid in pregnancy. The American Medical Association has called for a ban of ephedra in supplements.	May potentiate anesthetic effects. May affect blood pressure.	7 days. Discontinuation is especially important in patients awaiting organ transplantation or who may require oral anticoagulation postoperatively.
Valerian	Causes a significant decrease in sleep latency. Causes dose-dependent sedation and hypnosis.	Used for insomnia or anxiety.	Avoid concomitant use with barbiturates, alcohol, and benzodiazepines as excessive sedation can occur. Can cause "morning hangovers."	May potentiate sedation caused by anesthesia.	7 days. Abrupt discontinuation in patients who are physically dependent may cause benzodiazepine-like withdrawal. Taper over several weeks.

BPH, Benign prostatic hypertrophy; CNS, central nervous system; FDA, Federal Drug Administration; GABA, gamma aminobutyric acid; GERD, gastroesophageal reflux disease; GI, gastrointestinal; NSAIDs, nonsteroidal antiinflammatory drugs; PONV, postoperative nausea and vomiting; PMS, premenstrual syndrome; PSA, prostate specific antigen; MAOIs, monoamine oxidase inhibitors; MI, myocardial infarction; SSRI, selective serotonin release inhibitors, such as nefazodone, sertraline, or paroxetine; TMJ, temperomandibular joint; UTI, urinary tract infection; WBCs, white blood cells.

    C. Regulation of herbals in the United States
        1. In 1994, herbal medications were classified as dietary supplements in the Dietary Supplement Health and Education Act.
        2. This law exempts herbals from the safety and efficacy requirements that must be met by prescription and over-the-counter drugs.
          a. It requires no proof of efficacy, no proof of safety, and set no standards for quality control.
          b. It does require that supplements not promise a specific cure on the label.[54]
        3. There is no guaranty that the herb(s) listed on the packaging are actually present, that the ingredient is bioavailable, the dosing is appropriate, or whether the next bottle will have the same composition.
          a. The same herb marketed by different manufacturers can vary greatly.
          b. Herbs manufactured from outside the United States may contain heavy metals, pesticides, and even pharmaceuticals.
        4. The Food and Drug Administration must show that an herbal product is unsafe before it can be removed from the market.
        5. There is no mechanism for reporting of herbal adverse effects, or herbal and drug interactions; thus, they are grossly underreported.
    D. Regulation of herbals in Europe
        1. In Germany, France, the United Kingdom, and Canada, regulating agencies enforce standards of herb quality and safety assessment of manufacturers.[54]
        2. The German Commission E Monographs are a comprehensive study of herbals.
        3. Significant numbers of studies are being conducted in Germany, France, Japan, China, and India, but most will not be translated into English.
    E. Vitamins and dietary supplements
        1. Vitamins are complex, organic substances found in most foods that are essential for the normal function of the body.
        2. Dietary supplements correct a dietary deficiency.
        3. A number of commonly used vitamins and dietary supplements interact with perianesthetic drugs in similar ways to herbals (Table 20-2).
IV. Complementary therapies useful in perianesthesia
    A. Nursing and complementary therapy
        1. Nurses are in a unique position to create a union between conventional Western medicine and many complementary therapies.
        2. The integrative and holistic nature of nursing lends itself well to the esoteric nature of many complementary interventions.
        3. Forty-seven percent of state boards of nursing permit the practice of some CAMs (Arizona, Arkansas, California, Connecticut, Illinois, Iowa, Kansas, Louisiana, Maine, Maryland, Massachusetts, Mississippi, Missouri, New Hampshire, New York, Nevada, North Carolina, North Dakota, Ohio, Oregon, Pennsylvania, Texas, Vermont, and West Virginia).
        4. The practice of CAMs is under discussion in seven states (Delaware, District of Columbia, Georgia, Minnesota, New Jersey, New Mexico, and Washington).
        5. The remaining 40% of states have no formal position on CAMs (Alabama, Alaska, Colorado, Florida, Georgia, Hawaii, Idaho, Indiana, Kentucky, Michigan, Montana, Oklahoma, Puerto Rico, Rhode Island, South Carolina, Tennessee, Utah, Virgin Islands, Virginia, Wisconsin, and Wyoming).
        6. The five complementary therapies that follow are ones that could be practiced by nurses in the perianesthetic setting.
    B. Aromatherapy
        1. Is the use of essential oils (EO) for therapeutic or medical purposes
        2. Has been used throughout history in many cultures, including ancient Egypt in 3000 B.C.
        3. EOs are steam distillates from aromatic plants and can be used with massage, friction, inhalation, compresses, and baths.
        4. EOs can have sedative, stimulatory, analgesic, antispasmodic and antibacterial properties.

TABLE 20-2
■ Dietary Supplements

Dietary supplements	Actions	Uses	Side Effects	Perianesthetic Implications	Preoperative Discontinuation
Chondroitin	Usually given in conjunction with glucosamine. Contains glycosaminoglycans, which increase proteoglycan concentration, a substance that forms cartilage in the joints. Also reduces collagen breakdown. Also has antiinflammatory effects.	May improve joint pain and function in osteoarthritis.	Mild GI symptoms. Concomitant use with warfarin should be avoided.	None	Not necessary
Coenzyme Q$_{10}$	Is a fat-soluble chemical present in all tissue used to make ADP. Acts as an antioxidant, removing free radicals. Improves immune function.	Is used to treat cancer, heart failure, cardiomyopathy, hypertension, angina, and dysrhythmias.	Mild GI distress. Works synergistically with antihypertensives. Concomitant use with warfarin should be avoided. May diminish the effects of aspirin, NSAIDs, and other anticoagulants.	May augment hypotensive effects of anesthesia. May have anticoagulant effects.	2 weeks
Fish oil	Have antiinflammatory and antiembolus effects. Promote vasodilation. Reduce cholesterol production.	Used to treat coronary artery disease, hyperlipidemia, hypertension, and diabetes.	Belching, bad breath, heartburn, and nosebleeds. May increase bleeding time. Works synergistically with antihypertensives.	Anticoagulant effects due to inhibition of platelet aggregation. May augment the hypotensive effects of anesthesia.	2 weeks
Glucosamine	Usually given with chondroitin. Is an aminomonosaccharide, which stimulates the	May improve joint pain and function in osteoarthritis. Is slow acting; may have	Mild GI distress. Avoid if allergic to shellfish or iodine. May raise blood sugar levels.	None	Not necessary

	production of glycosaminoglycans, a component of cartilage. Also has antiinflammatory effects.	to take it for up to 2 months before benefits are seen.		
Melatonin	Is a hormone produced by the pineal gland during sleep. Is produced from tryptophan.	Used to treat insomnia, and sleeplessness caused by jet lag or working the night shift.	Headaches, vivid dreams or nightmares, and morning hangovers. Is contraindicated is severe mental illness or autoimmune disease.	May potentiate sedation.	24 hours
Vitamin C	Is an essential nutrient needed for collagen and tissue formation, hormone production, carbohydrate metabolism, and immune system function.	A wide variety of uses, including treatment and prophylaxis of colds, immune system stimulation, would healing, and periodontal disease.	Rare side effects. May cause GI distress.	May decrease the effects of heparin or warfarin.	Not necessary
Vitamin E	Is an essential fat-soluble vitamin. Acts as an antioxidant, binding to free radicals. Is a component of the immune system, maintains healthy eyes and skin, and promotes normal clotting.	A wide variety of uses, including diabetes, Alzheimer's disease, fibrocystic breast disease, immune system integrity, skin disorders, and menopause.	Rare side effects. As a fat-soluble vitamin, is stored in the liver.	Anticoagulant effects due to inhibition of platelet aggregation. May augment the hypotensive effects of anesthesia.	2 weeks
Zinc	Acts as an immunostimulant.	Used to decrease the symptoms and longevity of the common cold.	Do not give with immunosuppressants. May cause nausea and a bad taste.	None known	Not necessary

ADP, Adenosine triphosphate; GI, gastrointestinal; NSAIDs, nonsteroidal antiinflammatory drugs.

5. The effects of the EO depend on the therapeutic actions of the oil as well as the learned smell memory of the patient.
6. Inhaled peppermint and ginger can be used to treat postoperative nausea and vomiting.
7. Inhaled lavender, Roman chamomile, lemongrass, and rose can be used to treat pain.

C. Massage
   1. Is an ancient technique; a Chinese medical work written in 2760 B.C. contains descriptions of massage techniques
   2. Modern massage was developed by Henrik Ling from Sweden (1776-1839).
   3. Is a series of soothing and energizing stroking techniques that stimulates the muscles, increasing their ability to absorb nutrients and eliminate waste products
   4. Is a nonpharmacologic and holistic intervention
   5. Relieves muscle tension, stimulates the nervous system, enhances skin condition, improves circulation, aids digestion and intestinal function, increases mobility in joints, relieves chronic pain and especially low back pain, and reduces swelling and inflammation
   6. Has been used to ease childbirth; with asthmatic children to improve breathing; with terminally ill, homebound, and nursing home residents; and with preoperative and postoperative patients
   7. Do not use massage with fever, infections, open wounds, contagious skin conditions or diseases, phlebitis, or acute strains or sprains; wait 48 hours after a strain or sprain to massage.

D. Music
   1. Uses melody to affect changes in behavior, emotions, and physiology
   2. Lowers anxiety, provides distraction, promotes relaxation, and increases pain tolerance; helps the body release energy used for healing
   3. Has been utilized in the perioperative period, and many patients feel less anxious when listening to music before and after surgery
   4. A trained sound therapist uses a wide range of tools, including musical instruments, tapes, tuning forks, and machines that release sound waves at specific frequencies to help heal the body.

E. Relaxation therapy
   1. Encompasses a variety of stress-reduction techniques
   2. Can be done with yoga, meditation, guided imagery, hypnosis, positive suggestions, and breathing techniques
   3. Elicits a relaxation response, which results in reduced muscle tension, decreased blood pressure, heart rate, and respiration, and reduced oxygen consumption
   4. Surgical patients who use relaxation exercises recover more quickly, use less pain medication, have lower blood pressure, and have fewer postoperative complications than those who did not use them.

F. Therapeutic touch
   1. Was first developed in the early 1970s by Dolores Kreiger, PhD, RN, and psychic Dona Kunz
   2. Is based on an ancient technique called laying-on of hands
   3. Is similar to qigong
   4. The healing force of the therapist affects the patient's recovery.
   5. The practitioner scans the patient's energy field by moving their hands in a sweeping motion above the body, clears the energy field to blockages of energy, and facilitates the flow of energy from his or her hands to the patient's energy field.
   6. Can be used to promote relaxation and reduce stress, pain, anxiety, and restlessness—can also promote a sense of well-being
   7. Can be used in acute situations to treat sprains or muscle spasms, to sooth and relax, and to decrease heart rate and blood pressure
   8. Can enhance the onset of pain medications as well as the effectiveness

V. Brief definitions of selected complementary and alternative therapies

   A. Acupuncture

     1. Is based on traditional Chinese medical theory, and has been in existence for at least 2500 years

     2. Involves inserting thin-gauged needles into specific anatomical points in the body for therapeutic purposes

     3. Disrupted patterns of energy flow (qi) are rebalanced by acupuncture.

     4. Insertion points tend to correspond to areas where connective tissue is the thickest.

   B. Ayurvedic

     1. Ayurvedic medicine is traditional Hindu medicine, and was developed over 5000 years ago.

     2. Ayurveda means the "science of life."

     3. The physician prevents or treats diseases by restoring the balance of body, mind, and spirit with diet, exercise, meditation, herbs, massage, and controlled breathing.

   C. Balneotherapy involves the use of baths in the treatment of health conditions.

   D. Chiropractic

     1. Focuses on the relationship between bodily structure and function and how that relationship affects the preservation and restoration of health

     2. Uses spinal manipulation and adjustments to bring about healing

   E. Homeopathy

     1. Is a Western system of care based on the belief that very dilute substances are able to stimulate a healing response in the body

     2. Was developed by Samuel Hahnemann, a German physician who practiced medicine in the late 1700s

     3. Stimulates the body's defense mechanisms to cure symptoms by administering minute doses of medicinal substances; these same substances at higher doses would actually cause symptoms or disease

   F. Magnetic therapy

     1. Electromagnetic fields are invisible lines of force that are present in the Earth and are believed to be produced by electric currents flowing at the Earth's core.

     2. Often used to relieve pain

   G. Meditation

     1. Is a cultivation of the mind through quieting, and observing one's inner state

     2. Is learning to slow down and examine passing sensations in minute detail[56](p. 156)

     3. The practitioner allows pain, emotions, and bodily sensations to be experienced as a natural progression of life.

     4. Results in a reduction of stress activity and lowered heart rate, blood pressure, and respirations; evokes the "relaxation response"

   H. Naturopathy

     1. Arose in the late nineteenth century in America

     2. Works with natural healing forces within the body to restore health through nutrition, exercise, homeopathy, acupuncture, herbal medicine, hydrotherapy, massage, counseling, and/or pharmacology

   I. Osteopathic medicine

     1. Is a form of conventional medicine that emphasizes that diseases arise in the musculoskeletal system

     2. Its paradigm is that all of the body's systems work together, and a disturbance in one system may affect functioning in other body systems.

   J. Prayer

     1. Addresses a Supreme Being or a Higher Power and implies a relationship between the individual and the Higher Power

     2. The control of healing is given to a higher being.

     3. Resembles meditation, bringing similar benefits such as lowered blood pressure and a strengthened immune system

    K. Qigong

        1. Is pronounced chee kung

        2. Qi is an ancient term denoting the vital energy of the body, and gong is the skill to work with qi.

        3. Is part of traditional Chinese medicine

        4. Combines movement, meditation, and regulation of breathing to remove blockages that stop or slow the flow of qi and to ensure an equal balance of qi within the body

        5. Qigong masters can treat organ systems or body areas with or without physical contact

        6. Can be used to enhance the immune system, treat heart disease, stroke, hypertension, osteoporosis, cancer, and senility

    L. Reflexology

        1. Was practiced by Egyptians as early as 2330 B.C.

        2. Is a touch modality based on the principle that reflexes exist on each foot and hand that correspond to the glands, organs, and parts of the body

        3. Of the three different methods that exist (foot, hand, and zone therapy), the most commonly practiced is foot therapy.

        4. Used to reduce anxiety, stress and tension, and facilitate sleep

    M. Reiki

        1. Is a Japanese word denoting Universal Life Energy

        2. Is based on a belief that when spiritual energy is channeled through a Reiki practitioner, the patient's spirit is healed, which heals the body

    N. Yoga

        1. Is an East Indian practice that has existed for 5000 years

        2. The word *yoga* comes from the Sanskrit word *yui*, which means to unite

        3. A central belief of yoga is that a healthy body, mind, and spirit are needed for a healthy person.

        4. Involves stretching exercises, breathing control, and meditation

        5. Yoga training results in decreased sympathetic tone, decreased peripheral vascular resistance, improved cardiac output, and lowered blood pressure and heart rate.

            a. Can help many conditions, including diabetes, epilepsy, obesity, asthma, depression, osteoarthritis, and cardiovascular disease

VI. Websites For CATs

    A. National Center for Complementary and Alternative Medicine: http://www.nccam.nih.gov

    B. HerbMed: http://www.herbmed.org

    C. PubMed: http://www.ncbi.nlm.nih.gov/entrez/query

    D. Cumulative Index for Nursing and Allied Health Literature (CINAHL): http://www.cinahl.com

    E. The Nurse Healers–Professional Associates International and Therapeutic Touch: http://www.therapeutic-touch.org

    F. RJ Buckle Associates (aromatherapy): http://www.rjbuckle.com

    G. American Massage Therapy Association: http://www.amtamassage.org

BIBLIOGRAPHY

1. Ang-Lee MK, Moss J, Yuan CS: Herbal medicines and perioperative care. *J Am Med Assoc* 286(2):208-216, 2001.

2. Barnes J, Abbot NC, Harkness EF, et al: Articles on complementary medicine in the mainstream medical literature: An investigation of MEDLINE, 1966 through 1996. *Arch Intern Med* 159(15):1721-1725, 1999.

3. Buckle J: *Clinical aromatherapy in nursing.* London: Arnold, 1997.

4. Buckle J: Aromatherapy in perianesthesia nursing. *J PeriAnesth Nurs* 14(6):336-344, 1999.

5. Burns SB and Burns JL: Acupressure and massage. *J Altern Complement Med* 5(1):3, 1999.

6. Cherkin DC, Eisenberg DM, Shennan KJ, et al: Randomized trial comparing traditional Chinese medical acupuncture, therapeutic massage, and self-care education for

chronic low back pain. *Arch Intern Med* 161(8):1081-1088, 2001.

7. Chopra D: *Restful sleep.* New York: Three Rivers Press, 1994.

8. Cohen SM, Rousseau ME, Robinson EH: Therapeutic use of selected herbs. *Holist Nurs Pract* 14(3):59-68, 2000.

9. Crowe S, Fitzpatrick G, Jamaluddin MF: Use of herbal medicines in ambulatory surgical patients. *Anaesthesia* 57(2):203-204, 2002.

10. Crowley G: The science of alternative medicine. *Newsweek* 140(23):45-77, 2002.

11. Dumhoff A: New codes for CAM: HHs review could make them a reality. *Altern Ther Health Med* 8(4):32-36, 2002.

12. Eisenberg DM: Trends in alternative medicine use in the United States 1990-1997: Results of a follow-up national study. *J Am Med Assoc* 280(18):1569-1565, 1998.

13. Ekmekcioglu C: Balneotherapy: Soaking your stress away. *Choices Health Med* 1(1): 12, 2001.

14. Ernst E: Back to basics? How important is basic research in CAM? *Altern Ther Health Med* 7(5):30-32, 2001.

15. Foster DF, Phillips RS, Hamel M, et al: Alternative medicine use in older Americans. *J Am Geriatr Soc* 48(12):1560-1565, 2000.

16. Gottlieb B, editor: *New choices in natural healing.* New York: Bantam, 1997.

17. Grant KL: Patient education and herbal dietary supplements. *Am J Health Syst Pharm* 57(21):1997-2003, 2000.

18. Hodges PJ, Kam PC: The peri-operative implications of herbal medicines. *Anaesthesia* 57(9):889-899, 2002.

19. Jeffrey SLA, Belcher HJ: Use of arnica to relieve pain after carpal-tunnel release surgery. *Altern Ther Health Med* 8(2):66-68, 2002.

20. Kava: A supplement to avoid. *Consum Rep* 68(3):8, 2003.

21. Keenan P: Maternity massage. *Choices Health Med* 1(1):10-11, 2001.

22. Kim YH, Lichenstein G, Waalen J: Distinguishing complementary medicine from alternative medicine. *Arch Intern Med* 162(8):943, 2002.

23. Kreitzer MJ, Snyder M: Healing the heart: Integrating complementary therapies and healing practices into the care of cardiovascular patients. *Prog Cardiovasc Nurs* 17(2):73-80, 2002.

24. Kuhn MA, Winston D: *Herbal therapy and supplements.* Philadelphia: Lippincott, 2000.

25. Liebert MA: Managed care and complementary and alternative medicine: Lessons from the past and suggestions for the future. *J Altern Complement Med* 5(1):1-2, 1999.

26. Low Dog T, Riley D, Carter T: Traditional and alternative therapies for breast cancer. *Altern Therap Health Med* 7(3):36-46, 2001.

27. McKenna DJ, Jones K, Hughes K: Efficacy, safety, and use of *Ginkgo biloba* in clinical and preclinical applications. *Altern Therap Health Med* 7(5):70-92, 2001.

28. McKenna DJ: Black cohosh. *Choices Health Med* 1(1):7-8, 2001.

29. McKoy J: Complementary and alternative options in pain management. Opening Paindora's Box: A symposium on pain management at the Queen's Medical Center, Honolulu, Hawaii, 2002.

30. Mesienhelder JB, Chandler EN: Prayer and health. *Choices Health Med* 2(4):10-11, 2002.

31. Miller LG: Herbal medicinals. *Arch Intern Med* 158(9):2200-2211, 1998.

32. Mitzel-Wilkinson A: Massage therapy as a nursing practice. *Holist Nurs Pract* 14(2): 48-56, 2000.

33. Moss CA: Five-element acupuncture. *Choices Health Med* 2(4):25-7, 2002.

34. Moss TA: Herbal medicine in the emergency department: A primer for toxicities and treatment. *J Emerg Nurs* 24(6):509-513, 1998.

35. Myers CD, White BA, Heft MW: A review of complementary and alternative medicine used for treating chronic facial pain. *J Am Dent Assoc* 133(9):1189-1196, 2002.

36. National Center for Complementary and Alternative Medicine: What is complementary and alternative medicine (CAM)? Available at http://nccam.nih.gov/health/whatiscam. Accessed on December 28, 2002.

37. Norred CL, Brinker F: Potential coagulation effects of preoperative complementary and alternative medicines. *Altern Therap Health Med* 7(6):58-65, 2001.

38. Norred CL, Zamudio S, Palmer SK: Use of complementary and alternative medicines by surgical patients. *AANA J* 68(1):13-18, 2002.

39. North Hawaii Community Hospital Healing Services Department (producer): *Malama Ola: Keeping health and well being* [film]. Available from North Hawaii Community Hospital, 65-1123 Mamalahoa Hwy, Kamuela, HI 96743, 1997.

40. Office of Dietary Supplements, National Institutes of Health: Questions and answers about black cohosh and the symptoms of menopause. Available at http://ods.od.nih.gov/factsheets/blackcohosh.html. Accessed December 28, 2002.

41. Ornish D: Interview: Dean Ornish, MD. *Choices Health Med* 2(1):20-22, 2002.

42. Perry JJ: Therapies for surgery. *Choices Health Med* 2(2):12-13, 2002.

43. Prioreschi P: Alternative medicine in ancient and medieval history. *Med Hypotheses* 55(4):319-325, 2000.

44. Rich D: An alternative approach to hepatitis C. *Choices Health Med* 1(1):8, 2001.

45. Riley D, Berman B: Complementary and alternative medicine in outcomes research. *Altern Therap Health Med* 8(3):36-38, 2002.

46. Sancier KM: Medical qigong. *Choices Health Med* 2(4):22-23, 2002.

47. Smith R: Oriental medicine: First line of defense. Kamuela, Hawaii: Traditional Chinese Medical College of Hawaii, 2002. Available at http://www.ilhawaii.net/~chinese. Accessed on November 23, 2003.

48. Sparber A: State boards of nursing and scope of practice of registered nurses performing complementary therapies. *Online J Issues Nurs* 6(3), 2001. Available at http://www.nursingworld.org/ojin/topic15/tpc15_6.htm. Accessed on January 12, 2003.

49. Stengard PM: New model guidelines for the use of complementary and alternative therapies in medical practice. *Altern Therap Health Med* 8(4):44-47, 2002.

50. Tough SC, Johnston DW, Verhoef MJ, et al: Complementary and alternative medicine use among colorectal cancer patients in Alberta, Canada. *Altern Therap Health Med* 8(2):54-60, 2002.

51. Tsen LC, Segal S, Pothier M, et al: Alternative medicine use in presurgical patients. *Anesthesiology* 93(1):148-151, 2000.

52. Working to get ephedra banned. *Consum Rep* 68(2):6, 2003.

53. Weymouth KF: Healing touch program research and literature review. Unpublished manuscript. San Francisco, CA: Saybrook Graduate School and Research Center, 2001.

54. Winslow LC, Kroll DJ: Herbs as medicines. *Arch Intern Med* 158(20):2192-2199, 1998.

55. Wren KR, Kimbrall S, Norred CL: Use of complementary and alternative medications by surgical patients. *J PeriAnesth Nurs* 17(3):170-177, 2002.

56. Wren KR, Norred CL: *Complementary and alternative therapies.* Philadelphia: WB Saunders, 2003.

21 ■■■ The Mentally and Physically Challenged Patient

KATY FLANAGAN

■■ A disability refers to personal limitations that represent a substantial disadvantage to functioning in society. Patients with disabilities present significant challenges in providing quality nursing care. Perianesthesia standards for ethical practice require that quality care be given to all patients regardless of their disabilities. The Americans with Disabilities Act (ADA) of 1990 covers a person who has a physical or mental impairment that substantially limits one or more major life activities, a person who has a history or record of such impairment, or a person who is perceived by others as having such impairment. Under the ADA, health care facilities are required to provide the disabled with full and equal access of the facility's goods, services, programs, and activities.

The information in this chapter will assist the nurse in caring for the patient with a specific disability. The information on what is included in routine protocols for any patient, including those with disabilities, will be found in other chapters.

OBJECTIVES
At the conclusion of this chapter the reader will be able to:

1. List special considerations in interviewing the mentally challenged patient.

2. List the different stages of Alzheimer's disease and the manifestation of limitations in each stage.

3. State effective communication techniques to use with the hearing impaired.

4. Identify techniques to facilitate learning and reduce apprehension for the visually impaired patient.

5. Identify manifestations of selected physical disabilities and incorporate management of these symptoms and risks in the nursing plan of care.

I. The mentally challenged patient
   A. Communication considerations
      1. Communication—an act by means of which one person conveys to another his or her ideas, thoughts, needs, or feelings
      2. To communicate, a person must have some communication channel open to convey information to those around him or her.
      3. Communication involves
         a. Getting information to the brain
         b. Processing the information
         c. Transmitting the brain's response
      4. For the mentally or physically challenged patient, normal channels of communication may not be available.
      5. Mental ability may be impaired from birth or acquired as a result of disease or injury.

    a. Congenital defect
    b. Infectious process
    c. Trauma
    d. Manifestation of a medical problem
    e. Psychiatric disorder
  6. Level of impairment of developmentally disabled
    a. Mild
      (1) Slow learner
      (2) Rarely asks questions
      (3) Answers questions with a minimum of words
      (4) Can usually function at a 10-year-old level
    b. Moderate
      (1) Has little or no speech
      (2) Understands and can follow simple commands
      (3) Can learn simple tasks; may need supervision to perform
      (4) May be able to function at 2-year-old to 6-year-old level
    c. Severe and profound
      (1) May learn to perform simple self-care tasks with supervision
      (2) Shows basic emotional response
      (3) May cause self harm
      (4) May function at 0-year-old to 2-year-old level
  7. Cognitive considerations of the mentally challenged patient
    a. Degree of impairment will determine method of instruction.
    b. Simple words and phrases are more likely to be understood than complex words and ideas.
    c. Common traits
      (1) Short attention span
      (2) Decreased retention capability
      (3) Decreased sensory capability
    d. Instructions may be taken very literally.
      (1) May need to have basic concepts deconstructed to the essence
      (2) Instructions should build on this basic essence.
    e. Becomes confused and distracted easily
    f. Fearful of changes in environment, loss of familiar routine
  8. Mental status
    a. May be agitated
    b. May show aggression
    c. May not exhibit any response
    d. May have delusions, hallucinations, and/or paranoia
  9. Sensory function
    a. May have visual deficits
    b. May have auditory deficits
    c. May have asthenia   *loss of strength, any weakness*
  10. Communication problems
    a. Poor articulation, especially consonants
    b. More inarticulate when upset, frustrated, or discussing emotionally charged information
    c. May use words that he or she does not really understand
    d. May be eager to please and say what thinks interviewer wants to hear
    e. May need extra time to formulate answers
    f. May use sign language, read lips
    g. May use nonverbal forms of communication
B. Education implementation
  1. Determine the patient's strengths and weaknesses.
  2. Show respect to the patient.
    a. Do not talk down to the patient.
    b. Treat the patient according to age—do not treat adults as children.

     3. Be sensitive to nonverbal communication.

     4. Allow adequate time.

         a. Remain calm, relaxed, and unhurried.

         b. Wait at least 30 seconds to allow patients to respond to a question.

         c. May need to repeat information

         d. May need to reformulate the question

     5. Use the name to which the patient is accustomed.

     6. Be aware that some patients may have delusions, hallucinations, and/or paranoia.

         a. Approach in a calm, nonthreatening, reassuring manner.

         b. Avoid activities that may feed into abnormal thinking.

            (1) No sudden movement

            (2) Avoid standing too close.

            (3) Do not whisper or joke in patient's presence.

            (4) Do not show signs of impatience.

            (5) Do not touch the patient.

            (6) Challenge or agree with patient's delusions, hallucinations, or paranoia.

     7. Communicate slowly and clearly.

         a. Use open-ended questions.

         b. Be prepared to reword questions if the patient does not grasp the meaning of what is being asked.

     8. Encourage and allow patient independence according to abilities.

     9. Include family and caregiver in planning care and instructions as appropriate.

    10. Demonstration may be more effective than verbal explanations.

    11. Provide frequent reinforcement.

C. Preadmission, preoperative interview and management

     1. An in-person interview is preferable to a telephone interview.

         a. Nonverbal communication may be as important as verbal communication.

         b. Face to face may be the only way to communicate with the person.

         c. Allow adequate time for the interview and assessment.

     2. Determine the patient's functional ability and needs.

         a. Developmental assessment if appropriate

         b. Question the family and caregiver about the patient's abilities.

         c. Family's and caregiver's successful management techniques

         d. Use of assistive devices (i.e., glasses, braces, hearing aid)

         e. Effective means of communication; be alert to nonverbal communication

         f. Willingness and capability of family and caregiver to participate in preoperative preparation and postoperative care

     3. Determine the patient's, the family's, and caregiver's knowledge and expectations of the proposed procedure.

     4. Complete health history per protocol

         a. Cause of disability

            (1) At birth or acquired

            (2) Degree of disability

               (a) Retains self-determination capabilities

               (b) Caregiver shares decision making.

               (c) Durable power of attorney for health care

               (d) Legal guardian appointed

         b. Consider common health conditions associated with multiple disabilities.

            (1) Alimentary—dental caries, high arched palate, gum disease, facial asymmetry, mandible subluxation, jaw and tongue asymmetry, oral sensitivity, inadequate nutrition

            (2) Sensory—limited communication abilities, visual and hearing impairment

      (3) Cardiovascular—reduced cardiac and lung functions linked to spinal curvature, chronic respiratory infections, pneumonia, aspiration

      (4) Musculoskeletal—spinal curvatures such as scoliosis, hyperlordosis, hyperkyphosis, deformities of shoulders, elbows, wrists and hands, knees and feet, hypertonia, hypotonia, fluctuating muscular tone, athetosis

      (5) Skin—damage to skin integrity from pressure and incontinence

      (6) Elimination—urinary and fecal incontinence, urinary tract infection (UTI), constipation, urinary retention, bowel impaction

      (7) Central nervous—epilepsy, seizures

c. Past illnesses—especially those for which the patient was hospitalized

      (1) Coping mechanisms to handle illness-related stress

      (2) Length of recuperative period

      (3) Frequency of respiratory infections

      (4) Normal response to pain

      (5) Bladder function difficulties

      (6) Bowel function difficulties

d. Other health problems

      (1) Congenital heart defect

      (2) Diabetes—mellitus, insipidus

      (3) Seizures

        (a) Time of last seizure

        (b) Frequency of seizures

        (c) Description of seizures

      (4) Elicit if any other problems.

e. Medications

      (1) Current medication use

        (a) Prescription

        (b) Over-the-counter

        (c) Herbal preparations

        (d) Dietary supplements

      (2) Behavior changes caused by medications

      (3) Previous response to medications

f. Allergies

      (1) Medications

      (2) Environmental

      (3) Food

      (4) Latex

      (5) Tape

      (6) Type of reactions to allergies

g. Nutritional requirements and modifications

      (1) Special dietary restrictions

      (2) Food consistency

      (3) Preferences

      (4) Ability to swallow

      (5) Ability to eat independently or amount of assistance needed

h. Usual behavior

      (1) Patient's interaction with people and environment

      (2) Orientation to time and place

      (3) Emotional stability

        (a) Mood swings

        (b) Potential for violence

        (c) Panic attacks

        (d) Hallucinations, delusions, paranoia

      (4) State of consciousness

      (5) Language ability

5. Physical assessment per protocol
   a. Vital signs and oxygen saturation (vital signs usually within expected range for size and age)
      (1) Past history of vital sign instability
      (2) Past tendency for pronounced temperature deviations
   b. Body size
      (1) Obese
      (2) Emaciated
   c. Skin color and blemishes may provide clues to other illnesses.
      (1) Pallor may indicate anemia.
      (2) Uneven coloring and/or mottling may indicate poor neural functioning of the autonomic system.
      (3) Excessive pigmentation (freckles) could indicate pathology.
      (4) Multiple café au lait spots indicate neurofibromatosis (von Recklinghausen's disease).
      (5) Port wine stain on the face along the trigeminal nerve may indicate Sturge-Weber syndrome.
   d. Differences in skin temperature, skin turgor
   e. Defects of the craniofacial area
      (1) Anatomical deformities that interfere with intubation
      (2) Weakness of pharyngeal muscles
      (3) Large tongue
   f. Joint deformities
      (1) Pain on movement
      (2) Muscle strength
      (3) Involuntary movements
      (4) Altered stance, gait, or posture
      (5) Contractures
   g. Deficits in hearing or vision
6. Psychosocial assessment per protocol
   a. Anxiety
      (1) Fear of strange environment
      (2) Loss of independence
      (3) Change in daily routine
   b. Support system
      (1) Ensure competent and willing adult to assist with preoperative care and after discharge.
      (2) May need early social service referral for discharge care
7. Develop a plan of care based on the assessment of the patient's and caregiver's knowledge and needs.
8. Preoperative teaching per protocol and using techniques listed in prior sections
   a. Explain what will happen in simple terms.
   b. Explain what to expect preoperatively and immediate postoperatively.
   c. Determine the patient's regular schedule and incorporate that schedule into the hospital routine whenever possible.
   d. Include family and caregiver in the preoperative and postoperative preparations.
   e. Encourage the patient to bring some familiar comfort item from home.
   f. Demonstrate preoperative preparation or postoperative exercises and/or treatments and have the patient or caregiver do a return demonstration.
   g. Nothing by mouth (NPO) requirements—consider harm of extensive NPO time element to patient's emotional well-being.
   h. Medications to take or hold
      (1) Maintain regular dose schedule as much as possible.
      (2) Keep in mind the interactions with anesthesia of tricyclic antidepressants and monoamine oxidase (MAO) inhibitors when

giving instructions—seek clarification from the anesthesia provider if necessary.

    i. Pain scale (modify to suit patient's learning ability)

      (1) Demonstrate use of pain scale to patient.

      (2) Have patient return demonstration.

    j. Ensure that appropriate person will be available to sign necessary consents.

    k. Ensure arrangements for safe transport to and from the hospital.

    l. Ensure that there will be a responsible adult to assist with care after discharge.

  9. Complete preparation for admission per protocol

    a. Make referrals as necessary.

    b. Preoperative testing as ordered

    c. Document and communicate special needs to the perianesthesia staff.

  D. Day of admission—see Box 21-1.

  E. Preoperative holding and intraoperative—see Box 21-2.

  F. Phase I—see Box 21-3.

  G. Phase II—see Box 21-4.

  H. Postdischarge—see Box 21-5.

II. Alzheimer's disease (AD)

  A. Background information

    1. Alzheimer's is a complex progressive, ultimately fatal, disorder.

      a. Certain types of nerve cells in particular areas of the brain degenerate and die.

      b. Affected cells include cortical pathways involved in catecholaminergic, serotonergic, and cholinergic transmission.

      c. Advancing pathology leads to the classic clinical symptoms.

        (1) Memory loss

        (2) Changes in personality

        (3) Noticeable decline in cognitive abilities (including speech and understanding)

■ BOX 21-1
■ **ADMISSION PROCEDURE**

- Review data collected during preadmission interview.
- Verify compliance to preoperative instructions with patient, family, and caregiver.
- Verify safe transportation home and competent adult help at home.
- Verify consents are appropriately signed.
- Physical assessment (history and physical per policy)
- Provide emotional support to patient and family and caregiver.
- Institute appropriate nursing measures to decrease anxiety.
- Decrease stimulation in the waiting area.
- Limit number of personnel who interact with the patient.
- Allow family and caregiver to remain with the patient as long as possible.
- Allow patient to use assistive devices as long as possible.
- Consider preoperative medications to decrease anxiety.
- Consider applying eutectic mixture of local anesthetic (EMLA) cream at least 1 hour prior to IV insertion.
- Maintain a calm, unhurried, and accepting attitude.
- Call patient by name he or she is most familiar with.
- Allow patient to take comfort item to surgery if permissible.
- Prepare patient for procedure per protocol.
- Communicate patient's special needs to all members of the health care team (surgical, anesthesia, and postanesthesia care unit [PACU] team members).

(4) Loss of executive function (decision making)

(5) Losses impairing activities of daily living (dressing, eating, toileting, etc.)

2. Stages of progression

   a. Forgetful stage—changes in short-term memory, depression, conflict with others, expressive aphasia, frustration

   b. Confused stage—agnosia (inability to recognize common objects), decreased time sense, withdrawn, impaired reading abilities, difficulty managing daily activities (money, driving, cooking, cleaning), wandering, night walking, walking without lifting feet, belligerence, confusion, paranoia, agitation, delusions, aggression

■ BOX 21-2
■ PREOPERATIVE HOLDING AND INTRAOPERATIVE

- Whenever possible, have the PACU nurse meet the patient beforehand so that the patient will recognize and be comforted by a familiar face in an unfamiliar and frightening environment.
- Review collected data.
- Provide routine care per protocol.
- Provide emotional support.
- Use the name with which the patient is familiar.
- Reassure the patient you are with him or her; touch patient if it will provide comfort.
- Allow patient to keep comfort item.
- Whenever possible, allow patient to keep hearing aid, glasses, etc.
- Maintain normothermia.
- When moving patient, lift, rather than pull, especially if joint deformities are present.
- Communicate the patient's special needs to the PACU staff.

■ BOX 21-3
■ PHASE I

- Review collected data.
- Provide routine care per PACU protocol.
- Be alert for agitation, disorientation, or combative behavior.
- Minimize risk of aspiration.
- Observe for return of gag and swallowing reflexes.
- Elevate head of bed if not contraindicated.
- Suction as necessary.
- Position on side if not contraindicated.
- Provide for safety—use restraints for protection only as a last resort to prevent injury (refer to facility policy on restraint use).
- Assess frequently for pain and administer medication as indicated.
- Recognize patient may not be able to tell you pain is present.
- Be attuned to nonverbal communication.
- Provide emotional support.
- Use the name with which the patient is familiar.
- Provide reassurance to the patient that you are present.
- Allow use of comfort item if sent with a patient.
- Reorient patient to surroundings.
- Allow use of assistive devices as soon as possible.
- Have a family member and caregiver with the patient if possible.
- Communicate patient's special needs to phase II team.

■ BOX 21-4
■ **PHASE II**

- The patient may return to phase II directly from the operating room (fast-tracking).
- Patient may be disoriented, combative, or agitated.
- Review collected data.
- Provide routine care per protocol.
- Minimize risk of aspiration.
- Observe for return of gag and swallowing reflexes.
- Elevate the head of bed if not contraindicated.
- Suction as necessary.
- Position on side if not contraindicated.
- Use caution when giving liquids or solids.
- Assess for pain level per protocol.
- Use a pain scale that patient is familiar with.
- Medicate as needed.
- Use relaxation methods as appropriate.
- Document reactions to interventions.
- Provide emotional support.
- Allow family and caregiver to be with patient as soon as possible.
- Allow use of assistive devices as soon as possible.
- Reorient to surroundings.
- Prepare for discharge.
- Verify safe transportation home and competent adult to care for patient at home.
- Include family and caregiver when reviewing instructions; if a procedure is to be done at home, have patient or caregiver perform a return demonstration.
- Recognize the possible need to give instructions to protect operative site based on patient's psychological needs.
- Provide written as well as verbal home care instructions.
- Use large type if necessary for written instructions.
- It may be necessary to use a tape recorder if reading skills are inadequate.
- Obtain a phone number to reach the patient and caregiver for postoperative follow-up phone call.
- Give appropriate phone numbers so the patient and caregiver can obtain assistance if questions or problems arise at home.

■ BOX 21-5
■ **POSTDISCHARGE**

- Contact patient and caregiver within 24 hours of discharge.
- Identify yourself, and state purpose of the call.
- Identify compliance with postoperative instructions.
- Identify potential complications:
  - Unrelieved pain and nausea
  - Unexpected or excessive bleeding or swelling
  - Elevated temperature
  - Redness or drainage from operative site
  - Other adverse occurrences
- Refer to appropriate physician or agency as necessary.
- Complete postdischarge assessment per facility protocol.

      c. Demented stage—loss of ability to perform activities of daily lving (ADLs), decreased awareness, repetitive behaviors, decline in language ability

      d. End stage dementia—loss of purposeful mobility, loss of communication, dependence in ADLs, patient is at risk for

          (1) Contractures

          (2) Weight loss

          (3) Skin breakdown

          (4) Repeated infections

          (5) Aspiration

  3. Treatment—stabilize symptoms and minimize or prevent behavioral problems.

      a. Acetylcholinesterase inhibitor drugs temporarily delay worsening cognitive symptoms.

          (1) Tacrine (Cognex)

          (2) Donepezil hydrochloride (Aricept)

          (3) Rivastigmine (Exelon)

          (4) Galantamine (Reminyl)

      b. Vitamin E—may delay the progression from one stage to the next

          (1) Antioxidant properties

          (2) Doses prescribed range from 400 IU twice per day to 1200 IU twice per day.

      c. Behavioral modification for agitation

  4. Symptoms are exacerbated by

      a. Illness, disease

      b. Increased temperature

      c. Dehydration

      d. Medications, including anesthesia

      e. Tests, treatments

      f. Changes in routine

      g. Unfamiliar people, sights, sounds, smells

B. Preadmission and preoperative interview and management

  1. Patient may not be able to provide information.

  2. Determine the patient's level of ability with input from family and caregiver.

  3. Determine the patient's and family's understanding of Alzheimer's.

  4. Determine the family's willingness and ability to participate in preoperative preparation and postoperative care.

  5. Provide a safe, comfortable environment without distraction and allow enough time for interview and assessment.

      a. Include family and caregiver to decrease anxiety and agitation and increase compliance.

      b. Include the patient in discussions about his or her procedure.

          (1) Establish eye contact, talk in a low-pitched, reassuring tone of voice, use patient's name.

          (2) Speak slowly and clearly using short, simple sentences with familiar words.

          (3) Ask one question at a time.

          (4) Ask yes or no questions.

          (5) Allow 20-30 seconds for patient to answer question.

          (6) Give simple directions, one step at a time.

          (7) Because of patient's short-term memory loss, be prepared to repeat information frequently.

          (8) AD patients may respond to mood of situation more than words spoken.

          (9) Overstimulation of environment or pressure to answer questions may make patient more confused, agitated, aggressive.

         (10) Be alert to patient's nonverbal communication.

         (11) Do not leave patient alone as he or she may wander away.

6. Assessment per protocol
   a. Abilities and needs of the patient
      (1) Caregiver's and family's successful management techniques
      (2) Use of assistive devices
      (3) Effective method of communication
      (4) Normal daily routine for patient
   b. Degree of disability
      (1) Retains self-determination capabilities
      (2) Family shares decision making.
      (3) Has durable power of attorney for health care
      (4) Legal guardian appointed
7. Complete health history per protocol
   a. Swallowing problems
   b. History of aspiration
   c. Triggers for agitation
8. Physical assessment per protocol
   a. At risk for aspiration caused by
      (1) Decreased level of consciousness
      (2) Decreased cough and gag reflexes
      (3) Impaired swallowing mechanism
   b. Patients treated for AD with Vitamin E may be at increased risk of bleeding.
      (1) Observe for bruising.
      (2) Consult with primary care physician (PCP) about stopping or adjusting dosage prior to surgery
9. Psychosocial assessment per protocol
   a. Support system
      (1) Possible lack of support system related to
         (a) Personality changes
         (b) Altered behavior patterns
         (c) Depression
         (d) Inability to interact in an adult manner
         (e) Delusions
         (f) Socially unacceptable behavior
      (2) Consider early referral to social services for discharge planning.
      (3) Arrangements for safe transportation to and from the hospital
      (4) Arrangements for willing, competent adult in home for postdischarge care
   b. Anxiety—symptom for all stages of AD
      (1) One nurse as much as possible for continuity of care and familiarity
      (2) State name and purpose of encounter every time.
      (3) Orient patient frequently.
10. Develop a plan of care based on patient's and family and caregiver's knowledge and needs.
11. Preoperative teaching per protocol
    a. Include family and caregiver—patient is likely to forget instructions.
    b. Small amount of information at one time
    c. Give written as well as verbal instructions.
12. Complete preparation for admission per protocol
    a. Referrals as necessary
    b. Preoperative tests as ordered
C. Admission for procedure—see Box 21-1.
   1. Provide safe, calm, unhurried environment.
      a. Use one nurse for care and approach as outlined in previous section.
         (1) State name and what is happening every time.
         (2) Orient patient to surroundings frequently.
         (3) Explain actions before proceeding.

(4) If becomes agitated, pat or hold hand gently—avoid physical contact that could seem restraining.
  b. Keep bed low, side rails up, family and caregiver at bedside.
  2. Cognitive assessment
    a. Memory loss
    b. Confusion and disorientation
    c. Agitation
D. Preoperative holding and intraoperative—see Box 21-2.
  1. Use care when moving the patient.
    a. Lift rather than pull to protect skin.
    b. Protect bony prominences by positioning and use of padding.
  2. Restraints are likely to cause agitation.
    a. May need sedation prior to applying restraints necessary for procedure
    b. Will need distraction from restraints if awake
  3. Patient may be at risk for aspiration—more common in the later stages of AD.
    a. Elevate the head of the bed if possible.
    b. Suction as needed.
    c. Position on side if possible.
  4. AD patients may have an impaired cholinergic system—avoid anticholinergic medicines such as atropine and scopolamine that may result in untoward behavioral activity.
E. Phase I—see Box 21-3.
  1. Pain is frequently undertreated in AD patients because of cognitive disability.
    a. Pay attention to nonverbal clues.
    b. Observe carefully for response to pain medication.
  2. Increased risk of bleeding if has been on Vitamin E treatment
  3. May be agitated, combative, confused
    a. Repeated orientation to surroundings
    b. Use one nurse for care.
    c. Use nasal cannulas rather than mask.
    d. Turn down sound from bedside monitors.
    e. May need to wrap intravenous (IV) in gauze or put on stockinette sleeve
    f. If nasogastric tube in place, tape behind ear and fasten to gown's shoulder.
    g. Consider dehydration as contributing cause.
    h. Observe for bladder distension.
    i. Allow use of assistive devices as soon as possible.
    j. Return to area with family and caretaker as soon as possible.
    k. Avoid restraints if at all possible.
F. Phase II—see Box 21-4.
  1. May be at risk for aspiration
    a. May need to remind the patient to swallow
    b. Elevate the head of the bed if possible.
    c. Suction as needed.
    d. Position on side if not contraindicated.
    e. Use caution when giving liquids and solids.
  2. Patient may be confused, combative.
    a. Frequently orient patient to surroundings.
    b. Allow family and caregiver to be with patient.
    c. Allow use of assistive devices as soon as possible.
    d. Provide safe environment, nursing interventions as listed in prior sections.
  3. Pain is frequently undertreated in AD patients because of cognitive disability.
    a. Pay attention to nonverbal clues.
    b. Observe carefully for response to pain medication.

    4. Discharge
       a. Patient will benefit from returning to familiar environment as soon as possible.
       b. Verify safe transportation home.
  G. Postdischarge—see Box 21-5.

PHYSICAL DISABILITIES

    Physical disabilities may be manifest in many different ways. Persons with similar deficits will cope in different ways. It is important to treat each person as an individual, determining his or her method of coping and functional ability, and develop the plan of care based on the individual patient's needs.

  III. Hearing impairment
    A. Background information
      1. Estimate of 28 million of U.S. population has a hearing impairment
        a. Leading disability in America
        b. Affects 1 in 4 people between 65-74 years of age
        c. Affects 1 in 3 people over 75 years of age
      2. Definitions
        a. Deaf—people who are unable to hear or understand oral communications with or without the aid of amplification devices
        b. Hard of hearing—people with a hearing loss severe enough to necessitate use of amplification devices to hear oral communication
      3. Hearing deficit is not reflective of low intelligence.
      4. Not all hearing impaired people can read lips or use sign language.
      5. Only about 20% to 30% of words are readable on the lips.
    B. Techniques for effective communication with the hearing impaired in any setting
      1. Provide an environment for effective communication.
        a. Provide a quiet, distraction-free area.
        b. Provide adequate lighting.
        c. Provide interpreter if necessary.
        d. Supply a battery-powered microphone with earpiece if applicable.
      2. Get patient's attention before speaking.
        a. Approach within the patient's line of vision.
        b. Wave hand.
        c. Touch gently as to avoid startling the patient.
      3. Determine the patient's preferred method of communication.
        a. Hearing aid
        b. Lip reading
        c. Sign language
        d. Written messages
        e. Alphabet, picture, word or phrase board
        f. Combination of methods
      4. For lip reading and/or hearing augmented by hearing aids
        a. Sit or stand directly in front of the patient.
        b. Keep mouth visible when speaking.
        c. Do not chew gum or food.
        d. Maintain comfortable voice volume.
        e. Speak slowly and distinctly; do not exaggerate your pronunciation.
        f. Use smallest number of words to convey the message.
        g. Maintain eye contact.
      5. Working with an interpreter
        a. The interpreter is used to transmit information not to explain information or give opinions.
        b. Stand or sit across from the patient with the interpreter beside you.
        c. Speak at a normal tone and face the patient directly.

    d. Ask the patient, not the interpreter, to clarify information if not understood.

C. Preadmission and preoperative interview and management

  1. An in-person interview facilitates the patient's participation, especially if he or she relies on lip reading or gestures.

    a. Determine if an interpreter for sign language will be needed to communicate with the patient.

    b. Determine if the patient has access to a telecommunications relay service for phone messages.

  2. Incorporate communication techniques for hearing impairment.

  3. Include family member in preoperative visit if possible.

  4. Identify level and duration of disability.

    a. Totally deaf

    b. Able to hear with hearing aids in place

    c. Severe decrease in hearing

      (1) Is one ear better than the other?

      (2) Is hearing improved by using a supplemental microphone with earpiece?

  5. Provide adequate time for interview and assessment.

  6. Utilize patient's method of communication; provide an interpreter if necessary.

  7. Determine the patient's and family's knowledge and expectations of the proposed procedure.

  8. Assessment per protocol

    a. Abilities and special needs

    b. Willingness of family to participate in preparation for procedure and postoperative care

    c. Use of hearing aid or other assistive devices

    d. Be alert to nonverbal communication.

  9. Complete health history per protocol

 10. Physical assessment per protocol

 11. Psychosocial assessment per protocol

    a. Anxiety

      (1) Feeling of isolation because of disability

      (2) Fear of not understanding what is happening in a strange environment

    b. Support system

      (1) Arrangements made for safe transportation to and from hospital

      (2) Arrangements made for competent adult help after discharge

      (3) Arrangements to communicate messages to the patient

        (a) Prior to the procedure—time changes if necessary

        (b) Interpreter on hand day of surgery if needed

        (c) Follow-up postoperatively

      (4) If patient is primary caregiver of another person, have arrangements for help been made while patient recovers?

 12. Develop a teaching plan based on patient's and family's knowledge and needs.

 13. Preoperative teaching per protocol

    a. Verify that the patient understands instructions.

      (1) Ask the patient directly.

      (2) Repeat or reinforce information as necessary.

      (3) Provide written information to take home.

    b. Explain that family can be with patient as long as possible before surgery and as soon as possible after surgery.

    c. Hearing aid and/or assistive devices will be used as long as safely possible before surgery and returned as soon as possible after surgery.

    d. If patient wears a hearing aid, instruct to check hearing aid battery and that aid is clear of earwax before admission.

        14. Complete preparation for admission.
- **a.** Referrals made as necessary
- **b.** Preoperative tests as ordered
- **c.** Arrange for interpreter day of procedure if necessary.

        15. Document and communicate special needs to other members of perioperative team.

  D. Admission for procedure—see Box 21-1.
- **1.** Utilize communication techniques for hearing impairment.
  - **a.** Know patient's method of communication.
  - **b.** Provide interpreter if necessary.
  - **c.** Inform patient that hearing aid or communication device will be returned as soon as possible after surgery.

  E. Preoperatove holding and intraoperative—see Box 21-2.
- **1.** Utilize communication techniques for hearing impairment.
- **2.** If possible, avoid covering face with mask when speaking to patient.
- **3.** Allow use of hearing aid, communication, or other assistive devices if possible.
- **4.** Use gestures or written messages if necessary.

  F. Phase I—see Box 21-3.
- **1.** Approach patient in his or her line of sight.
- **2.** Gently touch patient to get his or her attention.
- **3.** If protective lubricant used, clear from patient's eyes.
- **4.** Return hearing aid or other assistive devices as soon as possible.
- **5.** Speak slowly and distinctly.
  - **a.** Remain in patient's line of vision when speaking.
  - **b.** Keep your mouth visible when speaking.
  - **c.** Recognize that the patient will hear and understand less when tired and ill.

  G. Phase II—see Box 21-4.
- **1.** Return hearing aid and assistive devices as soon as possible.
- **2.** Utilize communication techniques for hearing impairment.
- **3.** Recognize that the patient will hear and understand less when tired and/or ill.

  H. Postdischarge—see Box 21-5.

IV. Vision impairment
  A. Background information
- **1.** Estimated 10 million people affected in United States
  - **a.** Seventy percent of the estimate is age 65 or older.
  - **b.** Complete blindness—no vision
  - **c.** Legal blindness—unable to see at 20 feet what normal vision can see at 200 feet
  - **d.** Partially sighted—need adaptive methods to read and write
  - **e.** Hemiplegics—may have loss of half of visual field in each eye
  - **f.** Macular degeneration—loss of sight in the center vision field
- **2.** May or may not have other disabilities

  B. Preadmission and preoperative interview and management
- **1.** Identify yourself and state purpose of visit.
  - **a.** Use a normal tone of voice.
    - (1) Sense of hearing in a blind patient is often very acute.
    - (2) Ask the patient if they can hear you before speaking louder.
  - **b.** Provide a safe environment.
    - (1) If moving to another area, offer arm to patient.
      - (a) Patient takes arm from behind, just above the elbow.
      - (b) Expect the patient to keep a half step behind you so he or she can anticipate if a step is coming.
    - (2) Orient to environment.
      - (a) Give specific directions such as "straight in front of you" and "directly to your left."

(b) Introduce everyone in the room.
(c) Let the patient know what you are doing if there is silence in the room for awhile: "I need to write this down now."
  c. Assure patient his or her needs will be communicated to perianesthesia team members.
2. Identify level and duration of disability.
  a. Totally blind
  b. Partial vision
  c. Light perceptive
  d. Patient's management skills
3. Ask the patient how much assistance he or she needs and wants in performing ADLs.
4. Determine patient's and family's knowledge of proposed procedure.
5. Assessment per protocol
  a. Abilities, special needs
  b. Desired method of communication
    (1) Braille
    (2) Special glasses or contacts
    (3) Large print
    (4) Audiotape
    (5) Computer disc
  c. For other disabilities
6. Complete health history per protocol
7. Physical assessment per protocol
8. Psychosocial assessment per protocol
  a. Support system
    (1) Has competent adult who can assist at home after discharge
    (2) If the patient and/or caregiver is a primary caregiver for another person, have arrangements been made for someone else to provide care for that person?
    (3) Safe transportation to and from the hospital
  b. Anxiety
    (1) Isolation because of disability
    (2) Fear of being left alone
9. Develop plan of care based on patient's needs and knowledge.
C. Preoperative teaching and preparation per protocol
  1. Provide instructions.
    a. Verbal
    b. Preferred method to take home—consider making an audiotape
    c. Need for a safe environment at the facility
      (1) Side rails for safety; keep bed low
      (2) Call light will be within reach.
      (3) Encourage support person to be available to stay with patient the day of surgery.
    d. Assure patient of emotional support.
      (1) Explain what will happen preoperatively and in the immediately postoperative period.
        (a) Describe what surroundings will sound and feel like: "group room with curtain dividers," "cold," and so forth.
        (b) Explain who will be present in the different stages of care.
      (2) Availability of preoperative medications for relaxation
      (3) Assure patient that staff will be within calling distance.
  2. Prepare for procedure per protocol.
    a. Referrals as necessary
    b. Preoperative testing as ordered
  3. Document and communicate patient's special needs to perioperative team members.

    D. Admission for the procedure—see Box 21-1.
       1. Utilize communication technique in which patient is comfortable
          a. Verbal only, Braille, combination of methods
          b. Get patient's attention before speaking.
             (1) Speak in normal tone of voice.
             (2) Provide a quiet area to prevent distraction.
       3. Promote independence based on patient history.
       4. Provide description of new surroundings.
          a. Identify those present.
          b. Allow time and opportunity for patient to explore new environment.
       5. Include patient in discussions about his or her procedure.
       6. Inform patient that communication device will be returned as soon as possible after the procedure.
    E. Preoperative holding and intraoperative—see Box 21-2.
       1. Avoid confusion and too many people speaking at once.
       2. Let the patient know who is in the room.
       3. Let the patient know what is being done before touching him or her.
       4. Keep the environment safe.
          a. Use safety devices such as side rails and straps for stretchers.
             (1) Explain to patient where the devices are located.
             (2) Purpose of and how the straps feel before applying
          b. Have a means for the patient to call for assistance.
          c. Assure patient he or she will not be left alone.
   F. Phase I—see Box 21-3.
       1. Speak in a normal tone of voice.
       2. Touch patient gently to get his or her attention.
       3. Resume use of assistive devices if possible.
       4. Maintain calm, quiet environment to decrease confusion.
   G. Phase II—see Box 21-4.
       1. Speak softly and gently touch patient to get his or her attention.
       2. Use safety devices such as side rails.
          a. Keep call light within reach at all times.
          b. Allow family or caregiver in as soon as possible.
       3. Discharge—see Box 21-5.
          a. Provide clear discharge instructions.
             (1) Provide written copy of instructions for caregiver.
             (2) May need to provide audiotape of instructions
          b. Instruct caregiver on visual assessment of the operative site.
V. Speech impairment
   A. Background information
       1. Aphasia—language disorder that impairs the expression and understanding of language as well as reading and writing
          a. Occurs from damage to portions of the brain that are responsible for language
          b. Usually occurs suddenly—stroke or brain injury
          c. May develop slowly—brain tumor
          d. Patient may also suffer from
             (1) Dysarthria—difficult, poorly articulated speech
             (2) Apraxia—inability to correctly position and sequence speech muscles to produce understandable speech
             (3) Aphonia—loss of ability to produce normal speech sounds from vocal cords
       2. Mutism—inability to speak caused by a physical defect or emotional problem
       3. Neurological diseases can cause speech disorders.
          a. Parkinson's disease
          b. AD

           c. Stroke

           d. Brain tumors

      4. Malignant conditions may require the removal of speech apparatus.

           a. May use a voice synthesizer

           b. Laryngectomy patient may use controlled breathing or belching to speak.

B. Techniques for effective communication with the speech impaired

      1. Keep distractions to a minimum—turn off radio, television.

      2. Maintain a natural conversational manner appropriate for an adult.

      3. Include the speech-impaired person in conversations.

      4. Simplify language using short and simple sentences.

      5. Maintain a normal voice volume.

      6. Allow enough time for a response.

           a. Avoid correcting the person's speech.

           b. Encourage any type of communication.

                (1) Speech

                (2) Gestures

                (3) Pointing

                (4) Drawing

C. Preadmission and preoperative interview and management

      1. An in-person interview will be more effective than a telephone interview and will allow the patient a greater opportunity to participate.

      2. Use techniques for effective communication with the speech impaired.

      3. Determine the patient's effective means of communication.

           a. Use of assistive devices (i.e., glasses, hearing aid)

           b. Story board, writing tablet or slate

      4. Encourage, but do not pressure the patient to respond in whatever way he or she can.

           a. Encourage patient to write responses, if he or she can write and spell.

           b. Encourage the use of gestures if that is most effective means to communicate.

      5. Allow adequate time for the interview and assessment.

           a. Allow for differences in accuracy and articulation when soliciting patient's response.

           b. Present a relaxed attitude by mannerisms, patience, and acceptance.

           c. One person speaking at a time helps to decrease confusion.

           d. Ask direct questions requiring one-word answers.

      6. Encourage family and caregiver to be present.

           a. May better understand patient's gestures and speech patterns

           b. Continue to include patient in discussions.

      7. Complete health history per protocol

           a. Cause and duration of disability

           b. Concurrent diseases that contribute to speech impairment

      8. Physical assessment per protocol

      9. Psychosocial assessment per protocol

           a. Anxiety level—concern over ability to communicate with staff

           b. Support system

                  (1) Willingness of family and caregiver to be present the day of surgery to assist with communication

                (2) Arrangements made for patient to communicate with hospital staff from home concerning questions or changes

                    (a) Contact person via phone

                    (b) Internet and e-mail access

    10. Determine the patient's and family's knowledge of the proposed procedure.

    11. Develop a teaching plan based on the patient's and family's knowledge and needs.

        12. Preoperative teaching per protocol

           a. Use techniques for effective communication with the speech impaired.

           b. Give written instructions to review at home.

        13. Complete preparation for admission.

           a. Preoperative tests as ordered

           b. Referrals as necessary

           c. Document and communicate patient's special needs to perioperative team members.

    D. Day of procedure admission—see Box 21-1.

        1. Use techniques for effective communication with the speech impaired.

        2. Provide enough time for the patient to communicate concerns.

    E. Preoperative holding and intraoperative—see Box 21-2.

        1. Allow the patient to continue to use assistive devices as long as possible.

        2. Discuss with patient how he or she can make needs known or answer questions if he or she is without his or her normal communication tools.

           a. Squeeze hand—once for yes, twice for no.

           b. Raise hand if appropriate.

           c. Give patient a bell to ring.

        3. Reassure the patient that you are with him or her.

    F. Phase I—see Box 21-3.

        1. May be at higher risk for aspiration

           a. Observe for return of swallowing and gag reflexes.

           b. Position on side, if allowed, until return of gag and swallowing reflexes.

           c. Elevate head of bed after return of reflexes if not contraindicated.

           d. Suction as needed.

        2. Reduce apprehension.

           a. Reorient to surroundings.

           b. Provide means of communicating.

           c. Reunite patient and family as soon as possible.

    G. Phase I—see Box 21-4.

        1. Use techniques for effective communication with the speech impaired.

        2. Return assistive devices as soon as possible.

        3. Arrange for a contact person to phone or how to communicate with patient at home for postoperative follow-up.

    H. Postdischarge—see Box 21-5.

VI. Spinal cord injury

    A. Background information

        1. Classification

           a. Complete—total paralysis and loss of sensation below the zone of injury, resulting in quadriplegia or paraplegia

           b. Incomplete—with partial preservation of function below the zone of injury

           c. Measurement of functional ability—functional independence measurement (FIM)

             (1) Seven point scale measures 18 items in six categories; self-care, continence of bowel and bladder, mobility, locomotion, communication, and social cognition

             (2) Scale of 1 equals total dependence on caregiver

             (3) Scale of 7 indicates independence

        2. Consequences of level of injury

           a. C1 to C4—results in quadriplegia with complete loss of motor and sensory function from the neck down and loss of respiratory function

           b. C5—results in quadriplegia and loss of all functions below the upper shoulder level; the phrenic nerve is intact but not the intercostal muscles

           c. C6—results in quadriplegia and loss of all functions below the shoulders and upper arms, no use of intercostal muscles

        d. C7—results in incomplete quadriplegia with loss of motor control to parts of the arm and hand, and loss of sensation below the clavicle and parts of the arms and hands, no use of intercostal muscles

        e. C8—results in incomplete quadriplegia with loss of motor control to parts of the arms and hands and loss of sensation below the chest and part of the hands, no use of intercostal muscles

        f. T1 to T6—results in paraplegia with loss of motor function below the midchest, including the trunk muscles, and loss of sensation from the midchest downward, including the lower limbs; the phrenic nerve functions independently; there is some impairment of the intercostal muscles.

        g. T6 to T12—results in paraplegia with loss of motor control and sensation below the waist; there is no interference with respiratory function.

        h. L1 to L3—results in paraplegia with loss of most of the control of the legs and pelvic area, and loss of sensation to the lower abdomen and legs

        i. L3 to L4—results in incomplete paraplegia with loss of control and function of part of the lower legs, ankles, and feet

        j. L4 to S2—results in incomplete paraplegia with varying degrees of motor and sensory loss; can walk with braces or may use a wheelchair, and can be relatively independent

    3. May be at a higher risk for

        a. Cardiac arrhythmias and cardiac arrest

        b. Orthostatic hypotension (especially with an injury above level of T7)

        c. Autonomic hyperreflexia (possible only in an injury above the level of T6)

        d. Sleep apnea

        e. UTI

        f. Skin breakdown

        g. Spasticity

        h. Difficult pain management

B. Preadmission/preoperative interview and management

    1. Provide a comfortable space for the interview.

    2. Recognize that a physical disability alone does not affect intelligence.

        a. Refer to the patient as a person with a disability not as a disabled person.

        b. Speak directly to the patient.

        c. Ask the patient the type of physical assistance he or she prefers.

    3. Identify the level and duration of the disability.

    4. Determine patient's and family's management and coping strategies.

    5. Conduct interview and assessment per protocol.

        a. Physical abilities, special needs

        b. Use of assistive devices—braces, splints, ADL modifications

        c. Willingness and ability of family to participate in preoperative preparation and postoperative care

    6. Complete health history per protocol

        a. Cardiac arrhythmias and cardiac arrest

            (1) Electrolyte imbalance

            (2) Response to vagal stimulation

        b. Orthostatic hypotension—history of hypotension when the head of the bed is raised or when the patient is gotten out of bed

        c. Autonomic hyperreflexia—previous response to noxious stimulation of the sensory receptors

            (1) Urinary calculi

            (2) Severe bladder infections

            (3) Urinary retention

            (4) Operative incisions

    d. Pain

      (1) Spinal cord injury (SCI) pain most common type of pain in this population

        (a) Mild, tingling to severe, intractable

        (b) Usually unresponsive to standard pain treatments

      (2) Transitional zone pain

        (a) Felt at the level of injury

        (b) Bandlike pattern over the trunk or upper arms

      (3) Pain can be felt above or below the level of injury.

      (4) Pain management techniques patient has found most helpful

    e. Spasticity

      (1) A state of increased tonus in a weak muscle

      (2) Usually peaks 1.5 to 2 years after the injury

      (3) Gradual regression

    f. Pressure sores

      (1) Usual skin care routine

      (2) Positioning routine

    g. Bladder and bowel management—recognize increased risk for latex sensitivity if has indwelling catheter.

    h. Nutrition

      (1) Type of diet

      (2) Amount of assistance needed to eat

      (3) Mechanical consistency of foods

      (4) Methods used to prevent aspiration

7. Physical assessment per protocol

8. Psychosocial assessment per protocol

    a. Anxiety

      (1) Losing independence

      (2) Suffering greater disability caused by complications from procedure

      (3) Inadequate pain relief postoperatively

    b. Support system

      (1) Availability and willingness of responsible adult to provide care at home

      (2) Arrangements for safe transport to and from the facility

      (3) Referrals to social services if needed

        (a) Make arrangements for additional equipment in the home

        (b) May need home health care for postoperative discharge care

9. Develop a plan of care based on the knowledge and needs of the patient and family.

10. Preoperative instructions per protocol—include family and caregiver if possible.

11. Complete preparation for admission

    a. Preoperative test as ordered

    b. Referrals as necessary

    c. Document and communicate the patient's special needs to the perioperative team members.

C. Admission—see Box 21-1.

    1. Use latex precautions if the patient is on a bladder program or has indwelling catheter.

    2. Laboratory values within acceptable range

      a. Electrolytes, especially potassium

      b. Blood coagulation studies

      c. Urinalysis—evaluate for evidence of urinary tract infections (UTI)

D. Preoperative holding and intraoperative—see Box 21-2.

    1. Use latex precautions if necessary.

    2. Maintain normothermia.

3. Be aware of potential for
   a. Cardiac arrhythmias
      (1) Electrolytes, especially potassium within normal range
      (2) Avoid excessive vagal stimulation.
   b. Autonomic hyperreflexia symptoms
      (1) Hypertension
      (2) Superficial vasodilatation
      (3) Flushing
      (4) Profuse sweating
      (5) Piloerection (gooseflesh) occurring above the level of injury, often seen in patients with upper thoracic and cervical injuries
   c. Pain, paraesthesia, and hyperesthesia
   d. Spasticity
      (1) May result from a slight touch on the skin
      (2) Aggravated by cold or staying in one position for a prolonged period of time
4. Move patient with care, lifting rather than pulling.
5. Avoid pressure on bony prominences by positioning or use of padding.

E. Phase I—see Box 21-3
   1. Continue use of latex precautions if necessary.
   2. Keep patient warm.
   3. Be aware that even slight touch could trigger spasticity.
   4. Monitor for signs of bladder distension.
   5. Monitor for signs of autonomic hyperreflexia.
      a. Paroxysmal hypertension
      b. Pounding headache
      c. Vasodilatation
      d. Flushing
      e. Profuse sweating
      f. Piloerection
   6. Increased potential for orthostatic hypotension exists.
      a. Be cautious when elevating the head of the bed if the patient is a quadriplegic.
      b. Most often seen with patients sustaining injury above the T7 level
   7. Be aggressive with pain management.

F. Phase II—see Box 21-4.
   1. Keep patient warm without overheating.
   2. Be aware that light touch on the skin may trigger spasticity.
   3. Monitor for bladder distension.
   4. Monitor for autonomic hyperreflexia.
   5. Monitor for orthostatic hypotension.
      a. Be cautious when elevating the head of the bed of the patient.
      b. Provide assistance when increasing activity.
   6. Be aggressive with pain management.
   7. Return assistive devices as soon as possible.

G. Discharge—see Box 21-5.

VII. Traumatic brain injury
A. Background information
   1. Approximately 600,000 new traumatic brain injuries (TBI) occur in the United States each year.
      a. Nearly 100% of persons with severe head injury and two thirds of those with mild injury will be permanently disabled.
      b. Greatest cause of TBI is motor vehicle accidents.
      c. Most severe head injuries occur in adolescents and young adults.
   2. May have motor impairment
      a. Spasticity, tremors, ataxia
      b. Weakness

      c. Apraxia—the inability to perform a skilled motor act in the absence of paralysis

      d. Paralysis

      e. Poor breathing patterns

  3. May have sensory impairment

      a. Impaired sense of position

      b. Impaired spatial judgment

      c. Impaired vision, hearing, touch, smell, and taste

      d. Increased pain sensitivity

  4. May have communication impairment

      a. Aphasia—inability to communicate

      b. Dysarthria—defective articulation caused by motor deficits of the tongue or muscles used for speech

  5. May have cognitive impairment

      a. Impaired abstract thinking

      b. Impaired judgment

      c. Impaired generalization and planning abilities

      d. Impaired memory

      e. Decreased concentration ability

      f. Reduced tolerance for stress, irritability, impatience

B. Preadmission and preoperative interview and management

  1. An in-person interview may be more beneficial than a telephone interview; the patient may use nonverbal forms of communication.

  2. Provide a calm, quiet environment; limit stimulation factors.

  3. Include family and caregiver whenever possible.

  4. Allow adequate times for interview and assessment; recognize that the patient's attention span may be limited.

  5. Remember to include patient in the conversation.

  6. Complete health history per protocol

      a. Cause and duration of disability

      b. Type of limitations caused by disability

      c. Seizure activity, if appropriate

        (1) Manifestation of seizure

        (2) Frequency

        (3) Aura, triggers

  7. Assessment per protocol

      a. Abilities, special needs

        (1) Level reached on a rehabilitation scale

          (a) Rancho Los Amigos, a cognitive functioning scale; Level I—no response, total assistance, to Level X—modified independent

          (b) Disability Rating Scale (DRS)—point system to estimate general level of disability from none to extreme vegetative state

        (2) Patient's and family's or caregiver's successful management techniques

      b. Use of assistive devices

  8. Physical assessment per protocol

      a. Swallowing difficulty because of poor muscle control

      b. Positioning problems caused by paralysis, contractures, spasticity

  9. Psychosocial assessment

      a. Anxiety

        (1) Be alert to nonverbal communication.

        (2) Level of ability to cope with hospital environment

      b. Emotional lability

      c. Support system

        (1) Arrangements for safe transport to and from the facility

        (2) Willingness and ability of family to participate in preoperative preparation and postoperative care

      d. Make referrals as necessary.

10. Develop a plan of care based on the knowledge and needs of the patient and family.
11. Preoperative teaching per protocol
    a. Provide verbal and written preoperative instructions.
    b. Include family and caregiver in instructions if at all possible.
    c. Adjust teaching to patient's level of disability.
        (1) Recognize patient may have short attention span.
        (2) Patient may have short-term memory problems.
        (3) Use short clear instructions; do not use abstract ideas.
    d. Emphasize pain management.
        (1) Determine which pain scale is most appropriate for the patient.
        (2) After instruction, have patient demonstrate the use of the pain scale.
12. Complete preparation for admission
    a. Preoperative tests as ordered
    b. Referrals as needed
    c. Document and communicate special needs to the perioperative team members.
C. Admission—see Box 21-1.
    1. Limit stimulation in room.
D. Preoperative holding and intraoperative—see Box 21-2.
    1. Recognize that the patient may be emotionally labile.
    2. Provide a calm, quiet environment.
E. Phase I—see Box 21-3.
    1. If swallowing difficulty exists, minimize risk for aspiration.
        a. Observe for return of swallowing and gag reflexes.
        b. Suction as needed.
        c. Elevate the head of the bed if allowed.
        d. Position on side if not contraindicated.
    2. Allow use of assistive devices as soon as possible.
F. Phase II—see Box 21-4.
    1. Verify competent adult help at home after discharge.
G. Postdischarge—see Box 21-5.
VIII. Parkinson's disease (PD)
    A. Background information
        1. PD is a common slowly progressive neurological disease.
            a. Peak onset at age 55-60
            b. Affects men more than women: 55 men to 45 women
            c. Affects Caucasians more than people of color
            d. Progresses from diagnosis to major disability over 10-20 years
        2. Symptoms result primarily from loss of dopamine in the brain.
        3. Primary clinical symptoms
            a. Rigidity of the limbs—appreciated as stiffness of the joints simulating arthritis
            b. Tremor of the limbs—more prominent in the hands and is asymmetrical
            c. Bradykinesia of the limbs and body—most prominent and disabling symptom of PD
                (1) Difficulty initiating movement
                (2) Slowness in movement
                (3) Paucity or incompleteness of movement
            d. Postural instability—results from impairment of postural reflexes
                (1) Patient perceives as unsteadiness or lack of balance.
                (2) When patients trip, they are unable to stop falling or ease their fall.
        4. Secondary symptoms
            a. Difficulty walking resulting from a combination of bradykinesia and postural instability.
                (1) Short steps and shuffling gait
                (2) Festinating gait—a manner of walking in which speed increases to catch up with a displaced center of gravity

(3) Anteropulsion—be propelled forward, or backward (retropulsion)

(4) Freeze—a difficulty turning, and a tendency to stop abruptly and inexplicably

(5) Stooped posture

b. Masklike features

(1) Appears to be expressionless

(2) Stares straight ahead

(3) Has decreased blinking of eyes

c. Speech changes

(1) Difficulty initiating speech

(2) Difficulty coordinating expiration and articulation

d. Autonomic symptoms

(1) Drooling

(2) Excessive perspiration

(3) Constipation

(4) Orthostatic hypotension

(5) Dysphasia

e. Changes in behavior and mental ability

(1) Depression

(2) Slowness of information processing

(3) Social withdrawal

(4) Generalized apathy

(5) Dementia

f. General weakness and muscle fatigue

g. Hypersensitivity to heat

5. Treatment

a. Anti-parkinson drugs to restore dopamine or mimic dopamine's actions; partial list

(1) Levodopa

(2) Carbidopa and levodopa (Atamet, Sinemet)

(3) Dopamine agonists: Pergolide (Permax), pramipexole (Mirapex), ropinerole (Requip)

(4) Amantadine, anticholinergics

b. Surgical treatment

(1) Thalamotomy, pallidotomy

(2) Deep brain stimulation (DBS)

B. Preadmission and preoperative interview and management

1. An in-person interview affords the opportunity to observe the patient's abilities and interaction with family members.

2. Maintain a calm, unhurried, accepting attitude in a safe, comfortable environment.

a. Provide assistance with ambulation.

b. Recognize information processing may be slowed

3. Speak to the patient and encourage to respond in whatever manner he or she can.

a. PD does not affect patient's intelligence.

b. Respect patient's level of independence.

4. Include the family and caregiver in preoperative preparation when possible.

5. Assessment per protocol

a. Abilities and special needs of the patient

(1) Determine the patient's and/or family's understanding of Parkinson's disease.

(2) Length of time disease has been present

(3) Manifestations of PD

(4) Effects of PD on patient

(a) Patient's usual routine to cope with limitations

(b) Consider using PD's ADL scoring system.

(c) Patient's and family's successful management techniques

(5) Use of assistive devices

(6) Sleep disturbances

    b. Willingness and ability of family and caregiver to participate in preoperative preparation and postoperative care

6. Complete health history per protocol

7. Physical assessment per protocol

    a. Vital signs and oxygen saturation

    b. Muscle strength

    c. Location of tremors

    d. History of dysphagia

8. Cognitive assessment

    a. Memory loss

    b. Depression

    c. Information processing speed may be slowed down.

9. Psychosocial assessment per protocol

    a. Anxiety

        (1) Prominent feature in 40% of PD patients

        (2) Many PD patients have panic attacks.

        (3) Determine patient's coping mechanisms.

    b. Support system

        (1) Competent adult help at home after discharge

        (2) Arrangements made for safe transportation to and from the hospital

10. Develop plan of care based on the patient's and family's knowledge and needs.

11. Preoperative teaching per protocol

    a. Provide verbal and written preoperative instructions.

    b. Patients should be instructed to take normal PD medications the day of surgery.

        (1) Prevent muscle weakness and tremors that make self-care difficult.

        (2) Rigidity may contribute to a difficult intubation.

        (3) Rigidity predisposes to venous thrombosis.

12. Complete preparation for admission per protocol

    a. Referrals as necessary

    b. Preoperative testing as ordered

    c. Document and communicate patient's special needs to the perianesthesia team.

C. Admission—see Box 21-1.

1. Verify competent adult help at home after discharge.

2. Physical assessment per protocol

    a. Muscle strength

    b. Tremors, rigidity

    c. Swallowing problems

3. Prepare patient per protocol.

    a. Verify PD drugs have been taken as instructed.

    b. Drugs that exacerbate extra pyramidal symptoms should be avoided.

        (1) Metoclopramide

        (2) Droperidol

        (3) Phenothiazines

4. Provide emotional support for family and patient.

    a. Use measures to decrease anxiety.

    b. Provide safe environment.

        (1) Assist patient in getting out of bed.

        (2) Keep side rails up and bed position low.

        (3) Do not leave patient unattended.

    c. Maintain comfortable temperature.

    D. Preoperative holding and intraoperative—see Box 21-2.

        1. Recognize potential for aspiration.

        2. Avoid overheating.

        3. Recognize patient is a greater risk for hypotension and cardiac arrhythmias.

    E. Phase I—see Box 21-3.

        1. Patient at increased risk for aspiration because of difficult or ineffective swallowing

            a. Elevate head of the bed if allowed.

            b. Suction as necessary.

            c. Observe for return of gag and swallowing reflexes.

            d. Position on side if not contraindicated.

        2. Prevent overheating.

    F. Phase II—see Box 21-4.

        1. Patient at increased risk for aspiration because of difficult or ineffective swallowing

            a. Elevate head of the bed if allowed.

            b. Suction as necessary.

            c. Observe for return of gag and swallowing reflexes.

            d. Position on side if not contraindicated.

        2. Prevent overheating.

        3. Increased risk of orthostatic hypotension

            a. Ambulate gradually and with assistance.

            b. Evaluate vital signs after activity progression.

    G. Postdischarge—see Box 21-5.

IX. Multiple sclerosis

    A. Background information

        1. Multiple sclerosis (MS) is a chronic, unpredictable neurological disease that affects the central nervous system.

        2. In MS, myelin is lost in multiple areas, leaving scar tissue—sclerosis.

            a. Damaged areas—plaques or lesions

            b. Disrupts ability of the nerves to conduct electrical impulses to and from the brain

        3. Usually diagnosed between the ages of 20 and 50

        4. Two to three times as many women as men have MS.

        5. Clinical courses—each may be mild, moderate, or severe.

            a. Relapsing–remitting—clearly defined episodes of acute worsening of neurologic function followed by partial or complete remission free of disease progression

            b. Primary progressive—slow but nearly continuous worsening from onset; rates of progression vary over time with occasional plateaus or temporary minor improvements.

            c. Secondary progressive—initial period of relapsing–remitting disease followed by a steadily worsening disease

            d. Progressive–relapsing—steadily worsening disease from onset with clear acute flare-ups with or without recovery; periods between relapses have continuing disease progression.

        6. Symptoms are unpredictable; vary from person to person and from time to time in the same person

            a. Sensory—numbness, paresthesia, pain, dysesthesia, trigeminal neuralgia, Lhermitte's sign, chronic pain from other symptoms, decreased proprioception and sense of temperature, depth, and vibration

            b. Motor—paresis, paralysis, dragging of foot, dysphagia, spasticity, diplopia, bowel and bladder dysfunction (incontinence or retention)

            c. Cerebellar—ataxia, staggering, loss of balance and coordination, nystagmus, speech disturbances, tremors, vertigo

            d. Other symptoms—optic neuritis, impotence or decreased genital sensation, depression or euphoria, fatigue or decreased energy level

7. Factors that may cause a relapse
   a. Infections
   b. Trauma—accidental or planned (i.e., surgery)
   c. Pregnancy
   d. Undue fatigue or excessive exertion
   e. Overheating or excessive chilling or cold
   f. Emotional stress
B. Preadmission and preoperative interview and management
   1. Provide a comfortable, safe environment.
      a. Allow adequate time—patient fatigue may be a factor.
      b. Patient may need extra time to formulate questions and responses.
   2. Assessment per protocol
      a. Abilities, special needs
         (1) Determine level and duration of disease.
         (2) Determine patient's and family's understanding of MS.
         (3) Determine patient's and family's routine to minimize symptoms.
      b. Use of assistive devices
      c. Willingness and capability of family to participate in preoperative preparations and postoperative care
   3. Complete health history per protocol
      a. Identify previous events triggering relapses.
      b. Determine patient's response to physical and psychological stresses.
   4. Physical assessment per protocol
      a. Evaluate ability to swallow.
      b. Evidence of infectious process present
   5. Psychosocial assessment per protocol
      a. Anxiety
         (1) Surgery may cause relapse.
         (2) Loss of independence
      b. Support system
         (1) Competent adult help at home on discharge
         (2) Arrangements made for safe transport to and from the hospital
   6. Develop plan of care based on patient's and family's knowledge and needs.
   7. Preoperative teaching per protocol
      a. Provide verbal and written instructions.
      b. Include family in instructions if at all possible.
   8. Complete preparation for admission per protocol
      a. Make referrals as necessary.
      b. Preoperative tests as ordered
      c. Document and communicate special needs to the perianesthesia team.
C. Admission—see Box 21-1.
   1. Provide comfortable safe environment.
      a. Assist patient in getting out of bed if needed.
      b. Keep side rails up and bed in low position.
   2. Use measures to reduce stress.
      a. Explain what will be happening.
      b. Allow patient to verbalize concerns.
      c. Allow family to be with patient as long as possible.
      d. Allow use of assistive devices as long as possible.
      e. Allow extra time for patient to answer, or formulate questions.
   3. Avoid undue fatigue; provide periods of rest.
   4. Physical assessment per routine protocol
      a. Sensory deficit
      b. Motor deficit
      c. Cerebellar disturbances
D. Preoperative holding and intraoperative—see Box 21-2.
   1. Maintain normothermia.

      2. If swallowing deficits, may be at increased risk for aspiration

        a. Elevate head of bed if possible.

        b. Suction as needed.

        c. When possible, position on side.

  E. Phase I—see Box 21-3.

      1. Provide specialized care based on patient's symptoms.

      2. May be at higher risk for aspiration

        a. Elevate head of bed if not contraindicated.

        b. Suction as needed.

        c. Observe for return of swallowing and gag reflexes.

        d. Position on side if not contraindicated.

      3. Maintain normothermia.

      4. Reduce stress.

        a. Reorient patient to surroundings.

        b. Medicate for pain or anxiety as necessary.

  F. Phase II—see Box 21-4.

      1. Patient may be at increased risk for aspiration.

        a. Elevate head of bed if not contraindicated.

        b. Suction as needed.

        c. Observe for return of swallowing and gag reflexes.

        d. Position on side if not contraindicated.

      2. Provide comfortable, safe environment.

        a. Reorient patient to surroundings.

        b. Allow use of assistive devices as soon as possible.

        c. Assist patient with ambulation.

      3. Reduce stress.

        a. Reunite patient and family as soon as possible.

        b. Avoid fatigue; provide periods of rest.

  G. Postdischarge—see Box 21-5.

X. Myasthenia gravis

  A. Background information

      1. Myasthenia gravis (MG) is a chronic, progressive autoimmune disease causing voluntary muscle weakness.

      2. Two thirds of patients first present with ocular motor disturbances, ptosis, or diplopia.

      3. Most other patients first have oropharyngeal muscle weakness, difficulty chewing, swallowing, or talking.

      4. Severity of weakness fluctuates, being the most severe after prolonged use of affected muscles.

      5. As progression occurs, the patient may exhibit.

        a. Increased weakness of certain voluntary muscles

        b. Improvement of muscle strength with rest

        c. Dramatic improvement in muscle strength with use of anticholinesterase drugs

        d. Difficulty with speech

        e. Difficulty swallowing

        f. Respiratory insufficiency

        g. Drooping head

        h. Fatigue

        i. Bowel and bladder dysfunction

        j. Depression

        k. May develop myasthenia crisis (weakness from MG exacerbation) or a cholinergic crisis (weakness from too much anticholinesterase medication)

          (1) Acute respiratory difficulty

          (2) Acute motor weakness of voluntary muscles, including those for swallowing, speaking, and moving parts of the body

          (3) Treatment for either crisis is respiratory assistance

      6. Symptoms worsen with
        a. Emotional upset
        b. Systemic illness
        c. Viral respiratory infections
        d. Hypothyroidism and hyperthyroidism
        e. Pregnancy, menstrual cycle
        f. Drugs affecting neuromuscular transmission
        g. Increased body temperature

B. Preadmission and preoperative interview and management
    1. Provide a calm environment.
    2. Allow for periods of rest if necessary.
    3. Include family in preoperative preparations whenever possible.
    4. If patient has difficulty talking, provide with alternative communication tools.
    5. Assessment per protocol
      a. Patient's abilities and special needs
        (1) Determine patient's and family's understanding of myasthenia gravis.
        (2) Patient's successful management techniques
        (3) Use of assistive devices
        (4) If patient has had any myasthenia crisis episodes—treatment needed
      b. Willingness and capability of family to participate in preoperative preparation and postoperative care
    6. Complete health history per protocol
      a. Progression of disease
      b. Normal routine to avoid exacerbating factors
      c. Particularly note anticholinesterase medications patient is taking for myasthenia gravis.
        (1) Pyridostigmine—Mestinon, Neostigmine—Prostigmin
        (2) Cholinergic effects can be reversed by common perioperative medications such as mycin type antibiotics, aminoglycosides, nondepolarizing muscle relaxants, morphine, procainamide
    7. Physical assessment per protocol
      a. Respiratory assessment—ease of breathing, depth of respirations, auscultation
      b. Muscle strength—identify which muscles are involved with the disease
    8. Psychosocial assessment per protocol
      a. Anxiety
        (1) Determine patient's coping mechanisms.
        (2) Fear of respiratory difficulties during surgery and recovery
      b. Support system
    9. Develop a plan of care based on patient's and family's knowledge and needs.
    10. Preoperative teaching per protocol
    11. Complete preparation for admission per protocol
      a. Referrals as necessary
      b. Preoperative tests as ordered
      c. Document and communicate patient's special needs to the perianesthesia team.

C. Admission
    1. Physical assessment per protocol
      a. Respiratory function assessment
        (1) Auscultation
        (2) Observation
      b. Muscle strength—note which muscles are affected by the disease at this time.

    2. Monitor patient closely after any medication for signs of interaction with routine myasthenia gravis medications.

      a. Increased muscle weakness

      b. Decreased respirations

      c. Agitation

D. Preoperative holding and intraoperative—see Box 21-2.

    1. Observe for myasthenia crisis, manifested with

      a. Increased muscle weakness

      b. Respiratory distress

      c. Difficulty talking or swallowing

    2. Potential for aspiration

      a. Elevate head of bed if possible.

      b. Suction as necessary.

      c. Monitor for swallowing difficulty.

    3. At increased risk for infection

      a. Maintain aseptic technique.

      b. Use care to avoid skin tears.

        (1) Protect bony prominences by positioning and padding.

        (2) Use care when removing adhesive pads.

        (3) Lift, rather than pull, when moving patient.

    4. Maintain normothermia.

    5. Use measures to reduce stress.

    6. Monitor patient closely after any medication for signs of interaction with routine myasthenia gravis medications.

      a. Increased muscle weakness

      b. Respiratory difficulty

      c. Agitation

    7. Protect eyes from injury.

      a. Lubricant

      b. Tape eyelids closed.

E. Phase I—see Box 21-3.

    1. Patient at greater risk for aspiration

      a. Observe for return of gag and swallowing reflexes.

      b. Elevate head of bed if allowed.

      c. Suction as necessary.

      d. Watch for weakness in throat.

        (1) Difficulty speaking

        (2) Difficulty swallowing

      e. Position on side if not contraindicated.

    2. Patient at greater risk for respiratory distress

      a. Auscultation of lungs

      b. Observe respiratory pattern and effort.

      c. Monitor oxygen saturation.

    3. Patient at risk for myasthenia crisis

      a. Maintain normothermia.

      b. Monitor patient closely after any medication for signs of interaction with routine myasthenia gravis medications.

        (1) Increased muscle weakness

        (2) Respiratory difficulty

        (3) Agitation

      c. Observe for symptoms that may indicate crisis.

        (1) Acute respiratory distress

        (2) Acute motor weakness of voluntary muscles, including those for swallowing, speaking, and moving parts of the body

      d. Assess muscle strength frequently.

    4. Monitor vital signs and temperature frequently.

F. Phase II—see Box 21-4.
  1. Patient at risk for respiratory distress
    a. Auscultate lungs.
    b. Observe respiratory pattern and effort.
    c. Monitor oxygen saturation.
    d. Avoid fatigue.
  2. Patient at higher risk for aspiration
    a. Elevate head of bed.
    b. Suction as necessary.
    c. Assess for weakness of throat muscles.
    d. Position on side if not contraindicated.
    e. Exercise caution when giving fluids or solids.
  3. Patient at risk for myasthenia crisis—observe for symptoms that may indicate an impending myasthenia crisis.
    a. Acute respiratory distress
    b. Acute motor weakness of voluntary muscles, including those used for swallowing, speaking, and moving part of the body
  4. Monitor patient closely after any medication for signs of interaction with routine myasthenia gravis medications.
    a. Increased muscle weakness
    b. Respiratory difficulty
    c. Agitation
  5. Assess muscle strength frequently.
  6. Reduce psychological stress.
    a. Reorient patient to surroundings.
    b. Allow use of assistive devices as soon as possible.
    c. Allow family to be with patient as soon as possible.
  7. Keep patient comfortable.
    a. Have room at comfortable temperature—prevent overheating the patient.
    b. Medicate for pain or nausea and observe for desired or adverse medication reactions.
    c. Provide nourishment with care.
    d. Check for bladder distension.
G. Postdischarge—see Box 21-5.

BIBLIOGRAPHY

1. Alzheimer's Disease Education and Referral Center: Growing challenges of Alzheimer's disease in residential settings: communication: Changes over the course of the disease, 1999. Available at http://www.alzheimers.org/caregiving/challenge.htm. Accessed on December 14, 2002.

2. Alzheimer's Disease Education and Referral Center: Growing challenges of Alzheimer's disease in residential settings: Things to think about when you speak, 1999. Available at http://www.alzheimers.org/caregiving/challenge.htm. Accessed on December 14, 2002.

3. American Foundation for the Blind: An overview, 2002. Available at http://www.afb.org/diroverview.asp. Accessed on December 14, 2002.

4. Awakenings: Internet focus on Parkinson's disease. Primary care physicians: Rating scales. Available at http://www.parkinsonsdisease.com/pcp/rating.htm. Accessed on December 17, 2002.

5. Bonifazi W: Patience equals better care. *Nurs Spectrum,* Midwest ed. 11:10, 11, 2002.

6. Burns S: Sleep apnea syndrome in SCI. *Spinal Cord Inj Update* 10(1), 2001. Available at: http://depts.washington.edu/rehab/sci/updates/01w_sleep_apnea.html. Accessed on December 14, 2002.

7. Cardenas D: Pain and spinal cord injury: Causes and treatments. *Spinal Cord Inj Update* 10(2), 2001. Available at http://depts.washington.edu/rehab/sci/updates/01sum_pain_sci.html. Accessed on December 14, 2002.

8. Chapuis T: Parkinson's disease: Manifestations and management. *Clin Rev* 12(2): 62-68, 2002. Available at http://www.medscape.com/viewarticle/429892. Accessed on December 14, 2002.

9. Centre for Neuro Skills. Traumatic brain injury resource guide. Assessment scales. Available at http://www.neuroskills.com/index.html?main=tbi/rancho.shtml. Accessed on December 14, 2002.

10. Davis D, Northway R: Disability: Collaboration in primary care. *J Community Nurs Online.* 15:3, 2001. Available at http://www.jcn.co.uk/article.asp?ArticleID=328. Accessed on December 14, 2002.

11. US Department of Justice: First response to victims of crime who have a disability. Office for Victims of Crime, Pub No. NCJ 195500. Washington, DC: Department of Justice, 2002.

12. Howard J: Myasthenia gravis: A summary, 1997. Available at http://www.myasthenia.org/information/summary.htm. Accessed on December 14, 2002.

13. Irvin S: Sensorineural hearing loss after select procedures. *J PeriAnesthesia Nurs* 17:89-97, 2002.

14. National Institutes of Health: Facts about telecommunication relay services. NIH Pub. No. 94-3754, 2002. Available at http://www.nidcd.nih.gov/health/hearing/telecomm.asp. Accessed on December 14, 2002.

15. National Multiple Sclerosis Society: What is multiple sclerosis? 2002. Available at http://www.nationalmssociety.org/what%20is%20MS.asp. Accessed on December 14, 2002.

16. National Multiple Sclerosis Society: Symptoms. *MS Information Sourcebook.,* 2001. Available at http://www.nationalmssociety.org/sourcebook-symptoms.asp. Accessed on December 14, 2002.

17. National Institute on Deafness and Other Communication Disorders: Aphasia. NIH Pub. No. 97-4257, 1997. Available at http://www.nidcd.nih.gov/health/voice/aphasia.asp. Accessed on December 14, 2002.

18. Reth M: Managing Alzehimer's disease. *Natl Conf Gerontol Nurse Pract* 9:18-21, 2002. Available at http://www.medscape.com/viewarticle/443995. Accessed on December 14, 2002.

19. Saufl N: Special emotional, social, and cultural needs. In Burden N, DeFazio-Quinn DM, O'Brien D, et al, editors: *Ambulatory surgical nursing,* ed 2. Philadelphia: WB Saunders, 2000, pp 553-559.

20. Shepard S: Head trauma. *eMedicine,* 2002. Available at http://www.emedicine.com/med/topic2820.htm. Accessed on December 14, 2002.

21. Silver T, McKinley W: Functional outcomes per level of cord injury. *eMedicine,* 2002. Available at http://www.emedicine.com/pmr/topic183.htm. Accessed on December 14, 2002.

22. Snyder M: *A guide to neurological and neurosurgical nursing.* New York: Wiley, 1991.

23. *Standards of perianesthesia nursing practice*: Perianesthesia standards for ethical practice. Cherry Hill, NJ: American Society of PeriAnesthesia Nurses, 2002, p 9.

24. The Perspectives Network, Inc: What is an acquired brain injury? 2002. Available at http://www.tbi.org/html/faq_english.html. Accessed on December 14, 2002.

25. Whaley LF, Wong DL: *Nursing care of infants and children,* ed 5. St Louis: Mosby–Year Book, 1995.

26. Williams G: Mentally and physically challenged patient. In DeFazio-Quinn DM, *Ambulatory surgical nursing core curriculum.* Philadelphia: WB Saunders, 1999.

27. Ziolkowski L, Strzyzewski N: Perianesthesia assessment: Foundation of care. *J PeriAnesthesia Nurs* 16:359–370, 2001.

22 Transcultural Nursing

DONNA M. DEFAZIO QUINN

■ ■ ■

OBJECTIVES

At the conclusion of this chapter the reader will be able to:

1. Define transcultural nursing.

2. Describe nursing interventions for assessing culturally diverse patients.

3. Discuss the importance of communication as it relates to assessment of culturally diverse patients.

4. Discuss the significance of verbal and nonverbal communication in dealing with culturally diverse patients.

5. Describe the nutritional concerns of three ethnic groups.

I. Definitions
   A. Culture
      1. Integrated system of learned values, beliefs, and practices
      2. Characteristic of a society
      3. Guides individual behavior
         a. Thoughts
         b. Feelings
         c. Actions
   B. Transcultural nursing
      1. Integrates the concept of culture into all aspects of nursing
      2. A humanistic and scientific area of formal study and practice[10]
         a. Focuses on differences and similarities among cultures with respect to
            (1) Human care
            (2) Health (or well-being)
            (3) Illness
         b. Based on individual's:
            (1) Cultural values
            (2) Beliefs
            (3) Practices
   C. Cultural competence[7]
      1. Definition
         a. Dynamic, fluid, continuous process
         b. Individual or health care agency finds meaningful and useful care delivery strategies based on
            (1) Knowledge of the cultural heritage
            (2) Beliefs
            (3) Attitudes
            (4) Behaviors of those to whom care is rendered
      2. Health care professionals need to
         a. Utilize knowledge gained from conceptual and theoretical models of culturally appropriate care
      3. Cultural competence assists the nurse to devise meaningful interventions to promote optimal health among individuals regardless of race, ethnicity, gender identity, sexual identity, or cultural heritage.
II. Culture
   A. Values, norms, beliefs, and practices of a society
   B. Develops over time

      C. Learned responses, actions, words, and thoughts

      D. Passed down through the generations

      E. Not genetic in nature

      F. Guides behavior

      G. Affects health care practices

III. The Transcultural Nursing Society

      A. Founded in 1974

      B. Madeline Leininger, founder

      C. Publications on transcultural nursing

      D. Annual transcultural nursing conferences

      E. Certification available

IV. Major world views of health and illness

      A. Biomedical (scientific)

          1. Life regulated by biomedical and physical processes

          2. Health is absence of disease.

          3. Illness is alteration in structure and function of body.

          4. Treatment focuses on physical and chemical interventions.

      B. Magicoreligious (supernatural)

          1. All that exists is dependent on supernatural forces.

              a. Includes good and evil

          2. Health means person is blessed or favored by the supernatural.

          3. The cause of disease is mystical.

              a. Not based on scientific fact

              b. Foreign object or spirit enters the body.

              c. Sign of punishment or possession by the supernatural

          4. Treatment aimed at removing foreign object or spirit

      C. Holistic

          1. Everything governed by laws of nature

          2. Health achieved by adapting to constantly changing environment

          3. Illness is imbalance or lack of harmony between forces.

          4. Treatment aimed at restoring harmony or balance

V. Major sectors of health care

      A. Types

          1. Popular

          2. Folk

          3. Professional

      B. Characteristics

          1. Each explains and treats illness differently.

          2. Each defines who should be the health care provider.

          3. Each defines how the provider and patient should interact.

          4. Sectors used individually, in combination, or simultaneously

      C. Popular sector

          1. Lay; nonprofessional, nonfolk healer

              a. Define and treat illness.

          2. Determine if additional care is needed (folk or professional).

          3. Activities

              a. Self-care is administered using home remedies.

              b. Consult with family, friends, clergy, neighbors, others who have had same condition.

              c. Remedies include over-the-counter medications.

              d. Care provided by

                  (1) Self

                  (2) Family

                  (3) Friends

      D. Folk sector

          1. May be consulted when home remedies and self-care methods fail

          2. Ethnomedical and traditional

   3. Ethnomedical
      a. The study of non-Western, traditional, or folk medicine
      b. Encompasses cultural traditions, beliefs, and practices related to health and illness
      c. Not related to biomedical theory
   4. Characteristics
      a. Defines and removes supernatural causes
      b. Works to restore balance
      c. Strives to restore health and prevent illness
   5. Activities
      a. Holistic approach
      b. Treatment of illnesses caused by
         (1) Imbalances in individual, physical, social, and metaphysical environments.
         (2) Supernatural forces
      c. Treatment of
         (1) Culture-specific illnesses
         (2) Illnesses not controlled by home remedies or professional medicine
      d. Rituals
         (1) Incorporated to prevent illness, misfortune, and to enhance effects of biomedicine
   6. Acts as intermediary between popular and professional sectors
   7. May be the only sector consulted, depending on cause, signs, and symptoms
   8. Care provided by
      a. Folk healers
         (1) Secular
         (2) Sacred
         (3) Combination of both
E. Professional sector
   1. Types
      a. Biomedicine—United States
      b. Traditional Chinese medicine—China
      c. Ayurvedic medicine—India
   2. Goal: to define, treat, and prevent disease and illness
   3. May be consulted when home remedies or folk sector treatments are ineffective
   4. Initially consulted if acute trauma, surgery, or restoration of body part necessary
F. Use of different sectors
   1. Folk sector
      a. New immigrants and refugees use as primary source.
      b. Used by individuals from all socioeconomic groups
      c. Use dependent on cause of illness and availability of healers in other sectors
G. Nurse's role
   1. Understand why different sectors are used
      a. Enables nurse to explain better goals of nursing intervention and treatments
      b. Ensures patient understands advantages and disadvantages and potential incompatibilities of treatments from multiple sectors
VI. Traditional healers
A. Description
   1. Not part of popular or professional health sector
   2. Specialize in forms of healing characteristic of ethnomedicine
   3. Deal with secular, sacred, or both
   4. Combine methods from both sacred and secular

    B. Secular

      1. Use organic and technical means to treat conditions resulting from natural causes

      2. Types of healers

        a. Herbalist

        b. Bone setters

        c. Granny midwives

        d. Tooth extractors

        e. Injectionists

    C. Sacred

      1. Use nonorganic methods to treat supernatural and natural causes

      2. Nonorganic

        a. Semimystical and religious practices

        b. Influence mind and faith of individual

        c. Examples

          (1) Chants

          (2) Prayers

          (3) Rituals

          (4) Amulets—object worn or cherished to ward off evil or attract good fortune

        d. Types of healers

          (1) Sorcerers

          (2) Shamans

          (3) Spiritualists

          (4) Voodoo priests, priestesses

          (5) Diviners

    D. Nurse's role

      1. Determine if patient receiving treatment from traditional healer.

      2. Inform patient if traditional treatments and biomedical treatments are incompatible (see Table 22-1).

      3. Consult with traditional healer, if necessary, to ensure all have understanding of same goal: assisting the patient to recovery.

      4. Modify plan of care if no compromise is reached.

VII. Preoperative interview and nursing assessment

    A. Develop culture sensitivity.

      1. Clarify own culture and value systems.

        a. Reflect on actions, thoughts, communications, and beliefs of own culture.

      2. Examine personal negative opinions of different cultures.

      3. Increase awareness of other cultures through churches and schools.

    B. Do not project own views on patients through verbal and nonverbal communication cues (see Box 22-1).

      1. Verbal communication

        a. Voice quality

        b. Intonation

        c. Rhythm

        d. Speed

        e. Pronunciation used

      2. Nonverbal communications

        a. Facial expressions

        b. Gestures

        c. Posture

    C. Observe client's family and support system.

    D. Respect the patient.

      1. All cultures are unique.

      2. All individuals are unique.

■ TABLE 22-1
■ ■ Traditional Healers, Preparation, and Area of Practice

	Healer	Preparation	Practice
African American (southern urban)	Family members, especially grandmother	Word of mouth Practical experience	Secular: Common, everyday self-limiting illnesses that respond to home remedies Illness prevention
	Wise woman ("old day")	Practical experience of caring for and raising own children, grandchildren and other kin Develops reputation among family, friends, and neighbors of being knowledgeable about home remedies for common illnesses	Secular: Treatment and prevention of common, everyday illnesses Advice about child care and childrearing
	Herbalist	No formal training	Secular: Diagnose a variety of natural illnesses Dispense herbs to neutralize or eliminate harmful substances that impair the power of body to heal or protect itself
	Spiritualist	No formal training Power may be present at birth (twins) or given by God later in life Usually associated with fundamentalist Christian religion (Holy Ghost, Pentecostal)	Sacred: Cure illnesses sent by God as punishment Cure ailments beyond the power of biomedical practitioners (e.g., arthritis, hypertension, diabetes mellitus) Power of God is present in the body of the spiritualist and transferred to the ill person through laying on of hands Draws on the faith of the individual Sacred or secular: May combine laying on of hands with herbal therapy, massage, and life counseling
	Root doctor (root worker, conjure man or woman, voodoo priest or priestess)	Apprenticeship May be born with magical powers	Sacred or secular: Serves as intermediary between supernatural and natural worlds Enact or remove spells Counteract or protect against witchcraft or sorcery

Continued

■ TABLE 22-1 *Cont'd*
■ ■ **Traditional Healers, Preparation, and Area of Practice**

	Healer	Preparation	Practice
			Combine magical powers with use of herbs
			Read omens and signs and prescribe therapy or preventive measures
			Counseling and magical powers with use of herbs
African Caribbean (Haitian)	Family members, primarily female	Word of mouth generation to generation Practical experience	Secular: Prevention and treatment of common, everyday illnesses
	Doctor feuilles, bocars, dokte feuilles (leaf doctors, herbalists)	Apprenticeship training Hands-on experience Learn "formulas" for healing	Secular: Treats patients with herbs, roots, medicinal plants, and rituals Bone setting, burn treatments, and massage
	Droquistes	Apprenticeship	Secular: Make and sell potions to prevent or treat illnesses of natural causation
	Houngan (voodoo priest) Mambo (voodoo priestess)	Apprenticeship training in rituals Knowledge of prayers and herbal remedies from elders Long training in and study of mythology of spirits	Sacred or secular: Treatment of illnesses due to supernatural causation (angry voodoo spirits; dead ancestors; or magic, witchcraft, or sorcery) Treatment of illnesses that are long lasting or fail to respond to biomedicine
	Sages-femme, fam saj, matrone (lay midwife, wise woman)	Apprenticeship	Secular: Perform deliveries, prepartum and postpartum care, treats other "female" conditions related to reproduction Uses herbs, massage, rituals, baths, and diet
	Piqurestes (injectionists)	Training in missions and other medical facilities	Secular: Give injections, change dressings
Hispanic (Puerto Rican)	Family member, especially oldest female	Word of mouth Practical experience	Secular: Common everyday illnesses that respond to home remedies
	Curandero or curandera	Apprenticeship Gift from God	Sacred or secular: Knowledge of herbs, diet, massage, and ritual Commune with supernatural Conduct religious curing ceremonies

■ TABLE 22-1 *Cont'd*
■ ■ **Traditional Healers, Preparation, and Area of Practice**

	Healer	Preparation	Practice
	Partera (lay midwife)	Apprenticeship training from older female relatives	Secular: Prepartum and postnatal care, herbal remedies, massage, treatment of natural illnesses affecting women
	Yerbero (herbalist)	No formal training	Secular: Preventive and curative care Treats both ethnomedical and biomedical illnesses
	Santiguadore (sabador)	Apprenticeship	Secular: Massage and manipulation of body for illnesses affecting the musculoskeletal and gastrointestinal systems Treats both ethnomedical and biomedical illnesses
	Spiritualist (espiritualista, brujera, santero)	May be born with gift to foretell future Perfect skills through apprenticeship	Sacred: Prevention and diagnosis of illness due to magic, witchcraft, or sorcery; uses amulets, prayers, and other artifacts Some limited curative functions
Moslem (Iranian)	Family members, especially older women	Knowledge handed down generation to generation	Secular: Self-care measures such as bed rest, diet, herbs, home remedies, and childbirth assistance
	Dais (traditional midwife)	Apprenticeship Older women who have raised their own families	Secular: Prepartum and postpartum care Childbirth Newborn care Herbal therapies Massage
	Mullah (religious healer)	Religious training	Sacred: Prevention of illness via preparation of tawiz (amulet with verses from the Koran) Treat illnesses due to evil spirits Treat emotional problems, nervousness, excessive anxiety, and mental illness
	Injectionists	Self-taught	Secular: Administer medications prescribed by physicians Purchase and prescribe injectable medications on their own

Continued

■ TABLE 22-1 *Cont'd*
■ ■ **Traditional Healers, Preparation, and Area of Practice**

	Healer	Preparation	Practice
	Hakimji (traditional healer)	Apprenticeship	Sacred or secular: Combine procedures and medicines from Urani and Greco-Arabic medical traditions
	Bonesetters	Apprenticeship	Secular: Sets broken bones Treats sprains, strains, dislocations, and generalized body pains
Native American (Navajo Indian)	Family members	Knowledge handed down from generation to generation	Secular: Common everyday illnesses of natural origin Prevention of illness Herbal remedies
	Medicine man	Born with power to heal Acquire power to heal via vision or quest Apprenticeship with medicine man once power to heal is known	Sacred or secular: Diagnoses and treatment of supernatural or natural illness (meditation, trance state, divination, or star gazing) Use combination of herbs and curing ceremonies
	Diagnostician	As per medicine man	Sacred: Diagnose underlying cause of illness via divination
	Herbalists	Knowledge passed down generation to generation Apprenticeship	Secular: Diagnose and treat common illnesses of natural causation

From Luckman J, editor: *Saunders manual of nursing care.* Philadelphia: WB Saunders, 1997, pp 37-39.

E. Tips for effective communication
  1. Introduce yourself.
    a. Exhibit confidence; avoid arrogance.
    b. Shake hands if appropriate.
    c. Explain reason for your presence.
    d. Explain upcoming sequence of events (admission assessment, preoperative holding, intraoperative, postoperative).
  2. Avoid assuming where the patient comes from; the patient will tell you if he or she wants you to know.
  3. Show respect, especially to males.
    a. Males are often the decision makers.
    b. If patient is child or woman, male may be the one making decisions regarding care and follow-up.
  4. In some cultures it is customary for children to go everywhere with parents.
    a. Poorer families may not have child-care options available to them.
    b. Include children in perioperative experience.
  5. Understand traditional health-related practices.
    a. Do not show disapproval of them.
    b. If practice is potentially harmful, inform patient.

■ BOX 22-1
■ **VERBAL AND NONVERBAL COMMUNICATION**

Language or Verbal Communication
1. Vocabulary
2. Grammatical structure
3. Voice qualities
4. Intonation
5. Rhythm
6. Speed
7. Pronunciation
8. Silence

Nonverbal Communication
1. Touch
2. Facial expression
3. Eye movement
4. Body posture

Communications That Combine Verbal and Nonverbal Elements
1. Warmth
2. Humor

From Giger JN, Davidhizar RE: *Transcultural nursing: Assessment and intervention,* ed. 4. St Louis: Mosby, 2004, p 36.

6. Be cognizant of folk illnesses and remedies for the cultural population in your service area.
7. When possible, involve leaders of local groups.
   a. Leader may have understanding of problem.
   b. May be able to assist in offering acceptable interventions
   c. Ensure confidentiality is maintained.
8. Accept diversity as an asset, not a liability.
   a. Listening and verbal interactions need to be made with an appreciation of cultural differences (see Box 22-2).
9. Culturally sensitive interactions
VIII. Health habits
   A. Western
      1. Care providers
         a. Physician is most common care provider.
         b. Physician assistants
         c. Nurse practitioners
         d. Chiropractors
         e. Doctors of osteopathy
         f. Doctors of podiatry
      2. Causes for illness
         a. Genetic
      3. Toxins
         a. Cigarettes
         b. Asbestos
         c. Environmental
      4. Dietary
         a. Inappropriate diet
         b. Excessive fat intake
         c. Excessive alcohol intake
      5. Illness is treatable or curable.
      6. Focus on prevention of illness

■ BOX 22-2
■ **GUIDELINES: CULTURALLY SENSITIVE INTERACTIONS**

Nonverbal Strategies
- Invite family members to choose where they would like to sit or stand, allowing them to select a comfortable distance.
- Observe interactions with others to determine which body gestures (e.g., shaking hands) are acceptable and appropriate. Ask when in doubt.
- Avoid appearing rushed.
- Be an active listener.
- Observe for cues regarding appropriate eye contact.
- Learn appropriate use of pauses or interruptions for different cultures.
- Ask for clarification if nonverbal meaning is unclear.

Verbal Strategies
- Learn proper terms of address.
- Use a positive tone of voice to convey interest.
- Speak slowly and carefully, not loudly, when families have poor language comprehension.
- Encourage questions.
- Learn basic words and sentences of family's language, if possible.
- Avoid professional terms.
- When asking questions, tell families why the questions are being asked, the way in which the information they provide will be used, and how it might benefit their child.
- Repeat important information more than once.
- Always give the reason or purpose for a treatment or prescription.
- Use information written in family's language.
- Offer the services of an interpreter when necessary.
- Learn from families and representatives of their culture methods of communicating information without creating discomfort.
- Address intergenerational needs (e.g., family's need to consult with others).
- Be sincere, open, and honest and, when appropriate, share personal experiences, beliefs, and practices to establish rapport and trust.

From Wong DL, Hockenberry-Eaton M, Wilson D, et al: *Wong's essentials of pediatric nursing*, ed 6. St Louis: Mosby, 2001, p 124.

  B. Non-Western (folk medicine)
   1. Care providers
    a. Indigenous healers
     (1) Surgeons
     (2) Spiritualists
     (3) Herbalists
   2. Causes for illness
    a. Evil spirits
    b. Witches
    c. Dysfunction within the harmony of the body
 IX. Cultural beliefs of Asians (Chinese-Americans)
  A. Basis for health culture beliefs and practices is holistic.
   1. Oneness of all things with nature, the universe, and the divine
  B. Health
   1. Results when body works in rhythmic and finely balanced manner
   2. Body adjusts to external environment.
   3. Functions and emotions are in harmony.
  C. Traditional Chinese medicine (TCM)
   1. System of preventive medicine

2. Components
    a. Tao
        (1) Way of life, virtue, heaven, and death
        (2) Individuals should
            (a) Flow with nature.
            (b) Avoid excesses and extremes.
            (c) Maintain a middle position.
            (d) Practice moderation.
    b. Ch'i (vitality)
        (1) "Universal energy"
        (2) Fundamental concept of entire system of TCM
        (3) Origin of all disease
        (4) Health is balance of harmony in the flow of ch'i; illness results from imbalance.
    c. Yin and yang
        (1) Represents duality and unity of universe and Tao
        (2) Balance of yin and yang
            (a) The negative and positive energy forces
            (b) Gift from prior generations
            (c) Harmony and balance of physical and spiritual with nature
    d. Law of five elements
        (1) Association between external physical worlds and internal milieu of body
        (2) Includes fire, earth, metal, water, and wood
    e. Meridians and pulses
        (1) Invisible systems or pathways that carry ch'i through the body
        (2) Regulate organs, blood flow, and connect internal and external organs
        (3) Pulses
            (a) Present in each organ
            (b) Pulse indicates status of organ.
                (i) Balance
                (ii) Imbalance
            (c) No difference among pulses indicates perfect balance.
    f. Causative factors of disease
        (1) Internal
            (a) Excess or lack of emotion
            (b) Constitution
            (c) Anxiety
            (d) Irregularity of food and drink
        (2) External
            (a) Cold, heat, humidity, fire, dryness, dampness, and wind
        (3) Illness results from
            (a) Excess or deficiency of internal or external causative factors
            (b) Interruption in flow of ch'i
            (c) Loss of ch'i
            (d) Imbalance of yin and yang

D. Illness
  1. Prevented by
    a. Conforming with nature
    b. Wearing of jade charms to prevent harm
  2. Disruption of yin and yang energy forces caused by
    a. Overexertion
    b. Lying or sitting for prolonged periods
  3. Treatment
    a. Herbs such as ginseng
    b. Acupuncture

        c. Curing methods
          (1) Cold treatments
          (2) Hot treatments (moxibustion—application of heat to skin)
  E. Grief handled stoically and internalized
  F. Family
     1. Is valued
     2. Act as caregivers
     3. Respect and value elders
  G. Language and communication
     1. Mandarin is official language.
     2. Many dialects; not all are understood by other groups
     3. Silence is valued.
     4. Do not verbalize disagreements.
     5. Unacceptable to display affection to opposite sex in public
     6. Excessive eye contact may be interpreted as rude.
  H. Death
     1. Viewed as religious experience
  I. Medical conditions linked to Asians
     1. Thalassemia
     2. Lactose intolerance
  J. Medical care provided by healers
  K. Nursing implications
     1. Expect use of multiple sectors; attempt to accommodate alternative therapies.
     2. Patient will use self-care measures; support and encourage patient.
     3. Incorporate family in planning care.
     4. Patient tends to be submissive, quiet, and agreeable.
       a. Ability to maintain harmonious relationship supersedes disagreement.
       b. Impolite to disagree with authority figures
       c. Will say "yes" even when patient does not fully understand to prevent disruption in harmony
       d. Will not openly express pain
       e. Will not ask for assistance
     5. Do not draw large amounts of blood from patient.
       a. Blood contains ch'i
       b. Vital energy for TCM
     6. Avoid lengthy conversations and questioning of patient.
       a. May confuse patient or convey incompetence
       b. Combine health teaching with interactive techniques and demonstration.
X. Cultural beliefs of Hispanics (Puerto Rican-American)
  A. Basis for health culture beliefs and practices is holistic.
  B. Health
     1. Luck or gift from God
     2. Balance and harmony among mind, body, spirit, and nature
       a. Forces of "hot" and "cold," "wet" and "dry"
     3. Maintain equilibrium through
       a. Proper balanced diet
       b. Avoiding conflict
       c. Moderate lifestyle
       d. Sharing resources with others
       e. Honoring God
     4. Maintain health by
       a. Praying to God
       b. Consumption of herbs and spices
       c. Wearing amulets
       d. Keeping religious materials in home
       e. Proper conduct
       f. Proper nutrition

C. Illness
   1. Caused by God as punishment for misconduct
   2. Cause may be natural or supernatural
   3. Cause determined by
      a. Previous social behavior
      b. Religious behavior
   4. Spiritism
      a. Supernatural illness
      b. Cause is external force.
      c. Individual is "passive" instrument in treatment.
      d. Failure of patient to respond to biomedical treatment may confirm presence of supernatural cause.
D. Family
   1. Respect for one another is important.
   2. Plays key role in health care
   3. Strong sense of family, both nuclear and extended
      a. Needs of family supersede needs of individual
      b. Men are dominant providers; women are homemakers.
      c. Female health consultant is oldest female in family.
E. Treatment
   1. Medical care provided by Western and non-Western (healers)
   2. Healer (curandero)
      a. Cures hot illness with cold medicine and vice versa
      b. Uses massage and cleanings
      c. May use herbs and spices for prevention and healing
   3. Brujo
      a. Uses witchcraft for healing illnesses related to jealousy and envy
F. Medical conditions linked to Hispanics
   1. Diabetes mellitus
   2. Tuberculosis
G. Language and communication
   1. Primary language is Spanish.
   2. Direct confrontation considered rude and disrespectful
H. Death
   1. Predominantly Catholic
   2. Believe in heaven and hell
   3. Administration of sacraments of the sick is important.
I. Nursing implications
   1. Key cultural concepts
      a. Respect
         (1) Treat others and expect to be treated with dignity and respect.
            (a) Professional attire
            (b) Correct tone of voice
            (c) Professional image
            (d) Providing proper explanations for treatments
            (e) Answering all questions completely
            (f) Allowing patient opportunity to express his or her feelings
         (2) Personalismo: treating each patient as an individual
            (a) Establish rapport with patient initially.
            (b) Touch arm, shoulder, or back during interactions.
            (c) Allow patient opportunity to express concerns.
            (d) Take initiative to learn a few words in Spanish.
   2. Expect full physical for any complaint or problem.
   3. Very expressive, dramatic
      a. Cultural norm
   4. Difficult to express degree or location of pain
   5. Prefer Hispanic health care professional
      a. Understand and respect traditional health care beliefs

XI. Cultural beliefs of Native Americans (Navajo Indians)
  A. Basis of traditional Navajo health culture beliefs and practices is holistic.
    1. Health achieved by living in harmony with universe
    2. Individuals have spiritual and physical dimensions.
    3. Physical dimension
      a. Individuals treat bodies and nature with respect.
    4. Spiritual dimension
      a. Individuals participate in development of own potential through will or volition.
    5. World is governed by supernatural powers and holy people.
      a. Failure to honor supernatural results in lack of harmony.
      b. Harmony essential for good health
  B. Cultural traditions
    1. Emphasize cooperation rather than competitiveness
    2. Share and give to others.
    3. Continue to develop self throughout lifetime.
    4. Believe nature is more powerful than humans
    5. Respect elders.
    6. Welfare and security of family more important than individual success
    7. Strive to live in balance with nature.
  C. Health
    1. Harmony within self and environment
    2. Ability to survive under difficult circumstances
  D. Illness
    1. Caused by disharmony within self and environment
      a. Action of witches
      b. Disturbing physical world
      c. Angering the spirit world
      d. Failure to follow established rituals
      e. Not taking care of self
      f. Failure to observe moderation and balance in all things
      g. Being disrespectful
    2. Do not believe in infection, communicable agents, or physiologic processes
    3. Do not believe in germ theory
    4. Prevention by rituals
  E. Healing
    1. Occurs when ill person becomes one with holy people
    2. Establishes harmony with universe
  F. Treatment
    1. Biomedical and ethnomedical systems sought for treatment
    2. Medical care provided by Medicine Man
      a. Healing achieved only through ethnomedicine
      b. Healing cannot be separated from religion and individual spirituality.
      c. Chanting used at traditional healing ceremonies
        (1) Used to diagnose and restore balance
    3. Nature is powerful force.
    4. Medicine, rest, diet, isolation, and sweat baths
    5. Medications made of herbs and plants
    6. For medication to be effective, it must be administered according to proper ceremony.
  G. Family
    1. Should be included for nursing care
    2. Strong sense of community and extended family
  H. Prevention of illness
    1. Wearing of amulets to ward off illness or witchcraft
    2. Amulets can be bags of herbs, fetishes, or other symbolic objects that are believed to have curative or protective powers.

      3. Blessing occurs at important events.
        a. Enhance good fortune, happiness, and health
   I. Medical conditions associated with Native Americans
      1. Lactose intolerance
      2. Tuberculosis
   J. Language and communication
      1. Navajo or English
      2. Silence shows respect.
      3. Eye contact avoided

XII. Cultural beliefs of African-Americans
   A. Basis of health culture beliefs and practices is magicoreligious and holistic.
      1. Perceptions about health and illness come from popular, ethnomedical, and biomedical health culture.
      2. Little distinction between science and religion, or body and mind
      3. Good health equates to good fortune.
      4. Illness viewed as misfortune
   B. Health
      1. Is synonymous with good luck
      2. Is harmony with nature
   C. Illness
      1. Causes
        a. Disharmony with nature
        b. Demons
        c. Personal tragedy
      2. Classified as natural and unnatural
      3. Natural illness caused by failure to follow three laws of nature (God's law)
        a. Humans are bound by same laws of nature.
        b. Humans are to know, love, and serve God.
        c. Humans are to love each other.
      4. Unnatural illness caused by God withdrawing divine protection
        a. Makes person vulnerable to evil influences
        b. Devil is in control.
        c. Evil influences not responsive to treatment
      5. Individuals vulnerable to illness
        a. Elderly
        b. Young
        c. Women
        d. Unborn fetus
   D. Treatment
      1. Medical care by both Western and non-Western
      2. Cannot be separated from religious beliefs and practices
      3. Occurs around practice of religious ceremonies
      4. Prevention by
        a. Proper nutrition
        b. Adequate rest
        c. Taking care of relationship with God, nature, and others
   E. Family
      1. Strong family ties
      2. Extended family assists with health care
   F. Medical conditions linked to African-Americans
      1. Sickle cell anemia
      2. Hypertension

XIII. Cultural beliefs of Haitian-Americans (Caribbean)
   A. Basis of health culture beliefs is magicoreligious and holistic.
      1. Believe in healing power of Christian God
      2. Believe in traditional folk religion such as voodoo
        a. Maintaining health and recovery from illness depends on faith.

      b. Power of supernatural works in conjunction with traditional healers and biomedical health care providers.

      c. Usually seek biomedical care after appropriate rituals performed

  B. Health

    1. Ability to carry out activities of daily living

      a. Looks well

      b. Good appetite

      c. Shiny skin

      d. Bright eyes

      e. Good color

      f. Able to move about without pain

  C. Illness

    1. Natural

      a. Dominant illnesses

    2. Supernatural

      a. Rare

      b. Suspected when

        (1) Child becomes ill or dies.

        (2) Home remedies, biomedicine, or treatments from secular healers do not work.

        (3) Social conflict occurs prior to symptoms.

        (4) Sudden onset

        (5) Illness becomes life-threatening.

        (6) Other misfortunes occur at same time.

        (7) Occurs after one has good fortune; caused by envy and anger of others

  D. Family

    1. Rely on family, kin, and friends

    2. Usually use extended family

    3. Health care is home managed by grandmother, mother, or maternal aunt.

    4. Older siblings care for younger siblings.

  E. Nursing implications

    1. Patient may regard questions with suspicion.

      a. Keep questions to a minimum.

      b. Explain reason for questions.

      c. If health care practitioner asks too many questions, may be viewed as lacking competence

    2. Oral medications not so effective as parenteral

    3. View vitamin injections as important for maintaining blood

    4. Explain reason for all blood tests; very concerned about status of their blood

    5. Commonly use purgatives with castor oil

      a. Assess for signs and symptoms of dehydration, especially in children.

    6. Have difficulty expressing location of pain

      a. Have patient point to area.

      b. Give opportunity for patient to describe pain.

      c. Not accustomed to using pain rating scales to describe intensity

XIV. Cultural beliefs of White Americans or Anglo-Americans

  A. Basis of health culture beliefs and practices is scientific.

    1. Incorporate variety of self-care measures and home remedies

    2. Number of illness episodes brought to health care practitioner is limited.

    3. Faith in God

      a. Assists in protecting from illness

      b. Aids in recovery

      c. Assists in coping with illness

      d. May consider illness as punishment from God

    4. Supernatural causes

      a. Evil eye and curses

    B. Health

        1. Absence of illness

        2. Ability to function in acceptable manner

    C. Illness

        1. Interferes with ability to function in acceptable manner

        2. Experienced when

          a. Pain occurs.

          b. Changes in bodily feelings or functions occur.

        3. Most illnesses result from natural causes.

        4. Dominant theory is germ theory.

    D. Prevention

        1. Diet and nutrition

        2. Taking vitamins, minerals, and tonics

        3. Exercising

        4. Maintaining normal bowel function

        5. Moderate lifestyle

        6. Adequate sleep and rest

    E. Family

        1. Structure usually nuclear family only

        2. Spouse generally main health consultant

        3. Mother or wife primary caregiver

          a. Diagnoses illness when it occurs

    F. Nursing implications

        1. Wide variation among groups

        2. Some groups have difficulty expressing signs and symptoms.

        3. May not openly express pain

XV. Aspects of communication

    A. Factors that can have an effect on communication (see Box 22-3)

        1. Although communication is universal, styles and types of feedback may be unique to certain cultural groups.

    B. Communication techniques

        1. Use open-ended questions.

        2. Approach in nonthreatening manner.

        3. Allow time for patient's responses.

        4. Do not hurry through interview.

        5. Use professional interpreters whenever possible; patient may be more willing to give important health history information through stranger than family member (especially information regarding sexual matters).

■ BOX 22-3

■ **FACTORS INFLUENCING COMMUNICATION**

> **1.** Physical health and emotional well-being
> **2.** The situation being discussed and its meaning
> **3.** Distractions to the communication process
> **4.** Knowledge of the matter being discussed
> **5.** Skill at communicating
> **6.** Attitudes toward the other person and toward the subject being discussed
> **7.** Personal needs and interests
> **8.** Background, including cultural, social, and philosophical values
> **9.** The senses involved and their functional ability
> **10.** Personal tendency to make judgments and be judgmental of others
> **11.** The environment in which the communication occurs
> **12.** Past experiences that relate to the current situation

From Giger JN, Davidhizar RE: *Transcultural nursing: Assessment and intervention,* ed. 4. St Louis: Mosby, 2004, p 35.

      6. Avoid use of medical terms; use language appropriate to patient's level of understanding.

      7. Use language dictionary appropriate to culture.

      8. Use pictures and gestures.

      9. Speak slowly.

  C. Culture specific—verbal

    1. Chinese-Americans

      a. Soft tone

      b. Slow speech with silence at times

      c. Silence is valued.

    2. Hispanics

      a. Loud tone

      b. Rapid speech

    3. Native Americans

      a. Soft tone

      b. Slow speech with silence at times

    4. African-Americans

      a. Loud tone

      b. Rapid speech

  D. Culture specific—nonverbal

    1. Chinese-Americans

      a. Avoid eye contact.

      b. Discomfort expressed privately

      c. Avoid excessive touch.

    2. Hispanics

      a. Maintain eye contact.

      b. Discomfort expressed openly

      c. Tactile culture

    3. Native Americans

      a. Respect indicated by avoiding eye contact

      b. Respect indicated by periods of silence

      c. Discomfort expressed privately

      d. Light touch or hand passing

    4. Orthodox Jews

      a. Eye contact may have sexual connotation.

      b. Older male to female other than wife

      c. Tactile culture

    5. African-Americans

      a. Maintain eye contact (avoid prolonged eye contact).

      b. Open display of discomfort

XVI. Nutritional concerns

  A. Ethnic and religious food preferences

    1. Chinese-Americans

      a. Prefer rice with all meals

    2. Native Americans

      a. Usually consists of corn, beans, and squash

    3. African-Americans

      a. Prefer salted and spiced foods

      b. High intake of yellow and dark green leafy vegetables

    4. Hispanics

      a. Foods and illness have varying degrees of "hot" and "cold" (not related to temperature of food).

      b. Easier to digest hot foods—chili peppers, onions, garlic

      c. Cold foods include fresh vegetables, corn, beans, squash, tropical fruits.

    5. Jehovah's Witnesses

      a. No food that contains blood as an additive, such as lunch meats

      6. Seventh-Day Adventists
        a. Avoid meat or foods with shells.
        b. Avoid caffeine.
        c. Vegetarian diet encouraged
        d. Protein deficiency may need to be considered.
      7. Jews
        a. Consider pigs unholy or unclean
        b. Pork products not allowed
        c. Cannot mix meat with milk
        d. Kosher products
      8. Muslim
        a. No pork or food products made with pork
        b. No animal fat shortening
    B. Manner of preparation
      1. Identify any cultural preconditions.
    C. Frequency
      1. Identify any cultural requisites.
    D. Nursing implications
      1. Incorporate normal diet into postoperative plan of care.
      2. Consult with nutritionist if areas of concern are identified.
XVII. Spiritual and religious needs
    A. Practices pertaining to health care
      1. Availability of spiritual resources
      2. Pray before meals
      3. Religious articles made available
    B. Chinese
      1. Taoism
      2. Buddhism
      3. Islam
      4. Christianity
    C. Hispanics
      1. Catholicism
    D. Christian Science
      1. Prayer heals the body.
      2. Children treated by Christian Science practitioners only
    E. Jehovah's Witnesses
      1. Opposed to homologous blood transfusions
      2. May submit to autologous blood transfusions
      3. May refuse surgery if blood transfusion is required
      4. Do not partake in national holidays including Christmas
    F. Seventh-Day Adventists
      1. Belief that their bodies are temples of God
      2. Avoidance of meat, caffeine, drugs, tobacco, and alcohol
      3. May refuse foods with shells (lobster, crab)
    G. Nursing implications
      1. Be cognizant of patient's religious needs.
      2. Patient may request private time prior to procedure (preoperative holding).
XVIII. Perioperative nursing considerations
    A. Preoperative teaching
      1. Be alert and sensitive to cultural differences (see Box 22-4).
      2. Differences may
        a. Dictate type of teaching method based on patient's learning style
        b. Show variation in patient's educational needs
        c. Cause variation in patient's response to teaching
        d. Cause variations in patient's discharge plan
    B. Consent
      1. Decision for surgery may be made by head of family or group of elders in a religious community.

■ BOX 22-4
■ **GUIDELINES FOR RELATING TO PATIENTS FROM DIFFERENT CULTURES**

1. Assess your personal beliefs surrounding persons from different culture.
   - Review your personal beliefs and past experiences.
   - Set aside any values, biases, ideas, and attitudes that are judgmental and may negatively affect care.
2. Assess communication variables from a cultural perspective.
   - Determine the ethnic identity of the patient, including generation in America.
   - Use the patient as a source of information when possible.
   - Assess cultural factors that may affect your relationship with the patient and respond appropriately.
3. Plan care based on the communicated needs and cultural background.
   - Learn as much as possible about the patient's cultural customs and beliefs.
   - Encourage the patient to reveal cultural interpretation of health, illness, and health care.
   - Be sensitive to the uniqueness of the patient.
   - Identify sources of discrepancy between the patient's and your own concepts of health and illness.
   - Communicate at the patient's personal level of functioning.
   - Evaluate effectiveness of nursing actions and modify nursing care plan when necessary.
4. Modify communication approaches to meet cultural needs.
   - Be attentive to signs of fear, anxiety, and confusion in patients.
   - Respond in a reassuring manner in keeping with the patient's cultural orientation.
   - Be aware that, in some cultural groups, discussion concerning the patient with others may be offensive and may impede the nursing process.
5. Understand that respect for the patient and communicated needs is central to the therapeutic relationship.
   - Communicate respect by using a kind and attentive approach.
   - Learn how listening is communicated in the patient's culture.
   - Use appropriate active listening techniques.
   - Adopt an attitude of flexibility, respect, and interest to help bridge barriers imposed by culture.
6. Communicate in a nonthreatening manner.
   - Conduct the interview in an unhurried manner.
   - Follow acceptable social and cultural amenities.
   - Ask general questions during the information-gathering stage.
   - Be patient with a respondent who gives information that may seem unrelated to the patient's health problem.
   - Develop a trusting relationship by listening carefully, allowing time, and giving the patient your full attention.
7. Use validating techniques in communication.
   - Be alert for feedback that the patient is not understanding.
   - Do not assume meaning is interpreted without distortion.
8. Be considerate of reluctance to talk when the subject involves sexual matters.
   - Be aware that in some cultures sexual matters are not discussed freely with members of the opposite sex.
9. Adopt special approaches when the patient speaks a different language.
   - Use a caring tone of voice and facial expression to help alleviate the patient's fears.
   - Speak slowly and distinctly, but not loudly.
   - Use gestures, pictures, and play-acting to help the patient understand.
   - Repeat the message in different ways if necessary.
   - Be alert to words the patient seems to understand and uses them frequently.
   - Keep messages simple and repeat them frequently.
   - Avoid using medical terms and abbreviations that the patient may not understand.

■ BOX 22-4 *Cont'd*
■ **GUIDELINES FOR RELATING TO PATIENTS FROM DIFFERENT CULTURES**

10. Use interpreters to improve communication.
- Ask the interpreter to translate the message, not just the individual words.
- Obtain feedback to confirm understanding.
- Use an interpreter who is culturally sensitive.

From Giger JN, Davidhizar RE: *Transcultural nursing: Assessment and intervention,* ed. 4. St Louis: Mosby, 2004, p 35.

    2. Decision maker and patient must understand importance of surgery.
    3. Ensure consent forms signed appropriately, according to facility policy
  C. Body hair
    1. Shaving may violate some cultural beliefs and practices.
      a. Sikh religion (East India): forbids shaving of hair
      b. Greece: manhood is linked to body hair.
      c. Native Americans: body hair sign of health and strength
  D. Removal of jewelry
    1. Some cultures view as religious articles.
    2. Not permitted to be removed from body
      a. If site interferes with surgery, may consent to placement of article on another part of body
      b. May need to be secured (taped) on person prior to procedure
      c. Document presence of article in nursing record.
  E. Pain
    1. Emphasize that it is acceptable to express pain.
      a. Patient may not verbalize or may continue to deny pain.
      b. Incorporate nonverbal patient reactions into nursing assessment of pain.
      c. Medicate as necessary.
    2. Cultural belief to express stoic attitude toward pain
      a. Patient may refuse pain medication.
    3. Meditation
      a. Used by Eastern religions
      b. Relaxation techniques may be helpful in minimizing postoperative pain.
  F. Postoperative dietary needs
    1. Incorporate cultural food practices into dietary teaching for the postoperative patient.
  G. Geriatric considerations
    1. Nursing approach
      a. Elderly person is unique individual.
      b. Avoid imposing own attitude and belief toward aging on the patient.
XIX. Loss of privacy throughout perioperative experience
  A. History and physical (see Table 22-2)
    1. Use of touch during assessment: respect individual's cultural practice.
    2. Need to remove clothing: respect individual's cultural practice; accommodate patient's requests.
    3. Communication with physician regarding "taboo" topics
      a. Incorporate cultural practices into plan of care if appropriate.
  B. Exposure during perioperative experience
    1. Reinforce confidentiality; respect cultural practices; accommodate patient requests.
    2. Keep personnel to a safe minimum.
    3. Avoid overexposure.

TABLE 22-2

Culturally Sensitive Interview

Traditional Western Health Care History Model	Interview Example: Blending Explanatory Model and Traditional Model	Culture-sensitive Listening: Listening for Illness (Cultural Perception) and Disease (Biomedical Perception)
Introduction	Mr. Smith? Hi, I'm J. P., a primary care clinician. I will be working with you today. How would you like to be addressed? or What name would you like me to use?	In every culture, your name has special significance, and the way you are addressed may have great meaning. Never assume that it is acceptable to use the person's first name, or for them to use yours. Age, gender, and cultural norms all play a role in how individuals wish to be addressed.
Chief complaint	What brought you in today? (Ascertain what symptom is of concern.) What is the name of your problem?	Asking a patient to name the problem will give you clues to the patient's beliefs about the origin of the illness.
SYMPTOM ANALYSIS		
Onset/duration	When did it start? Can you think of anything that brought this on? What do you think caused your problem? Why do you think it started then? How long do you think it will last?	This will provide information about the patient's insight into the problem and may reveal underlying beliefs.
Location Frequency/chronology	What parts of your body are affected? How does it work in your body? How often do you notice it in your body? Have you noticed it before? Are you generally getting better? Worse? About the same? What is it like?	Actively listen to understand the patient's perception of the condition. This may add information regarding previous episodes and treatment modalities as well as patient expectations for treatment.

Quality	
Quantity	Is it dangerous?
	Will this last a long time? How much of a problem is it?
Aggravating or alleviating factors	Is there anything that makes it better? Makes it worse? (Ask about various common cultural practices.)	This shows interest and gives the patient permission to talk about the illness and his or her conceptualization of the condition.
Associated symptoms	Do you have any other symptoms with this? Is this causing any other problems in your body?	Again, this gives insight into the patient's perceptions.
Treatments tried	Have you talked with anyone else about this? Did they make any suggestions? Have you tried any other medicines or home remedies? Did these help? Are there any special remedies that you have been advised to try or that are recommended by your healers? Who recommended the remedies you have tried?	Knowing, understanding, and accepting culturally determined treatments and respecting those who utilize them often enables you to develop treatment plans that blend traditional healing measures with allopathic health care practices.
Effects on ADLs	What bothers you most about this illness? How has it affected your daily life?	Provides insight into the patient's illness and allows interpretation of the disease effects.
Patient perceptions	What do you think is going on? Is there anything you fear about your illness? What would you like me to do today?	Positions the clinician to better provide a culturally appropriate plan of care.
Conclusion	Is there anything else I should know or that you would like to tell me? What would you like me to do today?	Patients may or may not be able to tell you what they would like you to do. In some cultures, it may be presumptuous to tell a provider what to do or to express an opinion.

Show empathy, interest, and respect for the patient's concerns.
Encourage the patient to explain.

From Meredith PV, Horan NM: *Adult primary care.* Philadelphia: WB Saunders, 2000, p 72.

XX. Personal space
  A. Determined by individual cultures
    1. Close personal space
      a. Chinese-Americans
      b. Hispanics
      c. Native Americans
      d. African-Americans
    2. Distant personal space
      a. Whites

BIBLIOGRAPHY

1. Campesino M: Commentary: Problematic issues in cultural comparisons. *J Prof Nurs* 18(6):343-345, 2002.
2. Campinha-Bacote J: The process of cultural competence in the delivery of healthcare services: A model of care. *J Transcult Nurs* 13(3):181-184, 2002.
3. Chang MK, Harden JT: Meeting the challenge of the new millennium: Caring for culturally diverse patients. *Urol Nurs* 22(6):372-376, 390; quiz 377; 2002.
4. Cioffi RN: Communicating with culturally and linguistically diverse patients in an acute care setting. *Int J Nurs Stud* 40(3):299-306, 2003.
5. Dawood M, James J: Cross-cultural care: What are you afraid of? *Nurs Times* 97(40):24-25, 2001.
6. Geissler EM: *Cultural assessment,* ed. 2. St Louis: Mosby, 1998.
7. Giger J, Davidhizar RE: *Transcultural Nursing: Assessment and intervention.* St Louis: Mosby, 1999.
8. Kearns CJ, Meehan NK, Carr RL, et al: Using cross-cultural definitions of health care. *Nurse Pract* 28(1):61-62, 2003.
9. Krau SD: Working toward cultural competence in the workplace. *SCI Nurs* 19(4): 193-194, 2002.
10. Leininger M: Transcultural nursing: The study and practice field. *Imprint* 38(2):55-56, 1991.
11. Leininger M: Founder's focus: Transcultural nursing care makes a big outcome difference. *J Transcult Nurs* 14(2):157, 2003.
12. Luckman J, editor: *Saunders manual of nursing care.* Philadelphia: WB Saunders, 1997.
13. Martsolf DS: Cultural aspects of orthopaedic nursing. *Orthop Nurs* 18(2):65-71, 1999.
14. McEvoy M: Culture and spirituality as an integrated concept in pediatric care. *MCN Am J Matern Child Nurs* 28(1):39-43; quiz 44; 2003.
15. Narayanasamy A: Transcultural nursing: How do nurses respond to cultural needs? *Br J Nurs* 12(3):185-194, 2003.
16. Sharma SB, Smith MK: The importance of cultural assessment. *SCI Nurs* 19(4):177-180, 2002.
17. Stacciarini JM: Experiencing cultural differences: Reflections on cultural diversity. *J Prof Nurs* 18(6):346-349, 2002.
18. Wong DL, Hockenberry-Eaton M, Wilson D, et al: *Wong's essentials of pediatric nursing,* ed 6. St Louis, Mosby, 2001.

23 Immediate Preoperative Preparation

ROSE FERRARA-LOVE

OBJECTIVES

At the conclusion of this chapter the reader will be able to:

1. State goals of preoperative preparation.

2. Evaluate the alternatives to on-site visit to surgical center.

3. Identify essential components of preadmission assessment.

4. Explain how the psychological and emotional assessment of a patient will reduce anxiety on day of surgery.

5. Analyze the learning needs of ambulatory surgery patients.

I. Goals of preoperative preparation
   A. Collection of data through assessment and interview
      1. Nursing process
         a. Essential that initial assessment be complete and accurate
            (1) Nursing discharge plan is built on this information.
   B. Provision of accurate information to patient and family
      1. Physician and anesthesiologist primary sources of information
   C. Nurse has specific teaching role as a primary "information provider."
      1. Nurse's role is to clarify patient understanding of
         a. Procedure
         b. Anesthetic approach
         c. Expected outcomes
         d. Personal responsibilities
            (1) Comprehensive nursing instructions assist patient and family.
               (a) Understand and comply with preoperative preparations
               (b) Allow patient and family to prepare for postoperative home needs.
   D. Assurance of appropriate preoperative compliance
   E. Promotion of the wellness concept
   F. Provision of emotional support
      1. Encourage patients and families to express openly and honestly:
         a. Needs
         b. Emotions
         c. Concerns
             (1) Often inaccuracies or misinformation cause fear.
   G. Reduction of patient anxiety
      1. Done by providing clear explanations
      2. Opportunities for expressions of fears and emotions
         a. Induction of anesthesia smoother in calm persons
         b. Recovery is less stressful.

    H. Decreasing potential for complications
      1. Potential problems are identified prior to surgery.
      2. Promotes patient safety
      3. Ensures smooth-flowing operative schedule
        a. Fewer cancellations
   I. Provision of smooth flow of the surgery schedule
      1. Initial steps
        a. Selection
          (1) Based on
            (a) Type of planned surgery
              (i) Likelihood of complications
            (b) Potential for more complex surgery
            (c) Third-party reimbursement
        b. Scheduling
          (1) Based on comprehensive
            (a) History and physical
            (b) Emotional attitude
            (c) Available home support
  II. Scheduling concerns
    A. Surgery scheduling
      1. Based upon
        a. Surgeon
        b. Available time slots on the operative schedule
        c. Patient needs
          (1) Emotional
          (2) Physical
          (3) Urgency of surgical procedure
          (4) Personal and familial schedule
            (a) May not want to delay procedure for someone who is extremely apprehensive and nervous
          (5) Amount of time needed for day of surgery preparation
            (a) Patients with mobility problems or the elderly need extra time for preparation.
            (b) Children and diabetics need to maintain nutrition and medication schedules.
            (c) Patients who need extended postoperative observation should be done early in the day.
              (i) Patients undergoing general anesthesia tend to do better physiologically and psychologically when done early in morning.
            (d) Hospital-based ambulatory surgery centers must coordinate with main operating room schedule if operating rooms are integrated.
            (e) Preoperative policy may indicate time necessary between admission and start of surgery.
              (i) Completed preadmission work-up may require arrival time of only one hour prior to surgery.
            (f) Two or more hours may be needed if preoperative work-up has not been completed.
 III. Preoperative program alternatives
    A. On-site preadmission visits
      1. Formal preadmission program
        a. Necessitates extra trip for patient
        b. May be costly
          (1) Nursing hours
      2. Necessary space requirements

3. Advantages
   a. Patient satisfaction
   b. Fewer delays and cancellations
      (1) May also meet with anesthesiologist during this visit
         (a) History and physical may be completed by anesthesiologist including
            (i) American Society of Anesthesiologists (ASA) status
               [a] ASA-1. A healthy patient
               [b] ASA-2. Healthy patients with mild systemic disease (chronic bronchitis, moderate obesity, diet-controlled diabetes mellitus, mild hypertension, old MI) that are well controlled
               [c] ASA-3. Patients with severe systemic disease that limits activity but is not incapacitating (coronary artery disease with angina, insulin-dependent diabetes mellitus, morbid obesity, moderate to severe pulmonary insufficiency)
               [d] ASA-4. Patients with severe systemic disease that is incapacitating, a constant threat to life (organic heart disease with marked cardiac insufficiency, persisting angina, intractable dysrhythmias, advanced pulmonary, renal, hepatic, or endocrine insufficiency)
               [e] ASA-5. A moribund patient who is not expected to survive without the surgery (ruptured abdominal aortic aneurysm with profound shock)
               [f] ASA-6. A declared brain-dead patient whose organs are being removed for donor purposes
               [g] E. The suffix E is used to denote an emergency surgical procedure.
            (ii) Ambulatory surgery patients usually fall into the first three categories.
   c. Allow for adequate preparation.
      (1) Home
         (a) Caregiver present
         (b) Practice techniques
            (i) Crutch walking
         (c) Dressing changes
         (d) Emptying of drains or catheters
   d. Psychosocial
      (1) Address fears.
      (2) Provide for question and answer.
      (3) Opportunity to meet staff
         (a) Form relationship with staff
   e. Earlier recognition of potential complications or problems
      (1) Allows time for further evaluation or treatment without altering original surgery schedule
4. Scheduling issues
   a. Need for flexibility
      (1) Arrange convenient time for patients.
      (2) No need to take extra time off work
   b. Coincide with availability of anesthesiologist and nursing staff
   c. Coordinate diagnostic testing so only one trip is necessary.
B. The telephone interview
   1. Common means of preadmission assessment and instructions
      a. May be screening tool for identifying high-risk patients
         (1) Then requested to make personal visit to ambulatory surgery center (ASC) for further work-up

       b. Provides emotional and personal contact
         (1) Allows for question-and-answer session
         (2) Health history can be obtained.
           (a) Does not replace physical assessment
           (b) Supplies clues to patient's physical status and needs
         (3) Opportunity to provide instructions
           (a) Safety
           (b) Comfort
         (4) Contact day or evening prior to surgery.
           (a) Confirm arrival time.
           (b) Reinforce nothing by mouth (NPO) status.
           (c) Ensure transportation arrangements.
           (d) Medication instructions
    2. Disadvantages
       a. Complete physical assessment must be done on day of surgery.
       b. Timing of call is important.
         (1) Early enough to allow time to follow up on identified problems
         (2) Not too early that instructions are forgotten
       c. Phone calls may be to patient's place of employment.
         (1) Not conducive to teaching as patient may not be able to speak freely
           (a) May not be able to ask needed questions
           (b) Elicit best time to phone patient.
    3. Documentation and communication
       a. Information must be forwarded to other members of health team.
         (1) Indicates preoperative teaching and preadmission health history have been completed
  C. Preparation of patients at alternate sites
    1. Physician offices may provide ambulatory center with
       a. History and physical
       b. Diagnostic testing results
       c. Surgical consent
       d. Preoperative orders
       e. Evidence of preoperative teaching completed
  D. Admissions coordinator
    1. Responsible for preadmission of ambulatory surgery patients
       a. Secure paperwork and test results
         (1) Often from other facilities
       b. Experienced in preoperative preparation
         (1) Provides preoperative evaluation and teaching
       c. Liaison among the ASC, physicians, and other departments

IV. Documenting the preoperative assessment
  A. Format for documenting health history and physical assessment
    1. Completed prior to actual admission to ASC
    2. Differs from center to center
  B. Preanesthesia assessment
    1. May be completed by patient or family member
       a. Nontechnical form
       b. Easy to read, understand, and complete
    2. Allow space for nurse's objective findings
       a. Vital signs
       b. Physical assessment
       c. Emotional assessment
       d. Special instructions given to patient
       e. Name of responsible adult
       f. Time patient told to arrive on day of surgery
       g. Any other pertinent information
         (1) Medications to take on morning of surgery

  (2) What to bring to center

   (a) Type of clothing to wear

V. Preoperative instructions

 A. Steps in teaching process

  1. Assessing learning needs

   a. Nurse's ability to teach

   b. Patient's learning needs and readiness to learn

    (1) Patient's interest level

     (a) Attentiveness

    (2) Level of understanding

    (3) Ability to comprehend

    (4) Obstacles to learning

     (a) Language barrier

     (b) Sensory losses

  2. Planning a teaching approach

   a. Content and type of information

    (1) Provided at level of patient understanding

     (a) Avoid use of medical jargon.

     (b) Provide easy-to-understand explanations.

   b. Type of media

    (1) Learning and retention enhanced with more than one medium

     (a) Verbal and written instructions

      (i) Verbal instructions more personal and individualized

     (b) Encourage questions and feedback from patients.

     (c) Written instructions allow for reference later.

     (d) Audiotapes

     (e) Videotapes, slides, films

     (f) Charts

     (g) Hands-on demonstrations

     (h) Tour of facility

      (i) Useful for children

   c. Who will be involved?

   d. Environment

   e. Time frame

   f. Group versus one-on-one teaching

    (1) One-on-one most effective

     (a) More personal

    (2) Group more economical

 B. Implementing a teaching plan

  1. General information

   a. Arrival time

    (1) Varies for individual surgical center

   b. Diet

    (1) NPO restrictions

    (2) Smoking

     (a) Refrain from smoking for at least 8 hours or longer before surgery or per facility policy.

      (i) Reduces the amount of carbon monoxide in blood

       [a] Promotes better oxygenation during anesthesia

      (ii) Reduce upper airway irritation

      (iii) Reduces bronchospastic tendency

      (iv) Reduces gastric volumes

  2. Medication protocol

   a. Instructions usually given by surgeon or anesthesiologist regarding medications

    (1) Reinforced by nurse

    (2) Patients should follow usual medication routine at least until midnight prior to surgery.

        (a) Some drugs are continued up to the time of surgery
           (i) Cardiac drugs
          (ii) Antihypertensives
         (iii) Beta blockers
         (iv) Calcium channel blockers
          (v) Anticonvulsants
         (vi) Monoamine oxidase inhibitor (MAOI) antidepressants (Parnate, Nardil, Eutonyl)
            [a] Usually discontinued prior to anesthesia
            [b] Interaction between MAOIs and anesthetic drugs can result in a release of epinephrine and dopamine stores
        (vii) Anticoagulant therapy
            [a] Coumadin is often discontinued 48 hours prior to surgery
            [b] Clotting studies done immediately prior to surgery
            [c] Patients on long-term therapy must be monitored closely for signs of bleeding
            [d] Platelet function
            [e] Aspirin
              [i] Affects platelet adhesiveness for up to one week
              [ii] Discontinued 7 days prior to surgery
            [f] Dipyridamole (persantine) usually stopped 2 days prior to surgery
            [g] Indomethacin, vitamin E, tricyclic antidepressants, phenothiazines, furosemide, steroids also interfere with platelet function

C. Patient participation
   1. Encourage patients to ask questions.
   2. Obtain information necessary to personalize care.

D. Documenting the teaching
   1. Checklist format is efficient way to identify topics covered and patient's response to them.
   2. Special needs or problems should be charted to alert health care workers on day of surgery.
   3. Appropriate follow-up care can be completed.

VI. Consents

A. Surgical consents
   1. Must accurately identify procedure being performed
   2. Words and names should be spelled correctly.
      a. Avoid abbreviations.
      b. No blank areas
      c. No erasures
      d. No obliterations
      e. Language that is understood by patient
        (1) Changes or additions to consent should be written or typed clearly.
        (2) Person making change should initial change and date it.
        (3) Patient should also initial and date area that is changed.
          (a) Significant changes are best done with new consent form.
   3. Nurse's role in obtaining consent
      a. Actual consent for surgery occurs when the surgeon and patient agree to proceed.
      b. Explanation of the procedure, including risks, benefits, outcome, and potential complications, is surgeon's responsibility.
      c. Legal responsibility to obtain consent
        (1) Many institutions require that the nurse facilitate the process by obtaining patient's signature on consent form as well as witnessing that signature.
        (2) The nurse is not legally responsible for obtaining actual consent for surgery or treatment.

      d. According to the American Nurses Association
- (1) Nurse has moral and ethical obligation to ensure that the patient does not feel forced or pressured into treatment.
- (2) Patient receives accurate information that is understood by the patient.
- (3) Patient understands that consent can be withdrawn at any time.
- (4) Nurse ensures that the patient understands what is being done.
  - (a) If patient understands, the nurse may obtain signature on consent form and witness that signature.
  - (b) If patient does not indicate understanding or is unsure about other aspects of the surgery, inform surgeon prior to obtaining signature.
  - (c) Document incident and subsequent conversation in patient record.

  B. Special consents
- **1.** Anesthesia consents obtained by anesthesiologist.
- **2.** In some instances, additional consents may be required.
  - **a.** Sterilization procedures
  - **b.** Termination of pregnancy
  - **c.** Implantation of investigational devices
  - **d.** Photographing procedure
  - **e.** Exception is procedure done via video.
  - **f.** Laparoscopic procedures
  - **g.** Release of information to another physician and/or institution

VII. Patient Self-Determination Act

  A. Omnibus Budget Reconciliation Act of 1990
- **1.** Patient Self-Determination Act
  - **a.** Requires all individuals receiving medical care be given written information about their rights under state law
  - **b.** Decisions regarding medical care
    - (1) Right to accept or refuse treatment
      - (a) Medical or surgical
    - (2) Right to initiate advance directives
      - (a) Living will
      - (b) Durable power of attorney
      - (c) Right to direct end-of-life decisions
    - (3) Does not require that patients have living will or durable power of attorney, only that they be given this information
      - (a) Currently only hospitals, nursing homes, nursing facilities, and home health agencies are required to participate.
      - (b) Some freestanding surgical centers are supplying this information.

VIII. Health Insurance Portability and Accountability Act (HIPAA) Regulations

  A. Took effect in April 2003

  B. Involves three separate sets of rules to protect patients health information
- **1.** Transactions
- **2.** Security
- **3.** Privacy

IX. AM Admissions

  A. Response to increasing costs of hospitalization
- **1.** Large percentage of surgical patients are having diagnostic testing performed as an outpatient.
  - **a.** Patients are then admitted the morning of surgery.
    - (1) Following postanesthesia care, they are admitted to hospital room.
- **2.** Often require extensive preoperative work-up on morning of surgery
  - **a.** May be done as outpatient to facilitate morning admission
- **3.** Preoperative assessment
  - **a.** May be done as outpatient or by telephone interview

(1) History
(2) Physical
(3) Preoperative teaching
(4) Anesthesia evaluation

X. Immediate preoperative preparations
  A. General preparations
    1. Morning of surgery
      a. Physical and emotional support
        (1) Ensure privacy.
        (2) Family and friends
          (a) Directed to waiting room
          (b) Given approximate length of time for surgery completion
      b. Clothing and valuables
        (1) Hospital gowns
          (a) Some surgical centers allow patients to wear undergarments if they do not interfere with surgical site.
            (i) *No* nylon undergarments
        (2) Clothes are kept in patient lockers.
          (a) Some surgical centers place clothing in bags to be kept below stretcher and with patient throughout stay.
        (3) Women are usually asked not to wear makeup.
          (a) Especially mascara because of potential for eye irritation
          (b) Nail polish
            (i) Nearly all pulse oximeter manufacturers provide information regarding use with nail polish or artificial nails.
        (4) Valuables
          (a) Allow family members to keep any valuables.
          (b) Sensory aids
            (i) Beneficial to encourage adequate communication
          (c) If glasses, hearing aids, or dentures must be removed, they should be returned as soon as the patient is awake.
          (d) Label with patient's name and keep with patient's belongings.
  B. Reassess patient's understanding of procedure and preoperative instructions.
    1. Medication instructions
    2. NPO status
      a. Specifically water (if not taking medication)
      b. Hard candy
      c. Chewing gum
        (1) Many people seem confused about these items and maintaining NPO status.
        (2) Chewing gum and hard candy stimulates increased production of stomach juices.
    3. Vital signs
      a. If patient was seen prior to surgery, compare these measurements with preoperative visit.
    4. Significant changes in health history since preoperative visit
    5. Upper respiratory infections
      a. Pulmonary congestion
      b. Fever
    6. Nausea and vomiting
    7. Skin disruptions
      a. Specifically at surgical site
        (1) Shave preparation
        (2) Area of controversy

(3) Association of periOperative Registered Nurses (AORN) recommendation is that hair that does not interfere with surgery should be left intact.
   (a) Hair removal is often unnecessary.
   (b) Possibly harmful
   (c) Relationship between shaving and increased wound infection
      (i) Depilatories and clippers are often used instead of razors.
   (d) Less incidence of skin nicks
      (i) Lower postoperative skin infections
   (e) Incidence of increased infection from earlier shave preparations
   (f) Microscopic nicks serve as good medium for bacterial growth.
   (g) If shaving necessary, many surgeons now prefer it be done just prior to surgery.

C. Intravenous access
   1. Policies regarding intravenous access vary greatly from facility to facility.
   2. Insertion of venous access may be responsibility of admitting nurse.
      a. Nurse Anesthestist (CRNA)
      b. Intravenous team nurse
      c. Anesthesiologist
   3. Needle gauge
      a. Depends on patient needs
      b. Most ambulatory surgery patients will not require blood.
         (1) A 20 gauge is adequate.
         (2) A 22 gauge may be needed for elderly patients with small, fragile veins.
      c. AM admission patients, however, may be facing more complicated procedures.
         (1) Large-bore needle (18 gauge) for fluid and blood administration is recommended.

D. Medication protocol
   1. Goals of preoperative medications
      a. Reduce anxiety
      b. Reduce incidence of nausea and vomiting
      c. Decrease oral secretions
      d. Decrease potential for laryngospasm
      e. Related potential for aspiration
         (1) Decrease gastric acidity and volume
      f. Antibiotics
         (1) Prophylaxis for subacute bacterial endocarditis (SBE)
            (a) Generally given prior to dental, gastrointestinal, genitourinary, oral, and respiratory procedures
   2. Anesthesia preparations
      a. General anesthesia
      b. Regional anesthesia
      c. Monitored anesthesia care (MAC) anesthesia
         (1) Local sedation
   3. Provide emotional support during regional administration.
      a. Positioned so patient can see nurse
      b. Maintain eye contact.
      c. Hold hand if necessary.
      d. Supportive conversation
   4. Physical support
   5. Emergency equipment readily available
      a. Oxygen
      b. Suction
      c. Potential for complications
         (1) Drug reactions
         (2) Perforation of vessel or body cavity

       (3) Hemorrhage

       (4) Respiratory arrest

       (5) Cardiac arrest

E. Emotional support

  1. Provide emotional support while completing preparations.

  2. Calm, unhurried demeanor can help calm patient and reduce anxiety.

    a. Soft music

    b. Subdued lighting

    c. Warm colors

    d. Paintings on walls

      (1) Outdoor, nature settings

    e. Soothing voice

F. Documenting and reporting care

  1. Preoperative nursing care documented according to facility's policy

    a. Charting should be simple but complete.

      (1) Checklist, fill-in, graphs

      (2) Allow space for narrative documentation if needed.

    b. Include

      (1) Vital signs

        (a) Including height and weight

      (2) Allergies

      (3) Emotional assessment

      (4) Medications

        (a) Patient's own

        (b) Any administered for surgery

      (5) Special preoperative preparations needed

      (6) Specific and unusual findings

        (a) Bruises

        (b) Unsuccessful intravenous attempts

        (c) Reactions to medications

        (d) Disposition of valuables

        (e) Responsible adult for home transport

        (f) Infectious diseases

        (g) Positioning requirements

        (h) Prostheses

        (i) Hemiparesis

        (j) Presence of dialysis catheter

          (i) Use of unaffected arm for blood pressure and venipucture

        (k) Special requests of patient

          (i) Wearing religious medal

        (l) Where family is waiting

BIBLIOGRAPHY

1. Bogart J, editor: *Legal nurse consulting: Principles and practice.* Boca Raton, FL: CRC Press, 1998.
2. Boike L, Canala L, Kozminski K, et al: Development of an outpatient perioperative care record. *J Post Anesth Nurs* 10(3): 140-150, 1995.
3. Brumfield VC, Kee CC, Johnson JY: Preoperative patient teaching in ambulatory surgery settings. *AORN J* 64(6):941-946, 948, 951-952, 1996.
4. Burden N: *Ambulatory surgical nursing.* Philadelphia: WB Saunders, 2000.
5. Drain C: *The post anesthesia care unit: A critical care approach,* ed 3. Philadelphia: WB Saunders, 2002.
6. Dunn D: Preoperative assessment criteria and patient teaching for ambulatory surgery patients. *J PeriAnesth Nurs* 13(5):274-291, 1998.
7. Kerridge R, Lee A, Latchford E: The perioperative system: A new approach to managing elective surgery. *Anaesth Intensive Care* 23(5):591-596, 1996.
8. Knoerl DV, Faut-Callahan M, Paice J: Research utilization: Preoperative PCA teaching program to manage postoperative pain. *Medsurg Nurs* 8(1):25-33, 1999.
9. Lancaster KA: Patient teaching in ambulatory surgery. *Nurs Clin North America* 32(2):417-427, 1997.

10. Lisko SA: Development and use of video-taped instruction for preoperative education of the ambulatory gynecological patient. *J Post Anes Nurs* 10(6):324-328, 1995.

11. Lewis SM, Heitkemper MM, Dirksen SR: *Medical-surgical nursing: Assessment and management of clinical problems,* ed 5. St Louis: Mosby, 2000.

12. McCaffery M: Teaching your patient to use a pain rating scale. *Nursing* 32(8):17, 2002.

13. Palmerini J, Jasovsky D: Patient education: A guide for success. *Nurs Manage* 29(9):45-46, 1998.

14. Swan BA: Assessing symptom distress in ambulatory surgery patients. *Medsurg Nurs* 5(5):348-354, 1996.

15. Williams GD: Ambulatory surgery: Preoperative assessment and health history interview. *Nurs Clin North America* 32(2): 391-416, 1997.

CORE COMPETENCIES OF PACU NURSING

Fluid and Electrolyte Balance

KATHLYN CARLSON

OBJECTIVES
At the conclusion of this chapter the reader will be able to:

1. Identify three fluid compartments of the body.

2. Explain the volume and distribution of fluids in each body fluid compartment.

3. Differentiate between crystalloid and colloid.

4. Identify electrolyte imbalances and nursing management involved for each.

5. Identify procedures highly associated with nausea and vomiting.

  I. Perianesthesia issues

    A. Clinical status alters fluid status.

      1. Cell function requires an exquisite yet dynamic fluid and chemical balance.

      2. Normal required daily fluid intake is approximately 2 L.

        a. Stress, food and fluid restrictions, preexisting chronic conditions, acute illness or trauma, surgically induced losses, or medication effects alter normal fluid requirements.

        b. Extent of preoperative dehydration undervalued for patients with limited fluid reserves

          (1) Even healthy ambulatory surgery patient is mildly dehydrated, perhaps 5%, by nothing by mouth (NPO) restrictions.

          (2) Preanesthesia NPO rules relaxed: clear liquids permitted 2-4 hours preprocedure.

          (3) *Children* can become significantly dehydrated and hypoglycemic.

          (4) Percentage of body water less in *obese* patients: fat contains little water.

          (5) Percentage of body water decreases with *age:* muscle decreases, fat increases, kidneys less able to conserve fluid (concentrate) and regulate sodium

          (6) *Malnutrition* alters protein intake and use, so water balance altered

      3. Preoperative deficit, surgical blood loss replaced with an isotonic crystalloid solution

        a. Consider fluid spacing when managing fluid infusions.

          (1) *First spacing*: normal distribution of body fluids

          (2) *Second spacing*: excess accumulation of interstitial fluid (ICF) with edema, such as puffy eyelids, fingers, and ankles

          (3) *Third spacing*: fluid migration from vascular space (ECF) to areas normally with minimal or no fluid; also known as the *trancellular spaces.*

            (a) Examples: ascites, or bowel after peritonitis, injury or surgery

            (b) Depletes vascular circulation: hypovolemia, ongoing hypotension

B. *Before* the day of surgery, determine *stable* biochemical status, organ function.
  1. Clinically relevant laboratory tests are within normal limits.
    a. Selectively assess preoperative laboratory values only when warranted by a patient's health needs, medications, coexisting disease, and medical history, age, or physical examination (refer to Table 24-1).
      (1) If no new clinical events, lab results acceptable for 3-6 weeks
      (2) Some believe preoperative renal assessment with blood urea nitrogen (BUN) and creatinine indicated if elderly, systemic disease; uses nephrotoxic medications
      (3) Verify stable fluid status, update specific tests (potassium, glucose) on the day of surgery if indicated.
    b. For *ambulatory* surgery, no extensive physiologic fluid or electrolyte shifts.
      (1) No increased risk of perianesthetic crisis is foreseen.

■ TABLE 24-1
■ ■ **Clinical Indicators for Preanesthetic Laboratory Assessment**

Obtain Preoperative Test	To Assess
POTASSIUM* IF	
Potassium-depleting diuretics digoxin, especially with toxicity corticosteroids, preoperative colon preparation, or laxative	Hypokalemia: lethal cardiac dysrhythmia
Chronic renal failure	Acidosis, hyperkalemia: muscle weakness, including respiratory; metabolic dysfunction
ELECTROLYTE PANEL AND CHEMISTRIES IF	
Renal failure, diabetes, cardiopulmonary disease, chemotherapy	Hyperkalemia, acidosis, BUN, and creatinine increases potential for renal failure
	Renal function, acidosis
GLUCOSE* IF	
Diabetes mellitus	Baseline preoperative status when insulin dependent, recheck preoperatively
Chronic corticosteroid use	Possible hyperglycemia, need for insulin
HEMOGLOBIN, HEMATOCRIT	
Infants less than 1 year old	Normal physiologic anemia
Renal disease	Chronic anemia, suppressed RBC manufacture
Anticoagulants	Unrecognized bleeding potential and determine baseline status
Malignancy, radiation/chemotherapy	Suppressed bone marrow function, RBCs
Use of nonsteroidal antiinflammatories	Mild anemia
COAGULATION: PT/PTT/INR/PLATELETS†	
Chronic anticoagulation	Great risk of excessive or prolonged bleeding
Warfarin stopped at least 3-7 days preoperatively	Risk of intraspinal bleed if spinal anesthetic
	Verify return to normal parameters.
Chronic aspirin or nonsteroidal	Altered platelet function
Antiinflammatory drugs (NSAIDs)	Potential for prolonged postsurgical bleeding— unresearched, but risk presumed less likely if risk of intraoperative bleeding is low

*Some recommend potassium and glucose values be updated on day of surgery.
†PT, Prothrombin time; PTT, partial thromboplastin time; INR, international normalized ratio.

(2) Aged, American Society of Anesthesiologists (ASA) classification III and IV patients increasingly accepted

(3) Anticipated need for blood transfusion is a debatable issue.

   (a) Some surgeons transfuse autologous blood after liposuction.

   (b) Large blood loss often results in unplanned hospital admission.

(4) For preterm infants less than 60 weeks old, hematocrit less than 30% increases risk of apnea.

  c. "Routine" laboratory tests: need versus cost in *ambulatory* surgery

    (1) A controversial, well-scrutinized issue

    (2) *No* lab measures truly required for healthy, asymptomatic patients for either ambulatory or inpatient surgery

    (3) A battery of "routine" laboratory tests costly, medically unnecessary

    (4) Studies demonstrate even new abnormal lab findings in asymptomatic patients *rarely* cause surgery to be canceled.

    (5) False-positive abnormal results in healthy, asymptomatic patients create undue concern, increase costs, and/or cause surgical delays.

C. Postanesthetic hydration and chemical concerns

  1. Postoperative nausea and vomiting (PONV)

    a. Increases potential for hypovolemia

    b. Significantly delays discharge to home

    c. Increases cost of care

    d. Infants, children, and elderly patients dehydrate easily.

    e. Unrelenting, protracted vomiting can result in clinically significant chemical imbalances and hospital readmission.

    f. Highly associated with laparoscopy, strabismus correction, and ear surgery

  2. Replace preoperative deficit and surgical blood loss with an isotonic crystalloid solution and colloids as required.

  3. In PACU, measure and replace postoperative electrolytes, magnesium, calcium, particularly when intraoperative blood loss is high, fluid and colloid replacement is large (refer to Box 24-1).

II. Physiologic fluid homeostasis

  A. Fluid (solvent) facts

    1. Body water account for approximately 60% of total body weight (TBW).

    2. Percentage of water varies with percentage of body fat.

      a. Muscle: high water content

      b. Fat: low water content

      c. Female body contains a higher proportion of fat than male.

■ BOX 24-1
■ **TOXICITY OF REPLACEMENT IV SOLUTIONS**

Tonicity	IV Solutions
Isotonic: Osmolality 240-340 mOsm/L	0.9 normal saline (NS): 310 mOsm/L
Concentration of dissolved particles in ECF = ICF	5% dextrose in water (D_5W): 252 mOsm/L
	5% dextrose in one fourth NS (D_5 0.225 NS): 326 mOsm/L
	Lactated Ringer's (LR): 272 mOsm/L
Hypertonic: Osmolality >340 mOsm/L	5% dextrose in lactated Ringer's (D_5LR): 524 mOsm/L
ECF concentration > ICF	
Causes water to move from cell *to* serum to help maintain circulating blood volume	5% dextrose in one half normal saline (D_5 0.45 NS): 406 mOsm/L
	10% dextrose in water (D_{10}W): 505 mOsm
Hypotonic: Osmolality <240 mOsm/L	Half normal saline (0.45 NS): 154 mOsm/L
ECF concentration < ICF	
Causes water to move *from* serum into cells	

B. Body fluid compartments: volume and distribution
  1. *ECF* compartment
     a. Volume: approximately 28 liters—33% to 40% of adult's total body weight (TBW), nearly 75% of a young child's body weight
     b. Fluid circulating *outside* of cells, including
        (1) Intravascular fluid: fluid *within* plasma
            (a) Crucial for cardiovascular function
            (b) About one third of ECF volume or 8% of total body water
        (2) Interstitial fluid: fluid *between* cells
            (a) Returns to circulation via lymphatics
            (b) Controlled by capillary cell wall integrity, oncotic and hydraulic pressures
            (c) About two thirds of ECF volume or 20% of adult body water
        (3) Transcellular fluid: in saliva, glands, cerebrospinal, gastric
     c. Anesthetic medications dilate vasculature and expand ECF capacity.
        (1) Ease fluid overload and improve diastolic filling in the heart
        (2) If ECF volume insufficient, significant hypotension results
  2. *ICF* compartment
     a. Volume accounts for 66% to 75% of TBW.
     b. Fluid *within* cells
  3. Factors influencing water distribution: primarily regulated by *osmosis*
     a. Cell wall permeability (integrity)
     b. Serum sodium levels
     c. Cellular sodium pumps and large concentration gradients between ECF and ICF prevent major electrolytes in ECF and ICF from ever equalizing.
III. Physiologic particle (solute) homeostasis
  A. Physiologic balance critical for normal cellular function, including during the perianesthetic period
     1. Imbalances may result from
        a. Transient, mild respiratory acidemia related to anesthetic-induced hypoventilation and sedation
        b. Preoperative hypokalemia related to potassium-depleting bowel preparations or chronic medications such as diuretics or digoxin
        c. Physiologic stress related to surgery and a patient's anxiety alters homeostasis by increasing sodium and fluid retention
     2. Noncritical illness and brief, elective procedures mean significant electrolyte imbalance is uncommon in ambulatory surgery patients.
  B. Components (solute) distributed within body water
     1. *Electrolytes*: electrically active ions with either a positive or negative charge when dissolved in solution (refer to Box 24-1). *NOTE*: A measure of the *serum* (ECF) concentration of an electrolyte does not necessarily reflect the electrolyte content of intracellular electrolytes (ICF).
        a. Primary ECF electrolytes
           (1) *Cation:* positively charged ion
               (a) *Sodium (Na⁺)* reflects serum osmolality and regulates fluid balance.
               (b) Expect fluid imbalance if serum sodium increased *or* decreased.
               (c) Inverse relationship with serum potassium: if Na^+ rises, expect low K^+.
           (2) *Anion:* negatively charged ion
               (a) *Chloride (Cl^-)* competes with bicarbonate to combine with sodium.
               (b) *Bicarbonate (HCO_3^-):* immediately available acid-base buffer
        b. Primary ICF electrolytes: Cannot directly measure, reflected by ECF values. *NOTE*: Status of ICF electrolytes is not necessarily reflected by a laboratory measure of an electrolyte in the serum (ECF).
           (1) *Cations:* positively charged ions, critical for cardiac function
               (a) Potassium (K^+): poorly stored, deficits quickly if loss or low intake
               (b) Magnesium (Mg^+)

(c) Calcium (Ca^{++})

(d) Replace slowly, *always* in diluted solution, never intravenous (IV) push

(2) *Anions:* negatively charged ions

(a) Phosphorus (P), present in body fluid as phosphate (PO_4)

2. Undissolved, nonelectrolyte *particles:* sugar, urea, and protein are examples.

    a. Large, osmotically active molecules

    b. Influence movement of water across permeable cell membranes

3. *Buffers:* physiologic controls to regulate acids and bases

    a. Bicarbonate: immediate chemical buffer, present in ECF

        (1) Regulate (buffer) pH by accepting or releasing acidic hydrogen ions (H^+).

        (2) Maintain serum's chemical neutrality, specifically pH = 7.4: a mathematic representation of hydrogen ion (H^+) in ECF.

        (3) Maintain bicarbonate to carbonic acid ratio of 20 to 1 (see Chapter 25).

    b. Phosphate, hemoglobin, and protein: chemical buffers

        (1) Present in all body fluids to help maintain acid-base balance, coagulation

        (2) Proteins create colloid osmotic pressure to regulate fluid distribution

            (a) Low-protein conditions allow fluid to leak from vascular space (ECF) to ICF or transcellular (third) space

            (b) Low-protein conditions: hemorrhage (red blood cell [RBC] loss) malnutrition, severe infections, fistulae, and fluid imbalances

            (c) Need serum albumin level >4g/dl for adequate protein level

4. *Salts:* potassium chloride (KCl) is one example

  C. *Osmolality* indicates body's hydration status.

    1. Expresses the concentration of particles in serum, per kilogram

    2. Normal value is 280-294 milliosmols (mOsm)/Kg.

    3. Changes in osmolality sensed by baroreceptors at right atrium

        a. Osmolality high: ECF concentrated (*hypertonic*) patient is dehydrated.

        b. Osmolality low: ECF dilute (hypotonic) patient is overhydrated.

        c. Primarily adjusted by antidiuretic hormone (ADH)

        d. Total number of "osmotically active" particles in a solution

            (1) Determined by total of electrolyte and nonelectrolyte particles.

            (2) Creates *osmotic pressure* per liter of solution to maintain water in appropriate compartment

            (3) Serum sodium (Na^+) is the most important determinant.

                (a) Water "follows" sodium to equalize concentration and establish equilibrium.

                (b) When serum sodium elevated, water shifts into serum (ECF) by osmosis: *dilutes* sodium, normalizes osmolality.

                (c) When serum sodium is low, water shifts from serum by osmosis to *concentrate* sodium and normalize osmolality.

IV. Fluid and electrolyte equilibrium: regulators

  A. Water facts

    1. Water constantly seeks to establish equilibrium between ECF and ICF.

    2. *Osmosis* controls *fluid* movement between ECF and ICF.

    3. *Diffusion* governs *solute* distribution through a selectively permeable membrane.

    4. Fluid balance requires both normal volume of water *and* normal concentrations of particles in solution (refer to Table 24-2).

  B. Mechanisms of passive transport

    1. *Diffusion:* movement of *particles* in solution across a selectively permeable cell membrane from a concentrated solution toward a more dilute one

        a. Purpose: try to equalize concentration of *particles* between compartments

        b. Electrolytes are small; pass easily across cell walls

        c. Larger particles inhibited from crossing selectively permeable membrane

        d. Though individual ions move constantly, passively and randomly between ECF and ICF, net migration of ions is toward the dilute solution.

■ TABLE 24-2
■ ■ **Primary Electrolytes of the ECF and ICF***

ECF Ion	Normal Serum Value	Indicators	
		Deficit (hypo-)	Excess (hyper-)
Sodium (Na⁺) ■ Regulates ECF osmolality and vascular fluid volume ■ Active transport via sodium pump—to sustain high intracellular K⁺	135-145 mEq/L	*Hyponatremia* ■ <130 mEq/L, ↓ serum osmolality ■ Salt diluted by excess retained water ■ Bladder irrigations, electrolyte-free IVs, ADH oversecretion *Outcomes:* ■ Weak muscles ■ Confusion ■ Nausea/vomiting ■ Hypotension, seizure ■ Coma if <115 mEq/L	*Hypernatremia* ■ >145mEq/L, ↑ serum osmolality ■ Excess salt from water loss ■ Inadequate osmotic diuresis—poor fluid intake *Outcomes:* ■ Thirst ■ Flushed skin ■ Hypotension ■ Oliguria ■ Seizures, coma if extreme
Chloride (Cl⁻) ■ Preserve acid-base balance ■ rReciprocal: if Cl⁻ depleted, HCO₃⁻ rises ■ cCombines with sodium to maintain osmolality	96-106 mEq/L	*Hypochloremia* ■ <98mEq/L ■ Prolonged Cl⁻ loss: gastric suction, diuresis *Metabolic Alkalosis* ■ Patient hypoventilates.	*Hyperchloremia* ■ >108 mEq/L ■ Cl⁻ gain *Metabolic Acidosis* ■ Patient hyperventilates.
Bicarbonate (HCO₃⁻)	24-28 mEq/L	*Metabolic Alkalosis* ■ pH >7.45 ■ Patient hypoventilates>	*Metabolic Acidosis* ■ pH <7.35 ■ Patient hyperventilates. ■ Hyperkalemia occurs.
Osmolality (mOsm)	280-300 Osm/Kg	*Dehydration* ■ ECF concentrated	*Overhydration* ■ ECF dilute
Potassium (K⁺) ■ ECF content small ■ Potent effect on cell neuromuscular irritability ■ Acidosis, catabolism move K⁺ to serum ■ Insulin, glucose shift K⁺ back to cell	3.5-5.0 mEq/L	■ *Hypokalemia* ■ <3.5 mEq/L ■ Reflects ECF loss: diuretics, diarrhea, vomit, digitalis, bowel preps ■ If ECF depleted, ICF is also ■ Muscle weakness ■ Hypoventilation ■ Flaccid paralysis ■ Cardiac arrhythmias: more PVCs, U wave classic, conduction blocks ■ *Slow* KCl doses	■ *Hyperkalemia* ■ >5.0 mEq/L ■ *Gain in serum:* tissue lysis, acidosis from renal or diabetes—MALIGNANT HYPERTHERMIA CAN BE LETHAL ■ Muscle weakness ■ Hypoventilates ■ Paralysis ■ Arrhythmias: peaked T wave, wide QRS, asystole ■ Stat *insulin* carries K⁺ back to ICF ■ Dialyze renal patients. ■ Stop any K⁺ intake

■ TABLE 24-2 *Cont'd*
■ ■ **Primary Electrolytes of the ECF and ICF***

ECF Ion	Normal Serum Value	Indicators	
		Deficit (hypo-)	**Excess (hyper-)**
Magnesium (Mg⁺) ■ Promotes acetylcholine (ACh) release at neuromuscular junction ■ Regulates K⁺ ■ Opposes Ca⁺⁺	1.5-2.5 mEq/L	*Hypomagnesemia* ■ <1.5 mEq/L *Causes:* diarrhea, malabsorption, long-term vomiting, excess aldosterone *Signs:* ■ Neuromuscular irritability ■ Cardiac: long PR wide QRS, flat T ■ K⁺, Ca⁺⁺ and PO_4^-	*Hypermagnesemia* ■ >2.5 mEq/L *Causes:* $MgSO_4$, infusion, ketoacidosis, chronic renal failure *Signs:* ■ CNS depression, sedation, muscle weakness ■ Hypotension, bradycardia ■ If Mg⁺ >12, hypoventilation
Phosphate (PO_4^-) ■ Most stored in bone ■ Essential for energy &and acid-base balance ■ Inverse relationship with calcium: if PO_4^-↑, Ca⁺⁺↓ ■ Need parathyroid hormone (PTh) to excrete	1-2 mEq/L (3-4.5 mg/dl)	*Hypophosphatemia* ■ <1.5 mg/dl *Causes:* aspirin overdose, ketoacidosis, malabsorption, steroids, hypercalcemia *Outcome* ■ Energy depletion: weak muscle, seizures, cardio-respiratory failure	*Hyperphosphatemia* ■ >4.5 mg/dl *Causes:* ■ Laxative excess ■ Supplement in diet ■ Trauma *Outcome* ■ Cell death, renal failure, PTh decreases
Calcium (Ca⁺⁺) ■ Critical for impulse conduction, cardiac contraction, coagulation ■ Is stored in bone ■ Present in blood (ECF): ionized (50%), protein bound ■ Reciprocal relationship with phosphorus: when Ca⁺⁺↑, PO_4^-↓	4.5-5.3 mEq/L (8.5-10.5 mg/dl)	*Hypocalcemia* ■ <4.5 mEq/L *Causes:* low albumin, renal failure (chronic), hypoparathyroidism *Signs and symptoms:* tingling/weakness, twitching/tetany, low blood pressure /electrocardiogram change, postoperative laryngospasm	*Hypercalcemia* ■ >4.5 mEq/L *Causes:* immobility, malignancy, low PO_4^-, hyperparathyroidism *Signs and symptoms:* lethargy, short QT

*Electrolytes found in high concentration in ECF are in low concentration in ICF; similarly, the primary electrolytes of the ICF are present, but in low concentrations, in the ECF.

    e. Particle concentration dissolved in ECF or ICF determines water movement and balance.

    f. Solute concentration difference between areas is a *concentration gradient.*

  2. *Osmosis:* movement of *water* from a dilute space with few particles across a semipermeable membrane to a more densely concentrated space

    a. Purpose: try to equalize compartment concentrations

    b. Unequal numbers and size of particles in ECF and ICF water

      (1) Glucose, urea, and protein are large molecules that normally cannot pass from blood (ECF) through selectively permeable cell walls.

(2) Because of these large particles in the blood, ECF contains more particles, and is therefore more concentrated, than in cells (ICF).

(3) Water shift is constant though net movement of water is toward the ECF, preventing cells from becoming waterlogged, edematous, and bursting.

3. *Carriers* or facilitated diffusion: A substance (for example, insulin), abets diffusion of particle (for example, glucose) across the semipermeable membrane.

4. *Filtration*: transfer of water and dissolved substances through the semipermeable gradient via a *pressure* gradient from higher to lower pressure
   a. Pressure created by the weight of the solute-laden solution
   b. Glomerular filtration in kidney's nephron is an example: arterial blood pressure is greater than intrarenal pressure; this pressure gradient forces blood into the glomerulus for filtration.
   c. A force opposing osmosis

C. Mechanisms of pressure and energy
   1. *Active transport*
      a. Metabolic energy, adenosine triphosphate (ATP), consumed to move substances through semipermeable membranes
      b. Oxygen required
      c. Propels sodium-potassium pump, used after every neuromuscular action
         (1) During neuron "firing," sodium migrates through cell wall to ICF and potassium diffuses out of the cell.
         (2) Active transport pumps return sodium to ECF and potassium to ICF, their respective "normal" homes.
   2. *Osmotic pressure*: pressure exerted within a compartment by osmotically active particles in solution
      a. Differences in particle concentration between two compartments create a *concentration gradient*.
      b. Pressure across this gradient moves (redirects) water across the gradient to equalize water between cells or fluid compartments.
      c. After water equilibrates, the concentrations of particles in solution become equal, but the volume of water in the compartments may not be equal.
      d. Opposes interstitial fluid pressure.

D. *Oncotic pressure*
   1. Also called colloid osmotic pressure
   2. Colloids are large particles, such as protein, that normally cannot cross cell membrane.
   3. *Plasma colloid osmotic pressure:* primarily contained in serum and pulls fluid from interstitial space into capillaries across a *pressure gradient*

E. *Hydrostatic pressure*
   1. Pressure exerted by blood against blood vessel, capillary, walls
      a. Variable: with arterial and venous pressures, and vascular resistance in small venules and capillaries
         (1) Capillary hydrostatic pressure elevated with rise in arterial pressure or vessel resistance.
         (2) Low capillary resistance or low arterial pressure reduces capillary hydrostatic pressure.
   2. Primary reason fluid moves from vascular system to interstitial space
      a. Principle force of capillary filtration
      b. Greater at arterial capillary (32 mm Hg) than venous (15 mm Hg)
      c. Opposes osmotic pressure

V. Renal and hormonal regulators of blood volume
   A. Antidiuretic hormone (ADH): adjusts serum osmolality, concentrates electrolytes
      1. Prompts reabsorption or elimination of water, but not sodium, at the kidney's collecting tubules, thereby concentrating or diluting Na^+
      2. Released by the pituitary's posterior hypophysis in response even 1% to 2% increase or decrease in serum osmolality, as sensed by *osmoreceptors*

3. *Increased* ADH secretion: response to increased serum osmolality
   a. Prompts water reabsorption at kidney's collecting ducts: urine concentrates.
      (1) Specific gravity increases: more concentrated with dissolved solutes
      (2) Normal specific gravity: 1.010-1.025
   b. Secretion stimulated by stress such as pain, trauma, surgery, hypovolemia, opioids, hypoxia, or hypercapnia
4. *Decreased* ADH secretion: response to decreased serum osmolality
   a. Promotes water elimination through collecting ducts: urine dilutes
   b. Secretion halted by mechanical ventilation, pulmonary disease, such as pneumonia, or central nervous system pathology, such as cranial trauma, tumors, surgery, and infection
   c. *Diabetes insipidus* may follow pituitary hypophysectomy; observe for dilute, unconcentrated urine, thirst, and dehydration.
   d. Urine specific gravity decreases: fewer solutes dissolved in urine

B. *Atrial natriuretic peptide* (ANP)
   1. Secreted by cardiac atrium when stretched by increased venous return
      a. Circulating volume elevated
      b. Spurs excretion of sodium, followed by water excretion

C. *Renin-angiotensin:* regulates circulating blood volume and peripheral vascular resistance to sustain blood pressure
   1. Through feedback mechanisms to the nephron's distal tubule, baroreceptors at the juxtaglomerular sense blood flow changes (increased or decreased perfusion pressure) at the glomerulus changing glomerular filtration rate (GFR).
   2. *Renin* is released by the juxtaglomerular apparatus in nephron, which senses decreases in GFR. Renin release: kidney's effort to raise blood pressure and GFR
   3. *Angiotensin I* is released in response to rennin and converted to the potent vasoconstrictor *angiotensin II* at peripheral blood vessels and the lung.
   4. Reduction in GFR results from vasoconstriction; in other words, fluid volume status and renal perfusion stimulate *aldosterone* release from the adrenal cortex.

D. *Aldosterone:* primary mineralcorticoid hormone of adrenal cortex
   1. Acts at the kidney's renal tubule: actively increases total body water by regulating *sodium* reabsorption in response to serum osmolality
   2. Water migrates with sodium and is therefore retained.
   3. Aldosterone regulation does *not* alter ECF sodium concentration.
   4. Aldosterone regulates only about 2% of total body sodium, which sufficiently prevents hypovolemia and hypotension.
   5. Sodium retained, potassium or hydrogen ions excreted to maintain ion balance
   6. Decrease in aldosterone secretion excretes sodium and water, retains potassium

VI. Fluid imbalances (refer to Box 24-2)
A. Fluid spacing may be
   1. *Localized:* migration to single area or organ, as with a sprained ankle or blister
   2. *Multisystem:* postoperative migration to abdominal spaces after organ removal, repair of obstructions, or fluid leakage from sites of severe burns: third spacing
   3. Caused by
      a. *Decreased plasma proteins:* insufficient to maintain oncotic osmotic pressures and ECF fluid volumes—renal protein losses
      b. *Increased capillary permeability:* alteration from sepsis, allergic reaction, radiation, and trauma allows fluid leakage
      c. *Lymphatic blockage:* lymph system is an accessory route to return excess interstitial fluid and leaked proteins into vascular space.
   4. Related to anesthetic issues
      a. Anesthetic depth and medications, sepsis, or fever can mask fluid volume excess or deficit until the postoperative period.
      b. Rewarming after intraoperative hypothermia may cause peripheral vasodilation, thereby expanding the vascular compartment (ECF); transient but significant hypotension results, requiring fluid volume expansion

■ BOX 24-2
■ **REGULATORS OF FLUID AND ELECTROLYTE EQUILIBRIUM**

Diffusion:	Movement of *particles* such as potassium or calcium through a cell's permeable wall from an area of high concentration to a lower concentration
Osmosis:	Movement of *water* from a dilute solution toward a more concentrated fluid
Concentration gradient:	Difference in concentration (osmolality) between two solutions that promotes fluid or electrolyte movement
Osmotic pressure:	A physical force, determined by the number of particles in a solution (or its concentration) that causes water to move toward the concentrated solution
Oncotic pressure:	Osmotic force produced in vascular spaces by molecules such as plasma proteins
Antidiuretic hormone (ADH):	Hypothalamic hormone released by the posterior pituitary gland in response to increased serum osmolality; ADH regulates sodium concentration and thereby the passive movement of water toward sodium

   c. Spinal and epidural anesthetic techniques expand the ECF by dilating peripheral vasculature.
      (1) Vasopressors and fluid volume expansion is needed until anesthetic effects have resolved and normal vessel tone has returned, often well into the postanesthesia period.
      (2) Excess interstitial fluid and leaked proteins can flow back into vascular space.
5. Surgical shifts: third space fluid loss:
   a. Shifts begins immediately after massive trauma or surgery.
      (1) Capillary permeability increases.
         (a) Protein leaks from cell into inflamed or traumatized areas.
         (b) Fluid shifts through leaky cell walls from vascular to interstitial space.
      (2) Ongoing hypotension common
   b. Reabsorption phase: within 72 hours post injury or trauma
      (1) Injured tissues heal.
         (a) Capillaries repair: normal permeability restored
         (b) Lymph blockage clears.
         (c) Plasma proteins return to normal.
         (d) Capillary pressures, filtration, reabsorption restored
      (2) Fluid volume returns (shifts) to vascular compartment.
         (a) Urine volume increases as excess fluid excreted.
         (b) Low urine specific gravity
         (c) Fluid output *exceeds* intake.
         (d) Water weight loss
      (3) Monitor electrolytes homeostasis (refer to Box 24-1).
B. ECF volume deficit (hypovolemia): ECF shift to ICF, or total loss from body
   1. Caused by
      a. Abrupt decrease in fluid intake: NPO status
      b. Acute loss: blood loss (hemorrhage), fluid shifts caused by altered capillary membrane permeability, diuretics, excess fistula drainage, burns, vomiting, diarrhea
      c. Third spacing
   2. Assess and monitor
      a. Dehydration and hemoconcentration
         (1) Increased serum osmolality and sodium: thirst

(2) Impaired renal perfusion: oliguria (<15 ml/hour)
    (a) Low-volume concentrated urine, high specific gravity
    (b) Acute tubular necrosis (ATN) and renal failure if protracted
(3) Poor skin turgor: dry skin and mucous membranes
(4) Decreased cardiac output
    (a) Hypotension and tachycardia
    (b) Decreased central venous (CVP), pulmonary artery pressures
(5) Clear lung fields
(6) Inadequate cerebral perfusion: confusion, lethargy

3. Intervene and evaluate (refer to Boxes 24-3 and 24-4).
  a. Generous fluid replacement with isotonic solutions and/or colloid
  b. Treat underlying cause.
    (1) Return to operating room to reexplore, cauterize bleeding vessels, or repair anastamoses.
    (2) Replace large urine losses hourly, caused by diabetes insipidus, for example, and monitor electrolytes.

■ BOX 24-3
■ **SYMPTOMS ASSOCIATED WITH CHEMICAL AND FLUID IMBALANCES**

Symptom	Possible clinical significance
Cardiovascular	
Bounding pulse CVP, neck vein distention	Fluid overload, increased ECF
Weak or thready pulse	Dehydration, decreased ECF volume
Increased heart rate	May reflect fever, acidosis, or ECF volume deficit
Irregular pulse	Cardiac arrhythmia—may signal hypokalemia
Hypotension, orthostatic	ECF volume deficit
Respiratory	
Increased rate and depth	Anxiety with hyperventilation can prompt respiratory alkalosis.
	Perhaps compensation for retained carbon dioxide (acidosis)
Decreased rate and depth	Perhaps compensation for alkalosis and insufficient carbon dioxide
	Possible muscle weakness from hypermagnesemia or hypokalemia
	With somnolence, may signal oversedation
"Crackles" and rales at lung bases	Overhydration or cardiac congestion and failure
Neurologic	
Level of consciousness	Low or elevated sodium, dehydration, acid-base imbalance
Vertigo	ECF volume deficit
Muscle weakness	Severely elevated or low potassium, hypercalcemia, hypermagnesemia
	May reflect volume losses
Altered reflexes	Magnesium or calcium imbalance
Tingling	Hyperventilation with respiratory alkalosis
	Suspect calcium elevation
Excitability	Decreased calcium or magnesium
Skin	
Turgor at sternum	Dehydration if remains "tented" when pinched
	Not reflective of fluid status in elderly patients
Mucous membranes	Dryness may indicate ECF deficit.

■ BOX 24-4
■ **ECF VOLUME EXPANDERS**

Solution	Considerations
*Colloid**	Raise oncotic pressure in ECF
Synthetic fluids	Blood products refused, contraindicated
Hetastarch	Jehovah Witness beliefs
Dextran	High antibody titers: cannot cross-match
	Less expensive than blood products
	Caution: Can interfere with clotting
Albumin: 5%, 25%	
Blood products	Indicated by laboratory measures
	Anemia: Hemoglobin, hematocrit decrease
	Coagulopathy: Elevated INR, PTT
	Albumin decrease
*Crystalloid**	Restore circulating fluid volume, electrolytes
Hypertonic electrolyte solutions	Maintenance fluid: 100-200 ml/hour
Isotonic fluids	Operative: 1 to 2 L to rehydrate after NPO and replace
	surgical, insensible losses
	Critical hypovolemia, massive burns: replace up to 8-10 L
Hypotonic fluids	Rehydrate cells
	Hyperosmolar diabetes

*Preferred solution debatable: often colloids *and* crystalloids given in varying combinations

(3) Replace large fluid and electrolyte losses via surgical wound drains, nasogastric tube, vomiting, and diarrhea hourly,

C. ECF volume excess (hypervolemia): shift from ICF to ECF (serum) or *second spacing.*
  1. Caused by
    a. Fluid intake, either oral or parenteral, beyond physiologic tolerance
      (1) Renal failure: inability to excrete fluid
      (2) Congestive heart failure: circulatory overload
      (3) Remobilization of third space fluid 48-72 hours postoperatively
    b. Excess sodium intake
      (1) Intravenous sodium
      (2) Hyperaldosteronism: sodium retention
      (3) Seawater ingestion
    c. Sodium hemodilution: relative fluid excess
      (1) Intraoperative absorption of fluid through vascular "beds" during transurethral resection of prostate (TURP): confusion, hyponatremia, possibly seizures result
  2. Assess and monitor: overhydration, hemodilution, low osmolality
    a. Circulatory overload: observe
      (1) Increased CVP, pulmonary artery (PA) pressures
      (2) Congestive heart failure (CHF), pulmonary edema: respiratory compromise, rales, dyspnea, S3 heart sound
      (3) Peripheral edema: pitting edema at ankles, fingers, and eyelids
      (4) Jugular vein distention
      (5) Pleural effusion
      (6) Hypertension or hypotension, perhaps tachycardia
      (7) Renal perfusion
      (8) Skin: plump, moist, and perhaps weeping through pores
      (9) X-ray evidence of pulmonary congestion, enlarged cardiac silhouette
      (10) Hypoxia, hypercapnia per arterial blood gases, electrolyte measures
      (11) Mental status

3. Intervene and evaluate: Remove excess fluid, maintain electrolyte balance, unless hypernatremic.
    a. Treat underlying cause.
    b. Diuretics
    c. Fluid restriction

BIBLIOGRAPHY

1. Ard JL, Prough DS: Perioperative electrolyte and acid-base abnormalities. In Benumof JL, Saidman LG, editors:. *Anesthesia and perioperative complications*, ed 2. St Louis: Mosby, 1999, pp 503-535.
2. Chernecky C, Butler SW, Graham P, et al: *Real-world nursing survival guide: Fluids and electrolytes*. Philadelphia: WB Saunders, 2002.
3. Cowling GE, Haas RE: Hypotension in the PACU: An algorithmic approach. *J Perianesth Nurs* 17:159-163, 2002.
4. Ferrara-Love R: Immediate postanesthesia care. In Burden N, DeFazio Quinn DM, O'Brien D, et al, editors: *Ambulatory surgical nursing*, ed 2. Philadelphia: WB Saunders, 2000, pp 442-448.
5. Golembiewski JA, O'Brien D: A systematic approach to the management of postoperative nausea and vomiting. *J Perianesth Nurs* 17:364-376, 2002.
6. Goskowicz R: Complications of blood transfusions. In Benumof JL, Saidman LG, editors: *Anesthesia and perioperative complications*, ed 2. St Louis Mosby, 1999, pp 536-574.
7. Heitz UE, Horne MM, Webber KS: *Guide to fluid, electrolyte and acid-base balance*. St Louis: Mosby–Yearbook, 2001.
8. Krau SD: Selecting and managing fluid therapy. *Crit Care Nurs Clin North America* 10:401-410, 1998.
9. Litwack K: Perioperative fluid administration: Colloid or crystalloid. *Anesth Today* 8:15-18, 1997.
10. O'Flaherty JE, Berry FA: Anesthesia complications occurring primarily in the very young. In Benumof JL, Saidman LG, editors: *Anesthesia and perioperative complications*, ed 2. St Louis Mosby, 1999, pp 606-625.
11. Pandit UA, Pandit KS: Fasting before and after ambulatory surgery. *J Perianesth Nurs* 12:181-187, 1997.
12. Roth S, Gillesberg I: Injury to the visual system and other sensory organs. In Benumof JL, Saidman LG, editors: *Anesthesia and perioperative complications*, ed 2. St Louis: Mosby, 1999, pp 377-408.
13. Stark J: The interrelation between renal and cardiac function. *Crit Care Nurs Clin North America* 10:411-419, 1998.
14. Toto KH: Fluid balance assessment. *Crit Care Nurs Clin of North America* 10:383-400, 1998.
15. Woods S: Fluid and electrolyte homeostasis. In Kinney MR, Dunbar SB, Brooks-Brunn J, et al, editors: *AACN clinical reference for critical care nursing*, ed 4. St Louis: Mosby, 1998, pp 113-133.

CHAPTER

25 Acid-Base Balance

■■■ KATHLYN CARLSON

OBJECTIVES

At the conclusion of this chapter the reader will be able to:

1. Identify clinical situations suggesting need for arterial blood gases (ABGs).

2. Describe the components and values of ABGs.

3. Describe the steps in analysis of ABGs.

4. Identify acid-base imbalances and compensation mechanisms.

I. Acid-base concepts: Physiology of chemical balance
  A. Body cells: extremely sensitive to the chemical environment
    1. Cell wall protects environment to maintain life-sustaining, intracellular functions.
    2. Minor changes in acidity or alkalinity alter cellular function, cause cell death.
    3. Chemical imbalance affects electrolyte ionization and changes ion concentrations in solution.
    4. Carbonic acid (H_2CO_3), the body's dynamic chemical buffer system, compensates for moment-to-moment acid-base shifts to maintain acid-base "harmony" in a normal ratio of 20 base to 1 acid (see Table 25-1).
    5. Oxygen: critical component of acid-base balance; metabolism occurs even during oxygen lack, producing an acid environment.
    6. Adequate hemoglobin is a must for effective oxygen transport to cells.
    7. Extracellular fluid (ECF) is the accessible, and therefore measurable and treatable, body fluid to repair acid-base disharmony; semipermeable cell walls allow some equilibration of ions—therefore ICF is also affected.
    8. Carbon dioxide is more soluble in cool temperature; acidity increases.
  B. Perianesthesia concerns
    1. Acid-base disruption is relatively common among perianesthesia patients, whether preoperative or postoperative.
      a. Trauma, acute or chronic illness, surgical fluid shifts and anesthetic effects can disturb ability to sustain acid-base balance.
      b. The body of a healthy patient "automatically" compensates to sustain normal acid-base parameters.
      c. The perianesthesia nurse must recognize conditions that disrupt a patient's acid-base balance, understand ABG results, and quickly initiate nursing and ordered medical interventions.
      d. Acidosis is likely with hypothermia and hypoxia: *Warm* patients with active rewarming techniques and ensure *oxygenation*, supplementing if needed.
  C. Definitions
    1. Acid: A hydrogen ion (H^+) *donor* when a compound is in solution
      a. Reacts with a base to form an inert compound
      b. The body's primary acid is *hydrogen ion (H^+)*.
    2. Base: A hydrogen ion (H^+) *acceptor* when a compound is in solution
      a. Synonymous with the term *alkali*
      b. The body's primary base is bicarbonate (HCO_3^-).

TABLE 25-1

■ ■ Carbonic Acid Regulation of Acid-Base Balance

Immediate response as directed by *Henderson-Hasselbach equation*[*]:

Hydrogen	+	Bicarbonate	$\rightleftarrows$	Carbonic Acid	$\rightleftarrows$	Water	+	Carbon Dioxide
H^+	+	HCO_3^-	$\rightleftarrows$	H_2CO_3	$\rightleftarrows$	H_2O	+	CO_2

Acidic conditions (pH <7.35):
Bicarbonate ion is reabsorbed.
Recombines with hydrogen ion
Forms more carbonic acid

Alkalotic conditions (pH >7.45):

Bicarbonate ion excreted
Relative excess of hydrogen ion
Less carbonic acid is formed.

$H_2CO_3^-$ dissociates to water and CO_2.
Respiratory rate and depth increase.
CO_2 is exhaled (pCO$_2$↓).
pH restored (↑) toward 7.4

Respiratory rate and depth decrease.
CO_2 accumulates (p$_a$CO$_2$↑).
pH restored (↓) toward 7.4

[*]Henderson-Hasselbach equation: describes a dynamic buffer of body fluids. Hydrogen ion is regulated by combining with or dissociating from bicarbonate.

3. Acidosis: Abnormal *increase* of acid content within body fluids from accumulation of acid (H^+) or loss of base (HCO_3^-)
   a. May arise from respiratory or metabolic causes
   b. *Acidemia* refers to an acid condition in the blood.
4. Alkalosis: Abnormal *decrease* in acid content within body fluids from loss of acid (H^+) or accumulaton of base (HCO_3^-)
   a. *Alkalemia* refers to an alkaline status of blood.
D. Determinants of acid-base homeostasis
   1. pH: A mathematic calculation reflecting the concentration of hydrogen ion (H^+) in solution
      a. An abbreviation for "potential hydrogen"
      b. Is the negative logarithm of hydrogen ion in concentration
      c. Describes the relative balance between acids and bases in solution
      d. pH of a neutral, neither acid nor alkaline, solution is 7.0.
         (1) Increasing a solution's acidity (adding acid or H^+) *decreases* pH to <7.0.
         (2) Decreasing a solution's acidity (adding base by bicarbonate (HCO_3^-) or losing acid (H^+) *increases* pH to >7.0.
      e. Body's buffer systems normally maintain the pH of blood within a slightly alkaline range of 7.35-7.45.
      f. Definitive therapy is indicated when pH <7.15 or >7.60.
      g. Death is imminent at pH <6.90 or >7.90 if no intervention.
   2. Partial pressure of carbon dioxide (PaCO_2): Respiratory component, an *acid*
      a. Represents the partial pressure of carbon dioxide in *arterial* blood
      b. Dissolves in plasma to create carbonic acid (H_2CO_3): considered a nonfixed or volatile acid
      c. Regulated by *breathing* to exhale CO_2 (acid) from body
         (1) Encourage a groggy perianesthesia patient with a purely respiratory acidosis (elevated PaCO_2) to deep breathe; can correct this acid-base disturbance by exhaling excess carbon dioxide
      d. Residual muscle relaxant, sedation, and unresponsiveness may render the patient unable to follow the request to deep breathe; reintubation or positive pressure ventilation, manually or by mechanical ventilator, may be necessary.
         (1) A patient with severe metabolic acidosis will "automatically" compensate by increasing respirations to exhale excess acid in the form of carbon dioxide.
            (a) An example is the deep, regular Kussmaul respiration style in the patient with diabetic ketoacidosis.

3. Bicarbonate (HCO_3^-): Metabolic component
   a. Represents amount of HCO_3^- available to buffer acids
   b. Regulated at *kidney*: excreted or reabsorbed at the collecting tubule
   c. Influenced by amount of fixed (nonvolatile) acid
      (1) Infuse sodium bicarbonate to increase HCO_3^- levels and buffering capacity.
      (2) Correct other electrolyte disturbances.
4. Anion gap: Expressed as base excess (BE)
   a. Calculated difference between serum cations and anions
   b. Formula: Serum sodium value *minus* sum of bicarbonate and chloride

$$\text{Anion Gap} = Na^+ - (HCO_3^- + Cl^-)$$

   c. Normal anion gap = 8-16 milliosmoles per liter
   d. *Increased* anion gap: associated with metabolic acidosis
      (1) Ketoacidosis: diabetic, alcoholic, starvation
      (2) Lactic acidosis: hyoxia (anaerobic metabolism), shock, sepsis
      (3) Rhabdomyelosis: acute, massive tissue destruction
   e. *Normal* anion gap associated with metabolic acidosis: increased Cl^-
      (1) Diarrhea, intestinal or biliary fistulae
      (2) Excess intake of chlorine-containing acids
      (3) Excessive sodium chloride (NaCl) intake
5. Temperature: pH decreases (produces acidosis) as temperature decreases.
   a. PCO_2 decreases by 4.5% per degree centigrade.
   b. Hemoglobin, one of the body's acid-base buffers, accepts more hydrogen ions (H^+) in cool temperatures, so pH increases.
6. Oxygenation: PO_2, percent saturation and hemoglobin
   a. PO_2: measure of partial pressure of oxygen in arterial blood
   b. Oxygen loosely bound to hemoglobin or dissolved in blood
   c. *Oxyhemoblobin dissociation*: relationship between arterial PO_2 and oxygen bound to hemoglobin
      (1) PaO_2 >70 mm Hg is critical point: hemoglobin saturation is nearly 100%.
      (2) As PaO_2 dips <70 mm Hg, small decrease in PaO_2 correlates with large decrease in oxygen saturation as hemoglobin quickly releases oxygen to maintain tissue oxygenation.
         (a) When PaO_2 = 40 mm Hg, hemoglobin <80% saturated
         (b) Temperature, acidosis ($PaCO_2$) affect binding or release of oxygen to hemoglobin.

II. Primary acid-base imbalance
   A. Acidosis
      1. *Respiratory*: $PaCO_2$ >45 and pH <7.35
         a. Results from alveolar hypoventilation: failure to excrete carbonic acid
         b. Metabolic state normal
         c. Clinical causes
            (1) *Depression* of central respiratory centers
               (a) Effects of residual anesthetic agents, such as muscle relaxants that render the patient unable to breathe effectively
               (b) Consider pseudocholinesterase deficiency if respiratory effort ineffective after succinylcholine
               (c) Sedation from narcotics or hypnotic (intentional or as part of conscious sedation) or caused by overmedication.
               (d) Compression of medullary centers increases intracranial pressure:
                  (i) Edema from surgical intervention or trauma
                  (ii) Masses caused by lesions
                  (iii) Increased PCO_2, a potent vasoconstrictor
               (e) Hypothermia: Slows metabolism of depressant meds
               (f) Exhaustion from ineffective respiratory effort
            (2) Interference with *muscles* of respiration
               (a) Residual effects of neuromuscular blocking agents

(b) Pain causes splinting and limited chest expansion, more pronounced after thoracic and abdominal surgery.

(c) Physical limitation of chest expansion from tight chest binders, chest tubes and dressings, from burn eschar, kyphosis —humpback

(d) Obesity: lung expansion especially hampered in supine   spinal curvature position

(e) Neuromuscular diseases: myasthenia gravis, poliomyelitis

(f) Inadequate mechanical ventilation: rate or tidal volume too low to exhale carbon dioxide

  (3) Airway *obstruction*

(a) Oropharynx: secretions, relaxed tongue, pharyngeal edema, tracheal or subglottic stenosis

(b) Laryngospasm or bronchospasm

(c) Pulmonary aspiration

(d) Endotracheal tube (ET)

    (i) Malpositioned results in single lung ventilation.

    (ii) Blocked by secretions or kinks

  (4) Pulmonary *disease*

(a) Chronic obstructive pulmonary disease (COPD)

(b) Pulmonary fibrosis

(c) Atelectasis and pneumonia

(d) Asthma

d. Therapeutic interventions to correct

  (1) Stimulate! Stir up! Remind patient to breathe.

  (2) Ensure airway patency.

(a) Jaw lift, head reposition, suction, insert oral or nasal airway.

(b) Intubation if stimulation is ineffective

(c) Mechanical ventilation as needed

  (3) Provide oxygen.

  (4) Reverse muscle relaxants and/or sedatives or narcotics.

  (5) Mechanically rewarm a hypothermic patient.

2. *Metabolic:* HCO_3^- <22 and pH <7.35

a. Results from accumulated ionized acid (H^+) or depletion of base

b. Respiratory status normal, except as in compensation

c. Clinical causes

  (1) Acid *overproduction:* promotes *potassium* release from cells

(a) Ketoacidosis: diabetic or starvation

(b) Anaerobic metabolism: lactate production (acidosis)

(c) Renal failure, acute and chronic

(d) Muscle destruction: rhabdomyolysis

(e) Overdose: salicylic acid (aspirin) or ferrous sulfate (iron)

    (i) Salicylate metabolites increased fixed acids

    (ii) Directly stimulates respiratory chemoreceptors to cause hyperventilation

    (iii) Respiratory alkalosis predominates in adults.

    (iv) Metabolic acidosis predominates in infants, young children.

(f) Fevers caused by infection

  (2) Severe bicarbonate *loss*

(g) GI: diarrhea, small bowel or pancreatic fistulae

(h) Excessive doses: acetazolamide (Diamox) or ammonium chloride

d. Therapeutic interventions to correct

  (1) Encourage deep breathing (increase respiratory rate and depth) so carbon dioxide exhaled

  (2) Administer sodium bicarbonate, usually 50 mEq/kg.

  (3) Remonitor ABGs, K^+ retreat as needed: aim for slow resolution.

  (4) Give insulin to return potassium to cells as acidosis resolves.

(5) Monitor cardiac rhythm (electrocardiogram) for arrhythmia, peaked T waves.

(6) Frequently monitor vital signs, neurologic, respiratory status.

B. Alkalosis

1. *Respiratory*: $Paco_2$ <35 and pH >7.45

a. Results from alveolar *hyperventilation:* oversecretion of carbonic acid

b. Respirations increased, metabolic status normal

c. Clinical causes

(1) Psychogenic causes: pain, anxiety and panic

(2) Respiratory center overstimulation: Tumors at medulla or pons, surgical manipulation of brainstem

(3) Overzealous mechanical ventilation: rate, tidal volume too high

(4) Normal finding in pregnancy

d. Patient reports headache, dizziness, tingling, paresthesias.

e. Therapeutic interventions to correct

(1) Sedate or provide analgesia.

(2) Coach breathing: slow, regular, moderate depth.

(3) Emotional support and calming reassurance.

(4) Adjust mechanical ventilator settings to reduce rate, tidal volume.

(5) Monitor ABGs, labs, clinical status.

2. *Metabolic* HCO_3^- >26 and pH >7.45

a. Results from excessive loss of acid (H^+) or accumulation of bases

b. Respirations normal, though may be shallow as compensatory means

c. Clinical causes

(1) Excessive loss of highly acid HCl in upper gastrointestinal tract, or insufficient replacement: Protracted vomiting, gastric suction or lavage

(2) Excessive circulating bicarbonate (HCO_3^-):

(a) Chemical response relative to chlorine loss

(b) Overcorrection of acidosis with bicarbonate

(c) Overingestion of antacid or baking soda

(d) Overinfusion of lactated solution

(3) Overretention of base ions

(a) Diuretics: furosemide (Lasix) and thiazides

(b) Excessive administration of corticosteroids

(4) Systemic diseases: Cushing's syndrome, aldosteronism

d. Therapeutic interventions to correct

(1) Treat or eliminate cause.

(2) Monitor lab values, particularly hypokalemia as K^+ moves to cell.

(3) Observe clinical status, reporting confusion, muscle cramps, twitching, tingling.

III. Mixed acid-base imbalances

A. Inadequate compensation: several concurrent acid-base disorders

1. For example, if pH <7.35 + $Paco_2$ = 55 + HCO_3^- = 14, both respiratory and metabolic component cause acidosis.

a. Could occur in patient with chronic lung disease (chronic respiratory acidosis, usually compensated) who develops diarrhea with large HCO_3^- losses

B. pH change is dramatic with mixed acidosis or mixed alkalosis disorders.

C. pH change less severe if mixed acidosis-alkalosis: opposing disorders balance

IV. Physiologic compensation of acid-base imbalances

A. The body's natural effort to restore acid to base ratio toward 1:20 and pH toward 7.40

1. *Compensation* occurs when pH is within normal range.

2. *Partial compensation* results when $Paco_2$ or HCO_3^- changes but pH changes minimally.

3. Rarely overcompensates

B. Compensation for *respiratory acidosis* occurs slowly in *kidneys* over days.
  1. Reabsorption of bicarbonate ion (HCO_3^-)
  2. Excretion of hydrogen ion (H^+): acidic urine results.
C. Compensation for *respiratory alkalosis* occurs in *kidneys*.
  1. Excretion of bicarbonate ion (HCO_3^-)
  2. Retention of hydrogen ion (H^+): results in alkalotic urine
D. Compensation for *metabolic acidosis* occurs rapidly in *lungs* over minutes to days.
  1. Hyperventilation to *eliminate* carbon dioxide (CO_2)
E. Compensation for metabolic alkalosis
  1. Hypoventilation to *accumulate* carbon dioxide (CO_2)
V. Interpreting arterial blood gases (ABGs)
  A. Purpose for measuring ABGs
    1. Determine status of alveolar ventilation and arterial oxygenation.
      a. Determine acid-base status of patient.
      b. Guide respiratory and metabolic interventions.
      c. Must interpret in the context of the patient's clinical status
  B. Systematic ABG analysis: name the disorder
    1. Consider pH, the acidosis/alkalosis component—*normal: 7.35 to 7.45*
      a. If <7.35 (low), condition is *acidosis*
      b. If >7.45 (high), condition is *alkalosis*
      c. If in normal range, condition is "normal pH," and patient either has normal acid-base balance or acidosis or alkalosis is *compensated*.
    2. Next, consider $Paco_2$, the respiratory component—*normal: 35-45 mm Hg*
      a. If <35 mm Hg (decreased) and pH high, condition is *respiratory alkalosis*
      b. If >45 mm Hg (elevated) and pH low, condition is *respiratory acidosis*
      c. If normal, move on to consider HCO_3^- as cause of high or low pH.
    3. Then, consider HCO_3^-, the metabolic component—*normal: 22-26 mEq/L*
      a. If <22 mEq/L (low) and pH high, condition is *metabolic* acidosis
      b. If >26 mEq/L (high) and pH low, condition is *metabolic* alkalosis
    4. Consider Pao_2: Is patient hypoxic? *Normal: 80-100 mm Hg*
      a. If <80 mm Hg: Stimulate patient to increase respiratory effort, treat airway obstructon, pulmonary congestion, obstruction or bronchospasm, or measure hemoglobin level.
      b. If >100 mm Hg: Monitor status.
      c. If >150 mm Hg, adjust oxygen delivery.
      d. Is *percent saturation* >95%? Verify respiratory quality and adequacy of circulating hemoglobin to transport oxygen.
      e. Remember that hypoxemia contributes to acidosis.
    5. Determine abnormality and determine whether acute (primary abnormality) or compensated.
      a. Assess pH to identify the trend.
      b. If pH within normal range but not exactly 7.40
        (1) If pH is 7.35 to 7.39, leans toward acidosis
        (2) If pH is 7.41 to 7.45, leans toward alkalosis
      c. Determine processes $Paco_2$ and HCO_3^- as in steps 2 and 3 above.
        (1) *Primary* process: signified by component that supports leaning tendency of pH
        (2) Com*pensation:* signified by component that supports opposite tendency before treatment is initiated
      d. Now state your decision based on the ABG facts.
        (1) Does decision mesh with the patient's history or clinical status?
          (a) Respiratory acidosis or metabolic acidosis?
          (b) Respiratory alkalosis or metabolic alkalosis?
        (2) Report ABG results to physician; plan interventions.

BIBLIOGRAPHY

1. Agodoa L: Acute renal failure in the PACU. *J PeriAnesth Nurs* 17:377-383, 2002.
2. Ayrd JL, Prough DS: Perioperative electrolyte and acid-base abnormalities. In Benumof JL, Saidman LJ, editors: *Anesthesia and perioperative complications,* ed 2. St Louis: Mosby, 1999, pp 503-535.
3. Berry BE, Pinard AE: Assessing tissue oxygenation. *Crit Care Nurse* 22:22-40, 2002.
4. Czekaj LA: Promoting acid-base balance. In Kinney MR, Brooks-Brunn, et al, editors: *AACN clinical reference for critical care nursing,* ed 4. St Louis: Mosby, 1998, pp 135-145.
5. Gorgono AW: Fundamentals of acid-base balance. New Orleans: Department of Anesthesiology, Tulane University School of Medicine, 2003. Available at http://gasnet.med.yale.edu/acid-base. Accessed on January 1, 2003.
6. Heitz UE, Horne MM, Wevver KS, et al: *Guide to fluid, electrolyte and acid-base balance.* St Louis: Mosby, 2001.
7. O'Brien D: Acute postoperative delirium: Definitions, incidence, recognition, and interventions. *J PeriAnesth Nurs* 17:384-392, 2002.
8. Schlichtig R, Grogono AW, Severinghaus JW: Current status of acid-base quantitation in physiology and medicine. *Anesth Clin North America* 16:211-233, 1998.
9. Simpson PJ, Popat M: *Understanding anaesthesia,* ed 4. Boston: Butterworth/Heinemann, 2002.
10. Toto K: Fluid balance assessment. *Crit Care Nurs Clin North America* 10:383-400, 1998.

26 Anesthetic Agents and Adjuncts

LOIS SCHICK

■■■ Note: Dosage guidelines presented in this chapter are for healthy adults unless otherwise stated.

OBJECTIVES

At the conclusion of this chapter the reader will be able to:

1. Describe anesthetic options used.
2. Recognize the local anesthetics used for regional anesthesia.
3. Review the postanesthesia care unit (PACU) nursing care implications for patients who have received epidural and spinal anesthetics.
4. Differentiate between thiopental, methohexital, etomidate, ketamine, and propofol as intravenous (IV) anesthetics.
5. Identify the PACU nursing care implications for patients who have received benzodiazepines.
6. Identify common pharmacologic properties of opioids.
7. Describe the physiologic and pharmacologic differences between depolarizing and nondepolarizing muscle relaxants.
8. Define the mechanism of action of anticholinesterase reversal agents.
9. Describe the use of anticholinergic agents in anesthesia.
10. Recognize the mechanism of action of inhalation anesthetics.
11. Identify properties specific to each inhalation anesthetic.
12. Describe implications for the PACU nurse in caring for patients who have received inhalation agents.

I. Consider anesthesia as a continuum from an awake conscious state to an unconscious state (see Table 26-1).
   A. Awake
   B. Minimal sedation (anxiolysis)
      1. Patient remains conscious.
      2. Responds normally to verbal commands
      3. Ventilatory and cardiovascular functions are unaffected.
   C. Moderate sedation and analgesia or monitored anesthesia care (MAC)
      1. Drug-induced minimally depressed level of consciousness
      2. Patient maintains patent airway independently and continuously.
      3. Patient responds to verbal commands.
      4. Cardiovascular function is usually maintained.
      5. Patient does not lose consciousness.
      6. When provided by anesthesiologist, is known as MAC
   D. Deep sedation and analgesia
      1. Patient may sleep and may be aroused.
      2. Respond purposefully following repeated or painful stimulation
         a. Reflex withdrawal is not considered a purposeful response.

■ TABLE 26-1
■ ■ Continuum of Anesthetic Options

Awake-conscious	Awake/moderate Sedation	Moderate Sedation/deep Sedation	Deep Sedation	General Anesthesia
NONE	**LOCAL ANESTHESIA**			**Sedatives/hypnotics**
			Gaseous inhalation	
	Topical	**INTRAVENOUS**	**Anesthetic**	Etomidate (Amidate)
	EMLA	Droperidol	Nitrous oxide	Propofol (Diprivan)
		Anticholinesterases		**Intravenous barbiturates**
		Neostigmine	**Dissociative**	Thiopental
	REGIONAL	Edrophonium	Ketamine (Ketalar)	Methohexital
	IV regional blocks	Pyridostigmine		
	Bier			**Inhalation**
Oxygen		**Benzodiazepines**		Halothane
	Peripheral nerve block	Diazepam		Enflurane (Ethrane)
		(Valium)		
	Cervical plexus	Midazolam		Isoforane (Forane)
		(Versed)		
	Brachial plexus	Lorazepam		Desflurane
		(Ativan)		(Suprane)
	Digital			Sevoflurane (Ultane)
		Benzodiazepine		**Depolarizing**
	Intercostal	**antagonist**		**muscle relaxants**
	Lower extremity	Fluzamenil		Succinylcholine
				Nondepolarizing
	Sympathetic block	**IV OPIOIDS**		**muscle relaxants**
	Stellate ganglion	Morphine		Atracurium (Tracrium)
	Celiac plexus	Meperidine		Cisatracurium (Nimbex)
	Lumbar	Dilaudid		Curare (d-tubocurarine)
		Alfentanil		Doxacruium (Nuromax)
	Regional blocks	Fentanyl		Gallamine
	Caudal	Remifentanil		Metocurine
	Epidural	Sufentanil		Mivacurium
	Spinal			(Mivacron)
				Pancuronium (Pavulon)
				Pipercuronium
				(Arduan)
				Rocuronium
				(Zemuron)
				Vecuronium
				(Norcuron)
				Nondepolarizing muscle relaxant reversals
				Anticholinesterases
				Neostigmine
				Edrophonium (Enlon)
				Pyridostigmine
				Anticholinergics
				Atropine
				Scopolomine
				Glycopyrollate
				(Robinul)

See Table 26-3 for regional anesthetic medications.

   3. May require assistance in maintaining a patent airway
   4. Ability to independently maintain ventilatory function may be impaired.
   5. Cardiovascular function is usually maintained.
  E. General anesthesia
   1. Patient is not arousable.
   2. Ability to independently maintain ventilatory function is often impaired.
   3. Assistance to maintain a patent airway is often required.
   4. Positive pressure ventilation may be required because of depressed spontaneous ventilation or drug-induced depression of neuromuscular function.
   5. Cardiovascular function may be impaired.
   6. Reversible state providing
     a. Analgesia
     b. Sedation
     c. Appropriate muscle relaxation
     d. Appropriate control of autonomic nervous system
     e. Partial or complete loss of protective reflexes
 II. Pharmacokinetics and pharmacodynamics
  A. Pharmacokinetics
   1. Relationship between
     a. Dose of drug administration
     b. Concentration of drug delivered to site of action
   2. What the body does to the drugs (i.e., drug uptake, distribution, biotransformation, excretion of drugs)
     a. How the body
       (1) Absorbs
       (2) Distributes
       (3) Metabolize
       (4) Excretes
  B. Pharmacodynamics (i.e., additive, synergistic, antagonistic effect)
   1. Relationship between
     a. Concentration of drugs at site of action
     b. Intensity of effect produced
   2. What the drugs do to the body
III. Stages of anesthesia (see Figure 26-1)
  A. Stage I: Stage of anesthesia and amnesia
   1. Begins with initiation of anesthesia and ends with loss of consciousness
     a. Patient can follow simple commands.
     b. Protective reflexes remain intact.
  B. Stage II: Stage of delirium
   1. Starts with loss of consciousness and ends with disappearance of lid reflex
     a. Respirations irregular
     b. May be passed through quickly with newer anesthetic agents
  C. Stage III: Stage of surgical anesthesia
   1. Cessation of spontaneous respirations
     a. Absence of
       (1) Eyelash response
       (2) Blink
       (3) Swallowing reflexes
  D. Stage IV: Cessation of respiration to circulatory collapse
   1. Considered overdose of anesthetic
IV. Anesthesia options (see Table 26-3)
  A. Local and regional anesthetic agents
   1. Common property general facts

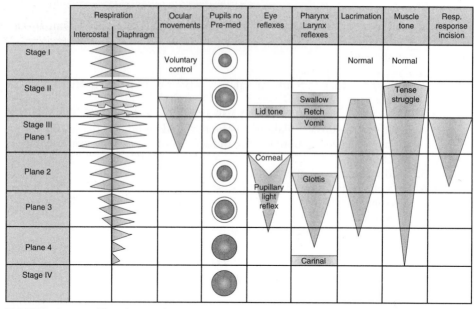

FIGURE 26-1 ■ The signs and reflex reactions of the stages of anesthesia. (From Drain CB: *Perianesthesia nursing: A critical care approach,* ed 4. St Louis: WB Saunders, 2003, p 277. Adapted from Gillespie NA: Signs of anesthesia. *Anesth Analg* 22:275, 1943.)

■ BOX 26-1
■ **SEQUENCE OF SPINAL RESOLUTION**

Order of Loss of Function
- Autonomic or sympathetic functions (vasomotor, bladder control)
- Sense of temperature
- Pain
- Touch
- Movement
- Proprioception (sense of body location)
  - Example: "Phantom response" is a response in which patients may ask you to straighten their legs when they are already straight. The last position the patients were in prior to the regional medications taking effect is that position they believe they are still in.
- Last blocked is first to recover.

Order of Return of Function
- Proprioception
- Movement
- Touch
- Pain
- Sense of temperature
- Autonomic or sympathetic functions (vasomotor, bladder control)

    a. Agents that impair conduction of neurally mediated impulses
    b. Two chemical groups
       (1) Esters: cocaine, procaine, chloroprocaine, tetracaine
       (2) Amides: prilocaine, lidocaine, mepivacaine, bupivacaine, etidocaine, ropivacaine, chirocaine
  2. Physiology: three major classes of nerves (see Table 26-2)
    a. A fibers: myelinated somatic nerves
    b. B fibers: myelinated preganglionic autonomic nerves

■ TABLE 26-2
■ ■ **Classification of Nerve Fibers**

Fiber Type	Myelin	Diameter (μm)	Function
Aα	+++	10-20	Motor neurons (efferent: to skeletal muscle)
Aβ	++	5-10	Touch, pressure, and proprioception neurons (afferent: from skin)
Aγ	++	5-10	Motor neurons (efferent: to muscle spindles)
Aδ	++	1-5	Pain (sharp/fast) and temperature neurons (afferent: from skin)
B	+	1-2.5	Preganglionic sympathetic neurons (efferent: to vascular smooth muscle)
C	±	0.5-1	Pain (dull/slow) and temperature neurons (afferent from skin) Postganglionic sympathetic neurons (efferent: to vascular smooth muscle)

        c. C fibers: lightly myelinated postganglionic autonomic nerves
        d. Pharmacodynamics
            (1) Impair conduction of impulses along axons
                (a) Effect mediated by blocking sodium channels
                (b) Communication between central nervous system (CNS) and peripheral nervous system is impaired.
                (c) Block is reversible and dose dependent.
            (2) Rank order of nerve fiber sensitivity to local anesthetic blockade
                (a) B > C and Aδ > Aγ > Aß > Aα
            (3) Rank order of nerve fiber diameters:
                (a) C < B < Aδ < Aß and Aγ < Aα (thinnest/least myelinated nerves blocked first)
            (4) Two separate pain-conducting pathways (both blocked by same tissue concentration of agent)
                (a) C fibers (slow pain)
                (b) Aδ fibers (fast pain)
        e. Pharmacokinetics (see Table 26-3)
            (1) Esters: hydrolyzed by plasma cholinesterase
            (2) Amides: metabolized in liver
      3. Esters
        a. Cocaine
            (1) First ester class drug used for clinical local anesthesia in 1884
            (2) Excellent topical anesthetic
            (3) Used for anesthesia and vasoconstriction in the nasal mucosa before nasotracheal intubation and during nasal operations
            (4) Sympathomimetic properties
                (a) Causes accumulation of synaptic norepinephrine
                (b) Inhibits reuptake of norepinephrine released from adrenergic nerve endings.
                (c) Increased synaptic norepinephrine thus facilitates sympathomimetic responses.
                (d) Warning: Cocaine can cause severe increases in heart rate and blood pressure.
            (5) CNS stimulant, especially cerebral cortex, because of accumulating synaptic norepinephrine.
            (6) Pyrogenic activity: potential side effect

■ TABLE 26-3
■ ■ **Local Anesthetics Used for Regional Techniques**

Drug	Onset	Duration (minutes)	Local	Topical	IV block	Peripheral	Epidural	Spinal
ESTERS								
Cocaine	Rapid	10-55	No	Yes	No	No	No	No
Procaine (Novocaine)	Slow	15-30	Yes	No	No	Yes	No	Yes
Chloroprocaine (Nesacaine)	Rapid	15-30	Yes	No	No	Yes	Yes	No
Tetracaine (Pontocaine)	Slow	120-240	No	Yes	No	No	No	Yes
AMIDES								
Prilocaine (Citanest)	Slow	60-120	Yes	No	Yes	Yes	Yes	No
Lidocaine	Rapid	60-120	Yes	Yes	Yes	Yes	Yes	Yes
Mepivacaine (Carbocaine)	Slow	45-90	Yes	No	No	Yes	Yes	No
Bupivacaine (Marcaine, Sensorcaine)	Slow	120-240	Yes	No	No	Yes	Yes	Yes
Etidocaine (Duranest)	Slow	240-480	Yes	No	No	Yes	Yes	No
Ropivacaine (Naropin)	Rapid	240-360	Yes	No	Yes	Yes	Yes	Yes
Levobupicaine (Chirocaine)			Yes	No	No	Yes	Yes	Yes

  (7) Administration route and dosage
    (a) Topical use as 4% to 10% solution for mucous membrane anesthesia, especially nasopharynx
    (b) No other uses because of side effects and toxicities
  (8) Pharmacokinetics
    (a) Well absorbed from all routes
    (b) Hydrolyzed by plasma cholinesterases
  (9) Drug interaction: Causes myocardium to be more responsive and sensitive to catecholamines.
  (10) Nursing considerations:
    (a) Potential for toxicity
    (b) High potential for abuse: powerful cortical stimulant
 b. Procaine (Novocaine)
  (1) First synthetic ester class local anesthetic (1904)
  (2) Administration route
    (a) Local infiltration
    (b) Peripheral nerve block
    (c) Spinal anesthesia
  (3) Pharmacokinetics
    (a) Absorption
      (i) Vasoconstrictors prolong local anesthetic action: slower absorption diminishes chance for systemic toxicity.
    (b) Metabolized by plasma cholinesterases, which include pseudocholinesterase (PChE)
 c. Chloroprocaine (Nesacaine)
  (1) Rapid onset, short duration, little systemic toxicity ester class drug

(2) Thrombophlebitis is frequent side effect.

(3) Notoriety of causing spinal neuropathy has limited its use.

    (a) Toxicity traced to bisulfite preservative and acidic pH of its solution

    (b) Toxic combination of preservative and acidic solution is now removed.

(4) Administration route

    (a) Local infiltration

    (b) Peripheral nerve block

    (c) Epidural anesthesia (lumbar and caudal routes)

(5) Pharmacokinetics: metabolized by plasma cholinesterases (including PChE)

(6) Pharmacodynamics: blocks sensory more than motor nerves

d. Tetracaine (pontocaine)

(1) Slow onset of analgesia, long duration, ester class drug synthesized in 1931

(2) Ten times more potent and toxic than procaine

(3) Causes extensive motor and sympathetic blockade

(4) Administration route

    (a) Topical anesthesia

        (i) Corneal

        (ii) Endotracheal topical anesthesia

    (b) Spinal anesthesia

        (i) Isobaric solutions: 2-3 hours spinal anesthesia

        (ii) Add epinephrine: 4-6 hours duration

(5) Pharmacokinetics

    (a) Readily absorbed from all routes

    (b) Metabolized by plasma cholinesterases (including PChE)

(6) Pharmacodynamics

    (a) Blocks sensory and motor nerves equally well

4. Amino-amides

a. Prilocaine (Citanest)

(1) Intermediate potency amino-amide class drug

(2) Duration: 60 minutes

(3) Less vasodilation than lidocaine

(4) Uses

    (a) Local

    (b) Peripheral nerve block

    (c) Intravenous

    (d) Epidural

    (e) Subarachnoid

b. Lidocaine

(1) Medium-acting local anesthetic of amide class

(2) Quick, potent, and longer lasting than procaine

(3) High incidence of sleepiness and dizziness

(4) IV lidocaine depresses laryngeal and tracheal reflexes.

(5) Notable antidysrhythmic properties on the myocardium

(6) When infiltrated as a local anesthetic, its vasodilator activity facilitates its rate of absorption.

    (a) Epinephrine (coadministered with lidocaine) decreases this vasodilation and absorption.

    (b) Mepivacaine (another local anesthetic, see Section c) does not have this vasodilator effect and thus can be a substitute for lidocaine with epinephrine when epinephrine's use is not desirable.

(7) Administration route and dosage

    (a) Local infiltration, 0.5% to 2% (with or without epinephrine)

    (b) Peripheral nerve block, 1% to 2% solutions (with or without epinephrine)

(c) Epidural anesthesia, 1.5% to 2% solutions
  (i) Average dose: 15 to 20 ml of 1.5% to 2% solution
  (ii) Duration: 0.75 to 1.5 hours
(d) Spinal anesthesia, hyperbaric, 1.5% or 5% solutions (with or without dextrose)
  (i) Average dose: 50 to 80 mg (1 to 1.6 ml)
  (ii) Duration: 0.75 to 1.5 hours
  (iii) Note: Because of a possible association with transient radicular irritation (TRI), it is now recommended that the 5% lidocaine solution be diluted with cerebrospinal fluid (CSF) to a final concentration of 2% before injection.
(e) Topical anesthesia, 2% jelly or 4% solution
(f) Intravenous (Bier) block, 40 to 50 ml of 0.5% solution
(8) Pharmacokinetics: metabolized by hepatic microsomal enzymes
(9) Pharmacodynamics: blocks sensory and motor nerves equally well
(10) Nursing considerations
  (a) Lidocaine (topical or IV) is useful in anesthetizing the trachea prior to intubation.
  (b) Topical or IV lidocaine will depress laryngeal and tracheal reflexes.
C. Mepivacaine (Carbocaine)
  (1) Medium-acting local anesthetic of amide class
  (2) Longer duration of action than lidocaine
  (3) Does not cause vasodilation as does lidocaine
  (4) Moderate potency and toxicity
  (5) Administration route and dosage
    (a) Local infiltration, 1% to 2% solutions
    (b) Peripheral nerve block, 1% to 2% solution
    (c) Epidural anesthesia (lumbar and caudal routes), 1% to 2% solutions
      (i) Average dose: up to 25 ml of 2% solution
      (ii) Duration: 1 to 2 hours
    (d) Not for use in spinal anesthesia
  (6) Pharmacokinetics: longer acting than lidocaine
  (7) Pharmacodynamics: similar to lidocaine (and other amide local anesthetics) except it does not cause vasodilation (alternative to lidocaine with epinephrine)
d. Bupivacaine (Marcaine, Sensorcaine)
  (1) High potency amino-amide
  (2) Long duration of action, 3 to 10 hours
  (3) Residual analgesia outlasts anesthetic effects
  (4) Cardiac toxicity—warning: Excessive dosing or accidental IV injection can cause ventricular dysrhythmias that are difficult to correct; do not exceed the maximally allowed dose (see Section 9, following).
  (5) Administration route and dosage
    (a) Epidural or caudal anesthesia, 0.25% to 0.5% solutions
      (i) Average dose: 15 to 20 ml of 0.5% solution
      (ii) Duration: 2 to 4 hours
    (b) Spinal anesthesia, 0.75% solution (with or without dextrose)
      (i) Average dose: 7.5 to 12 mg (1 to 1.6 ml)
      (ii) Duration: 2 to 4 hours
  (6) Pharmacokinetics: metabolized by hepatic microsomal enzymes
  (7) Pharmacodynamics: blocks sensory more than motor nerves
  (8) Uses
    (a) Local
    (b) Peripheral nerve block
    (c) Intravenous

(d) Epidural

(e) Subarachnoid

(9) Nursing considerations

(a) Has a prolonged anesthetic and analgesic action

(b) Frequently infiltrated during surgery as a postoperative analgesic for incision pain (analgesia lasts about 4 to 8 hours)

(c) May cause ventricular dysrhythmias when local anesthetic doses become excessive or are injected intravenously by accident. Treatment must be with bretylium or amiodarone. Lidocaine will be ineffective or may worsen condition.

e. Etidocaine (Duranest)

(1) High potency amino-amide of long duration

(2) Duration 5-10 hours

(3) Need high concentration for adequate sensory block

(4) Uses

(a) Local

(b) Peripheral nerve block

(c) Epidural

f. Ropivacaine (Naropin)

(1) High potency amino-amide

(2) Chemically similar to bupivacaine

(3) Produces less motor blockage than bupivacaine

(4) Duration as long as 12 hours

(a) Similar anesthetic properties to bupivacaine (i.e., both have more of an effect on sensory nerves than on motor nerves, although ropivacaine may have slightly less effect on motor nerves)

(b) Appears to be somewhat less cardiotoxic than bupivacaine, however, cardiotoxicity may still be of concern with slightly larger doses

(c) Preliminary clinical experience suggests a dosing schedule similar to that of bupivacaine.

(5) Uses

(a) Epidural

(b) Safe for obstetric use

g. Levobupivacaine (Chirocaine)

(1) Amino-amide local infiltrate

(2) Similar pharmacokinetic profile as bupivacaine

(3) Fast onset, moderate duration

(4) Used for surgical anesthesia and pain management cases

(5) May be administered in combination with epidural fentanyl or clonidine

h. Preservative-free morphine

(1) General facts

(a) Brand names: Duramorph, Astramorph, and others

(b) Used as an adjunct for neuroaxial (NA) anesthesia

(c) Epidural administration provides pain relief for extended periods.

(i) No loss of motor or sensory functions

(ii) Some dose-dependent decreases in sympathetic function may occur.

(iii) Respiratory depression is always possible but not likely if conservative doses are given.

(d) Onset occurs 15 to 60 minutes after NA administration; analgesia may last 12 to 36 hours.

(e) Initial adult dose is 2 to 5 mg.

(f) Delayed respiratory depression is possible.

(i) Patient should be monitored for 18 to 24 hours after administration, depending on dose given.

(g) Resuscitation equipment and naloxone should be available to counteract any potential respiratory depressant effects.

(h) Nausea and vomiting possible; need for antiemetics should be anticipated

V. Regional techniques
  A. General facts
    1. Anesthetic is injected into or around a nerve or nerve plexus.
      a. Requires a knowledge of anatomy
      b. Absorption of excessive doses can lead to systemic toxicity.
      c. Epinephrine-containing solutions will delay systemic absorption and thus decrease systemic toxicity.
  B. Topical
    1. Anesthetic is applied directly to:
      a. Skin
      b. Mucous membrane
      c. Urethra
      d. Nose
      e. Pharynx
    2. Systemic absorption occurs after application to mucous membranes.
      a. Increases the risk of toxicity if excessive doses are applied
        (1) Especially true of the vascular tracheobronchial tree
  C. Intravenous (Bier blocks)
    1. Produces anesthesia of the arm or leg
    2. Injection of large volumes of local anesthetic intravenously while the circulation to the extremity is occluded by a tourniquet
    3. Onset rapid, muscle relaxation profound
    4. Duration depends on tourniquet time inflation.
    5. Risk of toxicity when tourniquet released
    6. No analgesia after circulation restored
  D. Local infiltration and field blocks
    1. Anesthetic is injected directly into tissue.
    2. Field block: anesthetic injected into surrounding tissue
      a. Blocks transmission of sensory impulses
      b. Warning: epinephrine-containing solutions should not be infiltrated into confined areas (fingers, toes, ears, nose, penis); gangrene may develop.
    3. Peripheral nerve block: Specific site to block conduction
      a. Complications common to nerve blocks
        (1) Reaction to local anesthetic
        (2) Nerve damage
        (3) Failed block
        (4) Hematoma
      b. Infiltration—inject into tissue
      c. Field block—inject into surrounding tissues
      d. Cervical plexus block
        (1) Formed by first four cervical nerves
        (2) Common use for carotid endarterectomy
      e. Brachial plexus
        (1) Formed by anterior rami of C5-C8 and T1, which divide into three trunks to supply the shoulders and upper extremity
        (2) Three approaches
          (a) Interscalene used for shoulder
          (b) Supraclavicular anesthetizes entire plexus
            (i) Risk of pneumothorax
          (c) Axillary
            (i) Most popular
            (ii) Easy and safe
            (iii) Surgery procedures distal to elbow

    f. Distal nerve block of upper extremity
      (1) Can block median, ulnar, and radial nerves
      (2) May be used for isolated finger or toe procedures
    g. Intercostal blocks
      (1) Twelve pair of intercostal nerves supply the ribs and abdominal wall skin and skeletal muscles.
      (2) Used for postoperative pain after thoracic or abdominal surgery
      (3) Used for pain of rib fractures
      (4) Risk of pneumothorax and intravascular injection
      (5) May need to sedate patient for procedure
    h. Lower extremity block
      (1) Supplied by widely separated nerves
      (2) To block entire lower extremity requires blocks of the lumbar and sacral plexuses.
      (3) Unpopular because of multiple injections
      (4) Nerves blocked include
        (a) Sciatic
        (b) Femoral
        (c) Lateral femoral cutaneous
        (d) Obturator
        (e) Saphenous
      (5) Ankle blocks require five nerves around the circumference to be injected.
E. Sympathetic
  1. Stellate ganglion
    a. Used for diagnosis and treatment of reflex sympathetic dystrophies (RSD)
    b. Used for management of circulatory insufficiency in the upper extremity
    c. Signs of a successful block
      (1) Horner's syndrome — *contraction pupil   partial ptosis of eyelid*
        (a) Ptosis
        (b) Miosis — *contraction of pupils*
        (c) Anhydrosis *↓ sweat*
      (2) Ipsilateral nasal congestion *— on the same side*
      (3) Flushing of the conjunctiva and skin
      (4) Temperature increase in the ipsilateral arm and hand
    d. Common side effects
      (1) Sensation of a "lump in the throat"
      (2) Temporary hoarseness and dysphasia because of recurrent laryngeal block
      (3) Unpleasant effects of Horner's syndrome
      (4) Hematoma
  2. Celiac plexus block
    a. Used for relief of severe visceral pain (i.e., pancreatic cancer)
    b. Complicated technique
    c. May see
      (1) Orthostatic hypotension
      (2) Increased gastrointestinal motility with possible diarrhea
      (3) Vascular injury because of close proximity to aorta
      (4) Spinal block
  3. Lumbar sympathetic block
    a. Used for diagnostic, prognostic, and therapeutic purposes
    b. Used for long-term chronic pain syndromes by injecting phenol
    c. Complications include
      (1) Neuritis of the genitofemoral nerve
      (2) Kidney perforation

           (3) Subcapsular hematoma

           (4) Horner's syndrome

           (5) Somatic nerve damage

           (6) Subarachnoid injection

           (7) Intravascular injection

           (8) Perforation of disk

           (9) Stricture of the ureter

          (10) Infection

          (11) Ejaculatory failure

          (12) Chronic back pain

  F. Spinal anesthesia (intrathecal or subarachnoid block)

    1. Specific facts

      a. Anesthetic solution is injected into the intrathecal space.

        (1) Nerve roots and part of spinal cord anesthetized

        (2) Warning: Spinal cord usually ends at L1-L2 interspace; agent should be injected below this level to avoid possible cord trauma.

    2. Spinal—block nerve conduction in extremity or region of the body

    3. Systemic toxicity: rare because of small doses given

    4. Baricity (see Table 26-4)

      a. Addition of 5% to 10% glucose makes solution heavier than CSF.

        (1) Solution tends to "sink" within CSF according to pull of gravity.

        (2) Level of anesthesia influenced by body's position

        (3) Trendelenburg position will hasten cephalad spread of local anesthetic.

  G. Epidural anesthesia

    1. Specific facts

      a. Anesthetic solutions can be administered into the epidural space by

        (1) Single injection

        (2) Repetitive bolus injections (by catheter)

        (3) Continuous infusion (by catheter)

      b. Produces nerve root, spinal cord, and paravertebral nerve anesthesia

      c. Produces less sympathetic blockade than intrathecal (spinal) block

      d. Higher chance for systemic toxicity than spinal block

        (1) Greater amount of drug needs to be administered for epidural anesthesia (in contrast to spinal anesthesia).

        (2) Greater amount of drug administered is systemically absorbed.

      e. Epidural—agents into thoracic or lumbar epidural space

      f. Because of the procedural use of a larger needle, an increased risk for a more pronounced headache is present if an inadvertent dural puncture occurs.

    2. Indications

      a. Procedures on abdomen

      b. Procedures on lower extremity

      c. Treatment of chronic pain

■ TABLE 26-4
■ ■ **Baricity of Solution**

Type	Specific Gravity	Diluent	Uses
Hypobaric	<1.003	Distilled water	Perineal, rectal, and total hip arthroplasty procedures
Isobaric	1.003-1.009	CSF	Used when anesthesia required as a specific level (i.e., lower extremity surgery, fractured hips)
Hyperbaric	>1.009	Dextrose 10%	Most frequent use because solution settles to most dependent aspect of subarachnoid space

    H. Caudal—injection into sacral canal below dural sac
       1. Used in children and during labor
       2. Single shot for surgery below the diaphragm
       3. Continuous block for pain relief
   I. Neuraxial (NA) Anesthesia
       1. Common properties for spinal and epidural blocks (i.e., anesthetics)
         a. Typically used for surgical cases involving the abdomen, perineum, and the lower extremities
         b. Dermatomes
           (1) Used in the assessment of the evolution and extent of an NA anesthetic
           (2) Nerve roots exiting the spinal cord innervate the skin in contiguous sensory bands or stripes (1 to 2 inches wide); these bands arise posteriorly (from the spinal column) and typically radiate away laterally, anteriorly, or caudally (looking like zebra stripes, if they could actually be seen).
           (3) Each sensory stripe (dermatome) corresponds to a specific nerve root.
           (4) Each sensory stripe (dermatome) has been investigated, mapped, and standardized in such a manner as to portray the idealized person.
           (5) The anatomic relationships of representative dermatomes are listed below (see Figure 26-2).
              (a) Neck: C3
              (b) Clavicles: C5
              (c) Nipples: T4
              (d) Xiphoid: T6
              (e) Navel: T10
              (f) Groin: L1
              (g) Knees: L4
              (h) Dorsum of foot: L5
              (i) Lateral ankles: S1
       2. Evolution of an NA anesthetic
         a. The evolution of an NA anesthetic is influenced by a number of factors.
           (1) Amount of agent given (dose)
           (2) The volume of the solution
           (3) The position of the patient after injection (i.e., sitting, supine, Trendelenburg, reverse Trendelenburg)
           (4) The baricity of the solution (spinal blocks)
           (5) Anatomic and physiologic considerations
              (a) Height
              (b) Hormonal influences
              (c) Obesity
              (d) Coincident pregnancy
         b. After NA injection, the evolution of the anesthetic block is monitored closely (as it moves cephalad) by assessing the loss of sensation along the previously mentioned dermatomal levels (see Box 26-1).
         c. Assess the loss of sensation to "sharp" (point of a sterile needle) or "dull" (blunt hub of a sterile needle).
         d. NA anesthetic is noted to first take effect in the feet and then move cephalad (the degree of cephalad movement being influenced by the factors mentioned previously).
       3. Side effects
         a. Sympathetic blockade is more likely to be caused by a spinal rather than an epidural block.
           (1) Hypotension is more likely with a NA block higher than T6 (but less than T3) because such blocks tend to impair the sympathetic vasoconstrictor outflow from the spinal cord (T6 to L2) to the

blood vessels of the mesentery and lower extremities; this effect can lead to

(a) Reduction in venous tone
(b) Reduction in venous return to heart
(c) Decrease in cardiac filling and cardiac output
(d) Decrease in arterial blood pressure
(e) Reflex increase in heart rate
(f) Potential for a decrease in coronary blood flow
(g) Probable increase in myocardial oxygen consumption

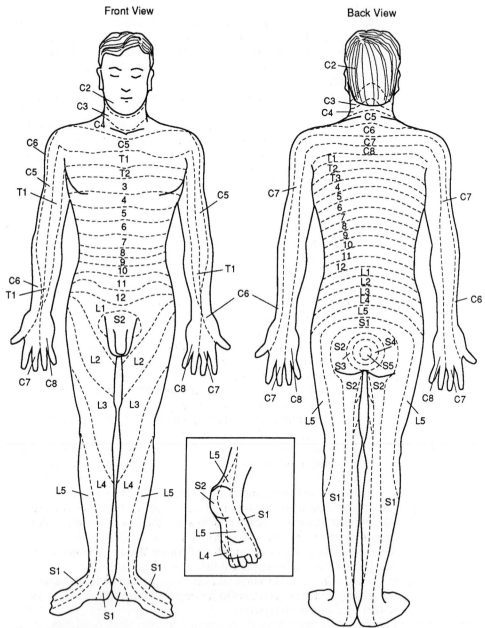

FIGURE 26-2 ■ Dermatomes. (From Cardona VD, Hurn PD, Mason PJB, et al: *Trauma nursing from resuscitation through rehabilitation,* ed 2. Philadelphia: WB Saunders, 1994, p 444.)

(2) Bradycardia is more likely with a block higher than T3 because such blocks tend to impair the sympathetic cardioaccelerator outflow (T1 to T4) to the sinoatrial (SA) and atrioventricular (AV) nodes of the myocardium; this effect leaves the cardiodecelerator effects of the vagus nerve (cranial nerve X) unrestrained.

    (a) Treat with atropine as needed.

    (b) Precautionary treatments that may be considered before the potential development of hypotension from sympathetic blockade include

        (i) Preblock fluid loading: use 20 to 25 ml/kg of normal saline or lactated Ringer's solution.

        (ii) Prophylactic administration of intramuscular (IM) ephedrine, 25 to 50 mg

        (iii) Not using excessive amounts of NA anesthetics

    (c) Treatment options for hypotension after there has been an excessive NA sympathetic block

        (i) Elevation of the patient's legs (this does not necessarily mean placing the patient in Trendelenburg position; under some circumstances, Trendelenburg position if initiated too early can worsen a high NA block)

        (ii) IV fluid boluses as needed to fill dilated venous capacitance vessels

        (iii) Vasopressors to support poor vascular tone (i.e., hypotension) until block resolves

            [a] Consider IV phenylephrine if heart is tachycardic (incremental IV doses of 100 mg).Caution: phenylephrine may cause reflex bradycardia.

            [b] Consider IV atropine if heart is bradycardic; incremental IV doses of 0.5 to 1 mg per advanced cardiac life support (ACLS) protocol.

            [c] Do not hesitate to use incremental doses of IV epinephrine if cardiovascular collapse appears imminent.

            [d] Consider infusion if cardiovascular depression has occurred.

            [e] Consider the placement of an arterial line for blood pressure monitoring if it is needed.

    (d) "High" sensory block

        (i) Block higher than T1 may cause severe cardiopulmonary collapse.

        (ii) Hydration, vasopressors and vagolytics, intubation, and cardiopulmonary resuscitation (CPR) may be needed as the NA blockade moves closer toward the brainstem.

        (iii) See following information on respiratory effects.

4. Neurologic complications

  a. Postdural puncture headache (PDPH)

    (1) Incidence

      (a) Directly related to size of hole made in dura by the spinal or epidural needle used: larger needles make larger holes.

      (b) Inversely related to age of patient: older patients are less likely to experience postdural puncture headaches.

      (c) With regard to spinal anesthesia, blunt (spreading tip) needles are less likely than sharp (cutting tip) needles to produce headaches; Whitacre, Sprotte, and Gertie-Marx needles are examples of the "blunt tip" category; Quincke needles are an example of the "cutting tip" type.

(2) Symptoms of a PDPH
  (a) The headache typically is felt in a frontal or occipital location or both (worsened by sitting or standing up); if it is to occur, it usually does so after 24 to 72 hours.
  (b) Associated symptoms include neck ache or stiffness (57%), backache (35%), and nausea (22%).
  (c) Less commonly associated symptoms include shoulder pain, blurred vision, vomiting, tinnitus, or auditory difficulties, and diplopia (i.e., cross-eyed, from a bilateral abducens nerve palsy).
  (d) The severity of the PDPH may be relieved by pressure on jugular veins or worsened by pressure on carotid arteries.
(3) Symptomatic treatment includes hydration, analgesics, and caffeinated beverages.
(4) Definitive treatment, if symptoms persist, includes an epidural blood patch that may be given 24 hours after a PDPH develops.
b. Adhesive arachnoiditis
  (1) Caused by introduction of foreign materials into intrathecal space
  (2) Results in chronic inflammation of the arachnoid
  (3) Progressive weakness and sensory loss of perineum or lower limbs
  (4) May advance to paraplegia
c. Cauda equina syndrome
  (1) May be caused by adhesive arachnoiditis
  (2) Persistent paresis of legs
  (3) Sensory loss in perineum
  (4) Bowel and bladder dysfunction
  (5) Effects usually permanent and may slowly deteriorate
  (6) In some cases, slow regression of symptoms occurs over months.
d. Peripheral nerve palsy is usually temporary but can be permanent from nerve root damage.
e. Septic meningitis
  (1) Symptoms appear within 24 hours of intrathecal contamination.
    (a) Fever
    (b) Headache
    (c) Neck rigidity
    (d) Kernig's sign: with the patient in the supine position, the thigh is flexed to a right angle with the trunk; Kernig's sign is present if the same-sided leg cannot be extended completely because of severe neck pain.
  (2) Good outcome if diagnosed early; must be treated immediately with antibiotics

5. Respiratory effects
  a. Effects on the ventilatory system increase as the NA block moves in the cephalad direction.
  b. First, the ability to cough is weakened from paralysis of the abdominal muscles; the inability to cough can impair the patient's capacity to clear airway secretions.
  c. Next, the progressive cephalad anesthesia of the intercostal nerves increasingly becomes impaired.
    (1) The intercostal *sensory* nerves and the patient's ability to perceive that he or she is breathing by the usual sensory cues from the skin (i.e., that the chest wall is moving normally with each breath)
    (2) The intercostal *motor* nerves and the patient's ability to take deep breaths (the patient's inspiratory capacity is also progressively lost).
    (3) Note: Some deprivation of chest wall sensation can be unavoidable under ordinary circumstances; reassurance is helpful in allaying patient anxiety.

(4) Warning: With a complete loss of chest wall sensation and patient complaints of increasing difficulty breathing, the possibility of a NA block progressing toward complete phrenic nerve paralysis (C3 to C5) should be suspected: emergent intubation of trachea may be immediately necessary!

    d. Finally, a high enough NA block to cause paralysis of the phrenic nerve (C3 to C5) is rarely seen if reasonable attention to technique is provided; however, if apnea does occur, patient will require assisted ventilation and possibly intubation to protect the airway from secretions or the aspiration of possible gastric contents.

J. Nursing interventions

  1. Hypotension is a common side effect.

  2. Have respiratory support equipment available.

  3. Assess residual block.

    a. Motor block can outlast some sensory blocks.

    b. Be careful standing patients.

    c. Motor assessment

      (1) Dorsi plantar flex (push down on gas pedal)

      (2) Invert and evert movement (windshield wiper movement of foot).

      (3) Extension

  4. Some resolution of block prior to discharge from PACU

  5. Appropriate discharge instructions should be given.

    a. Do not get up without assistance first few times.

    b. Patient may have long-acting local anesthetic drug on board so may not have return of complete sensation and motor ability.

VI. IV anesthetic induction agents

  A. Common properties

    1. General facts

      a. IV administration

      b. Good patient acceptance

      c. Quick onset

      d. Very brief duration

      e. Quick offset because of redistribution

      f. IV administration quickly and reversibly induces anesthesia.

        (1) CNS depression occurs.

        (2) Spontaneous ventilation is arrested.

        (3) Laryngeal reflexes are lost.

        (4) Increased risk for aspiration can occur.

      g. Patients generally recover within 5 to 10 minutes after a single dose.

      h. Specific agents have variable side effects, depending on circumstances.

    2. Elimination

      a. The amount of anesthetic agent distributed to each region of the body is directly proportional to the amount of blood each region receives; those regions receiving the greatest amounts of blood will be anesthetized first.

        (1) Highly perfused regions

          (a) Brain

          (b) Heart

          (c) Kidney

          (d) Liver

        (2) Moderately perfused regions

          (a) Muscle

          (b) Skin

        (3) Mildly perfused regions

          (a) Fat

          (b) Bone marrow

        (4) Poorly perfused regions

            (a) Tendons

            (b) Ligaments

            (c) Bone

  b. Although metabolism does occur for most of these drugs, plasma levels are initially reduced, primarily by redistribution (see the following).

  c. Redistribution occurs very quickly with IV induction agents.

      (1) On IV injection (single dose) the injected drug is diluted into the primary vascular space (i.e., central compartment—the concentration of drug in blood is now at its maximum).

      (2) Next (and very quickly) the central compartment distributes the drug first to those organs richly supplied by the vasculature.

         (a) Because the brain and heart are small, only minor amounts of drug are distributed here.

         (b) At this time the concentration of drug in the central compartment is still near its peak level.

         (c) Note that drug's effects on the CNS and cardiovascular system are now maximal.

      (3) As time proceeds, drug in the central compartment is redistributed into larger organs and tissue less richly supplied by the vasculature (i.e., muscle, skin, fat, and bone marrow).

         (a) If monitored, the concentration of drug in the vascular space would now appear to decline.

         (b) Clinically, the effects of the drug on the CNS and cardiovascular system begin to wane.

3. Respiratory effects

  a. Respiratory, laryngeal, and pharyngeal reflexes are blunted.

  b. Upper airway obstruction can be caused by relaxation of surrounding soft tissue muscle tone.

  c. Ventilatory depression is usually guaranteed.

4. Immune response effect

  a. Initial studies suggest that T-lymphocyte proliferations are inhibited by most of the induction agents (thiopental more than methohexital and etomidate, which have equal effect) except propofol.

  b. Propofol may be one of the least T-lymphocyte-inhibiting drugs to use for patients who are immunocompromised.

5. Nursing considerations

  a. Ventilation will need to be supported until the effects of these agents wear off.

  b. If gastric contents are present, the airway and lungs will need to be protected until the protective airway reflexes return.

      (1) Be vigilant.

      (2) Maintain proper positioning of airway.

      (3) Be prepared for immediate suctioning of the airway if vomiting occurs.

B. Thiopental

  1. General facts

    a. Brand name: Sodium Pentothal and others

      (1) Used as anesthetic IV induction agent

         (a) Generally rapid

         (b) Pleasant

      (2) Used for

         (a) Electroconvulsive therapy

         (b) Cardioversion

    b. Dose-dependent depression of CNS function: effects range from sedation through coma.

  2. Administration route and dosage

    a. Individuals with adequate cardiovascular stability

      (1) 2.5 to 5 mg/kg, titrated to effect

      b. Individuals without adequate cardiovascular stability
         (1) Induction dosage of thiopental must be reduced.
         (2) Consider alternate IV agents: etomidate or ketamine
      c. Respiratory impact
         (1) Decreased tidal volume
         (2) Apnea may occur.
         (3) Garlic taste
   3. Pharmacokinetics
      a. Onset: <30 seconds
      b. Duration: 5 to 10 minutes
      c. Metabolism
         (1) Hepatic microsomal enzymes
         (2) Chronic use causes predictable enzyme induction.
      d. Elimination
         (1) Termination of action is primarily by redistribution.
         (2) Multiple dosing saturates this process and will delay clinical recovery.
         (3) Thiopental is largely eliminated in urine as water-soluble metabolites.
   4. Pharmacodynamics
      a. Dose-dependent depression of CNS function
         (1) Depresses polysynaptic responses
         (2) Thought to potentiate effect of inhibitory neurotransmitter (GABA)
         (3) Important locus of depression is reticular activating system (required for wakefulness).
      b. Hyperalgesic effect at low blood levels; patient may perceive more pain
   5. Hepatic effects
      a. With liver disease metabolism is impaired, drowsiness is prolonged, and ventilation is depressed.
   6. Nursing considerations
      a. Reconstituted solution is very alkaline (pH >10) and incompatible with acidic solutions.
         (1) Infiltrated injections may need special attention: apply warm compresses.
      b. See yawning, hiccoughing, and possible laryngospasm.
C. Methohexital
   1. General facts
      a. Brand name: Brevital and others
         (1) Used as anesthetic induction agent
      b. Dose-dependent depression of CNS function: effects range from sedation through coma.
      c. Potency: twice that of thiopental
      d. Action: similar to thiopental at equianesthetic doses but has less effect on respiratory depression
   2. Administration route and dosage
      a. IV induction: 1 to 2 mg/kg
      b. Rectal doses
         (1) 20 to 30 mg/kg
         (2) Used in pediatric patients
         (3) Onset in about 7 minutes
         (4) Recovery usually begins in about 45 minutes.
   3. Pharmacokinetics: see Section VI.B.3 information on thiopental.
   4. Pharmacodynamics: see Section VI.B.4 information on thiopental.
   5. Nursing considerations
      a. Several side effects on injection: pain, myoclonus, hiccoughs
D. Etomidate
   1. General facts
      a. Brand name: Amidate
         (1) Used as anesthetic induction agent

      b. Agent of choice in patients with cardiovascular disease
      c. Excellent cardiovascular stability
         (1) Less likely to cause hypotension than thiopental
         (2) Heart rate and cardiac output tend to remain constant; negative inotropic effects are minimal.
         (3) Slight decrease in blood pressure possible because of slight peripheral vascular relaxation
      d. Dose-dependent suppression of adrenal steroidogenesis
         (1) Up to 24 hours after one induction dose
         (2) Also occurs after prolonged infusions
            (a) Use contraindicated in critically ill patients
            (b) May cause reversible adrenal insufficiency
      e. Dissolved in propylene glycol: pain and venoirritation may occur on injection.
  2. Administration route and dosage
      a. IV induction: 0.2 to 0.4 mg/kg
  3. Pharmacokinetics
      a. Onset: 15 to 45 seconds
      b. Duration: 3 to 12 minutes
      c. Metabolism: hepatic microsomal enzymes and plasma esterases; hydrolysis of this drug is nearly complete.
      d. Elimination
         (1) Action is terminated primarily by redistribution.
         (2) Rapid metabolism also contributes to prompt awakening.
         (3) Overall, clearance is five times faster than with thiopental.
  4. Pharmacodynamics
      a. Hypnotic without analgesic effect
      b. Unconsciousness occurs in 1 minute or less
  5. Cardiovascular effects: see general facts (preceding)
  6. Respiratory effects
      a. Dose-dependent hypoventilation and apnea
      b. Rapid return of spontaneous ventilation
  7. Skeletal muscle effects
      a. Myoclonus is occasionally seen on induction. *Twitching -Spasm muscle*
      b. Premedication with narcotic or benzodiazepine diminishes myoclonus.
  8. Nursing considerations
      a. Several side effects on injection
         (1) Dose-dependent suppression of adrenal function
            (a) Etomidate inhibits cortisol synthesis.
            (b) Circulating levels of cortisol are depressed.
            (c) Circulating levels of ACTH are increased.
            (d) Effects may last up to 24 hours after a single dose.
         (2) Myoclonus
         (3) Pain when rapidly injected into small vein
         (4) Nausea or vomiting is common.
      b. Use of etomidate infusions in intensive care units (ICUs) leads to adrenocortical suppression with increased morbidity and mortality.
         (1) Adrenal insufficiency possible
         (2) Use contraindicated in critically ill patients
E. Ketamine
  1. General facts
      a. Brand name: Ketalar
         (1) Used as anesthetic induction agent
      b. Intense analgesic properties
      c. Useful in minor surgical procedures
         (1) Burn debridement
         (2) Oral surgery where intense analgesia is necessary

  d. Related to phencyclidine, PCP, and LSD; vivid hallucinations are possible during and after surgery.
 2. Administration route and dosage
   a. IV doses
    (1) Induction: 1 to 2 mg/kg
     (a) Rapid onset
     (b) Recovery usually begins in about 5 to 10 minutes.
    (2) Maintenance: 0.5 to 1 mg/kg every 5 to 30 minutes
    (3) Infusion: 1 mg/kg per hour (may have fewer aftereffects)
   b. IM dose: 5 to 10 mg/kg
    (1) Onset within 3 to 5 minutes
    (2) Recovery usually begins in about 10 to 20 minutes.
 3. Pharmacokinetics
   a. Onset: 15 to 45 seconds
   b. Duration: 3 to 12 minutes
   c. Metabolism: occurs extensively by hepatic microsomal enzymes
   d. Elimination
    (1) Action is terminated primarily by redistribution.
    (2) Largely eliminated in urine
 4. Pharmacodynamics
   a. Depresses neocortex
   b. Produces excellent analgesia
   c. Stimulates limbic system
   d. Does not depress reticular activating system
   e. Produces dissociation of thalamoneocortical and limbic systems
   f. Produces dissociative anesthesia
    (1) No recollection of surgery
    (2) Patient appears to be awake.
    (3) Minimal respiratory depression
 5. CNS effects
   a. Increases cerebral blood flow; has been reported to increase intracranial pressure
   b. Emergence from anesthesia can be associated with delirium.
    (1) Alterations in mood and body image
    (2) Vivid dreams, sometimes progressing to hallucinations
    (3) Out-of-body experiences or psychomotor activity
   c. Recurrent illusions or flashbacks (may occur up to several weeks after anesthesia)
   d. Strategies to reduce or eliminate "emergence" phenomena
    (1) Use diazepam as premedicant.
    (2) Preoperatively mention possibility of dreams.
    (3) Recovery in dark, quiet environment has no beneficial effect.
 6. Cardiovascular effects
   a. Increases heart rate, blood pressure, and cardiac output (probably mediated by CNS effects)
 7. Respiratory effects
   a. Respiratory, laryngeal, and pharyngeal reflexes remain nearly normal.
   b. Spontaneous ventilation tends to be maintained.
   c. Ventilatory depression and obstruction indicate overdosage.
   d. Potential for *increased salivary gland secretion* may require patient premedication with an antisialagogue such as glycopyrrolate
 8. Skeletal muscle effects
   a. Usually causes increase in muscle tone
 9. Contraindications
   a. Hypertension
   b. Previous stroke
   c. Psychiatric disorders
   d. Elevated intracranial pressure

10. Nursing considerations
    a. Can produce vivid hallucinations in PACU; patient may need to be restrained or require benzodiazepine sedation.
    b. Incidence of delirium
       (1) Greater in adults than in children
       (2) Fifty percent of adults older than 30 years experience excitement and delirium.
    c. Preanesthetic visit should mention potential for dreamlike effects that may be experienced on emergence and during first day after ketamine exposure.
    d. Can produce irritability and compromise suck reflex in infants
F. Propofol
    1. General facts
       a. Brand name: Diprivan
          (1) Used as anesthetic induction agent
       b. Formulated in a milky white emulsion of glycerin, lecithin (from egg yolks), and soybean oil
          (1) Avoid in patients with allergy to eggs and soybean.
       c. May cause hypotension if injected too rapidly; more pronounced in hypovolemic patients
       d. No analgesic effects
       e. Rapid and alert emergence
       f. High incidence of pain on IV injection
          (1) Distal veins: 40%
          (2) Larger veins: 10%
          (3) IV lidocaine used to decrease this pain (usually 2% lidocaine is used)
       g. No preservatives: cannot be stored after opening ampules (opened ampules can support vigorous growth of microorganisms)
    2. Administration route and dosage
       a. IV doses
          (1) Reduce dosage in elderly, premedicated, and hypovolemic patients.
          (2) Induction: 1.5 to 2.5 mg/kg
          (3) Maintenance: vary infusion from 50 to 150 mcg/kg per minute.
             (a) Propofol can be used as primary anesthetic.
             (b) Narcotics and nitrous oxide may be added as adjuncts.
             (c) Infusion discontinued 10 to 15 minutes before case ends
    3. Pharmacokinetics
       a. Onset: 15 to 45 seconds
       b. Duration: 5 to 10 minutes
       c. Metabolism: extremely rapid
       d. Elimination
          (1) Action is terminated primarily by redistribution; prolonged administration, however, can saturate this process.
          (2) Largely eliminated in urine
          (3) Clearance 5 to 10 times faster than with thiopental
          (4) Clearance significantly greater than liver blood flow
    4. Nursing considerations
       a. Lower incidence of postoperative side effects
          (1) Less hangover
          (2) Less nausea and vomiting
          (3) Less psychomotor impairment
       b. Earlier ambulation and discharge after outpatient surgery
          (1) Time in PACU decreased
          (2) Outpatients ready to go home earlier
          (3) Patients resume day-to-day activities earlier.
          (4) Patients are more alert and drink fluids and eat earlier.
          (5) Patients often more responsive and in elevated mood

      c. Rapid emergence from anesthesia may hasten pain awareness.

        (1) Propofol does not provide any residual postanesthetic analgesic effect.

        (2) Intraoperative or postoperative analgesics may need to be administered.

   G. Benzodiazepines (see Section VIII.C)

     1. Diazepam (Valium)

     2. Midazolam (Versed)

     3. Lorazepam (Ativan)

VII. Intravenous opioid anesthetics

  A. Common properties

    1. General facts

      a. Synthetic opioids

        (1) Used as analgesic or anesthetic induction agents

        (2) Also used as premedicant: sedative, analgesic, or anesthetic adjunct

        (3) Intraoperative use will decrease requirement for general anesthesia.

    2. Pharmacokinetics

      a. Onset: rapid

      b. Duration of analgesia: 30 minutes

      c. Redistribution half-life: 15 minutes

      d. Metabolized by liver

      e. Elimination

        (1) Lower doses: termination of action primarily by redistribution; multiple doses or large doses will saturate this process; see information on intravenous anesthetic induction agents for more information on "redistribution" phenomena (see Section VI.A.2.c).

        (2) Higher doses: primarily by metabolism; various half-lives

          (a) Remifentanil: 0.25-0.33 hours

          (b) Alfentanil: 1.5 hours

          (c) Sufentanil: 2.5 hours

          (d) Fentanyl: 3.5 to 4 hours

          (e) Morphine 3-4 hours

          (f) Meperidine 3-4 hours

          (g) Hydromorphone (Dilaudid)

    3. Pharmacodynamics

      a. Appears to modulate intracellular production of cyclic adenosine monophosphate (AMP)

      b. May inhibit transmembrane calcium currents

        (1) Effect appears to be potentiated by calcium channel blockers.

        (2) Effect at presynaptic neurons may decrease release of neurotransmitters.

      c. Overall, opioids inhibit pain by modulating synaptic impulse transmission.

      d. Opioids decrease perception of and response to pain by

        (1) Effects at level of dorsal horn cells of spine

        (2) Activation of descending inhibitory pathways from brain stem

        (3) Altering emotional response to pain in limbic cortex

        (4) Opioids relieve continuous "dull" pain better than intermittent sharp pain.

    4. Side effects

      a. Miosis: stimulation of oculomotor nerve; reversed by naloxone, atropine, or glycopyrrolate

      b. Bradycardia: stimulation of vagus nerve is treatable with atropine or glycopyrrolate

      c. Muscle rigidity: alfentanil is worst offender; more pronounced when injected rapidly.

      d. Nausea and vomiting: use antiemetics.

  e. Hypotension
   (1) May be caused by bradycardia and/or a decrease in sympathetic tone
   (2) Exaggerated in patients who are anxious, hypovolemic, or in pain
  f. Delayed awakening
  g. Respiratory depression: background $Paco_2$ required to stimulate normal ventilation is increased.
 5. Nursing considerations
  a. Observe for respiratory depression in PACU.
   (1) Assess need for ventilatory support.
   (2) Naloxone should be readily available.
  b. Reduce doses in elderly and hypovolemic patients.
  c. Respiratory depression can outlast analgesic effect.
B. Morphine
 1. General facts
  a. "Gold standard" and other narcotics compared with it
  b. Use preservative-free for epidural and intrathecal doses.
  c. Mu receptor agent
 2. Administration route and dosage
  a. Guidelines for IV loading dose (titrated to effect)
   (1) Perioperative analgesia: 2-15 mg
    (a) Onset: 1-5 minutes
    (b) Peak analgesia at 20 minutes
    (c) Duration: 4 hours
   (2) Epidural anesthesia: 2-5 mg bolus
   (3) Intrathecal: 0.2-1.0 mg
  b. Histamine release resulting in
   (1) Hypotension
   (2) Pruritis
   (3) Wheezing
C. Meperidine
 1. General facts
  a. Brand name: Demerol
  b. Synthetic narcotic analgesic
 2. Administration route and dosage
  a. Guidelines for IV loading dose (titrated to effect)
   (1) Perioperative: used for shivering
    (a) Thought to act through a K receptor mechanism
    (b) Use 12.5-25 mg for postoperative shivering
    (c) Contraindicated in patients on monoamine oxidase (MAO) inhibitors
D. Hydromorphone
 1. General facts
  a. Brand name: Dilaudid
  b. Synthetic narcotic analgesic
 2. Administration route and dosage
  a. Guidelines for IV loading dose (titrated to effect)
   (1) Perioperative analgesia: 0.5-2.0 mg
    (a) Onset: <1 minute
    (b) Duration: 2-4 hours
    (c) Six times more potent than morphine
E. Alfentanil
 1. General facts
  a. Brand name: Alfenta
   (1) Used as analgesic and anesthetic adjuvant
  b. Synthetic narcotic analgesic
   (1) One tenth as potent as fentanyl
   (2) Ten times more potent than morphine

    2. Administration route and dosage
       a. Guidelines for IV loading dose (titrated to effect)
         (1) Perioperative analgesia: 10 to 25 µg/kg
         (2) Balanced anesthesia: 50 to 150 µg/kg
       b. Guidelines for continuous IV infusion (titrated to effect)
         (1) Perioperative analgesia: 0.25 to 1 µg/kg per minute
         (2) Balanced anesthesia: 0.5 to 3 µg/kg per minute

F. Fentanyl
   1. General facts
      a. Brand name: Sublimaze
        (1) Used as analgesic and anesthetic adjuvant
      b. Synthetic narcotic analgesic: 100 times more potent than morphine ←
      c. Duration of analgesia: 30 to 60 minutes
      d. Mu receptor agent
   2. Administration route and dosage
      a. Guidelines for IV loading dose (titrated to effect)
        (1) Perioperative analgesia: 1 to 3 µg/kg
        (2) Balanced anesthesia: 5 to 15 µg/kg
      b. Guidelines for continuous IV infusion (titrated to effect)
        (1) Perioperative analgesia: 0.01 to 0.03 µg/kg per minute
        (2) Balanced anesthesia: 0.03 to 0.1 µg/kg per minute

G. Remifentanil
   1. General facts
      a. Brand name: Ultiva
        (1) Used as analgesic and anesthetic adjuvant
      b. Synthetic narcotic with an extremely short half-life
      c. After an initial loading dose, the effects of this drug must be continued by continuous infusion.
      d. The abrupt discontinuation of infusions of this drug can cause the sudden onset of extreme pain and related adverse effects.
      e. Because remifentanil by itself cannot ensure unconsciousness, its exclusive use in general anesthesia is not recommended.
      f. Spinal or epidural use is not recommended because of the motor dysfunctions that might occur from its glycine vehicle (glycine is a spinal cord neurotransmitter).
   2. Administration route and dosage
      a. Guidelines for IV loading dose (titrated to effect)
        (1) Balanced anesthesia: 0.5 to 2 µg/kg
      b. Guidelines for continuous IV infusion (titrated to effect)
        (1) Balanced anesthesia: 0.25 to 0.5 µg/kg per minute
   3. Nursing considerations
      a. The sudden discontinuation of infusions of this drug after surgery may bring on the sudden onset of intense pain; the supplemental use of longer lasting analgesics must be anticipated and administered without delay.
      b. Because of its high potency, remifentanil not administered by nursing personnel

H. Sufentanil
   1. General facts
      a. Brand name: Sufenta
        (1) Used as analgesic and anesthetic adjuvant
        (2) Mu receptor agonist
      b. Synthetic narcotic analgesic
        (1) Is 500 to 1000 times more potent than morphine ←
        (2) Is 5 to 10 times more potent than fentanyl
      c. Used in balanced general anesthesia
        (1) For induction and maintenance
        (2) In major surgical procedures

       2. Administration route and dosage

          a. Guidelines for IV loading dose (titrated to effect)

             (1) Balanced anesthesia: 1 to 3 μg/kg

          b. Guideline for continuous IV infusion (titrated to effect)

             (1) Balanced anesthesia: 0.01 to 0.05 μg/kg per minute

VIII. Intravenous anesthetic adjuncts

    A. Droperidol

       1. General facts

          a. Brand name: Inapsine and others

             (1) In small doses this antipsychotic agent is widely used in anesthesia for its antiemetic properties.

          b. Moderate antiemetic effects; dose: 0.0625 to 0.125 mg IV

          c. Neuroleptic anesthesia (Innovar)

             (1) Combines properties of droperidol with those of fentanyl in a 50:1 mixture

             (2) Primary effects

                (a) Ataraxia

                (b) Some amnesia

                (c) Reduced motor movement

                (d) Patient arousable and responsive but indifferent

          d. Additional effects

             (1) Alpha adrenergic blocking activity produces vasodilation and mild to moderate hypotension.

             (2) Elevates threshold for myocardial dysrhythmias but may also prolong the QT interval

             (3) Anticonvulsant action

             (4) Slight respiratory depression

       2. Pharmacokinetics: Metabolized by the liver

       3. Pharmacodynamics: Works within the CNS as dopamine antagonist

       4. Side effects

          a. Dystonic reaction: Muscle spasm of face, neck, tongue, or upper back

             (1) Occurs in about 1% of patient population

             (2) May also be caused by metoclopramide

             (3) Treatment: diphenhydramine (Benadryl), 25 to 50 mg by slow IV

             (4) Alternate treatment: benztropine (Cogentin), 1 to 2 mg IV

          b. Postanesthetic dysphoria (internalized overwhelming fear)

             (1) May occur when droperidol (a psychotropic drug) is given alone without the beneficial effect of narcotics such as fentanyl

             (2) May occur if the beneficial effect of a coadministered narcotic wanes

             (3) Effect of droperidol usually persists longer than that of narcotics

             (4) Patients and their families may require some reassurance if the dysphoric effect occurs.

    B. Anticholinergics

       1. Atropine

          a. 0.5 to 1 mg IM or IV

          b. Inhibits salivary and respiratory tract secretions

          c. Causes bronchodilation

          d. Counteracts bradycardia and related dysrhythmias

          e. Given with antiacetylcholinesterase (anti-AChE) agents at end of general anesthesia·

          f. Crosses blood-brain barrier, causes CNS stimulation

          g. Can produce central anticholinergic syndrome

             (1) Restlessness, irritability, disorientation, delirium

             (2) Can be major cause of postoperative dysphoria

             (3) Central effects can be reversed by physostigmine.

       2. Scopolamine

          a. Same preoperative use as atropine

          b. Dose is 0.3 to 0.6 mg IM or IV

       c. Causes CNS depression, drowsiness, amnesia, euphoria, fatigue

       d. May cause paradoxical excitation

       e. Less effective at preventing bradycardia

       f. Higher incidence of postoperative dysphoria and delirium

       g. May cause short-term amnesia when given with morphine

    3. Glycopyrrolate (Robinul)

       a. Longer acting than atropine

       b. More potent antisialagogue than atropine

       c. Dose: 0.1 to 0.2 mg IM or IV

       d. More potent inhibitor of gastric acid secretion than atropine

       e. Does not cross blood-brain barrier

       f. Does not produce sedation

       g. Does not produce central anticholinergic syndrome

       h. More rapid postoperative awakening than with atropine

       i. Prevents bradycardia and less likely to cause tachycardia than atropine

C. Benzodiazepines

    1. General facts

       a. Administered by oral, IM, or IV routes

         (1) Absorbed from gastrointestinal tract

       b. Metabolized by hepatic oxidative microsomal enzymes; inactive metabolites excreted in urine

       c. Lack of analgesic properties

       d. Dose-related depression of ventilation

       e. Warning: ventilatory rate must be monitored closely after IV sedation; use pulse oximetry to confirm patient's return to normalcy.

       f. Exhibits amnestic, anxiolytic, hypnotic, and sedative properties

       g. Also exhibits anticonvulsant and muscle relaxant properties

       h. Bind to modulating sites on GABA receptors in CNS

       i. Leads to hyperpolarization of postsynaptic membranes; highest density of benzodiazepine receptors is in cerebral cortex, where there is an inhibitory effect on excitation of neurons.

         (1) Mild cardiovascular depressant effects: mild vasodilation

         (2) Minor direct myocardial depression

         (3) Greater effects from midazolam than from diazepam and lorazepam

       j. Skeletal muscle relaxation reflects action on spinal internuncial neurons.

         (1) Skeletal muscle tone reduced

         (2) Benzodiazepines do not reduce surgical requirements for muscle relaxants.

       k. Recovery of fine motor skills

         (1) More rapid with midazolam than with diazepam or lorazepam

       l. Can markedly attenuate cardiostimulatory effects of ketamine; also minimizes emergence sequelae of ketamine

    2. Diazepam

       a. Brand name: Valium and others

         (1) Used as a sedative and anesthetic adjunct

       b. Insoluble in water

         (1) Parenteral formulation contains propylene glycol; injection may be associated with venous irritation and pain.

       c. Dosing schedule

         (1) Sedation

           (a) IV: 2.5 to 5 mg

           (b) Orally (PO): 5 to 10 mg

         (2) Induction of general anesthesia: 0.25 to 0.5 mg/kg IV

         (3) Treatment of seizures: 0.10 mg/kg IV and titrate to effect

       d. Onset

         (1) IV: rapid

         (2) PO: 30 to 60 minutes

       e. Duration: IV, 15 minutes to 3 hours

       f. Low hepatic clearance rates: elimination half-life is 20 to 40 hours

  3. Lorazepam

       a. Brand name: Ativan

          (1) Used as sedative and anesthetic adjunct

       b. Insoluble in water

          (1) Parenteral formulation contains propylene glycol; injection may be associated with pain and venous irritation.

       c. Dosing schedule for sedation

          (1) IV: 1 to 2 mg

          (2) PO: premedicant, 0.05 mg/kg (not to exceed 4 mg)

       d. Onset

          (1) May be slow and somewhat unpredictable

             (a) May be marked lag between peak blood concentration and clinical effect

             (b) Clinical effect may be difficult to titrate.

          (2) IV: 5 to 20 minutes

          (3) IM: 0.5 to 2 hours

          (4) PO: 1 to 2 hours

       e. Duration

          (1) IV: 4 to 6 hours

          (2) IM: 8 hours

          (3) PO: 8 hours

       f. Elimination half-life is 10 to 20 hours.

  4. Midazolam

       a. Brand name: Versed

          (1) Used as sedative and anesthetic adjunct

       b. Water-soluble formulation

          (1) Minimal local irritation on injection

       c. Midazolam has a steep dose-response curve; careful titration very important.

       d. Dosing schedule

          (1) Sedation

             (a) IV: 1 to 4 mg

             (b) IM: 0.05 to 0.1 mg/kg

          (2) Induction of general anesthesia: 0.1 to 0.2 mg/kg IV

       e. Onset

          (1) IV: 15 minutes

          (2) IM: 10 to 30 minutes

       f. Duration

          (1) IV: 2 to 6 hours (induction dose)

          (2) IM: 1 to 2 hours

       g. Rapid and extensive hepatic metabolism and renal excretion; elimination half-life is 2 to 4 hours.

D. Benzodiazepine antagonist

  1. Flumazenil

       a. Brand name: Romazicon

          (1) Only drug available in this class

          (2) Specific benzodiazepine receptor antagonist

          (3) Blocks CNS effects of benzodiazepines

       b. Dosing schedule: IV doses of 0.1 mg increments to maximum of 1 mg

       c. Onset (IV): within 1 minute

       d. Duration: 1 to 2 hours

       e. Hepatic metabolism and renal excretion

          (1) Redistribution half-life: about 5 minutes

          (2) Elimination half-life: about 60 minutes

IX. Volatile inhalational anesthetics

    A. Common properties

        1. General facts

            a. Exist as liquids that evaporate at room temperature

            b. Amount of liquid evaporated is controlled by a device called a vaporizer.

            c. Concentration of vapor administered determines the patient's depth of anesthesia.

            d. The term *minimum alveolar concentration (MAC)* defines the concentration (vol%) of anesthetic vapor (at 1 atmosphere of pressure) that prevents skeletal muscle movement in 50% of the patients given a painful stimulus (surgical skin incision). The MAC is determined only after the anesthetic has had time to equilibrate throughout the body.

        2. Administration route and dosage

            a. "Simple" inhalational anesthesia

                (1) Volatile agent is used by itself with no adjuncts.

                (2) Either halothane or sevoflurane are used because they are pleasant smelling; these two agents are recommended for mask inductions and maintenance anesthesia.

                (3) Enflurane, isoflurane, and desflurane are used only for maintenance anesthesia because they are too irritating to inhale for mask inductions; with these agents general anesthesia is commenced with a short-acting IV induction agent (see Section VI).

            b. "Balanced" inhalational anesthesia

                (1) Intravenous adjuncts (narcotics, N_2O, muscle relaxants) are added to enhance the effects of the volatile agents, thus reducing the doses of the inhalational agents required.

        3. Pharmacokinetics

            a. Uptake into the capillary blood (from alveoli) is directly proportional to the lipid solubility of the anesthetic vapor.

            b. The amount of anesthetic agent distributed to each region of the body is directly proportional to the amount of blood each region receives; those regions receiving the greatest amounts of blood will be anesthetized first.

                (1) Highly perfused regions

                    (a) Brain

                    (b) Heart

                    (c) Kidney

                    (d) Liver

                (2) Moderately perfused regions

                    (a) Muscle

                    (b) Skin

                (3) Mildly perfused regions

                    (a) Fat

                    (b) Bone marrow

                (4) Poorly perfused regions

                    (a) Tendons

                    (b) Ligaments

                    (c) Bone

            c. Vapor elimination from various regions of the body (back to the lungs) is also determined by the regional rates of blood flow; elimination is slowest from the regions with the poorest blood supply.

                (1) Poorly perfused regions serve as storage sites for volatile anesthetics—the extent of this "storage" being a function of the time allowed these regions to absorb anesthetic agent and their size (i.e., obese patients have a larger capacity to store volatile anesthetics than slender patients).

4. Pharmacodynamics
   a. Dose-dependent central nervous system (CNS) depression
      (1) Several sites and mechanisms of action are under consideration; all of these are not completely understood.
      (2) Overall, it can be stated simply that general anesthetics "anesthetize" by impairing CNS synaptic transmission.
5. CNS effects
   a. Impairs CNS synaptic transmission
   b. Decreases cerebral metabolism
   c. Increases cerebral blood flow
      (1) Effect occurs within minutes.
      (2) Cerebral blood flow (CBF) is variably increased by each agent.
      (3) Intracranial pressure (ICP) is also variably increased.
      (4) Increases in intracranial swelling and ICP are serious concerns in cases involving head trauma; note that the above deleterious effects of volatile agents can be attenuated by intentionally hyperventilating the patient to achieve hypocarbia.
6. Cardiovascular effects
   a. Sensitization of the myocardium to dysrhythmogenic actions of catecholamines:
      (1) Halothane > isoflurane = enflurane
      (2) Ventricular ectopy, tachycardia, or fibrillation are all possible.
7. Respiratory (ventilatory) system
   a. Dose-dependent depression of spontaneous ventilation
   b. Dulls ventilatory responsiveness to hypoxemia and hypercarbia
   c. Obtunds laryngeal and pharyngeal reflexes
      (1) Some of the agents can be used to facilitate intubation (i.e., halothane and sevoflurane).
      (2) Depressed laryngeal reflexes increase the risk for aspiration (if gastric contents are present).
   d. Bronchodilation
      (1) There is a direct relaxing effect on bronchial smooth muscles.
      (2) All the volatile agents can be useful in unconscious patients, but only halothane and sevoflurane are useful in initiating anesthesia by mask (the others are too irritating to inhale by awake patients).
8. Renal effects
   a. Dose-dependent decreases in renal blood flow, glomerular filtration, and urine output can be offset by adequate prehydration.
9. Hepatic effects
   a. Dose-dependent reductions in total hepatic blood flow can lead to impaired hepatocyte oxygenation and a self-limiting form of hepatic dysfunction (can be more significant with halothane).
   b. Although all volatile anesthetics can cause a rare form of severe hepatitis, certain adults exposed to halothane appear to be at greater risk (see Section IX.B).
10. Gastrointestinal effects
    a. Relaxes smooth muscle and motility
11. Uterine effects
    a. Dose-dependent relaxation of uterine smooth muscle
       (1) Greater degrees of relaxation may cause greater amounts of uterine bleeding during cesarean sections.
       (2) A safe rule of thumb is to administer volatile anesthetics at a dose equal to 0.5 MAC (a dose that should only inhibit uterine contractility by about 80%); supplemental analgesia can be provided by the coadministration of nitrous oxide with oxygen in a 50:50 mixture (see Section X.A).

12. Drug interactions that *potentiate* the effects of volatile anesthetics (some of these drugs can also introduce some of their own unique problems)
    a. Acute ethanol intoxication
    b. Ketamine
       (1) May enhance the occurrence of dreams and hallucinations
       (2) When used in patients with asthma receiving aminophylline, it may induce seizures (i.e., combinations of ketamine and aminophylline can lower the seizure threshold).
    c. Nitrous oxide (see Section X)
    d. Narcotics (morphine, fentanyl, sufentanil)
       (1) Cause a dose-dependent desensitization in the normal ventilatory response to increases in plasma CO_2; narcotics upwardly reset the concentration of plasma CO_2 that is considered to be "normal" by the medullary chemoreceptors
       (2) Higher than normal concentrations of plasma CO_2 eventually will restore "normal" spontaneous tidal volumes, but this assumes that ventilation is sufficient in the meantime to maintain an adequate supply of oxygen.
       (3) As a consequence of this dose-dependent narcotic-induced hypercapnia, carbon dioxide levels will continue to rise until the catecholamines released trigger cardiac dysrhythmias or until the hypercapnia becomes so severe that the CNS becomes progressively depressed.
       (4) Patients who have received narcotics must be monitored closely to ensure that their ventilatory patterns are sufficient to maintain adequate oxygenation and exhalation of carbon dioxide; supplemental oxygen and ventilatory equipment must be available.
    e. Sedatives (benzodiazepines and barbiturates)
       (1) As with narcotics, sedatives decrease chemoreceptor sensitivities to plasma CO_2, but unlike narcotics, sedatives also depress the maximal response that can be achieved to increase ventilation (i.e., no increase in plasma CO_2 will ever be sufficient to stimulate the chemoreceptors enough to restore normal tidal volumes); thus the excessive use of sedatives (more so than narcotics) threatens a patient with irreconcilable hypercapnia.
       (2) Patients must also be monitored closely to ensure adequate oxygenation and exhalation of carbon dioxide; supplemental oxygen and ventilatory equipment must be supplied as needed.
    f. Acute tetrahydrocannabinol (marijuana) intoxication
13. Drug interactions that *antagonize* the effects of volatile anesthetics (increase the amount of volatile anesthetics required)
    a. Amphetamines
    b. Cocaine
    c. Chronic ethanol intoxication
    d. Naloxone
    e. Chronic tetrahydrocannabinol (marijuana) intoxication
14. Toxicities
    a. Respiratory depression
    b. Respiratory arrest (apnea)
    c. Cardiovascular depression
    d. Malignant hyperthermia: see following section.
15. Nursing considerations
    a. Impairment of spontaneous ventilation
       (1) CNS response to hypercapnia may be depressed.
       (2) CNS response to hypoxemia may be depressed.
    b. Depression of laryngeal and pharyngeal reflexes
       (1) Aspiration risks are increased. Warning: be vigilant!

      c. Volatile anesthetics have dysrhythmogenic effects (to varying degrees); these effects are worsened by the concomitant use of epinephrine (in mixture with local anesthetics).

      d. Volatile anesthetics offer no residual analgesic effect.

         (1) When general anesthesia is discontinued, a patient will awaken into an awareness of the pain of his or her surgery (unless IV analgesics, regional anesthetics, or local anesthetics are used before patient's emergence from general anesthesia).

         (2) The rapidity with which a patient awakens into pain is determined in part by how fast his or her anesthetic wears off (see nursing considerations for each specific volatile anesthetic).

      e. Be vigilant for malignant hyperthermia (see Chapter 28); its onset is sometimes delayed and may first be recognized in the PACU.

      f. Monitoring vital signs will trace the waning residual effects of anesthesia

      g. Monitoring urine output will assess the patient's volume status, renal blood flow, glomerular filtration rate, and the overall health of the kidney.

      h. Hypothermia

         (1) Results from marked intraoperative heat loss

         (2) May lead to marked peripheral vasoconstriction

            (a) If the skin appears blanched, suspect vasoconstriction.

            (b) If skin appears hyperemic, vasoconstriction is less likely.

         (3) Temperature of patient must be normalized.

            (a) Administer warmed IV fluids.

            (b) Use active rewarming methods (warmed blankets or air).

         (4) May lead to profound shivering

            (1) Increases oxygen consumption (important in anemic patients or in patient with poor pulmonary or cardiac reserve)

B. Halothane

  1. General facts

      a. Brand name: various manufacturers

         (1) Oldest agent currently in use; commonly used in pediatric anesthesia

      b. Its vapor is pleasant smelling and nonirritating.

         (1) Commonly used for mask inductions

         (2) Not likely to cause coughing and laryngospasm

         (3) Can be used for maintenance anesthesia

  2. Administration route

      a. Inhalation only

  3. Pharmacokinetics

      a. Metabolism: by hepatic microsomal enzymes

      b. Elimination

         (1) Unmetabolized drug: lungs (80%)

         (2) Metabolized drug: kidneys (20%)

  4. CNS effects

      a. Cerebral vasodilation

         (1) Greatest with halothane

         (2) Can induce an increase in ICP

         (3) Hypocapnia, if induced before exposure, will blunt the increase in ICP.

  5. Cardiovascular effects

      a. Myocardial depression: decreased heart rate, contractility, stroke volume, and cardiac output

      b. Systemic vasodilation: decreased systemic vascular resistance (SVR) by direct relaxant effect on vascular tone

      c. Impairs normal function of AV node

         (1) Bradycardia

         (2) Nodal rhythms

         (3) Wandering pacemaker

   d. Dysrhythmias
   (1) Sensitization of the myocardium (by volatile anesthetics) to exogenously administered epinephrine is the highest seen (i.e., greater in halothane than in isoflurane and desflurane, which are equal in effect but greater than enflurane).
      (a) Dose of exogenously administered epinephrine (e.g., found in some local anesthetics) should be kept to less than 2 µg/kg body weight
      (b) The above sensitization to epinephrine can be lessened by the coadministration of lidocaine.
 6. Renal effects
   a. Decreased renal blood flow and glomerular filtration may be offset by adequate prehydration.
 7. Hepatic effects
   a. Reversible reduction in hepatic blood flow is possible.
   b. Reversible decrease in hepatic function and self-limited hepatotoxicity is possible.
   c. Halothane hepatitis
      (1) Rare (1:20,000 to 200,000); less likely in children
      (2) Can lead to massive hepatic necrosis and death
      (3) Occurs 5 to 6 days after exposure
      (4) Risk factors may include enzyme induction, female gender, genetic predisposition, hypoxemia, hypermetabolic states, multiple exposures, middle age, and obesity.
      (5) Appears to be caused by the covalent binding of oxidative metabolites to liver parenchyma
         (a) The binding of these metabolites to the liver deranges its molecular architecture in such a way that the body does not recognize the liver as "self" anymore (thus, neoantigens are formed), and the immune system begins to attack the "nonself" liver with antibodies.
      (6) The disease presents with marked increases in serum alanine aminotransferase (ALT), aspartate aminotransferase (AST), and bilirubin; other findings include hepatomegaly, hepatic encephalopathy, fever, jaundice, malaise, and nonspecific gastrointestinal symptoms.
 8. Sympathetic nervous system effects
   a. Sensitizes heart to dysrhythmogenic action of catecholamines
 9. Skeletal muscle effects
   a. Causes mild relaxation
   b. Can augment overall effect of muscle relaxants
 10. Toxicities (by two different mechanisms)
   a. Self-limited mild hepatotoxicity (related to decreased blood flow) with presenting symptoms and signs of low-grade fever, nausea, lethargy, and mild transient elevations of liver aminotransferase enzymes (ALT, AST)
   b. "Halothane hepatitis" is a much rarer but more severe toxicity (see preceding Section IX.B.7).
 11. Drug interactions
   a. Adrenergic blockers
      (1) Hypotension as a result of decrease in heart rate and contractility
C. Enflurane
 1. General facts
   a. Brand name: Ethrane
      (1) Older agent used with decreasing popularity, in part because of its slow onset and offset of anesthetic action
   b. Volatile liquid with pungent and irritating odor
      (1) Not useful for mask inductions; may cause breath holding, coughing, and laryngospasm

(2) Used only for maintenance anesthesia after general anesthesia has been initiated with intravenous induction agents

c. In an unwanted reaction, enflurane can be degraded into carbon monoxide as it passes through the CO_2 absorbent of the anesthesia machine. Normally, enflurane passes through the anesthesia machine unchanged and does not interact with the soda lime or Baralyme of the CO_2-absorbing canisters. However, if enflurane is exposed to excessively dry soda lime or Baralyme, it can be chemically degraded and released as carbon monoxide gas.

2. Administration route
    a. Inhalation only
3. Pharmacokinetics
    a. More resistant to metabolism than halothane
    b. Some liver metabolism (2%)
    c. Metabolites excreted by kidneys
    d. Primarily eliminated as unchanged exhaled vapor (80% to 95%)
4. CNS effects
    a. Motor hyperactivity in 2% of patients
        (1) May see electroencephalographic (EEG) seizure patterns
        (2) May progress to tonic-clonic seizures
5. Cardiovascular effects
    a. Hypotension possible
        (1) Mild depression of cardiac output
        (2) Mild relaxation of vascular resistance
    b. Dysrhythmias
        (1) Stable heart rate
        (2) Sensitization of the myocardium (by volatile anesthetics) to exogenously administered epinephrine is minimal (i.e., greater with halothane than with isoflurane and desflurane, which are equal but greater than enflurane)
        (3) Dose of exogenously administered epinephrine (e.g., found in some local anesthetics) should be kept to less than 11 µg/kg body weight
6. Respiratory effects
    a. See Section IX.A.7.
7. Hepatic effects
    a. Less likely when compared with halothane but still may cause syndrome such as "halothane hepatitis" (see Section IX.B.7.c)
8. Skeletal muscle effects
    a. Promotes and potentiates neuromuscular blockade, although it is not a true nondepolarizing or depolarizing muscle relaxant (see following Section XI)
9. Drug interactions
    a. See Section X.A.12.
10. Nursing considerations
    a. May enhance seizure activity
    b. Patients are more hemodynamically stable than with halothane.
    c. Enflurane, which is slowly eliminated, is the most likely of all volatile anesthetics to produce a lingering CNS depressant effect in PACU.
D. Isoflurane
    1. General facts
        a. Brand name: Forane
            (1) Clinically useful anesthetic for maintenance of general anesthesia
        b. Volatile liquid with a strongly pungent and irritating odor
            (1) Not useful for mask inductions; may cause breathholding, coughing and laryngospasm
            (2) Used only for maintenance anesthesia after general anesthesia has been initiated with intravenous induction agents

      c. In an unwanted reaction, isoflurane can be degraded into carbon monoxide as it passes through the CO_2 absorbent of the anesthesia machine (see carbon monoxide discussion, Section IX.C.1.c.).

  2. Administration route and dosage

      a. Inhalation only

  3. Pharmacokinetics

      a. More resistant to metabolism than enflurane and halothane

      b. Eliminated primarily by exhalation as an intact molecule

      c. Some metabolism (0.2%) by liver

      d. Metabolites excreted by kidneys

  4. CNS effects

      a. See preceding Section IX.A.5.

  5. Cardiovascular effects

      a. Myocardial function only slightly affected

         (1) Weak negative inotrope

      b. Peripheral vasodilation

      c. Dysrhythmias

         (1) No bradycardia

         (2) Possible tachycardia

         (3) Sensitization of the myocardium (by volatile anesthetics) to exogenously administered epinephrine is less than that seen with halothane (i.e., greater effect with halothane than with isoflurane and desflurane, which are equal in effect but greater than enflurane)

            (a) Dose of exogenously administered epinephrine should be kept to less than 7 µg/kg body weight

  6. Respiratory effects

      a. See Section IX.A.7.

  7. Hepatic effects

      a. Historically, a possible carcinogenic effect was reported.

         (1) Original study and results not reproducible

         (2) Clinical use now widely accepted

  8. Skeletal muscle effects

      a. Promotes and potentiates neuromuscular blockade

  9. Toxicity: rare

 10. Drug interactions

      a. See Section IX.A.12.

 11. Nursing considerations

      a. Commonly used inhalational agent

      b. Postoperative shivering may be caused by increased heat loss from intraoperative vasodilation.

E. Desflurane

  1. General facts

      a. Brand name: Suprane

         (1) Newer clinically useful anesthetic for maintenance of general anesthesia

      b. Volatile liquid with pungent and irritating odor

         (1) Not useful for mask inductions; may cause breath holding, coughing, and laryngospasm

         (2) Used only for maintenance anesthesia after general anesthesia has been initiated with intravenous induction agents

      c. In an unwanted reaction, desflurane can be degraded into carbon monoxide as it passes through the CO_2 absorbent of the anesthesia machine (see carbon monoxide discussion, Section IX.C.1.c).

      d. Solubility in blood extremely low and similar to nitrous oxide

         (1) Allows for very fast onset and offset of CNS effects

  2. Administration route and dosage

      a. Inhalation only

3. Pharmacokinetics
   a. Extremely resistant to metabolism
   b. Most chemically inert of all volatile anesthetic agents
   c. Eliminated primarily by exhalation as an intact molecule
4. Cardiovascular effects
   a. May have coronary arteriolar vasodilator effects that promote "coronary steal" and myocardial ischemia; this concern is controversial clinically but should not be a problem perioperatively as long as the oxygen supply to the myocardium is maintained and its oxygen demand is minimized.
   b. During sudden increases in inspired gas concentrations, desflurane stimulates a transient sympathetically mediated increase in heart rate and blood pressure (to a lesser extent this is also observed with isoflurane); this response can be blunted by the preadministration of narcotics such as fentanyl.
   c. Dysrhythmias
      (1) Sensitization of the myocardium (by volatile anesthetics) to exogenously administered epinephrine is comparable to that seen with isoflurane (i.e., greater effect with halothane than with isoflurane and desflurane, which are equal in effect but greater than enflurane)
         (a) Dose of exogenously administered epinephrine should be kept to less than 7 μg/kg body weight.
5. Respiratory effects
   a. See Section IX.A.7.
6. Hepatic and renal systems
   a. Hepatic and renal blood flow appear to be well preserved.
7. Skeletal muscle effects
   a. Promotes and potentiates neuromuscular blockade
8. CNS effects
   a. Remarkably fast onset and offset of anesthesia
      (1) Solubility in blood is very low (as with nitrous oxide).
   b. Preliminary evidence suggests that desflurane at 1 MAC significantly increases CSF pressure more so than 1 MAC isoflurane.
9. Nursing considerations
   a. Commonly used for maintenance anesthesia in adults and in ambulatory surgery settings
   b. Extremely rapid onset and offset of CNS effects; rapid offset leaves no lingering analgesia; the requirement for supplemental analgesia must be anticipated.

F. Sevoflurane
   1. General facts
      a. Brand name: Ultane
         (1) Newest inhalational anesthetic
      b. Because of chemical configuration, it *cannot* be broken down into carbon monoxide even if it does pass through dry carbon dioxide absorbents (see preceding Section IX.C.1).
         (1) Sevoflurane *can*, however, be converted into other toxic products, including Compounds A and B (see following Section 10).
      c. Its vapor is pleasant smelling and nonirritating
         (1) Very useful for mask inductions
         (2) Also useful for maintenance anesthesia as long as certain criteria are followed (see following Section 10).
   2. Administration route
      a. Inhalation only
   3. Pharmacokinetics
      a. Up to 5% of administered dose is metabolized by liver.

4. Cardiovascular effects
   a. Has less potent coronary arteriolar vasodilator effects and does not appear to cause "coronary steal"
   b. During sudden increases in inspired gas concentrations, it does not result in transient sympathetically mediated increases in heart rate and blood pressure (i.e., unlike desflurane and to a lesser extent isoflurane).
   c. Dysrhythmias
      (1) Unlike the other volatile agents, sevoflurane does not appear to sensitize the myocardium to the dysrhythmogenic effects of exogenously administered catecholamines.
5. Respiratory effects
   a. Dose-dependent depression of ventilation
   b. Pleasant smelling and nonirritating; of all the volatile agents, it is least likely to cause coughing, breath holding, excessive salivation, or laryngospasm.
6. Hepatic and renal systems
   a. Hepatic and renal blood flow appear to be well preserved.
   b. Hexafluoroisopropanol, one of the metabolites, is conjugated in the liver with glucuronic acid and excreted by the kidney into the urine.
   c. Fluoride ion, the other metabolite, may be associated with renal impairment if allowed to accumulate (see following Section 10).
7. Skeletal muscle effects
   a. Promotes and potentiates neuromuscular blockade
8. CNS effects
   a. Solubility in blood is very low (as with desflurane and nitrous oxide).
      (1) Allows for fast onset and offset of CNS effects
      (2) Speed of onset and offset slightly slower than desflurane and nitrous oxide
   b. Is not associated with convulsive or epileptic activity (unlike enflurane)
   c. Causes minimal increases in intracranial pressure over the 0.5 to 1 MAC range
9. Toxicity of metabolites
   a. Fluoride ion can be nephrotoxic if levels are allowed to rise high enough.
      (1) The peak concentration of fluoride ion appears to be similar to that after enflurane use.
      (2) No clinical demonstration of nephrotoxicity has yet been described, even though moderately elevated plasma levels of fluoride ion have been seen.
      (3) Caution is advised in using sevoflurane in patients with known renal impairment.
   b. Hexafluoroisopropanol is potentially hepatotoxic if not eliminated rapidly by glucuronidation (beware in patients with hepatic disease); glucuronide metabolite is excreted by the kidneys (be wary in patients with renal impairment).
10. Breakdown product
    a. Sevoflurane can be broken down by exposure to Baralyme or soda lime; the rate of this breakdown is increased by certain conditions.
    b. Several breakdown products can be formed.
       (1) Compounds A, B, C, D, and E
       (2) Note, only compound A (and to a lesser extent compound B) is likely to be clinically relevant.
       (3) Compound A causes renal, hepatic, and cerebral damage in animal studies.

11. Nursing considerations
   a. Pediatric use is becoming more common and is competing with halothane usage.
   b. Adult use in ambulatory surgery settings is becoming more common.
   c. Least irritating of all the volatile agents used
   d. Extremely rapid onset and offset of CNS effects; rapid offset leaves no lingering analgesia; the requirement for supplemental analgesia must be anticipated.
   e. May not be useful in patients with hepatic or renal insufficiency

X. Gaseous inhalational anesthetic
   A. Nitrous oxide (N_2O)
      1. General facts
         a. Exists as a gas at atmospheric pressure
         b. Brand name: various manufacturers
            (1) Odorless to sweet-smelling inorganic gas
         c. Nonflammable but will support combustion
         d. Prominent analgesic effects
            (1) Reduces amount of volatile agents required
            (2) Analgesic effect is further enhanced by narcotics.
         e. Weak anesthetic effects
            (1) Is not potent enough to provide anesthesia
         f. Minimal muscle relaxant properties
      2. Administration route
         a. Administered by inhalation
         b. Clinically useful doses range between 50% and 70%.
            (1) Use of greater concentrations may cause hypoxia.
            (2) Clinical doses at 50% to 70% provide limited analgesic effects.
            (3) The limited analgesia provided may be enhanced by the coadministration of opioids.
      3. Pharmacokinetics
         a. Quick onset of effects occurs over minutes.
            (1) Quick onset is related to its very low solubility in blood.
            (2) Quick onset is also related to high concentrations used.
         b. Metabolism is negligible.
         c. Offset of effects
            (1) 5 to 10 minutes (assuming adequate ventilations)
            (2) Related to its very low solubility in blood
            (3) Assumes adequate ventilation of fresh oxygen into lungs
         d. Diffusion hypoxia and anoxia
            (1) When a N_2O-O_2 blend is being delivered into patients' lungs, the N_2O cannot accumulate in the alveoli more than the 50% to 70% being given; however, when the external delivery of N_2O is stopped, the entire amount of N_2O that accumulated within the patient can diffuse back into the alveoli at a concentration approaching 100% if the patient is poorly ventilated.
            (2) The back diffusion of N_2O dilutes alveolar O_2 and ultimately causes hypoxemia.
            (3) Accumulating alveolar N_2O must be ventilated out of lungs and replaced with a fresh supply of 100% oxygen.
      4. CNS effects
         a. Mild amnesia (incomplete CNS depression)
         b. Very good analgesic effects
         c. May increase CBF and ICP
      5. Cardiovascular system
         a. May initially increase heart rate, SVR, and cardiac contractility indirectly by evoking release of catecholamines

    b. However, it ultimately decreases heart rate, SVR, and cardiac contractility by a direct depressant effect.

      (1) Depressant effect is seen when catecholamine stores in sympathetic nerve endings are depleted because of prolonged hypovolemia, cardiac failure, shock, or trauma.

6. Pulmonary and ventilatory system

    a. Chemoreceptor response to hypercapnia decreased

    b. High inhaled concentrations (50% to 70%) are required for analgesia.

      (1) Must mix this agent with 100% oxygen, not air (21% oxygen)

      (2) Must be vigilant for possible development of hypoxemia

7. Uterine effects

    a. Does not alter contractility in doses used for analgesia

8. Untoward effects

    a. Diffusion hypoxia (see preceding Section 3.d)

    b. Nausea may be related to diffusion of nitrous oxide into middle ear.

    c. Undesirable expansion by N_2O of closed gaseous spaces (within the body) filled with nitrogen

      (1) Room air is approximately 80% nitrogen.

      (2) When nitrous oxide is introduced into the lungs, it (as do all gases) will begin to evenly distribute itself (through the bloodstream) throughout the body's fluid space, and also, into any collections of air or nitrogen.

      (3) As it moves down its concentration gradient into the blood and any collections of air, it will be met by the opposite movement of nitrogen down its concentration gradient (from the collections of air) toward the lungs full of nitrous oxide (and oxygen) but very little nitrogen.

      (4) Given enough time, these two gases will equilibrate down their gradients.

      (5) Because nitrous oxide is 34 times more soluble in blood than nitrogen, nitrous oxide equilibrates first and thus tends to expand any pockets of air trapped within the body until the nitrogen eventually equilibrates "out."

      (6) In the interim (while nitrogen is trying to leave), there can be a tremendous increase in the volume and pressure of these pockets of gases, which leads to the undesirable gaseous expansions.

      (7) Examples of trapped air that can expand (with consequent dilemmas) include middle ear (nausea, a ruptured tympanic membrane), small air pneumothoraces (tension pneumothorax), air emboli in blood (myocardial infarction, stroke), and air emboli in CSF (tension pneumoencephaly).

    d. Undesirable collapse of closed gaseous spaces (within the body) filled with nitrous oxide

      (1) The exact opposite of the preceding can occur after a patient has been under general anesthesia with nitrous oxide for a long period; in this case, an eardrum can be severely retracted until room air nitrogen equilibrates back into the gaseous vacuum left behind in the middle ear space after the nitrous oxide equilibrated "out."

9. Drug interactions

    a. Narcotics enhance analgesia and may enhance circulatory depression (see preceding Sections A.1.d and A.5.b).

10. Nursing considerations

    a. Be wary of diffusion hypoxemia in patients who have received intraoperative nitrous oxide; on their initial arrival in the PACU patients may have some degree of diffusion hypoxia if N_2O was not adequately eliminated from their bodies before their departure from the operating room.

    b. Be wary of the potential for increased nausea.

    c. Be wary of the potential for expanded or retracted pockets of air.

XI. Nondepolarizing muscle relaxants (NDMRS)
  A. Common properties
    1. Physiology of the neuromuscular junction (NMJ) (see Figure 26-3)
      a. Anatomy and physiology
        (1) Presynaptic nerve terminal
          (a) Releases "packets" of neurotransmitter
        (2) Neurotransmitter
          (a) Acetylcholine (ACh)
          (b) Transmits a chemical signal across the synaptic cleft
        (3) Synapse (synaptic cleft)
          (a) Extremely narrow, extracellular interconnection point between a nerve ending and a muscle cell
        (4) Postsynaptic ACh receptors (on muscle cells)
      b. Presynaptic activity
        (1) Impulse is conducted down the presynaptic neuron.
        (2) Presynaptic nerve ending is depolarized.
        (3) Nerve ending releases ACh into synapse.
      c. Synaptic activity
        (1) Released ACh diffuses across the synapse to postsynaptic receptors on muscle cell.
      d. Postsynaptic activity
        (1) ACh binds to receptors on muscle cell.
        (2) Postsynaptic membrane of muscle cell is depolarized.
        (3) Membrane depolarization triggers a mechanism within muscle cell that leads to contraction.
      e. Termination of skeletal muscle contraction
        (1) Impulses are no longer conducted down presynaptic neuron.
        (2) Presynaptic nerve ending repolarizes.
        (3) ACh release into synapse is reduced.
        (4) Cholinesterase in synapse hydrolyzes previously released ACh
        (5) Insufficient ACh remains in synapse to continue depolarization of the postsynaptic side of the neuromuscular junction.
        (6) Muscle cells return to noncontracted state.
    2. Pharmacokinetics
      a. Absorption
        (1) Poorly absorbed from gastrointestinal tract
        (2) Typically given by IV injection
        (3) Onset of paralysis by IV injection is 1 to 2 minutes.
      b. Elimination
        (1) First, redistribution occurs.
        (2) Next, hepatic or renal excretion or both

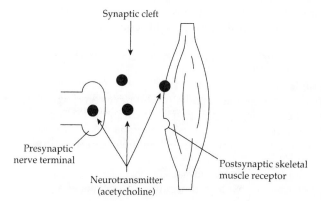

FIGURE 26-3 ■ Neuromuscular junction.

Synaptic cleft

Presynaptic nerve terminal

Neurotransmitter (acetycholine)

Postsynaptic skeletal muscle receptor

3. Pharmacodynamics
   a. NDMRs block the binding of ACh to postsynaptic receptors of skeletal muscle, impairing skeletal muscle contraction (see Figure 26-4).
      (1) NDMRs bind to postsynaptic receptors.
      (2) ACh is still released from presynaptic terminals.
      (3) However, NDMRs compete with ACh for postsynaptic receptor sites.
      (4) Degree of competition (i.e., the extent of muscle paralysis) depends on dose of NDMR given.
   b. Sequence of paralysis
      (1) Advances from fine to gross motor impairment (eyes → jaw → hands → limbs and neck → intercostal muscles → diaphragm)
   c. Sequence of recovery is in the *reverse* order of the sequence of paralysis.
   d. Reversal of NDMR effects
      (1) Various mechanisms lead to a "natural decay" in the concentration of NDMR within the synapse (thus restoring the ability of "naturally" released ACh to reach postsynaptic muscle receptors).
         (a) Redistribution
         (b) Metabolism
         (c) Renal excretion
         (d) Biliary excretion
      (2) Reversal can be enhanced or expedited by "pharmacologic intervention" to exaggerate amount of ACh "naturally" found within synapse during blocked neuromuscular transmission; increased amounts of ACh can compete more easily with NDMRs for postsynaptic muscle receptors (see Section XIII).
4. CNS effects
   a. NDMRs do not cross blood-brain barrier.
      (1) No CNS effects
      (2) Patient can be paralyzed and not speaking but be fully awake and alert!
5. Toxicity
   a. Ventilatory paralysis requires ventilatory support.
   b. *Recurarization* (i.e., reblockade) occurs when some condition or factor invigorates a previously attenuated neuromuscular blockade (this effect requires the presence of "subtherapeutic" amounts of NDMR that would not normally cause skeletal muscle paralysis).
      (1) Can be induced when respiratory acidosis occurs because of the injudicious use of narcotic analgesics
      (2) Can occur when long-acting NDMRs are "reversed" with short-acting NDMR reversal agents (see Section XIII)

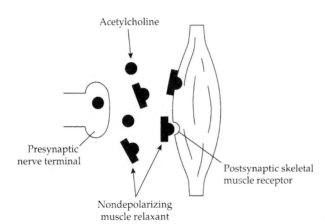

Acetylcholine

Presynaptic nerve terminal

Nondepolarizing muscle relaxant

Postsynaptic skeletal muscle receptor

FIGURE 26-4 ■ Nondepolarizing muscle relaxants compete with acetylcholine for skeletal muscle receptor site.

6. Interactions

    a. NDMR paralysis can be enhanced by drugs.

        (1) Aminoglycosides

        (2) Calcium channel blockers

        (3) Clindamycin

        (4) Lithium

        (5) Magnesium

        (6) Tetracyclines

        (7) Volatile anesthetics

    b. NDMR paralysis can be enhanced by physiologic imbalances.

        (1) Respiratory acidosis

        (2) Dehydration

        (3) Hypercapnia

        (4) Hypokalemia

        (5) Hyponatremia

        (6) Hypermagnesemia

        (7) Hypothermia

    c. NDMR paralysis can be antagonized by drugs.

        (1) NDMR reversal agents (increase synaptic ACh)

        (2) Caffeine

        (3) Epinephrine

        (4) Norepinephrine

        (5) Theophylline

    d. NDMR paralysis can be antagonized by physiologic imbalances.

        (1) Hypocapnia

        (2) Hyperkalemia

        (3) Hypernatremia

        (4) Respiratory alkalosis

7. Nursing considerations

    a. CNS

        (1) Never assume a paralyzed patient is asleep.

        (2) A paralyzed patient may be fully awake and feeling pain.

    b. Paralysis may be potentiated by many drugs or conditions (see preceding Section 6).

    c. Hypothermia

        (1) Can prolong recovery from a neuromuscular block

    d. Warning: watch for "reparalysis" in patients that may be inadequately reversed or may still have unacceptably high residual amounts of long-acting NDMRs.

        (1) Need to clinically assess each patient's muscle strength

        (2) Inquire as to *if, how much,* and *when* a long-acting NDMR was given.

        (3) Note: Be familiar with the long-acting NDMRs by name: doxacurium, pancuronium, pipecuronium, and tubocurarine.

B. Atracurium

1. General facts

    a. Brand name: Tracrium

        (1) Classified as an intermediate-acting NDMR

    b. Commonly used

    c. Drug spontaneously "self-destructs" systemically by a process known as Hoffman elimination.

        (1) No enzyme systems required

        (2) Occurs only in mildly alkaline solutions or blood at its normal pH of 7.4

        (3) Process can still occur when hepatorenal systems are impaired.

        (4) Hoffman elimination is slower and paralysis lasts longer if blood is acidotic.

    d. Drug can also be degraded by ester hydrolysis in an otherwise healthy patient.

Doxa
Pan
Pipe
turbo

    2. Administration route and dosage
      a. IV doses: 0.4 to 0.5 mg/kg for intubation
    3. Pharmacokinetics
      a. Onset: 3 to 5 minutes
      b. Duration: 20 to 35 minutes
      c. Elimination
        (1) Hoffman elimination normally eliminates 33% of a given dose with the production of two metabolites: laudanosine and a monoacrylate compound.
          (a) Laudanosine does not have NDMR properties, but in high concentrations has been shown to cause vasodilation, cerebral excitation, and seizure activity in animals.
          (b) Laudanosine is principally eliminated by the kidneys; theoretically it may accumulate in patients with renal failure.
        (2) Under normal conditions spontaneous recovery from paralysis can occur in 40 to 60 minutes.
        (3) Even with hepatic or renal system failure, complete recovery can still occur (albeit slower) by way of Hoffman elimination.
    4. Cardiovascular effects
      a. Histamine release may cause hypotension and tachycardia.
        (1) Depends on dose and rate of IV injection
        (2) More likely to occur if dose is injected rapidly
        (3) More likely to occur if dosage exceeds 0.4 to 0.5 mg/kg
    5. Effect of physiochemical extremes on elimination
      a. Hypothermia and acidemia may lengthen the time of paralysis by slowing Hoffman degradation.
      b. Hyperthermia and alkalemia may shorten the time of paralysis by hastening Hoffman degradation.
    6. Nursing considerations
      a. Eliminated by nonrenal and nonhepatic pathways
      b. Hypothermia and acidemia prolong paralysis and weakness.
      c. Residual paralysis or weakness is easily reversed with NDMR reversal agents.
C. Cisatracurium
    1. General facts
      a. Brand name: Nimbex
        (1) Classified as an intermediate-acting NDMR
      b. Is one of 10 stereoisomers of atracurium
      c. It is three times more potent than atracurium.
      d. In contrast to atracurium, it is primarily eliminated (80%) by the process known as Hoffman elimination.
      e. In sharp contrast to atracurium, it is not significantly degraded by nonspecific plasma esterases.
      f. Clinically, less laudanosine is generated.
      g. Overall it may offer advantages over atracurium when used during very long operations or in the ICU for patients being chronically ventilated (especially those with renal failure).
    2. Administration route and dosage
      a. IV doses: 0.15 to 0.2 mg/kg for intubation
    3. Pharmacokinetics
      a. Onset: 1.5 to 2 minutes
      b. Duration: 50 to 60 minutes
      c. Elimination
        (1) Hoffman elimination: 80% of a given dose
        (2) Plasma esterase hydrolysis: not significant
        (3) Renal and hepatic excretion: 20% of a given dose
        (4) Even with hepatic or renal system failure, complete recovery can still occur by way of Hoffman elimination.

4. Cardiovascular effects
   a. Histamine release is less of a concern than with atracurium.
5. Effect of physicochemical extremes on elimination
   a. Hypothermia and acidemia may lengthen the time of paralysis by slowing Hoffman degradation.
   b. Hyperthermia and alkalemia may shorten the time of paralysis by hastening Hoffman degradation.
6. Nursing considerations
   a. May be considered an improved form of atracurium
   b. Greater use for long operating room (OR) cases or mechanically ventilated ICU patients

D. Curare (d-tubocurarine, DTC)
1. General facts
   a. Brand name: various manufacturers
      (1) Classified as a long-acting NDMR
      (2) It is the oldest NDMR in clinical use.
      (3) Not commonly used clinically anymore as a primary NDMR
   b. Has the greatest potential of all NDMRs to release histamine
   c. Some preparations contain sulfite preservatives.
      (1) Ascertain sulfite presence in brand to be used.
      (2) Allergic reactions may occur in susceptible patients.
   d. Reversal of blockade should not be attempted unless some spontaneous recovery has begun (this point applies to all NDMRs, especially the long-acting NDMRs).
2. Administration route and dosage
   a. IV dose: 0.6 mg/kg for intubation
3. Pharmacokinetics
   a. Onset: 3 to 5 minutes
   b. Duration: 60 to 90 minutes
   c. Hepatic metabolism: not significant
   d. Biliary excretion (unchanged drug): 10% to 40%
   e. Renal excretion (unchanged drug): 45%
   f. Uptake: Some drug may be taken up into inactive tissue sites for a prolonged period (longer than 24 hours).
4. Cardiovascular effects
   a. Hypotension
      (1) Caused by release of histamine from mast cells
      (2) Amount of histamine released depends on the curare dose and its rate of injection.
      (3) Can be caused by the blockade of autonomic ganglia if the predominant autonomic tone is sympathetic
      (4) More pronounced in presence of hypovolemia
   b. Bradycardia and decreased contractility
      (1) Can be caused by the blockade of autonomic ganglia if the predominant autonomic tone is sympathetic
   c. Tachycardia
      (1) Can be caused by the blockade of autonomic ganglia if the predominant autonomic tone is parasympathetic
      (2) May be potentiated by a reflex response secondary to previously mentioned hypotension
5. Gastrointestinal effects
   a. Impaired peristaltic activity
      (1) Can be caused by the blockade of autonomic ganglia if the predominant tone is parasympathetic (peristaltic)
6. Side effects
   a. Secondary to histamine release
      (1) Wheals
      (2) Pruritus

(3) Erythema
(4) Hypotension
(5) Bronchospasm
(6) Bronchial and salivary secretions
(7) Decreased coagulability caused by concomitant release of heparin from mast cells
  b. Secondary to ganglionic blockade
(1) Affects many systems but is usually incomplete (see preceding)
7. Toxic effects
  a. Cardiovascular collapse
(1) Excessive histamine release
(2) Ganglionic blockade of a dominant sympathetic tone
  b. Some preparations contain benzyl alcohol preservatives.
(1) Toxicity may occur in neonates.
8. Nursing considerations
  a. Hypotension
(1) More profound in presence of hypovolemia
(2) Rehydrate and support blood pressure as needed.
  b. History of allergies, asthma, and/or anaphylactic reactions
(1) Avoid curare.
  c. Use not recommended in patients with renal disease
(1) Decreased renal elimination causes slower recovery from paralysis.
E. Doxacurium
  1. General facts
    a. Brand name: Nuromax
(1) Classified as a long-acting NDMR
    b. Most potent NDMR currently available: 2.5 to 3 times more potent than pancuronium
    c. Recommended for use during long surgical cases
    d. Useful in cases requiring cardiovascular stability (minimal drug-related changes in blood pressure and heart rate)
    e. Reversal of blockade should not be attempted unless some spontaneous recovery has begun (this point applies to all NDMRs, especially the long-acting NDMRs).
  2. Administration route and dosage
    a. IV dose: 0.04 to 0.08 mg/kg for intubation
  3. Pharmacokinetics
    a. Onset: 4 to 6 minutes
    b. Duration: 60 to 90 minutes
    c. Hepatic metabolism: unknown
    d. Biliary excretion (unchanged drug): unknown
    e. Renal excretion (unchanged drug): 70%
  4. Cardiovascular effects
    a. Does not cause clinically significant hemodynamic effects; slight decrease in heart rate, central venous pressure, or pulmonary artery pressure is possible
  5. Side effects uncommon but can include
    a. Flushing
    b. Urticaria
    c. Hypotension
    d. Bronchospasm
  6. Nursing considerations
    a. Very long-acting NDMR
    b. Elimination depends on renal and biliary excretion.
    c. Renal and hepatic disease slows recovery from paralysis.
    d. Requires adequate reversal or long spontaneous recovery period
(1) Warning: be watchful for a downward trend in minute ventilation in the PACU.

(2) A return of paralysis can be caused by the administration of inadequate amounts or inappropriate selections of NDMR reversal agents.

(3) A return of paralysis can also be caused by the administration of excessive amounts of this long-acting NDMR given too close toward the end of surgery.

(4) Note: Additional reversal agent may be required in PACU.

F. Gallamine
   1. General facts
      a. Brand name: various manufacturers
         (1) Classified as a long-acting NDMR
      b. Not commonly used clinically
      c. Substantial "vagolytic" (antimuscarinic) effect
         (1) May cause tachycardia
      d. Histamine release occurs only with excessive doses.
   2. Administration route and dosage
      a. IV dose: 3 to 4 mg/kg for intubation
      b. Not suitable for prolonged surgery because of its solubility in fat
         (1) Repetitive dosing may lead to accumulation of drug in fat tissue.
         (2) Weakness or paralysis may be prolonged in obese patients.
   3. Pharmacokinetics
      a. Onset: 3 to 5 minutes
      b. Duration: 60 to 90 minutes
      c. Hepatic metabolism: not significant
      d. Biliary excretion (unchanged drug): ~0%
      e. Renal excretion (unchanged drug): ~100%
   4. Drug interactions: same as with curare
   5. Nursing considerations
      a. Excreted entirely by kidneys
      b. Useful in patients with hepatic impairment
      c. Not useful in patients with renal impairment
      d. Moderate solubility in fat
         (1) Warning: reparalysis or prolonged weakness may occur in obese patients.

G. Metocurine
   1. General facts
      a. Brand name: various manufacturers
         (1) Classified as a long-acting NDMR
      b. Not commonly used anymore
      c. Small amount of histamine release (dose dependent)
   2. Administration route and dosage
      a. IV dose: 0.3 to 0.4 mg/kg for intubation
   3. Pharmacokinetics
      a. Onset: 3 to 5 minutes
      b. Duration: 60 to 90 minutes
      c. Hepatic metabolism: not significant
      d. Biliary excretion (unchanged drug): 1% to 2%
      e. Renal excretion (unchanged drug): ~43%
      f. Uptake: Some drug may be taken up into inactive tissue sites for a prolonged period.
   4. Cardiovascular effects: negligible
   5. Drug interactions: same as with curare
   6. Nursing considerations: same as with curare

H. Mivacurium
   1. General facts
      a. Brand name: Mivacron
         (1) Classified as a short-acting NDMR
      b. Administered as a continuous infusion or with frequent boluses

  c. Drug does not usually accumulate.

  d. Reversal of neuromuscular blockade is frequently not necessary.

  e. Succinylcholine (SCh) is still the best choice for emergency intubations.

 2. Administration route and dosage

  a. IV dose: 0.25 mg/kg for intubation (in two divided doses)

 3. Pharmacokinetics

  a. Onset: 2 to 3 minutes

  b. Duration: 12 to 20 minutes

  c. Metabolism: by plasma cholinesterase (PChE)

   (1) Typical homozygous PChE (most common variant)

    (a) "Normal" condition

    (b) No "abnormal" reduction in rate of PChE metabolism

   (2) Atypical heterozygous PChE

    (a) Not usually clinically significant

    (b) Mild reduction in rate of PChE metabolism

    (c) Small reduction in dosage may be required.

   (3) Atypical homozygous PChE

    (a) Clinically significant

    (b) Dosage reduction required

    (c) Occurs infrequently: 1:2500 patients

    (d) Seriously impairs metabolism and prolongs paralysis and weakness

    (e) "Abnormality" seriously impairs role of PChE metabolism.

   (4) Burn patients require reduction in dosage because of reduced levels of typical homozygous PChE.

   (5) Hepatic disease requires dosage adjustment because of decreased synthesis of typical homozygous PChE.

   (6) Full-term and postpartum women

    (a) Mild prolongation of paralysis and weakness may occur.

    (b) Patients have reduced levels of typical homozygous PChE.

    (c) Dosage adjustment not typically required

  d. Biliary excretion (unchanged drug): not significant

  e. Renal excretion (unchanged drug): not significant

 4. Cardiovascular effects

  a. Some histamine-related effects possible

   (1) Hypotension and tachycardia: determined by dose and rate of IV injection

 5. Side effects

  a. Apnea or hypoventilation

  b. Some related to histamine release

 6. Nursing considerations

  a. Short-acting NDMR

  b. Residual paralysis or weakness is not likely to be seen but is easily reversed with a little time or NDMR reversal agents.

  c. With prudent dosing, use of NDMR reversal agents is rarely needed in patients with typical homozygous PChE.

I. Pancuronium

 1. General facts

  a. Brand name: Pavulon and others

   (1) Classified as a long-acting NDMR

  b. Commonly used

  c. Potential histamine release with excessive doses

  d. Reversal of blockade should not be attempted unless some spontaneous recovery has begun (this point applies to all NDMRs, especially the long-acting NDMRs).

 2. Administration route and dosage

  a. Dose: 0.08 to 0.10 mg/kg for intubation

3. Pharmacokinetics
   a. Onset: 3 to 5 minutes
   b. Duration: 60 to 90 minutes
   c. Hepatic metabolism: 10% to 40%
   d. Biliary excretion (unchanged drug): 5% to 10%
   e. Renal excretion (unchanged drug): 80%
4. Cardiovascular effects
   a. Anticholinergic and vagolytic action may cause tachycardia.
   b. Sympathomimetic actions
      (1) Enhances release of norepinephrine from adrenergic nerve endings
      (2) Inhibits reuptake of norepinephrine from adrenergic nerve endings
      (3) Overall sympathetic effect may increase heart rate and blood pressure.
5. Nursing considerations
   a. Requires adequate reversal or a long spontaneous recovery period
      (1) Warning: Be watchful for a downward trend in minute ventilation in the PACU.
      (2) A return of paralysis can be caused by the administration of inadequate amounts or inappropriate selections of NDMR reversal agents.
      (3) A return of paralysis can also be caused by the administration of excessive amounts of this long-acting NDMR given too close toward the end of surgery.
      (4) Note: Additional NDMR reversal agent may be required in PACU.
J. Pipecuronium
   1. General facts
      a. Brand name: Arduan
         (1) Classified as a long-acting NDMR
      b. Recommended for use during prolonged surgery
      c. Recommended for cases requiring cardiovascular stability
      d. Reversal of blockade should not be attempted unless some spontaneous recovery has begun (this point applies to all NDMRs, especially the long-acting NDMRs).
   2. Administration route and dosage
      a. IV dose: 0.07 to 0.085 mg/kg for intubation
         (1) Onset within 5 minutes
         (2) Recovery usually begins in 45 to 120 minutes.
   3. Pharmacokinetics
      a. Onset: 3 to 5 minutes
      b. Duration: 60 to 90 minutes
      c. Hepatic metabolism: 10%
      d. Biliary excretion (unchanged drug): 20%
      e. Renal excretion (unchanged drug): 70%
   4. Cardiovascular effects
      a. Does not cause clinically significant hemodynamic effects
   5. Side effects
      a. Rash and urticaria: possibly related to histamine release
      b. Hypoventilation and apnea: caused by effects of residual NDMR
   6. Nursing considerations
      a. Long-acting NDMR
      b. Elimination depends on renal excretion; dose should be reduced in patients with renal impairment.
      c. Requires adequate reversal or a long spontaneous recovery period
         (1) Warning: inadequate reversal may have been given in OR.
         (2) Warning: watch for downward trend in minute ventilation.
         (3) Paralysis may recur once effect of reversal agent has worn off; additional reversal may be required in PACU.

  K. Rocuronium
1. General facts
    a. Brand name: Zemuron
        (1) Classified as a short-acting NDMR
    b. No histamine release
    c. Appears devoid of cardiovascular effects
    d. Very fast onset of muscle relaxation
    e. However, in certain situations SCh may still be the best choice for emergency intubations.
2. Administration route and dosage
    a. IV dose: 0.5 mg/kg for intubation
3. Pharmacokinetics
    a. Onset: 1 minute
    b. Duration: 15 to 20 minutes
    c. Metabolism: does not appear to be significant
    d. Elimination: unchanged by liver and kidney
4. Nursing considerations
    a. Similar to vecuronium: see following.
  L. Vecuronium
1. General facts
    a. Brand name: Norcuron
        (1) Classified as an intermediate-acting NDMR
    b. No histamine release (even at high doses)
    c. Generally speaking, no cardiovascular effects
        (1) Minimal, if any, effects on blood pressure and heart rate
        (2) Occasional reports of histaminelike reactions
2. Administration route and dosage
    a. IV dose: 0.08 to 0.1 mg/kg for intubation
3. Pharmacokinetics
    a. Onset: 3 to 5 minutes
    b. Duration: 20 to 35 minutes
    c. Hepatic deacetylation: 20% to 30%
    d. Biliary excretion (unchanged drug): 40% to 75%
        (1) Elimination can be prolonged with severe liver disease.
    e. Renal excretion (unchanged drug): 15% to 25%
4. Nursing considerations
    a. Lack of cardiovascular effects; useful in cardiac surgery
    b. Hepatobiliary excretion: prolonged effect with severe liver disease
XII. Depolarizing muscle relaxant (DMR)
  A. Succinylcholine (SCh) (only drug of this class in the United States)
1. General facts
    a. Brand names: Anectine, Quelicin, and Sucostrin
        (1) Classified as ultrashort-acting DMR
        (2) Very rapid onset and offset
        (3) Frequently used when intubating conditions are needed rapidly
    b. Warning: Its use in children is controversial and potentially dangerous; its use may be appropriate if the benefits of promptly intubating the trachea are greater than the risks of using SCh.
        (1) Note: If used in children, be wary of sudden cardiac standstill caused by a SCh-induced sudden release of intracellular skeletal muscle potassium (which abruptly establishes a hyperkalemic crisis and depolarizes all the contractile tissue of the heart); should this occur (in addition to any requisite basic life support) the hyperkalemic crisis is treated initially with titrated doses of calcium chloride (which helps to stabilize and repolarize the resting membrane potential of the cardiac cells) and subsequently with the administration of insulin, glucose, and bicarbonate (which helps pump extracellular potassium back into skeletal muscle cells).

   c. Warning: Contraindicated in patients after the acute phase (after 2 to 4 days) of certain types of neuromuscular injury (because of the potential for the release of life-threatening amounts of intracellular potassium from denervated skeletal muscle subsequently exposed to SCh)
      (1) Major burns
      (2) Multiple trauma
      (3) Upper motor neuron injury
      (4) Lower motor neuron injury
      (5) Cerebral vascular accidents
      (6) Extensive denervation of skeletal muscle
   d. Warning: May also be contraindicated in patients with chronic illnesses (after several days) because of an excessive release of intracellular potassium from skeletal muscle that has been in a state of chronic disuse
      (1) Disuse atrophy
      (2) Critical illness
      (3) Severe infection
      (4) Prolonged immobilization
      (5) Recent discontinuation of prolonged NDMR use in a critical care setting
   e. Warning: Use in children with muscular dystrophies or myotonias is particularly ill-advised; these children may be more likely to develop a life-threatening type of prolonged skeletal muscle spasm, or malignant hyperthermia (see Chapter 28).
2. Administration route and dosage
   a. Usually as single IV bolus
      (1) About 1-1.5 mg/kg for intubation
      (2) Infusion "titrated to effect" may be used to prolong relaxation.
   b. Phase I block (occurs after a brief single-dose exposure to SCh)
      (1) This is the type of neuromuscular paralysis typically associated with DMRs.
         (a) Caused by single doses of SCh not exceeding 3 mg/kg
         (b) Relaxant effect wears off quickly (usually within minutes) after SCh is rapidly metabolized and the neuromuscular junction completely repolarizes (see exceptions following, atypical PChE).
         (c) If a nerve stimulator is used minutes after administration of SCh, a brief sustained (tetanic) stimulation to the nerve of a muscle (being tested for recovery) will produce a contraction of *low* but *sustained* amplitude. Over time, as the effects of the DMR block continues to wear off, each subsequent tetanic stimulation (allowing for rest periods in between) will continue to produce *sustained* amplitudes of contraction (within each test) but with *increasing* amplitudes overall.
         (d) If an anticholinesterase drug is given during the drug recovery period (a practice not recommended), there will be an augmentation of the DMR block (now caused by an increase in synaptic ACh rather than SCh concentrations) and a return of neuromuscular paralysis; a brief tetanic stimulation will produce a sustained contraction of decreased (or no) amplitude.
   c. Phase II block (acts more as an NDMR block)
      (1) This is a type of neuromuscular paralysis similar to that caused by NDMR.
         (a) Occurs after a single bolus dose of >3 mg/kg or after a continuous infusion (total dose) of >7 mg/kg
         (b) The postsynaptic ACh receptor appears to change the way it interacts with SCh. SCh still binds to the ACh receptor, but

depolarization no longer occurs. Thus under the conditions of chronic exposure to SCh, the ACh receptor appears to protect itself (from continuing depolarization) by responding to SCh as if it were an NDMR. General anesthetics may facilitate this phenomenon.

(c) Note that the phase II relaxant effect of SCh does *not* wear off quickly and completely; thus prolonged apnea, slow recovery from paralysis, and prolonged intubation and mechanical ventilation may be observed.

(d) A brief tetanic stimulation to the nerve of a muscle recovering from a phase II block will produce contractions of *low* and *unsustained* amplitude. As the effects of the NDMR block wear off, each subsequent tetanic stimulation (allowing for rest periods in between) continues to produce *unsustained* amplitudes of contraction (within each tetanic period but with ever-increasing amplitudes overall. As the effects of phase II block completely resolve, the *unsustained* amplitudes (seen during a tetanic stimulation) ultimately become *sustainable*.

(e) If an anticholinesterase drug is given during the drug recovery period, there will be a beneficial antagonism of the phase-II block and a return of neuromuscular function; edrophonium, 0.1 mg/kg IV, may be used to briefly test whether a phase II type block exists (the effects of this small dose are short-lived if a phase I type block is actually present).

3. Pharmacokinetics
   a. Absorption
      (1) Must be given by IV or IM injection
      (2) Onset of paralysis after IV injection occurs in about 1 minute.
   b. Duration
      (1) Generally short (about 5 minutes), after a single intubating dose
      (2) Complete recovery normally occurs in about 15 minutes.
   c. Metabolism
      (1) Normally hydrolyzed by PChE
      (2) Not hydrolyzed by acetylcholinesterase (AChE)
      (3) Decreases in the quantity (concentration) or quality (i.e., molecular defects) of PChE will prolong the effects of an administered dose of SCh.
      (4) See following information on plasma cholinesterase.
   d. Renal excretion (unchanged drug): 10%

4. Plasma cholinesterase (PChE)
   a. Also called pseudocholinesterase
   b. Produced by liver
   c. Serum albumin and PChE levels
      (1) Tend to be directly related
      (2) Hypoalbuminemic patients tend to have PChE deficiency.
   d. Role of PChE
      (1) No clearly understood physiologic role
      (2) Responsible for metabolism of SCh, local anesthetics (esters), and trimethaphan (an antihypertensive medication)
   e. Typical homozygous PChE
      (1) Majority of population has this genetic variant.
      (2) SCh metabolized with rapid rate of ester hydrolysis
   f. Atypical heterozygous PChE
      (1) 4% of population
      (2) SCh metabolized with mildly reduced rate of hydrolysis
      (3) Mild prolongation of intraoperative apnea possible if SCh given

      g. Atypical homozygous PChE
         (1) 0.03% of population
         (2) SCh metabolized with severely reduced rate of hydrolysis
         (3) Severe prolongation of postoperative apnea possible if SCh given

  5. Acquired changes in plasma cholinesterase activity
      a. Decreased activity (decreased quantity of active enzyme molecules)
         (1) Advanced age
         (2) Renal failure
         (3) Malnutrition
         (4) Severe anemia
         (5) Severe hepatic disease
         (6) Bronchogenic carcinoma
         (7) Prolonged cardiopulmonary bypass
         (8) Postpartum period (levels lowest on third postpartum day)
         (9) Inquire as to the recent administration of NDMR reversal agents (i.e., neostigmine and pyridostigmine).
      b. Increased activity (increased quantity)
         (1) Obese have more activity than nonobese patients.
         (2) Whole blood, packed red blood cells (RBCs), and fresh frozen plasma (FFP) are an exogenous source of PChE.

  6. Pharmacodynamics
      a. SCh depolarizes the NMJ of skeletal muscle as endogenous ACh does (see Figure 26-5).
         (1) Normally, ACh binds to the nicotinic receptors of the NMJ, but this binding is short-lived because ACh is rapidly hydrolyzed by the presence of AChE.
         (2) SCh also binds to the nicotinic receptors of neuromuscular junction and, notably, does so more effectively; SCh's binding and depolarization of the NMJ lasts longer than that caused by ACh.
      b. Sequence of SCh-induced paralysis
         (1) Advances from fine to gross motor impairment
         (2) Eyes, jaw, and hands → limbs and neck → intercostal muscles → diaphragm
      c. Initial depolarization causes transient fasciculations.
         (1) May or may not cause postoperative myalgia
         (2) Myalgia can be reduced by pretreatment with small dose of NDMR.

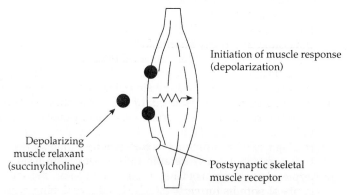

FIGURE 26-5 ■ Paralysis with succinylcholine: initiation of skeletal muscle response. First, depolarization initiates uncontrolled random contractions (fasciculations); then during the next several minutes, persisting receptor depolarization leads to muscle paralysis/relaxation.

(3) May transiently increase intraocular pressure (IOP) (possibly involves transient contraction or fasciculation of extraocular muscles)

(4) Use of SCh may cause extrusion of eye contents in "open globe" cases.

7. CNS effects
   a. Does not cross blood-brain barrier
      (1) No CNS effects
      (2) Patient can be paralyzed (and not speaking) but be fully awake and alert!

8. Cardiovascular effects
   a. Stimulation of vagal nuclei and nerve (the vagus nerve innervates the atria and the SA/AV nodes) leads to
      (1) Bradycardia and supraventricular dysrhythmias
      (2) "Digitalized patients" may manifest exaggerated bradycardia.
   b. Stimulation of sympathetic ganglia
      (1) Hypertension and tachycardia may follow usual doses because of the initial (phase I) effects of SCh on ganglionic nicotinic receptors.
   c. Inhibition of sympathetic ganglia
      (1) Hypotension and bradycardia may subsequently follow extremely high doses of SCh because of its phase II blockade of ganglionic nicotinic receptors.

9. Respiratory effect
   a. Ventilation must be artificially supported during muscle paralysis.

10. Gastrointestinal effects
    a. Increases intragastric and intraabdominal pressure
    b. But also increases lower esophageal sphincter pressure
       (1) Therefore risk of regurgitation is lower than expected.
       (2) "Aspiration precautions" should still be maintained.

11. Hepatic effects (none)

12. Renal effects
    a. Direct: not likely
    b. Indirect: excessive fasciculations may cause myoglobinuria; however, myoglobinuria is most likely seen in children or adults in whom malignant hyperthermia develops (see Chapter 28).

13. Histamine release
    a. Occasionally causes mild reaction: rash on arms and upper chest

14. Eye effect (transiently raises IOP)
    a. Contracts extraocular muscles
    b. Contraindicated in patients with eye injuries (i.e., "open globe") because the eye contents may be extruded during the initial SCh-induced fasciculations of the extraocular muscles

15. Induced hyperkalemia
    a. Depolarization of skeletal muscle causes release of intracellular potassium into the extracellular fluid (ECF).
       (1) Normally amounts to about 0.5 mEq/L
       (2) Effect peaks in 5 minutes; normalizes in 10 to 15 minutes
       (3) Excessive increases in serum potassium can cause cardiac arrest.
    b. As mentioned above, SCh-induced depolarization of denervated skeletal muscle causes a copious release of potassium into the ECF (effect is observed initially 2 to 4 days after denervation and is maximal after 14 days); this unusual release of potassium occurs because denervated skeletal muscle increases (i.e., "up regulates") its population of nicotinic receptors in the hope of "reestablishing contact" with its formerly attached and functioning nerve endings.
    c. Conditions that can lead to some form of skeletal muscle denervation
       (1) Severe burns
       (2) Denervation injuries
       (3) Massive muscle or soft tissue trauma

(4) Spinal cord injury (up to 6 months after initial insult)

(5) Upper motor neuron lesions: stroke, encephalitis

d. Muscle fasciculations

(1) Related to the wholesale depolarization of skeletal muscles throughout the human body

(2) Very small and judicious doses of NDMRs (administered before the use of SCh) are used by some clinicians to reduce these fasciculations.

16. Concurrent hyperkalemia

a. As stated previously, SCh releases potassium into the ECF.

b. The use of SCh may be inadvisable with some conditions.

(1) Renal disease

(2) Severe intraabdominal infections

(3) Patients experiencing congestive heart failure (CHF) or receiving digoxin

17. Toxic effects

a. Prolonged apnea

b. Cardiac arrest

c. Malignant hyperthermia (see Chapter 28)

18. Interactions

a. Enhancement of DMR effects by drugs

(1) Calcium channel blockers

(2) NDMR reversal agents inhibit PChE.

(a) Note: If SCh is administered in the PACU, a patient who has been given the NDMR reversal agent neostigmine or pyridostigmine (not edrophonium) can have an unanticipated period of prolonged muscle paralysis (see Section XIII).

b. Drugs that inhibit PChE can prolong the effects of SCh

(1) Trimethaphan

(2) Local anesthetic esters (procaine, chloroprocaine, and tetracaine)

c. DMR paralysis can be enhanced by physiologic imbalances.

(1) Respiratory alkalosis

(2) Hyperkalemia

(3) Hypermagnesemia

(4) Hypothermia

(5) Decreased renal function

(6) Dehydration

(7) Lithium pharmacotherapy

(8) Low quantity or abnormal quality of PChE

d. DMR paralysis can be antagonized by physiologic imbalances.

(1) Respiratory acidosis

(2) Hypokalemia

(3) Decreased peripheral perfusion

19. Nursing considerations

a. SCh has no effect on mentation; thus never assume that a paralyzed patient is asleep or pain free.

b. Malignant hyperthermia

(1) May or may not occur during anesthesia

(2) It may first manifest itself in the PACU.

c. Postoperative myalgia

(1) Caused by SCh-induced fasciculations

(2) Can be lessened by a very small dose of NDMR before SCh

d. If a slow recovery occurs from SCh-induced paralysis

(1) Check serum albumin level; if albumin low, PChE level may also be low.

e. Treatment of phase II block

(1) Careful clinical correlation required

(2) Reversal of paralysis is attempted with an anticholinesterase drug.

f. SCh use after patient has received an anticholinesterase drug

(1) Acceptable if SCh is used to treat postoperative laryngospasm

(2) Acceptable if SCh is used to reintubate patient in PACU

(3) Remember that relaxation of skeletal muscle will be prolonged if PChE is inhibited.

(4) Note: Neostigmine and pyridostigmine will inhibit PChE as well as AChE(see following Section XIII)

(5) Note: Edrophonium inhibits AChE but *not* PChE.

XIII. NDMR reversal agents (anticholinesterases)

A. Common properties

1. Physiology

   a. Physiology of neuromuscular junction (NMJ) (see Section XI.A.1)

   b. Released ACh depolarizes skeletal muscle by binding to postsynaptic nicotinic receptors at the NMJ.

      (1) Contraction of skeletal muscle is initiated in this manner.

      (2) Contraction ceases when neural release of ACh ends and when residual ACh in synapse is destroyed: such destruction of Ach is performed rapidly by a synaptic enzyme called acetylcholinesterase (AChE).

   c. NDMRs prevent released ACh from reaching the nicotinic receptors of skeletal muscle.

      (1) Molecules of NDMRs bind to and block these receptors.

      (2) Voluntary control of skeletal muscle contraction is thereby weakened or lost.

2. Pharmacodynamics

   a. NDMR reversal agents provide a means of overpowering the effects of NDMRs.

      (1) This is done by inhibiting synaptic AChE and thus increasing the synaptic levels of ACh.

      (2) Greater amounts of NDMR are displaced from nicotinic receptors as the synaptic concentration of ACh exceeds that of NDMR.

      (3) The return of neuromuscular control can be hastened as the synaptic concentration of ACh is artificially increased concurrent with the progressive reduction in the concentration of NDMR (by breakdown, metabolism, excretion, and discontinuing its administration).

   b. NDMR reversal agents exert a *desired* effect by increasing the synaptic levels of ACh at the nicotinic receptors of skeletal muscle.

   c. However, NDMR reversal agents exert an *undesired* effect by increasing the synaptic levels of ACh at muscarinic receptors in the following organs.

      (1) Eyes: miosis

      (2) Heart: bradycardia

      (3) Lungs: bronchospasm

      (4) Gastrointestinal tract: enhanced peristalsis

      (5) Secretory glands: enhanced secretions

   d. The undesired effects of NDMR reversal agents can be minimized by the coadministration of antimuscarinic agents (atropine or glycopyrrolate).

   e. If excessive doses of NDMR reversal agents are administered, an excessive increase in synaptic ACh will occur; this will result in synaptic depolarization (by ACh) and resulting skeletal muscle weakness.

3. CNS effects

   a. NDMR reversal agents have no direct effects (they do not cross blood-brain barrier).

4. Toxicities

   a. Minimal if dosed properly and combined with the appropriate antimuscarinic drug (see following Section VIII.B)

B. Neostigmine
  1. General facts
    a. Brand name: various manufacturers
      (1) Commonly used reversal agent for NDMRs
    b. Binds to synaptic AChE
      (1) Prevents AChE from breaking down ACh
        (a) Half-life of neostigmine-AChE binding: 30 minutes
        (b) Half-life of ACh-AChE binding: 42 microseconds
      (2) Synaptic levels of ACh accumulate.
        (a) Competitive antagonism between ACh and NDMR occurs.
      (3) Bound neostigmine eventually hydrolyzes spontaneously.
        (a) Thereafter AChE is available to bind more ACh.
    c. Inhibits PChE and will prolong the effects of other drugs metabolized by PChE
      (1) SCh
      (2) Mivacurium
      (3) Trimethaphan
      (4) Local anesthetic esters (i.e., procaine, chloroprocaine, and tetracaine)
  2. Administration route and dosage
    a. IV dose: 0.05 mg/kg
      (1) Must be given concurrently with IV glycopyrrolate (0.01 mg/kg)
      (2) Should not be given unless some spontaneous recovery of the NMJ is evident (assess motor strength before dosing)
  3. Pharmacokinetics
    a. Onset (IV injection)
      (1) 50% of peak activity within 3.5 minutes
      (2) 100% of peak activity within 7 minutes
    b. Duration: 60 minutes
    c. Metabolism: ester hydrolysis by AChE and PChE
    d. Excretion: renal (50%)
    e. Elimination: primarily renal (75%)
      (1) Metabolites from hydrolysis
      (2) Unchanged drug, small amount
  4. Pharmacodynamics
    a. Reversibly inhibits synaptic AChE
      (1) Dose-dependent increase in synaptic ACh
      (2) ACh competitively antagonizes presence of NDMRs.
    b. Alert: Neostigmine also reversibly inhibits PChE.
      (1) Effect may last up to 4 hours.
      (2) This will prolong the effects of drugs metabolized by PChE.
        (a) SCh
        (b) Mivacurium
        (c) Trimethaphan
        (d) Local anesthetics, esters
    c. Note: Excessive neostigmine can actually cause neuromuscular paralysis.
      (1) A "depolarization block" can occur (as with SCh).
      (2) Caused by the effects of excessive doses (>0.075 mg/kg)
        (a) Direct effects: in excessive doses neostigmine can directly depolarize nicotinic receptors.
        (b) Indirect effects: maximally increased levels of ACh in synapse may also cause a depolarization block of the NMJ.
  5. Cardiovascular effects
    a. Bradycardia
      (1) Caused by increased ACh at sites of vagal innervation: SA and AV nodes
      (2) Can profoundly lower heart rate and cardiac output

   b. Peripheral vasodilation may cause hypotension.
      (1) Caused by activation of vascular muscarinic receptors
 6. Drug combinations
   a. Neostigmine with atropine
      (1) Not a preferred combination
      (2) The onset and effect of atropine precedes that of neostigmine.
         (a) More tachycardia
         (b) More dysrhythmias
   b. Neostigmine with glycopyrrolate
      (1) Preferred combination for neostigmine
      (2) Onset time of glycopyrrolate better matches that of neostigmine.
         (a) Less tachycardia
         (b) Fewer dysrhythmias
      (3) In addition, neither drug crosses blood-brain barrier; therefore CNS effects are minimal.
 7. Nursing considerations
   a. Commonly used reversal agent for NDMRs
   b. Monitor vital signs and pulse oximetry (SpO$_2$) when reversal agents are given.
C. Edrophonium
 1. General facts
   a. Brand name: Enlon
      (1) Frequently used anticholinesterase for NDMRs
   b. Alert: Onset of effects is rapid; a profound increase in vagal tone (muscarinic tone) on the heart will occur if atropine is not coadministered; severe bradycardia, or even asystole, may result.
   c. It is good reversal agent if used correctly (atropine *must* be coadministered with edrophonium).
   d. Does not inhibit PChE (neostigmine and pyridostigmine will)
 2. Administration route and dosage
   a. Intravenously: 0.5 to 1 mg/kg
      (1) Not given unless some spontaneous recovery is evident
      (2) Given in combination with IV atropine (7 to 14 µg/kg)
 3. Pharmacokinetics
   a. Onset (IV injection)
      (1) 50% of peak activity within 0.5 minutes
      (2) 100% of peak activity within 1 minute
   b. Duration: 60 minutes
   c. Metabolism: conjugation to glucuronide
   d. Elimination: primarily renal (75%)
      (1) Tubular secretion
      (2) Metabolites from hydrolysis
      (3) Small amount of unchanged drug
 4. Drug combinations
   a. Edrophonium with atropine
      (1) Preferred combination for edrophonium
      (2) Onset time of atropine matches that of edrophonium.
         (a) Less bradycardia
         (b) Fewer dysrhythmias
         (c) Much less likely to see asystole
      (3) Atropine does cross blood-brain barrier.
   b. Edrophonium with glycopyrrolate
      (1) Potentially dangerous combination
      (2) Onset time of glycopyrrolate lags behind that of edrophonium: severe bradycardia, asystole, cardiovascular collapse can occur.
 5. Nursing considerations
   a. Formerly was not a popular reversal agent because it was not regarded as being very potent

(1) This was true historically; however, inadequate doses were given.

(2) Dosage should be 0.5 to 1 mg/kg (in combination with atropine).

b. Currently is used more

(1) Edrophonium is available in solution by itself (Enlon); use atropine concurrently.

(2) Edrophonium also comes premixed with atropine (Enlon Plus).

c. Alert: Edrophonium still not recommended for reversing a dense block; neostigmine (in combination with glycopyrrolate) will be more effective.

D. Pyridostigmine

1. General facts

a. Brand name: various manufacturers

(1) Less commonly used reversal agent for NDMRs

b. Less potent reversal agent than neostigmine; only 20% of the reversal activity of neostigmine

c. Duration of action (4 to 5 hours): 40% longer than that of neostigmine

d. Fewer muscarinic effects

e. Profound depression of PChE

(1) Longer lasting than neostigmine

(2) Will prolong effects of drugs metabolized by PChE

(a) SCh

(b) Mivacurium

(c) Trimethaphan

(d) Local anesthetics, esters

2. Administration route and dosage

a. IV dose: 0.25 mg/kg

(1) Not given unless some spontaneous recovery is evident

(2) Given in combination with IV glycopyrrolate (0.01 mg/kg); administer slowly to diminish side effects.

3. Pharmacokinetics

a. Onset (IV injection)

(1) 50% of peak activity in 4 minutes

(2) 100% of peak activity in 12 minutes

b. Duration: about 90 minutes

c. Metabolism: hydrolysis by AChE and PChE

d. Elimination: primarily renal (75%)

4. Drug combinations

a. Pyridostigmine with atropine

(1) Not a preferred combination

(2) Onset time of atropine precedes that of pyridostigmine.

(a) More tachycardia

(b) More dysrhythmias

b. Pyridostigmine with glycopyrrolate

(1) Preferred combination for pyridostigmine

(2) Onset time of glycopyrrolate better matches that of pyridostigmine.

(a) Less tachycardia

(b) Fewer dysrhythmias

(c) Neither crosses blood-brain barrier

5. Cardiovascular effects

a. Fewer autonomic side effects

b. Fewer dysrhythmias in elderly

6. Nursing considerations

a. Less commonly used NDMR reversal agent

b. Longer onset time than edrophonium or neostigmine

BIBLIOGRAPHY

1. Atlee J: *Complications in anesthesia.* Philadelphia: WB Saunders, 1999.
2. Barash P, Cullen B, Stoelting R, editors: *Clinical anesthesia,* ed 4. Philadelphia: Lippincott Williams & Wilkins, 2000.
3. Burden N, DeFazio Quinn D, O'Brien D, et al: *Ambulatory surgical nursing,* ed 2. Philadelphia: WB Saunders, 2000.
4. DeFazio-Quinn D: *Ambulatory surgical nursing core curriculum.* Philadelphia: WB Saunders, 1999.
5. Drain C: *Perianesthesia nursing: A critical care approach.* St Louis: Elsevier, 2003.
6. Faust R: *Anesthesiology review,* ed 3. New York: Churchill Livingstone, 2002.
7. Godden B, editor: *Core competency for perianesthesia nurses.* Cherry Hill, NJ: American Society of PeriAnesthesia Nurses, 2002.
8. Litwack K: *Core curriculum for post anesthesia nursing practice,* ed 4. Philadelphia: WB Saunders, 1999.
9. Miller R, editor: *Anesthesia,* ed 5. New York: Churchill Livingstone, 2000.
10. Roisen M, Fleisher L: *Essence of anesthesia practice,* ed 2. Philadelphia: WB Saunders, 2002.
11. Stoelting R: *Pharmacology and physiology in anesthetic practice,* ed 3. Philadelphia: Lippincott-Raven, 2000.
12. Stoelting R, Miller R: *Basics of anesthesia,* ed 4. New York: Churchill Livingstone, 2000.
13. Zaglaniczny K, Aker J: *Clinical guide to pediatric anesthesia.* Philadelphia: WB Saunders, 1999.

27 Moderate Sedation/Analgesia

MICHAEL KOST

OBJECTIVES

At the conclusion of this chapter the reader will be able to:

1. Define moderate sedation, deep sedation, and general anesthesia.

2. Identify the statutory, regulatory, practice guidelines, and promulgated professional standards of care for nurses administering moderate sedation and analgesia.

4. State the components of presedation patient assessment.

5. List sedative and analgesic medications, dosing guidelines, and nursing considerations associated with their administration.

6. Identify required monitoring parameters for the patient receiving moderate sedation and analgesia.

7. State postsedation monitoring requirements for the patient receiving sedation.

8. Identify risk management strategies used to reduce the incidence of complications associated with the delivery of sedative and analgesic medications.

SEDATION

I. Definitions
   A. Minimal sedation (anxiolysis)
      1. A drug-induced state during which patients respond normally to verbal commands. Although cognitive function and coordination may be impaired, ventilatory and cardiovascular functions are unaffected.
   B. Moderate sedation and analgesia ("conscious sedation")
      1. A drug-induced depression of consciousness during which patients respond purposefully to verbal commands, either alone or accompanied by light tactile stimulation. No interventions are required to maintain a patent airway, and spontaneous ventilation is adequate. Cardiovascular function is usually maintained.
   C. Deep sedation and analgesia
      1. A drug-induced depression of consciousness during which patients cannot be easily aroused but respond purposefully following repeated or painful stimulation. The ability to independently maintain ventilatory function may be impaired. Patients may require assistance in maintaining a patent airway and spontaneous ventilation may be inadequate. Cardiovascular function is usually maintained.
   D. Anesthesia
      1. Consists of general anesthesia and spinal or major regional anesthesia. It does not include local anesthesia. General anesthesia is a drug-induced loss of consciousness during which patients are not arousable, even with painful stimulation. The ability to independently maintain ventilatory function is often impaired. Patients often require assistance in maintaining a patent airway, and positive pressure ventilation may be required because of depressed spontaneous ventilation or drug-induced depression of neuromuscular function. Cardiovascular function may be impaired.

    E. Goals and objectives of moderate sedation and analgesia
        1. Maintain adequate sedation with minimal risk.
        2. Relieve anxiety.
        3. Produce amnesia.
        4. Provide relief from pain and other noxious stimuli.
        5. Overall goal: to allay patient fear and anxiety with a minimum of medication
        6. Mood alteration
        7. Enhanced patient cooperation
        8. Elevation of pain threshold
        9. Stable vital signs
        10. Rapid recovery
        11. Unconsciousness and unresponsiveness are not goals of moderate sedation and analgesia.
    F. Indications for moderate sedation and analgesia
        1. Diagnostic and therapeutic procedures that require anxiolysis and/or analgesia, widely utilized throughout healthcare facilities, particularly for
           a. Burn unit dressing changes
           b. Cardiology, Heart Station, Cardiac Catheterization Laboratory
           c. Cosmetic surgery
           d. Gastroenterology
           e. General surgery procedures
           f. Gynecology
           g. Ophthalmology
           h. Oral surgery
           i. Orthopedic procedures
           j. Pulmonary biopsy and bronchoscopy
           k. Radiology, interventional radiology
           l. Urology

II. Legal scope of practice issues
    A. An understanding of the definition and levels of sedation and adherence to the clinical criteria outlined are required for nurses to comply with legal scope of practice issues in many jurisdictions
        1. Legal scope of practice issues related to nursing are delegated and administered through state boards of nursing.
        2. It is imperative that nurses engaged in the administration of sedation ascertain their state board of nursing's formal position or policy statement delineating the role and responsibility of the nurse engaged in the delivery of sedation and analgesia.
        3. Most states have adopted guidelines. Some states, however, have not yet taken formal action on the issue or lack statutory authority to enact such legislation.

III. Joint Commission on Accreditation of Healthcare Organizations (JCAHO)
    A. JCAHO has taken an active role in the development of policies, standards, and intents related to the Standards and Intents for Sedation and Anesthesia.
        1. The Standards and Intents for Sedation and Anesthesia Care apply when patients receive, in any setting, for any purpose, by any route, moderate or deep sedation as well as general, spinal, or other major regional anesthesia.
    B. It is the obligation of each institution to develop appropriate protocols for patients receiving sedation.
    C. The JCAHO states
        1. Moderate or deep sedation and anesthesia are provided by qualified individuals.
        2. Sufficient numbers of qualified personnel are present during procedures using moderate or deep sedation and anesthesia.
        3. A presedation and preanesthesia assessment is performed for each patient before beginning moderate or deep sedation and before anesthesia induction.

4. Each patient's moderate or deep sedation and anesthesia care is planned.
5. Each patient's physiological status is monitored during sedation or anesthesia administration.
6. The patient's postprocedure status is assessed on admission to and before discharge from the postsedation or postanesthesia recovery area.

IV. Professional organizations
   A. In July 1991 the Nursing Organizations Liaison Forum in Washington, D.C., endorsed a position statement for the management of patients receiving intravenous sedation for short-term therapeutic, diagnostic, or surgical procedures.
      1. This position statement has been adopted by most professional nursing organizations.
   B. Professional organization guidelines, JCAHO Standards, and statutory regulations require policy development that prepares the nurse participating in the delivery of sedation to demonstrate.
      1. Knowledge of anatomy, physiology, cardiac dysrhythmias, and complications related to the administration of sedative agents
      2. Knowledge of the pharmacokinetic and pharmacodynamic principles associated with moderate sedation medications
      3. Presedation assessment and monitoring of physiologic parameters, including
         a. Respiratory rate
         b. Oxygen saturation
         c. Blood pressure
         d. Cardiac rate and rhythm
         e. Level of consciousness
      4. An understanding of the principles of oxygen delivery and the ability to use oxygen delivery devices
      5. The ability to rapidly assess, diagnose, and intervene in the event of an untoward reaction associated with the administration of moderate sedation
      6. Proven skill in airway management
      7. Accurate documentation of the procedure and medications administered
      8. Competency validation for training and education conducted on a regular basis

PRESEDATION ASSESSMENT AND PATIENT

I. Presedation assessment goals
   A. Identify preexisting pathophysiologic disease.
   B. Obtain baseline patient information.
   C. Take history and perform physical examination.
   D. Reduce patient anxiety through education and communication.
   E. Prepare a plan for the procedure.
   F. Obtain informed consent.

II. Components of presedation assessment
   A. Medical history
      1. Cardiac
         a. Angina
         b. Coronary artery disease
         c. Dysrhythmias
         d. Exercise tolerance
         e. Hypertension
         f. Myocardial infarction
      2. Pulmonary
         a. Asthma
         b. Bronchitis
         c. Dyspnea
         d. Exercise tolerance
         e. Cigarette smoking
         f. Recent cold or flu

3. Hepatic
   a. Ascites
   b. Cirrhosis
   c. Hepatitis
4. Renal
   a. Dialysis
   b. Renal failure
   c. Renal insufficiency
5. Neurologic
   a. Convulsive disorders
   b. Headaches
   c. Level of consciousness
   d. Stroke
   e. Syncope
   f. Cerebrovascular insufficiency
6. Endocrine
   a. Adrenal disease
   b. Diabetes
   c. Hyperthyroidism and hypothyroidism
7. Gastrointestinal
   a. Hiatal hernia
   b. Nausea
   c. Vomiting
8. Hematology
   a. Anemia
   b. Aspirin, nonsteroidal antiinflammatory drug (NSAID) use
   c. Excessive bleeding
9. Musculoskeletal
   a. Arthritis
   b. Back pain
   c. Joint pain

B. Nothing by mouth (NPO) status
   1. NPO Practice Guidelines[*] (American Society of Anesthesiologists and Anesthesia Patient Safety Foundation) fasting guidelines include:

Ingested Materials	Minimum Fasting Period[†]
Clear liquids[‡]	2 hours
Breast milk	4 hours
Infant formula	6 hours
Nonhuman milk[§]	6 hours
Light meal[∥]	6 hours

---

[*]These recommendations apply to healthy patients who are undergoing elective procedures. They are not intended for women in labor. Following the Guidelines does not guarantee a complete gastric emptying has occurred.

[†]The fasting periods apply to all ages.

[‡]Examples of clear liquids include water, fruit juices without pulp, carbonated beverages, clear tea, and black coffee.

[§]Since nonhuman milk is similar to solids in gastric emptying time, the amount ingested must be considered when determining an appropriate fasting period.

[∥]A light meal typically consists of toast and clear liquids. Meals that include fried or fatty foods or meat may prolong gastric emptying time. Both the amount and type of foods must be considered when determining an appropriate fasting period.

2. Emergent procedures require consideration of NPO status and the risk of gastric acid aspiration. Histamine blocking and gastrokinetic agents may be utilized to increase gastric acidity and decrease gastric volume.

PROCEDURAL CARE

I. Monitoring
   A. The monitoring process during the procedure includes
      1. Observation and vigilance
      2. Interpretation of data
      3. Initiation of corrective action when required
   B. Electrocardiogram (ECG)
      1. ECG monitoring during sedation procedures is required to detect
         a. Dysrhythmias
         b. Myocardial ischemia
         c. Electrolyte disturbance
         d. Pacemaker function
      2. Cardiac rhythm and dysrhythmias that may be encountered during the administration of moderate sedation include
         a. Sinus tachycardia (ST)
         b. Sinus bradycardia (SB)
         c. Sinus arrhythmia (SA)
         d. Premature atrial contractions (PAC)
         e. Supraventricular tachycardia (SVT)
         f. Atrial flutter
         g. Atrial fibrillation
         h. Junctional rhythm
         i. Premature ventricular contractions (PVC)
         j. Ventricular tachycardia (VT)
         k. Ventricular fibrillation (V-Fib)
      3. See Chapter 32 for description, ECG criteria, and treatment protocol for specific dysrhythmias.
   C. Noninvasive blood pressure
      1. Hypotension
         a. A decrease in systolic arterial blood pressure of 20% to 30%. Hypotension may be caused by a variety of factors including
            (1) Hypovolemia
            (2) Myocardial ischemia
            (3) Pharmacologic agents
            (4) Acidosis
            (5) Parasympathetic stimulation (pain, vagal stimulation)
         b. Treatment
            (1) Administer oxygen
            (2) Administration of a fluid challenge (300 to 500 ml crystalloid)
            (3) Correction of acidosis or hypoxemia
            (4) Relief of myocardial ischemia
            (5) Titration of sympathomimetic medications
            (6) Titration of inotropic agents
      2. Hypertension
         a. Systolic blood pressure greater than 140 mm Hg or a diastolic blood pressure greater than 90 mm Hg
         b. Increases bleeding
         c. Predisposes the patient to hemorrhage
         d. May lead to cardiac dysrhythmias
         e. Increases systemic vascular resistance
         f. Increases myocardial oxygen consumption
         g. Treatment

(1) Diuresis for fluid overload
(2) Noxious stimuli require analgesia or discontinuation of stimuli.
(3) Sympathetic nervous stimulation may require alpha and beta blockade.
(4) Myocardial ischemia requires nitrates and analgesia.
  D. Pulse oximetry
  1. Required for all sedation and analgesia procedures to monitor oxygenation status of the patient
  2. Provides a noninvasive, continuous monitoring parameter to assess the percent of hemoglobin combined with oxygen
  3. Pulse oximetry technology allows two light-emitting diodes (LEDs) to measure the intensity of transmitted light across the vascular bed.
  E. Capnography
  1. Consider using to monitor ventilatory status.
  2. Best monitor for measuring adequacy of ventilation
II. Procedural considerations
  A. All syringes labeled
  B. Emergency medications and equipment immediately available
  C. Adequate intravenous access established before the procedure

AIRWAY MANAGEMENT AND MANAGEMENT OF RESPIRATORY COMPLICATIONS

I. Evaluation of the airway
  A. Oral cavity inspection
  1. Loose, chipped, capped teeth
  2. Dental anomalies
    a. Crowns
    b. Bridges
    c. Dentures
  3. Obstruction to airflow
    a. Tumors
    b. Edema
    c. Inflammatory processes
  B. Temporomandibular joint examination
  1. Conducted with patient's mouth opened wide
    a. Normal distance between upper and lower central incisors is 4 to 6 cm
  2. Indications of reduced temporomandibular joint mobility
    a. A clicking sound when mouth is opened
    b. Pain associated with opening the mouth
    c. Reduced ability to open the mouth
  C. Physical characteristics
  1. The following physical characteristics may indicate the potential for difficult airway management.
    a. Recessed jaw
    b. Protruding jaw (hypognathous)
    c. Deviated trachea
    d. Large tongue
    e. Short, thick neck
    f. Protruding teeth
    g. High, arched palate
  D. Mallampati Airway Classification System (see Figure 27-1)
  1. Initially described in 1983, it offers the clinician a grading system for anticipation of difficult intubation.
  2. Examination is conducted while the patient's head is maintained in a neutral position and the mouth is opened 50 to 60 mm. Classes I to IV are based on anatomical areas visualized
    a. Class I: uvula, tonsillar pillars, soft and hard palate visualized
    b. Class II: uvula, hard and soft palate visualized

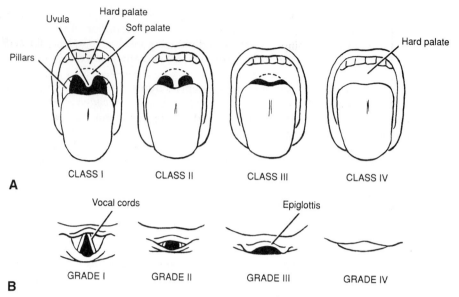

FIGURE 27-1 ■ Mallampati Airway Classification. (In Kost M: *Manual of conscious sedation.* Philadelphia: WB Saunders, 1998, p 80. From Mallampati SR: Clinical signs to predict difficult tracheal intubation [hypothesis]. *Can Anaesth Soc J* 30:316, 1983.)

      c. Class III: portion of uvula and hard palate visualized
      d. Class IV: portion of hard palate visualized
  II. Complications
    A. Sedative, hypnotic, and analgesic medications when used together have a potent synergistic effect.
    B. Decreased oropharyngeal muscle tone predisposes the patient to airway obstruction, leading to apnea and hypoxemia.
    C. Steps for restoration of airflow
      1. Lateral head tilt
      2. Chin lift
      3. Jaw thrust
      4. Nasal airway insertion
      5. Oropharyngeal airway insertion
      6. Endotracheal tube insertion
    D. Oxygen delivery devices: because of the respiratory depressant effects associated with the administration of sedative, hypnotic, or opioid medications, it is strongly recommended that supplemental oxygen be administered to all patients receiving sedation and analgesia (see Chapter 31).

PHARMACOLOGIC AGENTS

  I. Sedation and analgesia medications
    A. Benzodiazepines (see Chapter 26 for general facts, pharmacokinetics, and pharmacodynamics)
    B. Midazolam (Versed) sedation dosing guidelines are individualized and titrated to effect. Do not administer by rapid injection. Titration to effect means administration of drug until somnolence, nystagmus, or slurred speech occurs.
      1. Healthy patients: before the procedure, small increments (0.5 mg) of midazolam are administered over 2 minutes. Initial intravenous dose should not exceed 2.5 mg. Some patients may respond to as little as 0.5-1 mg.
      2. Adults 60 years of age or older: elderly, debilitated, chronically ill patients or patients with reduced pulmonary reserve require small incremental (0.25 to 0.5 mg) doses administered over 2 minutes. Initial dose should not exceed 1.5 mg. If additional sedation is required, it is imperative to wait

several minutes to evaluate the pharmacologic effect before administering additional sedation.

C. Diazepam sedation dosing guidelines: individualized and titrated to effect. Before the planned procedure, 1 to 2 mg of intravenous diazepam is titrated over a minute . Additional 1 mg increments may be administered over several minutes during the procedure. Additional time must be allowed to evaluate pharmacologic effect in geriatric or debilitated patients or patients with decreased cardiac output. Do not administer by rapid or single bolus injection. Extreme care must be exercised when administering diazepam concurrently with opioids.

D. Benzodiazepine antagonist: flumazenil (Romazicon)

1. Specific benzodiazepine antagonist. Reverses the central nervous system effects of benzodiazepines through competitive inhibition of the benzodiazepine receptor sites on the γ-aminobutyric acid (GABA) benzodiazepine receptor complex. The duration and degree of reversal is related to the total dose administered and plasma benzodiazepine concentration.

   a. Dosage: 0.2 mg administered intravenously over 15 seconds. If the desired level of consciousness is not obtained after waiting an additional 45 seconds, a further dose of 0.2 mg can be injected and repeated at 60-second intervals where necessary (up to a maximum of four additional times) to a maximum total dose of 1 mg). The dosage should be individualized based on the patient's response, with most patients responding to doses of 0.6 mg to 1 mg.

   b. Onset: 1 to 2 minutes; an 80% response will be achieved within 3 minutes of administration

   c. Duration: 40 to 80 minutes

   d. Resedation: patients who have responded to flumazenil should be carefully monitored (up to 120 minutes) for resedation.

E. Opioids

1. Opioids bind to specific opiate receptors located within the central nervous system: the mu, kappa, delta, and sigma receptor subtypes.

2. See Chapter 26 for general facts, pharmacokinetics, and pharmacodynamics.

3. Dosing guidelines

   a. Fentanyl: 1 to 2 μg/kg titrated in 25 μg increments

   b. Meperidine: 0.5 to 1 mg/kg titrated in 25 mg increments

   c. Morphine: 0.05 to 0.2 mg/kg titrated in 1 to 2 mg increments

F. Sedatives, hypnotics, and dissociative anesthetic agents

1. Sedative, hypnotic, and dissociative medications are added to deepen levels of sedation. The administration of these medications by registered nurses depends on statutory, regulatory, and recommended standards of care. Manufacturer recommendations generally advise that these agents be administered by anesthesia providers.

2. See Chapter 26 for general facts, pharmacokinetics, and pharmacodynamics.

II. Techniques of administration

A. The single-dose injection technique uses individual medications titrated slowly to effect. To establish an analgesic base, often opioids are administered before benzodiazepines. Two to three minutes before the procedure, intravenous opioids may be slowly administered to establish analgesia. Benzodiazepines are then added and titrated to patient effect.

1. Combining medications (narcotics, benzodiazepines, and hypnotics) reduces total dosage through synergistic action, assists the clinician in the maintenance of sedation and analgesia parameters, and provides rapid patient recovery.

B. Bolus techniques have been popular in oral surgery and gastroenterology. Based on a predetermined dosage (mg/kg), the entire dose or a large percentage is administered in one single injection.

1. The technique is particularly popular for administration of benzodiazepines. One advantage of this technique is its ability to rapidly provide a therapeutic plasma level immediately before the procedure.
2. Disadvantages associated with the bolus technique include respiratory depression, unconsciousness, chest wall rigidity, and cardiovascular depression. The bolus technique eliminates the safety features of slow titration, which assesses for patient response and clinical sedation end points (nystagmus, slurred speech).
3. Despite the speed with which a desired plasma concentration can be achieved, the risks associated with the bolus technique may outweigh the potential benefits. Small incremental doses allow therapeutic plasma levels to be reached slowly and produce the desired pharmacologic effect with a minimum of medication.

C. Continuous infusion techniques produce a constant medication plasma level. The continuous infusion technique avoids the fluctuations in medication plasma levels associated with the bolus technique. Continuous infusion is a popular sedative technique in critical care units for mechanically ventilated or agitated patients.
   1. Additional benefits include shorter recovery time, reduced medication requirement, and minimized side effects.
   2. Careful titration based on predetermined clinical endpoints (nystagmus, slurred speech, sedation) allows a rapid return to an alert state after the infusion is discontinued at the conclusion of the procedure.
   3. Continuous infusion techniques are extremely difficult to 'master' as a clinician, particularly in establishing a baseline level of sedation. When establishing baseline sedation levels, patients are predisposed to oversedation as the clinician is attempting to establish a desired level of sedation. This frequently results in patient's entering a state of deep sedation or general anesthesia.

POSTSEDATION RECOVERY

I. Monitoring
   A. Purpose
      1. Ensure return of physiologic function.
      2. Assess patient.
      3. Diagnose.
      4. Treat complications.
   B. Monitoring and discharge policies
      1. Required by accrediting bodies
      2. Recommended by professional organizations
   C. Dependent on
      1. Diagnostic or surgical procedure performed
      2. Length of procedure
      3. Preprocedure physiologic status
      4. Intraprocedural complications
      5. Medications administered
      6. Quantities of medications administered
   D. Documentation of recovery parameters
      1. Use of a postprocedure objective scoring tool (Aldrete). Objective parameters must assess
         a. Activity
         b. Respiration
         c. Circulation
         d. Level of consciousness
         e. Oxygenation
      2. Upon completion of the procedure, all patients must be monitored until all institution-approved discharge criteria are met. These discharge criteria must

be developed in conjunction with statutory, regulatory, and professional organization standards.

II. Postsedation
   A. Instruction
      1. Must be conducted in the presence of a responsible adult assuming care of the patient on discharge
      2. Written discharge instructions addressing medications, diet, and procedure-specific information must be reviewed with each patient.
      3. Sedation and analgesia discharge instructions identify medication used, side effects, and specific postprocedural guidelines to protect the patient.
   B. Sedation and analgesia postsedation follow up
      1. A mechanism to ascertain postprocedure status is recommended for patients discharged on the day of the procedure. Inpatient information may be gathered by the moderate sedation practitioner following the procedure. Methods of gathering data include the following
         a. Patient questionnaire
         b. Telephone interview
         c. Satisfaction survey
      2. The purpose of postsedation assessment is to evaluate the following
         a. Incidence of complications related to the administration of moderate sedation
         b. Delayed recovery
         c. Procedural complication rate
         d. Return to function

SEDATION RISK MANAGEMENT

I. **Strategies**
   A. Quality is broadly defined as the comprehensive positive outcome of a product. Achievement of excellence in health care requires quality care and service evaluation.
   B. The quality of sedation services is based on compliance with prescribed standards and recommended practice guidelines.
   C. Implementation of a successful moderate sedation program is based on the delivery of the highly technical aspects of care combined with positive outcomes.
   D. Unexpected events and complications may occur as a result of human error, periods of reduced observation, environmental factors, poor communication, haste, and lack of preparation. To prevent or reduce the number of adverse events, a risk reduction strategy should be implemented for all units and personnel engaged in the administration of moderate sedation. Individual injury prevention strategies include the following
      1. Development of a complete sedation plan
      2. Presedation preparation and patient assessment
      3. Application and use of required monitoring equipment
      4. Selection of appropriate pharmacologic medications and techniques
      5. Preparation and presence of emergency resuscitation equipment and personnel
      6. Preparation for specific procedures and locations
      7. Postsedation monitoring and discharge planning
   E. Ideally, individual risk reduction strategies prevent injury before an adverse incident or event takes place. Application of a risk management program on a department or institution basis requires development and implementation of mechanisms aimed at risk identification, analysis, and control. Creation of a moderate sedation database program as depicted in Figure 27-2 is essential. A coordinator guides input into the moderate sedation database. Once the database has been instituted, strategies to implement changes are used.

Conscious Sedation: Clinical Indicator Form

Patient Identification #_____ Age:_____ Date of Service:_____/_____/_____

Attending Physician: _____ Procedure:_____

CS Nurse: _____ Location:_____

MONITORING INDICATORS

A. Continuous ECG monitoring? ☐ Yes ☐ No
B. Continuous respiratory monitoring? ☐ Yes ☐ No
C. Continuous blood pressure monitoring? ☐ Yes ☐ No
D. Continuous pulse oximetry monitoring? ☐ Yes ☐ No
E. Continuous level of consciousness monitoring? ☐ Yes ☐ No
F. Continuous patient monitoring by nurse? ☐ Yes ☐ No

PREPROCEDURE INDICATORS

☐ Preprocedure assessment complete
☐ Incomplete informed consent/no signature
☐ Incomplete patient chart
☐ Incomplete labwork
☐ Medical consult required
☐ Noncompliance: NPO status
☐ Noncompliance: preprocedure medication instructions

PROCEDURE INDICATORS

☐ Respiratory depression
☐ Respiratory complication: stridor/laryngospasm/arrest
☐ Cardiovascular complications: cardiac arrest/ischemia/CHF/pulmonary edema
☐ Cardiovascular complications: hypotension/hypertension/dysrhythmias
☐ Level of consciousness: unresponsive/obtunded reflexes/agitation
☐ Medication: allergic reaction/wrong medication administered
☐ All medications administered as per facility policy
☐ Reversal agents administered (Flumazenil/Naloxone)

POSTPROCEDURE INDICATORS

☐ Prolonged somnolence
☐ Unexpected admission secondary to sedation
☐ Additional reversal agents administered (Flumazenil/Naloxone)
☐ Nausea/Vomiting: _____ times post discharge, current status:_____
☐ Evidence of postprocedure monitoring
☐ Documentation of discharge criteria
☐ Evidence of patient/family dissatisfaction
☐ Postprocedure follow-up complete

© 1996, Specialty Health Consultants

FIGURE 27-2 ■ Conscious sedation database program. (From Kost M: *Manual of conscious sedation.* Philadelphia: WB Saunders, 1998, p 236. Copyright 1996, Specialty Health Consultants.)

BIBLIOGRAPHY

1. Aldrete J: Postanesthesia recovery score revisited. *J Clin Anesth* 7:84, 1995.
2. American Nurses Association: Nursing liaison forum: Policy statement on conscious sedation. Washington, DC: American Nurses Association, 1991.
3. American Nurses Association: Policy statement on conscious sedation. Washington, DC: American Nurses Association, 1991.
4. American Society of Anesthesiologists Task Force on Sedation and Analgesia by Non-anesthesiologists: Practice guidelines for sedation and analgesia by non-anesthesiologists. *Anesthesiology* 96(4): 1003-1017, 2002.
5. Association of Operating Room Nurses: Standards, recommended practices and guidelines. Denver. *AORN J* 75:642-652, 2002.

6. Foster F: Conscious sedation...coming to a unit near you. Springhouse, PA: Springhouse Corporation, SpringNet, 2001.

7. Joint Commission on Accreditation of Healthcare Organizations: *Accreditation manual for hospitals: Revisions to anesthesia care standards comprehensive accreditation manual for hospitals.* Oakbrook Terrace, IL: Joint Commission on Accreditation of Healthcare Organizations, 2001.

8. Kost M: *Manual of conscious sedation.* Philadelphia: WB Saunders, 1998.

9. Kost M, Brown D, DeZayas B: The administration of conscious sedation by non-anesthesia personnel. *Anesth Today* 11(2):11–15, 2000.

10. OR Nurse Manager: Nurses uneasy about IV sedation for long cases. 6(3):1–4, 2000.

28 Thermoregulation

VALLIRE D. HOOPER

■ ■ ■

OBJECTIVES

At the conclusion of this chapter the reader will be able to:

1. Discuss the physiology of thermoregulation.

2. Identify two complications of altered thermoregulation in the perioperative setting.

3. Define unplanned perioperative hypothermia.

4. List three common causes of perioperative hypothermia.

5. Identify four adverse outcomes related to perioperative hypothermia.

6. Discuss phase specific recommendations for the prevention of perioperative hypothermia.

7. Discuss phase specific recommendations for the management of perioperative hypothermia.

8. Define the pathophysiology of malignant hyperthermia (MH).

9. Identify patients at risk for the development of MH.

10. Identify the signs and symptoms of MH.

11. Describe the treatment of MH.

THERMOREGULATION

I. Basic terms and definitions
  A. Thermal compartments
    1. Core thermal compartment
      a. Well-perfused tissues in which the temperature remains relatively uniform
      b. Consists of the organs of the trunk and head (not including skin and peripheral tissues of the trunk)
      c. Comprises 50% to 60% of the body mass
    2. Peripheral thermal compartment
      a. Consists of the arms and legs
      b. Temperature is nonhomogeneous and varies over time.
        (1) Temperature is usually 2-4° C lower than the core temperature in moderate environments.
        (2) Difference can be larger in more extreme thermal and/or physiologic circumstances.
          (a) Lower core-to-peripheral gradients
            (i) Warm environment
            (ii) Vasodilation in response to an increased metabolic heat (generated in the core)
          (b) Higher core-to-peripheral gradients
            (i) Cold environment
            (ii) Vasoconstriction in an attempt to shift metabolic heat to the core
  B. Temperature definitions
    1. Core temperature
      a. Temperature of the core thermal compartment
      b. Most accurate core temperature measurement sites
        (1) Pulmonary artery

(a) Obtained using a pulmonary artery (PA) catheter
(b) Considered most accurate as the artery brings blood directly from the core and its surroundings
(c) Affected by
(i) Large, rapid infusions of warmed or cold fluids
(ii) Respiratory cycles
(iii) Lower limb pneumatic compression devices
(2) Distal esophagus
(a) Best alternative to pulmonary artery site
(b) Affected by
(i) Active cooling phase of cardiopulmonary bypass
(ii) Surgery involving an open thorax or exposure of the diaphragm
(3) Nasopharynx
(a) Used to monitor brain temperature
(b) Not recommended with
(i) Substantial anticoagulation
(ii) When manipulation of the nasal mucosa is undesirable
(4) Tympanic membrane (see Figure 28-1)
(a) Preferred route of measurement by most perianesthesia nurses
(b) Correlation of readings to true core temperature measurements have shown mixed results in recent studies.
(c) Accuracy of the reading is dependent on
(i) Operator technique
(ii) Patient anatomy
(iii) Instrument used
c. Other temperature measurement sites can be used to estimate a core temperature (see Figure 28-2).
(1) Oral
(a) Site is dependable and safe in alert, oriented adults without mouth lesions.
(b) Temperature readings vary dependent on placement in the oral cavity (see Figure 28-3).
(c) Do not use in patients who are
(i) Unconscious
(ii) Disoriented

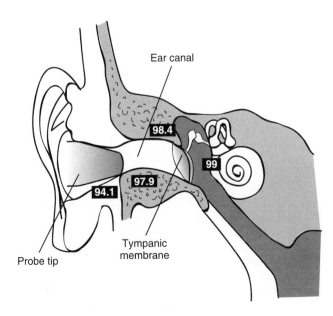

FIGURE 28-1 ■ Tympanic temperature monitoring. (From Nicoll LH: Heat in motion: Evaluating and managing temperature. *Nursing 2002* 32:s1-s12, 2002.)

Temperature Equivalency Chart

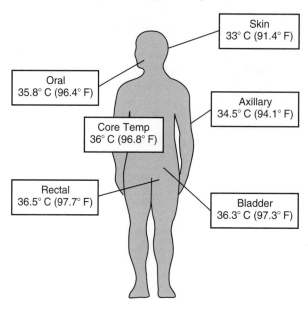

Conversion Formulas

$$F = C \times 9/5 + 32$$
$$C = F - 32 \times 5/9$$

Core Temperature Measurement Sites—Pulmonary artery, Tympanic membrane*, Nasopharynx, and Esophagus.
Sites that Estimate Core Temperature—Oral, axillary, skin, bladder and rectum*.

*Rectal temperatures are equal to core temperature when the patient is normothermic. Rectal temperatures become unreliable measurement when temperature flux is anticipated. (29)

*Accuracy of tympanic temperatures can vary depending on the instrument, operator, and the patient.

FIGURE 28-2 ■ Temperature equivalency chart. (From American Society of PeriAnesthesia Nurses: Clinical guideline for the prevention of unplanned perioperative hypothermia. In *ASPAN, 2002 standards of perianesthesia nursing practice.* Cherry Hill, NJ: American Society of PeriAnesthesia Nurses, 2002, p 57.)

        (iii) Shivering
        (iv) Having seizures
    (2) Axillary
    (3) Bladder
        (a) Subject to thermal lag in unsteady thermal states
        (b) Continuous urinary drainage required
        (c) Useful indicator of total body warming
    (4) Rectum
        (a) Subject to thermal lag in unsteady thermal states
        (b) Potential for probe to be inserted into stool
    (5) Skin
2. Normothermia: a core temperature of 36-38° C (96.8-100.4° F)
3. Hypothermia: a core temperature less than 36° C (96.8° F)
4. Hyperthermia: a core temperature greater than 38° C (100.4° F)

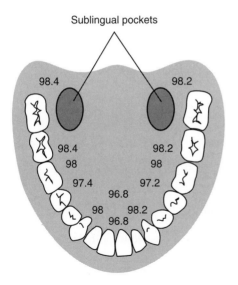

FIGURE 28-3 ■ Temperature variations in the oral cavity. (From Nicoll LH: Heat in motion: Evaluating and managing temperature. *Nursing 2002* 32:s1-s12, 2002.)

Hypothalamic "Thermostat"

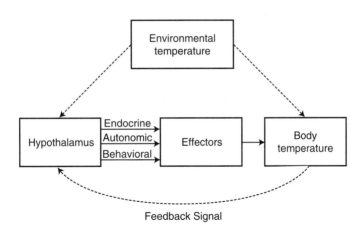

FIGURE 28-4 ■ The hypothalamic thermostat. (From Pressley TA: Temperature regulation, 2000. Available at http://phy025.lubb.ttuhsc.edu/Pressley/Course/Temp-Reg.htm. Accessed in March 2003.)

II. Thermoregulation physiology
   A. Most of the body's heat is provided by the basal metabolic rate.
      1. The core body temperature remains fairly constant.
      2. Skin and extremity temperatures may vary with environmental changes and thermoregulatory responses.
   B. Temperature regulation in conscious adults is mediated by the hypothalamus (see Figure 28-4) through a combination of behavioral and physiological responses.
      1. Hypothalamus
         a. Nestled at the base of the brain
         b. Primary temperature control center
            (1) Maintains normothermia by regulating heat loss with heat production

(2) Receives input via the spinal cord from thermoreceptors located in the
  (a) Skin
  (b) Nose
  (c) Oral cavity
  (d) Thoracic viscera
  (e) Spinal cord
c. Generates conscious and unconscious responses to maintain normothermia
2. Mechanisms of temperature regulation
  a. Behavior
    (1) Adding or removing clothing or covering
    (2) Changing location
    (3) Adjusting temperature of dietary intake
    (4) Adjusting environmental temperature
  b. Endocrine
    (1) Endocrine hormones are released in response to hypothalamic stimulation.
    (2) Initiates organ and tissue responses in all systems
  c. Autonomic
    (1) Changes in peripheral circulation
    (2) The peripheral shell may expand or contract in response to both peripheral and core temperature changes (see Figure 28-5).
C. Mechanisms of heat production and loss
  1. Mechanisms of heat production
    a. Body tissues produce heat in proportion to their metabolic rates.
      (1) Metabolism is the only natural internal source of heat.
      (2) Brain and major organs (the core thermal compartment)
        (a) The most metabolically active
        (b) Generate more metabolic heat than skeletal muscle at rest
      (3) Skeletal muscle can exceed the basal metabolic rate (BMR) by a factor of 10, but only briefly.
    b. Increased metabolism related to work or physical exercise

Relative Size of Insulating Shell

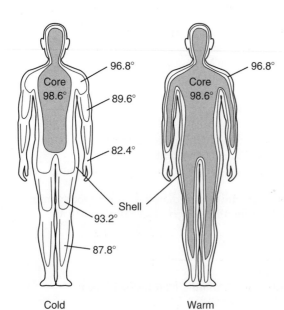

Cold

Warm

FIGURE 28-5 ■ Relative size of the insulating shell in response to temperature changes. (From Pressley TA: Temperature regulation, 2000. Available at http://phy025.lubb.ttuhsc.edu/Pressley/Course/Temp-Reg.htm. Accessed in March 2003.)

   c. Thermogenesis
   (1) Accomplished by shivering and nonshivering means
   (2) Nonshivering
      (a) A limited physiological response of the newborn infant to hypothermia
      (b) Involves the catabolism of brown fat, which is not coupled with adenosine triphosphate (ATP) formation
      (c) Releases energy in the form of heat
   (3) Shivering
      (a) Can increase heat production by up to 500%
      (b) Also accompanied by an increased metabolic rate and oxygen demand
2. Mechanisms of heat loss
   a. The physical processes controlling heat transfer between the body and the external environment are identical to the four mechanisms governing heat transfer in inanimate objects (see Figure 28-6).
   (1) Radiation
      (a) The loss of energy through radiant electromagnetic waves in the infrared spectrum
      (b) Involves no direct contact between the objects involved
         (i) Energy (or heat) radiates from the warmer object to a cooler one.
         (ii) Uncovered skin in the operative patient will radiate energy away from the patient, reducing the body temperature.
      (c) Accounts for 40% to 60% of all heat loss
      (d) Accentuated in the elderly and neonates
   (2) Convection
      (a) The loss of body heat by the means of transfer to the surrounding cooler air
      (b) There must be a temperature gradient between the body and surrounding air.
      (c) Heat transfer may occur in two ways
         (i) Passive movement
            [a] Warm air rises
            [b] May be seen in loss of body heat as a result of basic skin exposure
         (ii) Active movement
            [a] From a fan or wind blowing across the body surface
            [b] Can be facilitated by the laminar flow systems in an operating room (OR)
      (d) Accounts for 25% to 35% of heat lost and 10 kcal/hour

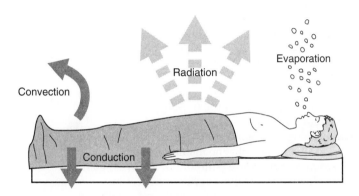

FIGURE 28-6 ■ Mechanisms of heat loss. (From Sessler DI: Perioperative heat balance. *Anesthesiology* 92:583, 2000.)

(3) Conduction
  (a) The transfer of heat energy through direct contact between objects
  (b) Heat loss in the perioperative setting may occur with contact with any of the following
    (i) Cold OR table
    (ii) Skin preparation solutions
    (iii) intravenous (IV) fluids
    (iv) Irrigants
    (v) Cold sheets and drapes
  (c) Causes the core body heat to move out to the cooler periphery
  (d) Accounts for up to 10% of heat loss
    (i) With IV fluid infusion, 16 kcal/hour loss
    (ii) With blood infusion, 30 kcal/hour loss
(4) Evaporation
  (a) The transfer of heat that occurs when a liquid is changed into a gas
  (b) Routes of heat loss
    (i) Perspiration (12-16 kcal/hour)
    (ii) Evaporation (12-16 kcal/hour)
    (iii) Exposed viscera during surgery or trauma
      [a] The larger the wound, the greater the heat loss
      [b] Can result in a 400 kcal/hour loss
  (c) May account for up to 25% of heat loss
b. Other routes of heat loss in the perioperative setting
  (1) Infusion of IV fluids that are cooler than the body temperature
    (a) A mass is added to the body that is cooler than the current body temperature.
    (b) The average body temperature falls.
    (c) Fluid exits the body as urine or blood after being warmed to the body temperature.
    (d) Net loss of heat energy occurs
  (2) Ventilation with dry gas
    (a) The gas is cooler than the body temperature.
    (b) Is warmed, heated, and humidified in the tracheobronchial tree
    (c) The gas, now warmed and saturated with water vapor, is exhaled at body temperature.
    (d) Significant heat energy loss may occur over time.
D. Physiological responses to changes in environmental temperature
  1. Cold environment
    a. Physiological goal is to minimize heat loss while maximizing heat production.
    b. Sympathetic stimulation
      (1) Increases thickness of the insulating shell through vasoconstriction
      (2) Stimulates nonshivering thermogenesis
      (3) Initiates piloerection
    c. Shivering thermogenesis initiated
    d. Long-term exposure also results in the release of thyrotropin-releasing hormone (TRH) from the hypothalamus.
  2. Hot environment
    a. Physiological goal is to maximize heat loss.
    b. Vasodilation shrinks the insulating shell.
    c. Sudomotor response (stimulation of sweat glands)
      (1) Regulates sensible evaporative heat loss
      (2) Increases activity of the cholinergic pathways
      (3) Critical for cooling in an environment that is hotter than the body
      (4) May also promote vasodilation

       d. Decreased heat production

       e. Long-term exposure

          (1) Increase in sweating capacity of sweat glands

          (2) Aldosterone-mediated increase in sodium retention

III. Perioperative thermoregulation

    A. Almost all patients receiving an anesthetic become hypothermic unless they are actively warmed.

      1. Usual temperature drop is 1-3° C.

      2. Temperature loss depends on

        a. Type and dose of anesthetic

        b. Amount of surgical exposure

        c. Ambient temperature

      3. Occurs because the normal physiological responses used to regulate the core temperature are impaired by the anesthetic agents

        a. Patient tends to become poikilothermic.

        b. The body takes on the temperature of the environment.

    B. Redistribution hypothermia occurs.

      1. Mechanisms of redistribution

        a. General anesthesia reduces the vasoconstriction threshold.

          (1) The threshold drops well below the normal core temperature.

          (2) Centrally mediated thermoregulatory constriction is inhibited.

        b. General and regional anesthesia also cause peripheral vasodilation.

          (1) Blood flow to the skin is increased.

          (2) Core heat is lost through peripheral tissues.

      2. Both mechanisms result in a core-to-peripheral redistribution of body heat (see Figure 28-7).

    C. Typical patterns of heat loss during a surgical case (see Figure 28-8)

      1. Core temperature drop of 1-1.5° C occurs during the first hour of surgery.

        a. Primarily caused by core-to-peripheral redistribution

        b. Affected by other factors

          (1) Initial body heat content

          (2) Body morphology

          (3) Amount of systemic heat loss

      2. Initial heat loss is followed by 2-3 hours of a slower, more linear drop.

        a. Metabolic rate drops 15% to 40% with the administration of general anesthesia.

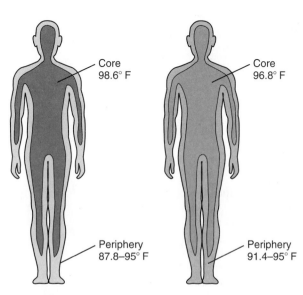

Core
98.6° F

Core
96.8° F

Periphery
87.8–95° F

Periphery
91.4–95° F

Vasoconstricted — Anesthesia ➔ Vasodilated

FIGURE 28-7 ■ Core-to-peripheral redistribution after the administration of anesthesia. (From Sessler DI: Perioperative heat balance. *Anesthesiology* 92:581, 2000.)

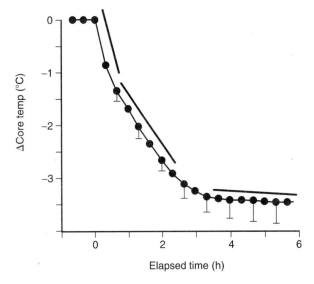

FIGURE 28-8 ■ Perioperative heat loss over time. (From Sessler DI: Perioperative heat balance. *Anesthesiology* 92:580, 2000.)

   b. Heat loss exceeds metabolic heat production.
   c. Heat loss is mediated by the four fundamental mechanisms of heat loss (see Figure 28-6).
      (1) Radiation
      (2) Convection
      (3) Conduction
      (4) Evaporation
3. Patient then enters a plateau phase where the core temperature stabilizes.
   a. Usually develops 2-4 hours into surgery
   b. Characterized by a constant core temperature
   c. May be passively or actively maintained
      (1) Passive plateau
         (a) Metabolic heat production equals heat loss without activating thermoregulatory defenses.
         (b) Most commonly seen in relatively small operations in which the patients are well covered with effective insulators
      (2) Active plateau
         (a) Patient becomes hypothermic enough to trigger thermoregulatory vasoconstriction.
         (b) Core temperature must drop to 34-35° C (93.2-95° F) for this to occur with most anesthetics.
   D. Postoperative return to normothermia
      1. Occurs when brain anesthetic concentration decreases enough to allow normal thermoregulatory responses to be triggered
      2. Can be impaired by residual anesthetics and postoperative opioids
      3. May take 2-5 hours
      4. Can be affected by
         a. Degree of hypothermia
         b. Age of the patient
IV. Planned perioperative hypothermia
   A. Hypothermia may be intentionally induced in some surgical cases to prevent intraoperative complications.
      1. Cardiac ischemia
      2. Cerebral ischemia
   B. Most common cases include
      1. Cardiac surgery requiring cardiopulmonary bypass
         a. Decreases amount of oxygen required by myocardial cells
         b. Slows metabolic demands

    2. Neurosurgical procedures

        a. Decreases intracranial pressure

        b. Decreases amount of bleeding

  C. Intentionally induced hypothermia has also been shown to be effective in the management of

    1. Acute stroke

    2. Perinatal asphyxia

    3. Neurologic outcome following cardiac arrest

    4. Severe head injury

V. Unplanned perioperative hypothermia (UPH)

  A. An unexpected core temperature decrease to less than 36° C (96.8° F) as a result of surgery

  B. May be present regardless of patient temperature if

    1. Patient complains of feeling cold

    2. Patient presents with common signs and symptoms.

        a. Shivering

        b. Peripheral vasoconstriction

        c. Piloerection *goose flesh*

  C. Risk factors

    1. Every patient undergoing surgery is at risk for developing UPH.

    2. Contributing risk factors include

        a. Extremes of ages

        b. Female sex

        c. Decreased ambient room temperature

        d. Length and type of surgical procedure

          (1) Longer procedures

          (2) Exposure of a large body cavity

        e. Cachexia *ill health, wasting poor nutrition*

        f. Preexisting conditions

          (1) Peripheral vascular disease

          (2) Endocrine disease

          (3) Pregnancy

          (4) Burns

          (5) Open wounds

        g. Significant fluid shifts

        h. Use of cold irrigants

        i. Use of general anesthesia

        j. Use of regional anesthesia

  D. Negative effects associated with UPH

    1. Patient discomfort related to

        a. Shivering

        b. An unpleasant sensation of being cold

    2. Adrenergic stimulation resulting in an increase in serum catecholamine levels

    3. Untoward cardiac events

        a. Increased catecholamines may cause myocardial ischemia.

        b. Cardiac function is directly impaired at temperatures less than 33° C (91.4° F)

        c. Threshold for arrythmias is around 31° C (87.8° F).

        d. Ventricular fibrillation likely at 30° C (86° F)

    4. Coagulopathy

        a. Platelet function is reduced.

        b. Clotting cascade is slowed.

        c. Blood loss increased

    5. Altered drug metabolism

        a. Elimination of injectable drugs prolonged

        b. Duration of anesthetic agents prolonged

      6. Impaired wound healing
        a. Tissue oxygenation decreased
        b. Immunity and collagen production impaired
        c. Infection rates increased
            (1) 19% in a hypothermic patient
            (2) 6 % in a normothermic patient
      7. Increased hospital costs
        a. Hypothermia of only 1.5° C below normal results in a $2500-$7000 increase in costs because of negative outcomes
        b. Elevated costs are related to
            (1) Increased length of stay in
                (a) Postanesthesia care unit (PACU)
                (b) Intensive care unit (ICU)
                (c) Hospital
            (2) Increased red blood cell (RBC), plasma, and platelet use
            (3) Increased need for mechanical ventilation
            (4) Management of adverse cardiac events
   E. Definitions
      1. Active warming measures
        a. Forced air convective warming
      2. Passive insulation
        a. Warmed cotton blankets
        b. Reflective blankets
        c. Circulating water mattress
        d. Socks
        e. Head covering
        f. Limited skin exposure
      3. Preventative warming measures: Initiation of passive insulation and/or active warming measures to maintain normothermia
   F. Perioperative patient management
      1. Preoperative (see Figure 28-9)

Thermal Management Flow Chart

Preoperative Patient Management
Identify patient's risk factors for hypothermia
Measure patient's temperature on admission
Determine patient's thermal comfort level (ask the patient if he/she is cold)
Observe for signs/symptoms of hypothermia (shivering, piloerection, and/or cold extremities)

Patient Normothermic
Institute preventative warming measures:
Passive insulation (apply warm cotton blankets, socks, head covering, and limit skin exposure)
Increase ambient room temperature (minimum 68°–75° F/20°–24° C)

Patient Hypothermic
Institute active warming measures:
Apply forced air warming system
Apply passive insulation
Increase ambient room temperature (minimum 68°–75° F/20°–24° C)

FIGURE 28-9 ■ Preoperative patient management. (From American Society of PeriAnesthesia Nurses: Clinical guideline for the prevention of unplanned perioperative hypothermia. In *ASPAN, 2002 standards of perianesthesia nursing practice.* Cherry Hill, NJ: American Society of PeriAnesthesia Nurses, 2002, p 55.)

     a. Assessment

       (1) Identify patient risk factors for UPH.

       (2) Measure patient temperature.

       (3) Determine patient's thermal comfort level.

       (4) Assess for other signs and symptoms of hypothermia.

     b. Interventions

       (1) Institute preventative warming measures for normothermic patients.

       (2) Institute active warming measures for hypothermic patients.

         (a) Also include passive insulation.

         (b) Consider warmed IV fluids.

     c. Outcome: patient will be normothermic before going to the OR.

  2. Intraoperative (see Figure 28-10)

     a. Assessment

       (1) Identify patient risk factors for UPH.

       (2) Measure patient temperature.

       (3) Determine patient's thermal comfort level.

       (4) Assess for other signs and symptoms of hypothermia.

       (5) Monitor intraoperative temperature according to national standards.

         (a) American Society of Anesthesiologists (ASA)

           (i) Appropriate body temperature should be maintained during the administration of all anesthetics.

           (ii) Every patient receiving anesthesia shall have temperature monitored when clinically significant changes in body temperature are intended, anticipated, or suspected.

Intraoperative Patient Management

Assessment

Identify patient's risk factors for hypothermia

Monitor patient's temperature (see guideline)

Determine patient's thermal comfort level (ask patient if he/she is cold)

Observe for signs/symptoms of hypothermia (shivering, piloerection, and/or cold extremities)

↓

Interventions

Passive insulation (apply warm cotton blankets, socks, head covering, and limit skin exposure)

Increase ambient room temperature (minimum 68°–75° F)

Institute active warming measures: apply forced air warming system

Warm fluids: intravenous and irrigants

Humidify and warm gases: anesthetic

↓

Expected Outcomes

The patient's core temperature should be maintained at 36° C (96.8° F) or above during the intraopertive phase unless hypothermia is indicated

---

FIGURE 28-10 ■ Intraoperative patient management. (From American Society of PeriAnesthesia Nurses: Clinical guideline for the prevention of unplanned perioperative hypothermia. In *ASPAN, 2002 standards of perianesthesia nursing practice.* Cherry Hill, NJ: American Society of PeriAnesthesia Nurses, 2002, p 55.)

(b) American Association of Nurse Anesthetists (AANA)
   (i) Body temperature shall be intermittently or continuously monitored and recorded on all patients receiving general anesthesia.
   (ii) The means to monitor temperature will be immediately available for use on all patients receiving local or regional anesthesia and used when indicated.
(c) If no anesthesia provider
   (i) The temperature shall be monitored at the beginning and end of the procedure.
   (ii) For cases longer than 30 minutes, serial temperatures will be obtained at least every 30 minutes.

b. Interventions
(1) Implement warming measures.
(2) Measures should include but are not limited to:
   (a) Passive insulation techniques
   (b) Increased ambient room temperature
      (i) Follow American Association of periOperative Registered Nurses (AORN) guidelines.
      (ii) 20-24° C (68-75° F)
   (c) Institute active warming measures.
   (d) Warm all fluids (IV and irrigants).
   (e) Humidify and warm anesthetic gases.

c. Expected outcome: The patient's core temperature will be maintained at 36° C or higher during the intraoperative period unless hypothermia is indicated for the procedure.

3. Postoperative patient management: Phase I PACU (see Figure 28-11)
a. Assessment
(1) Identify risk factors for UPH.
(2) Assess temperature on admission to phase I PACU.
   (a) If hypothermic, monitor serial temperatures at least every 30 minutes until normothermia is reached.
   (b) If normothermic, assess temperature prior to discharge and as ordered by the physician.
(3) Determine patient's thermal comfort level.
(4) Assess for signs and symptoms of hypothermia.

b. Interventions
(1) If normothermic
   (a) Institute preventative warming measures and passive insulation.
   (b) Increase ambient room temperature.
   (c) Assess patient's thermal comfort level every 30 minutes.
   (d) Observe for signs and symptoms of hypothermia.
   (e) Reassess temperature if patient's thermal comfort level decreases and/or if patient shows signs or symptoms of hypothermia.
   (f) Measure patient temperature prior to discharge.
(2) If hypothermic
   (a) Initiate active warming measures.
   (b) Apply passive insulation.
   (c) Increase ambient temperature.
   (d) Warm IV fluids.
   (e) Humidify and warm oxygen.
   (f) Assess temperature and thermal comfort level every 30 minutes until normothermia is reached.

c. Expected outcome
(1) Core temperature will be 36° C (96.8° F) or greater prior to discharge from PACU.
(2) All signs and symptoms of hypothermia will be resolved before discharge.

Postoperative Patient Management: Phase I PACU

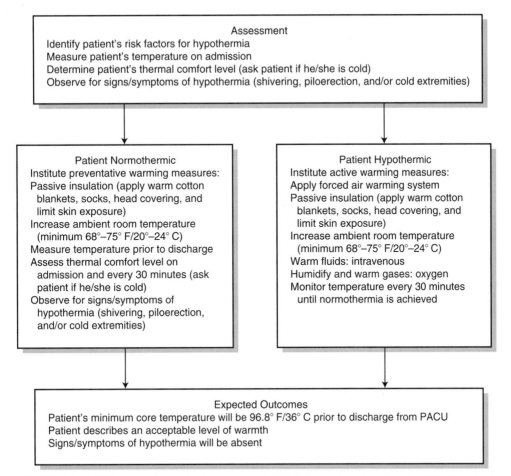

Assessment
Identify patient's risk factors for hypothermia
Measure patient's temperature on admission
Determine patient's thermal comfort level (ask patient if he/she is cold)
Observe for signs/symptoms of hypothermia (shivering, piloerection, and/or cold extremities)

Patient Normothermic
Institute preventative warming measures:
Passive insulation (apply warm cotton
  blankets, socks, head covering, and
  limit skin exposure)
Increase ambient room temperature
  (minimum 68°–75° F/20°–24° C)
Measure temperature prior to discharge
Assess thermal comfort level on
  admission and every 30 minutes (ask
  patient if he/she is cold)
Observe for signs/symptoms of
  hypothermia (shivering, piloerection,
  and/or cold extremities)

Patient Hypothermic
Institute active warming measures:
Apply forced air warming system
Passive insulation (apply warm cotton
  blankets, socks, head covering, and
  limit skin exposure)
Increase ambient room temperature
  (minimum 68°–75° F/20°–24° C)
Warm fluids: intravenous
Humidify and warm gases: oxygen
Monitor temperature every 30 minutes
  until normothermia is achieved

Expected Outcomes
Patient's minimum core temperature will be 96.8° F/36° C prior to discharge from PACU
Patient describes an acceptable level of warmth
Signs/symptoms of hypothermia will be absent

FIGURE 28-11 ■ Postoperative patient management: PACU. (From American Society of PeriAnesthesia Nurses: Clinical guideline for the prevention of unplanned perioperative hypothermia. In *ASPAN, 2002 standards of perianesthesia nursing practice*. Cherry Hill, NJ: American Society of PeriAnesthesia Nurses, 2002, p 56.)

      (3) Patient should verbalize an acceptable level of warmth.
      (4) Preventative warming measures and assessment for hypothermia will continue at whatever location to which patient is discharged.
   4. Postoperative patient management: Phase II PACU (see Figure 28-12)
     a. Assessment
      (1) Identify patient risk factors for UPH.
      (2) Measure patient's temperature on admission.
      (3) Determine thermal comfort level.
      (4) Assess for signs and symptoms of hypothermia.
     b. Intervention
      (1) If normothermic
        (a) Institute appropriate passive insulation.
        (b) Increase ambient room temperature.
        (c) Assess patient's thermal comfort level every 30 minutes.
        (d) Observe for signs and symptoms of hypothermia.
        (e) Reassess temperature if patient's thermal comfort level decreases and/or if patient shows signs or symptoms of hypothermia.

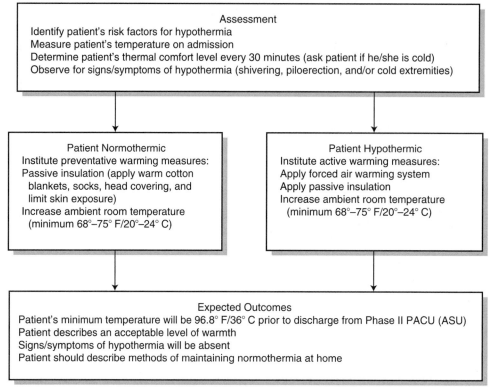

Postoperative Patient Management: Phase II PACU (ASU)

FIGURE 28-12 ■ Postoperative patient management: Phase II PACU. (From American Society of PeriAnesthesia Nurses: Clinical guideline for the prevention of unplanned perioperative hypothermia. In *ASPAN, 2002 standards of perianesthesia nursing practice.* Cherry Hill, NJ: American Society of PeriAnesthesia Nurses, 2002, p 54.)

   (f) Implement active warming measures if patient complains that he or she is cold or becomes hypothermic.
   (g) Instruct patient and/or responsible adult in methods to maintain normothermia at home.
   (h) Measure patient temperature prior to discharge.
   (2) If hypothermic
      (a) Initiate active warming measures.
      (b) Apply passive insulation.
      (c) Increase ambient temperature.
      (d) Consider warm IV fluids.
   c. Expected outcome
      (1) Patient's core temperature should be 36° C (96.8° F) or higher prior to discharge.
      (2) All signs and symptoms of hypothermia should be resolved.
      (3) Patient should verbalize an acceptable level of warmth.
      (4) Patient and/or responsible adult should be able to describe methods of maintaining normothermia at home.
VI. Malignant hyperthermia (MH)
   A. Definition of MH
      1. A hereditary abnormality of muscle metabolism caused by certain triggering agents and resulting in a life-threatening pharmacogenetic disorder

2. Patient must have specific genes for MH to occur.
   a. Relatives of patient who has had a MH crisis are at risk (siblings, parents, children).
   b. Inheritance by autosomal dominant pathway; risk diminishes as relationship to MH-susceptible person becomes further removed.
3. Characterized by muscular hypercatabolic reactions in which the level of intracellular calcium reuptake is impaired producing
   a. Muscle tetany
   b. Increased production of heat, carbon dioxide, and lactate

B. Incidence of MH
   1. More common in children
      a. Children: 1:15,000 anesthetics administered
      b. Adults: 1:20,000 to 1:50,000 anesthetics administered
   2. Many cases undetected
      a. Never anesthetized
      b. Short anesthetic period
      c. Effects of triggering agent may be modified by preceding it with use of nontriggering agents, such as thiobarbiturates, nondepolarizing muscle relaxants, or hypothermia.
      d. Many cases mild, not diagnosed

C. Mortality significantly reduced since availability of dantrolene in late 1970s
   1. Before 1970: 70%
   2. 1976: 28%
   3. Has remained 6% to 7% since the late 1980s
   4. Most deaths still occur in otherwise healthy children and adults.

D. Triggering agents
   1. Pharmacological
      a. Succinylcholine
      b. d-Tubocurarine (possible triggering agent)
      c. All volatile inhalation agents
         (1) Halothane
         (2) Enflurane
         (3) Isoflurane
         (4) Sevoflurane
         (5) Desflurane
      d. Intravenous potassium when given rapidly
      e. Possible triggers
         (1) Phenothiazines
             (a) Chlorpromazine
             (b) Prochlorperazine
         (2) Haloperidol
   2. Nonpharmacological
      a. Stress
      b. Sustained exercise
      c. Acute trauma
      d. Heat
      e. Pain
      f. Mental agitation
      g. Shivering

E. Safe anesthetic agents
   1. Nitrous oxide
   2. Opioids
   3. Barbiturates
   4. Droperidol
   5. Propofol
   6. Benzodiazepines
      a. Midazolam

      b. Diazepam

      c. Lorazepam

  7. Etomidate

  8. Ketamine

  9. Nondepolarizing skeletal muscle relaxants

      a. Vecuronium

      b. Atracurium

      c. Cisatracurium

      d. Pancuronium

      e. Mivacurium

      f. Rocuronium

      g. Doxacurium

      h. Pipecuronium

  10. Local anesthetics

      a. Amides

      b. Esters

F. Preoperative detection

  1. History

      a. Patient with previous MH episode obviously at risk

      b. Fifty percent of patients with MH have had previous anesthesia without a problem.

      c. Family member who has had MH crisis provides warning of possibility.

      d. History of any family member who died during surgery and anesthesia should be a red flag.

  2. Examination

      a. Usually reveals nothing

      b. Muscle weakness and myopathies associated with MH-like syndromes

         (1) Duchenne muscular dystrophy

         (2) Central core disease

         (3) Myotonia

         (4) Other unusual myopathies

  3. Laboratory tests

      a. Caffeine-halothane contracture test

         (1) Most reliable test for preoperative diagnosis

         (2) Few (about 12) hospitals in United States can perform this test.

         (3) Requires muscle biopsy

            (a) Must be performed at one of the testing hospitals

            (b) Cannot be mailed to testing center

         (4) Very costly

      b. Creatinine phosphokinase (CK)

         (1) Muscle enzyme

         (2) Unreliable diagnostic test for MH

         (3) Forty percent of MH patients have elevated CK.

         (4) Ten percent of normal people have elevated CK.

         (5) Other diseases produce elevated CK.

      c. Proposed tests currently under investigation

         (1) Molecular genetic testing

         (2) Nuclear magnetic resonance spectroscopy

         (3) Lymphocyte tests

         (4) Cultured muscle cells

G. Early signs and symptoms of MH

  1. Muscle rigidity

      a. Masseter muscle spasm after administration of succinylcholine

         (1) Intubation difficult

         (2) Indication to cancel anesthesia immediately in elective cases

         (3) Emergent cases may be carried out with nontriggering agents.

      b. Generalized rigidity
        (1) Definitive sign of MH
        (2) Begin MH treatment immediately.
  2. Tachycardia and dysrhythmia
    a. Very consistent and early sign of MH crisis
    b. Premature ventricular contractions, bigeminy common
    c. Sudden cardiac arrest resulting from hyperkalemia after succinylcholine in patients with muscle diseases
    d. Very nonspecific sign
  3. Cutaneous changes (inconsistent)
    a. Early generalized erythematous flush
      (1) Skin feels warm.
      (2) Core temperature may be normal.
    b. Later, skin becomes mottled followed by cyanosis.
  4. Tachypnea
    a. Results from increased CO_2 production
    b. If ventilation is controlled, increasing minute ventilation may mask rise of end tidal CO_2.
  5. Hyperkalemia
    a. Increased P_{CO_2}
    b. Acidosis
    c. Cardiac changes noted above
    d. Results from muscle membrane breakdown

H. Late signs and symptoms
  1. Pyrexia
    a. Temperature elevation
      (1) Hallmark of disease but often a late sign
      (2) Develops early if succinylcholine and volatile anesthetics used
    b. Rate of increase may be 1° F per 3 minutes
    c. Best measured by core temperature rise (e.g., nasopharyngeal, tympanic, bladder, rectal, axillary)
    d. Excessive heat production centered in skeletal muscle hypermetabolism
  2. Coagulopathy
    a. Disseminated intravascular coagulation (DIC)
    b. Venipuncture sites begin to bleed.
    c. Generally occurs after massive acidosis
      (1) Marked hyperthermia a nonspecific sign
  3. Rhabdomyolysis
    a. Result of muscle membrane breakdown
    b. Manifested first by brown or cola-colored urine
    c. Elevated levels of myoglobin in urine and serum
    d. Elevated CK levels (peak at 20 hours after event)
  4. Left ventricular failure (usually terminal event)
    a. Pulmonary edema
    b. Rales
    c. Frothy sputum
  5. Biochemical changes during MH
    a. Decreased pH secondary to CO_2 and lactic acidosis
    b. Increased P_{CO_2} (marked increase in CO_2 production)
    c. Decreased Pa_{O_2} (despite administration of 100% oxygen)
    d. Increased CK
    e. Increase in myoglobin in urine; hypercalcemia or hypocalcemia

I. Late diagnosis or unsuccessful treatment leads to death or permanent disability.
  1. Central nervous system (CNS) damage

          a. Coma

          b. Convulsions

          c. Permanent CNS damage

             (1) Paralysis

             (2) Blindness

    2. Renal failure resulting from myoglobinuria

        a. Caused by breakdown of skeletal muscle

        b. Clogs renal tubules, producing oliguria

    3. Recurrence of syndrome

        a. May recur several hours after initial successful treatment in as many as 25% of cases

        b. Patients must be monitored in an ICU and treated for at least 24-48 hours postoperatively.

    4. Muscle edema and weakness

  J. Treatment

    1. Immediate treatment

        a. Discontinue anesthesia and surgery immediately.

        b. Administer 100% oxygen

        c. Administer dantrolene (Dantrium) as soon as possible.

           (1) Dantrolene supplied in 20 mg vials and reconstituted with 60 ml preservative-free sterile water and shaking vigorously; warming bottle of solution may hasten mixing.

           (2) Recommended dose of dantrolene is 2.5 mg/kg body weight up to a total of 10 mg/kg; if syndrome not under control, even this limit may be exceeded. Administer by push initially; may be infused more slowly once syndrome under control.

           (3) Side effects of dantrolene include difficulty in walking, fatigue, muscle weakness, dizziness, blurred vision, nausea, and thrombophlebitis (late problems).

    2. Initiate patient cooling.

        a. Intravenous (IV) infusion of iced sodium chloride (NaCl)

        b. Surface cooling for all patients

           (1) Ice packs to groin, axillae, head

           (2) Cooling blankets

           (3) Immersion in container of ice

        c. Lavage stomach, bladder, and rectum with cold saline.

        d. Lavage peritoneal cavity with cold saline if open.

        e. Extracorporeal cooling by heart-lung machine in exceptional cases

        f. Discontinue cooling interventions when body temperature decreases to 38° C (100.4° F)

        g. In almost all situations, treatment with dantrolene, discontinuation of anesthetic combined with surface, stomach, and bladder lavage will be effective.

    3. Maintain fluid and electrolyte balance.

        a. Monitor arterial blood gases frequently.

        b. Monitor central venous pressure (CVP) or pulmonary artery catheter to guide fluid therapy as needed.

        c. Administer sodium bicarbonate as ordered to treat metabolic acidosis, 1 to 4 mEq/kg, on the basis of blood gas analysis.

        d. Use indwelling urinary catheter to monitor urine output.

        e. Administer IV fluids as ordered.

        f. Administer furosemide and mannitol as ordered.

        g. Administer glucose (or dextrose), insulin, and calcium as ordered for hyperkalemia.

    4. Monitor cardiac output.

        a. Maintain continuous cardiac monitoring.

        b. Treat ventricular dysrhythmias with procainamide or lidocaine (do not use calcium channel blockers).

    K. Follow-up after initial treatment

        1. Repeat dantrolene every 4 to 6 hours either IV or orally for up to 48 hours.

        2. Monitor patient for 24-48 hours postoperatively in an ICU to detect possible recurrence of MH.

        3. Monitor for the development of DIC.

        4. Follow CK for several days until normalized.

    L. Miscellaneous issues

        1. Ambulatory patients who are MH susceptible and have undergone uneventful surgery may be discharged after 4 hours in PACU.

        2. For inpatients, prominently label the patients' charts as "MH risk—do not use succinylcholine" because some MH patients who have required resuscitation have been given succinylcholine.

    M. Preparing for an MH crisis

        1. Maintain MH cart of all drugs and fluids required to treat acute MH episode (may share with operating room).

        2. Keep clear instructions with MH cart at all times.

        3. Develop a detailed MH crisis response plan specifying the roles of each staff member.

        4. Make sure MH treatment protocol is posted in highly visible place.

        5. Monitor and update education of all staff.

            a. Provide updates at least annually.

            b. Conduct mock MH crisis drills.

        6. Have dantrolene (at least 36 vials) immediately available (not in locked cabinet or stored in pharmacy).

        7. Have arterial blood gas (ABG) laboratory immediately available.

        8. Information sources

            a. Malignant Hyperthermia Association of the United States (MHAUS)

                (1) PO Box 1069, 39 East State St., Sherburne, NY 13460-1069

                (2) Phone

                    (a) 1-607-674-7901

                    (b) 1-800-98-MHAUS

                    (c) 1-800-MH-HYPER (MH hotline)

                (3) http://www.mhaus.org

            b. North American Malignant Hyperthermia Registry

                    (a) 1-888-274-7899

                    (b) http://naregistry.mhaus.org

VII. Syndromes resembling or mimicking MH

    A. Duchenne muscular dystrophy: X-linked disorder, therefore a syndrome of males. Onset is between age 2 and 8 years with muscle weakness progressing to death by late teens.

        1. Patients with muscular dystrophy who are too young to manifest signs of the disease may develop sudden, catastrophic hyperkalemia if given succinylcholine and/or a potent inhalation agent, which manifests as ventricular tachycardia and ventricular fibrillation; mild muscle rigidity and fever may also occur.

        2. Sometimes patients with muscular dystrophy may have catastrophic hyperkalemia develop after anesthesia with inhalation agents only, without succinylcholine.

            a. The first manifestation may be cardiac arrest in PACU.

        3. Diagnosis

            a. Sudden cardiac arrest in a child or young adult with no cardiac or pulmonary risk factors after anesthesia with succinylcholine and/or potent inhalation agents strongly suggests hyperkalemic arrest.

            b. Draw specimens for blood gas and potassium.

        4. Treatment

            a. Glucose and insulin, plus bicarbonate given intravenously

            b. For acute situations with ventricular tachycardia, calcium chloride or gluconate may be needed to prevent progression to ventricular fibrillation.

5. Follow up

    a. Evaluation by neurologist; muscle biopsy

B. Neuroleptic malignant syndrome: A disorder occurring in as many as 1.5% of patients receiving antipsychotic medications (e.g., clonazepine); not inherited; syndrome may occur during any time of therapy; usually occurs in hospital ward or as an outpatient.

    1. Signs and symptoms; signs similar to MH

        a. Fever

        b. Muscle tone increased

        c. Acidosis

        d. Rhabdomyolysis → *fatal disease characterized by destruction of skeletal muscle*

        e. Mental status changes

        f. Tachycardia, hypertension, and hypotension

    2. Treatment

        a. Cooling

        b. Dantrolene

        c. Bromocriptine (a dopamine agonist)

        d. Symptomatic therapy

    3. Testing

        a. No diagnostic test available

    4. Miscellaneous

        a. Electroshock therapy sometimes used for patients who cannot take phenothiazines

C. Endocrine disturbances

    1. Thyrotoxicosis

        a. Fever, tachycardia, hypertension, agitation, sometimes acidosis are cardinal signs.

        b. When occurring after anesthesia, may be confused with MH. However, no rigidity, little to no acidosis, no myoglobinuria

    2. Pheochromocytoma (the great mimicker)

        a. Hypertension, tachycardia, fever may be presenting signs. Crisis may be precipitated by anesthesia and surgery for unknown reasons.

        b. Some patients may have unexpected pulmonary edema after anesthesia.

        c. Dantrolene is of little or no value.

        d. Do not treat with beta-blockers only.

        e. Diagnosis very difficult acutely, requires urinary metanephrine levels, plasma catecholamine assays, and MRI

D. Hypoxic brain damage

    1. Periods of hypoxia, such as after cardiac arrest, can lead to hyperthermia in PACU because of hypothalamic dysfunction.

    2. Opisthotonic posturing and/or seizures occur.

    3. Patient usually fails to awaken

    4. Dantrolene may help with treatment of fever, but not specific.

    5. Muscle enzymes (CK) may be elevated because of seizures, posturing. Diagnosis requires high suspicion, CT scan.

    6. Treatment: mannitol, steroids

E. Ascending tonic-clonic syndrome: A rare syndrome occurring after radiologic contrast agent injected into CSF for myelogram, occurs usually with water-soluble contrast agent

    1. Signs

        a. Jerking movements of muscles in legs progress to whole body tonic activity.

        b. Patient loses consciousness and seizures develop. Seizures lead to hyperthermia.

        c. Signs usually begin within 1 to 2 hours of myelogram.

    2. Treatment is support of ventilation and vital signs. Dantrolene may help keep temperature normalized, but not a specific treatment.

        a. High mortality if not recognized and treated aggressively

BIBLIOGRAPHY

1. American Association of Nurse Anesthetists:. *Scope and standards for nurse anesthetists.* Park Ridge, IL: American Association of Nurse Anesthetists, 1998.

2. American Society of Anesthesiologists: Standards for basic anesthetic monitoring, 1998. Available at http://www.asahq.org/publicationsandservices/standards/02.pdf. Accessed in April 2003.

3. American Society of PeriAnesthesia Nurses: Clinical guideline for the prevention of unplanned perioperative hypothermia. In *ASPAN, 2002 standards of perianesthesia nursing practice.* Cherry Hill, NJ: American Society of PeriAnesthesia Nurses, 2002, pp 50-59.

4. Arndt K: Inadvertent hypothermia in the OR. *AORN J* 70:203-222, 1999.

5. Battin MR, Penrice J, Gunn TR, et al: Treatment of term infants with head cooling and mild systemic hypothermia after perinatal asphyxia. *Pediatrics* 111:244-251, 2003.

6. Caroff SN, Mann SC, Campbell EC: Neuroleptic malignant syndrome. *Adverse Drug React Bull* 209:799-802, 2001.

7. Craig JV, Lancaster GA, Taylor S, et al: Infrared ear thermometry compared with rectal thermometry in children: A systematic review. *Lancet* 360:603-609, 2002.

8. Eisenburger P, Sterz F, Holzer M, et al: Therapeutic hypothermia after cardiac arrest. *Curr Opin Crit Care* 7:184-188, 2001.

9. Ezri T, Szmuk P, Weisenberg M, et al: The effects of hydration on core temperature in pediatric surgical patients. *Anesthesiology* 98:838-841, 2003.

10. Fallis WM: Monitoring bladder temperatures in the OR. *AORN J* 76:467-489, 2002.

11. Fiedler MA: Thermoregulation: Anesthetic and perioperative concerns. *AANA J* 69:485-491, 2001.

12. Fortunato-Phillips N: Malignant hyperthermia: Update 2000. *Crit Care Nurs Clin North America* 12:199-210, 2000.

13. Georgiadis D, Schwarz S, Kollmar R, et al: Endovascular cooling for moderate hypothermia in patients with acute stroke: First results of a novel approach. *Stroke* 32:2550-2553, 2001.

14. Gupta AK, Al-Rawi PG, Hutchinson PJ, et al: Effect of hypothermia on brain tissue oxygenation in patients with severe head injury. *Br J Anaesth* 88:188-192, 2002.

15. Gurrera RJ: Is neuroleptic malignant syndrome a neurogenic form of malignant hyperthermia. *Clin Neuropharmacol* 25(4):183-193, 2002.

16. Haslego SS: Malignant hyperthermia: How to spot it early. *RN* 65(7):31-36, 2002.

17. Hooper V: Perioperative thermoregulation: A survey of clinical practices. Presented at Bethesda, MD: Consensus Conference on Perioperative Thermoregulation, American Society of PeriAnesthesia Nurses, 1998.

18. Hopkins PM: Malignant hyperthermia: Advances in clinical management and diagnosis. *Br J Anaesth* 85:118-128, 2001.

19. The Hypothermia After Cardiac Arrest Study Group: Mild therapeutic hypothermia to improve the neurologic outcome after cardiac arrest. *N Engl J Med* 346:549-556, 2002.

20. Jeran L, Hooper V: Thermoregulation. In *ASPAN, competency based orientation credentialing program.* Cherry Hill, NJ: American Society of PeriAnesthesia Nurses, 2002, pp 307-331.

21. Jurkat-Rott K, McCarthy T, Lehmann-Horn F: Genetic and pathogenesis of malignant hyperthermia. *Muscle Nerve* 23:4-17, 2000.

22. Kasai T, Hirose M, Takamata A, et al: Preoperative blood pressure and catecholamines related to hypothermia during general anesthesia. *ACTA Anaesthesiol Scand* 47:208-212, 2003.

23. Kasai T, Hirose M, Yaegashi K, et al: Preoperative risk factors of intraoperative hypothermia in major surgery under general anesthesia. *Anesth Analogue* 95:1381-1383, 2002.

24. Krieger DW, DeGeorgia MA, Abou-Chebl A, et al: Cooling for acute ischemic brain damage (cool aid): An open pilot study of induced hypothermia for acute ischemic stroke. *Stroke* 32:1847-1854, 2001.

25. Laptook AR, Corbett RJ: The effects of temperature on hypoxic-ischemic brain injury. *Clin Perinatol* 29:623-649, 2002.

26. Lien CA: Thermoregulation in the elderly. Available at http://www.asahq.org/clinical/geriatrics/thermo.htm. Accessed in March 2003.

27. Lien CA: The effect of anesthesia on thermoregulation in the elderly patient. *Curr Anesthesiol Rep* 2:473-481.

28. Longsayreepong S, Chaibundit C, Chadpaibool J, et al: Predictor of core hypothermia and the surgical intensive care unit. *Anesth Analogue* 96:826-833, 2003.

29. Mahoney CB, Odom J: Maintaining intraoperative normothermia: A meta-analysis of outcomes with costs. *AANA J* 67:155-164, 1999.

30. Malignant Hyperthermia Association of the United States: Clinical update 2000/2001: Managing MH. Available at http://www.mhaus.org. Accessed in April 2003.

31. Malignant Hyperthermia Association of the United States: Managing MH: Drugs, equipment, and dantrolene sodium. Available at http://www.mhaus.org. Accessed in April 2003.

32. Malignant Hyperthermia Association of the United States: Preventing malignant hyper-

thermia: An anesthesia protocol. Available at http://www.mhaus.org. Accessed in April 2003.

33. Malignant Hyperthermia Association of the United States: What is malignant hyperthermia? Available at http://www.mhaus.org. Accessed in June 2003.

34. Malignant Hyperthermia Association of the United States: Temperature monitoring in the perioperative period: Why, where, and how. Available at http://www.mhaus.org. Accessed in April 2003.

35. Malignant Hyperthermia Association of the United States: Testing for susceptibility to malignant hyperthermia. Available at http://www.mhaus.org. Accessed in April 2003.

36. Moran DS, Mendal L: Core temperature measurement: Methods and current insights. *Sports Med* 32:879-885, 2002.

37. Myrum P: Malignant hyperthermia. In *ASPAN, competency based orientation credentialing program*. Cherry Hill, NJ: American Society of PeriAnesthesia Nurses, 2002, pp 293-303.

38. Nicoll LH: Heat in motion: Evaluating and managing temperature. *Nursing 2002* 32: s1-s12, 2002.

39. Pressley TA: Temperature regulation, 2000. Available at http://phy025.lubb.ttuhsc.edu/Pressley/Course/Temp-Reg.htm. Accessed in March 2003.

40. Redmond MC: Malignant hyperthermia: Perianesthesia recognition, treatment, and care. *J PeriAnesth Nurs* 16:259-270, 2001.

41. Rosenberg H, Antognini JF, Muldoon S: Testing for malignant hyperthermia. *Anesthesiology* 96:232-237, 2002.

42. Sessler DI: Complications and treatment of mild hypothermia. *Anesthesiology* 95:531-543, 2001.

43. Sessler DI: Perioperative heat balance. *Anesthesiology* 92:578-596, 2000.

44. Tobin JR, Jason DR, Challa VR, et al: Malignant hyperthermia and apparent heat stroke. *J Am Med Assoc* 286:168-169, 2001.

45. Venes D: *Taber's electronic medical dictionary*, ed 19, 2001. Philadelphia: Davis. Available at http://www.tabers.com. Accessed in March 2003.

46. Welch TC: A common sense approach to hypothermia. *AANA J* 70 227-231, 2002.

29 Pain and Comfort Management

DINA A. KRENZISCHEK

OBJECTIVES

At the conclusion of this chapter the reader will be able to:

1. Define pain, commonly used terms, and types of pain.

2. Describe nociception: basic process of normal pain transmission.

3. Relate harmful effects of unrelieved pain.

4. Identify pain and comfort management in the perianesthesia settings, including special considerations and key concepts in analgesic therapy.

5. Categorize pharmacologic and nonpharmacologic interventions, including those for children and management of opioids complications.

6. Define comfort.

7. Identify context of comfort.

I. Pain
  A. Definition of pain
    1. Pain is whatever the experiencing person says it is, existing whenever he or she says it does.[15]
    2. Pain is unpleasant sensory and emotional experience associated with actual or potential tissue damage.[15]
  B. Types of pain
    1. Nociceptive pain—normal processing of stimuli that damages normal tissue or has the potential to do so if prolonged; usually responsive to nonopioids and/or opioids
      a. Somatic pain—is usually aching or throbbing in quality and is well localized
        (1) Arises from
          (a) Bone
          (b) Joint
          (c) Muscle
          (d) Skin
          (e) Connective tissue
      b. Visceral pain—arises from visceral tissue, such as the gastrointestinal (GI) tract and pancreas
    2. Neuropathic pain—abnormal processing of sensory input by the peripheral or central nervous system
      a. Treatment usually includes adjuvant analgesics.
      b. Centrally generated pain
        (1) Deafferentation pain—injury to either the peripheral or central nervous system
        (2) Sympathetically maintained pain—associated with dysregulation of the autonomic nervous system
      c. Peripherally generated pain
        (1) Painful polyneuropathies—pain is felt along the distribution of many peripheral nerves

(2) Painful mononeuropathies—usually associated with a known peripheral nerve injury, and pain is felt at least partly along the distribution of the damaged nerve

C. Definition of commonly used pain terms

1. Acute pain—usually elicited by the injury of body tissues and activation of nociceptive transducers at the site of local tissue damage; pain that extends until period of healing
2. Chronic pain—usually elicited by an injury but may be perpetuated by factors that are both pathogenetically and physically remote from originating cause: pain that extends beyond the expected period of healing (3-6 months since the initiation of pain)
3. Recurrent pain—episodic or intermittent occurrences of pain with each episode lasting for a relatively short period of time but recurring across an extended period of time
4. Transient pain—elicited by activation of nociceptors in the absence of any significant local tissue damage; this type of pain ceases as soon as the stimulus is removed (e.g., venipuncture)
5. Addiction—a behavioral pattern of psychoactive substance abuse; addiction is characterized by overwhelming involvement with the use of a drug, the securing of its supply, and a high tendency to relapse
6. Allodynia pain—caused by stimulus that does not normally provoke pain
7. Analgesia—absence of the spontaneous report of pain or pain behaviors in response to stimulation that would normally be painful
8. Central pain—initiated or caused by primary lesion or dysfunction in the central nervous system
9. Dysesthesia—an unpleasant abnormal sensation, whether spontaneous or evoked
10. Hyperalgesia—an increased response to a stimulus that is normally painful
11. Hypoalgesia—diminished pain in response to a normally painful stimulus
12. Hypochondriasis—an excessive preoccupation that bodily sensations and fears represent serious disease despite reassurance to the contrary
13. Malingering—a conscious and willful feigning or exaggeration of a disease or effect of an injury to obtain a specific external gain
14. Neuralgia—pain in the distribution of a nerve or nerves
15. Neurogenic pain—initiated or caused by a primary lesion, dysfunction, or transitory perturbation in the peripheral or central nervous system
16. Neuropathic pain—initiated or caused by a primary lesion or dysfunction in the nervous system
17. Noxious stimulus—a stimulus that is capable of activating receptors for tissue damage
18. Pain behavior—verbal or nonverbal actions understood by observers to indicate that a person may be experiencing pain and suffering
19. Pain relief—report of reduced pain after a treatment
20. Pain threshold—the least level of stimulus intensity perceived as painful
21. Pain tolerance level—the greatest level of noxious stimulation that an individual is willing to tolerate
22. Paresthesia—an abnormal sensation, whether spontaneous or evoked
23. Physical dependence—a pharmacologic property of a drug (e.g., opioid) characterized by the occurrence of an abstinence syndrome following abrupt discontinuation of the substance or administration of an antagonist; this does not imply addiction
24. Psychogenic pain—report of pain attributed primarily to psychological factors, usually in the absence of an objective physical pathology that that could account for pain
25. Suffering—reaction to the physical or emotional components of pain with a feeling of uncontrollability, helplessness, hopelessness, intolerability, and interminableness

26. Tolerance—a physiologic state in which a person requires an increased dosage of a psychoactive substance to sustain a desired effect

D. Nociception: Basic process of normal pain transmission
   1. Transduction—conversion of one energy from another.
      a. Process occurs in the periphery when a noxious stimulus causes tissue damage.
      b. The damaged cells release substance that activate or sensitize nociceptors.
      c. This activation leads to the generation of an action potential.
      d. Sensitizing substances released by damaged cells
         (1) Prostaglandins (PG)
         (2) Bradykinin (BK)
         (3) Serotonin (5-HT)
         (4) Substance P (SP)
         (5) Histamine (H)
      e. An action potential results from
         (1) Release of the preceding sensitizing substances (nociceptive pain) plus
         (2) A change in the charge along the neuronal membrane *or*
         (3) Abnormal processing of stimuli by the nervous system neuropathic pain plus
         (4) A change in the charge along the neural membrane
            (a) The change in charge occurs when Na^+ moves into the cell and other ion transfers occur.
   2. Transmission—the action potential continues from the site of damage to the spinal cord and ascends to higher centers; transmission may be considered in three phases.
      a. Injury site to spinal cord
         (1) Nociceptors terminate in the spinal cord.
      b. Spinal cord to brain stem and thalamus
         (1) Release of substance P and other neurotransmitters continues the impulse across the synaptic cleft between the nociceptors and the dorsal horn neurons.
         (2) From the dorsal horn of the spinal cord, neurons such as the spinothalamic tract ascend to the thalamus.
         (3) Other tracts carry the message to different centers in the brain.
      c. Thalamus to cortex
         (1) Thalamus acts as a relay station sending the impulse to central structures for processing.
   3. Perception of pain—conscious experience of pain
   4. Modulation—inhibitor nociceptive impulses
      a. Neurons originating in the brain stem descend to the spinal cord.
      b. Release substances that inhibit the transmission of nociceptive impulses
         (1) Endogenous opioid
         (2) Serotonin (5-HT)
         (3) Norepinephrine (NE) (Figure 29-1)

E. Harmful effects of unrelieved pain
   1. Endocrine
      a. Increase in the following
         (1) ACTH
         (2) Cortisol
         (3) Antidiuretic hormone
         (4) Epinephrine
         (5) Norepinephrine
         (6) Growth hormone
         (7) Catecholamines
         (8) Rennin
         (9) Angiotensin
         (10) Aldosterone
         (11) Glucagons
         (12) Interleukin

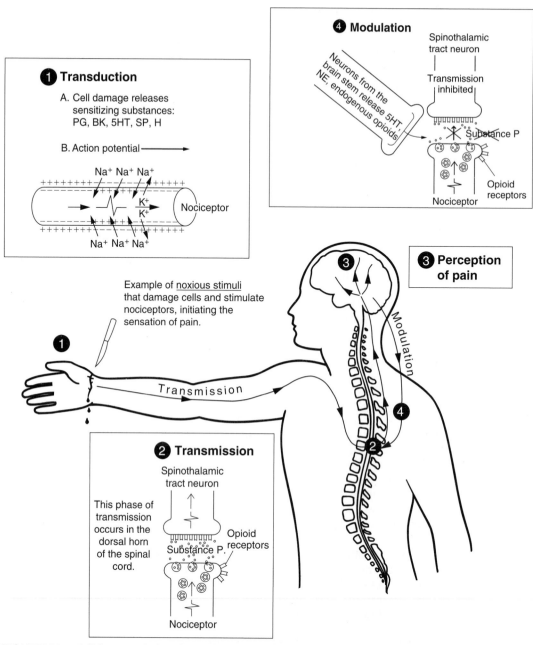

FIGURE 29-1 ■ Pain transmission. (From McCaffery M, Pasero C: *Pain: clinical manual.* St Louis: Mosby, 1999, p 21. Developed by McCaffery M, Pasero C, Paice JA.)

    b. Decrease in
       (1) Insulin
       (2) Testosterone
  2. Metabolic
    a. Gluconeogenesis
    b. Hepatic glycogenolysis
    c. Hyperglycemia
    d. Glucose intolerance
    e. Insulin resistance
    f. Muscle protein catabolism
    g. Increase lipolysis

3. Cardiovascular
   a. Increase in the following
      (1) Heart rate
      (2) Cardiac output
      (3) Peripheral vascular resistance
      (4) Systemic vascular resistance
      (5) Hypertension
      (6) Coronary vascular resistance
      (7) Myocardial oxygen consumption
      (8) Hypercoagulation
      (9) Deep vein thrombosis
4. Respiratory
   a. Decrease in flows and volumes
   b. Atelectasis
   c. Shunting
   d. Hypoxemia
   e. Decrease cough
   f. Sputum retention
   g. Infection
5. Genitourinary
   a. Decreased urinary output
   b. Urinary retention
   c. Fluid overload
   d. Hypokalemia
6. GI
   a. Decreased gastric motility
   b. Decreased bowel motility
7. Musculoskeletal
   a. Muscle spasm
   b. Impaired muscle function
   c. Fatigue
   d. Immobility
8. Cognitive
   a. Reduction in cognitive function
   b. Mental confusion
9. Immune
   a. Depression of immune response
10. Developmental
   a. Increase behavioral and physiologic response to pain
   b. Altered temperaments
   c. Higher somatization
   d. Infant distress behavior
   e. Possible altered development of the pain system
   f. Increase vulnerability to stress disorders
   g. Addictive behavior
   h. Anxiety states
11. Future pain
   a. Debilitating chronic pain syndromes
   b. Postmastectomy pain
   c. Postthoracotomy pain
   d. Phantom pain
   e. Postherpetic neuralgia
12. Quality of life
   a. Sleeplessness
   b. Anxiety
   c. Fear
   d. Hopelessness
   e. Increase thoughts of suicide

F. Pain and comfort management
  1. Preoperative phase—assessment
    a. Vital signs including pain and comfort goals (e.g., 0-10 scale)
    b. Medical history
      (1) Neurological status
      (2) Cardiac and respiratory instability
      (3) Allergy to medication, food and objects
      (4) Use of herbs
      (5) Motion sickness
      (6) Sickle cell
      (7) Fibromyalgia
      (8) Use of caffeine, substance abuse
      (9) Fear and anxiety
    c. Pain history
      (1) Preexisting pain
      (2) Acute, chronic pain level
      (3) Pattern
      (4) Quality
      (5) Type of source
      (6) Intensity
      (7) Location
      (8) Duration and time
      (9) Course
      (10) Pain affect
      (11) Effects on personal life
    d. Pain behaviors and expressions or history
      (1) Grimacing
      (2) Frowning
      (3) Crying
      (4) Restlessness
      (5) Tension and discomfort behaviors
        (a) Shivering
        (b) Nausea
        (c) Vomiting
      (6) Note that physical appearance may not necessarily indicate pain and discomfort or their absence.
    e. Analgesic history
      (1) Type
        (a) Opioid
        (b) Nonopioid
        (c) Adjuvant analgesics
      (2) Dose
      (3) Frequency
      (4) Effectiveness
      (5) Adverse effects
      (6) Other medications that may influence choice of analgesics
        (a) Anticoagulants
        (b) Antihypertensives
        (c) Muscle relaxants
    f. Patient's preferences for pain relief and comfort measures
      (1) Expectations
      (2) Concerns
      (3) Aggravating and alleviating factors
      (4) Clarification of misconceptions
    g. Pain and comfort acceptable levels
      (1) Patient and family (as indicated) agree on plan of treatment and interventions postoperatively.

    h. Comfort history
        (1) Physical
            (a) Warming measures
            (b) Positioning
        (2) Sociocultural
        (3) Psychospiritual
            (a) Spiritual beliefs and symbols
        (4) Environment
            (a) Music
            (b) Comfort objects
            (c) Privacy
            (d) Factors related to nausea and vomiting
  i. Educational needs
        (1) Consider age or level of education.
        (2) Cognitive
        (3) Language appropriateness
        (4) Barriers to learning
  j. Cultural language preference, identification of personal beliefs, and resulting restrictions
  k. Pertinent laboratory results
        (1) Prolonged prothrombin time (PT), partial thromboplastin time (PTT) to determine risk for epidural hematoma in patients with epidural catheter
2. Preoperative phase—interventions
  a. Identify patient.
  b. Validate physician's order and procedure.
        (1) Correct name of drug, dose, amount, route, and time
        (2) Validate type of surgery and correct surgical site as applicable.
  c. Discuss pain and comfort assessment.
        (1) Presence
        (2) Location
        (3) Quality
        (4) Intensity
        (5) Age
        (6) Language
        (7) Condition
        (8) Cognitive appropriate pain rating scale (Assessment method must be the same for consistency.)
            (a) 0 to 10
            (b) FACES scale
            (c) Comfort scale
  d. Discuss with patient and family (as indicated) information about reporting pain intensity using numerical or FACES rating scales and available pain relief and comfort measures.
        (1) Include discussion of patient's preference for pain and comfort measures.
  e. Implement comfort measures as indicated by patient.
        (1) Physical
        (2) Sociocultural
        (3) Spiritual
        (4) Environmental support
  f. Discuss and dispel misconceptions about pain and pain management.
  g. Encourage patient to take a preventive approach to pain and discomfort by asking for relief measures before pain and discomfort are severe or out of control.
  h. Educate on purpose of intravenous (IV) or epidural patient-controlled analgesia (PCA) as indicated.

    i. Educate about use of nonpharmacologic methods.
      (1) Cold therapy, relaxation breathing, music
    j. Discuss potential outcomes of pain and discomfort treatment approaches.
    k. Establish pain relief and comfort goals with the patient
      (1) A pain rating of less than 4 (scale of 1 to 10) to make it easy to cough, deep breathe, and turn
    l. Premedicate patients for sedation, pain relief, comfort.
      (1) Nonopioid
      (2) Opioid
      (3) Antiemetics
      (4) Consider needs of chronic pain patients.
    m. Arrange interpreter throughout the continuum of care as indicated.
    n. Utilize interventions for sensory impaired patients.
      (1) Device to amplify sound
      (2) Sign language
      (3) Interpreters
    o. Report abnormal findings including laboratory values among epidural patients.
      (1) Prolonged PT (>12.5 seconds.)
      (2) PTT (>35 seconds)
      (3) INR (>5)
      (4) Platelet (<150K per mm^3)
    p. Arrange for parents to be present for children.
  3. Preoperative phase—expected outcomes
    a. Patient states understanding of care plan and priority of individualized needs.
    b. Patient states understanding of pain intensity scale, comfort scale, and pain relief and comfort goals.
    c. Patient establishes realistic and achievable pain relief and comfort goals.
      (1) A pain rating of less than 4 (scale 0 to 10) to make it easy to
        (a) Cough
        (b) Deep breathe
        (c) Turn upon discharge
    d. Patient states understanding or demonstrate correct use of PCA equipment as indicated.
    e. Patient verbalizes understanding of importance of using other nonpharmacologic methods of alleviating pain and discomfort.
      (1) Cold therapy
      (2) Relaxation breathing
      (3) Music
  4. Postanesthesia phase I—assessment
    a. Refer to preoperative phase assessment, interventions, and outcomes data.
    b. Type of surgery and anesthesia technique, anesthetic agents, reversal agents
    c. Analgesics
      (1) Nonopioid
      (2) Opioid
      (3) Adjuvants given before and during surgery
      (4) Time and amount at last dose
      (5) Regional (e.g., spinal and epidural)
    d. Pain and comfort levels on admission and until transfer to receiving unit or discharge to home
      (1) Reassess frequently until pain or discomfort is controlled.
      (2) During sedation procedure (assess continuously)
    e. Assessment parameters
      (1) Functional level and ability to relax
      (2) Pain
        (a) Type
        (b) Location

           (c) Intensity

           (d) Use self-report pain rating scale whenever possible.

                (i) Age

                (ii) Language

                (iii) Condition

                (iv) Cognitively appropriate tools

                    [a] Quality

                    [b] Frequency (continuous or intermittent)

                    [c] Sedation level

        (3) Patient's method of assessment and reporting need to be the same during the postoperative continuum of care for consistency.

        (4) Self-report of comfort level using numerical scale (0 to 10 scale) or other   institutional approved instruments

        (5) Physical appearance

           (a) Pain and discomfort behaviors

           (b) Note: Pain behaviors are highly individual and the absence of any specific behavior (e.g., facial expression, body movement) does not mean the absence of pain.

        (6) Other sources of discomfort

           (a) Position

           (b) Nausea and vomiting

           (c) Shivering

           (d) Environment such as

                (i) Noise

                (ii) Noxious smell

                (iii) Anxiety

  f. Achievement of pain relief and comfort treatment goals.

  g. Age, cognitive ability, and cognitive learning method

  h. Status and vital signs

      (1) Airway patency

      (2) Respiratory status

      (3) Breath sounds

      (4) Level of consciousness

      (5) Pupil size as indicated

      (6) Other symptoms related to the effects of medications

      (7) Blood pressure

      (8) Pulse and cardiac monitor rhythm

      (9) Oxygen saturation

      (10) Motor and sensory functions post regional anesthesia technique

5. Postanesthesia phase I—interventions

  a. Identify patient correctly.

  b. Validate physician's order.

  c. Implement correct name of drug, dose, amount, route, and time.

  d. Include type of surgery and surgical site as applicable.

  e. Consider multimodal therapy.

  f. Pharmacologic (as ordered)

      (1) Mild to moderate pain—use nonopioids.

         (a) Acetaminophen

         (b) Nonsteroidal antiinflammatory drugs (NSAIDs)

         (c) Cox-2 inhibitors

         (d) All the patient's regular nonopioid prescription medications should be made available unless contraindicated.

         (e) May consider opioid

      (2) Moderate to severe pain.

         (a) Combine nonopioid and opioid.

      (3) Utilize the three analgesic groups appropriately.

         (a) Nonopioids (e.g., acetaminophen, NSAIDs, Cox-2 inhibitors)

            (i) Aspirin

            (ii) Ketorolac

     (iii) Ibuprofen
     (iv) Cox-2 inhibitors
    (b) Mu agonist opioids
     (i) Morphine
     (ii) Hydromorphone
     (iii) Fentanyl
    (c) Adjuvants
     (i) Multipurpose for chronic pain
      [a] Anticonvulsants
      [b] Tricyclic antidepressants
      [c] Corticosteroids
      [d] Antianxiety medication
     (ii) Multipurpose for moderate to severe acute pain
      [a] Local anesthetics
      [b] Ketamine
     (iii) Continuous neuropathic pain
      [a] Antidepressants
      [b] Tricyclic antidepressants
      [c] Oral or local anesthetic
     (iv) Lancinating (stabbing, knifelike pain) neuropathic pain
      [a] Anticonvulsant
      [b] Baclofen
     (v) Malignant bone pain
      [a] Corticosteroids
      [b] Calcitonin
     (vi) Postorthopedic surgery
      [a] Consider muscle relaxants if patient experiences muscle spasm.
    (d) Initiate and adjust regional infusions (PCA) as indicated and ordered, based on hemodynamics status.
     (i) Refer to institutional permissive procedure.
    (e) Nonpharmacologic interventions—use to complement, not replace, pharmacologic interventions
  f. Administer comfort measures as needed.
   (1) Physical
    (a) Positioning
    (b) Pillow
    (c) Heat and cold therapies
    (d) Sensory aids
     (i) Dentures
     (ii) Eye glasses
     (iii) Hearing aids
    (e) Use meperidine (Demerol) for shivering as ordered.
   (2) Sociocultural
    (a) Family and caregiver
    (b) Interpreter visit
   (3) Psychospiritual
    (a) Chaplain or cleric of choice
    (b) Religious objects and symbols
   (4) Environmental
    (a) Confidentiality
    (b) Privacy
    (c) Reasonably quiet room
   (5) Cognitive behavioral
    (a) Education and instruction
    (b) Relaxation
    (c) Imagery
    (d) Music

      (e) Distraction

      (f) Biofeedback

6. Postanesthesia phase I—expected outcomes
   a. Patient maintains hemodynamic stability including respiratory and cardiac status and level of consciousness.
   b. Patient states achievement of pain relief and comfort treatments goals (e.g., acceptable pain relief with mobility at time of transfer or discharge).
   c. Patient feels safe and secure.
   d. Patient demonstrates effective use of at least one nonpharmacologic method.
      (1) Breathing relaxation techniques
   e. Patient demonstrates effective use of PCA as indicated, and discusses expected results of regional techniques.
   f. Patient verbalizes evidence of receding pain level and increased comfort with pharmacologic and nonpharmacologic interventions

7. Postanesthesia phases II and III—assessment
   a. Refer to preoperative phase and phase I assessments, interventions, and outcomes data.
   b. Achievement of pain and comfort treatment goals and level of satisfaction with pain relief and comfort management.
   c. Pain relief and comfort management plan for discharge and patient agreement
   d. Educational and resource needs, considering age, language, condition, and cognitive appropriateness

8. Postanesthesia phases II and III—interventions
   a. Identify patient correctly.
   b. Validate physician's order.
   c. Implement correct name of drug, dose, amount, route, and time.
   d. Pharmacologic interventions (as ordered)
      (1) Nonopioid
         (a) Acetaminophen
         (b) NSAIDs
         (c) Cox-2 inhibitors
      (2) Mu agonist opioids
         (a) Morphine
         (b) Hydromorphone
         (c) Fentanyl
      (3) Adjuvant analgesics
         (a) Local anesthetics
   e. Continue and/or initiate nonpharmacologic measures from phase I.
   f. Educate patient, family, and caregiver
      (1) Pain and comfort measures
      (2) Untoward symptoms to observe
      (3) Regional or local anesthetic effects dissipating after discharge
         (a) Numbness
         (b) Motor weakness
         (c) Inadequate relief
   g. Discuss misconceptions and expectations, and implement plan of action satisfactory to patients.
   h. Address nausea with pharmacologic interventions or other techniques and discuss expectations.

9. Postanesthesia phases II and III—expected outcomes
   a. Patient states acceptable level of pain relief and comfort with movement or activity at time of transfer or discharge to home.
   b. Patient verbalizes understanding of discharge instruction plans.
      (1) Specific drug to be taken
      (2) Frequency of drug administration
      (3) Potential side effects of medication

        (4) Potential adjustments as applicable

        (5) Potential drug interactions

        (6) Specific precaution to follow when taking medication

           (a) Physical limitation

           (b) Dietary restrictions

        (7) Name and telephone number of the physician or resource to notify about pain, problems, and other concerns

    c. Patient states understanding or demonstrates effective use of nonpharmacologic methods.

        (1) Cold and heat therapy

        (2) Relaxation breathing

        (3) Imagery

        (4) Music

    d. Patient states achievement of pain and comfort treatment goals and level of satisfaction with pain relief and comfort management in the perianesthesia setting.

G. Methods for pain and comfort assessment

    1. Descriptive Pain Intensity Scales (AHCPR)

1	1	1	1	1	1
No pain	Mild pain	Moderate pain	Severe pain	Very severe pain	Worse possible Pain

    2. 0 to 10 Numerical Pain Intensity Scale (AHCPR)

0____ 1 ____ 2 ____ 3 ____ 4 ____ 5 ____ 6 ____ 7 ____ 8 ____ 9 ___ 10

No pain   Moderate pain   Most possible pain

    3. Visual Analog Scale (VAS) (printed with permission by Mosby)

_____

No Pain as bad as it
paincould possibly be

    4. Descriptive Pain Distress Scale (AHCPR)

1	1	1	1	1	1
None	Annoying	Uncomfortable	Dreadful	Horrible	Agonizing

    5. 0 to 10 Numeric Pain Distress Scale (AHCPR)

0____ 1 ____ 2 ____ 3 ____ 4 ____ 5 ____ 6 ____ 7 ____ 8 ____ 9 ___ 10

No pain   Distressing pain   Unbearable most pain

    6. Comfort Scale (printed with permission by Kolcaba)

0____ 1 ____ 2 ____ 3 ____ 4 ____ 5 ____ 6 ____ 7 ____ 8 ____ 9 ___ 10

No comfort   Moderately comfortable   Most comfortable

    7. FACES Scale (Figure 29-2)

    8. FLACC scale (Face, legs, activity, cry, consolability) (Figure 29-3)

    9. PACU Behavioral Pain Rating Scale (PBPRS) (Figure 29-4)

H. Special considerations

    1. Key principle: All patients deserve the best possible pain relief and comfort measures that can be safely provided.

    2. The following list is intended to emphasize important key elements of care in patients with special needs, but the list is not inclusive.

        a. Elderly patients

            (1) The principles of pain assessment and the pain assessment tools can be used in the same manner in cognitively intact elderly patients as in cognitively intact younger patients.

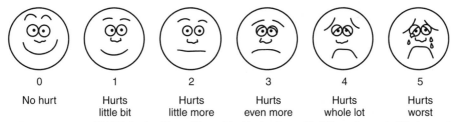

FIGURE 29-2 ■ FACES Scale. (From Wong DL, Hockenberry M, Wilson D, et al: *Whaley and Wong's nursing care of infants and children,* ed 7. St. Louis: Mosby, 2003. Printed with permission by Elsevier.)

FLACC

	0	1	2
Face	No particular expression or smile	Occasional grimace or frown, withdrawn, disinterested	Frequent to constant frown, clenched jaw, quivering chin
Legs	Normal position or relaxed	Uneasy, restless, tense	Kicking or legs drawn up
Activity	Lying quietly, normal position, moves easily	Squirming, shifting back and forth, tense	Arched, rigid or jerking
Cry	No cry (awake, or asleep)	Moans or whimpers, occasional complaint	Crying steadily, screams or sobs, frequent complaints
Consolability	Content, relaxed	Reassured by touching, hugging, talking	Difficult to console or comfort

FLACC Behavioral Pain Scale

    0 = Relaxed
  1–3 = Mile discomfort   When using this scale also use Self-report
  4–6 = Moderate pain   Watch awake patient 2–5 minutes
  7–10 = Severe discomfort   Watch sleeping patients 5 minutes

FIGURE 29-3 ■ FLACC Pain Assessment Tool. (From Pediatric Nursing, 1997, Volume 23, No.3, pp. 293-297. With permission of Jannetti Publications, Inc.

(2) Report of pain may be very different from younger patients because of physiologic, psychological, and cultural differences.

(3) Often suffer acute and chronic painful diseases

(4) Have multiple diseases

(5) Take many medications

(6) Prevalence of pain is two-fold higher in those over age 60 compared with those less than 60 years old.

(7) More than 80% suffer various forms of arthritis, and most will have acute pain at some time.

(8) More sensitive to both the therapeutic and toxic effects of analgesics
    (a) Various analgesics are influenced by age-induced changes.
        (i) Drug absorption
        (ii) Distribution
        (iii) Metabolism
        (iv) Elimination

(9) Prone to constipation when given opioid analgesic

(10) All NSAIDS must be used with caution because of the increased risk of
    (a) GI problems

(b) Renal insufficiency

(c) Platelet dysfunction

(11) More sensitive to analgesic effects of opioid drugs because elderly may experience a higher peak effect and longer duration of pain relief

(a) Recommended initial dose is 25% to 50%, with careful dose titration, and close monitoring of patient's responses.[15]

  b. Patients with known or suspected chemical dependency or history of such

(1) Patients usually experience traumatic injuries and a variety of health problems more often than the general population.

(2) Possible withdrawal from preexisting opioid use may stimulate sympathetic nervous system (restlessness, tachycardia, sleeplessness) caused by undertreated pain or opioid abstinence.

(3) The same principles of analgesia apply to all patients; focus on the immediate concern (i.e., managing pain or discomfort, not detoxification).

Instructions:

Ask the patient to self report pain. If unable, may use PBPRS.

If PBPRS is used:

1. Identify which behavior(s) are being demonstrated. Patient may demonstrate 1 or more pain behaviors with different intensities.

2. Identify the behavior that indicates the highest intensity of pain, for example, sounds 3 (severe-cries out or sobs). This correlates to self report of pain (Scale 1–10: 1–3 = mild, 4–6 = moderate, and 7–10 = severe).

3. Note: Pain behaviors are highly individual and the absence of any specific behavior (e.g. facial expression, body movement) does not mean the absence of pain.

Pain Behaviors	Definition
Restless: 0 = Relaxed 1 = Slightly .... 2 = Moderately .... 3 = Very	 Head turns to side Movements of upper/lower extremities (raising hands or lifting legs) Change of position >2× within 10 minutes, flapping extremities (1 or 2 legs or feet), pulling all covers (blanket), *or* attempts to get out of bed
Frowning/Grimacing: 0 = None 1 = Slight .... 2 = Moderate .... 3 = Severe	 Tightening of skin around the eyes Lowering and raising the eyebrows or closing eyes tightly Raising the upper lip, wrinkling the nose, stretching the lips horizontally, *or* opening of the mouth
Sounds: 0 = None 1 = Mild .... 2 = Moderate .... 3 = Severe	 Groans, moans softly Groans and moans loudly Cries or sobs
Muscle Tension: 0 = Relaxed 1 = Slight .... 2 = Moderate .... 3 = Severe	 Bracing (side rails and bed) or making closed fist Guarding hands, interlocking or pressing together, hyperextention of legs or pantar flexion (stationary), *or* rubbing abdomen (more than 2×/10 minutes) Bending knee (stationary)

FIGURE 29-4A ■ PACU Pain Behavioral Pain Scale. (A, Printed with permission by Johns Hopkins Hospital.)

Form 3.1 **Initial Pain Assessment Tool**

Date _____

Patient's Name _____ Age _____ Room _____

Diagnosis _____ Physician _____

Nurse _____

1. LOCATION: Patient or nurse mark drawing.

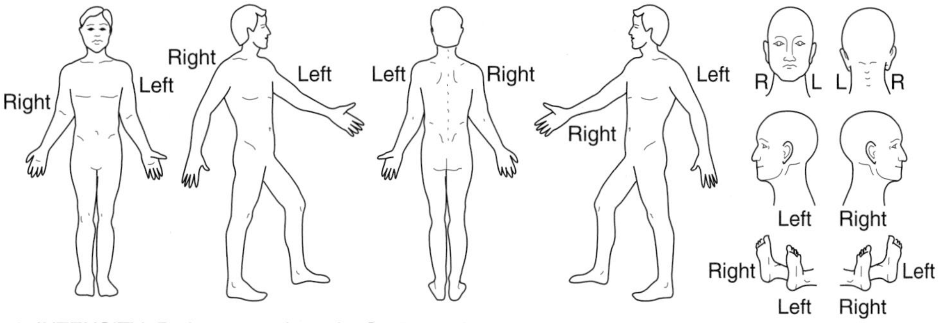

2. INTENSITY: Patient rates the pain. Scale used _____
   Present: _____
   Worst pain gets: _____
   Best pain gets: _____
   Acceptable level of pain: _____

3. QUALITY: (Use patient's own words, e.g., prick, ache, burn, throb, pull, sharp) _____
   _____

4. ONSET, DURATION, VARIATIONS, RHYTHMS: _____
   _____

5. MANNER OF EXPRESSING PAIN: _____
   _____
   _____

6. WHAT RELIEVES THE PAIN? _____
   _____
   _____

7. WHAT CAUSES OR INCREASES THE PAIN? _____
   _____
   _____

8. EFFECTS OF PAIN: (Note decreased function, decreased quality of life.)
   Accompanying symptoms (e.g., nausea) _____
   Sleep _____
   Appetite _____
   Physical activity _____
   Relationship with others (e.g., irritability) _____
   Emotions (e.g., anger, suicidal, crying) _____
   Concentration _____
   Other _____

9. OTHER COMMENTS: _____
   _____

10. PLAN: _____
    _____
    _____

FIGURE 29-4B ■ (B, From McCaffery M, Pasero C: *Pain: clinical manual*, p.60 © 1999, Mosby, Inc.)

(4) There is no evidence that withholding analgesics will increase the likelihood of recovery from addiction or that providing analgesics will worsen addiction.

(5) Patients with chemical dependency often require higher loading and maintenance doses of opioids to reduce intensity of postoperative pain to acceptable level.

(6) Provide nondrug interventions concomitantly with pharmacologic interventions.

(7) Consider requesting referral to an addiction specialist for ongoing care and rehabilitation after the acute pain period.

(8) Patients with chronic alcoholism who are actively drinking should be maintained on benzodiazepines or alcohol throughout the intraoperative and postoperative periods to prevent withdrawal reaction or delirium tremens.

c. Patients with concurrent medical conditions: Factors to consider

(1) In selecting analgesic for patients with concurrent medical condition, it is important to note whether the disorder produces either hepatic or renal impairment; the net result is drug accumulation.

(2) Elimination is decreased in patients with renal failure, and doses must be lowered or given less frequently.

(3) Careful planning is required for patients with respiratory insufficiency and chronic obstructive disease.

(4) Patients with psychiatric illness taking anxiolytics or other psychoactive drugs must be observed for drug interactions with pain medication taken.

d. Patient with shock, trauma, or burns

(1) Concern for cardiorespiratory instability is particularly important in the first hour of injury; it is recommended that incremental small intravenous doses of an opioid analgesic be carefully titrated and monitored.

(2) Damage to peripheral nerves may result in neuropathic pain that may require treatment with adjuvant analgesics, such as

(a) Tricyclic antidepressants

(b) Anticonvulsants

(c) Opioids

(d) Nonopioids.

e. Patients who have procedures outside of the operating room

(1) Only when immediate treatment of cardiorespiratory instability is required, or if a competent patient declines treatment, should analgesia be withheld for a painful procedure.

(2) No anesthetic or analgesic agent should be used unless the clinician understands the proper technique of administration, dosage, contraindications, side effects, and treatment of overdose.

(3) Regardless of the analgesic or adjuvant given, patients should be monitored closely according to institutional policy.

f. Pediatric patients

(1) Provide adequate and unhurried preparation of the child and family.

(a) Parental prediction of the child's response is highly correlated with the actual degree of distress.

(2) Manage preexisting pain optimally before beginning the procedure.

(3) Requires frequent assessment and reassessment of the presence, amount, quality, and location of pain.

(a) Focus on prevention and reducing anticipated pain because emotional distress accentuates the experience of pain.

(4) The inclusion of parents or caregiver is essential to pain assessment.

(a) Strategies for assessment should be tailored to the development level and personality of the child.

(5) Physiologic indicators may vary among children who are experiencing pain .

(a) The interpretation of physiologic indicators should be done.

(i) In the context of the clinical condition

(ii) In conjunction with other assessment methods

(6) Effective interaction is key to effective pain management.

    (a) Preferences of the child and family deserve respect and careful
        consideration.
    (b) The primary obligation is to ensure safe and competent care.
    (7) Environmental factors such as cold or crowded rooms or alarms on
        machines can escalate distress.
g. Site specific surgery
    (1) Dental surgery
        (a) Patient's anxiety is frequently disproportionate to the safety of the
            procedure.
            (i) A patient may benefit from behavioral or pharmacologic
                (anxiolytic) therapy.
        (b) Mild pain associated with uncomplicated dental care is well
            managed by oral administration of NSAID such as aspirin or
            ibuprofen.
            (i) This has shown delayed onset of postoperative pain and
                lessening of its severity.
        (c) Preoperative treatment such as ibuprofen and/or application of
            long-acting local anesthetic on more traumatic and intense
            procedure can delay onset of pain postoperatively.
        (d) Postoperative pain may require additional opioid in the
            nonsteroidal regimen such as codeine and alternative opioid such
            as oxycodone.
    (2) Radical head and neck
        (a) The nature of the operative procedure may dictate alternate routes
            for pain therapy.
            (i) Gastrostomy or jejunostomy instead of oral intake
        (b) Patient's ability to describe pain or response to analgesic
            intervention may be limited by the presence of
            tracheostomy.
        (c) Intraoperative positioning of the head and neck are critical.
            (i) Supportive devices such as protective padding may help
                minimize muscle spasm.
            (ii) Foam cushion can minimize decubitus.
        (d) Painful swallowing may require modification of diet, including
            liquid and soft foods and occasional use of topical anesthetics
            such as viscous lidocaine.
    (3) Neurosurgery
        (a) Patients undergoing an operation on the central nervous system
            frequently show abnormal neurologic signs and symptoms, such
            as pupillary reflexes and level of consciousness, which may be
            affected by conventional opioid analgesics.
        (b) Focus on the need to balance analgesia and provide appropriate
            neurological monitoring.
        (c) NSAIDs such as ketorolac may be considered because they have
            no effect on the level of consciousness or pupillary reflexes, but
            risk of coagulopathy or hemorrhage must be considered.
    (4) Thoracic surgery
        (a) Preexisting disease of the thoracic organs (i.e., chronic obstructive
            pulmonary disease) and prior medical treatment (i.e.,
            chemotherapy) are common.
        (b) Aggressive pain control in the form of epidural analgesia or
            neural blockade with local anesthetics after thoracic surgery
            improves pulmonary functions.
        (c) The use of opioids to reduce postoperative pain after thoracotomy
            is well documented.
        (d) The use of PCA has
            (i) Incrementally improved analgesia
            (ii) Increased patient satisfaction

(iii) Tendencies toward improved pulmonary function and early recovery and discharge

(5) Cardiac surgery

(a) Close observation is essential to distinguish postoperative pain originating in the chest wall and pleura from cardiac pain, which may be related to myocardial ischemia.

(b) Most cardiac operations involve a median sternotomy, and anesthetic induction of high dose of opioids is used.

(6) Upper abdominal surgery

(a) In preparation for surgery, choices of pain management must be reviewed with patient, and treatment for side effects and inadequate pain relief must be discussed.

(b) Patient will be educated that a scheduled postoperative opioid medication may be withheld in the event of side effects such as respiratory depression, nausea, and vomiting.

(c) Treatments and care plans will be discussed with patient.

(7) Lower abdominal surgery

(a) Pain management is based on the same principle as the upper abdominal surgery.

(b) Pain management related to active labor must be approached with special expertise and caution because of side effects that may impair fetal well-being.

(c) Epidural local anesthesia is beneficial in suppressing pain and surgical stress responses.

(d) Pain after procedures on the anus is particularly severe and requires adjunctive measures such as stool softeners, dietary manipulation, and local anesthetic suppositories for control.

(8) Back surgery

(a) Patients are frequently experiencing chronic pain and may be depressed, anxious, and irritable and have a tolerance level to opioid medications.

(b) Some procedures may limit the use of epidural and spinal delivery of pain medications.

(c) Patients can experience paraspinal muscle spasm—it is appropriate to add muscle relaxant to supplement conventional opioid therapy.

(d) Careful monitoring of neurologic functions

(9) Surgery on extremities

(a) A high degree of morbidity related to venous thromboembolitic complications must be considered.

(b) Pain control postoperatively should allow early ambulation and movement in the postoperative period.

(c) Pain therapy should not interfere with monitoring the patient's neurologic functions.

(d) Epidural analgesia allows early mobility and minimizes thromboembolic complications.

(10) Soft tissue surgery

(a) Patients having surgical procedures involving local soft tissue resections usually obtain pain control with oral opioids.

(b) Patients are anxious of the potential results of a small surgical biopsy and may need adjuvant drug or nondrug therapy.

h. Obstetric patients

(1) During pregnancy

(a) Analgesic considerations

(i) May increase vascular resistance or decrease placental flow

(ii) May cause transient or permanent harm to the fetus or infant

(b) Encourage the use of nondrug pain relieving measures and caution against the use of analgesics.

(c) Analgesics
   (i) Acetaminophen is safe for use in therapeutic doses.
   (ii) NSAIDs generally are not recommended.
   (iii) Opioid analgesics have long history of safely relieving perinatal pain.
      [a] Mu agonist meds are recommended.
         [1] Morphine
         [2] Hydromorphone
         [3] Fentanyl
         [4] Oxycodone
         [5] Hydrocodone
         [6] Meperidine is not recommended as first line opioid.
   (iv) Adjuvant analgesics are used to treat pain of neuropathic origin.
      [a] Local anesthetics
      [b] Antidepressants
      [c] Anticonvulsants
      [d] Corticosteroids
      [e] Benzodiazepines
   (v) Types of pain related to pregnancy
      [a] Round ligament pain (sides of the uterus)
      [b] Headache
      [c] Back pain
      [d] Pyrosis (heartburn)
      [e] Braxton Hicks contractions

(2) During childbirth
  (a) Labor pain is considered the most agonizing of pain syndromes.
  (b) Factors contributing to suffering
    (i) Lack of appropriate analgesics
    (ii) Lack of support person
    (iii) Hunger
    (iv) Fatigue
    (v) Low self-confidence
  (c) Nondrug methods
    (i) Relaxation
    (ii) Distraction
    (iii) Imagery
    (iv) Effleurage
    (v) Water heat
    (vi) Acupuncture
  (d) Analgesics
    (i) Mu opioid agonists are commonly used.
    (ii) Meperidine is not recommended.
    (iii) Local anesthetic bupivacaine is used most often for epidural analgesia and anesthesia.
    (iv) Benzodiazepines are recommended for muscle spasm only and their use for childbirth is not recommended.
  (e) Regional techniques used
    (i) Intrathecal analgesia
    (ii) Epidural analgesia and anesthesia
    (iii) Combined spinal-epidural analgesia

3. During postpartum
  a. Considerations: effective pain management is very important because clotting factors are elevated with high risk for thrombophlebitis.
  b. Pain relief should be directed toward maximizing patient's mobility.
  c. Bonding with baby is encouraged.

      d. Types of pain
- (1) Pain from uterine contractions
- (2) Episiotomy pain
- (3) Breast and nipple pain
- (4) Post–cesarean section pain

    4. During breast-feeding

      a. Secretion of medications into breast milk: considerations
- (1) High lipid solubility
- (2) Low molecular weights
- (3) The nonionized state

      b. Approximately 1% to 2% of the maternal dose of a drug is received by neonate.
- (1) It is recommended to take medications right before or after breast-feeding, which may minimize drug transfer.

      c. Analgesia acetaminophen is safe.
- (1) NSAIDs generally not recommended
- (2) Opioid analgesics: codeine, fentanyl, methadone, and morphine
- (3) Adjuvant analgesic for neuropathic pains

I. Key concepts in analgesic therapy

    1. Balanced analgesia

      a. Continuous multimodal approach in treating pain

      b. Considered as the ideal by experts

      c. Uses combined analgesic regimen, thereby reducing the likelihood of significant side effects from a single agent or method

      d. Opioid is commonly used in the balanced analgesia approach.
- (1) Administered preemptively as well as after the noxious event occurs

    2. Preemptive analgesia

      a. Involves an intervention implemented before noxious stimuli are experienced, which is designed to reduce the impact of these stimuli on the central nervous system (CNS)

      b. NSAIDs treatment is ideally used to reduce the activation and centralization of nociceptors.

      c. Local anesthetics are used to block sensory inflows.

      d. Opioids act centrally to control pain.

      e. Local anesthetics, primarily by sufficiently long regional blockade, are effective preemptive analgesia.
- (1) Indicated before painful procedures
- (2) Indicated whenever pain management is expected to be difficult

    3. Around the clock dosing (ATC)

      a. Two basic principles of providing effective pain management
- (1) Preventing pain
- (2) Maintaining a pain rating that is satisfactory to patients

      b. This is indicated whenever pain is predicted to be present for more than 12 or more hours out of 24.

      c. ATC dosing for continuous pain should be accompanied by provision of additional analgesic doses to relieve pain that exceeds or break through the ongoing pain.

      d. In PCA, the continuous infusion and clinician's administered rescue dose accomplish the same objective.

      e. ATC with short-acting mu agonist opioid analgesics is also used in breakthrough pain.
- (1) A transient and moderate to severe pain that increases above the pain addressed by the ongoing analgesics
- (2) The term is most often used in reference to patients with continuous cancer or chronic nonmalignant pain.

      f. Pain can have a sudden or gradual onset, and it can be brief or prolonged.

4. As needed (PRN) dosing
   a. Ordinarily, the patient requests analgesia.
   b. Effective PRN dosing requires active participation of patient.
      (1) Patient teaching is important to prompt patients to ask for medication before the pain is severe or out of control.
   c. Opioid analgesic is appropriate.
   d. ATC can be replaced with PRN dosing when acute pain is recovered and pain is resolved.
5. PCA
   a. An interactive method of pain management that permits patients to treat their pain by self-administering doses of analgesics
   b. Initiating PCA in the postanesthesia care unit (PACU) is recommended.
      1. To allow evaluation of patient's response to the therapy early in the postoperative course
      2. To prevent delays in analgesia on the nursing unit
   c. Types
      1. Subcutaneous
         (a) Indicated for patients who experience dose-limiting side effects with oral opioids or require parenteral opioids because of bowel obstruction but have limited IV access
         (b) Rarely used for acute pain management because onset is slow
            (i) It is used for children for intermittent bolusing after surgery.
         (c) Hydromorphone and morphine are most commonly used.
         (d) Methadone is not recommended because it causes irritation to the site.
         (e) Absorption and distribution vary depending on the placement of the needle and the patient's adipose tissue.
         (f) High concentration opioid formulations are used for infusion because infusion volumes must be limited.
            (i) Most patients can absorb 2 or 3 ml/hour.
            (ii) Some can absorb 5 ml/hour.
            (iii) Infusion pump must be able to deliver in tenths of milliliter (0.1 ml/hour).
         (g) Primary site of infusion
            (i) Left or right subclavicular anterior chest wall
            (ii) Left, right, or center abdomen
            (iii) Upper arms
            (iv) Thighs
            (v) Buttocks
      2. Intravenous
         (a) Most efficient when an immediate analgesic effect is required, such as for acute, severe escalating pain
            (i) Includes bolus
            (ii) Continuous infusion
            (iii) PCA
         (b) A steady state is better maintained with continuous infusion compared with the bolus method.
         (c) Duration of analgesia by bolus administration is dose dependent; the higher the dose, usually the longer the duration.
      3. Intraspinal analgesics (neuraxial):
         (a) Epidural—needle is inserted in the epidural space.
         (b) Intrathecal—needle is inserted in the subarachnoid space.
         (c) Catheters are removed after 2-4 days.
         (d) Long-term epidural and intrathecal catheters can be placed surgically (implanted) and tunneled subcutaneously to an implanted pump in a subcutaneous pocket in the abdomen.
            (i) Implanted catheters are easier to maintain, and risk of infection is less.

        (e) Contraindications for intraspinal use
- (i) Patient refusal
- (ii) Untreated sepsis, which could involve the site of injection
- (iii) Shock
- (iv) Hypovolemia
- (v) Coagulopathies

        (f) Contraindications to use of opioid analgesia
- (i) Contraindications to epidural catheter insertion
- (ii) History of adverse reactions to opioid medications
- (iii) Central sleep apnea
- (iv) Lack of familiarity of technique by patient caretakers

        (g) Potential complications
- (i) Total or high spinal blockade
- (ii) Intravenous injection
- (iii) Dural puncture resulting in a dural puncture headache
- (iv) Bleeding resulting in an epidural hematoma
- (v) Catheter problems including
  - [a] Migration of the epidural catheter
  - [b] Breakage of the catheter
  - [c] Infection

        (h) Analgesics commonly used
- (i) Fentanyl
- (ii) Sufentanil
- (iii) Morphine
- (iv) Hydromorphone
- (v) Ropivacaine
- (vi) Bupivacaine

    d. Special considerations for pediatric IV PCA
- (1) It is safe and effective and used commonly in children older than 5 years of age.
- (2) Parents and caregivers must be instructed not to press the PCA except the one designated as the child's pain manager.
- (3) The same patient selection guidelines and considerations for the use of PCA in adults apply to children.
- (4) The principles regarding starting dose estimates and titration for adults apply also to children.

J. Pharmacologic
1. Equianalgesic dose chart (Table 29-1)
2. Starting IV PCA prescription ranges for opioid naïve adults (Table 29-2)
3. Pediatric IV PCA dosing (Table 29-3)
4. Managing opioid-induced side effects
   - **a.** Constipation
     - (1) Stool softener
     - (2) Rectal exam to rule out impaction
     - (3) Disimpaction—administer rescue analgesia or tranquilizer prior to procedure.
   - **b.** Nausea and vomiting
     - (1) Titrate opioid doses slowly and steadily.
     - (2) Add or increase nonopioid or adjuvant for additional pain relief.
     - (3) Antiemetic
     - (4) Support use of relaxation techniques.
   - **c.** Pruritus
     - (1) Reduce opioid by 25% if analgesia is satisfactory.
     - (2) Add or increase nonopioid or nonsedating adjuvant for additional pain relief.
     - (3) Benadryl
     - (4) Naloxone as a last resource

■ TABLE 29-1
■ ■ **Equianalgesic Dose Chart**

Opioid	Parenteral (IM/SC/IV) (over ~4 h)	Oral (PO) (over ~4 h)	Onset (min)	Peak (min)	Duration* (h)	Half-life (h)
MU AGONISTS						
Morphine	10 mg	30 mg	30-60 (PO)	60-90 (PO)	3-6 (PO)	2-4
			30-60 (CR)[†]	90-180 (CR)[†]	8-12 (CR)[†]	
			30-60 (R)	60-90 (R)	4-5 (R)	
			5-10 (IV)	15-30 (IV)	3-4 (IV)*[‡]	
			10-20 (SC)	30-60 (SC)	3-4 (SC)	
			10-20 (IM)	30-60 (IM)	3-4 (IM)	
Codeine	130 mg	200 mg NR	30-60 (PO)	60-90 (PO)	3-4 (PO)	2-4
			10-20 (SC)	UK (SC)	3-4 (SC)	
			10-20 (IM)	30-60 (IM)	3-4 (IM)	
Fentanyl	100 µg/h parenterally and transdermally ≅; 4 mg/h morphine parenterally; 1 µg/h transdermally ≅ morphine 2 mg/24 h orally	–	5 (OT)	15 (OT)	2-5 (OT)	3-4[§];
			1-5 (IV)	3-5 (IV)	0.5-4 (IV)*[‡]	
			7-15 (IM)	10-20 (IM)	0.5-4 (IM)	
			12-16 h (TD)	24 h (TD)	48-72 (TD)	13-24 (TD)
Hydrocodone (as in Vicodin, Lortab)	–	30 mg[ǁ] NR	30-60 (PO)	60-90 (PO)	4-6 (PO)	4
Hydromorphone (Dilaudid)	1.5 mg[¶]	7.5 mg	15-30 (PO)	30-90 (PO)	3-4 (PO)	2-3
			15-30 (R)	30-90 (R)	3-4 (R)	
			5 (IV)	10-20 (IV)	3-4 (IV)*[‡]	
			10-20 (SC)	30-90 (SC)	3-4 (SC)	
			10-20 (IM)	30-90 (IM)	3-4 (IM)	
Levorphanol (Levo-Dromoran)	2 mg	4 mg	30-60 (PO)	60-90 (PO)	4-6 (PO)	12-15
			10 (IV)	15-30 (IV)	4-6 (IV)*[‡]	
			10-20 (SC)	60-90 (SC)	4-6 (SC)	
			10-20 (IM)	60-90 (IM)	4-6 (IM)	
Meperidine (Demerol)	75 mg	300 mg NR	30-60 (PO)	60-90 (PO)	2-4 (PO)	2-3
			5-10 (IV)	10-15 (IV)	2-4 (IV)*[‡]	
			10-20 (SC)	15-30 (SC)	2-4 (SC)	
			10-20 (IM)	15-30 (IM)	2-4 (IM)	
Methadone (Dolophine)	10 mg[#]	20 mg**	30-60 (PO)	60-120 (PO)	4-8 (PO)	12-190
			UK (SL)	10 (SL)	UK (SL)	
			10 (IV)	UK (IV)	4-8 (IV)*[‡]	
			10-20 (SC)	60-120 (SC)	4-8 (SC)	
			10-20 (IM)	60-120 (IM)	4-8 (IM)	
Oxycodone (as in Percocet, Tylox)	–	20 mg	30-60 (PO)	60-90 (PO)	3-4 (PO)	2-3
			30-60 (CR)[††]	90-180 (CR)[††]	8-12 (CR)[††]	4.5 (CR)
			30-60 (R)	30-60 (R)	3-6 (R)	
Oxymorphone (Numorphan)	1 mg	(10 mg R)	15-30 (R)	120 (R)	3-6 (R)	2-3
			5-10 (IV)	15-30 (IV)	3-4 (IV)*[‡]	
			10-20 (SC)	UK (SC)	3-6 (SC)	
			10-20 (IM)	30-90 (IM)	3-6 (IM)	
Propoxyphene[‡‡] (Darvon)	–	–	30-60 (PO)	60-90 (PO)	4-6 (PO)	6-12

Continued

■ TABLE 29-1 *Cont'd*
■ ■ **Equianalgesic Dose Chart**

Opioid	Parenteral (IM/SC/IV) (over ~4 h)	Oral (PO) (over ~4 h)	Onset (min)	Peak (min)	Duration* (h)	Half-life (h)
AGONIST-ANTAGONISTS						
Buprenorphine[§§] (Buprenex)	0.4 mg	–	5 (SL)	30-60 (SL)	UK (SL)	2-3
			5 (IV)	10-20 (IV)	3-4 (IV)*‡	
			10-20 (IM)	30-60 (IM)	3-6 (IM)	
Butorphanol[§§] (Stadol)	2 mg	–	5-15 (NS)[‖‖]	60-90 (NS)	3-4 (NS)	3-4
			5 (IV)	10-20 (IV)	3-4 (IV)*‡	
			10-20 (IM)	30-60 (IM)	3-4 (IM)	
Dezocine (Dalgan)	10 mg	–	5 (IV)	UK (IV)	3-4 (IV)*‡	2-3
			10-20 (IM)	30-60 (IM)	3-4 (IM)	
Nalbuphine[§§] (Nubain)	10 mg	–	5 (IV)	10-20 (IV)	3-4 (IV)*‡	5
			<15 (SC)	UK (SC)	3-4 (SC)	
			<15 (IM)	30-60 (IM)	3-4 (IM)	
Pentazocine[§§] (Talwin)	60 mg	180 mg	15-30 (PO)	60-180 (PO)	3-4 (PO)	2-3
			5 (IV)	15 (IV)	3-4 (IV)*‡	
			15-20 (SC)	60 (SC)	3-4 (SC)	
			15-20 (IM)	60 (IM)	3-4 (IM)	

May be duplicated for use in clinical practice.

From McCaffery M, Pasero C: *Pain: clinical manual*, ed 2, Mosby, St Louis, 1999, pp 241-243. Copyright © 1999, Mosby, Inc.

ATC, Around-the-clock; CR, oral controlled-release; h, hour; IM, intramuscular; IV, intravenous; μg, microgram; mg, milligram; min, minute; NR, not recommended; NS, nasal spray; OT, oral transmucosal; PO, oral; R, rectal; SC, subcutaneous; SL, sublingual; TD, transdermal; UK, unknown.

*Duration of analgesia is dose dependent; the higher the dose, usually the longer the duration.

†As in (e.g., MS Contin)

‡IV boluses may be used to produce analgesia that lasts approximately as long as IM or SC doses. However, of all routes of administration, IV produces the highest peak concentration of the drug, and the peak concentration is associated with the highest level of toxicity (e.g., sedation). To decrease the peak effect and lower the level of toxicity, IV boluses may be administered more slowly (e.g., 10 mg of morphine over a 15-minute period) or smaller doses may be administered more often (e.g., 5 mg of morphine every 1-1.5 hours).

§At steady state, slow release of fentanyl from storage in tissues can result in a prolonged half-life up to 12 h.

‖Equianalgesic data not available

¶The recommendation that 1.5 mg of parenteral hydromorphone is approximately equal to 10 mg of parenteral morphine is based on single dose studies. With repeated dosing of hydromorphone (e.g., PCA), it is more likely that 2-3 mg of parenteral hydromorphone is equal to 10 mg of parenteral morphine.

#In opioid-tolerant patients converted from continuous IV hydromorphone to continuous IV methadone, start with 10%-25% of the equianalgesic does.

**In opioid-tolerant patients converted to methadone, start PO dosing PRN with 10%-25% of equianalgesic dose.

††As in (e.g., Oxycontin)

‡‡65-130 mg = approximately 1/6th of all doses listed in this chart.

§§Used in combination with mu agonists, may reverse analgesia and precipitate withdrawal in opioid-dependent patients.

‖‖In opioid-naïve patients who are taking occasional mu agonists, such as codeine or oxycodone, the addition of butorphanol nasal spray may provide additive analgesia. However, in opioid-tolerant patients, such as those receiving ATC morphine, the addition of butorphanol nasal spray should be avoided because it may reverse analgesia and precipitate withdrawal.

    d. Mental confusion
        (1) Evaluate underlying cause.
        (2) Eliminate nonessential CNS acting medications (e.g., steroids).
        (3) Reduce opioid by 25% if analgesia is satisfactory.
        (4) Reevaluate and treat underlying process.
        (5) If delirium persists: trial of neuroleptic, switch to another opioid, switch to intraspinal route
        (6) Avoid naloxone.

■ TABLE 29-2
■ ■ **Starting IV PCA Prescription Ranges for Opioid-Naïve Adults***

Drug	Typical Concentration	Loading Dose	PCA Dose	Delay	Basal Rate	Hour Limit
Morphine	1 mg/ml	2.5 mg, repeat PRN	0.6-2.0 mg	5-10 min	0-1.25 mg/h	7.5-12.5 mg/h
Hydromorphone	0.2 mg/ml	0.4 mg, repeat PRN	0.1-0.3 mg	5-10 min	0-0.2 mg/h	1.2-2.0 mg/h
Fentanyl	10 μg/ml	25μg, repeat PRN	5-20 μg	4-8 min	0-10 μg	75-125 μg/h
Meperidine[†]	10 mg/ml	20 mg, repeat PRN	5-20 mg	5-10 min	0-10 mg/h[‡] NR	50-100 mg/h

From McCaffery M, Pasero C: *Pain: clinical manual*, ed 2, Mosby, St Louis, 1999.
To save time and prevent errors, tables with PCA prescription ranges commonly used for opioid-naïve patients with severe, moderate, and mild pain can be developed in advance. This table is an example for severe pain.
*Prescription ranges in this table are calculated for severe pain. Ranges for moderate pain are 50% of those for severe pain, for mild pain 25%.
[†]Should be used for very brief course, in patients who are allergic to the other opioids listed in this chart.
[‡]Accumulation of normeperidine can cause toxic CNS effects and is more likely to occur when meperidine is administered by continuous infusion.
H, hour; μg, microgram; *mg*, milligram; *min*, minute; *ml*, milliliter; *NR*, not recommended; *PRN*, as needed.
Information from American Pain Society (APS): Principles of analgesic use in the treatment of acute and cancer pain, ed 3, Glenview, IL, 1992, APS; Hunt RF, Abbott Laboratories, Hospital Products Division: Letter communication to Malcolm Cohen, MD, Mt. Sinai Medical Center, Miami Beach, FL, July 11, 1989.

■ TABLE 29-3
■ ■ **Pediatric IV PCA Dosing**

Opioid Analgesic	PCA Dose	Delay (lock-out)	Basal Rate
Morphine	10-30 μg/kg/dose	6-10 minutes	0-30 μg/kg/h
Fentanyl	0.5-1.0 μg/kg/dose	6-10 minutes	0-1.0 μg/kg/h
Hydromorphone (Dilaudid)	3-5 μg/kg/dose	6-10 minutes	0-5 μg/kg/h

From McCaffery M, Pasero C: *Pain: clinical manual*, ed 2, Mosby, St Louis, 1999.
h, hour; *kg*, kilogram; *μg*, microgram.
Information from Houck CS: The management of acute pain in the child. In Ashburn MA, Rice LF, editors: *The management of pain*, ed 3, New York: Churchill Livingstone, 1998, pp 651-666; Yaster M, Krane EJ, Kaplan RF, et al, editors: *Pediatric pain management and sedation handbook: Formulary*, St. Louis: Mosby, 1997.

   e. Sedation
      (1) Evaluate if related to sedation from opioid.
      (2) Eliminate nonessential CNS depressant medications.
      (3) Reduce opioid by 1% to 25% if analgesia is satisfactory.
      (4) Add or increase nonopioid or nonsedating adjuvant for additional pain relief.
      (5) Add stimulus during the day (e.g., caffeine).
   f. Respiratory depression
      (1) Monitor sedation level and respiratory rate.
      (2) Add or increase nonopioid or nonsedating adjuvants.
      (3) Decrease opioid by 25% if analgesia is satisfactory.
      (4) Stop opioid if patient is minimally responsive.

K. Nonpharmacologic and integrative therapies

   1. Cutaneous stimulation

 a. Definition: stimulation of the skin by such methods as heat, cold, and vibration

 b. Benefits: The potential benefits of cutaneous stimulation techniques range from

  (1) Making pain more tolerable to

  (2) Actual reduction of pain

 c. Various cutaneous stimulation methods include the use of

  (1) Heat

  (2) Cold

  (3) Vibration

  (4) A simple touch can be experienced as a therapeutic gesture of caring.

  (5) Other touch modalities are gaining popularity among patients who choose integrative therapies.

   2. Types

 a. Cold therapy

  (1) Cold tends to relieve pain faster and longer.

  (2) It decreases bleeding and edema.

  (3) Apply to site using

   (a) Waterproof bag with ice

   (b) Conventional cold pack

   (c) A commercial cold therapy device

   (d) Effective for

    (i) Surgical incisions

    (ii) Headache

    (iii) Muscle spasms

    (iv) Low back pain

  (4) Care must be taken to avoid tissue damage by providing appropriate protective covering.

  (5) Inspection of the skin to assess for potential tissue damage

 b. Heat therapy

  (1) Heat therapy may be useful in the following types of pain.

   (a) Muscle aches

   (b) Spasms

   (c) Low back pain

  (2) Care must be taken to avoid tissue damage by providing appropriate protective covering.

  (3) Care must be taken to inspect the skin for potential tissue damage.

 c. Vibration

  (1) It is a form of an electric massage.

  (2) It has a soothing effect.

  (3) Vibration with moderate pressure may relieve pain by causing

   (a) Numbness

   (b) Paresthesia

   (c) Anesthesia

  (4) Vibration may also change the character of the sensation from sharp to dull.

  (5) Handheld and stationary vibrators can be used.

 d. Touch modalities

  (1) Reiki techniques

   (a) Originating nearly 3000 years ago, Reiki is believed to balance energy and bring harmony to body, mind, and soul, and it is usually performed by a trained Reiki master.

   (b) Technique involves light touch over clothing beginning with the head and working down the body front and back.

   (c) Helpful in reducing stress and anxiety and promoting relaxation

   (2) Therapeutic touch
      (a) Introduced in 1979, unlike laying-on of hands, it does not require physical touch, and therefore its name can be misleading.
      (b) Practitioners of therapeutic touch believe that human beings are open energy systems and that the flow of energy between people is a natural and continuous event.
      (c) On this basis, the practitioner of therapeutic touch uses himself or herself to facilitate the healing that occurs during the treatment.
      (d) Provides
         (i) Calming response
         (ii) Decreased anxiety
         (iii) Promote sleep when used alone or with sedatives
      (e) Since physical touch is not necessary when doing therapeutic touch, it can ideally be used for patients with whom touch would be painful.
3. Relaxation techniques
   a. Definition: Relaxation is a state of relative freedom from both anxiety and skeletal muscle tension.
   b. Benefits
      (1) Not a substitute for appropriate pain management
      (2) May reduce anxiety
      (3) Decrease muscle tension
      (4) Promote the ability to sleep
   c. These techniques may be more beneficial when the patient receives preoperative instructions to practice relaxation techniques and is coached to use them during postoperative phase.
   d. To achieve the maximum stress reducing response from relaxation, researchers have suggested that a 20-minute technique be used three times a day.
   e. Types
      (1) Slow deep breathing: clench fists, breathe in deeply, and hold it a moment. Breathe out and let oneself go limp—then start yawning
      (2) Imagery: research showed a more effective approach to relaxation that reduces pain intensity.
         (a) Involves closing one's eyes to recall pleasant or peaceful experiences, calming places, or events
      (3) Superficial massage: Includes
         (a) Handholding
         (b) Rubbing a shoulder
         (c) Rhythmic application of pressure to skin and muscles
         (d) These may decrease pain, relax muscles, and facilitate sleep.
         (e) You must obtain patient's permission to be touched.
         (f) Common areas for massage include
            (i) Back and shoulders
            (ii) Hand or feet
         (g) It can communicate care and concern when verbal interactions are limited.
      (4) Music therapy
         (a) Patients can learn to use music for both distraction and relaxation.
         (b) Researchers who study music have found that patients who listen to music may have more satisfying hospital experiences.
         (c) Utilize soothing background music in the preoperative area.
         (d) Small portable tape players with headsets to help block out extraneous noises and promote relaxation
         (e) Establish a tape library with available music selections and relaxation tapes.
         (f) Encourage patient to request personal preferences.

(g) Study showed that patients who listened to music in the PACU reported their experience as significantly more pleasant than those who did not listen to music (Heitz, Symreng, Scamman, 1992).

4. Distraction
    a. Definition: sometimes referred to as cognitive refocusing; Attention and concentration are directed at stimuli other than pain.
    b. Benefits: Although, the effects as a method of pain management are unpredictable, it may
        (1) Decrease intensity of pain
        (2) Increase pain tolerance
        (3) Make more acceptable pain sensation
        (4) Improve positive mood
    c. Often beneficial in mild to moderate pain usually associated with a procedure
        (1) Peripheral IV insertion
        (2) Repositioning
    d. Distraction is used more effectively before pain actually begins.
        (1) Types
            (a) Music
            (b) Video games
            (c) Imagery
            (d) Prayer
            (e) Aromatherapy
            (f) Hypnotherapy
            (g) Humor

5. Nondrug approaches to pain management for children
    a. Distraction
        (1) Involve parent and child in identifying strong distractions.
        (2) Involve child in play: use radio, tape recorder, record player; have child sing or use rhythmic breathing.
        (3) Have child take a deep breath and blow it out until told to stop.
        (4) Have child blow bubbles to "blow the hurt away."
        (5) Have child concentrate on yelling or saying "ouch" by focusing on "yelling loud or soft as you feel it hurt; that way I know what's happening."
        (6) Have child look through kaleidoscope and ask to concentrate on the different designs.
        (7) Use humor such as watching cartoons, telling jokes or funny stories, or acting silly.
        (8) Have child read, play games, or visit with friends.
    b. Relaxation
        (1) Hold in a comfortable, well-supported position, such as vertical against the chest and shoulder.
        (2) Rock in a chair.
        (3) Repeat one or two words softly: "Mommy's here."
        (4) Ask child to take a deep breath and go limp like a rag doll.
        (5) Suggest child float like a balloon.
    c. Imagery for distraction or relaxation
        (1) Have child identify some highly pleasurable read or pretend experiences.
        (2) Have child describe details of the events.
        (3) Have child write down or record script.
        (4) Encourage child to concentrate only on the pleasurable event during the painful time.
    d. Cutaneous stimulation
        (1) Rhythmic rubbing
        (2) Pressure
        (3) Electric vibrator

      (4) Massage with hand lotion.

      (5) Powder or menthol cream

      (6) Application of heat and cold on the site before giving injection or application of ice to the site opposite the painful area

II. Comfort

  A. Definition: The immediate experience of being strengthened by having a need for relief, ease, and transcendence met in four contexts.

    1. Physical

    2. Psychospiritual

    3. Sociocultural

    4. Environmental

  B. Context of comfort

    1. Physical—pertaining to bodily sensations and homeostatic mechanisms that may or may not be related to specific diagnoses

    2. Psychospiritual—whatever gave life meaning for an individual and entailed self-esteem, self-concept, sexuality, and his or her relationship to a higher order or being

    3. Sociocultural—pertaining to interpersonal, family, and societal relationships including

      a. Finances

      b. Education

      c. Support

        (1) Family histories

        (2) Traditions

        (3) Language

        (4) Clothes

        (5) Customs

    4. Environmental—pertaining to external surroundings, conditions, and influences

BIBLIOGRAPHY

1. American Society of Anesthesiologists: What you should know about your patient's use of herbal medicines. Available at http://www.asahq.org/patientEducation/herbPhysician.pdf. Accessed in April 2001.

2. American Society of Anesthesiologists: What you should know about herbal and dietary supplement use and anesthesia. Available at http://www.asahq.org/patientEducation/herbPatient.pdf. Accessed in April 2001.

3. American Society of PeriAnesthsia Nurses: Resource 8: Agency for Health Care Research and Quality: Abbreviated acute pain management flowchart. In *2002 standards of perianesthesia nursing practice.* Cherry Hill, NJ: ASPAN, 2002.

4. Burden N, Quinn D, O'Brien D, Gregory-Dawes B: *Ambulatory surgical nursing,* ed 2. Philadelphia: WB Saunders, 2000.

5. DeFazio-Quinn D (ed): *Ambulatory surgical nursing core curriculum.* Philadelphia: WB Saunders, 1999.

6. Drain C: *The post anesthesia care unit: a critical approach to post anesthesia nursing,* ed 4. Philadelphia: WB Saunders, 2002.

7. Herdtner S: Using therapeutic touch in nursing practice. *Orthop Nurs* 19(5):77-82, 2000.

8. Heitz L, Symreng T, Scamman F. Effect of music therapy in the PACU: a nursing intervention. *J PeriAnesth Nurs* 7(1):22-31, 1992.

9. Joint Commission on Accreditation of Healthcare Organizations (JCAHO): Examples of compliance: Pain assessment and management. In *Joint commission resources.* Oakbrook Terrace, IL: JCAHO, 2002.

10. Kolcaba K, Wilson L: Comfort care: A framework for perianesthesia nursing. *J PeriAnesth Nurs* 17(2):102-114, 2002.

11. Kolcaba KY: A taxonomic structure for the concept of comfort. *Image* 23:237-240, 1991.

12. Kolcaba KY: Holistic comfort: Operationalizing the contruct as a nurse sensitive outcome. *ANS: Adv Nurs Sci* 15: 1-10, 1992.

13. Kolcaba KY: A theory of holistic comfort for nursing. *J Adv Nurs* 19:1178-1184, 1994.

14. Kolcaba KY: The comfort line website. Available at http://www3.uakron.edu/comfort/2002. Accessed in

15. Litwack K (ed): *Core curriculum for perianesthesia nursing practice,* ed 4. Philadelphia: WB Saunders, 1999.

16. McCaffery M, Pasero C: *Pain: Clinical manual.* St Louis: Mosby, 1999, pp 389-390, 404-421.
17. Merkel S, Shobha M. Pediatric pain: tools and assessment. *J PeriAnesth Nurs* 15(6):408-414, 2000
18. Merkel S, Voepel-Lewis T, Shayevitz J, et al: The FLACC: a behavioral scale for scoring postoperative pain in young children. *Ped Nurs* 23:293-297, 1997.
19. St. Marie B (ed): *American Society of Pain Management Nurses: core curriculum for pain management nursing.* Philadelphia: WB Saunders, 2002.
20. Wardwell DW, Engebretson J: Biological correlates of Reiki touch [SM] healing. *J Adv Nurs* 33(4):439-445, 2001.
21. Weeks J: JCAHO includes CAM (complimentary and alternative medicine) therapy. *Health Forum J* 45(2):33, 2002.

30 Hemodynamic Monitoring

SHERRIE L. SMARTT

OBJECTIVES

At the conclusion of this chapter the reader will be able to:

1. Identify surgical patients who might benefit from hemodynamic monitoring based on their risk of oxygen supply and demand imbalance.
2. Define the physiologic variables affecting cardiac function and link their interactions.
3. Discuss the principles of pressure monitoring and strategies to optimize accuracy.
4. Determine the indications, risks, complications, and perioperative considerations for specific hemodynamic monitoring, including arterial pressure, central venous pressure, and pulmonary artery pressure.
5. Identify normal waveform configurations for the preceding catheters.
6. Name the various ports of the pulmonary artery catheter, and list their functions.
7. Identify normal and calculated hemodynamic pressures, and link the clinical significance of alterations in surgical patients.
8. Compare and contrast the bolus and continuous cardiac output techniques for thermodilution cardiac output, and determine the significance of altered cardiac output states in surgical patients.
9. Define the function of SVo_2 and identify causes for variances.

   I. The goal of hemodynamic monitoring
     A. To assess and optimize the balance between oxygen supply and demand
  II. Indications
     A. Outcome must outweigh cost and potential for complications.
     B. High risk and/or hemodynamically unstable surgical patients
 III. Physiologic variables affecting cardiac function
     A. Cardiac output (CO)
       1. Definition: The amount of blood ejected from the ventricles measured in liters per minute
       2. CO = Stroke volume (SV) × Heart rate (HR)
       3. Influences on CO
         a. HR
         b. SV
           (1) Definition: The amount of blood ejected from the ventricle with each beat
           (2) Influences on SV
              (a) Preload (right and left)
                 (i) Definition: Filling volume of the ventricle at the end of diastole
                 (ii) Right-sided preload: central venous pressure (CVP) or right atrial pressure (RA)
                 (iii) Left-sided preload: left atrial pressure (LAP), pulmonary artery diastolic (PAD) pressure, pulmonary artery occlusion (wedge) pressure (PAOP) or pulmonary capillary wedge pressure (PCWP)

(iv) Influences on preload: Any condition that increases blood return to the heart or decreases ejection of blood from the heart, for example, pulmonary hypertension decreases the ability of the right ventricle (RV) to pump, thereby decreasing the ejection of blood from the RV and increasing RV preload; fluid infusions increase circulating blood volume thereby increasing right-sided and left-sided preload.

(b) Afterload (right and left)
  (i) Definition: The resistance, impedance, or pressure the ventricle must overcome to eject blood
  (ii) Affected by the volume and mass of the blood, the size and thickness of the ventricle, and the tone of the vascular beds
  (iii) Right-sided afterload: Pulmonary vascular resistance (PVR)
  (iv) Left-sided afterload = Systemic vascular resistance (SVR)
  (v) Influences on afterload: Any condition that increases the pressure required for the ventricle to eject volume. These conditions generally involve valve function or vascular tone but can also include blood viscosity, that is aortic stenosis would result in a narrowed outflow tract, increasing the pressure required for the left ventricle (LV) to eject blood and therefore increasing the left-sided afterload. Use of a vasodilator would relax the vessel beds and increase the diameter of the vessels, decreasing the pressure required for the ventricles to eject blood.

(c) Contractility
  (i) Definition: The inherent ability of the myocardial muscle fibers to shorten and contract regardless of preload or afterload
  (ii) Indirectly assessed through a calculated stroke work index

c. Atrioventricular (AV) synchrony
  (1) Definition: Coordinated contraction pattern between atria and ventricles
  (2) Influences on AV synchrony
    (a) Ischemia
    (b) Infarction
    (c) Conduction deficits
    (d) Dysrhythmia
  (3) Loss of synchrony decreases CO, blood pressure, and SV and increases LAP

IV. Hemodynamic evaluation of cardiac function
  A. Hemodynamic normal values (Table 30-1)
  B. Hemodynamic calculations (Table 30-2)

V. Limitations of hemodynamic monitoring
  A. Presumptions and assumptions
    1. Major presumption—pressure = Volume
      a. Right atrial pressure (RAP) = Right ventricular end-diastolic volume (RVEDV) = RV preload
      b. PAD = LAP = Pulmonary capillary wedge pressure (PCWP) = Left ventricular-end diastolic volume (LVEDV) = LV preload
    2. Reality
      a. The relationship between pressure and volume is curvilinear and is influenced by the compliance or ease of distensibility of the ventricle.

VI. Principles of pressure monitoring
  A. Utilizes a fluid-filled tubing system with a pressure transducer
  B. The mechanical impulse is transmitted from the tip of the catheter through the fluid to the transducer chip where it is converted from a mechanical signal to

■ TABLE 30-1
■ ■ **Hemodynamic Normal Values (Adult)**

Pressure	Value	Range
Right atrial pressure (RA)	Mean	2-6 mm Hg
Central venous pressure (CVP)	Mean	6-10 cm H_2O
Right ventricular pressure (RV)	Systolic	15-25 mm Hg
	Diastolic	0-8 mm Hg
Pulmonary artery pressure (PAP)	Systolic	15-25 mm Hg
	Diastolic	8-15 mm Hg
	Mean	10-20 mm Hg
Left atrial pressure (LAP)	Mean	6-12 mm Hg
Pulmonary artery occlusion pressure (PAOP)	Mean	6-12 mm Hg
Pulmonary capillary wedge pressure (PCWP)	Mean	6-12 mm Hg
Left ventricular end diastolic pressure (LVEDP)	Mean	6-12 mm Hg

From Lichtenthal PR: *Quick guide to cardiopulmonary care.* Irvine, CA: Edwards Lifesciences LLC, 1998, p 105.

■ TABLE 30-2
■ ■ **Hemodynamic Calculations (Adult)**

Pressure	Formula	Value
Mean arterial pressure (MAP)	$\dfrac{\text{Systolic BP} + 2\text{Diastolic BP}}{3}$	70-105 mm Hg
Cardiac output (CO) (L/min)	$HR \times SV$	4-8 L/min
Cardiac index (CI) (L/min/m^2)	CO/BSA	2.5-4.0 L/min/m^2
Stroke volume (SV)	$CO/HR \times 1000$	60-100 ml
Stroke index (SI)	SV/BSA or CI/HR	33-47 ml/beat/m^2
Left ventricular stroke work index (LVSWI)	$\dfrac{1.36 \times (MAP - PAOP) \times SI}{100}$	50-62 g-m/beat/m^2
Right ventricular stroke work index (RVSWI)	$\dfrac{1.36 \times (MPAP - RAP) \times SI}{100}$	5-10 g-m/beat/m^2
Systemic vascular resistance (SVR)	$\dfrac{MAP - RAP \text{ or } CVP \times 80}{CO}$	800-1200 dynes/sec/cm^5
Pulmonary vascular resistance	$\dfrac{RAP - PAOP(MPAP) \times 80}{CO}$	<250 dynes/sec/cm^5
Ejection fraction (EF)	$\dfrac{SV \times 100}{EDV}$ End diastolic volume	60-75% (left ventricle)
Body surface area (BSA)	Use Dubois chart.	1.5-2 m^2

From Lichtenthal PR: *Quick guide to cardiopulmonary care.* Irvine, CA: Edwards Lifesciences LLC, 1998, p 105.

an electronic signal and sent to the monitor through the transducer cable to be displayed as an electronic waveform on the monitor screen.

C. Optimizing accuracy of pressures
   1. Remove bubbles from tubing when priming.
   2. Utilize a continuous flush system with 300 mm Hg pressure to infusion bag.
   3. Eliminate tubing extensions if possible (use only nondistensible extension tubing).
   4. Level and zero transducer when indicated
      a. Position patient in 0-45° supine position (position of tolerance).

       b. Place air and fluid interface at the phlebostatic axis (fourth intercostal space, midchest) and open to air while activating the zero function on your bedside monitor (Figure 30-1).

       c. Transducer must be leveled and zeroed to atmospheric pressure initially and whenever the tubing is disconnected or changed.

       d. Allow 5 minutes after position changes before measuring pressures.

       e. Maintain as much consistency in patient's position as possible for measurement.

VII. Direct intraarterial pressure monitoring (arterial line) (AL)

  A. Allows for continuous observation of the patient's systemic blood pressure with calculation of the mean arterial pressure (MAP)

  B. Provides more accuracy than use of a sphygmomanometer during low cardiac output states

  C. Under optimal conditions, an indirect blood pressure (BP) will underestimate the systolic pressure and overestimate the diastolic pressure by about 5 mm Hg.

  D. Indications

    1. Cardiopulmonary bypass

    2. Procedures with potential for wide variation in blood pressure intraoperatively or postoperatively

      a. Carotid endarterectomy

      b. Aortic aneurysm resection

      c. Craniotomies

    3. Need for strict blood pressure control

    4. Multiple arterial blood gases or laboratory tests

    5. Titration of vasoactive medications (particularly those with an extremely short half-life, e.g., nitroprusside)

  E. Placement

    1. Site needs to be accessible and easily compressible in case of bleeding.

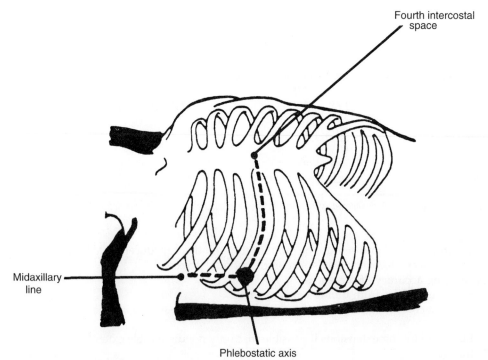

FIGURE 30-1 ■ Phlebostatic axis is an approximation of right atrium and is used for leveling air interface port of pressure monitoring system.

   2. Radial artery (most common)
     a. Allen test should be performed before insertion to assess for collateral ulnar flow.
      (1) Procedure
        (a) Compress both ulnar and radial arteries on one extremity while the patient repeatedly makes a tight fist to squeeze blood out of the hand.
        (b) Release compression of the ulnar artery to observe for reperfusion indicated by a blush of color.
        (c) Color should return within 5 to 10 seconds or radial artery should not be cannulated.
        (d) The test can be repeated on the radial artery for evidence of brisk perfusion.
   3. Femoral
     a. Most commonly seen with patients undergoing cardiac catheterization laboratory procedures
     b. Brachial artery (uncommon)
 F. Arterial pressure waveform; two components (Figure 30-2)
   1. Anacrotic limb: A sharp uprise in the tracing that reflects the outflow of blood from the ventricle and into the arterial system
   2. Dicrotic limb: Descending of the pressure tracing that reflects the decrease in the pressure during diastole. The beginning of diastole is seen as a small notch on the descending limb of the tracing caused by the closing of the aortic valve and is commonly called the dicrotic notch.
 G. Risks and complications
   1. Vascular compromise (e.g., thrombus, spasm)
   2. Disconnection: hemorrhage
   3. Accidental injection of drugs or air
   4. Infection
   5. Nerve damage
 H. Preoperative considerations
   1. Patient teaching
     a. Potential for extremity immobilization

Components of Arterial Pulse

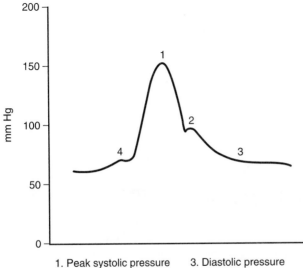

FIGURE 30-2 ■ Arterial pressure waveform. (From Headley JM: *Invasive hemodynamic monitoring: Physiological principles and clinical applications.* Irvine, CA: Edwards Lifesciences, 1996, p 55.)

1. Peak systolic pressure   3. Diastolic pressure
2. Dicrotic notch   4. Anacrotic notch

      b. Inform nurse if experience coldness, numbness, pain, or tingling

      c. May transfer to the receiving unit with AL in place

  I. Intraoperative and postoperative considerations

      1. Maintain aseptic technique (keep dead-ender caps on stopcock ports).

      2. Monitor pressures continuously (an AL should always be connected to the transducer cable and waveform displayed on the monitor).

      3. Assess and document appearance of site, immobilization, capillary refill of extremity, temperature and color of extremity.

      4. Document a monitor strip of the waveform in the chart to display waveform appearance.

      5. Always use luer lock connections.

      6. Level and zero transducer per standard

      7. Troubleshoot variances in the patient waveform. (Always assess the patient first when trouble-shooting a dampened waveform.) (Figure 30-3)

VIII. CVP monitoring

  A. Indications

      1. Rapid infusion of fluid or blood

      2. Inability to cannulate peripheral veins

      3. Administration of drugs that may cause peripheral sclerosis (i.e., potassium, epinephrine, norepinephrine, chemotherapeutic agents, aminoglycosides)

      4. Administration of hyperalimentation

      5. Access site for temporary transvenous pacing.

      6. Assessment of fluid status

  B. Placement

      1. The catheter is placed in a major vein leading to the superior vena cave (i.e., subclavian, internal jugular, femoral, or brachial vein).

      2. The side port of the pulmonary artery (PA) catheter introducer and the proximal port of the PA catheter can also be used as a central venous access.

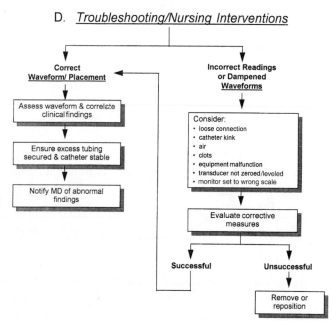

FIGURE 30-3 ■ Arterial pressure monitoring: Troubleshooting and nursing interventions.

C. Risks and complication
   1. Carotid artery puncture with insertion (internal jugular approach)
   2. Infection
   3. Thrombus or embolic event
   4. Air embolism
   5. Pneumothorax from insertion (subclavian approach)
D. Preoperative considerations
   1. Patient teaching
      a. Information regarding catheter insertion should be included in preoperative teaching and is part of informed consent.
      b. Differentiate whether lines will be placed in preoperative holding or after the induction of anesthesia.
   2. Intraoperative and postoperative considerations
      a. Obtain an order for a postinsertion chest x-ray to verify line placement and rule out complications.
      b. Maintain a sterile dressing per hospital standards for central lines.
      c. Intermittent readings via a water manometer are measured in centimeters of water (mm Hg × 1.36 = cm H_2O) (2 to 8 cm H_2O).
      d. Continuous readings via pressure transducer are measured in millimeters of mercury (2 to 6 mm Hg).
      e. Must be leveled and zeroed to phlebostatic axis
      f. Assessment and documentation
         (1) Pressures per unit standard
         (2) Location of catheter and appearance of site if visualized
         (3) Strip recording of waveform in chart (Figure 30-4)
            (a) Record waveform on two-channel recorder concurrently with electrocardiogram (ECG) to identify individual waves of waveform to ensure accuracy with increased respiratory artifact.
            (b) Record pressure at mean of the "a" wave at end-expiration (spontaneously breathing).
            (c) Record pressure at the mean of the "a" wave at end-inspiration (controlled mechanical ventilation).
      g. Troubleshooting and nursing interventions (Figure 30-5)
IX. Pulmonary artery pressure (PAP) monitoring (PA catheter)
   A. Indications
      1. Intraoperative risk that exceeds the cost and risk of complications of insertion of the catheter

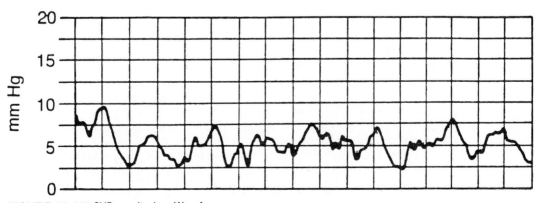

FIGURE 30-4 ■ CVP monitoring: Waveform.

D. _Troubleshooting/Nursing Interventions_

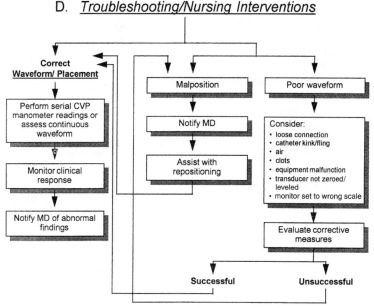

FIGURE 30-5 ■ CVP monitoring: Troubleshooting and nursing interventions.

    a. Perioperative monitoring of surgical patients with major preexisting systems dysfunction undergoing extensive operative procedures.
        (1) Thoracic or abdominal aortic aneurysms
        (2) Coronary artery bypass and valvular replacement
        (3) Extensive intraabdominal resections
        (4) Prolonged orthopedic procedures
        (5) Thoracic or abdominal aortic aneurysms
  2. Shock of severe or prolonged duration or unknown etiology
  3. Assessment of cardiovascular function and response to therapy in patients with complicated, unstable cardiovascular disease unresponsive to conventional therapy
  4. Use of mechanical assist devices (i.e., intraaortic balloon pump, ventricular assist device)
  5. Titration of cardioactive and vasoactive drugs
  6. Aspiration of air emboli in neurosurgical patients in the upright position intraoperatively
B. Placement
  1. Internal jugular and subclavian are preferred, but may also be placed in the brachial or femoral vein.
C. Catheter types (All catheters are flow directed thermal dilutional pulmonary artery catheters.)
  1. Garden variety—measures PAP, RAP, pulmonary artery occlusive pressure (PAOP) and allows for bolus thermodilutional CO computation
  2. Venous infusion port (VIP)—has extra venous infusion ports, generally exiting into the RA or RV
  3. Paceport—has an RV port for insertion of a ventricular pacing wire
  4. SVo_2—has a fiber optic tip which measures continuous mixed venous saturation in the PA (SVo_2)
  5. Continuous cardiac output (CCO)®—measures CCO by emitting random thermal energy impulses (Edwards Lifesciences)

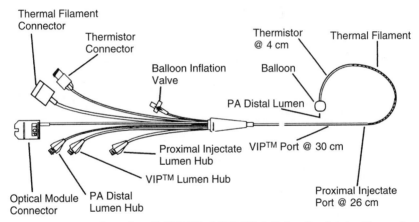

FIGURE 30-6 ■ Swan-Ganz® CCO/SVo₂/VIP® TD Catheter. Reprinted with permission from Edwards Lifesciences LLC, Irvine, CA.

6. CCOmbo®—measures continuous cardiac output plus mixed venous saturation (Edwards Lifesciences) (Figure 30-6)
7. CCOmbo V®—measures RV end-diastolic volume and RV ejection fraction (EF) as well as CCO and SVo₂ (Edwards Lifesciences)

D. Ports and measurements
   1. Distal port
      a. Exits at the tip of the catheter in the PA
      b. Measures PAP (systolic/diastolic/mean[S/D/M]), SVo₂, PAOP (PCWP)
      c. PAP systolic: 20 to 30 mm Hg; diastolic: <10 to 20 mm Hg; mean: >20 mm Hg
      d. PAOP: 6 to 12 mm Hg
      e. Infuse only pressurized saline or heparinized saline at 300 mm Hg.
      f. Indirectly reflects right (systolic) and left (diastolic) heart pressures in the absence of lung or valvular disease
   2. Proximal port
      a. Exits in the RA usually at the 26 to 30 cm mark
      b. Measures RA (CVP) and used for infusion of injectate with bolus CO
      c. RA: 2-6 mm Hg
      d. May be used for infusion although blood products and vasoactive drugs are discouraged
      e. Aspirate blood before performing bolus CO if using for infusion of medications (to prevent bolus of drugs).
   3. Balloon port or gate valve
      a. To obtain PAOP, inflate balloon with up to 1.5 ml of air for the 7.0 to 8.0 French catheters. (Generally, balloon volume is printed on the hub of the catheter.)
      b. Balloon should wedge with 1.25 to 1.5 ml of air. Allow syringe to passively refill, then lock gate valve when not in use.
      c. Do not inflate for more than 15 seconds or two respiratory cycles.
      d. Read pressure at end-expiration.
      e. PAOP should be within 2 to 5 mm Hg of PAD pressure.
      f. Indirectly reflects LAP and left ventricular end-diastolic pressure (LVEDP)

E. Waveforms (Figures 30-7 to 30-11)
F. Risks and complications
   1. Carries the same risks and complications of an AL and central venous line plus some unique to the PA catheter
      a. Pulmonary artery rupture
      b. Perforation of the RV

Right Atrial Waveform

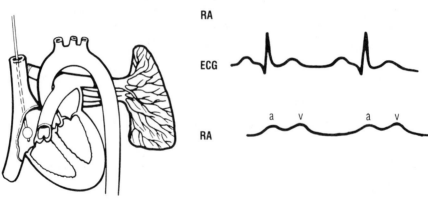

FIGURE 30-7 ■ Pulmonary artery waveforms: Right atrial waveform. (From Headley JM: *Invasive hemodynamic monitoring: Physiological principles and clinical applications.* Irvine, CA: Edwards Lifesciences LLC, 1996, p 23.)

Right Ventricular Waveform

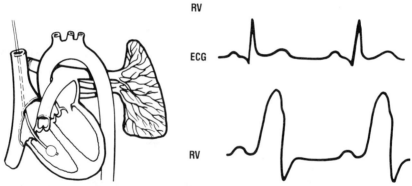

FIGURE 30-8 ■ Pulmonary artery waveforms: Right ventricular waveform. (From Headley JM: *Invasive hemodynamic monitoring: Physiological principles and clinical applications.* Irvine, CA: Edwards Lifesciences LLC, 1996, p 23.)

Pulmonary Artery Waveform

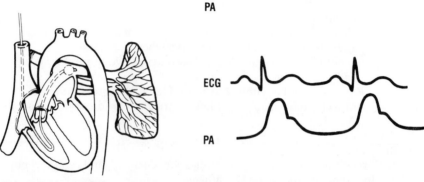

FIGURE 30-9 ■ Pulmonary artery catheter waveforms: Pulmonary artery. (From Headley JM: *Invasive hemodynamic monitoring: Physiological principles and clinical applications.* Irvine, CA: Edwards Lifesciences LLC, 1996, p 24.)

Pulmonary Artery Wedge Waveform

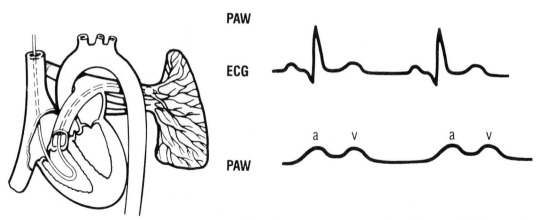

FIGURE 30-10 ■ Pulmonary artery catheter waveforms: Pulmonary capillary wedge. (From Headley JM: *Invasive hemodynamic monitoring: Physiological principles and clinical applications.* Irvine, CA: Edwards Lifesciences LLC, 1996, p 25.)

Normal Insertion Tracings

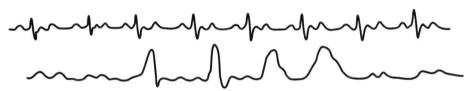

FIGURE 30-11 ■ Pulmonary artery catheter waveforms: Normal insertion tracings. (From Headley JM: *Invasive hemodynamic monitoring: Physiological principles and clinical applications.* Irvine, CA: Edwards Lifesciences LLC, 1996, p 25.)

    c. Dysrhythmias
    d. Electrical microshocks
    e. Catheter migration backward to RV or forward to wedged position
    f. Catheter knotting or kinking
    g. Balloon rupture
    h. Overwedging or failure to unwedge, resulting in pulmonary necrosis or infarction
G. Preoperative considerations
    1. Must have informed consent involving explanation of risks, alternatives and benefits
    2. Patient teaching
        a. Important to stress this is a diagnostic aid and does not assist the heart or lungs
        b. Generally inserted after the initiation of anesthesia
H. Intraoperative and postoperative considerations
    1. Ensure accuracy of measurements.
        a. Visualize waveform for normal configuration.
        b. Pressure readings
            (1) Read pressures end-expiration in the presence of spontaneous respiratory effort.
            (2) Read pressures end-inspiration when respiratory effort is completely controlled mechanically.

    c. Level air-water interface stopcock to the phlebostatic axis and zero transducer to atmospheric pressure initially and if tubing is opened to air or changed.

    d. Read pressures with the patient in the same position for consistency. Generally most accurate in a supine position with the head of bed < 45° upright

    e. Maintain catheter in position where balloon wedges with 1.25 to 1.5 ml of air.

    f. Remove all air bubble from tubing and maintain distal infusion fluids at 300 mm Hg.

    g. Discourage use of extra extension tubing.

  2. Assessment and documentation

    a. Measure and document hemodynamic parameters including calculated parameters upon insertion and per standard (initiation of vasoactive therapy or change in patient condition).

    b. Assess site for bleeding or hematoma. Mark and document size of hematoma in centimeters.

    c. Note and document centimeter markings at hub of catheter. (Thin markings are 10 cm, and thick markings are 50 cm.)

  3. Apply sterile central line dressing per hospital standard.

    a. Avoid taping across sheath covering external catheter.

  4. Maintain aseptic technique: Cover stopcock ports with sterile dead-ender caps.

I. PA catheter insertion in the postanesthesia care unit (PACU)

  1. Assemble all equipment (e.g., insertion supplies, catheter, monitor cables).

  2. Obtain permit if required.

  3. Instruct patient.

  4. Assess need for sedation.

  5. Prime transducer tubing (must be done prior to insertion).

  6. Monitor patient during procedure (BP, SpO_2, rhythm).

  7. Be prepared to inflate balloon.

  8. Cover site and obtain hemodynamic parameters quickly postinsertion.

  9. Obtain chest x-ray after insertion to verify placement and rule out complications.

  10. Document pressures and waveform strips in chart.

J. Clinical significance of alterations in hemodynamic pressures in surgical patients

  1. Elevated PAP (systolic) may be caused by any condition that directly or indirectly increases pressure and/or volume in the lungs or RV.

    a. Pulmonary hypertension

    b. LV failure and mitral stenosis

    c. Constrictive pericarditis

    d. Cardiac tamponade

    e. Congestive heart failure

    f. Atrial or ventricular septal defects

  2. Elevated PAP (diastolic) may be caused by any condition that directly or indirectly increases pressure and/or volume in the lungs or LV.

    a. LV failure

    b. Mitral stenosis

    c. Pulmonary hypertension

    d. Left-to-right shunts

  3. Elevated PAOP may be caused by any condition that increases pressure and/or volume in the LV.

    a. Constrictive pericarditis

    b. LV failure

    c. Mitral valve dysfunction

    d. Aortic insufficiency

        e. Fluid overload

        f. Ischemia

    4. Decreased PAP and PAOP may be caused by any condition or situation that decreases volume and/or pressure in the LV or decreases the pressure the LV must generate to open the aortic valve.

        a. Hypotension

        b. Hypovolemia

        c. Vasodilating drugs causing decreased afterload

X. Thermodilution cardiac output

  A. A method that applies indicator dilution principles, using temperature change as the indicator

  B. Direct measurement that indirectly reflects myocardial performance

    1. Bolus method

        a. A known amount of cool saline (generally 5 or 10 ml) is injected into the RA via the proximal port. This cooler solution mixes with and cools the surrounding blood, and the temperature is measured in the pulmonary artery by a thermistor bead on the tip of the catheter. The computer plots the change in temperature on a time-temperature curve.

    2. Continuous cardiac output (CCO)

        a. A special PA catheter contains a thermal filament between 14 and 25 cm from the distal tip. This filament emits a random thermal signal, resulting in a minute elevation in blood temperature downstream. The computer continuously cross correlates the input signal with the temperature change to produce a thermodilution washout curve. The computer continuously updates the CO data.

    3. Continuous wave Doppler probe

        a. Noninvasively measures thoracic electrical impedance via external electrodes placed on the neck and chest wall

  C. CO is 4-8 L/minute; cardiac index (CI) is 2.5-4 L/minute/m^2

  D. Indications

    1. Used for determination of calculated hemodynamic variables

    2. Perioperative fluid management

    3. Assessment of intraaortic balloon pump (IABP) therapy and positive end expiratory pressure (PEEP)

    4. Evaluation of effects of cardioactive drugs

    5. Indication for myocardial ischemia and infarction

  E. Techniques for accurate assessment

    1. Use accurately measured injectate volume (generally 10 ml for adults and 5 ml for children).

    2. Iced or room temperature (19-24°C) injectate can be used.

    3. Ice saline for injection if hyperthermic or in a high-flow state

    4. Use correct computation constant (packaged with catheter and based on catheter size and amount and temperature of injectate).

    5. Inject rapidly and smoothly within 4 seconds; wait 60 seconds between injections.

    6. Average three to five injections, preferably with results within 10% of each other.

    7. Perform injection during the same time in the respiratory cycle (end-expiration).

    8. Visibly inspect CO curve for technique and accuracy (Figures 30-12 and 30-13).

  F. Significance of CO and CI in surgical patients

    1. Low CO states

        a. Decreased or increased preload (e.g., hypovolemia or hypervolemia, hemorrhage, tamponade)

        b. Decreased myocardial contractility (e.g., drugs, myocardial infarction, LV failure, dysrhythmias)

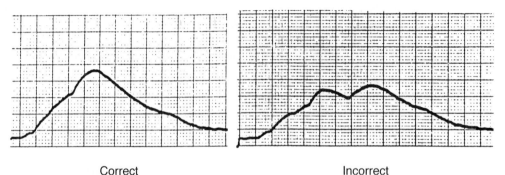

Correct   Incorrect

FIGURE 30-12 ■ Bolus CO waveform.

      c. Decreased or increased afterload (e.g., body temperature, valvular dysfunction, vasoconstriction or dilation, vasoactive drugs, loss of vascular neural control—spinal anesthesia)

    2. High CO states

      a. Hypervolemia

      b. Decreased afterload (e.g., vasodilatation, sepsis)

      c. High metabolic states (e.g., hyperthyroid states, pregnancy)

XI. Mixed venous oxygen saturation (SVO_2)

  A. Global measures of the end result of both oxygen delivery and consumption at the tissue level

  B. Oxygen leftovers (hemoglobin [Hgb] saturation) are measured via a fiber optic filament on the distal tip of the PA catheter utilizing reflective spectrophotometry.

  C. Sensitive, early indicator of oxygenation imbalances but not specific as to whether cause is associated with an oxygen supply or demand problem

  D. Necessary measurement for the calculation of oxygen delivery (Dao_2) and oxygen consumption (Vo_2) (Figure 30-14 and Table 30-3)

    1. Dao_2 definition: The amount of oxygen delivered to the tissues measured in milliliters per minute (normal ≈1000 ml/minute)

    2. Vo_2 definition: The amount of oxygen consumed by the tissues measured in milliliters per minute (normal ≈250 ml/minute)

    3. Oxygen demand definition: The amount of oxygen necessary to maintain aerobic metabolism. This is a dynamic variable dependent on the process of metabolism and is impossible to measure. We can indirectly support oxygen demand by assessing and optimizing Dao_2 and Vo_2

  E. Normal SVo_2 is 60% to 80%.

  F. Decreased SVo_2 (<60%) a result of

    1. Decreased oxygen delivered

      a. Lowered CO, lowered Hgb, or lowered Sao_2

    2. Increased oxygen consumption

      a. Increased cellular oxygen demand (e.g., fever, pain, shivering, seizing, injury, increased intracranial pressure)

  G. Increased SVo_2 >80%, result of

    1. Increased oxygen delivery

      a. Increased CO (e.g., hyperthyroidism, pregnancy, sepsis, vasodilatation)

    2. Decreased oxygen consumption

      a. Hypothermia, anesthesia, neuromuscular paralysis

    3. Faulty calibration of equipment

  H. Techniques for ensuring accuracy

    1. Calibrate PA catheter either before insertion (in vitro) or after insertion (in vivo) daily and with major changes in Hgb (2 g or more).

E. *Troubleshooting/Nursing Interventions*

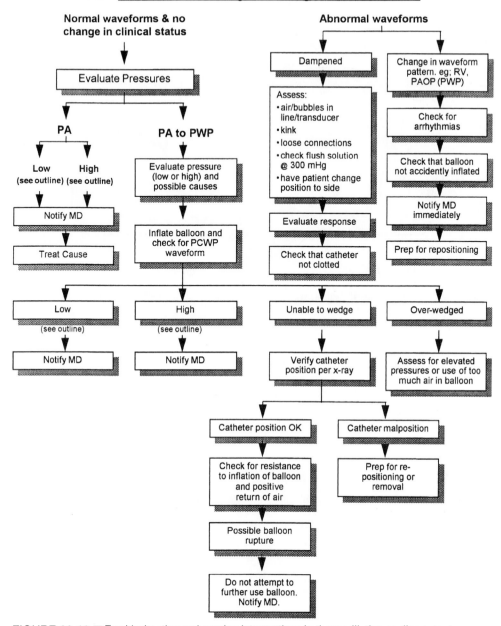

FIGURE 30-13 ■ Troubleshooting and nursing interventions in thermodilution cardiac output.

2. Withdraw blood sample for in vivo calibration from distal port very slowly (over 1-2 minutes) after discarding waste.
3. Maintain PA catheter position that requires 1.25-1.5 ml of air to wedge balloon.
4. Maintain PA catheter position for a signal quality index (SQI) of 1-2.

I. Clinical application of SVO_2
1. Assess for causes of a 5% change in SVO_2 that does not return to baseline within 5 minutes.
2. Differentiate between alterations in O_2 supply versus demand.

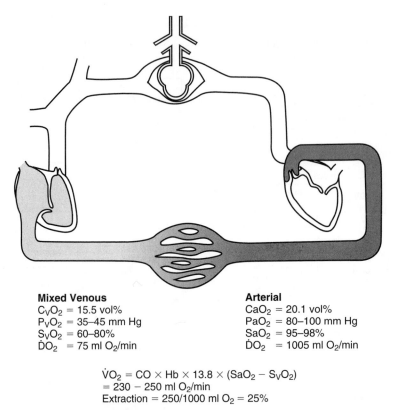

Mixed Venous
C_VO_2 = 15.5 vol%
P_VO_2 = 35–45 mm Hg
S_VO_2 = 60–80%
$\dot{D}O_2$ = 75 ml O_2/min

Arterial
CaO_2 = 20.1 vol%
PaO_2 = 80–100 mm Hg
SaO_2 = 95–98%
$\dot{D}O_2$ = 1005 ml O_2/min

$\dot{V}O_2$ = CO × Hb × 13.8 × (SaO_2 − S_VO_2)
= 230 − 250 ml O_2/min
Extraction = 250/1000 ml O_2 = 25%

FIGURE 30-14 ■ Normal oxygenation values. (From *Understanding continuous mixed venous oxygen saturation (SV)2): Monitoring with the Swan-Ganz® Oximetry TD System,* ed 2. Irvine, CA: Edwards Lifesciences LLC, 1996, p 8.)

■ TABLE 30-3
■ ■ **Oxygenation Parameters (Adult)**

Parameters	Equations	Normal Range
Partial pressure of arterial oxygen (Pao_2)		80-100 mm Hg
Partial pressure of arterial CO_2 ($PaCo_2$)		35-45 mm Hg
Bicarbonate (HCO_3)		22-28 mEq/L
pH		7.38-7.42
Arterial oxygen saturation (Sao_2)		95-100%
Mixed venous saturation (SVo_2)		60-80%
Arterial oxygen content (Cao_2)	(0.0138 × Hgb × Sao_2) + 0.0031 × Pao_2	17-20 ml/dl
Venous oxygen content (Cvo_2)	(0.0138 × Hgb × SVo_2) + 0.0031 × PVO_2	12-15 ml/dl
A-V oxygen content difference ($C(a-v)o_2$)	Cao_2 − Cvo_2	4-6 ml/dl
Oxygen delivery (Doa_2)	Cao_2 × CO × 10	950-1150 ml/min
Oxygen delivery index (Dao_2)	Cao_2 × CI × 10	500-600 ml/min/m²
Oxygen consumption (Vo_2)	($C(a-v)o_2$) × CO × 10	200-250 ml/min
Oxygen consumption index (Vo_2I)	($C(a-v)o_2$) × CI × 10	120-160 ml/min/m²
Oxygen extraction ratio (o_2ER)	[(Cao_2 − Cvo_2)/Cao_2] × 100	20-30%
Oxygen extraction index (o_2EI)	($Sao2$ − Svo_2)/Sao_2 × 100	20-25%

From Lichtenthal PR: Quick guide to cardiopulmonary care. Irvine, CA: Edwards Lifesciences LLC, 1998, p 106.

BIBLIOGRAPHY

1. Ahrens T: Hemodynamic monitoring. *Crit Care Nurs Clin North America* 11(1):19-31, 1999.
2. Bridges EJ: Monitoring pulmonary artery pressures: Just the facts. *Crit Care Nurse* 20(6):59-78, 2000.
3. Bryan-Brown CW, Dracup K: Doing the thing right: Assumptions and assessment in hemodynamic monitoring. *Am J Crit Care* 4(2):269-271, 1993.
4. Cathelyn JL, Samples DA: SVO_2 monitoring: Tool for evaluating patient outcomes. *Dimens Crit Care Nurs* 17(2):58-66, 1998.
5. Darovic G: *Hemodynamic monitoring: Invasive and noninvasive clinical application,* ed 3, St Louis: WB Saunders, 2002.
6. Dresden DG: Hemodynamic monitoring. In Litwack K, editor: *Core curriculum for perianesthesia nursing practice,* ed 4. Philadelphia: WB Saunders, 1998, pp 699-711.
7. Druding MC: Integrating hemodynamic monitoring and physical assessment. *Dimens Crit Care Nurs* 19(4):25-30, 2000.
8. Gawlinski A: Cardiac output monitoring. In Chulay M, Gawlinski A, editors: *Protocols for practice: Hemodynamic monitoring.* Aliso Viejo, CA: American Association of Critical-Care Nurses, 2001, pp 1-47.
9. Imperial-Perez F, McRaw M: Arterial pressure monitoring. In Chulay M, Gawlinski A, editors: *Protocols for practice: Hemodynamic monitoring.* Aliso Viejo, CA: American Association of Critical-Care Nurses, 2001, pp 1-35.
10. Jesurum JT: SVO_2 monitoring. In Chulay M, Gawlinski A, editors: *Protocols for practice: Hemodynamic monitoring.* Aliso Viejo, CA: American Association of Critical-Care Nurses, 2001, pp 1-48.
11. Keckeisen M: Pulmonary artery pressure monitoring. In Chulay M, Gawlinski A, editors: *Protocols for practice: Hemodynamic monitoring.* Aliso Viejo, CA: American Association of Critical-Care Nurses, 1998, pp 1-49.
12. Lichtenthal PR: *Quick guide to cardiopulmonary care.* Irvine, CA: Edwards Lifesciences, 1998.
13. McFetridge J, Sherwood A: Impedance cardiography for noninvasive measurement of cardiovascular hemodynamics. *Nurs Res* 48(2):109-113, 1999.
14. McMillen P: Calculating medication dosages. *Crit Care Nurse* 20(6):17-19, 2000.
15. Rice WP, Fernandez EG, Jarog D, et al: A comparison of hydrostatic leveling methods in invasive pressure monitoring. *Crit Care Nurse* 20(6):20-30, 2000.
16. Von Rueden KR, Turner JA: Advances in continuous, noninvasive hemodynamic surveillance. *Crit Care Nurs Clin North America* 11(1):63-75, 1999.

31 Respiratory Care

■ ■ ■   REX A. MARLEY and CAROLE A. RIES

OBJECTIVES

At the conclusion of this chapter the reader will be able to:

1. Describe risk factors for the development of postoperative hypoxemia.
2. Be knowledgeable regarding the performance features of the common oxygen therapy devices.
3. Describe the standard steps for proper aerosol administration for both small volume jet nebulizers and metered dose inhalers in the nonintubated patient.
4. List the indications and applications of various airway management devices.
5. Discuss the advantages and disadvantages of intermittent mandatory, assist and control, pressure support, and pressure control ventilation.
6. Identify extubation criteria for the postanesthesia care unit (PACU) patient.
7. Discuss the application of pulse oximetry and capnography.
8. Become knowledgeable about commonly encountered adverse respiratory events.

POSTOPERATIVE OXYGEN THERAPY

I. Indications for postoperative oxygen therapy
   A. To prevent and treat hypoxemia
   B. To decrease work of breathing
   C. To increase myocardial oxygen supply
   D. To decrease pulmonary hypertension
II. Risk factors for postoperative hypoxemia
   A. Patient age: <1 year and >60 years.
   B. Hypobaric conditions: High altitudes.
   C. Obesity: Especially males >120 kg and females >100 kg; high risk for obstructive sleep apnea (incidence: middle-aged men [4%] and women [2%])
   D. Cardiopulmonary disease: Preexisting chronic obstructive pulmonary disease (COPD) including asthma
   E. Smoking: Once smoking exceeds 8 to 10 pack years
   F. Duration of anesthesia: Surgeries lasting >1 hour
   G. Type of anesthesia: General anesthesia higher risk than regional techniques
   H. Order of risk by operative site from highest to lowest: (1) thoracic, (2) upper abdomen, (3) lower abdomen, (4) neck, extremities, head
   I. Abdominal distension: Contributes to atelectasis
   J. Pain: Splinting secondary to uncontrolled pain
III. Monitoring oxygenation
   A. Clinical signs of acute hypoxemia
      1. Anxiety; restlessness; inattentiveness
      2. Mental confusion
      3. Altered mental status
      4. Dyspnea
      5. Dimmed peripheral vision
      6. Diaphoresis
      7. Seizures; unconsciousness
      8. Cyanosis
      9. Increased cardiac output
      10. Increased stroke volume

11. Hypertension—early sign
12. Hypotension—late sign
13. Tachypnea (secondary to carotid body chemoreceptor stimulation and lactic acidosis)
14. Dysrhythmias
15. Tachycardia—early sign (secondary to sympathetic stimulation)
16. Bradycardia—late sign.

B. Pulse oximetry
   1. General principle of operation
      a. The sensor, usually placed on the patient's distal finger, consists of light-emitting diodes (LEDs) and a photodetector
      b. The LEDs emit two specific wavelengths of light, which are absorbed selectively by oxyhemoglobin and reduced hemoglobin (dyshemoglobins, e.g., carboxyhemoglobin and methemoglobin, are not measured).
      c. Ratio of oxyhemoglobin to total hemoglobin is then expressed in a percent (SpO_2).
      d. The partial pressure of dissolved oxygen in arterial blood (PaO_2) can be estimated from the SpO_2 by referring to the oxyhemoglobin dissociation curve (see Figure 31-1).
   2. Indications
      a. For the continual, noninvasive, and instantaneous SpO_2 determination
      b. Routine postoperative evaluation of oxygenation
      c. Evaluate efficacy of changes in supplemental oxygen therapy
   3. Factors influencing the accuracy of pulse oximetry

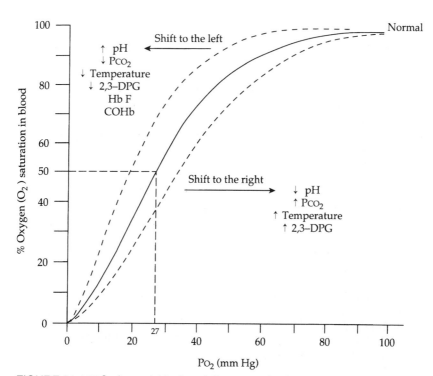

FIGURE 31-1 ■ Oxyhemoglobin dissociation curve, showing relationship between PaO_2 and SpO_2 and how that relationship can change (resulting in a rightward or leftward shift).

          a. Fingernail polish (e.g., blue, green, and black, interfere more than purple and red nail polish to produce falsely low readings).
            (1) Clear acrylic nails do not affect SpO_2.
          b. Venous pulsation (e.g., secondary to tricuspid valve regurgitation or venous engorgement) may yield falsely low readings.
          c. With deeply pigmented skin, falsely high readings may be recorded or unobtainable.
            (1) The finger probe will be more accurate than the ear probe.
          d. Exogenous and endogenous dyes (methylene blue greater effect than indocyanine green, which is greater than indigo carmine) will produce falsely low readings.
          e. Anemia (hematocrit <10%) yields falsely low readings at low oxyhemoglobin values.
          f. Reduced pulsatile component (i.e., secondary to hypotension, vasoconstriction, or hypothermia) yields inaccurate, unobtainable, or falsely low readings.
            (1) The ear probe is more accurate than finger probe in this instance.
          g. Hypoxemia (oxyhemoglobin saturations <75%) can give inaccurately low or high readings.
          h. Carboxyhemoglobinemia yields falsely high readings.
          i. Motion artifact yields falsely low readings.
          j. Methemoglobinemia yields falsely high readings at high oxyhemoglobin saturations and variable readings at low oxyhemoglobin saturations.
          k. Ambient light may yield falsely low readings.
          l. Incorrectly fitting probes yield falsely low readings.
     C. Arterial blood gas analysis—refer to Chapter 25.
  IV. Supplemental oxygen therapy
    A. Humidity and aerosol-generating devices
      1. Indications
        a. Delivery of gas to the intubated patient since the normal mechanism of humidifying inspired gas is bypassed
        b. Medication delivery
        c. Maintain mucous blanket stability
        d. Warm, humidified inspired gas
          (1) Accelerates recovery from hypothermia
          (2) Is therapeutic for upper airway inflammation
          (3) Blunts reactive airway response to cold inspired gas
          (4) Liquefies and mobilizes tenacious pulmonary secretions
      2. Types of humidifiers
        a. Bubble diffuser—provides approximately 20% relative humidity at body temperature
        b. Cascade—used with mechanical ventilators or continuous positive airway pressure (CPAP) masks; can provide up to 100% humidity
        c. Room humidifier (cool mist)—adds humidity to room air; can provide 100% humidity in a confined space
        d. Heat and moisture exchanger—a passive humidifier for short-term use in the intubated patient
          (1) When placed close to the artificial airway, exhaled heat and moisture are collected on this humidifier and returned to the patient during the following inspiration.
          (2) This device does not provide sufficient heat and humidity for long-term therapy.
      3. Types of aerosol generators
        a. Jet—a small volume nebulizer commonly used for the delivery of aerosolized medications
        b. Babington—a popular large volume nebulizer (e.g., Solosphere or Hydrosphere) capable of delivering a high-density mist with oxygen concentrations ranging from 21% to 100%.

   B. Oxygen therapy devices
   1. The appropriate device for individual patient use will be dependant upon the supplemental oxygen requirements of the patient and how well he or she tolerates a particular device.
   2. For higher inspired oxygen therapy requirements, combination therapy (e.g., nasal cannula in conjunction with a nonrebreathing mask or a double oxygen flowmeter setup) may be required. (Table 31-1)
V. Guidelines for postoperative oxygen therapy
   A. Supplemental oxygen therapy will be provided to treat and prevent hypoxemia as needed.
   B. Monitor patients continually with pulse oximetry while in PACU.
   C. If continual SpO_2 monitoring is unavailable, provide supplemental oxygen and spot check as needed plus upon arrival to and departure from PACU.
   D. Pulse oximetry and supplemental oxygen therapy should be available for patient transport from the operating room (OR) to the PACU as required.

■ **TABLE 31-1**
■ ■ **Common Oxygen Therapy Devices**

Device	FIO_2	O_2 Flow Rate	Comment
Nasal cannula	0.24-0.44	1-6 L/min	More comfortable, better tolerated; reservoir: nasopharynx; avoid O_2 flow rate >6 L/min since nasal irritation is likely and inspired oxygen increase is negligible
Simple O_2 mask	0.40-0.60	5-10 L/min	Oxygen flow rate should be at least 5 L/min to prevent a buildup of carbon dioxide within the mask.
Partial rebreathing mask	0.60-0.80	10-15 L/min	Adjust oxygen flow rate to keep reservoir bag partially inflated at peak inspiration to avoid room air entrainment.
Nonrebreathing mask	>0.80	>15 L/min	Leaflet valves closing both exhalation ports are not recommended because of the risks of suffocation.
Air entrainment mask	0.24, 0.28, 0.35, 0.40, 0.50	4 L/min for 0.24; 6 L/min for 0.28; 8 L/min for 0.35; 12 L/min for 0.40; 12 L/min for 0.50	Total gas flow (oxygen and air) should be sufficient to meet the patient's peak inspiratory flow requirements. The higher the FIO_2, the less room air is entrained, thus the need for higher oxygen flow rates.
Aerosol mask	0.28-0.98*	>8 L/min	When the FIO_2 exceeds 0.5, the total gas flow to the patient may be insufficient to prevent room air dilution.
Face tent	Variable; ↑→ 70% with close fit and sufficient O_2 flow*	>8 L/min	When the FIO_2 exceeds 0.5, the total gas flow to the patient may be insufficient to prevent room air dilution; good for patients with facial deformities and burns; used when the FIO_2 is not crucial.
Tracheostomy collar	0.28-0.98*	>8 L/min	When the FIO_2 exceeds 0.5, the total gas flow to the patient may be insufficient to prevent room air dilution.
T-piece with reservoir	0.28-0.98*	Sufficient to have continuous mist exiting from the reservoir tube	When the FIO_2 exceeds 0.5, the total gas flow to the patient may be insufficient to prevent room air dilution.

*Can deliver FIO_2 of 0.21 if used with compressed air instead of oxygen.

E. Patients at high risk for hypoxemia may require supplemental oxygen therapy for an extended time following surgery.

AIRWAY MANAGEMENT

I. Oropharyngeal airways

   A. Indications

      1. To treat supraglottic soft-tissue airway obstruction (e.g., relaxation of the soft palate, pharyngeal walls, or tongue in patients without a patent gag reflex)

      2. To prevent the patient from biting down and obstructing an endotracheal tube or laryngeal mask airway (LMA)

   B. Contraindications

      1. In the semiconscious patient, coughing, gagging, vomiting, or laryngospasm may be triggered from the oropharyngeal airway.

      2. Caution should be exercised in patients with extremely poor dentition or friable oropharyngeal tissue.

   C. Technique of insertion

      1. Sizing: An external landmark for estimating the proper length includes placing the airway along the cheek and measuring the distance from the corner of the mouth to the tragus of the ear.

      2. Insert right side up (consider employing a tongue blade to assist with displacing the tongue) or upside down and then rotate 180° into the proper position.

      3. Avoid trauma to the teeth, and confirm the tongue or lips are not sandwiched between the airway and teeth.

      4. Ensure that the tongue is not displaced back into the pharynx to contribute to further obstruction.

II. Nasopharyngeal airways

   A. Indications

      1. A temporary method to treat supraglottic soft-tissue airway obstruction (e.g., relaxation of the soft palate, pharyngeal walls, or tongue)

      2. Appropriate in the patient with upper airway obstruction who exhibits a clenched jaw, mouth trauma, tongue abnormality, or tooth pathology

      3. A nasopharyngeal airway is less stimulating and better tolerated in the semiconscious patient than the oropharyngeal airway

      4. In patients with persistent upper airway obstruction, consider employing both oropharyngeal and nasopharyngeal airways together.

   B. Contraindications

      1. Avoid the nasopharyngeal airway following tonsillectomy, adenoidectomy, or cleft palate repair.

      2. Insertion of the airway into the cranial vault may occur after basilar skull fracture.

      3. Use with caution in patients with coagulopathy or nasal deformities because nasal hemorrhage may result.

   C. Technique of insertion

      1. Use the larger nares for airway insertion.

      2. Sizing: The distal tip of the nasopharyngeal airway should rest just above the open epiglottis.

         a. An external landmark for estimating the proper length includes having the proximal end positioned at the nares and the distal tip placed at the tragus of the ear.

      3. Consider spraying a nasal vasoconstrictive agent (e.g., oxymetazoline) if appropriate.

         a. Laryngospasm may be a possibility should the liquid stimulate the vocal cords in the semiconscious patient.

      4. Lubricate the airway with a water-soluble lubricant (e.g., lidocaine gel) if the patient is awake.

     5. When inserting, point the bevel medially to prevent trauma to the turbinates.

     6. Advance the airway posteriorly (not upward toward the cribriform plate), parallel to the hard palate and beneath the inferior turbinate.

     7. If significant resistance is encountered, withdraw, rotate 90°, and readvance with gentle, steady pressure.

     8. Ease difficult passage by using a soft-suction catheter as an introducer.

     9. A flared proximal end or adjustable disk may be employed to limit insertion depth.

III. Laryngeal mask airway (LMA)

  A. Indications

     1. As a substitute for the facemask or endotracheal tube (when not indicated) during elective anesthesia in the spontaneously breathing patient

     2. To improve a difficult airway seal without endotracheal intubation as with the bearded or edentulous patient

     3. As an aide to endotracheal intubation (i.e., with the intubating LMA [LMA-Fastrach™]).

     4. Emergency ventilation when endotracheal intubation has failed

  B. Contraindications

     1. Patients with pharyngeal pathology interfering with its placement

     2. Patients with glottic or subglottic airway obstruction

     3. Extremely limited mouth opening (<1.5 mm) or neck extension

     4. When access to the airway is compromised (e.g., prone surgery)

     5. With low pulmonary compliance or high airway resistance (>20 cm H_2O)

     6. Presence of increased risk of regurgitation (e.g., morbid obesity, pregnancy, insufficient fasting interval, hiatal hernia, and intestinal obstruction)

  C. Technique of insertion

     1. Determine appropriate size.

       a. Use the largest size that will comfortably fit in the oral cavity.

       b. A bite block should be used while the LMA is in place.

     2. LMA insertion (Figure 31-2)

  D. Removal of the LMA

     1. The LMA should be removed in the supine or lateral position, with the patient deeply anesthetized or awake, but not at a halfway stage.

     2. The patient should be left undisturbed, with the exception of monitoring and providing supplemental oxygen, until reflexes are restored.

     3. Do not move the patient from the supine to lateral position unless an urgent reason exists (e.g., vomiting).

     4. Avoid suctioning with the LMA in place as this may provoke laryngospasm if the patient is light.

     5. If the LMA is to be removed with the patient awake, swallowing is usually a sign that it is safe to remove the device; deflate the cuff and simultaneously remove the LMA.

IV. Cuffed oropharyngeal airway (COPA): resembles a Guedel airway with an inflatable cuff along the distal half of its length and a 15-mm circuit adapter at the proximal end. The inflated cuff fills the pharynx and displaces the epiglottis and base of the tongue anteriorly.

  A. Indications

     1. As a substitute for the facemask or endotracheal tube (when not indicated) during elective anesthesia in the spontaneously breathing patient

     2. It has been used in the difficult-to-intubate patient.

  B. Contraindications: Similar to the LMA

  C. Technique of insertion: Similar to inserting an oropharyngeal airway

V. Support of the nonintubated airway: Airway maneuvers may be required to open an obstructed upper airway in the spontaneously breathing patient or to assist with ventilation in the patient not maintaining adequate minute ventilation. The oropharyngeal and nasopharyngeal airways may be indicated to assist with relieving upper airway obstruction.

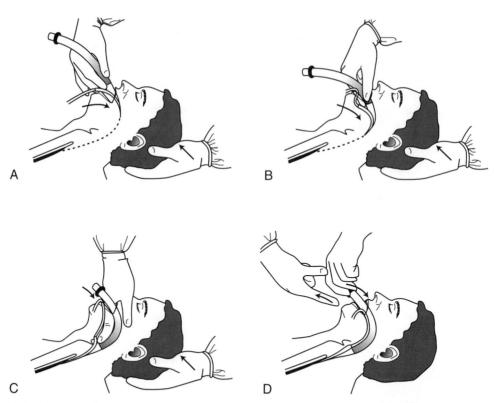

FIGURE 31-2 ■ Insertion technique for the LMA: *A,* With the head extended and the neck flexed, carefully flatten the LMA tip against the hard palate. To facilitate LMA introduction into the oral cavity, gently press the middle finger down on the jaw. *B,* The index finger pushes the LMA in a cranial direction following the contours of the hard and soft palates. *C,* Maintaining pressure with the finger on the tube in the cranial direction, advance the mask until definite resistance is felt at the base of the hypopharynx, not the flexion of the wrist. *D,* Gently maintain cranial pressure with the nondominant hand while removing the index finger. (From the LMA North America Inc., San Diego, CA.)

    A. Manual maneuver to open the airway: The goal is to lift the tongue away from the back wall of the pharynx thus opening an obstructed airway.
        1. Head tilt–chin lift
            a. Tilt the head back on the atlantooccipital joint while keeping the teeth approximated by placing the edge of one hand on the patient's forehead and two fingers of the other hand under the chin.
            b. The chin is lifted up while the head is tilted backward.
            c. Consider placing the adult patient in the "sniffing" position by elevating the head 1 to 4 inches above the level of the shoulders.
            d. Avoid the head tilt in patients suspected of having a neck injury.
        2. Jaw thrust
            a. Designed to open the airway while maintaining a neutral position in patients with suspected neck injury
            b. The teeth will have to be slightly opened to allow the mandibular teeth freedom to slide over the maxillary teeth as the mandible subluxes forward.
            c. The mandible is grasped bilaterally with the fingertips and lifted forward.
    B. Two-handed mask ventilation: Assisted ventilation will be required in the patient unable to maintain sufficient gas exchange.
        1. Select the appropriate size mask covering from above the nose to below the lower lip that allows a good seal between the mask and the patient's face; apply pressure to the mask sides with the thumb sides of the palms of both hands.

2. Employ the head tilt–chin lift or jaw thrust to open the airway; insert an oropharyngeal or nasopharyngeal airway as indicated; keep the mouth open if an airway is not utilized.
3. Interface the mask with a self-inflating bag connected with an oxygen source; a second rescuer should initiate manual ventilation with a tidal volume approximating 10 to 15 ml/kg over 1 to 2 seconds.
4. Cricoid pressure should be applied in the patient at risk for pulmonary aspiration of gastric contents.

VI. Tracheal intubation
 A. Indications
   1. Ensure an unobstructed airway
   2. Protect patient's airway from pulmonary aspiration of gastric contents
   3. To facilitate mechanical ventilation
   4. To enable suctioning of pulmonary secretions
   5. Provide conduit for medication delivery
   6. If it is feared that ventilation and intubation may later become impossible (i.e., acute epiglottitis)
   7. Airway adjunct for general anesthesia (e.g., thoracoabdominal surgery, remote access to the head, airway surgery in which secretions or blood might contaminate the trachea)
 B. Complications
   1. Suture lines may be disrupted if the patient coughs or strains on the tube.
   2. Postextubation laryngeal edema
   3. Negative pressure pulmonary edema
   4. Tachycardia, hypertension
   5. Bronchospasm in susceptible patients
   6. Hoarseness, pharyngitis
 C. Technique of insertion
   1. Equipment for laryngoscopy
     a. Oxygen source and self-inflating bag
     b. Face mask in various sizes
     c. Oropharyngeal and nasopharyngeal airways in various sizes along with tongue blades and lubricant
     d. Endotracheal tubes in various sizes
     e. Endotracheal tube stylet
     f. Intubating (Magill) forceps
     g. For endotracheal tube cuff inflation, 10 ml syringe
     h. Suction apparatus with tonsil tip suction catheter
     i. Two laryngoscope handles with fresh batteries
     j. Laryngoscope blades in various sizes: Common blades include the curved (Macintosh) and straight (Miller)
     k. Pillow, towel, blanket, or foam for head positioning
     l. Monitoring equipment: Electrocardiogram, pulse oximeter, blood pressure, and stethoscope

VII. The difficult airway
 A. Difficulty in endotracheal intubation is encountered in 1% to 3% of attempts depending on the intubator's experience.
 B. Failed intubation is encountered approximately 0.05% to 0.2% of time.
 C. The "can't intubate and can't ventilate" rate is 0.01%.
 D. The American Society of Anesthesiologists (ASA) has developed an algorithm for managing the difficult airway (Figure 31-3).

POSTOPERATIVE MECHANICAL VENTILATION

 I. Objectives of mechanical ventilation
 A. Physiological objectives

1. To support or manipulate pulmonary gas exchange (i.e., to maintain normal or deliberate hyperventilation or to maintain oxygen delivery at or near normal)
2. To increase lung volume: To prevent or treat atelectasis with adequate end-inspiratory lung inflation; to achieve and maintain an adequate functional residual capacity (FRC)
3. To reduce the work of breathing

B. Clinical objectives
1. Reverse acute respiratory failure
2. Reverse respiratory distress
3. Reverse hypoxemia
4. Prevent or reverse atelectasis
5. Reverse ventilatory muscle fatigue
6. Permit sedation and/or paralysis
7. Reduce systemic or myocardial oxygen consumption
8. Reduce intracranial pressure
9. Stabilize the chest wall

II. Ventilation modes
A. Assist-control: Patient initiates ventilation and is also guaranteed a backup rate; each breath, whether initiated by machine or patient, will have a predetermined volume; patient's inspiratory flow triggers a breath.
B. Intermittent mandatory ventilation (IMV, synchronized IMV [SIMV]): Ventilator delivers breaths at predetermined rate and volume; patient can breathe between machine breaths at his or her own rate and volume.
C. Pressure support ventilation: Patient initiates ventilation; each breath will have a predetermined amount of positive pressure added for support; can be used alone or with IMV; when used with IMV, machine breaths have a predetermined rate and volume, and spontaneous breaths have a predetermined pressure.
D. Pressure-controlled ventilation: Can be used either as can assist-control or IMV except breaths have a predetermined pressure (instead of a predetermined volume). This is used mainly for infants and adult respiratory distress syndrome (ARDS).

Difficult Airway Algorithm

1. Assess the likelihood and clinical impact of basic management problems:
A. Difficult ventilation
B. Difficult intubation
C. Difficulty with patient cooperation or consent
D. Difficult tracheostomy

2. Actively pursue opportunities to deliver supplemental oxygen thoughout the process of difficult airway management.

3. Consider the relative merits and feasibility of basic management choices:

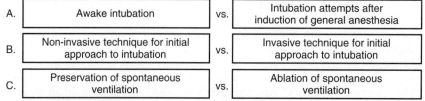

FIGURE 31-3 ■ American Society of Anesthesiologist's Difficult Airway Algorithm. (From American Society of Anesthesiologists Task Force on Difficult Airway Management: *Practice guidelines for management of the difficult airway.* American Society of Anesthesiologists, 520 N. Northwest Highway, Park Ridge, IL, 60068-2573.)

4. Develop primary and alternative strategies:

A.

Awake intubation

- Airway approached by non-invasive intubation
- Airway secured by surgical access*

Airway approached by non-invasive intubation →
- Succeed*
- FAIL

- Cancel case
- Consider feasibility of other options (a)
- Invasive airway access (b)*

B.

Intubation attempts after induction of general anesthesia

- Initial intubation attempts successful*
- Initial intubation attempts unsuccessful

From this point onwards consider:
1. Calling for help
2. Returning to spontaneous ventilation
3. Awakening the patient

- Face mask ventilation adequate
- Face mask ventilation not adequate

LMA adequate* ← Consider/attempt LMA → LMA not adequate or not feasible

- Non-Emergency Pathway
  Ventilation adequate, intubation unsuccessful
- Emergency Pathway
  Ventilation inadequate, intubation unsuccessful

- Alternative approaches to intubation (c)
- IF BOTH FACE MASK AND LMA VENTILATION BECOME INADEQUATE
- Call for help

- Successful intubation*
- FAIL after multiple attempts
- Successful ventilation*
- Emergency non-invasive airway ventilation (e)

FAIL

- Invasive airway access (b)*
- Consider feasibility of other options (a)
- Awaken patient (d)
- Emergency invasive airway access (b)*

---

*Confirm intubation with exhaled CO_2.

(a) Other options include (but are not limited to): surgery utilizing face mask or LMA anesthesia, local anesthesia infiltration or regional nerve blockade. Pursuit of these options usually implies that mask ventilation will not be problematic. Therefore, these options may be of limited value if this step in the algorithm has been reached via the Emergency Pathway.

(b) Invasive airway access includes surgical or percutaneous tracheostomy or cricothyrotomy.

(c) Alternative non-invasive approaches to difficult intubation include (but are not limited to): use of different laryngoscope blades, LMA as an intubation conduit (with or without fiberoptic guidance), fiberoptic intubation, intubating stylet or tube changer, light wand, retrograde intubation, and blind oral or nasal intubation.

(d) Consider re-preparation of the patient for awake intubation or canceling surgery.

(e) Options for emergency non-invasive airway ventilation include (but are not limited to): rigid bronchoscope, esophageal-tracheal combitube ventilation, or transtracheal jet ventilation.

FIGURE 31-3 *Cont'd*

III. Expiratory phase
   A. Positive end-expiratory pressure (PEEP): A small amount of positive pressure (typically 1 to 20 cm H_2O) is kept in the airways upon exhalation.
      1. Helps maintain alveoli diameter (increases FRC) for improved oxygenation.
      2. When used with spontaneous breathing (no set rate, volume, or pressure), this is called continuous positive airway pressure (CPAP).
      3. Goal: To enhance tissue oxygenation and maintain a Pao_2 >60 mm Hg, using an Fio_2 <0.4 while maintaining adequate cardiovascular function
      4. Complications
         a. Decreased venous return and cardiac output (i.e., with hypovolemia)
         b. Hypotension
         c. Untreated significant pneumothorax or tension pneumothorax
         d. Increased intracranial pressure
         e. Decreased urine output
         f. Barotrauma (in patients with [ARDS]).
IV. Monitoring of ventilation
   A. Capnography
      1. Represents the measurement of carbon dioxide partial pressure in exhaled gas ($PETco_2$)
      2. A graphic waveform is incorporated to display the pattern of gas exhalation.
      3. The most common methods of gas measurement are with infrared spectroscopy and mass spectroscopy.
      4. Under stable conditions, the $PETco_2$ approximates the $Paco_2$ with the values differing <10 mm Hg.
      5. Conditions of pulmonary hypoperfusion (e.g., pulmonary embolism, hypotension, hemorrhage, and cardiac arrest) will increase the gradient between arterial and end-tidal carbon dioxide values.
      6. Indications
         a. Monitoring adequacy of mechanical ventilation
         b. Assess intubation of the trachea versus the esophagus
         c. Monitoring the integrity of the mechanical ventilatory circuit and artificial airway
         d. Monitoring the adequacy of pulmonary and coronary blood flow (e.g., with cardiopulmonary resuscitation)
         e. Monitoring carbon dioxide production
      7. Nonintubated patient
         a. $PETco_2$ monitoring via devices (e.g., nasal prongs or masks) have been described in the nonintubated patient.
         b. Knowledge of the limitation of these devices is required; at the least, they may serve as an apnea monitor.
V. Criteria for routine "awake" extubation
   A. No indication to keep patient intubated
   B. Subjective clinical criteria
      1. Patient follows commands.
      2. Clear oropharynx and hypopharynx (e.g., no active bleeding, secretions cleared)
      3. Airway reflexes are recovered.
      4. Muscle relaxant is fully reversed (i.e., patient able to sustain a head lift for >5 seconds).
      5. Adequate pain control
      6. Minimal residual inhaled anesthetic agent
   C. Objective criteria
      1. Patient is hemodynamically stable.
      2. Tidal volume: >6 ml/kg
      3. Vital capacity: ≥10-15 ml/kg

      4. Maximum inspiratory pressure: ≤−20 cm H_2O
      5. Sustained tetanic contraction >5 seconds with peripheral nerve stimulator
      6. Respiratory rate <25 breaths per minute in the adult
VI. Routine tracheal extubation
    A. Patient meets weaning criteria (i.e., appropriate return of consciousness, spontaneous respiration, the resolution of neuromuscular block, and the ability to follow simple commands).
    B. Personnel and equipment available should reintubation become necessary
    C. Pharynx is suctioned to remove secretions.
    D. Increase inspired oxygen concentration to 100% for several minutes.
    E. Remove tape securing the endotracheal tube.
    F. Deflate the endotracheal tube cuff.
    G. Apply positive airway pressure or have the cooperative patient take a deep breath, then remove the tube.
    H. Suction the oropharynx again if secretions are present and the patient is unable to adequately expectorate.

ADMINISTRATION OF AEROSOLIZED MEDICATIONS

  I. Clinical indications for pharmacologically active aerosol therapy
    A. To relieve upper airway inflammation (i.e., glottic or subglottic edema or laryngotracheobronchitis)
    B. To provide topical anesthesia to the upper and/or central airway (i.e., for awake endotracheal intubation)
    C. To relieve vascular congestion (i.e., prior to nasopharyngeal instrumentation)
    D. To promote bronchodilation (i.e., treatment for reactive airway disease)
  II. Advantages of aerosol drug delivery
    A. Specific to desired site of action
    B. Smaller dosage necessary
    C. More effective drug response
    D. Rapid therapeutic onset of action
    E. Minimize systemic side effects
    F. Painless self-administration is possible by the patient.
  III. Disadvantages of aerosol drug delivery
    A. Failure to master the technique of aerosol drug delivery; insufficient knowledge of administration protocol
    B. Shorter duration of action in acute asthma
    C. Difficulty in dosage appraisal and reproducibility
  IV. Technique of aerosol delivery
    A. Assemble the necessary equipment.
    B. Explain the procedure and rationale to the patient.
    C. Position the patient in semi-Fowler's or sitting position as tolerated.
    D. Perform baseline monitoring (i.e., heart rate, breath sounds, blood pressure, oxyhemoglobin saturation, and respiratory rate).
    E. Considerations for the small-volume jet nebulizer
      1. Add appropriate medication to the reservoir.
        a. Standard amounts of normal saline to mix with the medication include 2 ml to 2.5 ml for children and 3 ml to 3.5 ml for adults if commercially prepared mixtures are unavailable.
      2. Driving gas (typically oxygen) flow rates should range between 6 L/minute and 8 L/minute.
        a. This promotes ideal aerosol particle size while keeping the treatment time to <10 minutes.
      3. Aerosolize medication only during inspiration, when permitted, to deliver more medication to the patient and less to the atmosphere.

    4. Periodically tap the sides of the nebulizer to return droplets back into the liquid reservoir.
        a. Once sputtering occurs, either the treatment is completed or additional medicated solution should be added to the nebulizers liquid reservoir.

  F. Considerations for the metered dose inhaler (MDI)
    1. Warming the MDI canister to body temperature will yield a particle size closer to ideal.
    2. Remove the protective cap and make sure no foreign objects are present in the mouthpiece.
    3. Vigorously shake the canister to mix the canister contents, then prime the canister by discharging it (three or four puffs should be wasted) if the unit has not been used during the previous 24 hours.
    4. Encourage the patient to exhale maximally.
    5. Instruct the patient to maintain his or her neck in a neutral position.
    6. MDI without a spacer: Position the MDI 2 cm to 4 cm from the patient's lips and aim the actuator mouthpiece at an open mouth and initiate inspiration after canister actuation.
    7. MDI with a spacer
        a. Position the patient's lips around the spacer's mouthpiece.
        b. Begin inspiration after canister actuation.
        c. Timing is not as critical when a spacer is used.
    8. Inspiration should continue slowly (may take 3 to 5 seconds) until maximal effort is achieved.
        a. Encourage the patient to then hold his or her breath for 10 seconds.
    9. Exhalation should then continue normally, and then wait 1 minute or longer before repeating the next prescribed puff.
    10. Replace the protective cap on the actuator mouthpiece after treatment completion to prevent foreign object contamination.

SELECT POSTOPERATIVE RESPIRATORY CARE ISSUES

  I. Bronchospasm
    A. Risk factors
      1. Endobronchial intubation
      2. Pulmonary edema
      3. Pulmonary embolus
      4. Pulmonary aspiration of gastric contents
      5. Pneumothorax
      6. Histamine release associated with medications
      7. Allergic or anaphylactic reactions to medications, latex, contrast media, or blood products
      8. Tobacco use
      9. History of bronchospasm
      10. Recent upper respiratory tract infection
    B. Signs and symptoms
      1. Prolonged expiratory time
      2. Wheezing
      3. Spontaneously breathing patients: Accessory muscle recruitment, labored ventilation, increased work of breathing
      4. Mechanically ventilated patients: high peak inspiratory pressure
    C. Management
      1. Determine the cause and treat (e.g., with endobronchial intubation, reposition the tube to terminate in the trachea).
      2. Remove source of laryngeal irritation if indicated.
      3. Implemented beta-2 agonist therapy.
      4. If ventilation is still compromised and labored after albuterol therapy, consider aminophylline loading dose and maintenance infusion.

     5. Bronchospasm resistant to beta-2 agonist therapy may improve with an anticholinergic medication (e.g., ipratropium bromide).

II. Laryngospasm

  A. Definition

    1. An exaggerated, prolonged protective closure reflex of the vocal folds

    2. Hypoxia and hypercarbia will result if the condition goes untreated.

    3. May occur secondary to stimulation from foreign body (e.g., oropharyngeal or nasopharyngeal airway) or secretions (e.g., saliva, blood, vomitus) on or around the vocal cords

    4. May also be secondary to airway irritation; accounts for 23% of all critical postoperative respiratory events in adults

  B. Risk factors: Foreign body or secretion stimulation of the vocal folds in association with a light plane (i.e., associated with emergence) of anesthesia

  C. Signs and symptoms

    1. Partial laryngospasm: High-pitched inspiratory stridor, thoracoabdominal dyscoordination, tracheal tug, and apprehension

    2. Complete laryngospasm: As described for partial laryngospasm except absence of stridor or air exchange

  D. Management

    1. Immediately remove source of irritation (i.e., gentle pharyngeal suctioning); consider lateral decubitus position to promote drainage.

    2. Gentle, positive pressure ventilation with bag-valve-mask with 100% supplemental oxygen; consider esophageal opening pressure of 18 to 20 cm H_2O and the likelihood of gastric insufflation.

    3. Anterior displacement of mandible.

    4. If these measures unsuccessful, succinylcholine 0.1 to 0.2 mg/kg (10 to 20 mg, adult) intravenously. Be prepared to assist ventilation with bag-valve-mask with 100% supplemental oxygen for 5 to 10 minutes.

    5. Lidocaine 1.5 mg/kg may be effective in preventing or minimizing partial laryngospasm.

    6. Consider endotracheal intubation.

      a. If unable to maintain adequate respiration with bag-valve-mask

      b. If ventilation required in patients at high risk of pulmonary aspiration of gastric contents, or

      c. With persistent, symptomatic partial laryngospasm

III. Negative pressure pulmonary edema

  A. Risk factors

    1. Upper airway obstruction (e.g., laryngospasm, upper airway mass, strangulation) when the patient attempts vigorous inspiratory efforts

    2. Sustained ventilatory efforts by the patient may generate high negative intrapleural pressures.

    3. Creates acute and marked increases in left ventricular preload and afterload

  B. Signs and symptoms

    1. Appearance of pink, frothy fluid, decreasing oxyhemoglobin saturation, wheezing, dyspnea, and increased respiratory rate.

    2. Chest radiograph: Diffuse, usually bilateral interstitial pulmonary infiltrates

  C. Management

    1. Supportive measures

      a. Relief of the obstruction and maintenance of a patent airway

      b. Supplemental oxygen

      c. Diuretics may be indicated in select cases.

      d. Recovery usually occurs rapidly within hours following surgery without intensive therapy.

    2. Mechanical ventilation with PEEP, or CPAP may be required in severe cases.

IV. Oxygen-induced hypoventilation: Select patients (i.e., severe COPD with attenuated response to the carbon dioxide drive to breathe; may hypoventilate and exhibit further respiratory acidosis when their PaO_2 is raised above 55 to 60 mm Hg)

  A. Risk factors: Include patients with

    1. A history of oxygen-induced hypoventilation

    2. COPD and chronic hypoventilation with presenting signs and symptoms of acute respiratory decompensation and deteriorating hypoxemia

    3. The "blue bloater" appearance, with peripheral edema from decompensated right-sided heart failure (cor pulmonale) along with hypercapnia and hypoxemia, but minimal or no dyspnea

    4. Sleep apnea syndrome, especially those with daytime hypoventilation and sleepiness (the "Pickwickian syndrome")

    5. Acute hypoxemia and hypersomnolence not secondary to sedative medications

  B. Signs and symptoms: If undetected initially, worsening hypercapnia and acidosis when exposed to preceding ambient levels of oxygen.

  C. Management

    1. Avoidance of this problem is ideal by

      a. Identifying high-risk patients in advance and

      b. Offering judicious use of supplemental oxygen therapy to maintain a target PaO_2 of 50 to 60 mm Hg with either nasal cannula or air entrainment mask

    2. Nasal cannula

      a. Initiate supplemental oxygen therapy at 1 L/minute oxygen flow rate.

      b. Increase the oxygen flow rate by 0.5 L/minute increments until the PaO_2 reaches at least 50 mm Hg.

    3. Air entrainment mask

      a. Set oxygen percentage at 24% or 28% initially at the manufacturer's recommended oxygen flow rate.

      b. Adjust the inspired oxygen concentration until the PaO_2 reaches at least 50 mm Hg.

    4. Progressive hypercapnia and respiratory acidosis are rare with overzealous supplemental oxygen therapy.

      a. Patient assessment should include arterial blood gas analysis to monitor these conditions.

V. Postextubation laryngeal edema: Secondary to irritation of the perilaryngeal tissues leading to edema formation

  A. Risk factors

    1. Patient age—especially <4 years.

    2. History of infectious or postextubation croup

    3. Anaphylactic reaction

    4. Inflammatory airway changes (e.g., upper respiratory tract infection)

    5. Surgery of head, neck, and oral cavity

    6. Surgery >1 hour

    7. Traumatic intubation or emergence

    8. Too large of endotracheal tube

  B. Signs and symptoms (Table 31-2)

  C. Management

    1. Begins with prevention

      a. Avoid endotracheal intubation when possible.

      b. Ensure smooth intubation.

      c. Avoid endotracheal intubation in children with upper respiratory tract infection when possible.

      d. Ensure audible leak around cuffless endotracheal tube at 25 to 35 cm H_2O airway pressure.

      e. Avoid endotracheal tube movement.

      f. Prevent coughing or bucking on endotracheal tube.

■ TABLE 31-2
■ ■ **Signs and Symptoms of Postextubation Laryngeal Edema**

Symptoms	Early	Late
Airway sound	Inspiratory stridor	Biphasic stridor
Appearance	Anxious, alert	Lethargic, obtunded
Breath sounds	Decreased bilaterally	
Cough	Barking, brassy	
Dysphagia	Difficulty swallowing, sore throat	
Heart rate	Sinus tachycardia	Bradycardia
Oxyhemoglobin saturation	Decreases with exhaustion	
Phonation	Dysphonia	Aphonia
Respiratory rate	Tachypnea	Bradypnea
Retractions	Suprasternal	Suprasternal, intercostals, subcostal
Voice changes	Hoarseness	

From Marley, RA: Postextubation laryngeal edema. *J PeriAnesth Nurs* 13(1):44, 1998.

2. Calm, reassuring support to alleviate fear and anxiety
3. Allow the child to assume position of comfort (e.g., high-Fowler's or in caregiver's lap).
4. Supplemental oxygen as indicated to prevent hypoxemia according to patient acceptance
5. Cool humidity in conjunction with supplemental oxygen therapy or room humidifier to soothe the inflamed laryngeal mucosa and thus minimize coughing
6. Aerosolized racemic epinephrine (topical vasoconstrictor)
    a. For moderate symptoms, 0.5 ml of 2.25% solution in 3 ml of normal saline
    b. May repeat in 30 minutes (up to three times) and every 2 to 4 hours, as needed
7. Dexamethasone 0.5 mg/kg intravenously every 6 hours as needed for moderate symptoms
8. Helium 80% and oxygen 20% via nonrebreathing mask to reduce airway resistance for severe symptoms
9. If severe symptoms persist
    a. Positive pressure ventilation with bag-valve-mask and supplemental oxygen synchronized to the patient's inspiratory effort
    b. Consider reintubation with smaller sized endotracheal tube.

VI. Pulmonary aspiration of gastric contents: Incidence of recognized clinical aspiration (bilious secretions or particulate matter in the tracheobronchial tree or presence of new infiltrate on postoperative chest radiograph) approximates 1.5 to 5 per 10,000 general anesthetics. Aspiration of sufficiently low gastric fluid pH (<2.5) places patients at risk for aspiration pneumonitis.

A. Risk factors
    1. Age extremes (<1 yr or >70 yr)
    2. Co-morbid diseases (e.g., diabetic gastroparesis)
        a. Central nervous system deficits
        b. Collagen vascular disease (e.g., scleroderma)
        c. Hepatobiliary and gastrointestinal diseases
        d. Renal dysfunction
        e. Pregnancy
        f. Recent oral intake
        g. Opioid administration
        h. Pain; anxiety and depression
        i. Gastrointestinal obstruction or dysfunction

  j. Obesity
  k. Depressed level of consciousness
  l. Previous esophageal dysfunction
  m. Head injury or neurologic dysfunction
  n. Lack of coordination of swallowing and respiration
  o. Ascites
  p. Procedures that increase intraabdominal pressure
B. Signs and symptoms: Depends on the severity of pulmonary aspiration
  1. Wheezing
  2. Rhonchi
  3. Hypoxemia
  4. Bilious secretions or particulate matter upon tracheal aspiration
  5. Presence of new infiltrate on postoperative chest radiograph
C. Management
  1. When regurgitation occurs, gastric contents should be removed from the pharynx by rapidly lowering the head, turning it to the side, and suctioning the pharynx with a tonsil-tip suction catheter.
  2. Support ventilation and oxygenation as required
  3. Suction trachea and bronchi (but do not instill saline). If particulate matter found or suspected, bronchoscopy is indicated to remove any large aspirated pieces.
  4. Prophylactic antibiotics and steroids are not warranted. Steroids may increase the risk of pulmonary infection by suppressing the immune response.
  5. Culture tracheal secretions; antibiotics if positive.
  6. Continue supportive respiratory therapy.
VII. Residual neuromuscular blockade: Incidence is up to 9% with intermediate-acting neuromuscular blocking agents (up to 50% with long-acting agents). Extubation of a partially paralyzed patient results in increased postoperative morbidity. Consequences of residual weakness include airway obstruction, hypoventilation, impaired ventilatory response to hypoxia, disturbed esophageal motility, and inability to handle vomitus.
A. Risk factors
  1. Use of long-acting neuromuscular blocking agents
  2. Not administering anticholinesterase reversal agents when indicated
  3. Plasma cholinesterase deficiency
  4. Atypical plasma cholinesterase
B. Signs and symptoms
  1. Air hunger
  2. Writhing
  3. Uncoordinated movements of the extremities
  4. Dysphagia (implies weakness of pharyngeal muscles)
  5. Spasmodic, paradoxical abdominal motion
  6. Impaired cough (occurs when vital capacity is 66% of normal)
  7. Hypertension
  8. Tachycardia
  9. Pupillary dilation
C. Management
  1. Is additional anticholinesterase indicated? Has the patient received the optimal dose of reversal agent?
  2. Ventilation: Support the airway and provide adequate ventilation as indicated. Consider whether the patient is at high risk for pulmonary aspiration of gastric contents.
  3. Sedation: Neuromuscular blocking agents do not alter the patient's level of consciousness. If the patient requires mechanical ventilation, provide sedation, analgesia, or amnesia as indicated.
  4. Evaluation: Assessing the need for continued ventilatory support and control of the airway will be required on an ongoing basis until the patient has sufficiently recovered from the neuromuscular blocking agents.

VIII. Opioid ventilatory depression: Opioid therapy is the primary vehicle for pain management in the surgical patient. Providing adequate and satisfactory pain relief with the least amount of risk is an important adjunct to patient recovery. Patient comfort and safety are essential and can be attained through proper monitoring and administration of opioids. Respiratory depression secondary to opioid administration occurs despite optimal patient care and must be diagnosed and managed appropriately.

  A. Risk factors
  1. Opioid naïve: A person who does not take opioids regularly may be expected to require less opioid than those who are exposed to potent analgesics.
  2. Chronic respiratory disease
  3. Liver or renal disease: Opioid elimination may be delayed in patients with severe liver or renal disease.
  4. Renarcotization: Naloxone has a duration of action approximating 30 to 45 minutes, which might be shorter than the duration of action of the administered opioid. It is possible for the patient that is treated with a long-acting opioid to exhibit recurrence of opioid ventilatory depression in this circumstance.
  5. Older patients: Secondary to prolonged drug elimination

  B. Signs and symptoms
  1. Mental obtundation
  2. Bradypnea
  3. Hypoxemia: May be a late sign especially in the patient receiving supplemental oxygen therapy
  4. Bradycardia
  5. Chest wall rigidity

  C. Management
  1. Prevention: Use of alternative pain relief methods (e.g., transcutaneous electrical nerve stimulation [TENS], massage therapy, distraction therapy) may lead to a reduced need for opioid therapy.
  2. Stir-up regimen: Tactile and verbal stimulation of the patient may be sufficient to maintain adequate spontaneous ventilation.
  3. Opioid antagonism (e.g., naloxone, naltrexone, nalmefene): Intravenous naloxone, 0.1 to 0.3 mg, in an average-sized adult, provides prompt reversal of opioid-induced ventilatory depression. Patient observation for renarcotization phenomenon should be employed. Intramuscular naloxone should be considered when longer-acting opioids have been administered.
  4. Ventilation: Short-term controlled ventilation may be indicated to normalize $PaCO_2$ until opioid antagonism therapy can be instituted.

BIBLIOGRAPHY

1. Benumof JL: *Airway management: Principles and practice*. St Louis: Mosby, 1996.
2. Fink JB, Dhand R: *Respiratory care clinics of North America: Aerosol therapy*. Philadelphia: WB Saunders, 2001.
3. Marley RA: Perioperative therapeutic aerosol administration. *AANA J* 63:165-175, 1995.
4. Marley RA: Postextubation laryngeal edema: a review with consideration for home discharge. *J PeriAnesth Nurs* 13:39-53, 1998.
5. Marley RA: Postoperative oxygen therapy. *J PeriAnesth Nurs* 13:394-412, 1998.
6. Pilbeam SP: *Mechanical ventilation: Physiological and clinical applications*. St Louis: Mosby, 1998.
7. Rau JL: *Respiratory care clinics of North America: Aerosolized drugs for the respiratory tract*. Philadelphia: WB Saunders, 1999.

OBJECTIVES

At the conclusion of this chapter the reader will be able to:

1. Describe the components of a detailed cardiovascular assessment, including normal and abnormal findings.

2. Identify possible cardiopulmonary complications occurring in the perioperative period.

3. Understand basic life support (BLS) and airway management in emergency situations.

4. Identify complicating and life-threatening dysrhythmias.

5. Understand the pharmacotherapy of drugs used in emergency situations.

6. Identify the indications, precautions, and techniques for defibrillation and cardioversion.

7. Compare the indications and perioperative considerations for various modes of temporary and permanent cardiac pacing.

8. Be familiar with the American Society of PeriAnesthesia Nurses' (ASPAN's) Standards of Nursing Practice specific to advanced cardiac life support (ACLS) (see Box 32-1).

9. Identify appropriate emergency drugs and equipment necessary in the postanesthesia care unit (PACU) for emergency care as identified by ASPAN (see Box 32-2).

I. Cardiac anatomy and physiology
   A. Structure and function (see Figure 32-1)
   B. Conduction system (see Figure 32-2)
      1. Sino-atrial (AV) node: pacemaker of the heart
      2. Internodal tracts and Bachmann's bundle
         a. Electrical pathways in atria
         b. Conducts impulse through atria and to the atrioventricular (AV) node
      3. AV node: impulse briefly delayed
      4. Ventricular conduction
         a. Bundle of His
         b. Left and right bundle branches
            (1) Deliver impulse to the Purkinje fibers
            (2) Fibers carry impulse to the ventricular muscle.
   C. Cardiac cycle
      1. Systole
         a. Isovolumetric contraction
            (1) Occurs when ventricular pressure is generated but has not exceeded vascular pressure
            (2) Pulmonic and aortic valves closed; tricuspid and mitral valves closed
            (3) Most oxygen using part of the cardiac cycle
         b. Systolic ejection
            (1) Ventricular pressure exceeds vascular pressure.
            (2) Pulmonic and aortic valves opened; tricuspid and mitral valves closed
            (3) Blood is ejected into the vasculature.

Drug information can change. Please refer to the disclaimer on page 111.

■ BOX 32-1
■ **STANDARD III STAFFING AND PERSONNEL MANAGEMENT (2002 ASPAN STANDARDS)**

"The professional perianesthesia nurse working in the Phase I setting will maintain a current Advanced Cardiac Life Support (ACLS) and/or Pediatric Advanced Life Support (PALS) provider status, as appropriate to the patient population served (Resource 6)."

Standard
An appropriate number of professional nursing staff with demonstrated competence are available to meet the individual needs of patients and families in each level of perianesthesia care based on patient acuity, census, and physical facility.

Rationale
Nursing care in perianesthesia settings is directed toward provision of direct patient care, supervision of care given by others, health teaching, and patient advocacy. The expertise of professional perianesthesia nurses is necessary to provide safe, quality care to patients in this environment.

Outcome
Staffing patterns reflect an adequate number of professional nursing staff with appropriate competencies to provide safe, quality nursing care.

Criteria
- Staff function within written job performance descriptions (see Resources 11 and 12, *Competency Based Orientation and Credentialing Book, A Competency Based Orientation and Credentialing Program for Unlicensed Assistive Personnel in the Perianesthesia Setting, and the Position Statement on Unlicensed Assistive Personnel*)
- Staff receive regularly scheduled performance appraisals.
- Staffing is based on patient acuity, census, and physical facility.
  - A competent perianesthesia professional nurse is present* at all times to provide direct care and/or supervision.
  - Preanesthesia assessment is performed by an RN competent in preanesthesia nursing.
  - Two licensed nurses, one of whom is an RN competent in phase I postanesthesia nursing, are present* whenever a patient is receiving phase I level of care.
  - Two competent personnel, one of whom is an RN competent in phase II postanesthesia nursing, are present* whenever a patient is receiving phase II level of care.
  - An RN competent in phase III postanesthesia nursing must be present* whenever a patient is receiving phase III level of care.
- Staffing patterns will reflect ASPAN's Patient Classification/Recommended Staffing Guidelines (Resource 3).
- A written plan for orientation and ongoing continuing education exists to validate and maintain competency.
  - New staff members demonstrate competency in the performance of responsibilities as defined in the job description.
  - Staff members participate in annual perianesthesia nursing competency validation and continuing educational opportunities.
  - The professional perianesthesia nurse working in the phase I setting will maintain a current Advanced Cardiac Life Support (ACLS) and/or Pediatric Advanced Life Support (PALS) provider status, as appropriate to the patient population served (Resource 6).

*ASPAN defines "present" as being in the particular place where the patient is receiving care.
From American Society of PeriAnesthesia Nurses: *2002 Standards of Perianesthesia Nursing Practice*, Cherry Hill, NJ: American Society of PeriAnesthesia Nurses, 2002.

■ BOX 32-2
■ **RESOURCE 6 EMERGENCY DRUGS AND EQUIPMENT (2002 ASPAN STANDARDS)**

This list is not meant to be all-inclusive. Refer to current ACLS and PALS protocols for dosing requirements.

A. Adult
1. Adenosine
2. Aminophylline
3. Amiodarone hydrochloride
4. Amrinone
5. Atenolol
6. Atropine sulfate
7. Calcium chloride
8. Calcium gluconate
9. Dextrose
10. Digoxin
11. Diltiazem hydrochloride
12. Dobutamine hydrochloride
13. Dopamine hydrochloride
14. Epinephrine hydrochloride
15. Esmolol
16. Flumazenil
17. Furosemide
18. Isoproterenol
19. Lidocaine hydrochloride
20. Methylprednisolone sodium succinate
21. Magnesium sulfate
22. Metoprolol
23. Naloxone hydrochloride
24. Nitroglycerine
25. Norepinephrine bitartrate
26. Procainamide hydrochloride
27. Propranolol hydrochloride
28. Sodium bicarbonate
29. Vasopressin
30. Verapamil hydrochloride
31. Sodium nitroprusside
32. Succinylcholine chloride

B. PALS emergency drugs
1. Adenosine: 6 mg/2 ml vials/syringes
2. Amiodarone hydrochloride
3. Atropine sulfate: prefilled syringes 0.1 mg/ml (5 ml, 10 ml) or 1 mg/ml (1 ml)
4. Calcium chloride 10%: prefilled syringes 100 mg/ml (10 ml)
5. Epinephrine hydrochloride: prefilled syringes 1:10,000 (0.1 mg/ml) 10 ml
6. Epinephrine hydrochloride (1:1000) should be available for ET and high-dose IV infusion (1 mg/ml): syringes 1 ml, or vial 30 ml
7. Dextrose 25%: 50 ml vial of D50 and dilute
8. Dopamine hydrochloride: 40 mg/ml (5 ml)
9. Dobutamine hydrochloride: 25 mg/ml (10 ml) or 12.5 mg/ml (20 ml)
10. Isoproterenol hydrochloride: 0.2 mg/ml (5 ml)
11. Lidocaine hydrochloride: 1%: prefilled syringes 10 mg/ml (5 ml), 20 mg/ml and
12. Vials: 40 mg/ml, 100 mg/ml, 200 mg/ml
13. Naloxone: vials 0.4 mg/ml (1 ml) or 1 mg/ml (2 ml)
14. Norepinephrine: for IV infusion only.
15. Sodium bicarbonate: prefilled syringes of 8.4% solution 1 mEq/ml (50 ml or 10 ml) or 0.5 mEq/ml of 4.2% (10 ml)

■ BOX 32-2 *Cont'd*

■ **RESOURCE 6 EMERGENCY DRUGS AND EQUIPMENT (2002 ASPAN STANDARDS)**

16. Sterile normal saline: 10 ml vials (preservative free)
17. Sterile water: 10 ml vials (preservative free)
18. One ml or tuberculosis syringes to mix medications

C. Emergency supplies
  1. Portable defibrillator (adult and pediatric pads/paddles)
  2. External cardiac pacing
  3. Defibrillator pads or gel
  4. Electrodes (include pediatric and diaphoretic)
  5. Gloves (sterile and nonsterile)
  6. Personal protective equipment
  7. Oral airways: assorted sizes including pediatric
  8. Nasal airways: assorted sizes including pediatric
  9. Laryngoscope
 10. Extra bulb
 11. Blades: straight and curved (include size appropriate for pediatrics)
 12. Endotracheal tubes (various sizes including pediatric, cuffed, and uncuffed)
 13. Expired CO_2 detector
 14. Stylet (adult and pediatric)
 15. Magill forceps
 16. Yankeur suction handle
 17. Regular suction catheters (assorted sizes)
 18. Syringes: assorted sizes
 19. Assorted needles
 20. IV catheters
 21. IV solutions: Dextrose 5% in water, normal Saline: 100 ml, 250 ml, and 500 ml
 22. IV tubings: standard and infusion regulator
 23. Central vein catheter set
 24. Sterile gloves
 25. Alcohol swabs
 26. Betadine swabs
 27. Tincture of benzoin
 28. Sponges—sterile 4×4, 2×2
 29. Medication labels
 30. Cardiac arrest documentation forms
 31. Arterial blood gases kit
 32. Tape
 33. Foley catheter supplies
 34. Nasogastric tubes/supplies

D. Additional pediatric needs
  1. Assorted needles: 18, 20, 22, and 25 gauge
  2. Butterfly: five eighths inch, 25 gauge (winged infusion needle)
  3. Lumbar puncture needles: three and one half inch, 19, 20, and 22 gauge
  4. Minidrip tubing
  5. Volume control chamber
  6. Syringes: tuberculosis and 50 ml
  7. Arm restraints
  8. Wrist restraints
  9. Interosseous needles: 18 gauge

E. Sterile packs
  1. Cutdown
  2. Tracheostomy
  3. Suture set

Continued

■ BOX 32-2 *Cont'd*
■ **RESOURCE 6 EMERGENCY DRUGS AND EQUIPMENT (2002 ASPAN STANDARDS)**

> **4.** Emergency tonsil set
> **5.** Pediatric: Infant gauge tray with assorted feeding tubes
> **6.** Central line

STRUCTURE AND FUNCTION OF THE HEART

Structure of the Heart:
The heart is located in the mediastinum, the space in the thoracic cavity between the lungs and above the diaphragm. It is a cone-shaped, hollow, muscular, contractile organ weighing about 300 gm (11 ounces).

Four vessels provide for blood flow into and out of the heart.

Superior vena cava drains blood from the upper body into the right atrium.

Coronary sinus drains blood from the cardiac veins into the right atrium.

Aorta carries blood from the left ventricle into the systemic circulation.

Inferior vena cava drains blood from the lower body into the right atrium.

Each side of the heart contains 2 chambers: the atrium and the ventricle.
Atrium: The atrium is a thin-walled upper collecting chamber.
Ventricle: The ventricle is a thick-walled lower pumping chamber.
The septum, a muscular wall, separates the chambers on the right side of the heart from those on the left side.

Four valves control blood flow through the heart.
Pulmonary valve: between the right ventricle and the pulmonary artery
Aortic valve: between the left ventricle and the ascending aorta
Mitral valve (bicuspid valve): between the left atrium and ventricle
Tricuspid valve: between the right atrium and ventricle

The heart consists of 3 layers of tissue:
Epicardium: The epicardium is a thin, transparent structure that covers the outer surface of the heart.
Myocardium: The myocardium is the middle layer and the contracting muscle of the heart, consisting of striated muscle fibers interlaced into bundles.
Endocardium: The innermost layer, the endocardium consists of thin endothelial tissue that lines the inner chambers and the heart valves.

Functions of the Heart:
The pumping action of the heart is the result of muscles in the heart's chambers alternately contracting and relaxing. Contraction of the heart chambers is called systole. Diastole is the relaxation of the heart chambers with resultant dilation and filling.

1 The heart collects deoxygenated blood from the venous system and pumps it to the lungs for reoxygenation. The right atrium receives deoxygenated blood from the body via the superior and inferior vena cava and from the heart muscle via the coronary sinus and pumps it through the tricuspid valve into the right ventricle. The right ventricle, a flat muscular pump, receives deoxygenated blood from the right atrium and pumps it through the pulmonary valve, against low resistance, into the pulmonary artery and into the lungs.

2 The heart pumps oxygenated blood into the systemic circulation, which carries it to the cells. The left atrium receives oxygenated blood from the lungs, via the pulmonary veins, and pumps it through the mitral valve to the left ventricle. The left ventricle, the heart's largest, most muscular chamber, receives oxygenated blood from the lungs via the left atrium and pumps it through the aortic valve against high systemic pressure into the aorta and into the systemic circulation.

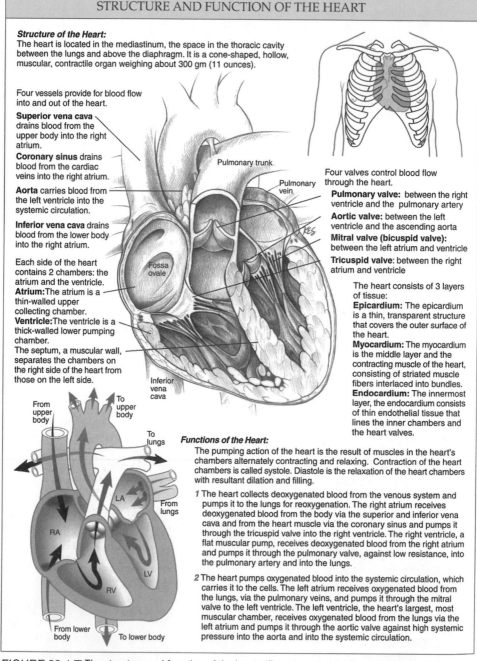

FIGURE 32-1 ■ The structure and function of the heart. (From Luecke LE, Mancine ME: Caring for people with cardiovascular disorders. In Luckman J, editor: *Saunders manual of nursing care.* Philadelphia: WB Saunders, 1997, p 982.)

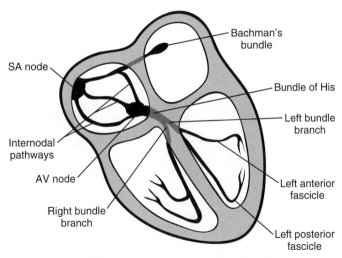

FIGURE 32-2 ■ The conduction system. (From Van Riper S, Luciano A: Basic cardiac arrhythmias: A review for postanesthesia care unit nurses. *J PeriAnesth Nurs* 9(1):3, 1994.)

    2. Diastole
        a. Ventricular relaxation
           (1) Ventricular pressure is less than vascular pressure.
           (2) Mitral valves open: ventricles fill passively
           (3) Pulmonic and aortic valves shut
        b. Provides for myocardial perfusion and ventricular filling
  D. Functional properties of cardiac muscle
    1. Excitability: ability of a nerve to produce an action potential
    2. Automaticity: spontaneous depolarization and generation of an action potential
    3. Conductivity: ability to conduct electricity
    4. Refractoriness: resistance to stimulation while heart is still contracting from an earlier stimulus
    5. Contractility: ability to shorten when stimulated
    6. Extensibility: ability to stretch when heart fills with blood during diastole
    7. Rhythmicity
        a. Ability to function with a definite rhythm
        b. Stimulation—transmission—contraction—relaxation
    8. Irritability: ability to be stimulated
  E. Effects of anesthesia on the heart
    1. Tachy and brady dysrhythmias
    2. Decreased contractility and cardiac output
II. Vascular structure and function
  A. Structure (see Figure 32-3)
  B. Function
    1. Arteries
        a. Transport oxygenated blood from the heart to the tissues
        b. Exception: pulmonary artery transports deoxygenated blood from the right ventricle to the lungs.
    2. Capillaries: thin-walled structure allows for the exchange of nutrients and wastes between the blood and cells.
    3. Veins
        a. Transport deoxygenated blood from the tissues to the right side of the heart

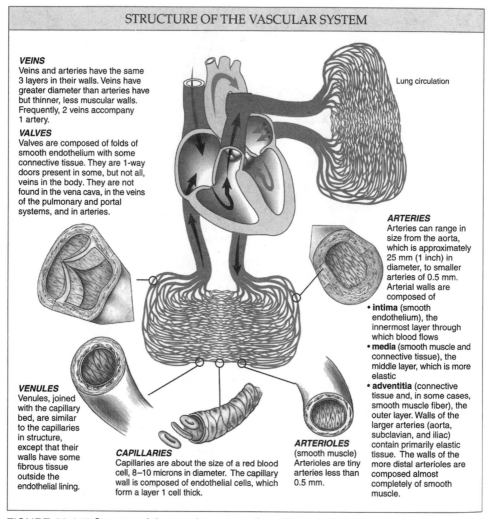

STRUCTURE OF THE VASCULAR SYSTEM

VEINS
Veins and arteries have the same 3 layers in their walls. Veins have greater diameter than arteries have but thinner, less muscular walls. Frequently, 2 veins accompany 1 artery.

VALVES
Valves are composed of folds of smooth endothelium with some connective tissue. They are 1-way doors present in some, but not all, veins in the body. They are not found in the vena cava, in the veins of the pulmonary and portal systems, and in arteries.

Lung circulation

ARTERIES
Arteries can range in size from the aorta, which is approximately 25 mm (1 inch) in diameter, to smaller arteries of 0.5 mm. Arterial walls are composed of
- **intima** (smooth endothelium), the innermost layer through which blood flows
- **media** (smooth muscle and connective tissue), the middle layer, which is more elastic
- **adventitia** (connective tissue and, in some cases, smooth muscle fiber), the outer layer. Walls of the larger arteries (aorta, subclavian, and iliac) contain primarily elastic tissue. The walls of the more distal arterioles are composed almost completely of smooth muscle.

VENULES
Venules, joined with the capillary bed, are similar to the capillaries in structure, except that their walls have some fibrous tissue outside the endothelial lining.

CAPILLARIES
Capillaries are about the size of a red blood cell, 8–10 microns in diameter. The capillary wall is composed of endothelial cells, which form a layer 1 cell thick.

ARTERIOLES
(smooth muscle) Arterioles are tiny arteries less than 0.5 mm.

FIGURE 32-3 ■ Structure of the vascular system. (From Turner J: Caring for people with peripheral vascular and lymphatic disorders. In Luckman J, editor: *Saunders manual of nursing care.* Philadelphia: WB Saunders, 1997, p 1092.)

  b. Exception: pulmonary vein transports oxygenated blood from the lungs to the left atrium.
  c. Approximately 75% of total blood volume is found in the venous system at any given time.
  d. Venous return is controlled by several factors.
   (1) Valves (see Figure 32-4)
       (a) Prevent backflow of blood, allowing flow to occur only in the direction toward the heart
       (b) Become incompetent when vein walls have been overstretched by excessive venous pressure
   (2) Venous elasticity
       (a) Venous walls are less elastic than arterial walls, thus allowing distention or pooling to occur.
       (b) This is known as venous capacitance.
   (3) Intrathoracic pressure
       (a) Negative intrathoracic pressure enhances flow into the heart by decreasing resistance.

NORMAL AND ABNORMAL VALVES

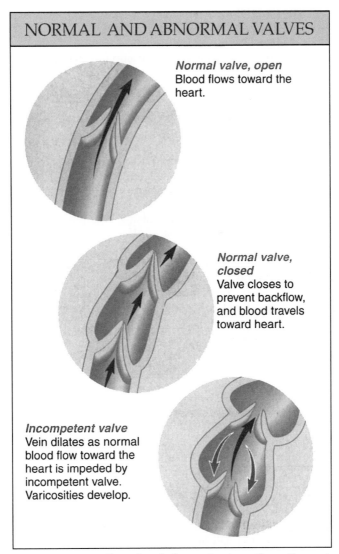

Normal valve, open
Blood flows toward the heart.

Normal valve, closed
Valve closes to prevent backflow, and blood travels toward heart.

Incompetent valve
Vein dilates as normal blood flow toward the heart is impeded by incompetent valve. Varicosities develop.

FIGURE 32-4 ■ Normal and abnormal valves. (From Turner J: *Caring for people with peripheral vascular and lymphatic disorders.* In Luckman J, editor: *Saunders manual of nursing care.* Philadelphia: WB Saunders, 1997, p 1093.)

        (b) Positive intrathoracic pressure reduces flow into the heart by increasing resistance.
    4. Arteriovenous anastomoses: channels where arterioles and venules connect without capillaries
C. Control of blood flow
    1. Neural control
        a. Baroreceptors and chemoreceptors (stretch receptors) on the aortic arch and internal carotid sinus and in the right atrium
           (1) Sense changes in blood flow
           (2) Send messages to the vasomotor center in the medulla
           (3) Stimulate the sympathetic nervous system (SNS) or parasympathetic nervous system to respond
               (a) Low flow: Epinephrine and norepinephrine are released.
               (b) Causes vasoconstriction, increased heart rate, and contractility

(c) High flow: Acetylcholine released

(d) Causes vasodilation

2. Humoral control

a. Also stimulated by the SNS in reaction to changes in blood flow, as well as other substances in the body

(1) Low-flow states

(a) Adrenocorticotropic hormone (ACTH) released: Leading to sodium and water reabsorption in renal tubules and increased intravascular volume

(b) Renin-angiotensin-aldosterone system stimulated: Marked constriction of peripheral arteries

(c) Antidiuretic hormone released: Increased water reabsorption in the renal tubules resulting in increased intravascular volume

(2) High-flow states

(a) Bradykinin (plasma protein): Potent vasodilator

(b) Histamine: Vasodilator released following mast cell injury

3. Local control: autoregulation

a. Blood vessels' ability to respond to tissue needs by dilating or constricting

b. Utilized mainly by arterioles as a result of

(1) Decreased oxygen availability

(2) Increased metabolic demand at the tissue level

III. Assessment and management

A. Preoperative baseline assessment

B. Cardiac-focused assessment

1. Chest pain

a. Stable

b. Unstable

2. Dyspnea (most common symptom of organic heart disease)

3. Paroxysmal nocturnal dyspnea

4. Syncope

5. Unexplained weakness or fatigue

6. Weight loss or gain

7. Dependent edema

8. Orthopnea

9. Coughing at night (assess for ACE inhibitor use)

10. Hemoptysis

11. Rapid heartbeat or palpitations

12. Nocturia

13. Intermittent claudication

C. Peripheral vascular focused assessment

1. Skin

a. Turgor

b. Edema

c. Compare temperature at different sites.

d. Inspect for lesions or ulcerations.

e. Determine history of slow wound healing.

f. Inspect for varicose veins: visibly engorged, palpable subcutaneous veins.

g. Differentiate between venous and arterial insufficiency.

(1) Arterial insufficiency: Loss of hair, pallor, and translucent, waxy appearance of skin

(2) Venous insufficiency: Skin thickened, reddish-brown pigmentation, and ulceration

2. Vasculature and circulation

a. Arterial

(1) Capillary refill

(a) Brisk: <3 seconds

(b) Sluggish: >3 seconds

(2) Bruits: Low-pitched blowing sound from turbulent flow
    (a) Indicative of atherosclerosis
    (b) Assess with bell of stethoscope at carotid and femoral arteries and abdominal aorta
(3) Determine strength of peripheral pulses.
    (a) Absent: 0
    (b) Diminished: +1
    (c) Normal, easily palpated: +2
    (d) Increased, strong: +3
    (e) Bounding: +4
(4) Neurovascular assessment: Five Ps, indicative of arterial insufficiency
    (a) Pain
    (b) Pulselessness
    (c) Pallor
    (d) Paresthesia
    (e) Paralysis
    (f) Ankle-brachial index (ABI): Inexpensive, noninvasive, bedside assessment of arterial perfusion (atherosclerosis)
        (i) Obtain the brachial blood pressure in both arms (use the higher systolic pressure for the calculation).
        (ii) Obtain the ankle blood pressure in the questionable extremity.
        (iii) Divide the systolic ankle pressure by the systolic brachial pressure.
        (iv) Index >0.95, normal perfusion
        (v) Index <0.90, early asymptomatic disease, difficulty with wound healing, increased risk for cardiovascular event (i.e., myocardial infarction [MI] or death)
        (vi) Index <0.60, wound probably will not heal, more advanced atheroma, greater risk for cardiovascular event or death
        (vii) Index >1.2, indicative of venous disease

b. Venous
(1) Superficial thrombophlebitis: subcutaneous cords with overlying erythema
(2) Deep vein thrombosis (DVT)
    (a) Silent at onset
    (b) Shooting pain at moment of embolism, with numbness and weakness followed by signs of ischemia
    (c) Homan's sign
        (i) Positive: pain in popliteal fossa and upper posterior calf on dorsiflexion of foot
        (ii) Helpful but not specific for DVT

D. Preexisting disease states
  1. Atherosclerotic heart disease
  2. Diabetes
  3. Hypertension
  4. Chronic obstructive pulmonary disease (COPD)
  5. Previous MI
  6. Congestive heart failure (CHF)

E. Specific allergies
  1. Shellfish
  2. Iodine
  3. Contrast media

F. Cardiac auscultation
  1. Normal heart sounds
    a. S1 (first heart sound)
      (1) Represents closure of tricuspid and mitral AV valves

        (2) Occurs at the end of atrial contraction and with the onset of ventricular contraction

        (3) Loudest at the apex

        (4) Slightly longer and lower pitch than S2

        (5) Occurs as the ventricles contract; almost synchronous with the carotid pulse

    b. S2 (second heart sound)

        (1) Caused by closure of the pulmonic and aortic valves at the end of ventricular contraction

        (2) Signals the beginning of diastole

        (3) Loudest at the base

        (4) Higher pitch than S1, so is louder and transmits better

    c. Split heart sounds

        (1) Split S1: occurs if right and left AV valves do not close at precisely the same time

        (2) Split S2: occurs if semilunar valves do not close simultaneously

        (3) Slight time variance normal; wide variance in time between right and left sided valve closure possibly related to conduction defects or obstruction to flow

2. Extra heart sounds

    a. S3 (ventricular gallop, Figure 32-5)

        (1) Immediately follows S2; sounds like "lubb-dup-up" or "Ken-tuc-ky"

        (2) Dull and low-pitched

        (3) Best heard at the apex with the bell of the stethoscope and the patient in the left lateral position

        (4) Occurs when the AV valves open and atrial blood rushes into the ventricles

        (5) Usually indicates decreased compliance of the ventricles commonly associated with heart failure

        (6) May also indicate mitral or tricuspid AV valve incompetence

    b. S4 (atrial gallop, Figure 32-6)

        (1) Immediately precedes S1; sounds like "la-lubb-dup" or "Ten-nes-see"

        (2) Very low pitch

        (3) Best heard at the apex with the bell of the stethoscope

        (4) Produced by atrial contraction when the ventricle is resistant to filling

        (5) Heard in patients with

            (a) Increased resistance to ventricular filling as seen in hypertension and mitral stenosis

            (b) Increased stroke volume as seen with severe anemia and hyperthyroidism

            (c) Delayed conduction between the atria and ventricles

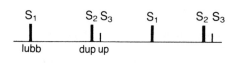

FIGURE 32-5 ■ Auscultated cadence of the third heart sound. (From Darovic GO, Marriott HJL: Physical assessment of the cardiovascular system. In Darovic GO, editor: *Hemodynamic Monitoring: Invasive and noninvasive clinical application,* ed 3. Philadelphia: WB Saunders, 2002, p 106.)

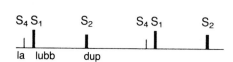

FIGURE 32-6 ■ Auscultated cadence of the fourth heart sound. (From Darovic GO, Marriott HJL: Physical assessment of the cardiovascular system. In Darovic GO, editor: *Hemodynamic Monitoring: Invasive and noninvasive clinical application,* ed 3. Philadelphia: WB Saunders, 2002, p 106.)

    3. Murmurs

      a. Caused by increased turbulence or blood flow through the heart

      b. Causes

        (1) Stenosis: Valves will not open properly

        (2) Regurgitant (incompetent, insufficient): Valves will not close properly to prevent backward flow of blood.

        (3) Presence of a congenital defect between chambers

        (4) Dilated heart chamber

        (5) Other

          (a) Increased blood flow: pregnancy, hyperthyroidism

          (b) Decreased blood viscosity

      d. Murmur description should include

        (1) Primary location related to valve where best auscultated

        (2) Area of radiation or site of maximum intensity

        (3) Timing as related to cardiac cycle

        (4) Pitch

        (5) Configuration or shape as determined by intensity over time

        (6) Quality

          (a) Blowing

          (b) Rumbling

          (c) Musical

          (d) Harsh

          (e) Intensity

        (7) Intensity (loudness)

          (a) Grade I: very faint, heard only after a period of intent listening

          (b) Grade II: Quiet and faint, but heard immediately upon placing the stethoscope on the chest

          (c) Grade III: Moderately intense

          (d) Grade IV: Loud, associated with a thrill

          (e) Grade V: Very loud, can be heard with the stethoscope partially off the chest wall

          (f) Grade VI: Very loud, can be heard with the entire chest piece just removed from the chest wall

    4. Pericardial friction rub

      a. Occurs if the pericardium becomes inflamed

      b. Is a scratchy "to-and-fro"; should be heard with each heartbeat

      c. Best auscultated with patient sitting upright and leaning forward

G. Laboratory studies

    1. Arterial blood gases as indicated

    2. Cardiac enzymes and markers (if history significant for myocardial ischemia) (see Table 32-1)

      a. Creatine kinase–MB isoenzyme (CK-MB) (cardiac specific)

        (1) Normal within 3 days: compromised ability for late diagnosis of MI

        (2) >10-13 U/L or >3% to 5% total CK activity

      b. Biochemical markers cardiac troponin I (cTnI) and cardiac troponin T (cTntT)

        (1) Efficient for late diagnosis of MI

        (2) Remain elevated for 7-10 days: compromise ability to diagnose recurrent infarction if used alone.

    3. Electrolytes critical to cardiac function (potassium, sodium, magnesium, calcium)

    4. Coagulation profile: prothrombin time, partial thromboplastin time, international normalized ratio (PT, PTT, INR)

H. Noninvasive diagnostic studies

    1. Chest x-ray

    2. Electrocardiogram (ECG)

      a. Twelve-lead ECG

      b. Determines or detects

Marker	Onset of Elevation (hr)	Peak Elevation (hr)	Return to Normal (days)
Troponin I (cTnI)* Normal <3.1 ng/ml	Within minutes	1	7-10
CK 12-80 U/L males; 10-70 U/L females	3-6	12-24	24-48
CK-MB (cardiac specific) 0% to 3% total CK	4-8	18-24	3
LDH 45-90 U/L	24-72	72-96	10-14
LDH$_1$ (cardiac specific) 20% to 30% total LDH	12-24	48	10-14
LDH$_1$ to LDH$_2$ ratio <1 (i.e., LDH$_2$ >LDH$_1$)	12-24	48	10-14

*Considered most diagnostic of myocardial injury.

      (1) Disturbances of rate, rhythm, or conduction
      (2) Ischemia or infarction
      (3) Electrolyte abnormalities
      (4) Anatomic orientation of heart
      (5) Chamber enlargement
      (6) Drug toxicity

  3. Echocardiography
    a. Ultrasonic exam
    b. Detects abnormalities of anatomy and/or motion and blood flow

  4. Radionuclide imaging
    a. Utilizes radioactive tracer injected into the bloodstream (thallium-201 [TI-201] or technetium-99m [Tc-99m]).
    b. May be performed at rest or with exercise stress or pharmacologic vasodilation
      (1) Infarction scintigram: Detects regional perfusion deficits that represent areas of ischemic or infarcted cardiac muscle
      (2) Angiography: Assesses ventricular size, volume, ejection fraction and wall abnormality
      (3) Positron emission tomography (PET): Uses biologically active radiopharmaceuticals to distinguish dysfunctional but viable myocardium from infarcted tissue.

  5. Exercise electrocardiography (stress testing)
    a. Most widely used method for assessing the presence and severity of coronary artery disease (CAD)
    b. The observation, measurement and recording of the ECG, blood pressure (BP), and heart rate (HR) in response to progressively increasing, graded levels of work
    c. May combine or utilize pharmacologic stressing for individuals unable to perform physically

I. Invasive diagnostic studies
  1. Cardiac catheterization: Fluoroscopically guided placement of catheters in the heart to measure intracardiac pressures, valve function, and oxygen saturation.

          a. Angiography: Injection of radiographic contrast material into cardiac chambers (ventriculography), coronary arteries, valve roots (aortography) or great vessels

      2. Electrophysiology studies (EPS): Fluoroscopically guided intracardiac placement of catheters to assess spontaneous function, responses to stress, and vulnerability to induced tachyarrhythmias

          a. Diagnostic modality for characterizing arrhythmic disorders, stratifying risk, and directing therapy for chronic arrhythmic disorders

      3. Endomyocardial biopsy: Acquisition of a small piece of myocardium for microscopic analysis utilizing a specially designed catheter

          a. Diagnostic technique for evaluating cardiac failure of unknown cause and response to cardiac transplantation

   J. Medications

      1. Types

      2. Dosages

      3. Consult with anesthesia or surgeon as to necessity of taking cardiac and antihypertensive medications the morning of surgery.

      4. If unable to obtain consult, have patient bring medications with him or her the morning of surgery.

   K. Determination of cardiac risk

      1. Goldman's Multifactorial Cardiac Risk Index (see Tables 32-2 and 32-3)

      2. Detsky's Multifactorial Index (see Tables 32-4 and 32-5)

IV. Cardiovascular operative procedures

   A. Coronary artery revascularization (see Chapter 39 for detailed discussion)

   B. Valvular repair or replacement (see Chapter 39 for detailed discussion)

   C. Permanent pacemaker implantation

      1. Indications

          a. Complete heart block

          b. Symptomatic bradycardia associated with sinus node dysfunction or second-degree heart block

          c. Acute MI with persistent, advanced second or third degree heart block

---

■ TABLE 32-2
■ ■ **Goldman's Multifactorial Cardiac Risk Index**

		Points
History	Myocardial infarction within 6 mo	10
	Age over 70 years	5
Physical examination	S3 gallop or jugular venous distention	11
	Important aortic stenosis	3
Electrocardiogram	Rhythm other than sinus or sinus plus APBs* on last preoperative electrocardiogram	7
	More than 5 PVCs per minute at any time preoperatively	7
Poor general medical status	Pao$_2$ <60 mm Hg, Paco$_2$ >50 mm Hg, K$^+$ <3.0 mEq/L, HCO$_3$ <20 mEq/L, BUN >50 mg/dl (18 mmol/L), Creatinine >3 mg/dl (260 mmol/L), abnormal SGOT, signs of chronic liver disease, patient bedridden from noncardiac causes	3
Intraperitoneal, intrathoracic, or aortic surgery		3
Emergency operation		4
Total:		53

From Goldman L, Caldera D, Nussbaum SR, et al: Multifactorial index of cardiac risk in non-cardiac surgical procedures. *N Engl J Med* 197:848, 1977.
*APB, atrial premature beat

■ TABLE 32-3
■ ■ **Prediction of Perioperative Cardiac Complications by Points in the Goldman Index**

	Point Total	Cardiac Death (%)	Other Life-threatening Complications* (%)
Class I	0-5	0.2	0.7
Class II	6-12	2.0	5.0
Class III	13-25	2.0	11.0
Class IV	≥26	56.0	22.0

From Goldman L, Caldera D, Nussbaum SR, et al: Multifactorial index of cardiac risk in non-cardiac surgical procedures. *N Engl J Med* 197:848, 1977.
*Nonfatal MI, CHF, and ventricular tachycardia.

■ TABLE 32-4
■ ■ **Detsky's Multifactorial Index**

Coronary artery disease	MI within 6 mo	10
	MI more than 6 mo previously	5
	Canadian Cardiovascular Society Angina:	
	▪ Class III	10
	▪ Class IV	20
Alveolar pulmonary edema	Within 1 wk	10
	Ever	5
Valvular disease	Suspected critical aortic stenosis	20
Arrhythmias	Rhythm other than sinus or sinus plus APBs on last preoperative electrocardiogram; more than 5 premature ventricular contractions at any time prior to surgery	5
Poor general medical status		5
Emergency operation		10

From Detsky A S, Abrams HB, McLaughlin JR, et al: Predicting cardiac complications in patients undergoing non-cardiac surgery. *J Gen Intern Med* 1:213, 1986.

■ TABLE 32-5
■ ■ **Likelihood Ratios of Perioperative Cardiac Complications* by Points in the Detsky Index**

Class (points)	Major Surgery	Minor Surgery	All Surgery
I (0-15)	0.42	0.39	0.43
II (15-30)	3.58	2.75	3.38
III (>30)	14.93	12.20	10.60

From Detsky AS, Abrams HB, McLaughlin JR, et al: Predicting cardiac complications in patients undergoing non-cardiac surgery. *J Gen Intern Med* 1:213, 1986.
*Defined as MI, pulmonary edema, ventricular tachycardia, or fibrillation, new or worsening CHF, and coronary insufficiency.

      d. Recurrent syncope associated with hypersensitive carotid sinus syndrome

      e. Advanced block with atrial fibrillation or flutter and symptomatic slow ventricular rate

      f. Symptomatic bradycardia secondary to pharmacologic therapy

  2. Pacing modes (see Table 32-6)

      a. Single chamber

          (1) AAI

          (2) VVI

      b. Dual chamber

          (1) DDD

  3. Implantation

      a. May be same day procedure; overnight hospital stay more typical

      b. Preoperative considerations

          (1) Education and informed consent

              (a) Postprocedure restrictions

              (b) Anticoagulants discontinued for several days (may have to initiate heparin therapy for patients with prosthetic valves)

          (2) Laboratory tests: Chemistries and coagulation studies

          (3) Chest x-ray

          (4) Antibiotics (preoperative and postoperative)

      c. Intraoperative considerations

          (1) Catheterization laboratory or operating room (OR)

          (2) Local anesthesia with mild sedation

          (3) Inserted through right or left subclavian or jugular vein

          (4) Pulse generator placement below the clavicle in a pocket between the pectoral muscle fascia and the overlying subcutaneous tissue

              (a) Depends on patient factor such as previous surgeries (e.g., mastectomy, history of radiation, central line placement, infection, dermatitis, vein occlusion or patient hobbies and dominant hand)

      d. Postoperative considerations

          (1) Complications

              (a) Perforation of the subclavian vein or right ventricle

              (b) Pneumothorax

              (c) Pacemaker failure

              (d) Electromagnetic interference (EMI): any signal, biologic or nonbiologic, that that is detected by the pacemaker and results in rate alteration or sensing abnormalities; possible causes are

               (i) Welding equipment

               (ii) Store security equipment: Maintain safe distance. Do not lean on equipment.

■ TABLE 32-6
■ ■ **Three-Position Pacemaker Code**

Chamber Paced	Chamber Sensed	Mode of Response*
V = Ventricle	V = Ventricle	I = Inhibited
A = Atrium	A = Atrium	T = Triggered
D = Atrium and ventricle	D = Atrium and ventricle	D = Atrial triggered and ventricle inhibited
0 = None	0 = None	0 = None

*Inhibited = Will not pace on sensing spontaneous cardiac activity.
Triggered = Delivers stimulus just after spontaneous depolarization and resets timing immediately on sensing spontaneous cardiac activity.

(iii) Cellular phones: Hold on ear opposite generator.

(iv) Microwave ovens are considered safe for use.

(e) Pacemaker syndrome: Hemodynamic compromise with VVI pacing as a result of intermittent loss of AV synchrony

(i) Reprogram pacemaker or replace generator.

(f) Cross-talk: Inappropriate sensing of output in dual-chamber pacemakers from one lead by the other with inhibition of pacing

(i) Reprogram pacemaker.

(f) Pacemaker-mediated tachycardia: A circular reentrant tachycardia induced by an ectopic ventricular impulse that is conducted retrograde to the atria in dual-chamber pacemakers with atrial sensing

(i) Apply a magnet over the pulse generator to disable atrial sensing.

(ii) Reprogram pacemaker.

(g) Infection

(i) Frequently produce fistula formation and chronic infection until removal of the pulse generator and as much of the leads as possible is accomplished

(2) Nursing care and follow-up

(a) Bed rest for 6 to 12 hours

(b) Limited arm movements on affected side

(c) Limited activity requiring vigorous arm movement for several weeks (e.g., golf, tennis)

(d) Written and verbal instruction regarding descriptive information and pacemaker identification (patient is given a temporary wallet card)

(e) Device registered with manufacturer for patient notification in the event of device recall

(f) Comprehensive pacemaker performance evaluation

D. Cardioverter-defibrillator implantation (ICD)

1. Indications[1]

a. Cardiac arrest not the result of a reversible cause

b. Spontaneous sustained ventricular tachycardia (VT) or ventricular fibrillation (VF)

c. Syncope of undetermined origin with clinically relevant, hemodynamically significant sustained VT or VF

d. Nonsustained VT with CAD, prior MI, left ventricular dysfunction and inducible VF or sustained VT at electrophysiology (EP) study not suppressed by a class I antiarrhythmic

2. ICD therapies

a. All currently used ICDs have the ability to defibrillate, cardiovert, and provide antitachycardia and antibradycardia pacing.

b. Preoperative considerations

(1) Same as for pacemaker except

(a) May be hospitalized preoperatively because of cardiac arrest or sustained VT

(b) Potential for significant lifestyle changes (e.g., driving) because of the possibilities of injury with syncope or working in an area with electromagnetic interference

(c) Education regarding possibility of discomfort with cardioversion

c. Intraoperative considerations

(1) Transvenous implantation in catheterization laboratory or OR

(2) Local anesthesia and sedation and analgesia; occasional need for deep sedation or general anesthesia

(3) External defibrillation patches are placed on the chest before draping patient.

(4) Implantation site determination same as for pacemaker; generator occasionally placed in the abdomen

(5) Early complications

(a) Difficult or unobtainable venous access

(b) Pneumothorax

(c) Tamponade

(d) Excessive defibrillation threshold (DFT)

(e) Refractory VF

d. Postoperative considerations

(1) Nursing care and follow-up

(a) Bed rest for 6 to 18 hours in a monitored setting

(b) Standard transthoracic defibrillation in the event of sustained VT or VF. Do not place paddles directly over generator.

(c) Limited arm movement on affected side

(d) Chest x-ray

(e) Discharge day of or day after implantation.

(f) Written and verbal instructions regarding device description (temporary identification card given), activity restrictions and instructions for what to do if device is discharged

(i) Driving typically restricted for 6 months

(ii) MRI prohibited

(2) Late complications

(a) Lead dislodgment

(b) Pocket hematoma

(c) Poor wound healing

(d) Worsening of arrhythmia

(e) Anxiety and depression: Early psychological intervention suggested for patients identified with significant anxiety and emotional distress

E. AV shunt placement and revision

1. Purpose: provide a permanent, internal vascular access for prolonged or long-term dialysis

2. Description

a. Surgically constructs an arteriovenous (AV) fistula

b. Brings arterial blood flow pressure into the vein that will be used for dialysis

(1) Significantly increases rate of venous flow to greater than 200 ml/minute

(2) Allows for completion of dialysis in a reasonable length of time (3-4 hours)

c. Minimum mortality rates

d. Technical failure rate of 10% to 15%

3. Preoperative care

a. Physical assessment issues

(1) Respiratory

(a) Common coexisting disease processes

(b) Pneumonia

(c) Pulmonary edema

(d) Uremic pleuritis

(e) Assess for

(i) Shortness of breath (SOB)

(ii) Orthopnea

(iii) Paroxysmal nocturnal dyspnea (PND)

(2) Gastrointestinal (GI)

(a) Common coexisting disease processes

(b) Delayed gastric emptying
(c) GI bleeding
(d) Assess for
    (i) Regurgitation
    (ii) Nausea and vomiting (N/V)
    (iii) Early satiety
(3) Hematology
    (a) Common coexisting disease processes
    (b) Anemia
    (c) Bleeding diathesis
    (c) Assess for
        (i) SOB
        (ii) Bruising
(4) Genitourinary (GU) and endocrine (ENDO)
    (a) Common coexisting disease processes
    (b) Oliguria or anuria
    (c) Uremia
    (d) Electrolyte and acid-base imbalance
    (e) Diabetes
    (f) Assess for
        (i) Weight (baseline and highest)
        (ii) Hiccoughs
        (iii) Anorexia
        (iv) N/V
        (v) Diarrhea
        (vi) Loss of skin integrity
(5) Central nervous system (CNS)
    (a) Common coexisting disease processes
        (i) Encephalopathy
        (ii) Seizures
        (iii) Neuropathy
        (iv) Perform musculoskeletal assessment.
  b. Recommended diagnostic studies
    (1) Chest x-ray (CXR)
    (2) Platelet count
    (3) BUN and creatinine
    (4) HCO_3
    (5) Blood glucose
  c. Determine nondominant arm.
    (1) Shunt should be easily accessible.
    (2) Should be placed on nondominant arm when possible
        (a) Allows for easy self-cannulation for home dialysis patients
        (b) Allows for increased patient ease with performance of daily activities
4. Intraoperative concerns
  a. Types of internal vascular accesses
    (1) Internal AV fistula
        (a) Creation of an actual fistula
        (b) Not available for immediate use; wound healing must occur and edema subside
        (c) Usually not accessible for weeks to months after surgery
    (2) Internal graft AV fistula
        (a) Straight or looped natural or synthetic graft
        (b) Placed in arm or thigh
        (c) Preferred for obese individuals
    (3) Internal AV graft with external access device
        (a) External access port is attached to AV graft.
        (b) Alleviates need for repeated needle insertions

    b. Common graft locations
- (1) Wrist
  - (a) "Snuff-box" fistula: Antebrachium-cephalic vein to radial artery
- (2) Forearm: radial, ulnar, or brachial artery to antecubital or brachial vein
- (3) Upper arm: brachial artery above elbow to basilic or axillary vein

    c. Anesthesia techniques
- (1) Monitored anesthesia care (MAC)
- (2) Regional
- (3) General

    d. Estimated blood loss (EBL): 25 to 100 ml

    e. Length of case: 1 to 2 hours

5. Postanesthesia priorities: Phase I PACU

    a. Avoid venipuncture, BP measurements, and injections in surgical arm.

    b. Assess for graft AND shunt patency.
- (1) Gently palpate for trill.
- (2) Auscultate for bruit.

    c. Elevate surgical arm to decrease swelling.

    d. Avoid circumferential dressings, arm bands, on surgical arm.

    e. Maintain adequate hydration.
- (1) Maintains blood pressure
- (2) Protects patency of graft

    f. Assess for bleeding. apply pressure dressing for profuse bleeding.

    g. Monitor for complications.
- (1) Thrombosis
- (2) Infection
- (3) Aneurysm
- (4) Steal syndrome
  - (a) Ischemic pain related to vascular insufficiency as a result of fistula formation
  - (b) Assess for
    - (i) Diminished pulses
    - (ii) Pallor
    - (iii) Pain distal to graft site
  - (c) Surgical revision or additional procedures required when this syndrome occurs

    h. Report any suspected or actual complications to physician.

6. Postanesthesia priorities: Phase II

    a. MAC and regional patients may be admitted directly to phase II.

    b. Continue phase I level of care.

    c. Pain management
- (1) Oral analgesia usually effective
- (2) Average discharge pain score: 1 to 2 (0 to 10 scale)

    d. Discharge teaching
- (1) Keep operative arm elevated for several days.
- (2) Avoid any venipuncture, BP measurements, and injections in operative arm.
- (3) Avoid wearing constrictive clothing, wristbands on operative site.
- (4) Instruct patient how to palpate for a thrill.
- (5) Instruct patient in assessment for and management of possible complications.

7. Postanesthesia priorities: Phase III

    a. Autogenous fistulas must adequately heal before being used for dialysis.
- (1) Blood flow increases with time.
- (2) Venous wall must adequately thicken to prevent tears and infiltration during dialysis.
- (3) Maturation time varies from 3 to 6 weeks.
- (4) Fistula should not be used for 3 weeks to avoid aneurysm formation.

        b. Teach importance of rotating injection sites when puncturing for dialysis.
           (1) Prevents aneurysm formation
           (2) Prevents shredding and eventual breakdown of shunt material
        c. Instruct patient that AV hemodialysis accesses have finite lifespan; replacements and revisions are common.
        d. Support patient on waiting list for renal transplantation.
           (1) Optimal therapy for end stage renal disease (ESRD)
           (2) Waiting time varies considerably.

V. Cardiac complications
    A. Hypotension
        1. Definition: systolic blood pressure >20% below baseline
        2. Assessment findings
           a. Low blood pressure
           b. Decreased urine output (oliguria to anuria)
           c. Tachycardia, tachypnea
           d. Pale, cool, clammy extremities
           e. Disorientation to unconsciousness
           f. Nausea
           g. Chest pain
        3. Potential causes
           a. Decreased intravascular volume
           b. Left ventricular failure
           c. Decreased vascular tone
           d. Exhaustion of catecholamines (e.g., prolonged pain)
        4. Treatment
           a. Oxygen therapy
           b. Assess and replace intravascular volume.
           c. For ventricular failure—coronary vasodilators, decrease afterload, inotropic support
           d. Maximize vascular tone—discontinue vasodilators, administer vasoconstrictive agents.
           e. Pain management
        5. Prevention through monitoring of preoperative, intraoperative, and postoperative volume status and titration of vasoactive and cardiac medications.
    B. Hypertension
        1. Definition: BP >20% to 30% above baseline blood pressure
        2. Assessment findings
           a. Elevated blood pressure
           b. Signs of sympathetic stimulation
           c. Headache with extreme elevations
           d. Decreased level of consciousness (LOC) with disruption of cerebral autoregulation and cerebral hemorrhage
           e. Signs of ventricular failure and pulmonary edema with long-standing elevations (>190/100 for 3 hours or more)
        3. Potential causes
           a. Preexisting disease
           b. CNS damage
           c. Cardiovascular impairment
           d. Excess catecholamine production (e.g., pain, emotional stress)
           e. Hypoxemia and hypercarbia
           f. Endocrinopathies
           g. Hypothermia
           h. Excess intravascular volume
           i. Sudden withdrawal or overdose of medications
           j. Visceral distention
           k. Preeclampsia

   4. Treatment
      a. Assess for and alleviate cause.
         (1) Restart antihypertensives.
         (2) Maximize cardiac function.
         (3) Pain and stress management
         (4) Maximize respiratory function.
         (5) Rewarming
         (6) Correct fluid overload (fluid restriction and diuretics).
         (7) Decrease visceral distention (Foley catheter, nasogastric tube).
   5. Prevention
      a. Assess for potential causes early.
      b. Patients to take antihypertensives on day of surgery
C. Cardiac dysrhythmias
   1. Causes
      a. Disturbances in automaticity—speeding and slowing
      b. Disturbances in conduction—too slow or fast
      c. Combinations of altered automaticity and conduction
   2. Normal ECG (Figure 32-7)
      a. P wave—represents origination of impulse in sinus node; abnormality indicates impulse origination in some other area of heart; atrial depolarization.
      b. PR interval—represents conduction through atria and AV node and into bundle of His.
      c. QRS complex—represents conduction through bundle branches; ventricular depolarization
      d. T wave—ventricular repolarization
   3. Rhythm assessment
      a. Electrode placement
         (1) Lead I: Positive left arm; negative right arm
         (2) Lead II: Positive left leg; negative right arm
         (3) Lead III: Positive left leg; negative left arm
      b. Evaluate rate
         (1) Bradycardia (<60 beats per minute [bpm])
         (2) Tachycardia (>100 bpm)
      c. Evaluate regularity.
         (1) R-R interval
         (2) P-P interval

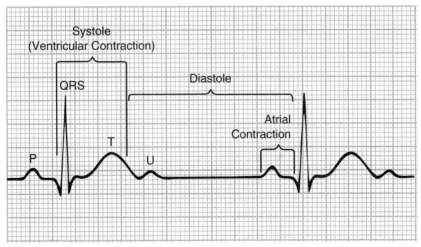

FIGURE 32-7 ■ Normal ECG. (From Grauer K: *A practical guide to ECG interpretation,* ed 2. St Louis: Mosby, 1998, p 4.)

  d. Evaluate P waves.
      (1) Presence: Does a P wave precede every QRS complex?
      (2) Morphology: Do all the P waves look alike?
      (3) Relationship to QRS complex
          (a) P-R interval (normal 0.12-0.20 seconds)
          (b) Length and consistency
  e. Evaluate QRS complex.
      (1) Width (normal = 0.12 seconds)
4. Dysrhythmia recognition and treatment
  a. Ventricular fibrillation (Figure 32-8)
      (1) Description
          (a) ECG with no organized rhythm
          (b) No cardiac output
          (c) Coarse or fine refers to amplitude
      (2) ECG criteria
          (a) Rate: rapid and too disorganized to count
          (b) Rhythm: irregularly irregular
          (c) No P wave, QRS complex, ST segment, or T wave
      (3) Treatment
          (a) Initiate primary and secondary assessment.
          (b) Immediate defibrillation: 200, 300, 360 joules
          (c) Vasopressin, 40 units intravenously (IV) (single dose only), or
              epinephrine, 1 mg IV or by endotracheal (ET) tube (twice the IV
              dose)
          (d) Defibrillate with 360 joules.
          (e) Consider antiarrhythmics.
              (i) Amiodarone, 300 mg IV
              (ii) Lidocaine, 1 to 1.5 mg/kg IV or by ET tube (twice the IV dose)
              (iii) Magnesium, 1-2 g IV
              (iv) Procainamide, 20-50 mg/minute up to 17 mg/kg total
          (f) Resume attempts to defibrillate.
          (g) Continue epinephrine 1 mg IV every 3-5 minutes, followed by
              cardiopulmonary resuscitation (CPR) and defibrillation. May
              initiate epinephrine 10-20 minutes after single dose of
              vasopressin
  b. Pulseless electrical activity (PEA; electromechanical dissociation)
      (1) Description: can be any rhythm on ECG (except VT/VF); however,
          no pulse and no blood pressure can be detected.
      (2) Treatment
          (a) Initiate primary and secondary assessment.
          (b) Assess for and treat reversible causes (five Hs and five Ts).
              (i) Hypovolemia
              (ii) Hypoxia
              (iii) Hydrogen ion–acidosis
              (iv) Hyperkalemia, hypokalemia

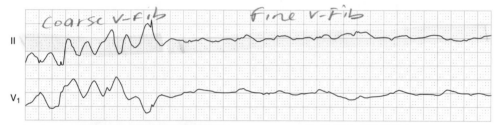

FIGURE 32-8 ■ Coarse ventricular fibrillation degenerating into fine ventricular fibrillation. (From Paul S: Interpreting basic cardiac rhythms. In Paul S, Hera J, editors: *The nurse's guide to cardiac rhythm interpretation.* Philadelphia: WB Saunders, 1998, p 144.)

(v) Hypothermia

(vi) Tablets (drug overdose, accidents)

(vii) Tamponade, cardiac

(viii) Tension pneumothorax

(ix) Thrombosis, coronary

(x) Thrombosis pulmonary (embolism)

(c) Epinephrine, 1 mg IV or by ET tube (twice the IV dose); repeat every 3-5 minutes.

(d) Atropine, 1 mg IV (if PEA rate is slow); repeat every 3-5 minutes to a total dose of 0.04 mg/kg.

c. Asystole (Figure 32-9)

(1) Description

(a) Total absence of ventricular electrical activity

(b) No pulse or blood pressure

(2) ECG criteria: complete absence of activity; "flat line"

(3) Treatment

(a) Initiate primary and secondary assessment.

(b) Transcutaneous pacing

(c) Epinephrine, 1 mg IV or by ET tube (twice the IV dose); repeat every 3-5 minutes.

(d) Atropine, 1 mg IV (if PEA rate is slow); repeat every 3-5 minutes to a total dose of 0.04 mg/kg.

(e) Consider withholding or ceasing resuscitative efforts.

d. Bradycardias

(1) Sinus bradycardia (Figure 32-10)

(a) Description: characterized by decrease in heart rate caused by slowing of sinus node; may be a result of sinus node disease, increased parasympathetic tone, or drug effects (beta-blockers, digitalis)

(b) ECG criteria

(i) Rate: <60 bpm

(ii) Rhythm: regular

(iii) P waves: upright

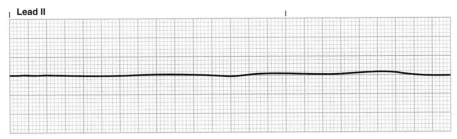

FIGURE 32-9 ■ Asystole. (From Huszar RJ: *Pocket guide to basic dysrhythmias*, ed 3. St Louis: Mosby, 2002, p 28.)

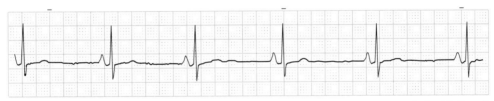

FIGURE 32-10 ■ Sinus bradycardia. (From Paul S: Interpreting basic cardiac rhythms. In Paul S, Hera J, editors: *The nurse's guide to cardiac rhythm interpretation*. Philadelphia: WB Saunders, 1998, p 62.)

        (c) Treatment—if symptomatic, consider
           (i) Atropine, 0.5 to 1 mg IV to a total of 0.03 mg/kg
           (ii) Transcutaneous pacing
           (iii) Dopamine, 5-20 μg/kg/minute
           (iv) Epinephrine, 2 to 10 μg/minute
           (v) Isoproterenol, 2 to 10 μg/minute

(2) First-degree block (Figure 32-11)
    (a) Description: Delayed conduction through the AV node between the atria and ventricles
    (b) ECG criteria
        (i) Regular rhythm
        (ii) P wave followed by QRS
        (iii) Prolonged PR interval (>0.20 sec)
        (iv) QRS normal
    (c) Treatment: None, does not result in symptoms

(3) Second-degree type I: Wenckebach block (Figure 32-12)
    (a) ECG criteria
        (i) Ventricular rate less than atrial rate
        (ii) Rhythm usually irregular
        (iii) P waves normal and followed by QRS except for dropped beat
        (iv) PR interval gets progressively longer until ventricular beat is dropped.
        (v) QRS normal
    (b) Treatment: None; generally not symptomatic; look for underlying cause and monitor rhythm.

(4) Second-degree type II Mobitz block (Figure 32-13)
    (a) ECG criteria
        (i) Ventricular rate less than atrial rate
        (ii) Rhythm regular or irregular (block may be variable)
        (iii) P waves normal and PR interval consistent for conducted beats
        (iv) Intermittent P wave not followed by a QRS
        (v) QRS normal
    (b) Treatment
        (i) Same as symptomatic sinus bradycardia except avoid atropine and utilize transcutaneous pacing or sympathomimetic drugs (prevents progression to a higher-grade block).

(5) Third-degree block (Figure 32-14)
    (a) Description: atrial and ventricular asynchrony, total loss of electrical conduction between the atria and ventricles
    (b) ECG criteria
        (i) Ventricular rate, 40 to 60 bpm; atrial rate, 60 to 100 bpm
        (ii) P wave normal, QRS may be normal or widened.
        (iii) P waves and QRS unrelated to each other

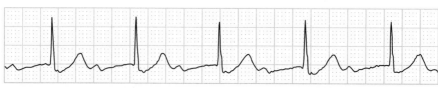

FIGURE 32-11 ■ First degree AV block. (From Paul S: Interpreting basic cardiac rhythms. In Paul S, Hera J, editors: *The nurse's guide to cardiac rhythm interpretation.* Philadelphia: WB Saunders, 1998, p 176.)

        (c) Treatment
           (i) Same as symptomatic sinus bradycardia, except avoid atropine and utilize transcutaneous pacing or sympathomimetic drugs

    e. Narrow complex tachyarrhythmias

      (1) Evaluate patient for serious signs and symptoms caused by tachycardia.

      (2) If unstable: Sedation and synchronized cardioversion
        (a) 100 joules
        (b) 200 joules
        (c) 300 joules
        (d) 360 joules

      (3) Have available at bedside.
        (a) SpO$_2$ monitor
        (b) Suction device
        (c) IV line
        (d) Intubation equipment

      (4) Attempt to slow and diagnose rhythm via
        (a) Vagal maneuvers
        (b) Adenosine, 6 mg IV push followed by fluid bolus (12 mg dose may be repeated twice).

Lead II

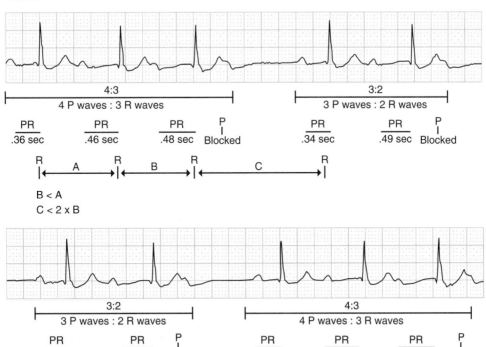

(continuous strip)

FIGURE 32-12 ■ Second degree type I (Wenckebach) block. (From Paul S: Interpreting basic cardiac rhythms. In Paul S, Hera J, editors: *The nurse's guide to cardiac rhythm interpretation.* Philadelphia: WB Saunders, 1998, p 177.)

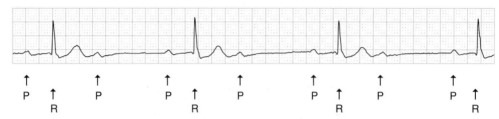

FIGURE 32-13 ■ Second degree type II block. (From Paul S: Interpreting basic cardiac rhythms. In Paul S, Hera J, editors: *The nurse's guide to cardiac rhythm interpretation.* Philadelphia: WB Saunders, 1998, p 181.)

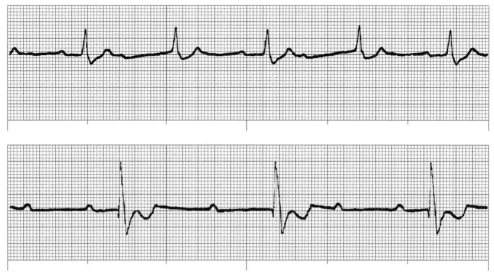

FIGURE 32-14 ■ Third degree AV block. (From Aehlert B: *ECG's made easy.* St Louis: Mosby, 1995, p 144.)

(5) Sinus tachycardia (Figure 32-15)—characterized by normal-looking QRS, rate greater than 100, regular rhythm, upright P waves in leads I, II, and AVF; evaluation and treatment of causes usually sufficient to resolve (pain, hypoxemia, hypovolemia)

(6) Junctional tachycardia (Figure 32-16)

   (a) Rate >100 with normal-looking QRS and P waves either absent, inverted, or following the QRS complex

   (b) Best treated by pharmacologic suppression of the AV node. Avoid DC cardioversion.

   (c) Assess for drug effects (often related to digoxin toxicity).

(7) Paroxysmal supraventricular tachycardia (Figure 32-17)

   (a) Rate >100 with normal-looking QRS and regular rhythm; sudden onset frequently initiated with a premature beat

   (b) Synchronized cardioversion effective in those with poor EF; often converts with adenosine; may utilize medications (calcium channel blockers, beta-blockers) to slow rate

(8) Multifocal atrial tachycardia (Figure 32-18)

   (a) Characterized by a rate >100 and at least three different morphologies of the P wave; normal-appearing QRS

   (b) Best treated with medications to slow rate; avoid cardioversion.

   (c) Typically have underlying pulmonary disease

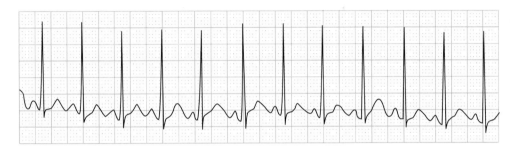

FIGURE 32-15 ■ Sinus tachycardia. (From Paul S: Interpreting basic cardiac rhythms. In Paul S, Hera J, editors: *The nurse's guide to cardiac rhythm interpretation.* Philadelphia: WB Saunders, 1998, p 61.)

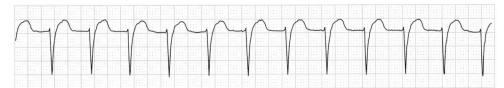

FIGURE 32-16 ■ Junctional tachycardia. (From Paul S: Interpreting basic cardiac rhythms. In Paul S, Hera J, editors: *The nurse's guide to cardiac rhythm interpretation.* Philadelphia: WB Saunders, 1998, p 113.)

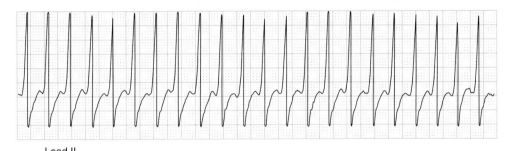

Lead II

FIGURE 32-17 ■ PSVT. (From Paul S: Interpreting basic cardiac rhythms. In Paul S, Hera J, editors: *The nurse's guide to cardiac rhythm interpretation.* Philadelphia: WB Saunders, 1998, p 115.)

    (9) Select slowing agents according to origin of tachycardia and pumping ability of myocardium.
        (a) Amiodarone, 150 mg/100 ml D_5W over 10 minutes, followed by 1 mg/minute infusion for 6 hours, and then 0.5 mg/minute for a maximum daily dose of 2 g
        (b) Beta-blocking agents
        (c) Calcium channel blocking agents
        (d) Digoxin
   (10) Atrial fibrillation and flutter (Figures 32-19 and 32-20)
        (a) Atrial fibrillation—atrial rate too rapid to be counted; no organized atrial activity, therefore no P waves; irregular ventricular rhythm; normal QRS unless aberrant conduction present
        (b) Atrial flutter—atrial rate usually 300 but may range from 220 to 350, atrial rhythm regular, ventricular rhythm usually regular but may be irregular, P waves resemble flutter and sawtooth waves
        (c) Determine if duration >48 hours.

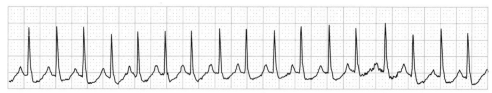

FIGURE 32-18 ■ Multifocal atrial tachycardia. (From Paul S: Interpreting basic cardiac rhythms. In Paul S, Hera J, editors: *The nurse's guide to cardiac rhythm interpretation.* Philadelphia: WB Saunders, 1998, p 83.)

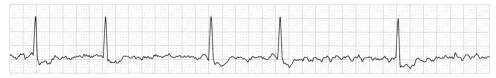

FIGURE 32-19 ■ Atrial fibrillation. (From Paul S: Interpreting basic cardiac rhythms. In Paul S, Hera J, editors: *The nurse's guide to cardiac rhythm interpretation.* Philadelphia: WB Saunders, 1998, p 87.)

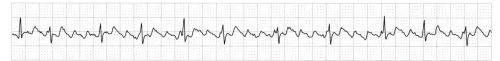

FIGURE 32-20 ■ Atrial flutter. (From Paul S: Interpreting basic cardiac rhythms. In Paul S, Hera J, editors: *The nurse's guide to cardiac rhythm interpretation.* Philadelphia: WB Saunders, 1998, p 85.)

        (d) Slow rate with appropriate agent depending on myocardial contractility

        (e) Initiate anticoagulation.

        (f) Synchronized cardioversion only if unstable

   f. Wide complex

      (1) Ventricular tachycardia (Figure 32-21); description: three or more beats of ventricular origin in a row with a rate greater than 100 bpm

      (2) ECG criteria

        (a) Rate: 100 to 220 bpm

        (b) Rhythm: usually regular

        (c) P waves: difficult to detect

        (d) QRS complex: wide and bizarre

        (e) Monomorphic: Regular with consistent appearance to complex

        (f) Polymorphic: Complexes are inconsistent and may be related to a prolonged Q-T interval resulting in a thick and thin spindle pattern. Commonly referred to as torsades de pointes (Figure 32-22)

   g. Premature ventricular complex (PVC)

      (1) Abnormal QRS usually wider than 0.12 seconds, full compensatory pause (Figure 32-23); indicative of ventricles firing prematurely; may occur isolated or in pairs (couplets) (Figure 32-24); may also occur from different foci in ventricles (multifocal/multiformed) (Figure 32-25); may occur every other beat (bigeminy) (Figure 32-26); every third beat (trigeminy), or every fourth beat (quadrigeminy); occurring too close to T wave may result in VT or VF (Figure 32-27)

5. Defibrillation and cardioversion
   a. Defibrillation
      (1) Indications
          (a) Ventricular fibrillation—initial intervention
          (b) Pulseless ventricular tachycardia—initial intervention
      (2) Technique
          (a) Confirm dysrhythmia.
          (b) Apply conductive gel to electrodes if necessary or use saline or gelled pads.

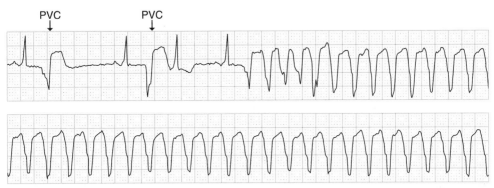

FIGURE 32-21 ■ Ventricular tachycardia. (From Paul S: Interpreting basic cardiac rhythms. In Paul S, Hera J, editors: *The nurse's guide to cardiac rhythm interpretation.* Philadelphia: WB Saunders, 1998, p 138.)

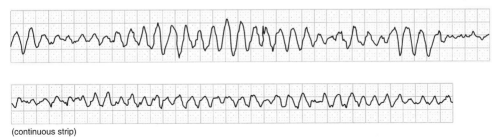

(continuous strip)

FIGURE 32-22 ■ Torsades de pointes degenerating into ventricular fibrillation. (From Paul S: Interpreting basic cardiac rhythms. In Paul S, Hera J, editors: *The nurse's guide to cardiac rhythm interpretation.* Philadelphia: WB Saunders, 1998, p 141.)

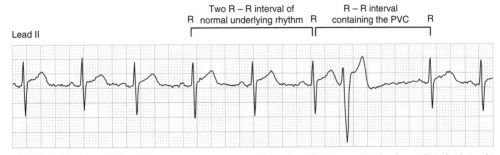

FIGURE 32-23 ■ PVCs with compensatory pause. (From Paul S: Interpreting basic cardiac rhythms. In Paul S, Hera J, editors: *The nurse's guide to cardiac rhythm interpretation.* Philadelphia: WB Saunders, 1998, p 132.)

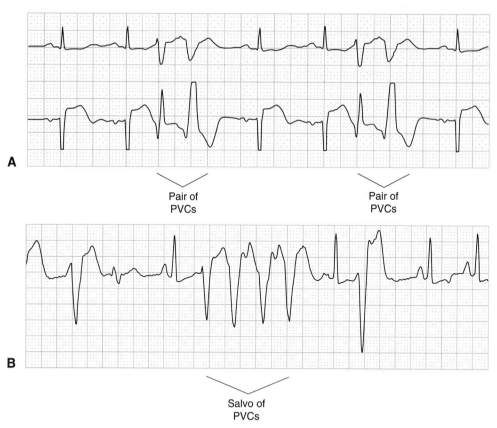

FIGURE 32-24 ■ Ventricular pairs (couplets). (From Paul S: Interpreting basic cardiac rhythms. In Paul S, Hera J, editors: *The nurse's guide to cardiac rhythm interpretation.* Philadelphia: WB Saunders, 1998, p 131.)

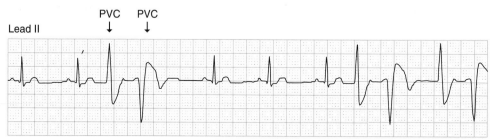

FIGURE 32-25 ■ Multiformed (multifocal) PVCs. (From Paul S: Interpreting basic cardiac rhythms. In Paul S, Hera J, editors: *The nurse's guide to cardiac rhythm interpretation.* Philadelphia: WB Saunders, 1998, p 132.)

    (c) Turn on defibrillator.
    (d) Select energy level.
       (i) Adults: 200 joules for adult, if ineffective; progress to 300, then 360 joules
      (ii) Pediatrics: 2 joules/kg of body weight; progress to 4 joules/kg if ineffective.
    (e) Charge defibrillator.
    (f) Apply paddles to chest.
       (i) One paddle just below right clavicle on chest

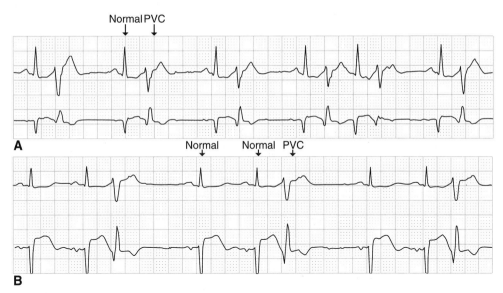

FIGURE 32-26 ■ **A,** Ventricular bigeminy. **B,** Ventricular trigeminy. (From Paul S: Interpreting basic cardiac rhythms. In Paul S, Hera J, editors: *The nurse's guide to cardiac rhythm interpretation.* Philadelphia: WB Saunders, 1998, p 133.)

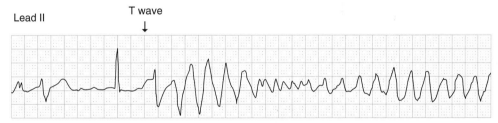

FIGURE 32-27 ■ R on T phenomenon. (From Paul S: Interpreting basic cardiac rhythms. In Paul S, Hera J, editors: *The nurse's guide to cardiac rhythm interpretation.* Philadelphia: WB Saunders, 1998, p 134.)

    (ii) One paddle to left of nipple in midaxillary line
    (iii) Use 25-lb paddle pressure on both paddles.
   (g) Clear personal contact with patient verbally and visually.
   (h) Deliver countershock.
   (i) Evaluate rhythm and pulse.
   (j) Repeat as necessary; select energy level.
  (3) Precautions
   (a) Know how defibrillator works in advance of need.
   (b) Defibrillation most effective when done promptly
   (c) Clear area to avoid delivering shock to others.
   (d) Always confirm rhythm and pulse before and after shock.
 b. Cardioversion
  (1) Indications
   (a) Treatment of choice for hemodynamically unstable tachydysrhythmias
    (i) Ventricular tachycardia
    (ii) Supraventricular tachycardias ⟵
  (2) Technique
   (a) If patient is conscious, consider sedation or analgesia; provide explanation.

      (b) Procedure is same as with defibrillation except

        (i) Unit is set on synchronous mode.

          [a] Adults: Initial setting is 50-100 joules; advance to 200, 300, and 360 joules if ineffective.

          [b] Pediatrics: Initial setting is 0.5-1.0 joules/kg of body weight; advance to 2 joules/kg if ineffective.

    (3) Precautions

      (a) Same as defibrillation

      (b) Recognition that ventricular fibrillation may occur

        (i) Turn off synchronous mode, charge unit to defibrillation energy level, and defibrillate.

        (ii) Prepare to initiate CPR.

      (c) Monitor per institutions sedation and analgesia policy.

6. Cardiac pacing

  a. Temporary pacing

    (1) Single chamber: Use of a pulse generator to provide electrical stimulation of either the atria or the ventricle to produce an action potential resulting in myocardial contraction

      (a) Indications

        (i) Intermittent AV nodal dysfunction or sinus bradycardia

        (ii) Suppression of ventricular ectopy

    (2) Dual chamber: Sequential pacing of the atrium and ventricle

      (a) Indications

        (i) Hemodynamically compromised patients with AV nodal dysfunction

    (3) Rapid atrial pacing: Delivery of pacing discharges at rates of up to 800 beats per minutes resulting in atrial overdrive

      (a) Indications

        (i) Paroxysmal atrial tachycardia or atrial flutter

    (4) Transcutaneous: Electrical energy delivered utilizing a defibrillator with pacing capabilities via gel pads applied to the chest wall in the anterior and posterior (preferred) or sternal and apex position

      (a) Indications: Emergency treatment of symptomatic bradycardic dysrhythmias

    (5) Transvenous: Pacing wires are inserted through a central venous access (i.e., femoral, subclavian, internal jugular or brachial).

      (a) Indications: Short-term therapy or bridge to permanent pacer implantation

      (b) Removal

        (i) Turn off generator

        (ii) Gently apply continuous tension to wires and remove in one continuous motion. Stop if resistance felt.

        (iii) Maintain digital pressure at insertion site until hemostasis achieved. Apply dressing.

        (iv) Observe rhythm, pulse and BP, insertion site and distal extremity every 15 minutes four times, then every 30 minutes two times.

    (6) Epicardial: Application of pacing wires to the surface of the epicardium via a surgical incision; most commonly done related to cardiac bypass or valvular surgery

      (a) Removal

        (i) Day before discharge

        (ii) Put patient in supine position and apply gentle traction after severing the skin suture.

        (iii) If unable to remove with gentle traction, swab entry site with antiseptic solution and cut wire off at skin while applying gentle traction on wires.

        (iv) Complications: cardiac tamponade

(v) Assess patient at 5 minute, 15 minute, and 30 minute intervals after removal.

(7) Precautions and common problems (Table 32-7)

(a) Direct stimulation of myocardium resulting in VF

(i) Insulate external pacing wire with needle cap, finger cot, or nonconductive tape and secure to chest when not in use.

(ii) Protect wire from moisture.

(b) Failure to pace or capture: Absent pacer spikes or spikes that are not followed by a QRS complex (Figure 32-28)

(i) Examine all pacing wire connections.

(ii) Increase milliamps.

(iii) Replace battery and/or pacing generator.

(iv) Assess for metabolic and acid/base abnormalities.

(v) Inform physician and prepare to support patient with transcutaneous pacing and pharmacologic agents (may be caused by pacer wire fracture or detachment from myocardium).

(c) Failure to sense (Figure 32-29): Undersensing of inherent patient complexes (pacer spikes occurring closely adjacent to or on inherent complexes) or oversensing (inhibition of pacer spikes in relation to movement or artifact)

(i) Adjust sensitivity setting while observing rhythm.

(ii) Change battery and/or pulse generator.

(iii) Undersensing: Conversion from unipolar to bipolar or vice versa

Cardiac Pacing

b. Permanent (see previous discussion in cardiac procedures)

(1) Indications

(a) Complete heart block

(b) Symptomatic bradycardia associated with sinus node dysfunction or second-degree heart block

(c) Acute MI with persistent, advanced second or third degree heart block

(d) Recurrent syncope associated with hypersensitive carotid sinus syndrome

(e) Advanced block with atrial fibrillation or flutter and symptomatic slow ventricular rate

(f) Symptomatic bradycardia secondary to pharmacologic therapy

---

■ TABLE 32-7
■ ■ **Troubleshooting Temporary Pacemakers**

Problem	Actions
Failure to capture	1. Check lead connections.
	2. Check lead placement by X-ray if transvenous.
	3. ↑ mA.
	4. Change battery.
	5. Reposition patient.
	6. Prepare to switch from transvenous to transcutaneous if applicable.
Failure to sense	1. ↑ sensitivity.
	2. Change battery.
Failure to pace	1. ↓ sensitivity.
	2. Switch to asynchronous mode.
	3. ↑ rate.

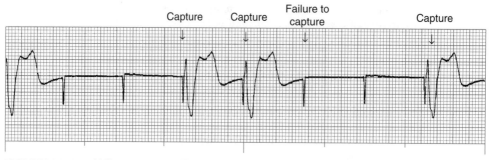

FIGURE 32-28 ■ Failure to capture. (From Aehlert B: *ECG's made easy*, 2nd ed. St Louis: Mosby, 2002, p 183.)

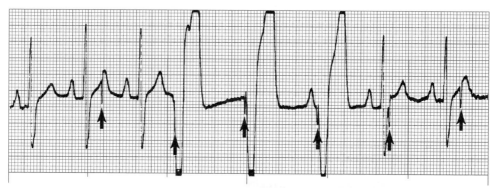

FIGURE 32-29 ■ Failure to sense. (From Aehlert B: *ECG's made easy*, 2nd ed. St Louis: Mosby, 2002, p 184.)

Cardiac Complications Continued

D. Hemorrhage
   1. Definition: loss of intravascular volume
   2. Assessment findings
      a. Visible blood on dressings, in drains, emesis
      b. Restlessness
      c. Swelling at surgical site
      d. Hypotension and signs of hypovolemia (*tachycardia*)
      e. Ear, nose, and throat—frequent swallowing, hemoptysis, vomiting blood
      f. Abdominal—increased girth, abdominal pain and hardness
   3. Potential causes
      a. Loss of vascular integrity
      b. Coagulation disorders
   4. Treatment
      a. Stop active bleeding.
      b. Support circulation—transfusion usually not indicated unless hemoglobin <7 or hematocrit <21, or unless autologous blood available or patient is symptomatic (patients with cardiac dysfunction will need transfusion earlier because of the increased need for oxygen carrying capacity)
      c. Patient comfort measures—decrease anxiety, keep warm, pain management
   5. Prevention
      a. Assess for bleeding disorders preoperatively.
      b. Assess for medications that interfere with coagulation and discontinue prior to surgery (include over-the-counter and herbal preparations).

           c. Maintain normothermic body temperatures.

           d. Investigate all elevations in HR for cause (i.e. pain, stress response, bleeding).

           e. Monitor closely postoperatively for unexplained or excessive bleeding.

    E. Peripheral circulatory compromise

        1. Definition: decreased or absent blood flow to an extremity

        2. Assessment findings

           a. Color changes of extremity (pale, flushed to blue)

           b. Swelling if obstructed venous return

           c. Diminished or absent pulses

           d. Delayed or absent capillary refill

           e. Pain, paresthesia

        3. Potential causes

           a. Bandage, splint, cast too tight

           b. Occurrence of thrombus or embolus

        4. Treatment

           a. Relieve restriction to blood flow by loosening constricting bandages.

           b. Possible return to surgery for thrombectomy or embolectomy

        5. Prevention

           a. Use caution when applying circumferential bandages.

           b. Evaluation of surgical site extremities

    F. MI (See Chapter 39 for discussion on CAD and MI)

    G. CHF

        1. New York Classifications of Heart Failure (Table 32-8)

        2. Preoperative considerations

           a. Weight gain may indicate worsening failure.

           b. Prone to electrolyte imbalances

           c. Must have preoperative ECG and chest x-ray

        3. Intraoperative considerations

           a. Prone to dysrhythmias

           b. Preload sensitive

               (1) Myocardial function dependent upon sufficient volume status

               (2) Prone to pulmonary edema with volume overload

           c. May develop myocardial ischemia with small to moderate loss of hemoglobin

---

■ TABLE 32-8
■ ■ **New York Heart Classification of Cardiovascular Disease**

Class Subjective	Assessment	Prognosis
I	Normal cardiac output without systemic or pulmonary congestion: asymptomatic at rest and on heavy exertion	Good
II	Normal cardiac output maintained with a moderate increase in pulmonary-systemic congestion; symptomatic on exertion	Good with therapy
III	Normal cardiac output maintained with a marked increase in pulmonary-systemic congestion; symptomatic on mild exercise	Fair with therapy
IV	Cardiac output reduced at rest with a marked increase in pulmonary-systemic congestion; symptomatic at rest	Guarded despite therapy

From Killip T, Kimball JT: Treatment of myocardial infarction in a coronary care unit. A two year experience with 250 patients. *Am J Cardiol* 20:457, 1967.

4. Postoperative considerations

    a. Phase I

        (1) Tachycardia may indicate decreased cardiac output.

        (2) Narrowing pulse pressure may be an indication of decreasing stroke volume.

        (3) Monitor ECG closely for changes consistent with myocardial ischemia.

        (4) Monitor fluid status closely.

    b. Phase II

        (1) Teaching to include signs and symptoms of heart failure

        (2) Instruct in daily weight and need to contact physician for weight gain of three pounds or more.

VI. Basic life support–airway management and CPR

Note: Consider patients DNR/DNI status (see Box 32-3).

    A. Establish unresponsiveness.

    B. Call for assistance; activate emergency system in your PACU.

    C. Open airway with head-tilt and chin lift, and assess for breathing: look, listen, and feel for chest and air movement.

    D. If patient is not breathing, give two breaths over 2 seconds each (two puffs if an infant <1 year); child 1 to 8 years, use appropriately smaller volumes.

        1. Bag-valve-mask (Ambu bag)

        Ventilate over 1.5 seconds with oxygen and 2 seconds without oxygen.

        2. Mouth to mask or appropriate barrier device

            a. If an infant, both nose and mouth are covered.

            b. Determine that airway is patent by observing chest rise.

                (1) If no movement noted, reposition airway, and attempt to ventilate again; if unable to ventilate, suspect obstruction; attempt to remove obstruction by finger sweep of mouth, suctioning, and abdominal thrusts (for an infant, no blind finger sweep is used, and chest compressions replace abdominal compressions to relieve obstruction).

    E. Once it is confirmed that patient is being ventilated, check for pulse (location: carotid artery in adults and children; brachial artery in infants).

        1. If pulse is present, ventilate patient once every 3 seconds for an infant or child and once every 5 seconds for an adult; if pulse is not present, initiate CPR.

■ BOX 32-3
■ **AMERICAN SOCIETY OF PERIANESTHESIA NURSES POSITION STATEMENT ON THE PERIANESTHESIA PATIENT WITH A DO-NOT-RESUSCITATE ADVANCE DIRECTIVE (ASPAN 1996)**

"The American Society of PeriAnesthesia Nurses (ASPAN) recommends that at the time of surgery and prior to receiving any anesthetic medication, a patient with an active do-not-resuscitate advance directive must reconsider this designation and reclarify wishes about resuscitation during the perianesthesia period.

To limit potential for ethical dilemmas, the patient's informed consent will include discussion of the advance directive, living will, or physician order that specifies do-not-resuscitate (DNR) or do-not-intubate (DNI) during a candid and well-documented conversation with physicians and appropriate significant other(s).

Each facility establishes and communicates a policy that identifies resources and procedures that detail the management of a patient's DNR/DNI status during the perianesthesia period."

From American Society of PeriAnesthesia Nurses: *Standards of Perianesthesia Nursing Practice.* Thorofare, NJ: American Society of PeriAnesthesia Nurses, 2002.

    F. CPR: process of combining ventilation and external chest compression as means to reverse or prevent cardiac and/or respiratory arrest

        1. Infant

            a. Compress 0.5 to 1 inch with two fingers one finger-width below the nipple line on the sternum at a rate of 100 compressions per minute.

            b. If two rescuers, may use both thumbs over the sternum with hands encircling chest

            c. Compression to ventilation ratio: 5:1 until intubated then 3:1 in the newborn; pause for ventilation until intubated.

        2. Child

            a. Compress 1 to 1.5 inches with the heel of one hand over the lower half of the sternum at a rate of 100 compressions per minute.

            b. Compression to ventilation ratio: 5:1 for one or two rescuer(s); pause for ventilation until intubated.

        3. Adult

            a. Compress 1.5 to 2 inches with two hands over the lower half of the sternum at a rate of 100 compressions per minute.

            b. Compression to ventilation ratio: 15:2 for one or two rescuer(s); pause for ventilation until intubated.

    G. Apply automated external defibrillator (AED) (if available).

        1. Power on the AED.

        2. Attach AED electrodes to patient's bare chest.

            a. Wipe off medication ointments.

            b. Avoid permanent pacer if possible.

            c. Dry off chest if wet.

            d. May need to quickly shave chest

        3. Analyze rhythm (do not touch the patient).

        4. Shock if advised (up to three times).

            a. *Do not touch the patient* or bed.

        5. If no shock advised, resume CPR for 1 minute and then reanalyze rhythm.

VII. Advanced cardiac life support: Adult and pediatric (ACLS/PALS) (see Box 32-1)

    A. ACLS universal algorithm

        1. Initiate BLS including early defibrillation.

        2. Airway: Consider placing an airway device (ET tube, combitube, laryngeal mask airway [LMA]).

        3. Breathing: Primary assessment for airway device placement (auscultation)

        4. Breathing: Secondary assessment for airway device placement (end-tidal CO_2, esophageal detector)

        5. Breathing: Secure tube.

        6. Breathing: Reassess effectiveness of ventilation.

        7. Circulation: Establish IV access if not present.

        8. Circulation: Identify rhythm, and administer appropriate drug regimen per appropriate algorithm.

        9. Differential diagnosis: Search for treatable, reversible causes.

    B. PALS universal algorithm

        1. Assess for responsiveness, and initiate BLS if no pulse.

        2. Pulse present

            a. Because of poor outcomes for pediatric pulseless cardiac arrest, emphasis must be placed on detection and treatment of respiratory failure and arrest and shock.

            b. Investigate and treat suspected cause.

                (1) Trauma

                (2) Special resuscitation circumstances

                (3) Arrhythmias

                    (a) Bradycardia

                    (b) Tachycardia

   3. Pulse absent
      a. Investigate and treat suspected cause.
         (1) VF and VT
         (2) PEA
         (3) Asystole
   C. Drug administration in emergency situation
      1. Know the drugs to be given; this is the principle of continuing education and ACLS repeat evaluation.
      2. IV drugs require circulation, either CPR or an effective, independent rhythm, and blood pressure of greater than 60 mm Hg systolic.
      3. IV drugs require an IV line; some require a central line; get IV access early in emergency situation in the largest vein possible.
      4. In absence of IV line, certain medications may be given by an ET tube, including lidocaine, epinephrine, atropine, and naloxone (some people remember these drugs with the acronym LEAN, because this word is spelled by the first letters of the drugs).
      5. If medications are given by an ET tube, they should be diluted into 10 ml of saline or distilled water, given as distally as possible, and followed with immediate Ambu bagging to force medications into lungs; double the IV dose when administering per ET tube.
      6. IV infusions of vasoactive medications—recommend arterial line placement to monitor blood pressure changes.
      7. Route, dosage, and time of all medications given should be documented along with patient response and associated rhythm; use of an arrest record can facilitate documentation.
      8. Refer to 2002 ASPAN Standards Resource 6 for detailed recommendations related to adult and pediatric emergency drugs and supplies (see Box 32-2).
VIII. Cardioactive drugs
   A. Inotropic agents
      1. Epinephrine
         a. Mechanism of action
            (1) Alpha and beta activity (beta greater than alpha) resulting in increased systemic vascular resistance (SVR), BP, automaticity, HR, coronary and cerebral blood flow, myocardial contraction, and myocardial oxygen consumption
         b. Indications
            (1) Drug of choice in asystole, PEA
            (2) Circulatory shock
         c. Dosage and route
            (1) Adult
               (a) Dose: 1 mg of 1:10,000 solution IV every 3 to 5 minutes
               (b) Double dose by ET tube
               (c) Infusion, 4 mg/250 ml D_5W; start at 1 µg/min and titrate to effect.
            (2) Pediatric
               (a) IV and intraosseous (IO): 0.01 mg/kg of 1:10,000 solution every 3 to 5 minutes
               (b) ET tube: 0.1 mg/kg
         d. Precautions
            (1) Not compatible with sodium bicarbonate
            (2) Excessive effects can produce ischemia, hypertension, and ventricular ectopy.
      2. Norepinephrine
         a. Mechanism of action: alpha 1–agonist, alpha 2–agonist, and beta 1–agonist (alpha greater than beta) resulting in increased myocardial contractility and vasoconstriction
         b. Indication: hemodynamically significant hypotension that does not respond to epinephrine or dopamine

    c. Dosage and route

        (1) IV infusion: 1-4 mg/250 ml D_5W. Begin at 2 μg/minute, and titrate to desired effect.

    d. Precautions

        (1) Strict BP monitoring requires use of arterial line.

        (2) Increases myocardial oxygen needs

        (3) May precipitate dysrhythmias

        (4) Ischemic necrosis if extravasation occurs; *cannot be infused through a peripheral line*

3. Dobutamine

    a. Mechanism of action: Potent beta 1–agonist, mild beta 2–agonist resulting in increases cardiac output, HR, and possible peripheral and coronary vasodilation

    b. Indications

        (1) Pulmonary congestion and low cardiac output with systolic BP of 70 to 100 mm Hg and no sign of shock

    c. Dosage and route

        (1) Infusion, 500 mg in 250 ml D_5W

        (2) 2-20 μg/kg per minute; titrate to effect (limit dose so that HR does not exceed >10% of baseline)

    d. Precautions

        (1) May cause tachycardia, arrhythmias

        (2) Myocardial ischemia at high doses

        (3) May exacerbate hypotension

4. Milrinone lactate (Primacor)

    a. Mechanism of action: Phosphodiesterase III inhibitor that results in dose-dependent positive inotrope and vasodilator with minimal chronotropic response, decreases pulmonary capillary wedge pressure (PCWP) and systemic vascular resistance (SVR) and increases cardiac output (CO)

    b. Indications

        (1) Severe heart failure or cardiogenic shock (not adequately responsive to standard therapy)

    c. Dosage and route

        (1) IV infusion: 50 mg/250 ml normal saline

        (2) Loading dose of 50 μg/kg over 10 minutes, then infusion of .375 to .750 μg/kg per minute for 2-3 days; titrate to effect.

    d. Precautions

        (1) Ventricular dysrhythmias

        (2) Hypotension

5. Dopamine

    a. Mechanism of action: Dose dependent beta 2–agonist, alpha 1–agonist, and alpha 2–agonist, and dopaminergic agonist.

        (1) Dose of 2 to 5 mcg/kg per minute: Dopaminergic stimulation may cause vasodilation of renal, mesenteric, and cerebral arteries.

        (2) Dose of 5 to 10 mcg/kg per minute: Beta 1 stimulation results in increased cardiac output (beta 1 effects), mild to moderate peripheral vasoconstriction (alpha effects)

        (3) Dose of 10 to 20 mcg/kg/min: stimulation result in profound increase in peripheral vasoconstriction (alpha 1 effects) and myocardial contractility and HR (beta 1 effects)

    b. Indications

        (1) Hemodynamically significant hypotension; systolic of 70-100 mm Hg with signs of shock

        (2) Symptomatic bradycardia if atropine ineffective and in the absence of a pacer

    c. Dosage and route

        (1) Infusion, 400 or 800 mg in 250 ml D_5W, NS or LR

(2) Begin at lowest appropriate dose for intended receptor stimulation and titrate to blood pressure, urine output, and signs of organ perfusion

d. Precautions

(1) May result in extreme tachycardia leading to severe dysrhythmias especially if hypovolemic; *always optimize volume status first.*

(2) Increases myocardial oxygen consumption at high doses

(3) Tissue necrosis if extravasation occurs

(4) Incompatible with sodium bicarbonate

6. Digitalis

a. Mechanism of action: Cardiac glycoside that also increases AV block and enhances vagal tone, which slows impulse conduction and prolongs the effective refractory period

b. Indications

(1) Atrial fibrillation

(2) Paroxysmal supraventricular tachycardia

(3) Congestive heart failure

c. Dosage and route (varies with ventricular rate, urgency, patient age, body size, and renal function)

(1) IV: Loading dose of 10 to 15 µg/kg lean body weight

(2) Nonemergency situation, oral

d. Precautions

(1) Toxicity

(a) Arrhythmias—all types

(b) Nausea, vomiting, diarrhea

(c) Visual disturbances—yellow halos

(d) More common with hypokalemia, hypomagnesemia, and hypocalcemia

(2) Treatment may require temporary pacemaker.

(3) Avoid electrical cardioversion unless condition is life threatening. Use lower currents (10 to 20 joules).

B. Beta-blocking agents

1. Mechanism of action

a. Block effect of catecholamines on beta-receptors

b. Decrease heart rate, blood pressure, contractility

2. Indications

a. Suspected MI and unstable angina in the absence of complications

b. Adjunctive agent with fibrinolytic therapy

c. Supraventricular tachydysrhythmias (PSVT), atrial fibrillation or flutter

d. Hypertension

3. Precautions

a. May cause severe hypotension especially if given concurrently with calcium channel blocking agents.

b. Avoid use in bronchospastic disease, symptomatic heart failure, and severe abnormalities in cardiac conduction.

c. Monitor cardiac and pulmonary status vigilantly.

4. Metoprolol (beta 1 selective)

a. Dose: initial IV dose, 5 mg slow IV at 5 minute intervals to a total of 15 mg; oral regimen to follow IV dose: 50 mg twice per day for 24 hours, then increase to 100 mg twice per day if tolerated

5. Atenolol (beta 1 selective)

a. Dose: 5 mg slow IV (over 5 minutes). Wait 10 minutes, then give second dose of 5 mg slow IV (over 5 minutes). In 10 minutes, if tolerated, may start 50 mg orally; then 50 mg twice a day.

6. Propranolol (beta 1 and beta 2 stimulation)

a. Dose: Total dose, 0.1 mg/kg divided in to 3 equal doses at 2-3 minute intervals. Do not exceed 1 mg/minute.

7. Esmolol
   a. Dose: 0.5 mg/kg over 1 minute, followed by a continuous infusion at 0.05 mg/kg per minute; titrate to effect; short half-life: 2-9 minutes (maximum: 0.3 mg/kg per minute)
8. Labetalol (alpha and beta 1 selective)
   a. Dose: 10 mg IV push over 1-2 minutes; may repeat or double dose every 10 minutes to a maximum of 150 mg; may be given as an infusion of 2-8 mg/minute after initial bolus. Do not repeat boluses if infusion initiated.
C. Calcium channel blocking agents
   1. Mechanism of action: Slow conduction and increase refractoriness in the AV node by blocking the movement of calcium into the cells
   2. Indications
      a. Termination of reentrant arrhythmias
      b. Control of ventricular response in atrial fibrillation and flutter and multifocal atrial tachycardia
   3. Precautions
      a. Do not use for wide-QRS tachycardias of unknown origin.
      b. Avoid use in patients with Wolff-Parkinson-White syndrome, sick sinus syndrome, or AV block without a pacemaker.
      c. May cause severe hypotension especially with concurrent beta-blocking agent use
      d. May exacerbate CHF with severe left ventricular failure
   4. Diltiazem
      a. Dose: 15 to 20 mg (0.25 mg/kg) IV over 2 minutes; may repeat in 15 minutes at 20 to 25 mg (0.35 mg/kg) over 2 minutes; may use as an infusion at 5 to 15 mg/hour titrated to HR
   5. Verapamil
      a. Dose: 2.5 to 5.0 mg IV bolus over 2 minutes (give doses over 3 minutes for older patients)
      b. Second dose in 15 to 30 minutes (if needed): 5 to 10 mg; maximum dose: 20 mg
      c. Alternate dosing: 5 mg bolus every 15 minutes to total dose of 30 mg
D. Antidysrhythmic agents
   1. Lidocaine
      a. Mechanism of action: Class IB antiarrhythmic; stabilizes the cell membrane by blocking the movement of sodium into cardiac conducting cells; suppresses ventricular dysrhythmias and elevates fibrillation threshold; also has a local anesthetic property
      b. Indications: Ventricular ectopy (VF/VT) and symptomatic premature ventricular contractions (PVCs)
      c. Dosage and route
         (1) Adult
            (a) Initial: 1 to 1.5 mg/kg IV or by ET tube every 3 to 5 minutes; repeat doses: 0.5 to 0.75 mg/kg every 5 to 10 minutes to a maximum of 3 mg/kg
            (b) Infusion: 2 g/500 ml normal saline at 1 to 4 mg/minute
         (2) Pediatric: 1 mg/kg IV, IO, ET tube
      d. Precautions
         (1) Excessive doses cause myocardial and circulatory depression.
         (2) Toxicity
            (a) Drowsiness, disorientation, twitching
            (b) Extreme toxicity can result in seizures.
   2. Amiodarone
      a. Mechanism of action: Class III antiarrhythmic agent with complex effects on sodium, potassium, and calcium channels as well as alpha-blocking and beta-blocking properties; prolongs the action potential duration

Amiodarone

   b. Indications
      (1) Ventricular rate control of rapid atrial arrhythmias in patients with compromised cardiac contractility and preexcited atrial arrhythmias
      (2) VT or VF
      (3) Hemodynamically stable VT
      (4) Adjunct to electrical cardioversion of PSVT and atrial tachycardia
   c. Dosage
      (1) Adult
         (a) VF or pulseless VT: 300 mg IV push; may be followed by 150 mg IV if defibrillation ineffective after first dose
         (b) Stable VT or atrial arrhythmias: 150 mg in 200 ml D_5W over 10-15 minutes followed by an infusion 1 mg/minute for 6 hours, then 0.5 mg/minute to a maximum daily dose of 2 g
      (2) Pediatric: 5 mg/kg bolus IV or IO
   d. Precautions
      (1) May cause hypotension and bradycardia
      (2) Infusion must be mixed in D_5W in a glass bottle.
      (3) Comes in glass ampule; use filter needle to aspirate
      (4) Can cause pulmonary fibrosis with extended use
  3. Procainamide
   a. Mechanism of action: Class IA antiarrhythmic; stabilizes cell membrane and decreases rates of conduction through the conducting system and ventricular tissue
   b. Indication
      (1) Recurrent VT and VF and antidysrhythmic of choice for stable monomorphic VT with an ejection fraction >40%.
   c. Dosage and route
      (1) Adult
         (a) IV: 20 to 50 mg/minute to a total of 17 mg/kg
         (b) Infusion: 2 g in 500 ml normal saline at 1 to 4 mg/minute
      (2) Pediatric: 15 mg/kg over 30 to 60 minutes
   d. Precautions: Stop drug if
      (1) Dysrhythmia is suppressed (IV bolus).
      (2) QRS complex widens by 50% of original width.
      (3) Hypotension develops.
  4. Magnesium sulfate
   a. Mechanism of action: Reduces sinoatrial (SA) node impulse formation, prolongs myocardial conduction time
   b. Indications
      (1) Hypomagnesemia
      (2) Ventricular dysrhythmias: VF and VT (drug of choice for torsades de pointes)
   c. Dosage and route
      (1) Adult
         (a) Cardiac arrest: 1 to 2 g of a 50% solution
         (b) Torsades de pointes: 1 to 2 g diluted in 100 ml D_5W over 5 to 60 minutes
           Follow with infusion of 0.5 to 1 g/hour for up to 24 hours
      (2) Pediatric: 20 to 50 mg IV or IO, maximum of 2 g over 10 to 20 minutes
   d. Precautions
      (1) Hypotension
      (2) Caution with renal failure
  5. Adenosine
   a. Mechanism of action: Depresses AV and sinus node activity (supraventricular); terminates reentry dysrhythmias (tachydysrhythmias)
   b. Indication: first line for narrow-complex SVT

    c. Dosage and route: (in the most central vein possible)
      (1) Adult
        (a) Rapid bolus of 6 mg over 1 to 3 seconds followed by 20 ml saline flush
        (b) Repeat a 12 mg dose in 1 to 2 minutes; may repeat in 1 to 2 minutes.
      (2) Pediatric
        (a) Dose of 0.1 mg/kg IV or IO (maximum first dose: 6 mg)
        (b) May double and repeat dose once (maximum second dose: 12 mg)
    d. Precautions
      (1) Short half-life (<5 seconds) may result in recurrent SVT
      (2) Less effective in patients taking theophylline
      (3) Side effects: chest pain, flushing, dyspnea are transient.
  6. Ibutilide
    a. Mechanism of action: Class III antiarrhythmic; prolongs the action potential duration and increases the refractory period of cardiac tissue
    b. Indications: Acute pharmacologic conversion of atrial fibrillation or flutter or as an adjunct to electrical cardioversion
    c. Dose
      (1) Adults, ≥60 kg: 1 mg IV over 10 minutes; dose may be repeated in 10 minutes
      (2) Adults, ≤60 kg: 0.01 mg/kg over 10 minutes
    d. Precautions
      (1) High incidence of polymorphic VT
      (2) Continuous monitoring for minimum of 4 to 6 hours
      (3) Optimize potassium and magnesium levels before initiating.
      (4) Patients with impaired left ventricle (LV) function at higher risk for proarrhythmia tendencies
E. Vagolytic agents
  1. Atropine
    a. Mechanism of action: Parasympatholytic resulting in increased automaticity, AV conduction, and vagolysis
  2. Indications
    a. Initial treatment for symptomatic bradycardia
    b. May be beneficial in asystole after epinephrine
    c. May be beneficial in symptomatic bradycardia and bradycardic PEA
  3. Dosage and route
    a. Adult
      (1) Dose of 0.5 to 1 mg IV every 3 to 5 minutes to a total of 0.03 to 0.04 mg or 2 to 3 mg by ET tube
    b. Pediatric
      (1) Dose of 0.02 mg/kg (minimum single dose: 0.1 mg); may repeat once.
  4. Precautions
    a. Tachycardia that may result in ischemia or infarction
    b. Excessive dosing, ventricular fibrillation, or ventricular tachycardia
F. Vasodilators
  1. Nitroglycerin
    a. Mechanism of action: Relaxes vascular smooth muscle resulting in dilation of coronary arteries and decreased systemic vascular resistance (especially in venous smooth muscle)
    b. Indications
      (1) Drug of choice with angina pectoris or acute MI
      (2) Drug of choice with congestive heart failure
    c. Dosage and route
      (1) Sublingual with angina: 0.3 to 0.4 mg; may repeat in 5 minutes to three-dose total

   (2) IV infusion: 50 mg in 250 ml D_5W; start at 10 to 20 µg/minute and titrate in 5 to 10 µg/minute increments to effect every 5 to 10 minutes
d. Precautions
   (1) Hypotension
   (2) Bradycardia
   (3) Recommend arterial line monitoring for infusion therapy.
   (4) Must be given by infusion pump
2. Sodium nitroprusside
   a. Mechanism of action: Potent, rapid-acting arteriolar and venous vasodilator resulting in a decrease in right and left ventricular filling (preload) and peripheral arterial resistance (afterload)
   b. Indications
      (1) Hypertensive crisis
      (2) Emergency treatment of heart failure
      (3) Pulmonary edema
   c. Dosage and route
      (1) IV infusion: 50 mg/250 ml D_5W
      (2) Begin at 0.15 µg/kg/minute; titrate to effect (higher doses may be needed). Average dose is 3 mcg/kg/min.
   d. Precautions
      (1) Requires arterial line monitoring
      (2) Can cause profound hypotension resulting in ischemia or infarction
      (3) Elderly patients more sensitive to effects
      (4) Metabolized to thiocyanate (cyanide toxicity)
      (5) Keep infusion protected from light (foil wrap).
      (6) Must be given by infusion pump
G. Vasopressors
   1. Epinephrine (see discussion in inotropic agents in Section VIII.A)
   2. Dopamine (10 to 20 µg/kg/minute, see discussion in inotropic agents in Section VIII.A)
   3. Norepinephrine (see discussion in inotropic agents in Section VIII.A)
   4. Vasopressin
      a. Mechanism of action: Naturally occurring antidiuretic hormone;. acts as a nonadrenergic peripheral vasoconstrictor at unnaturally high doses by directly stimulating smooth muscle.
      b. Indications
         (1) VF, pulseless VT
         (2) Vasodilatory shock
      c. Dose: 40 units IV push times one dose or an infusion titrated for effect
      d. Precautions
         (1) Extreme vasoconstriction may provoke myocardial ischemia and angina.
         (2) Not recommended for responsive patients with CAD
H. Sodium bicarbonate
   1. Mechanism of action: reacts with hydrogen ions to form water and CO_2 to buffer metabolic acidosis
   2. Indications
      a. Known, preexisting hyperkalemia
      b. Known, preexisting bicarbonate-responsive acidosis (i.e., diabetic ketoacidosis, tricyclic or cocaine overdose)
      c. Prolonged resuscitation after defibrillation, effective CPR, intubation, hyperventilation with 100% oxygen, epinephrine, and antidysrhythmics
   3. Dosage and route
      a. Initial dose of 1 mEq/kg, then 0.5 mEq/kg every 10 minutes

4. Precautions

    a. Sodium bicarbonate produces CO_2 and will worsen respiratory acidosis; CO_2 is also a negative inotrope; sodium bicarbonate causes oxyhemoglobin saturation curve to shift to left, decreasing oxygen release into plasma.

    b. Utilize blood gas analysis for monitoring if available.

BIBLIOGRAPHY

1. ACC/AHA guidelines for implementation of cardiac pacemakers and antiarrhythmia devices. *JACC* 31(5):1175-1209, 1998.

2. Aehlert B: *ECG's made easy.* St Louis: Mosby, 1995.

3. American Heart Association in Collaboration with International Liaison Committee on Resuscitation: Guidelines 2000 for cardiopulmonary resuscitation and emergency cardiovascular care: International consensus on science, part 3. Adult basic life 32. *Circulation* 102(8 Suppl):I22-59, 2000.

4. Ahrens TS, Martin NK, Powers C, et al: Angina pectoris and myocardial infarction. In Ahrens TS, Prentice D, editors: *Critical care certification: Preparation, review, and practice exams,* ed 4. Stamford, CT: Appleton & Lange, 1998, p 63.

5. Burden N: The surgical specialties—part 2: Gynecologic and obstetric, urologic, orthopedic and podiatric, general, and cardiovascular surgical procedures. In Burden N, editor: *Ambulatory surgical nursing.* Philadelphia: WB Saunders, 1998, p 502.

6. Chung MK: Cardiac surgery: Postoperative arrhythmias. *Crit Care Med* 28(10): N136-N144, 2000.

7. Detsky AS, Abrams HB, McLaughlin JR, et al: Predicting cardiac complications in patients undergoing non-cardiac surgery. *J Gen Intern Med* 1:213, 1986.

8. Finkelmeier BA: Cardiac rhythm disorders. In Finkelmeier BA, editor: *Cardiothoracic surgical nursing.* Philadelphia: Lippincott, 2000, pp 47-58.

9. Finkelmeier BA: Diagnostic evaluation of cardiac disease. In Finkelmeier BA, editor: *Cardiothoracic surgical nursing.* Philadelphia: Lippincott, 2000, pp 87-96.

10. Finkelmeier BA: Cardiac arrhythmias. In Finkelmeier BA, editor: *Cardiothoracic surgical nursing.* Philadelphia: Lippincott, 2000, pp 303-316.

11. Finkelmeier BA: Temporary pacing and defibrillation. In Finkelmeier BA, editor: *Cardiothoracic surgical nursing.* Philadelphia: Lippincott, 2000, pp 317-326.

12. Finkelmeier BA: Cardiovascular medications. In Finkelmeier BA, editor: *Cardiothoracic surgical nursing.* Philadelphia: Lippincott, 2000, pp 327-340.

13. Finkelmeier BA: Complications of cardiac operations. In Finkelmeier BA, editor: *Cardiothoracic surgical nursing.* Philadelphia: Lippincott, 2000, pp 341-356.

14. Gahart BL, Nozareno AR: *Intravenous medications: A handbook for nurses and allied health professionals,* ed 18. St Louis: Mosby, 2002.

15. Goldman L, Caldera D, Nussbaum SR, et al: Multifactorial index of cardiac risk in non-cardiac surgical procedures. *N Engl J Med* 197:848, 1977.

16. Hazinski M, Cummins RO, Field JM: *Handbook of emergency cardiovascular care for healthcare providers.* Dallas, TX: American Heart Association, 2000.

17. Heffline M: Cardiopulmonary care and emergency port. In Quinn DM, editor: *Ambulatory surgical nursing core curriculum.* Philadelphia: WB Saunders, 1999, pp 167-196.

18. Hicks FD: The cardiac surgical patient. In Litwack K, editor: *Core curriculum for post anesthesia nursing practice,* ed 3. Philadelphia: WB Saunders, 1995, p 243.

19. Huszar RJ: *Pocket guide to basic dysrhythmias,* ed 3. St Louis: Mosby, 2002.

20. Ide B: Cardiovascular system. In Thompson JM, McFarland GK, Hrisch JE, et al, editors: *Mosby's clinical nursing,* ed 5. St Louis: Mosby, 2002, pp 29-142.

21. Kennedy MM: Patient assessment: Cardiovascular system cardiac history and physical examination. In Hudak CM, Gallo BM, Morton PG, editors: *Critical care nursing, A holistic approach.* Philadelphia: Lippincott, 1998, p 198.

22. Kristt AM: The peripheral vascular surgical patient. In Litwack K, editor: *Core curriculum for post anesthesia nursing practice,* ed 3. Philadelphia: WB Saunders, 1995, p 279.

23. Kruse J, Finkelmeier BA: Permanent pacemakers and implantable cardioverter-defibrillators. In Finkelmeier BA, editor: *Cardiothoracic surgical nursing.* Philadelphia: Lippincott, 2000, pp 221-241.

24. Lee J, Lee PC: *Cardiology at a glance.* New York: McGraw-Hill, 2002.

25. McCance KL, Huether SE: *Pathophysiology: The biologic basis for disease in adults and children,* ed 3. St Louis: Mosby, 1998.

26. Noland L: Renal system. In Thompson JM, McFarland GK, Hrisch JE, et al: *Mosby's*

clinical nursing, ed 5. St Louis: Mosby, 2002, pp 857-916.

27. Rollant PD, Ennis DA: The renal system. In Rollant PD, Ennis DA, editors: *Medical-surgical nursing.* St Louis: Mosby, 2001, pp 237-265.

28. Seifert PC: *Cardiac surgery: Perioperative patient care.* St Louis: Mosby, 2002.

29. Yao AC: Cardiovascular disorders. In Finberg L, editor: *Saunders manual of pediatric practice.* Philadelphia: WB Saunders, 1998, pp 91-95.

33 Neurologic Care

PAMELA E. WINDLE

OBJECTIVES

At the conclusion of this chapter the reader will be able to:

1. Describe the pathophysiology of increased intracranial pressure (ICP).

2. Describe the nursing neurologic assessment.

3. Discuss potential causes associated with changes in pupillary size.

4. Explain the medical and nursing management of the patient with increased ICP.

5. Discuss the 5-point system used to assess muscle strength.

▪▪ Neurologic assessment in the postanesthesia care unit is essential to gain complete understanding of the patient's response to surgery and/or identify potential complications that may have occurred. The nervous system controls many processes; thus it can indirectly influence many body functions. Neurologic assessment and patient monitoring is a key component of postanesthesia care unit (PACU) nursing care for all surgical patients; especially those with surgeries involving the head and spinal cord. Timely identification of abnormal findings is crucial to prevent untoward outcomes.

NEUROLOGIC ASSESSMENT

I. Baseline status: necessary to determine improvement or deterioration in patient's condition
   A. Levels of consciousness (LOC)
      1. Full consciousness
         a. Awake, alert, and oriented to time, place, and person
         b. Able to express ideas verbally or in writing
         c. Comprehends spoken words
      2. Confusion
         a. Disoriented to time, place, or person
         b. Shortened attention span
         c. Difficulty with memory
         d. Difficulty in following commands
         e. Bewildered easily
         f. Alterations in perception of stimuli
         g. Hallucinations; agitated, restless, and irritable
         h. Increased confusion at night
      3. Lethargy
         a. Oriented to time, place, and person
         b. Very slow and sluggish in speech, mental processes, and motor activities
         c. Responds to painful stimuli
      4. Obtunded
         a. Arousable with stimuli, drowsy
         b. Responds verbally with a word or two
         c. Follows simple commands when stimulated
      5. Stupor
         a. Lies quietly, with minimal spontaneous movement

   b. Unresponsive except to vigorous and repeated stimuli
   c. Responds appropriately to painful stimuli
 6. Coma
   a. Sleeplike state with eyes closed
   b. Unresponsive to stimuli
   c. Does not make any verbal sounds
B. Assessment technique
 1. Arouse patient to maximum level of wakefulness.
 2. Begin by calling patient by familiar name.
 3. If no response, shake patient vigorously.
 4. If no response, apply noxious stimuli, being careful not to injure patient.
   a. Nail bed pressure
   b. Supraorbital pressure
   c. Pinching trapezius muscle
   d. Sternal pressure
 5. Assess orientation to environment.
   a. Ask alert, verbal patient to tell you where he or she is.
   b. Use yes or no questions to assess intubated patients
   c. For patients who may be confused, give choices similar to yes or no questions for intubated patients (i.e., "Is this place a hospital? Is this place your home?").
   d. Loss of orientation begins with loss of time, then place, then person.
   e. Avoid using "squeeze my hand" to assess strength or ability to follow commands.
     (1) Patients with diffuse cerebral injury, particularly frontal lobe problems, retain strong hand grasp reflex similar to infant.
     (2) Give patient a single step command (e.g., "Show me two fingers").
     (3) If you do ask patient to squeeze your hand, also ask patient to let go of your hand.
   f. Assess for behavioral changes such as restlessness, irritability, combativeness
C. Pupillary reactivity (Figure 33-1)
 1. Oculomotor nerve (CN III) and brainstem control pupil size and reaction.
 2. Sluggish pupils indicate pressure on CN III, which runs parallel to brainstem.
 3. Assessment technique (Figure 33-2)
   a. Observe size, shape, equality, and reaction to light.
   b. Assess and compare pupils bilaterally.
   c. Record pupil size as small, medium, or large unless reference is available to measure exact size
 4. Be aware of effect of anesthetic agents and preoperative medications on pupil size and reactivity.
   a. Constricting agents (miotic)
     (1) Opiates and narcotics
     (2) Cholinergic agents
       (a) Optical miotics (pilocarpine)
       (b) Neostigmine bromide (Prostigmin)
       (c) Barbiturates
       (d) Edrophonium chloride (Tensilon)
       (e) Pyridostigmine bromide (Mestinon)
   b. Dilating agents (mydriatic)
     (1) Anticholinergic agents

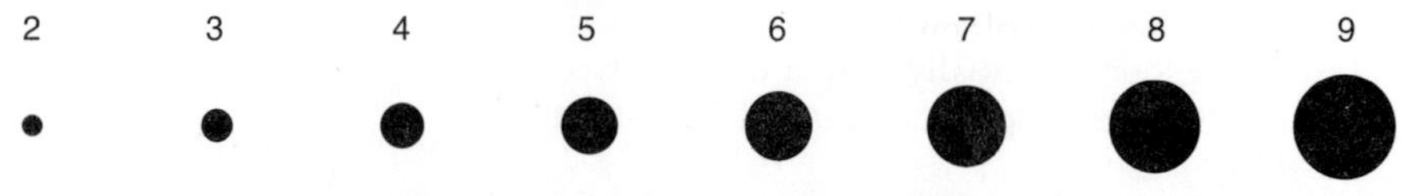

| 2 | 3 | 4 | 5 | 6 | 7 | 8 | 9 |

FIGURE 33-1 ■ Pupil gauge (millimeters).

In assessing pupillary size using either descriptive terms or a gauge, each pupil is assessed individually and then the findings for each pupil are compared. This is very important because pupils are normally equal.

Descriptive Term	Definition	Findings
Pinpoint 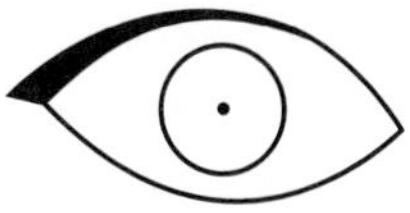	The pupil is so small that it is barely visible or appears as small as a pinpoint.	Seen with opiate overdose, pontine hemorrhage, ischemia.
Small 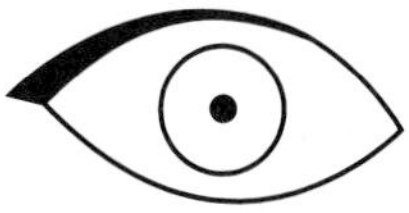	The pupil appears smaller than average, but larger than pinpoint.	Seen normally if the person is in a brightly lit place; also seen with miotic ophthalmic drops, opiates, pontine hemorrhage, Horner's syndrome, bilateral diencephalic lesions, and metabolic coma.
Midposition 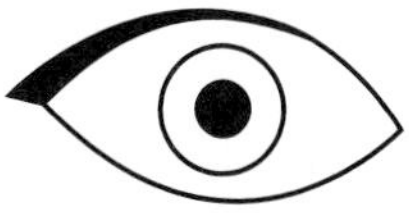	When the pupil and iris are observed, about half of their diameter is iris and half is pupil.	Seen normally; if pupils are midposition and nonreactive, midbrain damage is the cause.
Large 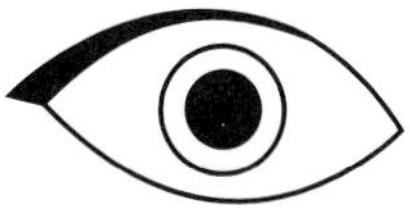	The pupils are larger than average, but there is still an appreciable amount of iris visible.	Seen normally if room is dark; may be seen with some drugs, such as amphetamines; glutethimide (Doriden) overdose; mydriatics; cycloplegic agents; and some orbital injuries.
Dilated 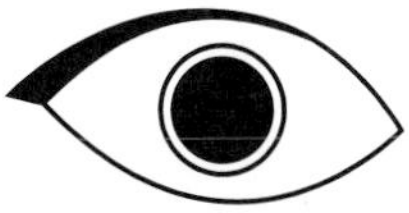	When the pupil and iris are observed, one is struck by the largeness of the pupil with only the slightest ring of iris, which is barely visible.	Abnormal finding; bilateral, fixed, and dilated pupils are seen in the terminal stage of severe anoxia-ischemia or at death.

FIGURE 33-2 ■ Assessing pupillary size. From Hickey JV: *The clinical practice of neurological and neurosurgical nursing,* 5th ed. Lippincott, 2003, p 171.

        (a) Atropine sulfate
        (b) Naloxone hydrochloride
        (c) Scopolamine
    c. Topical mydriatics
    d. Adrenergic agents
      (1) Catecholamines
        (a) Dobutamine (Dobutrex)

(b) Dopamine (Intropin)
(c) Epinephrine (Adrenalin)
(d) Isoproterenol (Isuprel)
(e) Norepinephrine (Levophed)
(2) Noncatecholamine agents
(a) Ephedrine
(b) Metaraminol (Aramine)
(c) Phenylephrine (Neo-Synephrine)
5. Pupil size can be altered by direct eye trauma or congenital malformations.
6. Any new change in pupil size or reactivity should be reported to physician at once (Figure 33-3).

(Note: Compare findings with previous assessment data, document, and report new findings to the physician.)

OCULOMOTOR NERVE COMPRESSION

Observation

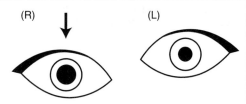

One pupil (R) is larger than the other (L), which is of normal size. The dilated pupil (R) does not react to light, although the other pupil (L) reacts normally. Ptosis may be seen in the dilated pupil.

Interpretation

A dilated, nonreactive (fixed) pupil indicates that the control for papillary constriction is not functioning. The parasympathetic fibers of the oculomotor nerve control papillary constriction. The most common cause of interruption of this function is compression of the oculomotor nerve, usually against the tentorium or posterior cerebral artery.

Action

Compare with data from previous assessments. If the dilated pupil is a new finding, it should immediately be reported to the physican, because the process of rostral-caudal downward pressure must be treated without delay. In this situation, changes in LOC, motor function, sensory function, and possible vital signs would be expected.

BILATERAL DIENCEPHALIC DAMAGE

Observation

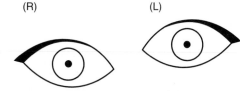

On examination, the pupils appear small but equal in size, and both react to direct light, contracting when light is introduced and dilating when light is withdrawn.

Interpretation

The sympathetic pathway that begins in the hypothalamus is affected. Because both pupils are equal in size and respond equally to light, the damage is bilateral. Therefore, it can be assumed that there is bilateral injury in the diencephalons (thalamus and hypothalamus). Because metabolic coma can also result in bilaterally small pupils that react to light, this diagnostic possibility must be ruled out.

Action

Compare findings with previous assessments to determine change. Consider metabolic coma by reviewing blood chemistry findings and other data. For example, diabetic acidosis may result in a metabolic coma because of a high blood glucose level.

FIGURE 33-3 ■ Common abnormal pupillary responses. From Hickey JV: *The clinical practice of neurological and neurosurgical nursing,* 5th ed. Lippincott, 2003, p 174-175.

HORNER'S SYNDROME

Observation

(R)   (L)

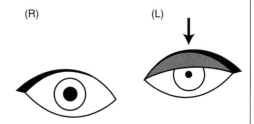

One pupil (L) is smaller than the other (R), although both pupils react to light. The eyelid on the same side as the smaller pupil (L) droops (ptosis). Inability to sweat (anhidrosis) on the same side of the face as the ptosis is common. The symptoms of a small reactive pupil, ptosis, and anhidrosis combine to form Horner's syndrome.

Interpretation

There is an interruption of the ipsilateral sympathetic innervation to the pupil that can be caused by hypothalamic damage, a lesion of the lateral medulla, or the ventrolateral cervical spinal cord, and, sometimes, by occlusion of the internal carotid artery.

Action

If this is a new finding, it should be reported.

MIDBRAIN DAMAGE

Observation

(R)   (L)

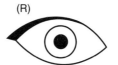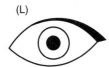

Both pupils are at midposition and nonreactive to light.

Interpretation

With midposition, nonreactive pupils, neither sympathetic nor parasympathetic innervation is functional. This finding is often associated with midbrain infarction or transtentorial herniation.

Action

Compare findings with previous assesment data. Consider also changes in other components of the assessment. The pupils should be evaluated in conjunction with other neurologic assessments. Report new findings to the physician.

PONTINE DAMAGE

Observation

(R)   (L)

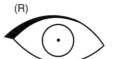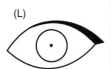

Very small (pinpoint), nonreactive pupils are seen.

Interpretation

This finding indicates focal damage of the pons, often due to hemorrhage or ischemia. *Bilateral* pinpoint pupils may occur from opiate drug overdose, so this possibility should be ruled out.

Action

Compare findings with previous assessment data. Report findings to the physician immediately. Other changes in neurological status, such as decreased LOC and respiratory abnormalities, would be expected.

FIGURE 33-3 ■ *Cont'd*

    D. Motor function

      1. Voluntary motor movement controlled by fibers originating in frontal lobes of cerebral cortex

      2. Fibers descend through brainstem; most cross and continue to spinal cord.

      3. Assessment technique for alert patient

        a. Test strength of all muscle groups against resistance and gravity.

          (1) Strength scale

            (a) 5 points: full strength, no deficit or weakness

            (b) 4 points: able to lift extremity against gravity and maintain position without wavering

            (c) 3 points: able to lift extremity against gravity, but wavers and cannot sustain

            (d) 2 points: able to slide along support surfaces such as bed or chair

            (e) 1 point: flicker or trace movement

            (f) 0 point: no movement

        b. Upper extremities: palmar (pronator) drift method

          (1) Ask patient to close eyes and extend arms in front, with palms up.

          (2) Paretic arm will slowly drift downward and palm will turn upward.

        c. Muscle strength assessed by testing active, passive, and active resistive movement

          (1) Upper extremities

            (a) Grasp: have patient squeeze your first and second fingers, compare right with left.

            (b) Extension: patient extends arms in front with palms up, eyes closed; observe for arm drift, indicating mild weakness.

          (2) Lower extremities

            (a) Leg lift: lying in bed, able to lift one leg at a time to clear bed and hold without wavering; compare left with right

          (3) Trunk

            (a) Able to sit on side of bed independently

          (4) Sensory (always compare right and left sides and test with patient's eyes closed)

            (a) Touch: eyes closed, identifies where touched; test opposite side to see if each side "feels the same"

          (5) Pain and temperature: eyes closed, identifies if pinprick is sharp and back of pin is dull, or identifies ice chip as cold

      4. Assessment technique for unconscious patient: apply noxious stimuli and observe response.

        a. Purposeful movement, such as pushing away stimulus, indicates intact neuraxis.

        b. Localization of gross location of stimulus indicates cortical dysfunction.

        c. Check for Babinski's sign, an indicator for disease along the voluntary motor pathways.

        d. Nonpurposeful responses indicate dysfunction deeper in cerebral hemispheres and midbrain area.

          (1) Incomplete removal of stimulus

          (2) Slight movement without moving away from stimulus

          (3) Withdrawal of only the part stimulated

          (4) Lower extremities flex at knees

        e. Decorticate posturing (flexion response)

          (1) Occurs with disruption of corticospinal pathways

          (2) Loss of cerebral cortex influence over movement

        f. Decerebrate posturing (extension response)

          (1) Indicates damage in deeper cerebral hemispheres and upper brainstem

          (2) Indicative of severe brain dysfunction with poor prognosis

    E. Reflexes that reflect integrity of neuraxis

      1. Oculocephalic reflex (doll's eyes)

     a. Can only be elicited in patients with depressed LOC
     b. Alert patients override reflex
     c. Tests integrity of brainstem between CN III and CN VIII
     d. Technique
       (1) Hold patient's eyes open.
       (2) Briskly turn patient's head side to side.
       (3) Pause to assess eyes on each side.
     e. Interpretation
       (1) Normal (doll's eye reflex present)
         (a) Conjugate eye deviation to direction opposite direction head is turned; eyes move in orbits.
         (b) In comatose patient, indicates brainstem is intact between CN III and CN VIII
       (2) Abnormal (doll's eye reflex absent)
         (a) Disconjugate eye movements
         (b) Eyes move with head; eyes do not move in orbits.
         (c) Eyes appear fixed, like painted eyes of a china doll.
         (d) Indicative of severe lesion in brainstem
         (e) Contraindicated in actual or suspected cervical injuries
  2. Oculovestibular reflex (cold calorics)
     a. Provides information about integrity of brainstem and connections to cerebral cortex
     b. Contraindicated in patients with ruptured tympanic membrane
     c. Technique
       (1) Assess integrity of tympanic membrane.
       (2) Cold water (50 ml) slowly injected into external auditory canal
       (3) Observe eye movement (two phases).
         (a) Normal: eyes initially deviate to side of stimulus, followed by rapid component of nystagmus deviating toward opposite side.
         (b) Common in brainstem; poor prognosis
 F. Vital signs
  1. Changes usually seen late in clinical course; should not be relied on to signal impending neurologic clinical problems
  2. Observe for widening pulse pressure: systolic blood pressure increases while diastolic pressure decreases.
  3. Observe for changes in respiratory rate and rhythm.
  4. Observe for Cushing's triad (reflex), a sign of increased ICP.
     a. Increased systolic blood pressure
     b. Decreased diastolic blood pressure
     c. Decreased pulse rate (bradycardia)
  5. Assessment of cranial nerve function may be needed, depending on underlying neurologic problem.
 G. Documentation
  1. Variety of assessment tools available, but most include parameters of Glasgow Coma Scale
  2. Frequency of neurologic assessment may be dictated by unit protocol and patient condition.
     a. Report abnormal findings to physician.
     b. Be alert to subtle changes in any of the above parameters.
  3. Give specific descriptions of stimulus used and resulting response of patient.

DYNAMICS OF INCREASED ICP

 I. Monro-Kellie hypothesis: skull is closed container with fixed volume of blood, CSF, and brain tissue contained within nondistensible skull.
  A. Contents of skull
   1. Blood: 10%

      2. CSF: 10%

      3. Brain tissue: 80%

  B. Volume-pressure relationship (elastance)

      1. Small increases in volume more readily compensated for in uninjured or noncompromised brain

      2. Increases in volume over extended period of time more readily compensated for than comparable volume over shorter period of time

      3. Little room in skull for slack

      4. In traumatized or injured brain even small increases in volume can produce drastic elevations in ICP.

  C. Compensatory mechanisms: increase in one intracranial volume must be compensated for by a decrease in one of the remaining volumes.

      1. Displacement and reduction of CSF volume

      2. Reduction in blood volume

      3. Displacement of brain tissue

  D. Normal intracranial pressure

      1. 0 to 15 mm Hg—with invasive monitoring

      2. 50 to 150 mm H_2O with external manometer

  E. Causes of increased ICP

      1. Abnormal production, circulation, or absorption of CSF

         a. Hydrocephalus

            (1) Communicating

            (2) Noncommunicating

         b. Congenital abnormalities: hydrocephalus, Arnold-Chiari malformation

         c. Obstructive masses: tumors, abscesses

      2. Increase in intracranial blood volume

         a. Hemorrhage

         b. Hyperthermia: increases metabolic demands and thus blood volume

         c. Venous drainage impairment

         d. Hypercapnia—increases in $Paco_2$ or H^+ levels

         e. Vascular abnormalities

             (1) Aneurysms

             (2) Arteriovenous malformations (AVMs)

         f. Vasodilating drugs

             (1) Anesthetic gases

                (a) Halothane

                (b) Enflurane

                (c) Isoflurane

                (d) Nitrous oxide

                (e) Sevoflurane

                (f) Desflurane

             (2) Some antihypertensives

             (3) Some histamines

      3. Increase in brain tissue volume

         a. Tumors

         b. Infectious processes

         c. Edema

      4. Other

         a. Respiratory: Intubation, positive end-expiratory pressure (PEEP), increased airway pressure

         b. Body positions: Trendelenburg, prone, extreme hip flexion, neck flexion

         c. Coughing

         d. Isometric muscle exercises

         e. Valsalva maneuver

         f. Noxious stimuli

         g. Emotional upset

      h. Seizure activity

      i. Rapid eye movement (REM) sleep or arousal from sleep

      j. Clustering care activities

  F. Autoregulation: ability of cerebral circulation to maintain relatively constant cerebral blood flow and pressure needed to provide oxygen and nutrients to brain tissue

    1. CPP

      a. Determines cerebral blood flow

      b. CPP = Mean arterial blood pressure (MABP) – ICP

      c. Interpretation of CPP values

        (1) 70 to 100 mm Hg: normal

        (2) 60 mm Hg: provides minimally adequate blood supply

        (3) <50 mm Hg: autoregulation begins to fail

        (4) <40 mm Hg: cerebral blood flow decreases by 25%

        (5) <30 mm Hg: incompatible with life: neuronal hypoxia and cell death

    2. Invasive ICP monitoring needed to calculate CPP

    3. CPP calculation should be part of neurologic assessment.

  G. Clinical presentation of signs of increased ICP

    1. Depends on location, cause, and degree of compensation

    2. Damage to brain tissue

      a. Tissue ischemia as a result of decreased cerebral blood flow

      b. Brain structures compressed by increasing pressure

    3. Symptoms

      a. Deterioration in LOC

      b. Pupillary dysfunction

      c. Changes in motor status

      d. Changes in vital signs: Cushing's triad (reflex)

      e. Seizures

      f. Headaches

      g. Vomiting

      h. Papilledema

      i. CN palsies

      j. Sensory changes

      k. Impaired brainstem reflexes

  H. Herniation syndromes: increasing pressure causes displacement of brain tissue (Figure 33-4)

    1. Transcalvarial herniation

      a. Occurs at surgical incision site or through site of gunshot or stab wound or fracture site

    2. Cingulate herniation

      a. One of cerebral hemispheres displaced laterally across midline, with blood vessels and tissue compressed

    3. Central transtentorial herniation

      a. Downward displacement of cerebral hemispheres through tentorial notch located at level of tentorium cerebelli, which separates cerebellum from cerebral hemispheres

    4. Uncal (lateral) herniation

      a. Displacement of medial tip of temporal lobe (uncus) through tentorium, compressing midbrain

      b. Most common herniation syndrome

    5. Infratentorial herniation

      a. Compression of brainstem, cerebellum

      b. Medullary collapse

II. Medical interventions

  A. Direct: remove cause.

  B. Indirect

    1. Maintain patent airway.

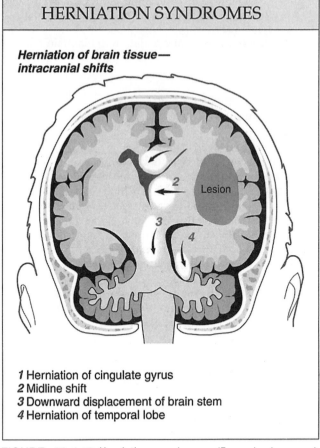

FIGURE 33-4 ■ Herniation syndrome. (From Luckmann J: *Saunders manual of nursing care.* Philadelphia, WB Saunders, 1997, p 675, Figure 18-23.)

2. Maintain normal fluid and electrolyte balance.
   a. Adequate fluid management with saline, to avoid dehydration and hypotension
   b. Serum osmolarity kept between 290 and 320 mOsm/kg
   c. Monitor serum glucose, electrolytes.
3. Avoid administration of narcotics.
4. Give diuretics.
   a. Osmotic diuretics: mannitol
      (1) Draws water from extracellular space of edematous brain into plasma
      (2) Does not cross blood-brain barrier
      (3) Can cause fluid and electrolyte imbalances
      (4) Furosemide (Lasix)
         (a) Thought to decrease cerebrospinal fluid (CSF) production
         (b) Decreases systemic fluid volume
         (c) Manage rebound effect of mannitol
5. Administer corticosteroids.
   a. Controversial with head trauma or cerebral infarction with edema, but useful with brain tumors
   b. Dosage tapered before discontinued
6. Initiate therapeutic hyperventilation.
   a. Maintain P_{CO_2} between 27 and 33 mm Hg
   b. Should be done with mechanical ventilation

  c. Short-term use recommended (<72 hours); not for prophylaxis.

  d. Manual hyperventilation with Ambu recommended only emergently for patients with "pressure signs" until ventilator available

 7. Reduce cerebral stimulation and metabolic demand.

  a. Control pain

  b. Maintain normothermia: if using hypothermia blankets, prevent shivering, which will increase metabolic demands and ICP.

  c. Control seizures with phenytoin sodium.

  d. Control hyperactivity with sedation.

  e. Neuromuscular blockade for severe agitation

 C. Ventriculostomy to drain CSF

 D. Operative decompression: surgical removal of tip of temporal lobe, portion of frontal lobe, or portion of cranial bone

III. Nursing interventions

 A. Goals

  1. Protect patient at risk from sudden increases in ICP.

  2. Prevent permanent brain damage.

   a. Maintenance of patent airway

   b. Ongoing neurologic assessment

 B. Positioning

  1. Elevate head of bed 30° to 45°.

  2. Maintain head in neutral position with sandbags or Philadelphia collar.

  3. Avoid prone position.

  4. Patients with infratentorial craniotomies may be positioned flat or slightly elevated.

 C. Prevent Valsalva maneuver by having patient exhale.

 D. Prevent isometric muscle contraction by assisting patient in turning.

 E. Avoid clustering of nursing activities—space nursing care to give patient frequent rest periods, which decreases stimulation.

IV. ICP monitoring

 A. Purpose

  1. Monitor trends in ICP.

  2. Measure cerebral perfusion pressure (CPP).

  3. Test intracranial compliance.

 B. ICP monitoring techniques

  1. Intraventricular catheter: inserted through anterior horn of lateral ventricle on nondominant side

   a. Most accurate measurement of ICP

   b. Allows for sampling of CSF

   c. Intrathecal administration of medications

   d. Use as ventriculostomy to decrease increased ICP.

   e. Increased risk of infection and hemorrhage

   f. Catheter placement difficult with small ventricles

  2. Subarachnoid bolt (Richmond or Becker bolt): inserted into subarachnoid space through cranial burr hole

   a. Less risk of infection

   b. Placement is easier and can be used in patients with small ventricles.

   c. Inability to sample CSF and test compliance

   d. Does not allow for intrathecal administration of medications

   e. Questionable reflection of actual ICP

  3. Epidural or subdural sensors or catheters: inserted into epidural or subdural space

   a. Easily inserted

   b. Decreased risk of infection

   c. Brain or subarachnoid space not penetrated

   d. Questionable reflection of actual ICP because of pressure from adjacent dura

   e. Inability to sample CSF

[handwritten marginal note: Plastic surgery in order to establish communication between the floor of the 3rd ventricle of the brain and the Cistern Interpeduncularis]

4. Fiber optic transducer-tipped catheter
   a. Easily inserted and requires small hole
   b. Versatile: can be inserted into ventricles, subarachnoid space, brain parenchyma, subdural space
   c. Zero balancing required only at time of insertion
   d. Decreased risk of infection
   e. Does not allow for CSF sampling or drainage
   f. Periodic replacement of probe may be necessary.
   g. Expensive
C. ICP waveforms
   1. Mechanism is transmission of pressure to transducer that converts pressure waves into waveform visible on oscilloscope.
D. Nursing considerations
   1. Strict aseptic technique
   2. Observe for leaks and breaks in system.
   3. Close observation of waveforms
   4. Troubleshooting of dampened waveforms
   5. Recalibration of system according to unit protocol
   6. Never irrigate system.
   7. Calculation of intracranial compliance is physician's responsibility.
   8. Removal of system is physician's responsibility.

NEUROLOGIC COMPLICATIONS

I. Headache
   A. Migraine (may be triggered by many factors involved with surgical procedures)
      1. Careful history should reveal method of treatment.
      2. Analgesics, narcotics, serotonin
      3. Ice or cool cloth to head or back of neck
      4. Treat mild hypoglycemia.
      5. Maintain fluid intake (nausea and vomiting may occur).
   B. Muscle tension (may be related to surgical position)
      1. Neutral head position
      2. Massage and topical creams
      3. Encourage range of motion of neck and shoulders.
      4. Relaxation techniques (deep breathing, etc.)
II. Seizures
   A. Classification
      1. Generalized
         a. Generalized tonic-clonic
            (1) Description:
               (a) Tonic phase: lasts 1 to 2 minutes: the patient is rigid, with increased muscle tone.
               (b) Clonic phase: usually lasts 1 to 2 minutes; the patient has jerking movements that gradually slow, then stop; usually breathing stops for 30 seconds to 1 minute.
               (c) Post-ictal phase: patient does not remember seizure, is confused, usually wants to sleep, may be combative when stimulated.
            (2) Medical emergency: notify physician immediately.
               (a) Lasts more than 5 minutes
               (b) One seizure occurs after another (status epilepticus).
            (3) Treatment
               (a) Do not restrain.
               (b) Do not force anything into the mouth.
               (c) Turn to side.
               (d) Protect from self-harm and the environment, put pillow under head, remove harmful objects.

(e) Padded "bite" may be placed between molars if patient opens mouth.

(f) May use oxygen if available

(g) Suction as needed; do not force into mouth.

(4) Assessment

(a) What was patient doing when seizure started?

(b) What was the first indication that a seizure had begun (confusion, jerking in any part of the body, etc.)?

(c) Length of seizure

(d) Physical appearance (body position, limb movement)

(e) Bowel or bladder incontinence

(f) Obtain stat glucose and electrolytes.

b. Absence: more common in children

(1) Description

(a) Short (several seconds) of blinking spells

(b) May occur 30 or greater times per day

(2) Medical concern if number of seizures reduces quality of life

2. Partial

a. Complex partial (temporal lobe)

(1) Description

(a) Appears awake, but confused

(b) May turn to examiner when name called

(c) Automatisms: repetitive activity, not goal-oriented, such as rubbing, rocking, pulling, pulling at clothes or bed linens

(d) Activity is not goal oriented.

(2) Medical emergency: notify physician immediately.

(a) If no history of epilepsy

(b) If lasts more than 5 minutes

(c) If one occurs after another

(d) Obtain stat glucose and electrolytes.

(e) Observe closely for secondary generalization.

(3) Treatment

(a) Do not restrain; patient may become hostile and perceive intervention as a threat.

(b) Redirect activity or ambulation by placing barriers (i.e., close doors, place chairs in his/her path).

(4) Assessment

(a) What was patient doing just prior to seizure?

(b) Length of time seizure lasts

(c) Automatisms

(d) Was patient able to speak?

III. Stroke (cerebrovascular accident [CVA])

A. Definition: A neurologic syndrome with gradual or rapid, nonconvulsive onset of neurologic deficits that last for over 24 hours. This occurs when the oxygen supply to a localized area is interrupted, leading to neural tissue destruction, then brain damage.

B. Description

1. Third leading cause of death

2. Risk increases with age (two thirds occur after age 65).

3. Affects more than 40% of the population over age 80

C. Classification

1. Ischemic (cerebral infarction)—85%

a. Thrombotic (most common)

(1) May progressively worsen over time

b. Embolic

(1) Sudden onset

2. Hemorrhagic—15%

a. Subarachnoid

b. Intracerebral

    D. Transient ischemic attacks (TIAs)
  1. Temporary focal or retinal deficits
  2. Caused by vascular disease that can clear completely in less than 24 hours
  3. Shorter and reverses completely within 1 hour
  4. Most important warning signs of stroke

    E. Warning signs
  1. Loss of strength and/or sensation, usually on one side of the body
  2. Decreased vision, dimness of vision, loss of vision in one eye, double vision
  3. Difficulty talking or understanding speech
  4. Difficulty swallowing
  5. Severe headache
  6. Sudden dizziness, nausea, and/or vomiting

    F. Treatment
  1. Stat brain computerized axial tomography CAT scan uncontrasted
  2. Maintain normotension for cerebral perfusion (do not overtreat elevated blood pressure).
  3. Neuroassessment every 15 to 30 minutes
  4. Elevate head of bed (HOB) to 30° to maintain venous outflow.
  5. Position to facilitate oral secretions drainage; avoid hip flexion and prone position.
  6. Turn every 2 hours.
  7. Chest physical therapy and range of motion exercises
  8. Maintain normothermia.
  9. Monitor level of sensation.
  10. Patch one eye at a time to control diplopia.
  11. Provide tactile stimuli to affected hands and limbs with decreased sensation.
  12. Avoid activities that increase ICP.

DIAGNOSTIC TOOLS

  I. Neuroimaging techniques

    A. Skull series
  1. Indications
     a. Fractures
     b. Skull erosions
     c. Deviated pineal gland — *pine cone shaped · in brain*
  2. No contraindications — *major site of melatonin synthesis*

    B. Cerebral angiography (conventional and magnetic resonance angiography [MRA])
  1. Purpose
     a. To detect abnormalities of cerebral circulation
     b. To locate lesions distorting cerebral vessels
  2. Indications
     a. Cerebral vascular abnormalities
     b. Aneurysms
     c. Arterovenous malformations (AVMs)
     d. Visualization of cerebral arteries and veins
  3. Contraindications
     a. Allergy to contrast dye

    C. Radionuclide scan
  1. Uses gamma scintillation counter and injection of radioisotope
  2. Radioisotope uptake increased in pathologic tissue
  3. Indications
     a. Brain tumors or masses
     b. Cerebral infarction
     c. Headaches

        d. Seizure disorders

        e. Other major neurologic disorders

    4. Contraindications

        a. Uncooperative patient

        b. Pregnancy

D. Computed tomography (CT) scan

    1. Noninvasive test, but contrast media may be injected to facilitate visualization of vasculature

    2. Provides clear, cross-sectional brain images

    3. Uses computer reconstruction

    4. Contrast media, gadolinium, may be used for enhancement.

    5. Contraindications

        a. Uncooperative patient

        b. Allergy to contrast dye or shellfish

E. Magnetic resonance imaging (MRI)

    1. Tomography technique using magnetic properties of protons in body tissues

    2. High-resolution images are very clear.

    3. Indications: any neurologic condition

    4. Contraindications

        a. Pregnancy

        b. Uncooperative patient

        c. Any metallic implants (e.g., pacemakers, orthopedic devices, clips)

    5. Sedation may be required because of claustrophobic nature of scanner.

F. Myelogram

    1. Visualization of the spinal column and subarachnoid space for suspected lesion

    2. Injection of contrast dye via lumbar or cisternal puncture into the subarachnoid space

    3. Keep head slightly elevated for 4-6 hours to prevent dye from migrating into the cerebrum.

G. Positron emission tomography (PET) scan

    1. Uses principles of CT scan and radionuclide scanning

    2. Evaluation of biochemical brain substances

    3. Maps metabolic brain activity

    4. Expensive

    5. Indications—limited diagnostic purposes

        a. Psychiatric disorders

        b. Epilepsy

        c. Alzheimer's disease

        d. Cerebrovascular disease

        e. Cerebral injuries

H. Evoked potentials

    1. Measure changes in brain's electrical activity in response to variety of sensory stimulation (visual, auditory, somatosensory)

    2. Indications

    3. Neuromuscular disorders

    4. Cerebrovascular disease

    5. Head and spinal cord injury

    6. Tumors

    7. Peripheral nerve disease

I. Other diagnostic tools

    1. Lumbar puncture

    2. Electrocardiogram (ECG)

    3. Electroencephalogram (EEG): assists in diagnosis of seizure activity, brain death.

    4. Echoencephalogram: detects shifts of midline structures

    5. Radiographs of other body systems as indicated

    6. Cerebral blood flow studies

    7. Electromyogram (EMG)

8. Laboratory testing
   a. Blood
   b. Urine
   c. Cultures (as needed)
   d. CSF studies

BIBLIOGRAPHY

1. American Association of Neuroscience Nurses: *Clinical guidelines series: Intracranial pressure monitoring*. Chicago: American Association of Neuroscience Nurses, 1997.
2. American Heart Association: Available at http://www.americanheart.org. Accessed on December 9, 2003.
3. Back Bubble: Available at http://www.backpainrelief.com. Accessed on December 9, 2003.
4. Cammermeyer M, Appledorn C: *AANN's Core Curriculum for Neuroscience Nursing*, ed 3. Chicago, American Association of Neuroscience Nurses, 1996.
5. Chipps E, Clanin N, Campbell V: *Neurologic disorders*. St Louis: Mosby–Year Book, 1992.
6. DeFazio Quinn D: *ASPAN's ambulatory surgical nursing core curriculum*. Philadelphia, WB Saunders, 1999.
7. Hickey J: *The clinical practice of neurologic and neurosurgical nursing*. ed. 4. Philadelphia: Lippincott, 2002.
8. Litwack K: *Core curriculum for post anesthesia nursing practice*. ed 3. Philadelphia, WB Saunders, 1995.
9. Luckmann J: *Saunders manual of nursing care*. Philadelphia, WB Saunders, 1997.
10. Marshall BA, Miller RH: *Essentials of neurosurgery: A guide to clinical practice*. New York: McGraw-Hill, 1995.
11. Medtronic Sofamor Danek: Available at http://sofamordanek.com. Accessed on December 9, 2003.
12. National Institute of Neurologic Disorders and Stroke: NINDS brain and spinal tumors age. Available at http://www.ninds.nih.gov/health_and_medical/disorders/brainandspinaltumors.htm. Accessed on December 9, 2003.
13. Neck Reference: Available at http://www.neckreference.com. Accessed on December 9, 2003.
14. Spinal Cord Injury Information Network: Available at http://www.spinalcord.uab.edu. Accessed on December 9, 2003.

34 Hematologic Care

KATHLYN CARLSON

OBJECTIVES

At the conclusion of this chapter the reader will be able to:

1. Evaluate normal and abnormal laboratory values and initiate appropriate nursing interventions as needed.

2. Describe the nursing care of a patient with a hematologic disorder.

3. Describe the nursing interventions of a patient with a disorder in hemostasis.

4. Discuss the nursing responsibilities associated with blood and blood component transfusions.

5. Identify the types of transfusion reactions and the appropriate nursing interventions.

▪▪ This chapter covers common blood dyscrasias in the areas of hematology and hemostasis. It is a broad presentation of the clinical signs, laboratory results, and nursing interventions for each area. For a detailed account of specific disease entities and syndromes, refer to the bibliography at the end of this chapter.

I. Perianesthesia issues relate to hematology
   A. Preoperative clinical assessment with laboratory tests
      1. Alterations affect outcomes, especially oxygenation and hemostasis.
         a. Critically assess potential for anemia and coagulopathy: review clinical indications and medical history.
         b. No established minimum value for presurgical hemoglobin
         c. Routine laboratory screening, though low cost, is neither required nor recommended for every preoperative patient.
            (1) When preoperative hemoglobin low, continuing with surgery-as-planned decided by acuity of anemia, patient's cardiopulmonary response, and surgical urgency
         d. Preoperative hemoglobin selectively recommended for
            (1) Neonates to detect physiologic anemia
            (2) Elderly patients and menstruating women
            (3) Patients with bone marrow suppression, malignancy, or genetically determined anemic conditions
         e. Preanesthetic screening may uncover unrecognized coagulopathy: documented coagulation disorder seldom appropriate for surgery in the nonacute ambulatory setting,
   B. Transfusion is not innocuous; there are potential risks.
      1. Though commonly given, particularly to intensive care unit (ICU) patients, complications cannot be overlooked or minimized.
         a. Hemolytic allergic reactions
         b. Acute lung injury
         c. Transfusion-transmitted: human immunodeficiency virus (HIV), cytomegalovirus (CMV), viral infections such as hepatitis
            (1) *Hepatitis* not detected by donor testing: long "seronegative" period; most (>90%) transmitted hepatitis is hepatitis C
            (2) *Cytomegalovirus (CMV):* Carried by 60% of donors

(3) Especially threatening to the immunosuppressed; occurs 3-6 weeks posttransfusion of large amounts of fresh blood

(4) *Bacterial contamination*: in blood bank–stored units can cause severe septicemia—mortality nearly 50% because of endotoxins

2. Weigh against serious anemia risk: oxygen deficit, decreased perfusion.

   a. If mild: palpitations, tachycardia, new ejection murmur
   b. If severe: stroke, myocardial infarction
   c. No specific minimum hemoglobin or hematocrit to trigger transfusion decision, especially for critically ill patients

3. Metabolic effects of stored blood: a 35-42 day "shelf life"

   a. Toxic enzymes from dead white blood cells (WBCs) and platelets "significant" after 14 days of storage
   b. Hypocalcemia: ionized calcium binds with citrate used to preserve stored blood
   c. Aging blood results in
      (1) Hyperkalemia: potassium released from cell lysis
      (2) Acidosis
      (3) Independent risk factors for multiple organ failure
   d. Postoperative infection and immunosuppression risk
      (1) May not be evident for months posttransfusion
      (2) After spinal fusion, joint replacement, transfusion associated with iatrogenic wound infection, longer hospital stay, and more days of fever, antibiotic therapy
      (3) Tumor recurrence linked to transfusion, unproven

C. Autologous transfusion: alternative to banked blood

   1. Patient predonates units of own blood.
   2. Reinfusion of salvaged blood shed into surgical field
   3. Patients may be ineligible for presurgical donation because of weight or age restrictions, anemia, or cardiac conditions.

II. Hematology components: Blood cells and clotting factors

A. Hemoglobin: carried on red blood cells (RBCs). (refer to Box 34-1)

   1. RBC physiology
      a. Critical transporter of oxygen to tissues
         (1) Carried on hemoglobin molecule to tissues
         (2) Normally concave on both sides (biconcave)
         (3) Proportion (percentage) in total blood volume is hematocrit.
      b. Produced in bone marrow and removed by the spleen
      c. Production stimulated by erythropoietin, which is produced by the kidney
      d. Life span is approximately 120 days.

   2. *Anemia*: Hemoglobin or RBC deficit; hematocrit reduction
      a. Cardiovascular symptoms vary with hemoglobin level and acuity of cell loss. Weakness and fatigue common.
      b. Assess and suspect acutely low hemoglobin if
         (1) Low *oxygen saturation* (SpO_2), particularly if intraoperative blood loss was significant
         (2) *Hypotension*, perhaps noted by orthostatic changes when head of bed raised or ambulatory surgery patient stands
         (3) *Tachycardia*, likely a compensatory way to sustain cardiac output and sustain normal blood pressure
            (a) A multipurpose indicator representing a response by sympathetic nerves of the autonomic system
            (b) Consider hypovolemia, with or without low hemoglobin, heart rate increases.
            (c) Stress, anxiety, and fever normally raise heart rate.
            (d) Patients who cannot respond with tachycardia

■ BOX 34-1
■ **HEMATOLOGY NORMAL* LABORATORY VALUES**

Red blood cells (RBCs)	*Male:* 4.5 to 6.2 million per microliter *Female:* 4 to 5.5 million per microliter
Hemoglobin (Hgb)	*Male:* 14 to 18 grams per deciliter (g/dl) *Female:* 12 to 16 g/dl
Hematocrit (HCT):	proportion of RBCs in circulating blood volume *Male:* 40% to 52% *Female:* 37% to 47%
White blood cells (WBCs): 5000 to 10,000 per microliter	*Differential:* Segmented neutrophils: 40% to 60% Band neutrophils: 0 to 3% Lymphocytes: 20% to 40% Monocytes: 4% to 8% Eosinophils: 1% to 3% Basophils: 0 to 1% Nucleated red blood cells: 0
Platelets: 150,000 to 400,000 per microliter	
Prothrombin time (PT): 11-13 seconds Usually expressed as International Normalized Ratio (INR): 1.0	
Partial thromboplastin time (PTT): 25-37 seconds	

*Guidelines only: normal values vary with clinical laboratory.

      (i) Patients on beta-blocker medications
      (ii) Patients with transplanted hearts, which are denervated and so lack autonomic responses
   c. Causes of hemoglobin deficit
     (1) *Loss*
      (a) Hemorrhagic: usually acute as in trauma, surgical loss, gastrointestinal, uterine, nasal, vascular
      (b) Hemodilution from fluid volume expansion
        (i) Normal during pregnancy
        (ii) Replacement with non-RBC colloid or crystalloids
      (c) Researchers implicate laboratory draws (phlebotomy) as source of accumulated blood loss especially for ICU patients: up to 40-70 ml daily
     (2) *Inadequate RBC production*
      (a) Insufficient vitamin B_{12} (intrinsic factor) needed for erythropoiesis
        (i) Postgastrectomy
        (ii) Pernicious anemia
      (b) Endocrine factors: insufficient erythropoietin production, as in chronic renal failure, Addison's disease, thyroid diseases
      (c) Liver disease: drug or alcoholic induced
      (d) Aplasia: bone marrow suppression with decreased hemoglobin, RBC, WBC, platelet levels
        (i) Malignancy: infiltration of marrow
        (ii) Chemotherapy
        (iii) Chemical or radiation exposure: dose dependent
        (iv) Medications: phenytoin, chloramphenicol
      (e) Inflammatory conditions: Rheumatoid arthritis, autoimmune diseases such as lupus erythematosus
        (i) About 15% of asymptomatic HIV positive patients are anemic.
      (f) Genetic predisposition: mutation or recessive traits

      (i) Alters a link in the chain of hemoglobin formation
      (ii) Produces hemolytic anemias such as
          [a] Sickle cell anemia (refer to Box 34-2)
              [1] Affects 1% of African-Americans
              [2] Hypoxia, fever, acidosis spur RBC change from biconcave to sickled.
              [3] Severe pain: joints, limbs, abdomen
              [4] Jaundice, ischemia, organ infarction
          [b] Thalassemia (Cooley's)
              [1] Major: early death, altered growth
              [2] Minor: Few symptoms, hemoglobin <12
          [c] Spherocytosis

■ BOX 34-2
■ **SICKLE CELL ANEMIA: PREDISPOSED BY HEREDITY**

Genetic Characteristics
Specific stimuli cause RBCs to alter shape and function.
Forms abnormal HbS rather than normal HbA
Trait carried by 10% of African-Americans
Fewer than 1% of African-Americans develop disease.

Clinical Concerns
Abnormal HbS cell forms have decreased affinity for oxygen.
Oxygen deficit causes cells to change shape and sickle.
Sickled cells rupture or clog small vessels.
Sickling crisis stimulated by
    Altered temperature: fever or cold
    Acidosis and hypoventilation
    Dehydration

Clinical Outcomes
Sluggish peripheral circulation
    Thrombosis, organ infarction
    Cerebral changes, altered renal function, cardiopulmonary compromise
    Limb ulcerations, necrosis
Ischemic pain, especially at limbs, joints, bones, and abdomen
Infection susceptibility

Nursing Responsibility: Prevention
Ensure *oxygenation:* Prevent hypoventilation, acidosis.
    Monitor respiratory quality, rate, and depth.
    Provide supplemental oxygen; titrate to oxygen saturation.
    Adequately reverse muscle relaxants.
    Position patient for effective lung expansion.
    Early mobility
Promote peripheral circulation: minimize vasoconstriction.
    Maintain normothermia.
    Ensure adequate hydration to reduce blood viscosity.
    Regularly assess limb, organ ischemia.
        Limit peripheral blood stagnation.
        Monitor renal labs, urine volume.
Reduce stress.
    Analgesia: manage pain.
    Antibiotics: prevent or control infection.
    Calming environment

[1] RBCs are spherical rather than biconcave disks; survival reduced to 14 days

(3) *Destruction* of RBCs: Normal vitamin B_{12} levels

(a) Pharmaceuticals, burns: destroys or impairs function

(b) Excessive physical stress

(c) Hemolysis: cell trauma, destruction, or consumption

(i) Defective prosthetic heart valves or blood pumps

(ii) Infection: bacterial or viral

(4) *Inadequate intake* of folic acid or iron

(a) Malnutrition: dietary lack, alcoholism, chronic anorexia

(b) Malabsorption as a result of ileal disease, surgical resection

d. Perianesthesia nursing interventions and evaluation related to *anemia*

(1) Need sufficient RBC numbers and hemoglobin level to bind oxygen for delivery to tissues

(2) No absolute minimum hemoglobin measure established, though acute loss may cause more hemodynamic instability than chronic deficit

(a) Hemoglobin of 9–10 g/dl is desired.

(b) Anesthesia may be safely administered to patients with hemoglobin of 6–7 g/dl, such as

(i) Patients with chronic renal failure whose erythropoietin is suppressed

(ii) Acutely ill Jehovah Witnesses who refuse blood on religious principles

(c) Acute anemia is unlikely in ambulatory surgery setting.

(3) Fully saturate circulating hemoglobin.

(a) Monitor oxygen saturation, ensure adequate oxygenation, limit oxygen demand.

(i) Stimulate the sedated patient!

(ii) Position the patient for optimal lung expansion.

(iii) Deliver supplemental oxygen by mask or nasal cannula, with or without humidity.

(iv) Provide analgesia to promote deep breathing.

(v) Reduce stress: provide anxiolytics if safe.

(vi) Remember hypoxia alters acid-base balance.

(b) Measure hemoglobin.

(i) Particularly if oxygen saturation decreases

(ii) Monitor postoperative blood and volume losses from drains, dressings, suction.

(iii) Prevent profound hypotension.

[a] Increase preload and support cardiac output: hydrate with crystalloid, colloid if necessary.

[b] Anticipate orthostatic effects: gradual position changes to upright, noting BP and heart rate.

[c] Transfuse if ordered by physician per facility protocol.

3. *Polycythemia*: exaggerated RBC, hemoglobin, hematocrit, WBC production

a. *Increased RBC production* unrelated to erythropoietin level

(1) Blood volume and viscosity profoundly increased: cause unknown

(2) Hypertension, vein engorgement, cardiac arrhythmia, thrombosis, tissue hypoxia can result.

(3) One form (P vera) occurs in adults over 60 years, primarily men.

b. *Physiologic response* by bone marrow as

(1) Adaptive response to altitude: normal compensation to environment

(2) Pharmaceutical response to parenteral erythropoietin given to patients with chronic renal failure

(3) Compensatory response to "perceived" hypoxemia associated with chronic cardiopulmonary conditions

(a) Valvular or structural cardiac anomalies impede cardiac outflow and therefore oxygen delivery to tissue.

        (b) Pulmonary obstructive diseases such as asthma, emphysema

        (c) Pulmonary hypertension, pheochromocytoma

   c. Assessment, intervention, evaluation

      (1) Laboratory tests: Hemoglobin >18 g/dl, hematocrit >54%, RBCs, WBCs, platelets elevated

      (2) Symptoms: Ruddy complexion, headache, weakness, angina, palpitations, hypertension, splenomegaly, claudication, phlebitis

      (3) Treatment: Chronic anticoagulation, splenectomy, phlebotomy

B. Leukocytes: White blood cells (WBCs)

  1. Physiology: mediate immune response with assorted WBC cell types.

  2. *Leukocytosis: increased* WBC production up to 100,000/microliter and anemia

    a. *Appropriate* inflammatory response to "invasion" by foreign substances or infection

    b. *Pathologic* response: bone marrow proliferation, elementary WBCs

      (1) *Acute lymphocytic leukemia* (ALL)

        (a) Affects children, with pain, fatigue, bleeding, enlarged lymph nodes, liver, spleen

      (2) *Chronic lymphocytic leukemia* (CLL)

        (a) Affects men over age 50 with enlarged spleen and neck lymph nodes

      (3) *Acute myelocytic leukemia* (AML)

        (a) Characterizes 80% of all adult leukemias

        (b) Produces fever, bruising, pallor, joint pain, fatigue, enlarged liver, spleen

      (4) *Hodgkin's disease*

        (a) Enlarged lymph nodes, starting at neck, axilla

        (b) Afflicts adults <20, >45 years with fever, night sweats, weight loss, fatigue, liver and spleen enlargement

      (5) *Lymphoma:* Burkitt's lymphoma, lymphosarcoma, sarcoma

        (a) Lymph node, spleen enlargement, jaundice

      (6) *Multiple myeloma*

        (a) Affects adults over age 70 years with bone pain, fractures, bleeding and bruising

    c. Perianesthesia interventions and evaluation

      (1) Increase oxygen delivery with supplemental oxygen.

      (2) Prevent tissue damage, bruising.

        (a) Use soft-tipped suction catheters.

        (b) Position gently; pad stretcher side rails if indicated.

        (c) Apply pressure; monitor venous, arterial puncture sites.

      (3) Transfuse blood components as ordered.

      (4) Prevent infection: respect protective isolation precautions when WBC, platelets dangerously low.

        (a) Provide postanesthesia care unit (PACU) care in operating room or patient's room per hospital policy rather than PACU.

  3. *Leukopenia:* production *reduced* to fewer than 5000/mm^2 of blood

      (1) Bone marrow suppression by disease, immunosuppression, radiation, toxins, or drugs

      (2) Patient safety may require protective isolation to prevent exposure to iatrogenic infection.

  4. Perianesthesia nursing assessments and interventions

      (1) Report deviation from normal parameters.

        (a) Preadmission tests might be first recognition of infection or leukemia.

        (b) Leukopenia and unusual bruising may coexist with anemias and platelet dysfunction.

      (2) Obtain accurate history: ask pointed preanesthetic questions.

        (a) Fevers, with or without chills?

        (b) Easy bruising or bleeding?

(c) Increased fatigue?
(d) Pain, especially in joints?
(3) Think "protection."
(a) Avoid pressure to skin and joints, and provide soft surfaces against skin.
(b) Prevent hematoma during venipuncture and suctioning.
(c) Isolate as required: infectious versus protective.
III. Coagulation: A chain of events to ensure hemostasis
  A. Physiology: Clotting is an intricate balance that requires
    1. Adequate *liver function* to produce a cascade of interrelated clotting factors which circulate until activated
    2. Functional *platelets*, normal *calcium*, and specific *enzymes*
      a. Platelets "plug" injury site
      b. About 66% circulate for their 7-10 day life span, rest in spleen
      c. Aspirin renders platelets less "sticky."
    3. *Vascular integrity* ensures a smooth, "healthy" endothelial wall for
      a. Adherence of a platelet plug bound by a fibrin clot
      b. Appropriate local constriction to limit local blood flow
    4. Synergy among a host of clotting factors (proteins) along the coagulation pathway
      a. Coagulation factors (refer to Box 34-3)
        (1) Vitamin K–dependent factors are factors II, VII, IX, X.
        (2) Platelets affect factor XIII.
      b. Naturally occurring coagulation inhibitors include alpha-1 antitrypsin, Protein C, antithrombin 3.
      c. Clotting pathways

■ BOX 34-3
■ COAGULATION PATHWAYS AND CLOTTING FACTORS

Pathway:	*Extrinsic*	*Intrinsic*
Response:	*Tissue*	*Within blood*
Activates:	Thromboplastin (factor III)	Circulating clotting factors
Result:	*Prothrombin* (made in liver) converted to *thrombin* via plasma proteins, enzymes and clotting factors	and platelets
	Fibrin forms from thrombin	+ Platelets aggregate, form plug

Clotting factors:
Activated in specific points in clotting sequence

Factor I	Fibrinogen
II	Prothrombin
III	Tissue thromboplastin
IV	Calcium ions
V	Proaccelerin
VII	Prothrombin conversion accelerator
VIII	Antihemophilic factor/von Willebrand factor
IX	Christmas factor (autoprothrombin II)
X	Stuart factor (autoprothrombin I)
XI	Plasma thromboplastin antecedent
XII	Hageman factor (enzyme)
XIII	Fibrin-stabilizing factor

    (1) *Extrinsic pathway*: triggered by tissue injury; thromboplastin released and a sequence of events leading to fibrin clot formation

    (2) *Intrinsic pathway*: occurs within blood; proenzyme (factor VII) activated, spurs a cascade of clotting factors

   a. Fibrin

    (1) Strands of structural support for platelet plug; formed when fibrinogen activated

    (2) Effect limited to injury site to prevent massive coagulation

B. Laboratory assessments of coagulation (refer to Box 34-1)

 1. Prothrombin time (PT): assesses conversion of prothrombin to thrombin and factors I, II, V, VII, X.

  a. Specific monitor for Coumadin, which affects the external coagulation pathway

  b. If prolonged: significant bleeding risk during surgery, trauma, or soft tissue injury and *must* correct preprocedure

   (1) Liver disease, vitamin K deficiency

   (2) Fibrinogen, prothrombin, clotting factors V, VII, X

  c. Clinical *interventions* to correct abnormal lab values

   (1) Vitamin K injections

   (2) Fresh frozen plasma

 2. Partial thromboplastin time (PTT): assesses intrinsic coagulation pathway

  a. Monitor if administering heparin.

  b. Detects alteration in clotting factors I, II, V, VIII, IX-XII

 3. Thrombin time (TT): assesses thrombin activity to stimulate fibrin creation at coagulation's final stage

  a. Prolonged by fibrinogen (factor I) deficiency

 4. Platelet count: number, shape, and size of circulating platelets

  a. Surgical bleeding is rare if numbers are 100,000 or greater.

  b. Anticipate spontaneous bleeding if platelet numbers <20,000.

  c. *Aspirin* alters function for the 7-day life of a platelet.

  d. nonsteroidal antiinflammatories (NSAIDs) alter platelet function, with recovery within 2 days.

C. Coagulopathies: acquired or hereditary disorders of clotting sequence

 1. *Idiopathic immune thrombocytopenia purpura* (ITP): characterized by spontaneous bleeding

  a. Autoimmune disorder: active antiplatelet antibodies and profoundly *reduced platelet* numbers, causing epistaxis, petechiae, bruising

  b. Acutely affects young children after immunization or viral infection with chicken pox, mumps, or measles

  c. Chronic ITP affects adults, primarily women, under age 50.

 2. *Disseminated intravascular coagulopathy* (DIC): clotting factor consumption in response to surgery, pregnancy toxemia, sepsis, cancer, trauma, or multiple transfusions

  a. Simultaneous active bleeding and intravascular (capillary) clotting: PT, PTT elevated, platelets, fibrinogen decreased

  b. Reflects severe, overwhelming response to organ system crisis

  c. Occurrence in ambulatory surgery setting is highly unlikely.

 3. *Hereditary* coagulopathies

  a. *Hemophilia*: sex-linked clotting factor deficiency affecting men

   (1) Hemophilia A: clotting factor VIII lacking

    (a) Significant bleeding into tissues and joints if active factor VIII is <5%

    (b) PTT prolonged and PT normal

   (2) Hemophilia B (Christmas disease): clotting factor IX lacking

    (a) Prevents formation of stable clots; regular infusions of cryoprecipitate or fresh frozen plasma (FFP) likely

    (b) Intraoperative *FFP* needed to support factor IX

    (c) PTT, PT, and TT all within normal limits

   b. *Von Willebrand's* disease: common disorder affecting men and women
      with mucous membrane bleeding, epistaxis, mild bruising
      (1) Defective von Willebrand factor (vWF),
         (a) Reduced activity of factor VIII: PTT increased
         (b) Platelet "stickiness" impaired, numbers adequate
      (2) Preoperative therapies
         (a) Desmopressin (DDAVP) can increase vWF
         (b) Cryoprecipitate in scheduled twice daily doses
 D. Perianesthesia nursing assessments and interventions
   1. Preanesthesia
      a. Identify at-risk patients: coagulation risk and bleeding history
         (1) Risk of intraspinal or epidural hematoma increases if an
             anticoagulated patient receives regional anesthesia.
         (2) Undetected coagulopathy can underlie persistent postsurgical bleeding.
      b. Document date and time of most recent anticoagulant medication.
         (1) Coumarins and heparin
         (2) Aspirin, NSAIDs
         (3) Chemotherapy agents that suppress bone marrow
      c. A patient with a significant bleeding disorder is an unlikely candidate for
         outpatient surgery with discharge home.
   2. Postanesthesia
      a. Observe often for insidious bleeding.
         (1) Always look *under* the patient as well as at the wound itself.
         (2) Increasing abdominal girth after laparoscopic procedures
         (3) An obese patient can accumulate a lot of blood in the abdomen before
             distention or tenderness is evident.
         (4) Oozing and bruising from incisions or venipuncture sites
      b. Link vital signs and oxygenation changes with bleeding potential.
         (1) Continuously monitor oxygen saturation, observe respiratory quality.
             Persistently low SpO_2 may indicate undetected hemoglobin loss.
         (2) Measure hemoglobin: Anemia often associated with coagulopathy
         (3) Support blood pressure with adequate fluid volume.
            (a) Maintain IV patency and limit venipuncture.
            (b) Consider central or arterial line for laboratory sampling.
         (4) Transfuse selected blood components as indicated per physician order.
IV. Transfusion physiology: Blood cell compatibility
 A. Blood and blood components
   1. Whole blood: 1 unit = 500 ml with hematocrit of 36% to 40%
      a. Used if profound bleeding or desired component unavailable
      b. Contains RBCs, plasma, WBCs, and platelets
   2. Packed red blood cells: 1 unit = 250-300 ml with hematocrit of 70%-80%
      a. Most commonly transfused component: used to restore oxygen carrying
         capacity
      b. Contains red blood cells, nonfunctional WBC and platelets, but minimal
         plasma
      c. *Washed* red blood cells contain 10% white cells and platelets but lose 20%
         of RBC volume, must be transfused within 24 hours
         (1) Purpose
            (a) Decrease sensitization to human leukocyte antigens (HLA)
            (b) Minimize febrile and allergic transfusion reactions from plasma or
                leukocyte antibodies, platelets, or proteins
            (c) Pretransplant renal patients or those with sodium, potassium, or
                citrate restrictions
      d. *Frozen washed* red blood cells: RBCs, 2% WBCs, and platelets
         (1) Purpose
            (a) Bone marrow transplant recipient
            (b) Autologous transfusion: elective surgery
            (c) Clinically significant Immunoglobulin A (IgA) antibodies

3. Platelet concentrates: 1 pack = 50-300 ml
   a. Restore clotting ability: infuse through microaggregate filter
   b. Treats
      (1) Leukemia
      (2) Disseminated intravascular coagulopathy (DIC)
      (3) Bleeding caused by thrombocytopenia
      (4) Platelet suppression caused by chemotherapy or radiation
4. Fresh frozen plasma (FFP): 1 unit = 125-260 ml
   a. Unconcentrated plasma containing all coagulation factors except platelets
   b. *Must* be ABO compatible; use within 24 hours after thawing
   c. Treats
      (1) Coagulation deficiencies secondary to liver disease
      (2) DIC
      (3) Antithrombin 3 deficiency
      (4) Dilutional coagulopathy after massive blood replacement
5. Cryoprecipitate antihemophilic factor (Cryo)
   a. Concentrated factors derived from FFP, *must* be ABO compatible
   b. Contains
      (1) Fibrinogen
      (2) Factors VIII C, VIII vWF, XII
   c. Use within 6 hours after thawing to treat
      (1) Hemophilia A
      (2) DIC
      (3) Von Willebrand's disease
      (4) Obstetric complications
      (5) Fibrinogen deficiency
6. Serum albumin: 5% solution = up to 500 ml; 25% solution = up to 100 ml
   a. Sterile product containing 96% albumin, 4% globulin, and other proteins
   b. Obtained from pooled plasma, heat treated to inactivate hepatitis virus
   c. Treats
      (1) Hypovolemia: expands plasma volume
      (2) Hypoproteinemia
7. Plasma protein fraction (Plasmanate, PPF) 1 unit = 50, 250, or 500 ml
   a. Contains 88% albumin, 12% globulins, but *no* coagulation factors
   b. Obtained from pooled plasma, heat treated to inactivate hepatitis virus
   c. Treats
      (1) Hypovolemia: a volume expander
      (2) Hypoproteinemia

B. Four major blood types A, B, AB, O
   1. A or B antigens or both carried on surface of red blood cells
   2. Form blood type A, B, or AB (refer to Table 34-1)
      a. Blood type AB is the "universal recipient" because it produces no antibodies.
      b. Blood type O is the "universal donor."
      c. Plasma also carries naturally occurring antibodies to antigens not present on the red cell.

■ TABLE 34-1
■ ■ **Red Cell Blood Type and Compatibility**

Patient Blood Type	Compatible Donor	Antigen	Antibody
A	A or O	A	B
B	B or O	B	A
AB	AB or A, B, O	AB	None
O	O only	NONE	AB

C. Rh type: Determined primarily by the D antigen
   1. Positive or negative antigen carried on surface of red blood cells
      a. Rh⁺ (positive for the D antigen) occurs in over 80% of people
      b. Rh⁻ (negative for the D antigen) occurs in less than 20%
   2. If Rh⁺, must receive Rh⁺ cells; if Rh⁻, must receive Rh⁻ cells
   3. Detection crucial to prevent
      a. Significant antibody stimulation from multiple transfusions: makes crossmatching for future transfusions difficult.
      b. Hemolytic disease of newborn antibodies produced in Rh⁻ woman pregnant with Rh⁺ fetus
         (1) Give *RhoGAM* per physician order to Rh⁻ mother to prevent hemolysis of a future baby's blood whether after full-term birth, miscarriage, or abortion
V. Administering blood and blood products
   A. Why transfuse? Indications
      1. Restore circulating volume
      2. Increase oxygen transport to tissues
      3. Replace coagulation factors or correct bleeding
      4. Replace granulocytes or treat sepsis
   B. Accuracy required to ensure *patient safety;* for *every* blood component
      1. Verify correct patient and blood component: *follow facility policy.*
      2. *At patient's bedside,* two (2) licensed staff simultaneously match information on patient, blood component, and blood bank compatibility label.
         a. Patient name and hospital identification number
         b. Donor number on blood product
         c. ABO and Rh type
         d. Expiration date of component
      3. Report any identification discrepancy to blood bank *immediately* and delay transfusion.
      4. Prepare to transfuse.
         a. Prime blood tubing with *normal saline;* cover filter in drip chamber.
            (1) D₅W is hypotonic and causes hemolysis.
            (2) Ringer's lactate contains calcium, can initiate coagulation.
            (3) Change blood tubing and filter after every 2 units: filter traps clots and coagulant debris.
            (4) *Never* add medications to a unit of blood or piggyback into tubing—this includes narcotic analgesics delivered by patient-controlled analgesia (PCA).
         b. Gently mix contents and examine unit carefully for bubbles, plasma discoloration.
         c. Explain procedure and transfusion need to patient.
         d. Verify intravenous (IV) is patent, nonreddened; an 18 or 19 gauge catheter is best.
         e. Before starting transfusion, measure and document patient's temperature, blood pressure, vital signs, and heart rate.
         f. Keep patient warm for comfort.
            (1) Use blood warmer, particularly if transfusing multiple units.
            (2) Apply warm blankets, active rewarming device.
            (3) Note: new onset chilling, shivering signals a transfusion reaction; immediately stop blood transfusion
         g. Start infusion slowly, and remain with patient for initial 15-20 minutes of infusion: document vital signs and observe for of transfusion reaction.
         h. Frequently monitor infusion and patient response.
            (1) Rate: 30 minutes to 4 hours according to acuity, patient tolerance
               (a) Apply pressure bag to rapidly administer cells or volume.
               (b) FDA regulations require a transfusion be completed within 4 hours.

(2) Document vital signs if clinical change and after infusion.

   i. Should a transfusion reaction occur, notify blood bank, surgeon, and anesthesiologist, and follow established protocols of institution.

C. Transfusion complications

  1. Hemolytic reaction a severe reaction caused by

    a. *ABO incompatibility:* immediate hemolysis of red blood cells after infusion of the first few milliliters of blood

    b. *Human clerical error:* patient or blood component not properly identified and matched; usual cause of hemolytic reactions

    c. Reason for 1999 JCAHO Sentinel Event Alert on transfusion safety: mortality up to 10%

    d. Assessment and observations

      (1) Burning sensation along vein receiving transfusion

      (2) Sudden fever to >104° F (40° C) and chills

      (3) Hypotension, hematuria, and hemolysis: with

        (a) Hematuria, flank pain and renal failure

        (b) Dyspnea, tachypnea, tachycardia, palpitations, substernal pain

      (4) Abnormal bleeding or DIC

    e. Be especially vigilant with the anesthetized or sedated patient.

      (1) Immediately report unexplained, significant oozing.

      (2) Patient cannot report pain, anxiety.

      (3) Difficult to distinguish hypotension caused by transfusion reaction from hypotension caused by hypovolemic shock

      (4) Muscle relaxant may limit shivering response.

    f. Intervention and evaluation

      (1) Stop transfusion *immediately*!

      (2) Assess and document patient clinical condition.

      (3) Infuse normal saline and inform physician.

      (4) Complete transfusion reaction profile and return

        (a) Facility's investigation form to blood bank

        (b) Intact set of blood component unit, tubing, and accompanying IV fluid to blood bank

        (c) Blood samples (one red and one lavender top) to blood bank

        (d) Urine sample for urine hemoglobin to laboratory

      (5) Simultaneously treat patient per physician orders.

        (a) Acetaminophen for fever

        (b) Benadryl for itching

        (c) Cautious fluid management

        (d) Furosemide if needed for diuresis

        (e) Frequently monitor and document patient response.

  2. Delayed hemolytic transfusion reaction

    a. Usually occurs several days after transfusion: transfused cells have antigen to which recipient has been previously sensitized

    b. Causative antibodies: Anti-E, Anti-C, Kidd system

    c. Assessment

      (1) Unexplained fever

      (2) Definite hemoglobin decrease 2-10 days posttransfusion

      (3) Positive direct Coombs' test, elevated bilirubin

  3. Pyrogenic (febrile) transfusion reaction

    a. *Not* hemolytic: Onset 1 hour into transfusion, may last 8-10 hours

    b. Causes

      (1) WBC or platelet antibodies

      (2) Contaminating pyrogenic bacteria

      (3) Pregnancy or previous transfusion

    c. Assessment and intervention

      (1) New onset chills with fever, increase 2° F.

      (2) Flushed skin, headache, tachycardia

(3) Hemolysis: Bacteria replicate quickly even when refrigerated—symptoms after infusion of first 50 ml of blood

(4) Severe hypotension, abdominal, extremity pain

(5) Hematuria, DIC, and renal failure

  d. Intervention and evaluation

   (1) Stop transfusion! Early signs parallel early hemolytic reaction.

   (2) Begin transfusion reaction investigation.

   (3) Antipyretics (acetaminophen) and antihistamine for itching (diphenhydramine)

   (4) Fluids to support blood pressure and urine volume; monitor airway

 4. Allergic transfusion reaction

  a. Hypersensitivity response: accounts for 1% to 3% of transfusion reactions

  b. Occurs as a result of *antibodies* to donor blood foreign proteins, often in a patient with significant allergy history

  c. Develop urticaria with hives, itching

  d. Assessment and intervention

   (1) *Stop transfusion!* Reaction may progress unpredictably.

   (2) Assess for glottal edema.

   (3) Give IV antihistamine (Benadryl).

BIBLIOGRAPHY

1. Brown M: Red blood cell transfusion in critically ill patients. *Critical Care Nurse* 20:1-14, 2000.
2. Bryan, S: Hemolytic transfusion reaction: Safeguards for practice. *J PeriAnesth Nurs* 17:399-403, 2002.
3. Burden, N, Odom, J: Patients with special medical needs. In Burden, N, DeFazio-Quinn, DM, O'Brien, D, et al, editors: *Ambulatory Surgical Nursing,* ed 2. Philadelphia: WB Saunders, 2000, pp 608-611.
4. Carson, JI, Altman, DG, Duff, A, et al. Risk of bacterial infection associated with allogenic blood transfusion among patients undergoing hip fracture repair. *Transfusion* 39:694-700, 1999.
5. Goskowicz, R: Complications of blood transfusion. In Benumof JL, Saidman LJ, editors: *Anesthesia and perioperative complications,* ed 2. St Louis: Mosby, 1999, pp 536-574.
6. Hebert, P, Wells, G, Blajchman, MA, et al: A multicenter, randomized, controlled clinical trial of transfusion requirements in critical care. *N Engl J of Med* 340:409-417, 1999.
7. Murphy, P, Heal, MN, Blumberg, N: Infection or suspected infection after hip replacement surgery with autologous or homologous blood transfusions. *Transfusion* 31:212-217, 1991.
8. Triulzi, DJ, Vanek, K, Ryan, DH et al: A clinical and immunologic study of blood transfusion and postoperative infection in spinal surgery. *Transfusion* 32:517-524, 1992.
9. Zallen, G, Offner, P, Moore, E, et al: Age of transfused blood is an independent risk factor for postinjury multiple organ failure. *Am J Surg* 178:570-572, 1999.

35 Immediate Post-operative Assessment

ROSE FERRARA-LOVE

OBJECTIVES

At the conclusion of this chapter the reader will be able to:

1. Plan the focus of nursing care for the ambulatory surgery patient.

2. Characterize ways to ensure patient satisfaction in the ambulatory surgery setting.

3. Explain staffing ratios for phase I and phase II postanesthesia care unit (PACU).

4. Identify key points of anesthesia report upon arrival in PACU.

5. Demonstrate initial patient assessment parameters.

6. Describe extubation criteria in the PACU.

7. Discuss causes of hemodynamic changes in the PACU.

8. Examine causes of alterations in level of consciousness after anesthesia.

9. Assess patient readiness for transfer from phase I to phase II following spinal or epidural anesthesia.

10. Compare PACU scoring systems.

I. Immediate postanesthesia care—phase I
   A. Focus of care
      1. Observe patient's physiologic status, and intervene appropriately in a way that encourages uneventful recovery from anesthesia and surgery
      2. Provide safe environment for the patient experiencing limitations in physical, mental, and emotional function.
      3. Avoid or immediately treat complications in the immediate postanesthetic period.
      4. Uphold the patient's right to dignity, privacy, and confidentiality.
      5. Encourage a sense of wellness and self-confidence needed for early discharge.
   B. Patient outcome (see Table 35-1)
      1. Return to consciousness.
         a. Avoid heavy sedation.
            (1) Possible overnight admission
            (2) Prolongs recovery period
      2. Encourage self-care.
         a. Promotes self-confidence
         b. Promotes sense of wellness, not illness
      3. Maintain patient dignity.
         a. Use patient's name.
         b. Maintain eye contact.
         c. Use therapeutic touch.
            (1) Includes voice, tone, facial expressions, for example.
      4. Resolution of effects of major regional anesthesia
      5. Patient satisfaction
         a. Provide privacy.
         b. Early reunion with family and responsible others

■ TABLE 35-1
■ ■ **Patient Outcome Grid: Postanesthesia Care Unit**

Potential and Actual Problems/ Nursing Diagnosis	Outcome Goals: The Patient will be able to:	Nursing Interventions Knowledge Base	Resources
Ineffective airway clearance Potential for aspiration Ineffective breathing patterns, respiratory depression R/T • Sedation • Anesthesia • Positioning • Pain • Increased secretions • Nausea/Vomiting	Maintain normal respiratory parameters (rate, depth, ease, clarity of breath sounds) Maintain clear airway Avoid aspiration Maintain adequate oxygenation of tissues Avoid symptoms of hypoxia Perform effective cough and deep breathing exercises	Knowledge of effects of anesthetics, analgesics, sedatives, and muscle relaxants and associated drug interactions Airway maintenance techniques Apply stir-up regimen. Administer oxygen per protocol. Continuous assessment of respiratory status Timely report of untoward symptoms to anesthesiologist/surgeon Provide adequate hydration and safe positioning. Identify preexisting respiratory disease and individualize care appropriately.	Physiologic monitoring equipment at each bedside Adequate staffing patterns to ensure proper nurse-to-patient ratio Immediate access to anesthesia provider Comprehensive anesthesia report before transfer of patient ASPAN Standards of Perianesthesia Nursing Practice Facility policies regarding interventions for cardiovascular/respiratory problems Oxygen and suction at each bedside Immediate access to emergency equipment • Crash cart • Resuscitator bag/valve device • Ventilator • Airway maintenance supplies • Drugs
Potential alteration in tissue perfusion Cardiovascular instability	Maintain normal cardiovascular parameters, avoiding hypertension and hypotension Demonstrate expected postoperative arousal and mental status Demonstrate normal parameters of peripheral circulation	Assess all parameters of vital signs in ongoing fashion, including heart rate and rhythm, BP. Assess mental status and progression. Check peripheral pulses, color, and sensory adequacy in ongoing fashion. Timely report of untoward symptoms to anesthesiologist/surgeon Maintain adequate fluid balance and hydration.	

Continued

TABLE 35-1

Patient Outcome Grid: Postanesthesia Care Unit—*Cont'd*

Potential and Actual Problems/ Nursing Diagnosis	Outcome Goals: The Patient will be able to:	Nursing Interventions Knowledge Base	Resources
Altered skin integrity R/T surgical wound Potential for infection at surgical site	Experience appropriate and uncomplicated wound healing	Use aseptic technique. Enhance circulation of surgical wound site. Maintain adequate hydration. Avoid constricting bandages at surgical site. Assess surgical site throughout PACU stay.	Standard precautions Personal protective equipment and sterile dressing supplies Intravenous fluids Antibiotics if ordered
Altered skin integrity R/T pressure points, positioning	Avoid skin breakdown R/T pressure, tape, constricting bandages	Position patient using appropriate padding to avoid pressure points. Encourage stir-up regimen. Assess skin around tape for reaction—report to physician and/or change tape if necessary. Avoid constricting bandages in PACU. Assess full body throughout PACU stay.	Frequent position changes, assessment of skin Nonallergic tape Padding, pillows, foam, and so on for padding
Anxiety R/T unfamiliar surroundings, isolation from family or responsible adult, potential diagnosis or surgical outcome	Express reduced anxiety. Display calm demeanor Verbalize needs R/T family, emotional support Maintain CV and R parameters within normal limits	Block sights/sounds of other areas of PACU whenever possible. Encourage/allow family presence in PACU. Provide emotional support and answers to patient questions within boundaries of nursing. Assess patient's orientation. Monitor and oversee patient care while patient is vulnerable to environment.	Policy allowing families/responsible adult to visit in PACU Cubicle curtains to reduce view of PACU Separation of ambulatory and critical care patients in PACU

Altered thought process and/or memory loss R/T sedation/anesthesia	Display/verbalize appropriate orientation to surroundings and situations Avoid self-injury R/T altered thought patterns Rely on RA who understands nature of patient's temporarily altered thought patterns and responsibility for patient care	Provide frequent affirmations of orientation to time, place, and events. Assess patient's orientation. Monitor and oversee patient care while patient is vulnerable to environment.	Pharmaceutical literature outlining effects of anesthesia and sedative medications Predetermined PACU discharge criteria that include assessment of mental status *ASPAN Standards of Perianesthesia Nursing Practice*
Alterations in comfort: pain	Express acceptable comfort level Maintain normal CV and R parameters	Administer appropriate analgesics. Position patient for comfort. Apply cold therapy as ordered. Provide positive reinforcements and encourage philosophy of wellness throughout process. Encourage appropriate pace for increased activities.	Physician's orders for analgesics Analgesic medications Knowledge of nursing interventions for comfort Positioning and support of body areas Breathing exercises Positive reinforcement of comfort
Alterations in comfort: nausea and vomiting	Express acceptable comfort level Avoid vomiting and retching	Encourage appropriate pace for oral intake of fluids. Administer antiemetics as needed. Provide positive reinforcement and encourage philosophy of wellness throughout process.	Physician's orders/prescriptions for antiemetics Intravenous fluids Literature R/T reducing GI symptoms Appropriate food and beverages—avoid acid-producing juices, spicy, or difficult-to-digest foods.
Self-care deficit	Display sufficient level of alertness and self-care for safe discharge to phase II PACU	Provide comprehensive nursing care modified to patient's abilities. Assess patient for ability to turn, move, sit up, and call for assistance before transfer.	PACU discharge criteria

Continued

■ TABLE 35-1

■ Patient Outcome Grid: Postanesthesia Care Unit—*Cont'd*

Potential and Actual Problems/ Nursing Diagnosis	Outcome Goals: The Patient will be able to:	Nursing Interventions Knowledge Base	Resources
Actual or perceived, loss of privacy or dignity	Express content at level of privacy provided Maintain dignity and sense of self-esteem	Support patient's right to privacy and dignity. Promote unit philosophy that demands support of patient's right to privacy. Explain and demonstrate to patient that privacy and dignity will not be invaded while patient is asleep or sedated. Provide privacy. ● Curtains ● Blankets ● Clothing that covers the patient Allow patient as much decision-making as is possible in the PACU setting.	Surroundings that are friendly, family focused, private, and apart from view of other patients or staff Patient Bill of Rights Patient linens that provide adequate cover Cubicle curtains
Risk of hemorrhage	Maintain blood volume at normal level Avoid hypertension	Ensure availability of intravenous solutions. Observe surgical site for signs of bleeding and report to physician. Administer anxiolytic and/or antihypertensive medications as ordered.	Blood bank contract and policies for rapid availability of blood products for freestanding ambulatory surgery unit Antihypertensive agents Anxiolytic medications

Nursing Diagnosis	Expected Outcomes	Nursing Interventions	Resources
Alterations in health that can complicate postanesthesia care	Provide preoperative information about any medical factors present Have complied with instructions to optimize medical status before day of surgery Experience no complications R/T prior medical status	Encourage patient to provide accurate information regarding health status and practices before surgery. Assess patient's physical status frequently. Use active listening and observe for clues to patient's health status. Review record, and receive comprehensive report from anesthesia provider. Individualize patient care R/T prior health status.	Structured preoperative time frame for physical and historical assessment Books and literature on patient assessment and various medical conditions Primary care physician available to assist in optimizing patient health status before and after surgery
Risk of injury R/T environment, equipment, positioning, medications, emergence delirium	Remain free from allergic reactions, burns, skin breakdown or pressure points, falls, or nerve or joint injuries Complete PACU course without complications or injury	Position patient according to acceptable standards of care and individual needs using proper body mechanics for staff and patients. Ensure that side rail remains in up position. Lock stretcher while patient is on it and during transfers. Observe patient at all times. Keep only current patient's chart at bedside. Check emergency call bell system and emergency equipment periodically. Reinforce patient's orientation to time and place. Identify symptoms of emergence delirium and appropriate actions, interventions.	Patient record Competency-based nursing practice *ASPAN Standards of Perianesthesia Nursing Practice* Manufacturer's instructions for proper use of equipment Appropriate positioning supplies ● Pillows ● Padding ● Foam sheeting Ongoing program of preventative maintenance of equipment Policy on enacting Safe Medical Devices Act Gentle restraint policy

Continued

■ TABLE 35-1

■ **Patient Outcome Grid: Postanesthesia Care Unit—*Cont'd***

Potential and Actual Problems/ Nursing Diagnosis	Outcome Goals: The Patient will be able to:	Nursing Interventions Knowledge Base	Resources
Hypothermia Discomfort R/T cold	Maintain normal body temperature Verbalize comfort with temperature Avoid shivering	Assess and document patient *temperature on* admission and periodically in PACU. Keep patient covered as fully as possible, including head and neck areas. Apply warm blankets or warm forced air warming equipment, especially on patients at high risk for hypothermia (infants, frail elderly).	*ASPAN Standards of Perianesthesia Nursing Practice* Warming cabinets with blankets and solutions Forced warmed air heating blankets Thermometers
Discomfort R/T thirst	Express comfort	Nursing interventions to moisten mouth Water or ice orally as soon as possible postoperatively	Policy that encourages appropriate early interventions for thirst

From Burden N, Quinn D, O'Brien D, et al: *Ambulatory surgical nursing.* Philadelphia: WB Saunders, 2000, pp 416-419.
CV, cardiovascular; *R,* respiratory; *R/T,* related to; *PRN,* as needed; *PACU,* postanesthesia care unit; *GI,* gastrointestinal; *BP,* blood pressure; *ASPAN,* American Society of PeriAnesthesia Nurses.

II. Equipment and environmental concerns
   A. Suggested 1.5 beds available for each operating room
      1. Two beds per OR suite may be needed for
         a. Short procedures
         b. Pediatric cases
   B. Physical environment
      1. Well-lighted area
      2. Visibility of all patients in the PACU from any area
      3. Freestanding facility
         a. Access from PACU to lobby waiting area for family members
      4. Hospital-based facility
         a. Situated between operating room (OR) suite and phase II area
            (1) Separate rooms or sections are recommended for phase I and phase II areas.
               (a) Provides ease in progression from OR to phase II
      5. Amenities
         a. Bathrooms
         b. Changing and dressing areas
         c. Bedside chair
         d. Room for family member or responsible other to visit
         e. Diversionary materials
            (1) Current magazines, radio, television, videos, for example.
         f. Noninstitutional decor
            (1) Promotes sense of wellness
               (a) Wallpaper
               (b) Draperies
               (c) Greenery
               (d) Windows
               (e) Wall decorations
               (f) Supplies in modern cabinets
   C. Emergency preparation
      1. Emergency call system
      2. Emergency equipment and medications
III. Policies, procedures, and staffing
   A. Policy manual per institutional guidelines
      1. Address broad range of nursing duties and administrative practice specific to PACU.
      2. Annual review of policies
      3. Staff participation in ongoing revision
   B. Outside certifying bodies
      1. Joint Commission for Accreditation of Healthcare Organizations
      2. Accreditation Association for Ambulatory Health Care, Inc. (AAAHC)
      3. American Association for Accreditation of Ambulatory Surgery Facilities (AAAASF)
      4. American Hospital Association
      5. State Health Department
      6. Third-party payers
         a. Medicare
         b. Medicaid
         c. Insurance companies
   C. Staffing ratios
      1. Determine full-time equivalent staffing (FTEs) needs of unit.
      2. ASPAN Standards of PeriAnesthesia Nursing Practice, 2002
         a. Phase I
            (1) Class 1:2—one nurse to two patients who are
               (a) One unconscious, stable without artificial airway and over the age of 9 years; and one conscious, stable, and free of complications

    (b) Two conscious, stable, and free of complications

    (c) Two conscious, stable, 11 years of age and under; with family or competent support staff present

   (2) Class 1:1—one nurse to one patient

    (a) At the time of admission, until the critical elements are met

    (b) Requiring mechanical life support and/or artificial airway

    (c) Any unconscious patient 9 years of age and under

    (d) A second nurse must be available to assist as necessary.

   (3) Class 2:1—two nurses to one patient

    (a) One critically ill, unstable, complicated patient

  b. Phase II

   (1) Class 1:3—one nurse to three patients

    (a) Over 5 years of age within one half hour of procedure or discharge from phase I

    (b) Age 5 years of and under within one half hour of procedure or discharge from phase I level of care with family present

   (2) Class 1:2—one nurse to two patients

    (a) 5 years of age and under without family or support staff present

    (b) Initial admission of patient postprocedure

   (3) Class 1:1—one nurse to one patient

    (a) Unstable patient of any age requiring transfer

  c. Phase III

   (1) Class 1:3/5—one nurse to five patients

    (a) Patients awaiting transportation home

    (b) Patients with no caregiver

    (c) Patients who have had procedures requiring extended observation or interventions.

     (i) Potential risk for bleeding

     (ii) Pain management

     (iii) Postoperative nausea and vomiting (PONV)

IV. Transfer of the patient to a PACU

 A. Transporting teams responsible for patient until responsibility accepted by PACU nurse

  1. Anesthesia report

   a. History

   b. Medications

   c. Anesthetic agents and doses

    (1) Untoward responses

     (a) Treatment

     (b) Result

   d. Vital signs

  2. Circulating nurse report

   a. Surgery performed

   b. Preoperative status

    (1) Emotional

    (2) Psychosocial

   c. Laboratory results

  3. Medical record

   a. Provides information not included in verbal report

  4. Deferring verbal report

   a. Patient's condition is unstable.

    (1) Immediate safety ensured by all participants before report provided

V. Initial patient assessment and care planning

 A. Systems assessment

  1. Usually rapid initial head-to-toe assessment

        a. Focus on vital functions
- (1) Airway
- (2) Circulatory

    2. Comprehensive assessment (see Box 35-1)

    3. Subjective assessment
- **a.** Patient's input
  - (1) Alertness
  - (2) Lucidity
  - (3) Orientation
  - (4) Motor abilities
    - (a) Sensory and motor control following regional anesthesia
  - (5) Comfort level
  - (6) Presence of nausea

    4. Assessments are ongoing.
- **a.** Concurrent with nursing interventions

VI. Respiratory adequacy

  A. Assessment

    1. Auscultation of breath sounds

    2. Assessment of chest expansion
- **a.** Ease and depth of respirations
- **b.** Use of accessory muscles
- **c.** Skin and mucous membrane color

    3. Administration of oxygen
- **a.** Considered standard following heavy sedation or general anesthesia
- **b.** Face mask
  - (1) Simple
  - (2) Aerosol
- **c.** Nasal canula

    4. Body's oxygen demand increases with
- **a.** Shivering
  - (1) By 400% or more
- **b.** Pain
- **c.** Anxiety
- **d.** Hypotension
- **e.** Hypertension
- **f.** Dysrhythmias
  - (1) Tachydysrhythmias
  - (2) Bradydysrhythmias
- **g.** Rapid fluctuations in intravascular volume
- **h.** Thromboembolic events
- **i.** Left ventricular failure
- **j.** Catecholamine release

  B. Monitoring equipment

    1. Primary
- **a.** Eyes and ears
  - (1) Observation
  - (2) Auscultation
  - (3) Palpation

    2. Mechanical
- **a.** Respirometer
  - (1) Detect lung volumes
    - (a) Tidal volume
    - (b) Vital capacity
  - (2) Negative inspiratory force (NIF) meter
    - (a) Least amount of negative force to initiate inhalation
- **b.** Arterial blood gas analysis (ABGs)
  - (1) Invasive, often painful arterial blood sample for analysis

■ BOX 35-1
■ **DIFFERENTIAL DIAGNOSIS OF POSTANESTHESIA COMPLICATIONS**

Restlessness
Hypoxemia ($\downarrow$ SpO$_2$)
Pain
Hypotension
Bladder distention/urinary retention
Emotional response
Shivering/feeling of being cold
Hypercarbia ($\uparrow$ CO$_2$)
Emergence delirium
GI distress/distention
Psychotropic effects of preoperative medications
$\uparrow$ Intracranial pressure, intracranial event

Hypotension
Decreased preload
    Hypovolemia from prolonged fasting or inadequate fluid replacement
    Excessive urinary or third-space losses, bleeding
    Peripheral vasodilation ($\downarrow$ resistance) (i.e., effects of major regional anesthesia)
Effects of sedative and narcotic drugs
Decreased myocardial contractility
    Effects of anesthetic drugs
    Perioperative cardiac event (i.e., MI)
    Preexisting cardiac disease
Orthostatic effects of progressive ambulation

Hypertension
Pain, surgical stimulation
Hypoxemia ($\downarrow$ SpO$_2$)
Bladder distention/urinary retention
Shivering, vasoconstriction caused by hypothermia
Preexisting disease (i.e., hyperthyroidism, essential hypertension, renal disease)
Emergence delirium, emotional response
Hypercarbia ($\uparrow$ CO$_2$)
Retching or vomiting
Fluid overload
Effects of medications (i.e., vasopressors, naloxone, ketamine, anticholinergics, cocaine, ephedrine, epinephrine)

Dysrhythmias
Pain
Hypoxemia ($\downarrow$ SpO$_2$)
Perioperative myocardial infarction
Catecholamine release
Metabolic changes (i.e., acidosis, alkalosis)
Preexisting disease
Hypercarbia ($\uparrow$ CO$_2$)
Failure of artificial pacemaker
Side effects of perioperative medications
Electrolyte imbalance (potassium, calcium, magnesium)

Tachycardia
Pain
Hypovolemia
Emergence delirium
Fever (i.e., malignant hyperthermia)

▨ BOX 35-1
▨ **DIFFERENTIAL DIAGNOSIS OF POSTANESTHESIA COMPLICATIONS**

Hyperthyroidism
Effects of medications (i.e., glycopyrrolate, atropine)

Bradycardia
Oculocardiac reflex
Stimulation of baroreceptors
Hypoventilation, especially in children
Cardiac effects of heavy athletic activity
Sedative, anesthetic drugs
Effects of medication (i.e. neostigmine, narcotics)

Respiratory Depression
Inadequate airway
Splinting, secondary to pain
Pulmonary congestion
Positioning, especially in the obese
Prolonged neuromuscular blockade
Mechanical failure of equipment (ventilator, bag/valve/mask)
Preexisting disease, chronic obstructive pulmonary disease (COPD), reactive airway

From Burden N, Quinn D, O'Brien D, et al: *Ambulatory surgical nursing.* Philadelphia: WB Saunders, 2000, pp 413.

    c. Pulse oximeter
       (1) Measures ratio of oxygenated hemoglobin to the total amount of
           hemoglobin and expresses it as a percent of saturation
           (a) Analyzes color of blood with two light-emitting diodes and a
              photodetector
       (2) Noninvasive
           (a) Detects oxygen saturation of hemoglobin in circulating blood
           (b) Sensitive to changes in blood content oxygen; heralds hypoxic
              event before clinical signs
           (c) Considered "standard of care" monitoring in anesthesia and
              PACU settings
       (3) Advantages
           (a) Simplicity
           (b) Noninvasive
           (c) Continuous display
           (d) Sensitivity to changes in blood oxygen levels
           (e) Ability to be applied to all ages
           (f) Relatively low expense
       (4) Disadvantages
           (a) Motion at sensor site
           (b) Low perfusion of the arterial bed being monitored
              (i) Hypothermia
              (ii) Hypotension
              (iii) Large doses of vasopressors
           (c) Significant dysrhythmias
           (d) Carbon monoxide or methemoglobin in the blood
           (e) Severe anemia
              (i) Hemoglobin level less than 5 g per dl
           (f) Venous pulsation
              (i) Sensor is too tight.
           (g) Electrical interference

(h) Interference from ambient or extrinsic light sources

    (i) Circulation intravenous dyes

(5) Complications

    (a) Burns and blisters

        (i) Usually on infants and children

    (b) Pressure necrosis

d. Capnography

    (1) Monitors exhaled carbon dioxide

        (a) End-tidal CO_2

    (2) Intraoperative monitoring of patients under general anesthesia

        (a) Used in PACU for critically ill patients

        (b) Used with sedation and analgesia

C. Respiratory complications (see Chapter 36 for other complications)

  1. Apnea

    a. Requires aggressive ventilatory support

      (1) Symptoms may be masked by general anesthesia

        (a) Lethargy

        (b) Confusion

        (c) Restlessness

        (d) Anxiety

        (e) Dysrhythmias

        (f) Cyanosis

        (g) Decreased Pa_{CO_2}

          (i) May lead to respiratory acidosis

        (h) Hypertension followed by hypotension

        (i) Decreased urinary output

  2. Treatment

    a. Pharmacologic cause

      (1) Narcotics

        (a) Intravenous narcotic antagonist—naloxone (Narcan)

          (i) 1 µg/kg (0.01 mg/kg)

            [a] Repeated 5-10 minutes

          (ii) Side effects

            [a] Cessation of analgesia

            [b] Agitation

            [c] Hypertension

            [d] Noncardiogenic pulmonary edema

            [e] Atrial and ventricular dysrhythmias

            [f] Cardiac arrest

      (2) Muscle relaxants

        (a) Depolarizing muscle relaxant

          (i) Succinylcholine (Anectine)

          (ii) Short acting

            [a] Not pharmacologically reversed

            [b] Action is self-limiting; effects usually dissipated before admission to PACU

          (iii) "Phase II block"

            [a] Mimic characteristics of nondepolarizing blockade in *large* doses >3 mg/kg

            [b] Requires pharmacologic reversal

        (b) Nondepolarizing muscle relaxants

          (i) Reversed with anticholinesterase agents (neostigmine, pyridostigmine, edrophonium)

            [a] Can cause vagal reactions (specifically bradycardia)

            [b] Usually administered in combination with a vagolytic agent (atropine or glycopyrrolate)

        (c) Reparalysis (or recurarization)

          (i) Major cause of respiratory depression

(ii) Inadequate pharmacologic reversal
   [a] Effects of muscle relaxant extend beyond effects of reversal agent
(iii) Other factors include *(Resp depression causes)*
   [a] General anesthetics
   [b] Hypothermia
   [c] Antidysrhythmics (quinidine, procainamide, and calcium channel blockers)
   [d] Respiratory acidosis
   [e] Metabolic alkalosis
   [f] Hypokalemia
   [g] Hypocalcemia
   [h] Local anesthetic agents (including lidocaine given as antidysrhythmics by intravenous [IV] drip or bolus postoperatively)
   [i] Furosemide IV in doses of 1 mg/kg
   [j] Dehydration
   [k] Hyponatremia
   [l] Antibiotics, particularly mycins and aminoglycosides

3. The intubated patient
   a. Nursing care
      (1) Constant nursing observation
      (2) Administration humidified oxygen
         (a) Compensates for bypassed upper airway
         (b) Provides moisture to artificially inspired air
      (3) Protect patient from aspiration by maintaining cuff inflation.
         (a) Position patient properly.
         (b) Suction as appropriate.
      (4) Ensure proper position of endotracheal tube by
         (a) Auscultation of breath sounds
         (b) Observation of symmetrical chest expansion
      (5) Provide emotional support and explanations to awakening patient.
      (6) Evaluate for signs of sufficient recovery to allow for safe extubation.
   b. Extubation criteria
      (1) Return of muscle strength after muscle relaxants
         (a) Equal hand grasps
         (b) Able to initiate head lift from bed and sustain at least 5 seconds
      (2) Respiratory parameters
         (a) Tidal volume at least 5 ml/kg
         (b) Vital capacity at least 15-20 ml/kg
         (c) Negative inspiratory force of 20-25 cm water pressure
      (3) Patient should respond appropriately to questions.
         (a) "Yes" or "no" head movements
         (b) Other forms of communication
            (i) Sign or picture board
            (ii) Writing
         (c) Protrude the tongue
         (d) Open eyes widely
      (4) Swallow and cough reflexes present
      (5) Regular respiratory pattern >10 breaths per minute
      (6) After extubation, close observation for hypoventilation
         (a) Presence of endotracheal tube may have stimulated patient to remain awake and breathing adequately

VII. Circulatory adequacy (see Chapter 36 for other complications)
   A. Cardiac status
      1. Constant assessment of pulse for rate, rhythm, amplitude
         a. Weak, absent, or irregular pulses
            (1) Hypovolemia

(2) Decreased cardiac output
(3) Myocardial ischemia
    (a) Prior cardiac compromise
        (i) Increased risk of cardiac complications postanesthesia
    (b) Cannot measure myocardial oxygenation directly
        (i) Clinical symptoms
    (c) Electrocardiogram (ECG) changes
    (d) Chest pain
    (e) Change in skin color
    (f) Diaphoresis
    (g) Gastrointestinal (GI) sequelae
(4) Acute myocardial infarction (MI)
    (a) Previous MI single most important risk factor for perioperative patient
        (i) Nonurgent surgery should be delayed until at least 6 months post-MI to reduce perioperative morbidity
    (b) Early signs of perioperative acute infarction or ischemia
        (i) ECG changes
        (ii) T wave inversion and ST segment depression of 1 mm or more below baseline indicative of ischemia
    (c) ST elevation indicates actual myocardial injury.
    (d) Later presence of Q wave of 0.03 sec. is definitive for infarction and tissue necrosis.
        (i) Subjective changes described by patient
        (ii) Anginal pain (often constant)
    (e) Nausea, vomiting
    (f) Diaphoresis
    (g) Feeling of impending doom or dying
        (i) Silent MI
        (ii) Only 25% patients who have MIs in the postoperative period experience typical anginal pain.
    (h) Most often seen in elderly, diabetic, and hypertensive patients
(5) Cardiac dysrhythmias
(6) Local pathology of the artery in extremity in question
b. Bounding pulses
  (1) Excitement
  (2) Hypertension
  (3) Fluid overload
2. Assess elderly especially for
  a. Uncompensated congestive heart failure
  b. Pulmonary edema
3. Cardiac monitoring
  a. Alarm parameters established
    (1) Alarm system should be activated.
  b. Lead II monitoring typically used in PACU
    (1) Superiority in dysrhythmia detection
    (2) No information on inferior areas of heart
        (a) Right coronary artery supply

■
■■ Note: ST segment and T wave changes are not absolutely diagnostic of an acute MI. They may be caused by digitalis therapy, hypothermia, electrolyte abnormalities, or dysrhythmias. These changes should be considered as one parameter of the diagnosis, which supports clinical evaluations and diagnostic enzyme tests.
VIII. Fluid and electrolyte balance
  A. Most ambulatory surgery procedures not associated with significant alterations in fluid and electrolyte status
    1. Average adult requires 2200 ml of fluid each day.

      a. Most ambulatory surgery patients can compensate for fasting and intraoperative fluid status.

      b. Those who cannot maintain homeostatic balance are

        (1) Small children

        (2) Debilitated adults with the following disease processes

          (a) Renal

          (b) GI

          (c) Endocrine

          (d) Cardiovascular

        (3) Elderly

        (4) Particularly thin or emaciated

  2. Other factors related to fluid and electrolyte disturbance

      a. Stress

        (1) Fear

        (2) Anxiety

          (a) Retention of water and sodium

      b. GI disturbances

        (1) Nausea and vomiting

        (2) Nasogastric suctioning

        (3) Bowel preparation

          (a) Loss of sodium and potassium

      c. Excessive bleeding

B. Blood administration

  1. Usually not common in the ambulatory setting

      a. Used to treat unexpected hemorrhage

      b. Significant blood loss may be expected.

        (1) Lipolysis

        (2) Lipectomy

  2. Autologous blood donation

      a. More than 5% of blood donations are autologous.

        (1) Several units are donated weeks before surgery.

          (a) Fresh, unfrozen blood can be stored up to 42 days.

            (i) Depends on local blood bank policies

          (b) Last unit must be drawn 72 hours before surgery.

            (i) Allow for regeneration of patient's blood volume.

          (c) Other criteria for autologous donation

            (i) Cardiovascular stability

              [a] No recent significant cardiac disease

            (ii) Between 12 and 75 years of age

            (iii) No history of seizures in adult life

            (iv) Minimal hemoglobin level of 11 g/dl

              [a] Hematocrit 34 %

            (v) No active infections

            (vi) No bone marrow cancer

            (vii) Availability of adequate venous access for blood collection

          (d) Low body weight may prevent withdrawal of full unit.

            (i) Does not preclude autologous donation

          (e) Although self-donated, autologous units are crossmatched.

            (i) Increases chance of clerical error during processing

  3. Transfusion precautions

      a. No difference in policies for autologous or allogeneic transfusion

        (1) Secure blood from blood bank.

        (2) Identify patient.

        (3) Identify blood bag.

          (a) Two nurses usually identify patient and blood.

            (i) One nurse and another professional is acceptable.

              [a] Certified registered nurse anesthetist (CRNA)

              [b] Physician

(4) Initiate transfusion.
   (a) Monitor patient throughout.
      (i) Include temperature in assessment.
(5) Respond to any untoward reactions.
   (a) Volume overload
   (b) Bacterial contamination
   (c) Air emboli
   (d) Hypotension
      (i) Bacterial contamination
   (e) Venous emboli
   (f) Hypocalcemia
      (i) Citrate intoxication
   (g) Hypersensitivity to plastics or stabilizers in tubing and bag
   (h) Anaphylaxis and hemolytic reactions
      (i) Urticaria (hives)
   (i) Chest tightness or pain
   (j) Dyspnea
   (k) Hyperthermia
   (l) Wheezing
      (i) Discontinue infusion immediately.
   (m) Maintain patent IV with new tubing and solution.
   (n) Notify physician.
   (o) Monitor vital signs.
   (p) Administer oxygen.
   (q) Diphenhydramine (Benadryl) IV is antihistamine of choice.
   (r) Protocol may require urine and blood specimens sent to blood bank with tubing and remaining blood in bag for analysis.
b. Securing blood products may be more difficult in freestanding surgical center.
   (1) Need contract with local blood bank
   (2) Procedure for rapid procurement when needed
      (a) Transfer of blood products must be efficient to address emergencies.
4. Other options for transfusion
   a. "Priming" bone marrow during autologous harvesting by adding erythropoietin
   b. Intraoperative blood salvage (IBS)
      (1) Blood lost by patient is processed by centrifugation and returned to patient.
         (a) Often approved by Jehovah's Witness patients provided blood not processed outside of operating room
   c. Autotransfusion devices
      (1) Blood from patient drains into collecting bag and transfused directly to the patient
         (a) Collection of blood for 2-4 hours and transfused over 2 hours
         (b) Often used with total joint replacements and cardiac surgery
C. Artificial blood sources
   1. Basic property of blood is oxygen and carbon dioxide transport and hemodynamic stability.
   2. Two types of substitutes under development
      a. Perfluorochemical emulsions (PFC)
         (1) Chemically inert liquids
         (2) High solubility for gases
         (3) Advantages
            (a) High O_2 solubility
            (b) Inert liquid
            (c) Adequate supply

      (4) Disadvantages
         (a) Long tissue half-life
         (b) Short vascular half-life
            (i) Less than 19 hours
         (c) Higher than normal P_{O_2} level is needed
         (d) Little is known about toxic effects.
   b. Hemoglobin solutions
      (1) Hemoglobin purified and reduced to a powder
         (a) Mixed with saline and infused
      (2) Advantages
         (a) Ability to carry oxygen at normal P_{O_2} levels
      (3) Disadvantages
         (a) Toxicities and impurities from residual red cell membrane (stroma)
            (i) Effects predominately renal
         (b) Vasoconstriction
         (c) Short vascular half-life
         (d) Uncertain supply

D. Nonblood volume substitutes
  1. Volume expanders
    a. Dextran
      (1) Synthetic plasma substitute
      (2) Advantages
         (a) Administered through standard IV tubing
         (b) Relatively inexpensive
         (c) Readily available
         (d) No risk of disease
      (3) Disadvantages
         (a) Hypersensitivity reactions
            (i) Usually in first 30 minutes of infusion
         (b) Interfere with platelet function
            (i) Transient prolongation of bleeding time
         (c) Certain methods of typing and crossmatching have been affected by dextran.
    b. Hetastarch (Hespan)
      (1) Artificial colloid
      (2) Inexpensive
      (3) Derived from cornstarch
         (a) Closely resembles human glycogen
      (4) Available in 6% in 0.9% sodium chloride solution
      (5) Minimal coagulation effects
      (6) Less likely to produce allergic reactions

E. Oral intake
  1. Preferred in ambulatory surgery patients
    a. Encouraged once patient is awake and sufficiently alert
      (1) All protective reflexes are present.
      (2) No nausea
    b. Raising patient's head promotes easy swallowing without choking.
    c. Appropriate fluids
      (1) Water and ice
      (2) Avoid citrus juice, coffee.
         (a) May cause nausea and vomiting
  2. Continue IV fluids until oral intake is tolerated.

F. Urinary status
  1. Average daily output of 600 ml is necessary to excrete waste products of metabolism.
    a. Optimal amount to ensure kidney function and adequate hydration is 30 ml/hour.

        b. Urine production can decrease as a result of
- (1) Hypovolemia
- (2) Hypothermia
- (3) Body's reaction to stress

2. Urinary retention
- **a.** Spinal and epidural anesthesias
- **b.** Surgical manipulation
- **c.** Use of local anesthetics surrounding structures
  - (1) Assess bladder for distention particularly after
    - (a) Urinary procedures
    - (b) Inguinal herniorrhaphy
    - (c) Gynecologic procedures
      - (i) Palpable in lower pelvis
    - (d) Firm, domed area above pubis
- **d.** Other symptoms of bladder distention
  - (1) Restlessness
  - (2) Lower abdominal pain
  - (3) Hypertension
  - (4) Tachycardia
  - (5) Anxiety
  - (6) Tachypnea
  - (7) Diaphoresis
    - (a) May mimic hypoxic symptoms
- **e.** May require catheterization

3. Urination may be required for home discharge.
- **a.** Discharge from phase I to phase II may be done if not uncomfortable and not distended.
- **b.** Allow patient to use bathroom if sufficiently recovered.

IX. Temperature regulation
- **A.** Normothermia
  - **1.** Hypothalamus
    - **a.** Regulatory center
      - (1) 98.6° to 99.5° F (36° to 37.5° C)
  - **2.** Major sites of heat production
    - **a.** By-product of metabolism
      - (1) Muscles
        - (a) Twenty-five percent of body heat production
      - (2) Liver
        - (a) Fifty percent of body heat production
      - (3) Glands
        - (a) Fifteen percent produced by brain
  - **3.** Heat loss mechanisms in surgery
    - **a.** Conduction of heat from body to cold surfaces it touches
    - **b.** Convection—heat loss to air current
    - **c.** Radiation—electromagnetic energy loss to colder objects in room
      - (1) Accounts for 65% heat loss
    - **d.** Evaporation from skin during preparations and through respiratory system and urine
- **B.** Hypothermia—core body temperature <95° F (35° C)
  - **1.** Patient factors affecting body temperature in surgery
    - **a.** Patient weight
      - (1) Thin patients lose more heat and generate less heat than heavier counterparts.
    - **b.** Length of surgical exposure of skin and internal structures
    - **c.** Site of surgery
      - (1) Peritoneal exposure significantly increases heat loss.
    - **d.** Intravenous infusion of room temperature fluids
    - **e.** Cool irrigants and skin preparation solutions

    f. Ambient room temperature

      (1) Constant air circulation increases environmental effect of cool room temperature.

        (a) Children—6 months to 2 years

          (i) Greater degree of heat loss

            [a] Larger body surface area compared with muscle mass

          (ii) OR temperature 76° F

            [a] Higher for newborns and premature babies

        (b) Elderly

          (i) Shrinking muscle mass and decreasing subcutaneous fat layer

            [a] Less able to conserve heat

2. Anesthesia factors

  a. Depress thermoregulatory center

  b. Neuromuscular relaxants stop muscle activity.

    (1) Also prevent shivering

  c. Inhalation agents

    (1) Respiratory heat loss from unarmed oxygen and inhalation gas delivery

3. Prevention of heat loss

  a. Increasing room temperature

  b. Heated blankets

  c. Warmed irrigation and preparation fluids

  d. Foil blankets to prevent radiation of patient's body heat

  e. IV fluid warmers

  f. Respiratory circuits

    (1) Provide for heat conservation

  g. Head covering for patient

    (1) More than 50% of body heat may be lost as radiation from scalp.

4. Benefits

  a. Decrease in oxygen requirements

    (1) Protect body tissues from hypoxemia

5. Drawbacks

  a. Slows metabolic rate

    (1) Effects of medications greatly enhanced

      (a) Active drug remains in body longer.

      (b) Less drug needed to produce desired effect

6. Treatment in PACU

  a. Observation

    (1) Cyanosis of extremities

      (a) Vasoconstriction of distal vessels

        (i) Physiologic response to conserve heat

      (b) May preclude accurate oxygen saturation measurements by pulse oximetry

    (2) Dysrhythmias

      (a) Secondary to hypothermia

    (3) Reparalysis (or recurarization)

      (a) Dose of reversal agents in hypothermic patient is no longer effective when metabolic rate increases in response to warmer temperature.

  b. Warming measures

    (1) Heated blankets

    (2) Forced air heat

    (3) Radiant heat

    (4) Warmed IV fluids

    (5) Covering head and upper torso

C. Shivering

  1. Major mechanism of heat production

  2. Spontaneously without known cause in normothermic patient

      3. Uncomfortable and unpleasant for the awakening patient

      4. Untoward effects

        a. Hypertension

        b. Self-injury

          (1) Operative site

          (2) Teeth

        c. Increase in oxygen demands

          (1) Four to five times normal

        d. Prolonged PACU time

          (1) Expense in additional PACU time, supplies, and medications

        e. Diffuse muscle aches for days after surgery

          (1) Intensity of muscle activity

            (a) Should be reported to phase II nurse for postoperative instruction regarding analgesia unrelated to surgical site

     5. Treatment

        a. Oxygen therapy

          (1) Observe for signs of hypoxia.

        b. Medications

          (1) Narcotics

            (a) Meperidine (Demerol)

              (i) Eighty percent effectiveness with 12.5-25 mg IV doses

          (2) Opiate agonist–antagonist analgesic

            (a) Butorphanol tartrate (Stadol)

              (i) Ninety-five percent effective within 5 minutes

  D. Hyperthermia

     1. Malignant hyperthermia (MH)

        a. Serious, hypermetabolic state

          (1) Genetic in origin

          (2) Triggered by certain anesthetic agents and muscle relaxants

            (a) For more detailed information, see Chapter 23.

X. Level of consciousness

  A. Unconscious patients should never be left unattended.

     1. Protective reflexes absent

     2. Cognitive abilities absent

        a. Patients totally dependent upon PACU nurse for protection from the environment

  B. Accepted that hearing is first sense to return upon awakening

     1. Speaking to the patient in calm, low tones helps arouse and orient semiconscious patients.

        a. Periodic, frequent attempts should continue until the patient responds except in

          (1) Signs of upper airway irritation

            (a) Gagging, coughing

               (i) Administer oxygen.

            (b) Position to avoid aspiration.

            (c) Allow to awaken slowly without intervention to decrease risk of laryngospasm.

          (2) Use of ketamine

            (a) Severe hallucinations can follow administration.

               (i) If ketamine-induced delirium occurs

               (ii) Diazepam (Valium), 5-10 mg IV

            (b) Thiopental, 50-75 mg IV

        b. Avoid extraneous noises (laughter, personal conversations, etc.).

          (1) May be distorted and confuse or agitate awakening patient

  C. Emergence delirium (emergence excitement)

     1. Signs and symptoms

        a. Restlessness

        b. Thrashing of extremities

      c. Combativeness

      d. Crying

      e. Moaning

      f. Screaming

      g. Irrational talking

      h. Disorientation

  2. Causes

      a. Preoperative medications

        (1) Scopolamine

      b. Pain

      c. Bladder distention

      d. Feelings of suffocation during awakening

      e. Possible cerebral hypoxia

      f. Psychological preoperative preparation

        (1) Fear of surgery

          (a) Body disfigurement

            (i) Children and adolescents particularly

        (2) Surgical diagnosis

  3. Untoward effects

      a. Self-injury

        (1) Limbs

        (2) Tongue

      b. Straining or opening suture lines

      c. Dislodging IV lines

      d. Self-extubation

  4. Treatment

      a. Gentle physical restraint

        (1) Total physical restraint may increase agitation.

        (2) May need several nurses or other personnel

      b. Pharmacologic treatment

        (1) Narcotics

          (a) Meperidine

          (b) Fentanyl with droperidol (Innovar)

          (c) Morphine

          (d) Methadone

        (2) Physostigmine (Antilirium)

          (a) Use is controversial as reversal agent to end episode of emergence delirium.

          (b) Useful in reversing effects of scopolamine or other anticholinergic drugs

            (i) Dose in 1 mg increments, IV, slowly

            (ii) Do not exceed 3 mg total.

          (c) Can cause severe bradycardia

D. Delayed awakening

  1. Causes

      a. Impaired metabolism, ventilation, circulation as a result of

        (1) Type and amount of preoperative medication

          (a) Benzodiazepines

          (b) Neuroleptic agents

          (c) Narcotics

          (d) Barbiturates

        (2) Intraoperative medications

          (a) Inhalation agents

          (b) Narcotics

          (c) Barbiturates

        (3) Other drugs self-administered prior to anesthesia

          (a) Cimetidine

          (b) Lidocaine

(c) Antihypertensives

(d) Monoamine oxidase inhibitors (MAOIs)

(e) Antidepressants

(4) Hypothermia

(5) Malignant hyperthermia

(6) Metabolic diseases

(7) Cardiovascular pathology

(a) Hypertension

(b) Hypovolemia

(c) Myocardial ischemia

(8) Respiratory inadequacy

(a) Narcotic induced

(b) Pathologic in nature

(9) Increased intracranial pressure

(10) Cerebrovascular accident (CVA)

(11) Undiagnosed intraoperative seizure

(a) Embolism

XI. Positioning

A. Ensure proper body alignment.

1. Provide comfort and safety.

a. Lateral positioning

(1) Prevention of aspiration

(2) Support patient's head and neck.

(3) Position extremities to avoid damage to nerves, tendons, and muscles.

(a) Avoid hyperextension of joints.

(i) Can result in pain and damage to joint structure

(4) Opposing skin surfaces should be separated with padding.

(5) Prolonged unconsciousness or immobility

(a) Provide gentle passive range of motion.

(b) Frequent repositioning

2. Promote cardiovascular and respiratory homeostasis.

a. Reposition slowly to avoid compromise.

(1) Reassess after repositioning.

3. Special surgical-specific positioning

a. Extremities

(1) Elevated above heart level

(a) Prevents bleeding and edema

(i) Promotes healing

(b) Decreases pain

b. Plastic surgery

(1) Fowler's position

(a) Head, face, neck, breast

(i) Promotes healing

(b) Prevents bleeding

c. Eye and ear surgery

(1) Usually surgeon specific

XII. Operative site

A. Assess wounds and/or dressings.

1. Bleeding

a. Frank bloody drainage

b. Rapid filling of collection systems

c. Bruising

d. Skin discolorations

e. Swelling

(1) Indicative of hematoma formation

f. Excessive swallowing following ear, nose, and throat (ENT) procedures

(1) Subjective complaints of drainage in back of throat

       g. Heavy vaginal flow

       h. Excessive hematuria

  2. Intraabdominal

       a. May not appear until blood loss is significant

       b. Signs and symptoms

         (1) Apprehension

         (2) Hypotension

         (3) Tachycardia

         (4) Splinting

         (5) Abdominal pain

         (6) Tenderness and rigidity

         (7) Pallor

         (8) Diaphoresis

  3. Laparoscopic procedures

       a. Particular risk for occult bleeding

         (1) Potential for laceration or inadvertent burning of abdominal vessels and organs

  4. Treatment

       a. Reduce or stop any excessive bleeding.

         (1) Manual pressure

         (2) Elevation of site if possible

         (3) Specific protocols

           (a) Ice or cool compresses to surrounding area

           (b) Increase IV infusion rate.

           (c) Sedation

           (d) Pressor agents

           (e) Blood replacement

             (i) Colloids

             (ii) Blood products

           (f) Oxygen therapy

           (g) Resuturing incision or packing body cavity

             (i) Sterile supplies should be readily available.

           (h) May return to OR

             (i) Consent must be obtained from family member.

               [a] Sedated patients cannot sign legal document.

       b. Airway involvement

         (1) Constant reassurance

         (2) Position appropriately.

         (3) Gentle suction of mouth

           (a) Do not place suction catheter near site of hemorrhage.

XIII. Peripheral circulation

  A. Surgically involved extremity assessment

    1. Circulatory compromise

       a. Constriction

         (1) Encircling bandage

           (a) ACE wrap

           (b) Cast

         (2) Thrombus

         (3) Embolus

         (4) Internal pressure

           (a) Hemorrhage

    2. Peripheral pulses

       a. Palpated bilaterally for presence, strength, symmetry

         (1) Numerical description

           (a) Absent—0

           (b) Weak and thready—1+

           (c) Normal—2+

           (d) Full and bounding—3+

      b. If not palpable

        (1) Reposition extremity and palpate pulse site again.

        (2) May need a Doppler ultrasound stethoscope (DUS)

          (a) Noninvasive

          (b) Uses sound-wave frequency to detect movement of red blood cells in underlying vessels

   3. Pulse oximeter

     a. Visual depiction of pulse strength on affected extremity

   4. Skin color and nailbed color

     a. Vasoconstriction in hypothermic patient may mimic cyanosis resulting from more severe causes.

     b. Blanching or redness from an intraoperative tourniquet may persist.

       (1) Evaluate for resolution of tourniquet-related symptoms.

   5. Capillary refill

     a. Quick return of color to nailbed or distal area of skin blanched by pressure

       (1) Normally occurs in 3-5 seconds

       (2) Helpful when dressing on extremity eliminates visual evaluation of all but tips of digits

XIV. Analgesia

  A. Pain

   1. Complex phenomenon

     a. Stimulation of nociceptors

       (1) Free nerve endings throughout body

         (a) Chemical

         (b) Thermal

         (c) Mechanical (surgical)

       (2) Impulses transmitted via spinal cord

         (a) Afferent nerve fibers

       (3) Brain

         (a) Consciously perceived as pain

   2. Personal experience

     a. Variable between people

       (1) Variable within same people at different times

     b. Emotional impact of pain

       (1) Preoperative counseling

         (a) General description of what can be expected

         (b) Direct relationship between preoperative education and decreased analgesic needs

           (i) Less fear

           (ii) Decreases feelings of powerlessness

           (iii) Earlier ambulation

             [a] Analgesia will be given.

         (c) Discharge will not be attempted without adequate pain relief.

     c. Pain-relieving techniques

       (1) Proper body mechanics

         (a) Body alignment

         (b) Positioning

       (2) Encouragement of patient's efforts

     d. Soothing conversation

     e. Hand holding

       (1) Pain often exacerbated by fear and anxiety

     f. Massage

     g. Awake patients

       (1) Positive encouragement of relaxation

         (a) Distraction

           (i) Imagine pleasant visions, sounds, and smells.

         (b) Guided imagery

         (c) Counting

        (d) Rhythmic breathing
      (2) Requires
        (a) Patient acceptance
        (b) Nursing skills
        (c) Preoperative discussion and practice
   h. Local infiltration
   i. Explanations of local anesthesia if surgeon routinely does so
3. Transcutaneous electrical nerve stimulator (TENS)
   a. Stimulation of cutaneous afferent nerve pathways
      (1) Inhibit perception of pain
        (a) Possible release of endorphins attach to opiate receptors and block transmission of painful stimuli
        (b) Usually used for chronic pain
          (i) Does have postsurgical applications
4. Operative site affects pain levels
   a. More discomfort
      (1) Thoracic
      (2) Abdominal
      (3) Rectal
   b. Less discomfort
      (1) Breast
      (2) Scrotal
      (3) Chest wall
      (4) Extremity
5. Anesthesia technique
   a. Regional
      (1) Usually longer period of analgesia
   b. Local anesthetic infiltration
      (1) Effective in reducing surgical site pain
   c. Intraoperative narcotics
6. Social issues
   a. Culture affects pain tolerance.
      (1) Nervous or anxious people
      (2) Those with particularly protective families
        (a) Difficulty in managing pain
7. Pain is subjective.
   a. No one knows how much pain the patient is really having.
   b. Objective observations are only clues.
      (1) Vital signs
        (a) Hypertension
        (b) Tachycardia
        (c) Tachypnea
      (2) Restlessness
      (3) Facial expression
      (4) Splinting
      (5) Posturing
      (6) Mood
      (7) Voice
      (8) Refusal to be repositioned
   c. Nurses' role is not to judge patient's pain.
      (1) Assess thoroughly.
        (a) Location
        (b) Intensity
          (i) Pain scale rates patient's perception of pain intensity.
            [a] Numerical (0-10)
            [b] Faces (smiling–crying)
            [c] Colors (blue–red)
        (c) Type

   (2) Provide appropriate interventions.
    (a) Relieve discomfort.
  8. Other sources of postoperative pain
   a. Bladder distention
   b. Uncomfortable positioning
   c. Joint pain
    (1) Arthritis
    (2) Gout
   d. Decubitus ulcers
   e. Preexisting diseases
   f. Placement of intravenous catheters
   g. Drainage tubes
    (1) Chest tubes
    (2) Jackson-Pratt
    (3) Autotransfusion
   h. Gastric distention
   i. Postoperative complications
    (1) Embolic events
    (2) Myocardial ischemia or infarction
    (3) Pulmonary ischemia
    (4) Hemorrhage
    (5) Ruptured viscus
 B. Ambulatory surgery expectations
  1. Analgesic needs will be met.
  2. Discourage use of "pain."
   a. Focus on "discomfort."
    (1) Different connotation
    (2) Fits philosophy of wellness
     (a) Exception is patient in extreme pain.
     (b) May seem unfeeling or trite to use "discomfort"
 C. Untoward effects if inadequate analgesia
  1. Respiratory dysfunction
   a. Secondary to wound splinting
   b. Shallow respirations
    (1) Respiratory acidosis
  2. Tachycardia
  3. Hypertension
  4. Increased peripheral resistance
  5. Increased cardiac output
  6. Increased myocardial oxygen demand
  7. Gastric stasis
   a. Paralytic ileus
   b. Increased incidence of nausea and vomiting
    (1) Increased risk of aspiration
  8. Endocrine and metabolic changes
 D. Analgesics
  1. Assessment prior to administration
   a. Often awakening from general anesthesia
    (1) Poorest inherent pain relief
    (2) Patient psychologically less able to handle pain
     (a) Compared with wakefulness and full control capacity
    (3) Magnified in half-awake state
    (4) Restless
     (a) Cause may be hypoxia.
   b. Naloxone (Narcan)
    (1) Administered as reversal agent
    (2) Also reverses analgesia

(a) Additional narcotics may produce additive effects once Narcan wears off.

2. Challenge
   a. Provide adequate analgesia without oversedation.
      (1) Smallest effective dose
      (2) Incremental administration favored
      (3) Narcotics
         (a) Most effective treatment in PACU
         (b) Following general anesthesia
            (i) Close observation for potential cumulative effects
         (c) Respiratory depression
         (d) Prolonged somnolence
         (e) Nausea and vomiting
   b. Dosage
      (1) Individual calculation essential
         (a) Patients vary significantly in
            (i) Weight and height
         (b) Age
         (c) Sensitivity to drug actions
         (d) Personal need or desire for certain level of comfort
         (e) Medication history
            (i) Rarely takes any medications so usually require smaller doses
         (f) Heavy alcohol, tobacco, or drug use
            (i) May decrease effectiveness of pharmacologic therapy through mechanism called enzyme induction
         (g) Causes increased production of hepatic enzymes
   c. Metabolism (biotransformation)
      (1) Converts lipid-soluble drugs into water-soluble usually inactive metabolites
         (a) Allows excretion through renal tubules
         (b) Hepatic microsomal enzymes responsible for most metabolic changes
            (i) Chronic increase in hepatic enzymes increases rate of drug metabolism.
            (ii) Increased doses are needed to produce therapeutic effect.

3. Routes of administration
   a. Choice depends on patient's individual experience with pain and response to medication.
   b. Transdermal and nasal agents
      (1) Still under clinical trials
      (2) May have widespread application in ambulatory surgery
   c. Intravenous agents
      (1) Rapid onset of action
      (2) Rapid onset of side effects
         (a) Apparent in PACU
      (3) Fentanyl
         (a) One hundred times more potent than morphine
         (b) Effective, rapid-acting
         (c) Produces minimal sedative hangover
            (i) Give in small incremental doses.
            (ii) Single 50 µg (1 ml) usually appropriate for average-weight adult
         (d) Potential for respiratory complications
         (e) Does not evoke histamine release
         (f) Minimal cardiovascular changes
            (i) Can cause bradycardia
            (ii) Usually avoided with pulse rate <50

           (g) Action

               (i) 30-60 minutes with IV administration

           (h) Up to 3 hours with IM administration

        (4) Patient-controlled analgesia (PCA)

           (a) Infusion pump method of intravenous postoperative narcotic pain control

           (b) Usually reserved for inpatient use

           (c) Manufacturers are developing miniaturized, battery-operated, or completely disposable systems for home and outpatient use.

    d. IM administration

        (1) Usually ordered out of habit for hospitalized patients

        (2) May be incompatible with goals of

           (a) Rapid analgesia

               (i) Studies have shown that one third of patients given IM narcotics usually continue with moderate to severe pain.

           (b) Quick arousal

               (i) IM administration accompanied by sedative effects

               (ii) Increased hypotensive and respiratory depression

                  [a] Requires longer observation period

           (c) Rapid ambulation

           (d) Rapid discharge

        (3) Other IM medications

           (a) Hydroxyzine (Vistaril, Atarax)

           (b) Phenothiazine derivatives

               (i) Promethazine (Phenergan)

           (c) Potentiate narcotic effects

               (i) Use cautiously in ambulatory surgery patients.

               (ii) Significant sedation

               (iii) Have antiemetic and anxiolytic properties

    e. Oral

        (1) Once believed only method for ambulatory surgery

           (a) Increasing complexity of ambulatory surgery procedures; oral analgesics not always sufficient

           (b) Providing immediate and effective pain relief important aspect

               (i) Preventing severe pain easier than controlling it

           (c) Produces effective serum levels after administration of IV medication

           (d) Nonsteroidal antiinflammatory drugs (NSAIDs)

               (i) Ibuprofen

               (ii) Ketorolac

                  [a] May cause gastric irritation

                  [b] Can interfere with coagulation mechanism

  4. Opioid agonist–antagonist

    a. Pentazocine (Talwin), Butorphanol tartrate (Stadol), Nalbuphine (Nubain)

        (1) Reduces pain when given without previous narcotics

        (2) When given in presence of narcotics

           (a) Antagonistic characteristics reverse narcotic effect resulting in

               (i) Pain

               (ii) Anxiety

               (iii) Loss of sedation

        (3) Contraindicated in chronically narcotic-dependent

           (a) Causes severe withdrawal symptoms

  5. NSAIDs

    a. Ketorolac tromethamine (Toradol)

        (1) Parenteral agent

(2) IV route
    (a) Dosage: 15-60 mg, depending on weight
(3) IM
    (a) Dosage: 30-90 mg, depending on weight
        (i) Effective as 12 mg morphine or 100 mg meperidine
(4) Few side effects
    (a) Nausea, dyspepsia, drowsiness, and GI pain
        (i) Occur in 3% to 9%
    (b) Edema, diarrhea, dizziness, headache, tinnitus, peptic ulcer, sweating, and injection site pain
        (i) Occur in <3%
    (c) Respiratory function not altered
    (d) No significant cardiovascular effects
(5) Often given with narcotic to obtain added analgesic benefits
    (a) Does not produce additive effects with narcotic administration
(6) No potential of addictive abuse
    (a) Ideal for narcotic-addicted patient
(7) Liver metabolism
(8) Renal excretion
    (a) Fifty percent excreted unchanged
    (b) Use with caution in patients with kidney or liver dysfunction and the elderly.
(9) Onset of action: 10 minutes
(10) Peak effect
    (a) Reached in 45-90 minutes
    (b) Approximate duration of 6 hours
        (i) Administering ketorolac 45-60 minutes prior to the end of surgery in the operating room helps prevent pain of an injection.

XV. Nausea and vomiting
  A. Primary goal is to prevent rather than treat.
    1. Obtain history of postoperative nausea and vomiting.
    2. Prophylactic
      a. Histamine blockers
      b. Antiemetics
  B. Nausea subjective
    1. Often difficult to describe
    2. Unpleasant
    3. May or may not result in retching or vomiting
  C. Other predisposing factors
    1. Obesity
      a. Usually increased gastric volumes
    2. Hiatal hernia
    3. Type of surgery
      a. Laparoscopy
      b. Ovum retrieval
      c. Abdominal procedures
      d. Pediatric strabismus
      e. Orchiopexy
      f. ENT
        (1) Results from blood entering the stomach
    4. Anesthetic technique
      a. Regional and local anesthetic approaches lower incidence.
      b. Nitrous oxide implicated as significant causative factor
        (1) Gravitates to any air-filled area of stomach and bowel
          (a) Abdominal distention and pressure
        (2) Collects in middle ear affecting vestibular system

      c. Propofol (Diprivan)
        (1) Anesthetic agent for induction and maintenance
          (a) Low (1% to 3%) incidence of nausea and vomiting
            (i) Dose of 10 mg may be beneficial as antiemetic agent.

D. Vomiting
   1. Complex occurrence
      a. Involves skeletal muscles and autonomic nervous system
      b. Reflex
   2. Direct stimulation of vomiting center
      a. Located near the dorsal nucleus of the vagus nerve in the medulla
      b. Chemoreceptor trigger zone (CTZ)
        (1) Three afferent nerve pathways
          (a) Cortical
            (i) Emotional
              [a] Stress, depression, and fear
            (ii) Organic
              [a] Hypoxia
              [b] Pain
              [c] Hypotension
              [d] Increased intracranial pressure
              [e] Hypovolemia
            (iii) Sensory
              [a] Sights and smells of OR or PACU
          (b) Visceral
            (i) Viscera and vagal nerve
              [a] Delayed gastric emptying
              [b] Abdominal distention
              [c] Handling abdominal contents during surgery
              [d] Pneumoperitoneum for laparoscopic procedures
              [e] Primary GI disorders
              [f] Cardiac disease
          (c) Vestibular
            (i) Tremors
            (ii) Motion
              [a] Patient with strong history of motion sickness may
                 have vomiting caused by vestibular afferent activity
            (iii) Otitis media
            (iv) ENT procedures
            (v) Anesthetics and narcotics
        (2) Response to stimulation via efferent nerve pathways (see Figure 35-1)
          (a) Respiratory center
            (i) Diaphragm
          (b) GI tract
            (i) Upper abdominal muscles

E. "Central vomiting"
   1. Direct effect on CTZ
   2. Decreased cerebral blood flow
   3. Circulating drugs
      a. Narcotics
      b. Inhalation agents
      c. Intravenous anesthetic agents
      d. Amphetamines
      e. Cardiac glycosides
      f. Ergot rates
      g. Chemotherapeutic agents

F. Nursing interventions
   1. No single approach to prevention or treatment of nausea and vomiting
      effective because of diverse etiology

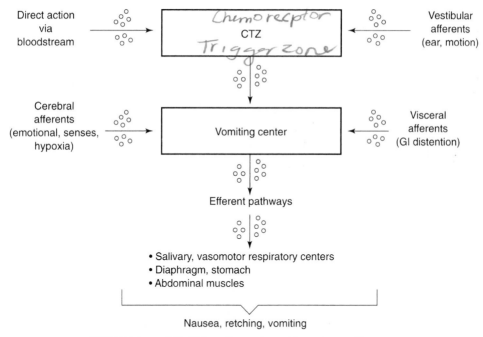

FIGURE 35-1 ■ Multiple pathways to and from the emetic center.

   2. In unconscious patient, protection of airway
      a. Avoid aspiration of stomach contents.
   3. Provide positive reinforcement to relieve anxiety.
   4. Avoid sights, smells, or conversations near the patient that could stimulate nausea or vomiting.
   5. Move and ambulate patient slowly.
   6. Allow patient to awaken slowly without aggressive stimulation.
   7. Maintain endotracheal tube cuff until extubation.
   8. Provide adequate analgesia.
   9. Use caution with oral intake.
      a. Avoid coffee, citrus juices.
   10. Limit irritation of upper airway.
      a. Reduce gagging.
      b. Limit secretions.
      c. Remove artificial airways as soon as possible.
      d. Gentle oral suction for blood and other secretions
   11. Provide privacy for the patient who is vomiting.
      a. Reassure to avoid embarrassment.
   G. Antiemetic agents
      1. Should reduce GI symptoms without oversedation
      2. Agents that block responsible receptors most effective
         a. Droperidol (Inapsine)
         b. Chlorpromazine (Thorazine)
         c. Trimethobenzamide (Tigan)
            (1) Dopamine antagonists suppress CTZ activity
         d. See Table 35-2 for additional antiemetic agents and their properties.
XVI. Progression of care
   A. Orientation
      1. Frequent orientation to surroundings
      2. Explanations
         a. Link with reality
         b. Aid in return of cognitive abilities

TABLE 35-2
■ Antiemetics

Group/Drug	Action/Uses	Dosage Ranges/Routes for Adults	Side Effects/Special Notes
PHENOTHIAZINES			
Prochlorperazine (Compazine)	Antiemetic, anxiolytic, tranquilizer	PO, 5-10 mg; IM, 5-10 mg deep IM; rectal, 25 mg; IV, 5-10 mg slowly—use great caution to prevent hypotension	Orthostatic hypotension, ECG changes, tachycardia, extrapyramidal reactions, sedation, pseudoparkinsonism, EEG changes, dizziness, ocular changes, blurred vision, dry mouth, constipation, urinary retention
Chlorpromazine (Thorazine)	Antiemetic, anxiolytic	IM, (deep) 12.5-25 mg	Orthostatic hypotension, tachycardia, ECG changes, seizures, sedation, extrapyramidal reactions, urine retention, dry mouth, constipation, neuroleptic malignant syndrome
Promethazine (Phenergan)	Anti–motion sickness, anticholinergic	IM (deep), 12.5-25 mg (reduce with CNS depressants)	Hypertension, hypotension, sedation, drowsiness, dry mouth; *never give* epinephrine to treat hypotension caused by promethazine because it could further lower blood pressure
OTHERS			
Trimethobenzamide (Tigan)	Antiemetic—depresses CTZ, sedative, weak antihistamine	PO, 250 mg; IM, 200 mg (deep IM), onset in 15 minutes, lasts 2-3 hours; rectal, 200 mg	Hypotension, seizures, drowsiness, coma, diarrhea
Benzquinamide (Emete-con)	Antiemetic	IM (preferred), 50 mg, onset in 15 minutes, peak, 15 minutes; lasts 3-4 hours; IV, 25 mg very slowly, decrease dose if patient on pressor agent or on epinephrine-like drug or in cardiac patient	Sudden rise in blood pressure and transient dysrhythmias (PVCs, PACs, and atrial fibrillation), hypotension, drowsiness, anorexia, dry mouth, urticaria, rash, diarrhea

Drug	Action	Dose	Side effects
Ondansetron (Zofran)	Depresses CTZ and $5HT_3$ receptor	PO, 16 mg, 1 hour prior to anesthesia induction; IV, 4 mg undiluted over 2-5 minutes	Diarrhea, constipation, musculoskeletal pain, urine retention, chest pain, injection site reaction, fever, hypoxia
Droperidol (Inapsine)	Potent tranquilizer (neuroleptic agent), anxiolytic, potentiates narcotics and CNS depressants	IV 0.625-1.25 mg (reduce dose when given with narcotics or CNS depressants), onset 3-10 minutes, peak 30 minutes, lasts 3-6 hours	Hypotension, tachycardia, laryngospasm, bronchospasm, extrapyramidal effects, drowsiness, hyperactivity
Dimenhydrinate (Dramamine)	Antiemetic, anti-motion sickness Depressant action on hyperstimulated labyrinthine function	IM, 50 mg; IV (dilute), 50 mg in 10 ml, slowly over at least 2 minutes; IV infusion, 50-100 mg in 500 ml solution	Palpitations, drowsiness, headache, dizziness, confusion, nervousness, insomnia (especially in children), blurred vision, dry mouth
Metoclopramide (Reglan)	Increases gastric motility	IM, 10 mg (5-20 mg range) onset	Restlessness, anxiety, suicidal ideation, seizures, hallucinations, transient hypertension, hypotension
Hydroxyzine (Vistaril, Atarax)	Antiemetic, anxiolytic Potentiates narcotics	IM, 25-10 mg (deep), decrease up to one half when given with CNS depressants (12.5-50 mg IM); do not give IV or subcutaneously	Drowsiness, dry mouth, marked discomfort at injection site
Diphenhydramine (Benadryl)	Competes for H1 receptor site	IM (deep), 10-50 mg; IV, 10-50 mg; PO, 25-50 mg	Palpitations, hypotension, tachycardia, dry mouth, epigastric distress, drowsiness, vertigo, sedation, dizziness, restlessness, seizures, diplopia, blurred vision, urinary retention, thickening of bronchial secretions
Scopolamine (Transderm-Scop)	Anti-motion sickness, antimuscarinic activity Acts on vestibular pathway and directly on vomiting center	One patch behind the ear 4 hours before surgery delivers 0.5 mg over 72 hours.	Palpitations, tachycardia, paradoxical bradycardia, disorientation, restlessness, hallucinations, dry mouth, blurred vision, dilated pupils; wash hands before and after application to avoid unintentional contact with the drug

    B. Operative site

       1. Monitor for

         a. Hemorrhage

         b. Swelling

         c. Compression of extremities

    C. Movement and ambulation

       1. Gradual

         a. Elevate head of bed slowly.

         b. Exercise extremities.

         c. Sitting on edge of bed or carrier

         d. Sitting in recliner

         e. Ambulation

            (1) With each level assess

              (a) Vital signs

                 (i) Specifically hypotension

              (b) Dizziness

              (c) Nausea

              (d) Faintness

            (2) If any symptoms occur, progress is slowed or reversed until symptoms subside.

XVII. Emotional and psychological support

    A. Ideally begun with preoperative visit and assessment

    B. PACU nurse first line with normalcy after surgery and anesthesia

       1. Use of positive language promoting wellness and self-sufficiency

         a. Address fears patient expresses.

            (1) Pathology or surgical outcome

            (2) Family or friends waiting

            (3) Returning home with no nursing or medical attention

            (4) Ability to deal with pain at home

            (5) Concern with family's ability to deal with postoperative needs

         b. Assure that anything said or done in the PACU is kept confidential.

    C. Encourage family and friends in care discussions.

       1. Family visitation in PACU fosters self-care model.

         a. Reduces anxiety and stress level

         b. May reduce length of stay

       2. Prolonged PACU stay should be communicated to the family to reduce their anxiety.

XVIII. Special needs of patients after local and regional anesthesia; nursing care after epidural and spinal anesthesia (see Chapter 26 for more information)

    A. Many patients undergoing brachial plexus, intravenous, periorbital, or other regional blocks may bypass phase I completely.

    B. Patients undergoing central regional blocks (epidural and subarachnoid or spinal) are admitted to phase I until major effects of the anesthesia have passed.

       1. Complications following epidural or spinal

         a. Hypotension

            (1) Vasodilation of large portion of vasculature

              (a) Blood pools in lower extremities.

              (b) Arteries and arterioles not able to constrict

                 (i) Compensatory mechanism lost

            (2) Maintain IV fluids.

              (a) Until full motor and sensory functions return

            (3) Aggressive therapy includes ephedrine 10-25 mg, IV, diluted and given slowly.

         b. Tachycardia

         c. Bradycardia

         d. Hypothermia

            (1) Peripheral dilation

(2) Warm carefully.
  (a) Can potentiate vasodilation
    (i) Result in hypotension
e. Pressure injury
  (1) Maintain proper body alignment.
  (2) Elevate heels from mattress.
f. Unnoticed trauma to tissue
  (1) Gentle passive range of motion
  (2) Repositioning
g. Epidural hematoma
  (1) Hemorrhage at injection site rare
    (a) Internal pressure from hematoma can result in permanent neurologic damage.
      (i) Rapid onset of neurologic deficit after the lock has resolved
    (b) Severe back pain
    (c) Surgical intervention must occur within 12 hours to prevent permanent damage.
h. High or total spinal
i. Postdural puncture (spinal) headache

C. Spinal anesthesia
  1. Technically easier and less time-consuming
  2. Appropriate for ambulatory surgery patients

D. Epidural anesthesia
  1. Ability to control titration of medication through a continuous catheter
  2. Low incidence of foreign or infectious material into cerebrospinal fluid (CSF)

E. Resolution of anesthetic effects
  1. Sensation generally returns first to areas most distal to the site of injection.
    a. Return of neurologic function is reverse to the sequence it was lost.
      (1) Autonomic control may return prior to movement and sensation, then usually in this order.
        (a) Proprioception (location of extremity in relation to the body) is usually first to return.
        (b) Pressure
        (c) Movement
        (d) Touch
        (e) Pain
        (f) Temperature
        (g) Sympathetic functions
          (i) Vasomotor
          (ii) Bladder control
  2. Dermatome levels (see Figure 26-2)
    a. Major landmarks
      (1) T4—sensation at nipple line
      (2) T10—sensation at umbilicus
      (3) L2 and L3—raising knee
      (4) L4 and L5—flexion of the knee
      (5) S1 and S2—dorsiflexion of the foot

F. High or total spinal anesthesia
  1. Upper extremities and/or respiratory cardiac functions are involved.
    a. Incidence is rare.
    b. May be caused by
      (1) Increased intrathecal pressure from coughing or straining
      (2) Too rapid injection or too large a volume injected
      (3) Positioning of the patient in head-down inclination before anesthetic agent has set at intended spinal level
  2. Treatment
    a. Usually instituted in OR

        b. Mechanical ventilation
          (1) Oxygen therapy
        c. Intravenous fluids
        d. Vasopressors
        e. Atropine or glycopyrrolate
          (1) Treatment of bradycardia
        f. Emotional support
  G. Autonomic innervation and urinary bladder tone
     1. Bladder distention may occur.
        a. Decreased bladder muscle tone after sympathetic blockade
          (1) Restlessness
          (2) Hypotension
          (3) Bradycardia
          (4) May or may not feel suprapubic pain
            (a) Depends on level of sensory block
        b. Treatment simple
          (1) Have patient void if possible.
          (2) Insert urinary catheter to drain bladder.
          (3) Provide specific instructions for bladder care.
            (a) When to phone or return for follow-up care if not voided by specific time
              (i) Use patient's language.
  H. Postdural puncture headache
     1. Cause
        a. Leakage of CSF through dural puncture site
          (1) Decrease in intrathecal pressure allows traction on pain-sensitive intracranial sensors.
          (2) Will usually appear within a few hours of the puncture
            (a) More likely becomes evident after 1 or 2 days
              (i) May take as long as 6 days to occur
            (b) Pain usually occipital
              (i) May also occur in frontal or vertex areas or behind the eyes
              (ii) More intense when patient sits up or stands, moves head, flexes neck, or coughs
            (c) Relieved with abdominal pressure
     2. Other signs of CSF leakage
        a. Neck muscle aches
        b. Double vision
        c. Other types of visual disturbances
        d. Auditory difficulties
     3. Occurrence is rare.
     4. Prevention may be accomplished with use of
        a. Small-gauge needles
        b. Conical-tipped needles (*example:* Whitacre)
          (1) Spread or split rather than cut dural fibers
        c. "Wet tap"
          (1) Inadvertent dural puncture with a large-bore needle
            (a) Prevent flow of CSF into epidural space.
              (i) Anesthesiologist injects saline into epidural space prior to removal of the needle to increase epidural pressure.
            (b) Blood patch may also be performed.
     5. Treatment
        a. Several hours of recumbent position not effective in preventing postspinal headaches
        b. Analgesics
        c. Subdued lighting
        d. Limited noise

       e. Aggressive hydration
          (1) Intravenous
          (2) Oral if tolerated
       f. Abdominal binder
          (1) Increases epidural venous plexus pressure
       g. IV caffeine may be effective treatment.
       h. Severe or unrelenting headache
          (1) Epidural blood patch
             (a) Patient's own blood (10 ml) is injected into epidural space surrounding original dural puncture.
                (i) Clots around puncture site
             (b) Stops CSF leak
             (c) Immediate relief of headache usually occurs.

XIX. Documentation of care
    A. Charting formats should provide ease of documentation and accommodate.
      1. Typically short procedures
      2. Frequent admissions
      3. Rapid turnover
    B. Form should allow check off documentation and charting by exception.
    C. Narrative notes should focus on individual patient responses.
      1. Specific descriptions of operative site
      2. Associated information
    D. Vital signs easily documented and readable
    E. Scoring parameters easily understood

XX. Discharge from a PACU—phase I
    A. Anesthesiologist usually responsible for discharge from phase I
      1. Internal policy may require physician's attendance for discharge at time of readiness.
      2. Predetermined criteria from the medical staff may allow the PACU nurse to discharge patients.
    B. Discharge criteria
      1. Written criteria should address parameters of physical and cognitive recovery.
      2. Appropriate to the unit or location to which patient is transferred
      3. Numeric scoring systems provide objective methods with which to evaluate and describe patient's condition.
        a. Used upon admission, throughout the PACU stay, and at discharge
        b. Aldrete Scoring System
          (1) Measures five parameters with scoring ranges from 0-2
             (a) Activity
             (b) Respiration
             (c) Circulation
             (d) Consciousness
             (e) Color
          (2) Score of 9 or 10 is generally required for PACU phase I discharge
             (a) May not reach this score for preexisting conditions
                (i) Paraplegic or quadriplegic
                (ii) Raynaud's disease
                  [a] Persistent peripheral cyanosis
             (b) Criticism of inclusion of color and ignoring blood pressure
                (i) Color is subjective finding affected by
                  [a] Surrounding wall or curtain color
                  [b] Type of lighting
                  [c] Mucous membrane color not indicative of oxygenation
             (c) Table 35-3 shows the Aldrete Modified Phase I PACU Scoring System.

■ TABLE 35-3
■ ■ **Aldrete's Modified Phase I Postanesthesia Scoring System**

Patient Index	Standard	Score
Activity	Patient is able to move...	
	4 extremities*	2
	2 extremities*	1
	0 extremities*	0
Respiration	Patient is....	
	able to deep-breathe and cough	2
	dyspneic or limited breathing	1
	apneic, obstructed airway	0
Circulation	Patient's BP⋊	
	±20% of preanesthesia value	2
	±20% to 49% of preanesthesia value	1
	±50% of preanesthesia value	0
Consciousness	Patient is....	
	fully awake	2
	arousable (by name)	1
	nonresponsive	0
Oxygen saturation	Patient's SpO_2.....	
	>92% on room air	2
	>90% with supplemental O_2	1
	<90% even with supplemental O_2	0

From Burden N, Quinn D, O'Brien D, et al: *Ambulatory surgical nursing.* Philadelphia: WB Saunders, 2000, pp 470. Adapted with permission from Aldrete JA, Kroulik D: A post-anesthetic recovery score. *Anasthesia Analgesia* 49:924-933, 1970.
*Voluntarily or to command

    c. REACT Scoring System
      (1) Respiration
      (2) Energy (movement)
      (3) Alertness
      (4) Circulation
      (5) Temperature
  4. Scoring systems are limited and do not address many important aspects of patient's condition (see Table 35-4).
    a. Presence of nausea and vomiting
    b. Pain
    c. Emotional status
    d. Chills and shivering
    e. Condition of operative site
      (1) Hemorrhage
      (2) Edema
    f. Fluid status
    g. Urinary status
    h. Cognitive abilities
    i. Peripheral circulation
    j. Temperature
      (1) These parameters must also be considered in the decision for PACU discharge.
  5. After spinal or epidural anesthesia
    a. Return of strength and sympathetic innervation must be evaluated.
      (1) Depending on facility policy, patients may be transferred to phase II with continued bed rest until spinal effects resolved.

■ TABLE 35-4
■ ■ Postanesthesia Discharge Scoring System

Patient Index	Standard	Score
Vital signs	Patient's BP....	
	within 20% of preoperative value	2
	20-40% of preoperative value	1
	>40% of preoperative value	0
Ambulation	Patient is able to ambulate...	
	gait steady; no dizziness	2
	with assistance	1
	inadequately, dizziness present	0
Nausea/vomiting	Patient's experience of nausea/vomiting is....	
	Minimal	2
	Moderate	1
	Severe	0
Pain	Patient's pain level is....	
	Minimal	2
	Moderate	1
	Severe	0
Surgical bleeding	Bleeding from operative site is...	
	Minimal	2
	Moderate	1
	Severe	0

Modified from Chung F, Chan VW, Ong D. A post-anesthetic discharge scoring system for home readiness after ambulatory surgery. *J Clin Anesth* 7:500-506, 1995.
Note: Total possible score is 10; patients scoring ≥9 are considered fit for discharge from phase II.

      (2) Most PACUs require patients to have return of movement and sensation prior to discharge.
    b. Ensuring the absence of orthostatic hypotension may be main criterion.
      (1) Safe discharge with a <10% drop in mean arterial pressure in response to two tests
        (a) Checking blood pressure in both sitting and supine positions
C. Transfer and report
  1. Comprehensive assessment prior to discharge
    a. Condition of operative site
    b. Vital signs
    c. Level of consciousness
    d. Comfort
  2. Skin care
    a. Remove any antiseptic solutions.
      (1) Avoid skin irritation.
      (2) Prevents staining of clothing
    b. Blood or surgical drainage should be removed.
      (1) Aesthetic reasons
      (2) Safety of patients, family, and staff
      (3) Emotional reasons
  3. Surgical site
    a. Dressing dry and intact
    b. Wound drainage bags emptied
    c. Urinary drainage bags emptied
  4. Personal dignity
    a. Patient's sensory aids returned
      (1) Eyeglasses

(2) Dentures

(3) Hearing aid

5. Complete report to phase II nursing staff

   a. Operative course

      (1) Include medications for blood pressure, heart rate, and so forth

   b. PACU course

      (1) Physician's orders completed in phase I

      (2) Medications administered

         (a) Antibiotics

         (b) Analgesics

XXI. Focusing on "success"

  A. Often difficult to measure and define

    1. Four focus points in PACU nursing care

      a. Catalyst who helps the patient return as closely and rapidly as possible to preoperative condition and to their families

      b. Being totally attentive for potential complications and helping to avoid them whenever possible

      c. Discharging the patient as awake, pain-free, and nausea-free as possible

      d. Ensuring that each patient is treated with dignity and as a person who is important and special

XXII. Special considerations in PACU care

  A. Medical support

    1. Individual facilities differ in the chain of medical responsibility involved with the patient.

      a. Anesthesiologist

         (1) The American Society of Anesthesiologists (ASA) Standards for Postanesthesia Care provide definite statements in that regard.

      b. Surgeon

  B. Quality improvement practices

    1. Involvement in ongoing clinical studies and identify valuable trends affecting current and future patient care

    2. All members of the anesthesia team should be involved in quality improvement.

    3. Evaluation of nursing care occurs both at discharge and during follow-up contact.

  C. The PACU as a treatment and anesthesia site

    1. Considered an excellent location because it is fully equipped

      a. ECG monitors

      b. Noninvasive blood pressure monitors

      c. Pulse oximetry

      d. Oxygen

      e. Suction

      f. Emergency equipment

    2. Often PACUs are used at sites for therapeutic procedures.

      a. Pain clinic procedures

         (1) Epidural steroid injections

         (2) Stellate ganglion blocks

         (3) Other sympathetic blocks

      b. Electroconvulsive shock therapy (ECT)

      c. Blood transfusions

      d. Chemotherapy

    3. Administration of local or regional anesthesia prior to surgery

    4. PACU nurse's role

      a. May act as physician assistant

         (1) Secure further supplies

         (2) Apply solutions or drapes

         (3) Adjust equipment

         (4) Reposition patient

b. Patient supporter
  (1) Emotional support
c. Monitor patient
  (1) Vital signs
  (2) Monitor pattern
  (3) Response to procedure

BIBLIOGRAPHY

1. Aldrete JA: Modifications to the postanesthesia score for use in ambulatory surgery. *J PeriAnesth Nurs* 13(3):148-155, 1998.

2. American Society of PeriAnesthesia Nurses: ASPAN Standards of PeriAnesthesia Nursing Practice. Cherry Hill, NJ: American Society of PeriAnesthesia Nurses.

3. Anonymous: *Documenting postoperative transfer. Nursing* 32(3), 2002.

4. Bennett J, Wren KR, Haas R: Opioid use during the perianesthesia period: Nursing implications. *J PeriAnesth Nurs* 16(4): 255-258, 2001.

5. Burden N, editor: *Ambulatory surgical nursing.* Philadelphia: WB Saunders, 2000.

6. Cowling GE, Haas RE: Hypotension in the PACU: An algorithmic approach. *J PeriAnesth Nurs* 17(3):159-163, 2002.

7. DeFazio-Quinn DM, editor: *The nursing clinics of North America: Ambulatory surgery.* Philadelphia: WB Saunders, 1997.

8. Despotis GJ, Goodnough LT: Transfusion considerations in the surgical patient: Current risks and specialized blood products. *Curr Rev Post Anesth Care Nurse* 22(14), 2000.

9. Drain C: *The Post Anesthesia Care Unit: A Critical Care Approach to Post Anesthesia Nursing.* Philadelphia: WB Saunders, 2002.

10. Farrell M, Johnson T, O'Neil L, et al: Care tracker: A new approach to nursing care in ambulatory settings. *Nurs Adm Q* 23(1): 72-81, 1998.

11. Hudack CM, Gallo BM, Morton PG: Cri*tical care nursing: Holistic approach,* ed 7. Philadelphia: Lippincott, 1998.

12. Janikowski D, Rockefella CA: Awake and talking: Ambulatory surgery and conscious sedation. *Nurs Econ* 16(1):37-43, 1998.

13. Joint Commission on Accreditation of Healthcare Organizations: *Comprehensive accreditation manual for hospitals.* Oakbrook Terrace, IL: Joint Commission on Accreditation of Healthcare Organizations, 1996.

14. Kartlet MC: Malignant hyperthermia: Considerations for ambulatory surgery. *J PeriAnesth Nurs* 13(5):304-312, 1998.

15. Kervin MW: Residual neuromuscular blockade in the immediate postoperative period. *J PeriAnesth Nurs* 17(3):152-158, 2002.

16. Kriby RR: Airway emergencies revisited. *Curr Rev Post Anesth Care Nurse* 22(15), 2000.

17. Kleinpell RM: Improving telephone follow-up after ambulatory surgery. *J PeriAnesth Nurs* 12(5):336-340, 1997.

18. Knowles R (1996) Standardization of pain management in the postanesthesia care unit. *J PeriAnesth Nurs* 11(6):390-398.

19. Knoerl DV, Faut-Callahan M, Paice J, et al: Research utilization: Preoperative PCA teaching program to manage postoperative pain. *Medsurg Nursing* 8(1):25-33, 36, 1999.

20. Kreger C: Getting to the root of pain: Spinal anesthesia and analgesia. *Nursing* 31(6):36, 2001.

21. Lattavo K: Pinpointing postoperative hypoxemia. *Nursing* 32(10), 2002.

22. Lewis SM, Heitkemper MM, Dirksen SR: Medical-surgical nursing: Assessment and management of clinical problems, ed 5. St Louis: Mosby, 2000.

23. MacDonald AJ, Cullen BF: Drug interactions in anesthesia. *Curr Rev Post Anesth Care Nurse* 22(8), 2000.

24. Macres SM, Richeimer S: Review of acute postoperative pain management. *Curr Rev Post Anesth Care Nurse* 21(6), 1999.

25. Marley RA, Moline BM: Patient discharge from the ambulatory setting. *J Post Anesth Nurs* 11(1):39-49, 1996.

26. McCaffery M: Teaching your patient to use a pain rating scale. *Nursing* 32(8):17, 2002.

27. Mecca RS: Prolonged unconsciousness after anesthesia. *Curr Rev Post Anesth Care Nurse* 23(1), 2001.

28. Mecca RS: Postanesthesia care after ambulatory surgery: How much progress have we made? *Curr Rev Post Anesth Care Nurse* 22(17), 2000.

29. Mecca RS: Systemic hypotension after surgery. *Curr Rev PeriAnesth Nurse* 21(12), 1999.

30. Norris J: *Nursing 97 drug handbook.* Springhouse, PA: Springhouse, 1997.

31. Nelson TP: Postoperative nausea and vomiting: Understanding the enigma. *J PeriAnesth Nurs* 17(3):178-187, 2002.

32. Ouellette SM: Perioperative management of the hypertensive patient. *Curr Rev PeriAnesth Nurse* 21(14), 1999.

33. Redmond MC: Malignant hyperthermia: Perianesthesia recognition, treatment, and care. *J PeriAnesth Nurs* 16(4):259-270, 2001.

34. Reed C: Care of postoperative patients with pulmonary edema. *J PeriAnesth Nurs* 11(3):164-169, 1996.

35. Saar L: Use of a modified postanesthesia recovery score in phase II perianesthesia period of ambulatory surgery patients. *J PeriAnesth Nurs* 16(2):82-89, 2001.

36. Warner ME: Risks and outcomes of perioperative pulmonary aspiration. *J PeriAnesth Nurs* 12(5):352-357, 1997.

37. White PF: What is new in ambulatory anesthesia. *Curr Rev PeriAnesth Nurses* 21(15), 1999.

38. White PF: Role of nonpharmacologic techniques in treatment of pain and emesis. *Curr Rev PeriAnesth Nurses* 22(18), 2000.

36 Perianesthesia Complications

KATHLYN CARLSON

OBJECTIVES
At the conclusion of this chapter the reader will be able to:

1. Discuss three potential airway complications that may occur in the immediate postanesthesia period.
2. Describe the signs and symptoms associated with pulmonary edema.
3. Discuss the signs, symptoms, and treatment of a patient with suspected pseudocholinesterase deficiency.
4. Identify two common causes of hypovolemia in the immediate postoperative setting.
5. Identify three risk factors that predispose a patient to postoperative nausea and vomiting (PONV).

■■■ In the perianesthesia setting, patient complications can occur at any time. Postanesthesia care (PACU) nurses need to assess continually the patient's status to identify potential complications. Being able to identify and treat untoward reactions is paramount to ensure positive patient outcomes.

I. Perianesthesia issues: Professional practice
  A. Adhere to standards of perianesthesia nursing practice.
    1. Framework for delivering professional care
    2. Developed by the American Society of Perianesthesia Nurses (ASPAN)
    3. Continually amended as nursing practice evolves and patient needs change
    4. Compendium of specific care standards, resources, position statements
      a. Recommended nurse-patient ratios
      b. Educational competencies
      c. Primary patient care reference for preanesthesia and postanesthesia assessment
      d. Phase I, phase II, phase III discharge criteria
  B. Safety related to sedation or anesthesia for every procedure
    1. Precarious balance between nurse-monitored sedation and analgesia and deeper anesthesia
      a. *Every* patient at risk for respiratory or cardiovascular compromise
      b. Signs of hypoxia not always obvious; must monitor with
        (1) Pulse oximeter, cardiac and blood pressure monitors, respiration
        (2) All alarms *on*
        (3) Correlate monitor data with nurse's astute clinical assessments.
    2. Perianesthesia nurse's role: *complication "sleuth"*
      a. Witness and stand by: *consider every patient to have a potential complication!*
      b. *Never* leave stretcher side of unresponsive, intubated, patient with airway.
      c. Protect from injury while sedated.
        (1) Corneal abrasion if rubbing eyes
        (2) Falls if tries to leave stretcher while agitated, disoriented
        (3) Bumps, lumps, and bruises if waves uncontrollable, nerve-blocked extremity
          (a) May hit head, nose (or nurse)

(b) Impair extremity circulation if dent and compress a still-drying cast on stretcher's side rail

(4) Hearing loss after cardiac bypass, assorted medications

d. Complacence has no place in *any* phase of postanesthesia care.

e. Every nurse's norm: knowledgeable assessment and clinical preparation

f. Maintain nurse to patient ratios outlined in ASPAN Standards

3. At risk for minutes to hours, even after briefest procedures, medication exposure

a. May require 1:1 nursing care, if only for a few minutes

b. Transport from procedure area or operating room (OR) raises risk: attention shifts from acute monitoring to navigating corridors

c. Without constant stimulation, patient can arrive in phase I PACU less responsive, hypoxic, or vomiting.

4. Challenge: ensure *equivalent* monitoring in every setting, every hour.

a. Potpourri of procedural settings

(1) Outpatient ambulatory centers

(2) Interventional radiology, cardiovascular, gastroenterology suites

(3) Physician and dental offices

(4) Stretcher side in emergency department, intensive cae unit (ICU), or postanesthesia units

b. Daytime or overnight, scheduled surgery, or emergency on call

(1) Standard: recommends that two licensed nurses be present whenever a patient is recovering in PACU phase I.

(2) At least one nurse must be competent to deliver the sometimes critical level of postanesthesia care.

C. Education: Ensure clinical competency.

1. Nurses from varied clinical backgrounds asked to monitor conscious sedation

2. Knowledgeable, competent registered nurse is patient's best advocate.

a. For minutes or hours, sedated adult or child dependent upon assessment skills, attentiveness, competence for his or her very life

b. Recognizes "recovery" from even briefest anesthetic exposure could actually take longer than the procedure.

c. Upholds standards of care

d. Orchestrates interventions

e. Applies specific discharge criteria

(1) Plans education

(2) Judges discharge readiness from every phase of perianesthesia care

3. Prepares patient for discharge during *pre*operative education and during every clinical assessment in PACU by discussing

a. Potential for sore throat and even hoarseness after endotracheal (ET) intubation or even laryngeal mask airway (LMA)

b. Advises patient to report potential airway related consequences

(1) Vocal cord palsy with dysphonia, ongoing hoarseness

(2) Swallowing difficulty: dysphagia to uvular bruising

c. Instruct about potential for shoulder pain after laparoscopic procedures.

d. Ongoing evaluation of surgical limb and ways to report problems

e. Pain management strategies after leaving perianesthesia care areas

4. Integrates ASPAN Standards into patient education and nurse competency

D. Discharge: When is it time to leave? (Tables 36-1 and 36-2)

1. Nurse assesses using critical judgment, intuitive experience, objective criteria.

2. "Rigorous" application of ASPAN or facility's discharge criteria at *each* phase

a. Pain managed to tolerable level (Table 36-3)

b. Airway patent, vital signs stable, euthermic

c. Conscious, mobile, surgically stable

3. Readiness or length of stay in any postprocedural area *not* time-dependent

4. Timing important to patient's confidence about managing at home

■ TABLE 36-1
■ ■ **Criteria for Discharge: PACU Phase I**

The perianesthesia nurse must assure a patient meets these discharge criteria when considering discharge from PACU phase I.
Document:
  Airway is patent, ventilation adequate, protective reflexes intact
  Temperature, color, vital signs, and oxygen saturation stable
  Consciousness at preprocedural baseline and muscles strong
  No overt bleeding; tubes, drains, and catheters patent
  Neurovascular function intact
  Pain, nausea, and anxiety managed to moderate levels

■ TABLE 36-2
■ ■ **Criteria for Discharge: PACU Phase II**

Nurse considerations and patient milestones prior to discharge from PACU phase I
Anesthesia: Patient remains in a postanesthesia environment for
  ▪ Minimum of 2 hours after the final dose of sedation
  ▪ Minimum of 1 hour after reversal with a narcotic or benzodiazepine antagonist
Document: Vital sign, muscle strength and respiratory function
    Swallowing and oral intake
    Pain management and interventions
    Neurovascular status related to position and procedural sites
    Discharge instructions reviewed with patient and care partner; patient receives a written and signed copy
    Safe transportation home with responsible adult.
Education and discharge instructions:
  Provide physician and facility phone numbers for emergency contact to report: extreme pain, fever, increased bleeding.
  Distinguish conditions to report to the physician from "normal" postanesthesia or postsurgical sensations or observations.
  Emphasize to family that, although the patient appears alert and functional, sedation impairs thought, judgment and reactions.
  For 24 hours, avoid:
  ▪ Leaving the patient alone
  ▪ Driving, operating equipment, or alcohol consumption
  ▪ Making important or legal decisions
Procedural requirements.
Interventional cardiology:
  Protocols vary with the procedure. If no wound oozing or hematoma, monitor cardiac rhythm for 2 to nearly 24 hours.
Interventional radiology: Oncology patients need prolonged postprocedure care, up to 6 hours, to manage vomiting or pain aggravated by procedure.
Endoscopy: No requirement for extensive observation
    Discharge home when airway reflexes recover, fluids are tolerated, and discharge criteria after sedation are met.

     E. Documentation: critical communication
        1. Anesthesia report: safe transfer of care (Table 36-4)
           a. From anesthesia provider, either an anesthesiologist or certified registered nurse anesthetist (CRNA) to registered nurse
           b. PACU nurse accepts responsibility for patient only after procedural and anesthesia information conveyed, emergent concerns resolved.
        2. Written or computerized record
           a. Convey patient's stable progressive transition from sedation to wakefulness

■ TABLE 36-3
■ ■ **Comfort: Managing Acute Pain**

Strategies and nurse approaches related to acute pain management in PACU

CRITICAL NURSING BEHAVIORS
Describes physiology of pain, including pathways and receptors
Identifies physiologic responses to pain and stress
Discusses effective, research-based pain interventions promoted identified by the Agency for Health Care Policy and Research (AHCPR)
Describes purposes, side effects and complications of analgesic medications
  ▪ Synergistic effects of postanesthesia doses on anesthetic medications
  ▪ Required assessments after administering narcotics or sedatives in PACU
  ▪ Appropriate doses of oral and intravenous analgesics
Suggests preemptive measures to attenuate pain
  ▪ Coaches relaxation techniques and breathing
  ▪ Adds music (though identified as an inconsistently useful tool)
  ▪ Ice to surgical sites or warmth to ease uterine cramping
  ▪ Identifies adjunctive medications and contraindications
  ▪ Incorporates a calming voice and behaviors, therapeutic touch, and an attitude of nonjudgment
Interacts with patient to
  ▪ Accept mild pain as a "norm"
  ▪ Begin doses of oral "take-home" medication preceded by crackers and fluids
  ▪ Encourage rest and tincture of time for pain to abate
  ▪ Balance pain relief with encouragement to progress toward activity

---

■ TABLE 36-4
■ ■ **Admission to Phase I: Content of Report**

Expected communications from anesthesia provider during admission to PACU

Communicate	Mutually Assess
Patient's name and age	Airway patency
Preoperative medical history	Breathing quality
Anesthetic technique and duration	Cardiovascular stability

Intraoperative Medications, Times, Doses	Determine and Manage
Sedatives, narcotics, relaxants	Consciousness
Reversal medications	Pain
Antibiotics, steroids, adjunctives	Muscle strength
Fluid balance	Wounds and drains
	Critical procedural events

---

      b. Inform all caregivers of events, complications, consultations, and interventions.
      c. Demonstrates patient meets medico-legal requirements, discharge criteria
      d. Must be complete, accurate, legible
   F. Trends
      1. *Fast tracking*: caution advised if bypassing phase I care
         a. Quick alertness, cardiorespiratory stability after short-acting sedatives
         b. Careful patient selection crucial to success
            (1) American Society of Anesthesiologists (ASA) I or II preferred
            (2) Patients with preexisting disease most at risk
         c. Must meet ASPAN criteria for phase I discharge when *leaving OR*

    2. High patient *volumes* and *acuity* promote rushing patients.

        a. Pushing a patient too quickly from phase I care can result in a hypotensive, listless, vomiting patient in phase II.

        b. Nurse's positive attitude can nudge reluctant patient toward lounge chair, food, and home.

    3. Nurses stand firm, resist pressure to speed care.

        a. Rely on discharge criteria, not political or peer pressure, to guide clinical decisions.

        b. Enter discussions and meetings armed with ASPAN standards.

        c. Garner support for positions from other professionals.

II. Critical postanesthesia assessments

  A. Anesthesia assessment priorities: during admission, then throughout PACU stay

    1. *Simultaneous* overview of organ systems and responses during admission

        a. Respiratory effort, oxygen saturation: artificial airway? Intubated?

        b. Cardiac rate, rhythm and vital signs: hypotensive?

        c. Awareness, level of consciousness and ability to move: rousable?

        d. Pain severity and anxiety: agitated or calm? Implement pain scale?

        e. Residual effect of local anesthetic blocks, regional anesthetics

            (1) Motor and sensory dermatome levels after spinal or epidural block

            (2) Regional block renders extremity numb and difficult to control.

                (a) Block effect provides wonderful pain management.

                (b) Safety concern: protect from flailing, floppy extremity.

        f. Thermoregulation: temperature and comfort

    2. Determine need for 1:1 nursing care according to ASPAN standards.

    3. Repeat assessment at regular intervals according to standards and policies.

  B. *Surgery*-specific observations

    1. Integrity of dressings or visible suture lines, any drainage

    2. Position, patency, and function of every monitoring line and wound drain

    3. Abdominal girth, distention, nausea

    4. Neurologic and neurovascular status

        a. Consciousness, respiratory effort, pupil size and equality, seizures, posturing, and movement after intracranial surgeries

            (1) Stimulus required to elicit response

                (a) Spontaneous?

                (b) Touch or voice?

                (c) Sternal rub?

            (2) Degree and quality of response

            (3) Improvement or decline during PACU observation

        b. Capillary refill, sensation, motion, strength after spinal, orthopedic, peripheral vascular procedures

            (1) Pulses, color, motion, sensation, temperature

                (a) Shoulders to fingertips

                (b) Hips to toes

            (2) Doppler assessment if circulation or pulse quality questionable

                (a) Cool or vasoconstricted extremity

                (b) May be normally diminished if peripheral vascular disease

            (3) Is any deficit new or present preprocedure worse or improved?

        c. Impairment related to surgical position or events

            (1) *Vision impairment* reported after hypotensive episodes

            (2) *Skin damage* at pressure points: redness, blisters, breaks

            (3) *Peroneal nerve compression* after legs in stirrups

                (a) Numbness or tingling after urologic, gynecologic procedures

            (4) *Ulnar nerve* stretch while are extended and muscle relaxed

                (a) Numbness, tingling, perhaps weakness

        d. Impairment related to procedure

            (1) Intravenous (IV) infiltration, medication extravasation, arterial monitoring lines can interrupt circulation distal to line insertion site.

(2) Edema or bleeding in surgical extremity can impair circulation.

(3) Tight casts, splints, and wraps can restrict venous return.

(4) *Compartment syndrome:* uncommon crisis

    (a) Increased pressure in extremity's fascial compartments

    (b) Perfusion impaired: muscle and nerve ischemia result.

    (c) *Prompt* pressure released lest tissue necrosis result

        (i) Surgical fasciotomy

        (ii) Remove or split cast.

        (iii) Monitor for hyperkalemia after muscle destroyed.

    (d) Report immediately: extreme pain unrelieved by narcotics, paresthesia or paralysis, pallor, or pulselessness of limb.

5. Genitourinary status

    a. Bladder distention: urge to void? Verify time of last void.

    b. Catheter patency, urine color, clarity, volume, clots

    c. Titrate flow of bladder irrigation systems.

    d. Bladder ultrasound to assess bladder volumes

    e. Determine necessity of urination before discharge.

        (1) Consider increasing IV fluid rate to promote bladder volume.

        (2) Instruct to strain urine for particles after lithotripsy.

6. Obtain, report, and review necessary x-rays, laboratory assessments.

    a. Chest x-ray to verify placement of new central lines, endotracheal tube

    b. Spinal or extremity x-rays per surgeon orders

    c. Arterial blood gases if patient intubated mechanically ventilated

    d. Serum glucose in diabetics

    e. Hemoglobin if significant blood loss during procedure

    f. Electrolytes if extended surgery with multiple transfusion, extensive muscle destruction

C. Clearly document all assessments and events according to facility style and policy.

    1. Observed deficits, physician consultations, orders

    2. Outcomes of interventions

    3. Times of each assessment, intervention

        a. Increase frequency of assessments when deficit or compromise.

        b. Every change in clinical status, improvement or decline: airway

        c. Airway removal, monitoring line insertion, laboratory and x-ray results

III. Airway integrity (Table 36-5)

  A. Complications heralded by

    1. Hypoxia: oxygen desaturation, decreasing Po_2: insufficient *delivery*

        a. Po_2 less than 60 mm Hg per arterial blood gas

        b. Monitored oxyhemoglobin saturation <90%

        c. Reduced respiratory rate, depth, effort

        d. Oversedation: limited consciousness reduces stimulus to breathe.

        e. Restlessness: still anesthetized patient may actually be disoriented, "air hungry."

            (1) May indicate return of narcotic or muscle relaxant effect

            (2) Always ensure adequate oxygenation and ventilation before sedating.

            (3) *Only* provide judicious, sparing analgesia until patient alert.

        f. Cardiovascular status varies: hypertension to hypotension, arrhythmias.

        g. "High" spinal blockade

    2. Hypercarbia: respiratory acidosis, increasing Pco_2

    3. Factors that may increase airway risk

        a. Anatomy: limit chest expansion, diaphragm, respiratory muscle movement.

            (1) Obesity or pregnancy

            (2) Neck: large and/or short neck

            (3) Receding chin, "no" jaw

            (4) Upper abdominal surgery

            (5) History of obstructive sleep apnea, often linked to obesity

■ TABLE 36-5
■ ■ **Respiratory Assessment**

Assessments and perianesthesia nurse competencies related to respiratory evaluation

CRITICAL NURSING BEHAVIORS
Never leaves patient unattended
Lists signs and symptoms of respiratory depression
Stimulates wakefulness, movement and deep breathing
Assesses ventilation
　Monitors oxygen saturation
　Auscultates lungs and observes chest movement
　Provides supplemental oxygen as appropriate
Positions patient for effective respiratory effort and chest expansion
　Slight head and chest elevation, particularly if patient is obese
　Ensures adequate blood pressure and patent airway
Plans interventions for airway obstruction
　Demonstrates mandibular lift (jaw support) for airway patency
　Suctions airway with proper technique before extubation and as needed
　Inserts oral or nasal airway when appropriate
　States indications for endotracheal reintubation
　Secures ET tube and demonstrates use of bag-valve-mask device
　Describes criteria for extubation readiness
Describes physiology and interventions for renarcotization, recurarization, pseudocholinesterase
deficiency and pulmonary edema
　Monitors and provides oxygen
　Obtains and prepares appropriate medications and emergency equipment
　Remains within sight near the patient's head
　Uses touch and soft, reassuring words
Prepares equipment for positive pressure airway support or mechanical ventilation
Consults anesthesiologist and communicates airway status
Documents events and interventions

---

   b. Poor muscle tone
    (1) Medication effects: narcotics, muscle relaxants
    (2) Neuromuscular diseases
     (a) Myasthenia gravis
     (b) Quadriplegia
   c. Facial, throat swelling
    (1) Anaphylaxis
    (2) Surgical manipulation
    (3) Edema
  B. *Obstruction*: interrupted patency—an emergency in any PACU
   1. *Soft tissue obstruction*: oropharynx blocked to air entry
    a. Slippage of tongue or foreign body (loose teeth) most common cause
    b. Common when patient very sedated: airway reflexes blunted
    c. Snoring signals partial airway obstruction
     (1) Reposition or elevate head, or turn patient to side-lying position.
     (2) Jaw support, or insert oral or nasal airway until patient awake
    d. Rocking, asynchronous chest movements indicates total obstruction.
     (1) No chest expansion, no air entry audible with auscultation
     (2) Flaring nostrils, tracheal tug, abdominal, accessory muscles
     (3) Muscle relaxation or reintubation if jaw support ineffective
   2. Risk
    a. Hypoventilation or even apnea
    b. Vomiting and aspiration, especially if

(1) Peptic ulcer or hiatal hernia

(2) Obese or pregnant

3. Nursing responsibility

   a. *Never* leave the bedside of the sedated, inadequately breathing patient.

   b. *Be prepared*: sudden, silent vomiting, airway obstruction, apnea, wild disorientation can occur at any (unexpected) moment.

   c. Ask a colleague to contact help or obtain supplies, medications.

   d. Open airway.

      (1) Turn patient to side.

      (2) Mandibular extension or jaw thrust

      (3) Insert artificial nasal or oral airway.

      (4) Backward tilt of head

      (5) Towel roll under shoulders

C. *Laryngospasm* and airway edema

   1. Spasm of laryngeal muscles with partial or complete closure

      a. Stridor: high-pitched, crowing respirations indicates partial.

      b. Absent breath sounds indicates total obstruction.

   2. Airway spasm precipitated by irritants or allergy

      a. Blood, vomitus, mucous on vocal cord

         (1) Suction well before extubation.

         (2) Reduce stimulation of extubation: remove ET tube or LMA while deeply anesthetized or wait until fully awake.

      b. Smoking, chronic obstructive pulmonary disease (COPD), airway irritability, history of asthma (bronchospasm)

      c. Airway trauma: procedure, long or difficult intubation or LMA.

         (1) *Never* remove LMA while patient deeply sedated, unresponsive.

         (2) Premature extubation or LMA removal predisposes patient to airway spasm plus aspiration, coughing, retching, obstruction.

         (3) Procedures: frequent suctioning, laryngoscopy, difficult intubation

      d. Postintubation croup common among children

      e. Coughing, upper respiratory infection

   3. May be able to speak, indicating partial closure

      a. Auscultate lungs for wheezes, air entry; monitor oximetry.

      b. Constant nurse presence and assessment

      c. Coach calmness, slow breathing; perhaps hyperextend head.

         (1) Elevate head or stretcher; provide humidified oxygen.

         (2) Racemic epinephrine inhalations reduce swelling.

         (3) Lidocaine, Decadron injections to reduce inflammation

         (4) Edema symptoms may recur: observe several hours later.

      d. Consult anesthesia provider, immediately if total obstruction.

         (1) Provide 100% oxygen by positive pressure ventilation.

         (2) Low (subparalytic) dose of succinylcholine to relax laryngeal muscles, then reintubate per anesthesia provider.

         (3) Steroids and/or lidocaine may be ordered to reduce airway irritation and swelling.

D. *Bronchospasm*

   1. Event

      a. Constriction of bronchial smooth muscle

      b. Closure of small pulmonary airways with edema, increased secretions

      c. Reaction caused by stimulating airway irritants

         (1) Allergic response: airway and vascular response

             (a) Occurs within 3 minutes after IV injection

             (b) Sensitivity to medications, chemicals, latex

         (2) Aspiration

         (3) Intubation or endotracheal suctioning

      d. Response more likely if preexisting COPD, asthma

   2. Symptoms

    a. Wheezing, often shallow, "noisy" respiration

    b. Decreased oxygen saturation, dyspnea

  3. Intervention

    a. Increase oxygen delivery; consider humidified source.

    b. Remove the irritant.

    c. Therapy with inhaled aerosol of bronchodilator like albuterol, or offer patient's personal inhaler

    d. Severe responses: add muscle relaxants, lidocaine, epinephrine, hydrocortisone to relax airway passages.

E. *Pulmonary edema:* pink frothy sputum, dyspnea, wheezing, rales, hypoxia

  1. *Noncardiac* origin: sudden onset in young, healthy patients

    a. Etiology: upper airway obstruction, rapid naloxone injection

      (1) A strong patient's effort to breathe against closed glottis

      (2) Negative pressure increases within chest cavity.

      (3) Sharp increase in hydrostatic pressure pulls water to lungs.

    b. Symptoms

      (1) Decreased lung compliance

      (2) Chest x-ray findings

        (a) Normal heart size

        (b) No congestive heart failure

  2. *Cardiac* origins: maximized cardiac compliance

    a. Etiology

      (1) Fluid overload

      (2) Ischemic heart disease, cardiomyopathy

      (3) Ventricular failure and/or cardiac valve dysfunction

      (4) Increase in pulmonary capillary permeability

        (a) Sepsis

        (b) Critical multisystem illness

        (c) Debilitation: cancer, liver failure

      (5) Anaphylaxis or transfusion reaction

    b. Symptoms

      (1) Tachycardia

      (2) Dyspnea

      (3) Tachypnea

      (4) Confusion

      (5) Wheezing

        (a) Rales

        (b) Crackles

      (6) Decreased blood pressure

      (7) Paroxysmal nocturnal dyspnea

  3. Intervention: treat cause.

    a. Evaluate chest x-ray: pulmonary infiltrates; reintubation, mechanical ventilation to maintain oxygen.

    b. Morphine boluses relax patient and pulmonary vasculature.

    c. Diuretics if cardiac origin—not deemed useful if noncardiac

    d. Monitor hemodynamics.

    e. Reduce hypoxemia.

    f. Upright position

    g. Oxygen administration

F. *Pulmonary embolus (PE):* blood flow obstruction in pulmonary vessels

  1. Likely causative factors in perianesthesia period

    a. Thrombus as a result of perioperative venous stasis and immobility

    b. Fat embolism after pelvic or long-bone fracture and/or surgery

    c. Hypercoagulability conditions, dehydration, or damaged vessels

  2. Symptoms and assessment

    a. Acute onset of pleuritic chest pain

    b. Tachypnea, tachycardia, agitation, apprehension

    c. Hemoptysis, hypoxia, and hypotension likely

    3. Intervention
       a. Correct hypoxia, cardiovascular instability.
       b. Prompt anticoagulation, initially with heparin
       c. Prophylactic prevention: elastic hose, sequential compression

G. *Aspiration pneumonitis*: *Prevention* most prudent therapy!
    1. Always a potential, albeit rare complication among the sedated or anesthetized
    2. Inhalation of gastric contents as a result of
       a. Full stomach: residual gastric volume, especially if particulate
       b. Acidic gastric contents
       c. Inability to protect airway: inhibited airway reflexes
       d. Obesity, pregnancy, hiatal hernia
       e. Diabetic: gastroparesis
       f. Upper abdominal surgery
       g. Laryngeal mask airway (LMA)
         (1) Aspiration an underreported complication
         (2) If malpositioned, coughing, straining on LMA risk is increased.
         (3) Potential greater when placed by the inexperienced
       h. Trauma patients
    3. Inhalation of blood or foreign body
       a. Loose teeth
       b. Trauma during oropharyngeal manipulation or surgery
    4. Assessment
       a. Coughing, wheezing, hypoxia, hypercarbia, tachypnea
       b. Bronchospasm or atelectasis, particularly if foreign body
       c. Heart rate changes, arrhythmias, hypotension
    5. Interventions
       a. *Prevent* by reducing risk.
         (1) Ensure nothing by mouth (NPO) status of recommended duration.
         (2) Side-lying position for sedated or obtunded patients
         (3) Rapid sequence induction for at-risk patients
       b. Chest x-ray to document infiltrates
       c. Ensure airway patency; turn sedated patient to side.
       d. Provide humidified oxygen; intubate if necessary.
       e. *Constant* observation: never step away from bedside monitor.
       f. *Count* minute respiratory rate; observe depth.
       g. Stimulate patient toward consciousness, deep breathing.
       h. Frequently assess vital signs and act to maintain stability.
       i. Continuously monitor oxygen saturation, even after PACU discharge.
       j. Bronchoscopy if foreign body, large particles
       k. Steroids controversial; antibiotic use only if indicated
       l. Histamine antagonists
         (1) Antacids
         (2) Antiemetics therapy
         (3) H2 receptor blockers
           (a) Cimetidine
           (b) Ranitidine
           (c) Famotidine

H. *Hypoventilation*: ineffective respiratory *effort*
    1. Results in
       a. Decreased oxygen saturation (Po_2), which may be first sign
       b. Subdued respiratory rate, depth, effort
       c. Obliterated airway protective gag and cough reflexes
       d. Increased risk of pulmonary aspiration
       e. Decreased level of consciousness: minimal responsiveness
       f. *Hypercarbia*: increasing Pco_2
         (1) Compounds unresponsiveness

(2) Respiratory acidosis: if unresolved, even less responsiveness, cardiac arrhythmia, unstable blood pressure result.

2. Contributing origins
   a. Associated conditions
      (1) Obesity or pregnancy
      (2) Lengthy or upper abdominal surgeries, procedures
      (3) Prolonged exposure to muscle relaxants, narcotics doses
   b. *Hemoglobin* loss
      (1) Reduces hemoglobin available to transport oxygen
      (2) Consider low hemoglobin when patient pale, oxygen saturation low, and/or tachycardia is persistent.
   c. *Renarcotization*: residual narcotic or sedative effect
      (1) Recurrence of extreme somnolence, poor ventilation
      (2) Caused by gradual migration of narcotics and sedatives from tissues back into bloodstream
      (3) Consider titrating a narcotic or benzodiazepine antagonist.
         (a) Dramatically reverses narcotic effect
         (b) Expect quick wakefulness, pain, agitation, tachycardia.
         (c) Extend observation period at least 30 minutes.
         (d) Opioid half-life is longer than single dose of antagonist.
   d. *Reparalysis* or *recurarization: protracted muscle weakness*
      (1) Neuromuscular blockade recreated
      (2) Residual nondepolarizing muscle relaxants in tissue "outlive" effects of anticholinesterase (reversal) medications.
      (3) Migrate into bloodstream and recreate weakness
      (4) Muscles uncoordinated, weak, "floppy"
      (5) Respirations shallow, gaspy; chest expansion minimal
      (6) Awake patients panicked, anxious, restless
      (7) Often pain despite weakness: no analgesia in muscle relaxants
      (8) May need additional reversal doses, respiratory support, even temporary intubation
   e. *Pseudocholinesterase deficiency: genetic* absence or lack
      (1) Insufficient amount of the intrinsic enzyme needed to hydrolyze succinylcholine, the depolarizing muscle relaxant
         (a) Normally breaks down within 3-5 minutes
         (b) Affects 1 in 2500 to 1 in 2800 individuals
         (c) Patient may be unaware of genetic predisposition until *after* receiving succinylcholine.
      (2) Prolonged duration of succinylcholine effect in patients with abnormal or low levels of plasmacholinesterase
         (a) Liver disease, malnutrition, severe anemia
         (b) Pregnancy, end-stage renal disease, acidosis
      (3) Unreversible muscle weakness ("floppy") and apnea
      (4) Requires mechanical ventilation to support respiration
         (a) Necessary until muscle strength gradually returns
         (b) Psychological support, information, sedation
      (5) Constant vigilance: patient alert, fearful, feels pain
      (6) Educate patient and family to reveal before next anesthetic.
      (7) Physician may recommend laboratory measure of dibucaine levels.
   f. *Pneumothorax:* air entry into pleural space
      (1) Acute chest pain, dyspnea, reduced or absent breath sounds in affected area from deflation of lung, lobe, or pleural bleb
      (2) Caused by
         (a) Alveolar rupture from mechanical ventilation
         (b) Surgical chest procedures that invade pleura
         (c) Central line placement
         (d) Complication of interscalene, intercostal, brachial plexus nerve blocks

(3) *Tension pneumothorax:* after air entry into chest, intrapleural pressure increases and lung deflates; heart and great vessels pulled toward the intact lung
   (a) Hypoxia and inability to ventilate
   (b) Decreased venous return, hypotension, tachycardia
(4) Monitor oxygenation; elevate head of bed.
(5) Serial chest x-rays
   (a) If <20% deflation, observe.
   (b) If >20% or patient symptomatic, insert chest tube.
      (i) Treat cardiopulmonary complications.

3. Care of intubated, perhaps ventilated, patient
   a. Verify effective placement of endotracheal tube.
      (1) Auscultate breath sounds.
         (a) Bilateral air entry all lobes
         (b) Clear sounds without rhonchi
      (2) Continuous monitoring of oxygen saturation with pulse oximetry
      (3) Sample arterial blood gases.
         (a) As basis to assess adequacy of ventilator settings
         (b) Determine acidosis.
   b. Periodically suction via ET tube to clear secretions: sterile technique.
   c. Sedate, relax to minimize stress of awareness while intubated.
      (1) Propofol infusion: sedation, quick consciousness within minutes
      (2) Precedex infusion: short-term sedation without respiratory depression. Use sanctioned for up to 24 hours only
      (3) Paralytics: muscle relaxants used to prevent activity, gagging on ET tube
      (4) Narcotics, analgesics *must* be given.
         (a) Sedatives, muscle relaxants offer no pain reduction.
         (b) Torture for patient to be responsive with light sedative but in pain and unable to indicate by movement or communication
   d. Be aware of sedation goals.
      (1) Deep sedation if intubated for days
      (2) Light sedation allows for regular, brief wake-up intervals to assess neurologic status.
   e. Stir up regimen
      (1) Every 10-15 minutes
         (a) Deep breathe
         (b) Cough
         (c) Turn from side to side.
   f. Extubation criteria
      (1) Return of muscle strength after muscle relaxants
         (a) Equal hand grasps
         (b) Able to initiate head lift from bed and sustain at least 5 seconds
      (2) Respiratory parameters
         (a) Tidal volume at least 5 ml/kg
         (b) Vital capacity at least 15-20 ml/kg
         (c) Negative inspiratory force of 20-25 cm water pressure
      (3) Patient should respond appropriately to questions.
         (a) "Yes" or "no" head movements
         (b) Other forms of communication
            (i) Sign or picture board
            (ii) Writing
         (c) Protrude the tongue
         (d) Open eyes widely
      (4) Swallow and cough reflexes present
      (5) Regular respiratory pattern >10 breaths per minute
      (6) After extubation, close observation for hypoventilation
         (a) Presence of endotracheal tube may have stimulated patient to remain awake and breathing adequately.

■ TABLE 36-6
■ ■ **Cardiovascular Assessment**

Assessments and perianesthesia nurse competencies related to cardiovascular evaluation

CRITICAL NURSING BEHAVIORS
Assesses cardiac and breath sounds and documents peripheral pulses
Discusses causes, physiologic responses, and interventions for hypotension
Increases frequency of blood pressure monitoring
    Identifies factors that alter vasoconstrictive reflexes and heart rate
    Infuses a small bolus (up to 250 ml) of crystalloid
    Observes for significant or ongoing blood loss.
    Consult anesthesiologist and surgeon
Describes causes, physiologic responses and interventions for hypertension
    Increases the frequency of blood pressure monitoring
    Identifies patients at risk and procedural or anesthesia-related causes
    States actions and effects of pharmacologic interventions (nifedipine, labetalol, esmolol, hydralazine,
      nitroprusside, nitroglycerin)
Identifies causes and interventions for common cardiac rhythms

---

IV. Cardiovascular stability (Table 36-6)
    A. Hypotension: consider an array of possible causes to plan interventions.
        1. Evidence: clinical signs of *hypoperfusion*
            a. Measured blood pressure 20% to 30% below baseline
            b. Mean arterial pressure (MAP) <65
            c. Initially, compensate with peripheral vasoconstriction unless sepsis.
                (1) Pale, cool, clammy skin ("cold" shock)
                (2) Warm extremities and hypotension suggest sepsis ("warm" shock).
                (3) Tachycardia: may precede blood pressure decrease
            d. Perfusion deficits as cardiac output continues to fall: *act quickly* to restore.
                (1) Nausea, sometimes vomiting
                (2) Dizziness
                (3) Confusion or even loss of consciousness if extreme
                (4) Chest pain, arrhythmias if susceptible or preexisting cardiac disease
                (5) Oliguria and metabolic acidosis if hypotension uncorrected
            e. Consider hypoxia, hypoglycemia, electrolyte imbalance as causes: measure.
                (1) Hypomagnesia, hypocalcemia alter contractile strength of cardiac muscle.
                (2) Acidosis exacerbates electrolyte disturbance (Table 36-7).
            f. Consider allergic response: accompanied by angioedema, urticaria
            g. Prompt, aggressive fluid resuscitation: multiple methods to calculate need
                (1) Improve cardiac output and therefore contractility first.
                (2) *Calculate overall fluid replacement* by "3 in 1" rule (Table 36-8).
                    (a) Replace 300 ml isotonic fluid rapidly for every 100 ml shed blood.
                (3) Infusion of 500 ml saline bolus; then assess, repeat
                (4) Vasopressin infusion may augment response to vasopressor medications; improves survival outcomes in critically ill.
        2. *Colloid versus crystalloid* controversy
            a. No studies clearly indicate improved outcomes with *either* therapy.
            b. To restore circulating volume and improve blood pressure, most perianesthesia patients need only boluses of isotonic fluid.
            c. Measure hemoglobin: does patient need blood transfusion?

■ TABLE 36-7
■ ■ **Severe Metabolic Acidosis**

Quickly intervene when hypotension and hypoxia occur in critically ill patients: inadequately treated hypoperfusion and hypoxia contribute to worsening metabolic acidosis.

Normals	Severe Acidosis
pH: 7.35 to 7.45	<7.20
HCO_3: 22-26 mEq/L (ABG)	<22
Total CO_2: 24-32 (chemistry panel)*	
Anion Gap: 8-12 mEq/L[†]	>13 mEq/L as HCO_3^- ions are depleted when used to buffer acids

Acidotic Conditions	Clinical Signs	Interventions
Lactic acidosis	Hyperkalemia	*CORRECT CAUSE*
Ketoacidosis	Cardiac contractility decreases	▪ Perfusion
▪ Diabetic	Pulmonary resistance increases (edema)	▪ Oxygenation
▪ Uremic	Poor catecholamine response	▪ Monitor ABG
▪ Starvation	Ventricular fibrillation more likely	*Titrate NaHCO₃*
Aspirin intoxication	Hyperventilation	▪ Controversial in therapy; few studies report improved outcomes, though usually ordered
	Decreased muscle energy	
	▪ Weakens respiratory strength	
	Somnolence	

*Total CO_2 = Bicarbonate (HCO_3^-) + Dissolved CO_2 + H_2CO_3; total CO_2 should nearly equal HCO_3.
[†]Anion gap: Guide to acidosis severity
Calculation: primary *cations* less primary *anions*
$(Na^+) - (Cl^- + HCO_3^-)$

---

    d. Critically or chronically ill may respond to colloid (albumin, hetastarch, or needed blood components) to increase osmotic effect in vascular system (extracellular fluid).

  3. Often transient, mild, but must plan response to profound low blood pressure

    a. *Orthostatic (postural) hypotension*

      (1) In ambulatory surgery or procedural areas, may not be evident until patient sits or stands

      (2) Peripheral vessels incompetent: remain vasodilated from effect of anesthetic medications

      (3) Monitor blood pressure as patient changes position, walks

    b. Continued effect of *spinal or epidural* (regional) anesthetic

      (1) Remaining vasodilation from sympathetic block

        (a) Increases relative size of vascular compartment

        (b) Peripheral pooling of blood

      (2) Most likely after high residual motor and sensory block

        (c) Respiratory compromise above level T4

        (d) Symptoms, hypotension, heat loss persist until blockade recedes.

      (3) Nursing intervention: remain at stretcher side.

        (a) Generous fluid volumes to fill expanded vascular space

        (b) Reclining, foot-elevated position

        (c) Consult anesthesia provider.

        (d) Explain situation, support emotionally, observe constantly.

      (4) Give vasopressors: epinephrine or neosynephrine.

      (5) Monitor oxygen saturations; observe respiratory quality.

        (a) Recognize hypoventilation.

        (b) Intubate, mechanically ventilate if hypoventilation persists.

■ TABLE 36-8
■ ■ **Treating Hypotension: Fluid Replacement**

Guide to approximate fluid replacement requirements

Goal	Action	Outcome
Increase preload	Volume replacement: Rapidly!	First priority
Also increases contractile force	Rate guide: 300 ml per 100 ml fluid loss*	MAP >65† Lower heart rate
Restore hemoglobin	Laboratory measure if persistent hypotension	
Clinical shock if 20% loss of circulating volume*	Transfuse according to physician orders. Patient history and clinical status Increase oxygen-carrying capacity.	Improve O_2 delivery. Less hypoxia Less acidosis pH toward 7.4
	Initiate vasopressors.	*Only* after fluid volume replaced!
Delivery oxygen	Find most effective method.	Raise oxygen saturation.

*Fluid replacement examples:

IF	THEN REPLACE
1. Blood loss ~800 ml Heart rate <100/min BP normal	Up to 2400 ml isotonic *crystalloid*
2. Blood loss ~1500 ml Heart rate >100 and BP normal	About 4500 ml isotonic *crystalloid*
3. Blood loss >2000 ml Heart rate >140 per minute Hypotensive Tachypneic, oliguric	About 6000 ml *crystalloid* + transfuse

†*MAP,* Mean arterial pressure
Calculation: Diastolic blood pressure + 1/3 (systolic BP - diastolic BP)
DBP + 1/3(SBP - DBP)

    c. *Hypothermia*: rewarm slowly, cautiously.
        (1) Initially, vasoconstrictive responses caused by cold temperature
           (a) Masks inadequate circulating fluid volumes
        (2) Peripheral vessels dilate as temperature normalizes.
           (a) Relative vascular space increases.
           (b) Blood pressure plummets.
    d. *Sepsis*
        (1) Consider if hypotension does not resolve after fluid, .rewarming
        (2) More likely after urologic procedures, preexisting infection, intraabdominal leaks, gastrointestinal death, trauma
        (3) Massive peripheral vasodilation
           (a) Low vascular resistance
           (b) Maintains large vascular space
        (4) Provide copious fluid volumes, antibiotics, vasopressors.
        (5) Act quickly to normalize blood pressure, electrolytes.
        (6) Close, even 1:1 observation in PACU, then consider ICU
    e. *Cardiogenic causes*
        (1) New onset periprocedural myocardial infarction
        (2) Cardiac tamponade
        (3) Embolism
        (4) Inability to respond with tachycardia, vasoconstriction
           (a) Medication effects: negative inotropics and chronotropics

    4. *Hypovolemia:* intravascular volume deficit
      a. *Most common cause* of hypotension, particularly in perianesthesia areas
        (1) Procedure-related bleeding
        (2) Insufficient replacement of fluid volume, considering
          (a) Intraoperative blood loss
          (b) NPO duration
          (c) Insensible losses
      b. Assessment indicators
        (1) Hypotension: *always* ask, "Is patient hypovolemic?"
        (2) Compensatory tachycardia
        (3) Significant *bleeding*: check
          (a) Wound drains
          (b) On or under dressings, splints, casts
          (c) Increasing abdominal girth after abdominal procedures
          (d) Hematuria or blood in emesis
          (e) Vascular integrity after orthopedic surgery
        (4) Cumulative losses from sampling for laboratory measures
        (5) Coagulopathy
          (a) Preprocedural condition
          (b) Aspirin, anticoagulants not stopped preoperatively
          (c) After multiple transfusions
          (d) May require Vitamin K, platelets, cryoprecipitate, fresh frozen plasma or Desmopressin (DDAVP), Amicar to treat
      c. Intervention: treat underlying cause.
        (1) Assess fluid volume status in all perianesthesia phases.
          (a) Transfuse with packed red cells if hemoglobin <7-9 g/dl.
          (b) Individual patient with cardiac disease may need transfusion at higher hemoglobin (Hgb).
          (c) *Autologous*: predonated by patient
          (d) *Directed*: donated to patient by a known "other" of same blood type
          (e) *Banked blood*: donated by unknown
        (2) *Always* provide oxygen if patient hypotensive and/or bleeding.
        (3) Fluid, blood product replacement according to calculated need
        (4) Early treatment of acidosis particularly if large blood loss
        (5) Return to operating room for reexploration of surgical site.
        (6) Elevate legs to increase venous return (preload).
B. Hypertension
    1. At least 20% increase above baseline or greater than 150/90, can cause
      a. Surgical bleeding
      b. Cardiac ischemia or failure
      c. Do not discharge from PACU until adequately treated.
    2. Causes in perianesthesia units
      a. Preexisting high blood pressure: *most common* postprocedural cause
        (1) Encourage patient to take antihypertensives before procedure.
      b. Inadequately treated pain, anxiety, or delirium
      c. Full, distended bladder
      d. Following vascular surgeries: carotid endarterectomy, cardiac surgery
      e. Fluid overload
      f. Preeclampsia among pregnant patients
      g. Hypothermia and shivering
    3. Treat by alleviating cause.
      a. Antihypertensives
        (1) Labetalol: peripheral vasodilation, heart rate reduction
        (2) Nitroprusside: peripheral vasodilation, reduces afterload
        (3) Hydralazine: relaxes arterioles
      b. Diuresis, bladder emptying
      c. Rewarming: promote vasodilation.
      d. Manage pain, anxiety.

4. *Autonomic dysreflexia*: sudden, dramatic blood pressure (BP) ↑ elevations
   a. Unimpeded discharge of sympathetic neurons
   b. Paraplegic or quadriplegic patients
   c. Prompted by stimulation
      (1) 'Oscopy procedures
      (2) Surgical manipulation
      (3) Full bladder: verify catheter patency.
      (4) Distended colon
      (5) Increased muscle spasm
   d. Symptoms
      (1) Severe, vessel-rupturing hypertension to 250/150
         (a) Seizures or stroke
         (b) Cardiac arrest
         (c) Surgical bleeding
      (2) Above level of spinal cord injury
         (a) Profuse sweating, flushed skin
         (b) Throbbing headache
      (3) Below injury level
         (a) Pale skin, gooseflesh
   e. Quick interventions
      (1) Empty bladder.
         (a) Void or catheterize.
         (b) Straighten tubing kinks.
      (2) Treat pain: morphine sulfate.
         (a) Markedly relaxes patient
         (b) Dilates peripheral vasculature
      (3) Vasodilating medications: nitroprusside, labetalol
      (4) Elevate head of bed.
C. Cardiac arrhythmias
   1. *Supraventricular tachycardia:* common, usually self-limiting
      a. Heart rate 100-140/minute often a normal compensatory response to
         (1) Surgical stress response
         (2) Pain and/or anxiety
         (3) Bladder distension
         (4) Hypovolemia or low hemoglobin (anemia)
         (5) Fever
         (6) Reflexive response to medications
            (a) Muscle relaxant reversal: glycopyrrolate
            (b) Vasoactive medications: nitroprusside, dopamine
      b. *Malignant hyperthermia*
         (1) Unexplained, ultrarapid tachycardia
         (2) Every PACU must be prepared with a protocol, supplies, personnel education to respond promptly to this anesthesia crisis.
   2. *Sinus bradycardia*: common, usually benign
      a. Heart rate less than 60 beats per minute
         (1) Especially among young, healthy athletes
         (2) Sleepy, under-stimulated patients
         (3) Expected response when using beta-blocking medications
         (4) Response to anesthetic medications: sinus and junctional
      b. No treatment unless
         (1) Dangerously low blood pressure
         (2) Progressive heart block
            (a) New or chronic cardiac disease
            (b) *Atropine* increases sinus firing and atrioventricular (AV) conduction.
            (c) Pacemaker for persistent, symptomatic blocks
      c. *Vagal nerve stimulation*: profound bradycardia, even asystole

(1) Normally sustains heart rate balance: opposes acceleration tendencies

(2) Undeterred stimulation as a result of

   (a) Valsalva: straining at stool or urination

   (b) Vomiting and retching

(3) Likely results in

   (a) Nausea

   (b) Profound hypotension

   (c) Dizziness, lethargy, even unconsciousness

(4) Intervene with

   (a) Recumbent flat position

   (b) Close monitoring of vital signs, cardiac rhythm, alertness

   (c) Medications as indicated per anesthesia provider or protocols

   (d) Defer transfer from PACU.

      (i) May occur when moving about in phase II; consider return to phase I care.

3. Premature ventricular contractions may

   a. Be benign, normally occurring

   b. Reflect hypokalemia, acidosis, hypercapnia: assess labs

   c. Indicate hypoxia: supplement oxygen, stimulate groggy patient

   d. Suggest cardiac ischemia

4. Atrial fibrillation or flutter

   a. Often a chronic condition, especially among elderly surgical patients

   b. Report to physician.

      (1) New onset: could reflect

         (a) Fluid overload in cardiac sensitive patient

         (b) Perianesthesia cardiac concern

      (2) Rapid, uncontrolled ventricular response

      (3) Physical decompensation

         (a) Associated with significant hypotension or hypertension

         (b) Chest pain

         (c) Respiratory changes: dyspnea, pulmonary congestion

D. Chest pain: *presume cardiac cause until excluded!*

   1. At-risk patients

      a. Preexisting cardiac disease

      b. Obesity

      c. Diabetes

      d. Debilitation

   2. Assess subjective description.

      a. Pleural versus angina, sharp versus pressure

      b. Location: jaw, chest, left arm, radiation to neck, back

      c. Notice accompanying diaphoresis, nausea, dyspnea

      d. Associated cardiac arrhythmias or blood pressure instability

   3. Differentiate

      a. Gas, especially post laparoscopy, colon surgery

      b. Referred surgical pain

      c. Pleural causes: pneumothorax, pleural effusion, pneumonia

      d. Gastrointestinal (GI) causes: reflux esophagitis, ulcer, pancreatitis

   4. Interventions

      a. Monitor rate and rhythm, obtain 12-lead electrocardiogram (ECG), compare with preoperative ECG

      b. Decrease myocardial work, and manage complications.

         (1) Relieve pain, and consider morphine for vasodilating benefits.

         (2) Antianginal (nitroglycerin), arrhythmia, blood pressure therapies

         (3) Adequate oxygenation and hydration

      c. Laboratory tests: serial troponins, cardiac enzymes

      d. Peripheral vascular integrity

      e. Reposition patient, offer antacids, which may relieve noncardiac pain

V. GI issues
  A. Nausea and vomiting
    1. All too common, miserable, resistant anesthesia outcome
      a. Alters patient reports of satisfaction with procedure
      b. Sedation increases aspiration risk.
      c. Persistent retching, recurrent emesis increase pain, dehydrate.
      d. May result in unplanned hospital admission after procedures, ambulatory surgery
    2. Physiology: narcotics, sedatives can trigger brain's emetic center.
      a. Retching controlled by vomiting center in medulla
      b. Vomiting center receives input from
        (1) Cerebral cortex: olfactory, visual, emotional stimuli
        (2) GI tract
        (3) Vestibular system
        (4) Chemoreceptor trigger zone (CTZ)
    3. Risk factors for developing PONV
      a. Predisposing factors
        (1) Female gender
        (2) Motion sickness or vestibular problems
        (3) Delayed gastric emptying or pressure
          (a) Morbid obesity
          (b) Early pregnancy
          (c) Gastroparesis: neurologic diseases, diabetes
          (d) Abdominal distention for laparoscopy
        (4) Increased gastric volume
          (a) Full stomach, insufficient duration of NPO restrictions
          (b) Anxiety
        (5) Hypotension, bradycardia: sudden, unexpected emesis
        (6) Severe pain
        (7) Dehydration: include NPO duration in fluid replacement, calculation.
      b. Specific surgical procedures highly associated with nausea
        (1) Laparoscopic procedures, particularly gynecologic
        (2) Strabismus surgery, primarily children
        (3) Middle ear procedures
      c. Anesthetic techniques
        (1) Inhalant anesthetics (gases): nitrous oxide, volatile agents
        (2) IV medications
          (a) Ketamine and etomidate
          (b) Narcotics, particularly meperidine, morphine
      d. Intervention: no panacea, "wonder" therapy
        (1) Prevention most effective treatment
          (a) Assess risk indicators.
          (b) Hydration! Generous IV fluid replacement
          (c) Avoid brisk head movement, restlessness.
          (d) Provide adequate analgesia; position for comfort.
          (e) Encourage deep breathing, relaxation.
        (2) Avoid gastric distention.
          (a) Restrictive oral fluids until nausea passes
          (b) Oral hygiene: many complain of anesthetic "taste."
          (c) Ensure patent nasogastric tube.
        (3) Medicate: preemptive combinations, particularly if high risk or history of postoperative nausea and vomiting (PONV).
          (a) Anticholinergics: scopolamine patch behind ear
          (b) Serotonins: ondansetron (Zofran) or cousin dolasetron (Anzemet)
          (c) Butyrophenones: droperidol (Inapsine)
            (i) Only limited use recommended for outpatients because of unpleasant extrapyramidal effects, also drowsiness
          (d) Steroids: dexamethasone (Decadron)

(e) Sedatives: propofol (Diprivan) has antiemetic properties.
(f) Phenothiazines
  (i) Prochlorperazine (Compazine): per rectal suppository, particularly if outpatient with resistant nausea
  (ii) Chlorpromazine (Thorazine)
(g) Antihistamines
  (i) Hydroxyzine (Vistaril, Atarax)
  (ii) Diphenhydramine (Benadryl)
(h) Benzamide
  (i) Metoclopramide (Reglan)
(4) Adjunctive methods to reduce dizziness, nausea
  (a) Acupressure antiemetic wrist bands
  (b) Power of suggestion
  (c) Hydration: up to 2000 ml for even minor procedures
(5) May vomit after discharge despite interventions
  (a) Persist up to 48 hours after discharge from phase I
  (b) Oral fluids and food too soon actually increase likelihood.
  (c) For patients discharged home, advise
    (i) Rest
    (ii) Nonnarcotic medications if possible
    (iii) Gradual increases in fluid intake: "treat yourself as though you had the flu."
    (iv) Contact physician for unrelenting vomiting.

B. GI perfusion: remember the gut!
  1. Potential for GI ischemia an overlooked consideration for critically ill patients
    a. Mesentery not directly visible for assessment
      (1) Absent bowel sounds may mean dead or poorly perfused gut.
      (2) Involve gastroenterology assessment quickly in sepsis.
    b. Crucial concern when evaluating sepsis, especially if
      (1) Unresolving hypotension, progressive acidosis
      (2) Trauma, pancreatitis, burns: potential for GI dysfunction high
    c. No specific, convenient measure to assess viability of GI tissue
      (1) GI often not treated until symptomatic—perhaps too late
        (a) Outcome worse the longer septic patient is hypotensive with low mean arterial pressure (MAP)
        (b) Alcoholism history increases risk of GI ischemia.
          (1) Poorly functioning liver
          (2) Immunosuppressed
      (2) *Kupffer cells*: critical to protecting "gut"
        (a) Immune (phagocytic) cells in liver kill bacteria released from "gut."
        (b) If unhealthy gut, more endotoxins circulate through liver, then seed other organs.
        (c) Impaired Kupffer cells predispose to sepsis, pulmonary failure (acute respiratory distress syndrome [ARDS])
        (d) Liver function tests only reflect injury, not systemic function: rise only if cell death.
      (3) *Tonometry studies* cumbersome at bedside but recommend:
        (a) Improve oxygen delivery, cardiac output *before* acidosis
        (b) Survival from sepsis increased if maintain oxygenation
  2. Prevent multisystem organ failure (MSOF) or dysfunction (MSOD).
    a. Per tonometry studies, prevent MSOF if perfuse gut
    b. Recommend *postpyloric* tube feedings to maintain viability and structural integrity of microvilli in small bowel cell walls.
      (1) If not stimulated, microvilli flatten.
      (2) Can occur even if NPO for 4 days
      (3) Bypass stomach when inserting feeding tube.
      (4) Infuse high glutamine solution, even in small amount.

■ TABLE 36-9
■ ■ **Safe Emergence: Delirium and Delayed Response**

Assessments and perianesthesia nurse competencies related to emergence delirium and delayed arousal after anesthesia

CRITICAL NURSING BEHAVIORS
Discerns hidden causes of agitation, especially hypoxia, undetected internal hemorrhage, or acidosis
Identifies physiologic possibilities for delayed emergence from anesthesia and appropriate nursing and medical interventions
Explains physiologic influence of medications used to calm the restless patient or to stir the slow to respond patient
- Medicates only when oxygenation is adequate
  - Hysostigmine, an anticholinesterase medication, penetrates the blood brain barrier to increase neuromuscular acetylcholine: quickly transforms agitation to calm
  - Titrates midazolam, lorazepam, narcotics to treat pain
  - Narcotic or benzodiazepine antagonists to reverse sedation
  - Medications to correct physiologic imbalance
Quickly transforms agitation to calm
Describes rationales to assure the agitated patient's safety while restless
- Always remains with the patient and frequently assesses oxygenation
- Loosely applies limb restraints; aware that limiting movement may increase fear, disorientation, and agitation
- Protects sensitive corneas from abrasion by flailing hands that rub eyes
- Involves family members
- Parents calm a wild child.
- A familiar voice might help reorient a patient with visual, hearing, intellectual, or emotional impairment.
Describes rationales to ensure safety of a patient with delayed arousal
- Always remains with the patient
- Closely monitors oxygenation, airway patency, and respiratory quality
- Frequently attempts to arouse patient
- Consults physicians as appropriate when sedation persists
- Rewarms a hypothermic patient; considers other medical possibilities

---

VI. Neurologic concerns and anesthesia
   A. Delayed emergence: slow to arouse, failure to return to preanesthetic baseline
      1. Consider multiple possible reasons and treat the cause (Table 36-9).
         a. Understimulated patient: actively stimulate at regular intervals!
            (1) Touch, shake, and call to patient.
            (2) Remain at stretcher side: Do not leave unresponsive patient unattended!
            (3) Know patient's neurologic baseline, medical history, laboratory results.
         b. Assess adequate ventilation and oxygenation.
            (1) Poor ventilation will only extend arousal period.
            (2) Hyperventilation
               (a) May be normal response: effort to exhale volatile (gas) anesthetics—observe, may rouse soon.
               (b) If diabetic, consider superelevated hyperglycemia and acidosis.
            (3) *Hypercarbia* (increased P_{CO_2}) impairs consciousness, extends sedation.
            (4) *Hypoxia* (decreased P_{O_2}) deprives tissues of oxygen, produces acidosis.
            (5) Monitor oxygen saturation, *deliver oxygen*, consult anesthesiologist.
            (6) Extended unresponsiveness: draw arterial blood gasses (ABG).
         c. Hypothermia
            (1) Cold body temperatures delay metabolism of medications.
            (2) Gradually rewarm while monitoring vital signs: prevent hypotension.

       d. Prolonged action of anesthesia medications: most likely cause

         (1) Ongoing neuromuscular blockade: is patient awake but unable to move?

         (2) Observe pupils: pinpoint constriction suggests continued narcotic effect.

         (3) Has sufficient time elapsed for medication metabolism and elimination?

         (4) Consider reversing narcotics, benzodiazepines, muscle relaxants.

       e. Metabolic causes: correct imbalances

         (1) Hypoglycemia or hyperglycemia: measure blood glucose!

         (2) Electrolyte imbalance

         (3) Preexisting reasons: hepatic, renal, Cushing's disease, hypothyroidism

       f. Organic dysfunction

         (1) Perioperative myocardial infarction? Assess per 12-lead ECG.

         (2) Cerebrovascular issues: stroke, seizure, intracerebral hemorrhage?

         (3) Air embolism related to surgical procedure

           (a) Cardiopulmonary bypass during heart surgery

           (b) Sitting position during cervical (neck) surgery

         (4) Craniotomy: new hematoma?

   B. Emergence delirium: "Waking up wild!" (Table 36-9)

     1. *Suspect hypoxia first!*

       a. Ensure adequate ventilation, oxygenation before giving *any* sedation.

       b. Patient may move but remain anesthetized, disoriented, air hungry.

         (1) Residual muscle relaxants: unable to "get enough air"

         (2) Narcotics, sedatives: hypercarbia from ineffective respiratory effort

         (3) Electrolyte or acid-base imbalance, hemoglobin deficiency

       c. Agitation may signal cerebral hypoxia.

       d. Consider severe anemia: Is patient bleeding actively?

         (1) Consider procedural blood loss according to preanesthetic hemoglobin.

         (2) Measure hemoglobin: adequate to transport oxygen to tissues?

     2. *Transient* restless, agitated, confused, or dysphoric arousal

       a. Squirmy, crying, strongly pushing away caregiver common in children, teens

       b. Normal response to pain, urgent call of a full bladder when not fully awake!

       c. Untoward response: fewer than 10% of all surgical patients

         (1) History may indicate prior occurrence with anesthetic exposure.

         (2) Confluence of multiple medications

           (a) Dreams, hallucinations when adults receive ketamine

           (b) Extrapyramidal effects caused by droperidol

           (c) Anesthetics and medications to treat organic brain syndrome

         (3) Continuation of preprocedural *anxiety* about life or procedure

       d. Signals chronic alcoholism: consult physician.

         (1) Drinkers often underestimate consumption.

         (2) When *was* the last drink? Is patient also tachycardic?

         (3) Consider delirium tremens (DTs): arrange for close observation after PACU discharge, initiate sedation protocol, often with lorazepam (Ativan), per order.

       e. Signals substance abuse, either legal or illicit

     3. Consider systemic causes.

       a. Acute dilutional hyponatremia: measure serum sodium.

         (1) May absorb intraoperative irrigant after transurethral resection of prostate (TURP), also known as "TURP Syndrome"

         (2) Women after hysteroscopy

       b. Hypotension: inadequate oxygen delivery

   c. Sepsis
   d. Hypothermia: unable to express feeling cold and slows medication elimination

4. Safety: irrational, agitated, thrashing patient is usually extremely strong.
   a. Constant presence of nurse required to ensure safe passage through this stage
   b. Often multiple personnel needed at bedside to restrain patient, keep on stretcher, avoid bodily injury to patient and nurse.
   c. Remain calm, speak softly to connect with and reorient patient.
      (1) Encourage, guide patient toward stillness.
      (2) When you can interact with patient, ask questions to assess.
         (a) Breathing: "getting enough air?"
         (b) Pain: presence and severity
         (c) Awareness of situation: does patient recall having procedure, know who, where he or she is?
         (d) Feeling cold?
      (3) Though tempting, overwhelming patient with forceful restraint and loud commands serves only to further agitate.
      (4) Carefully apply limb restraints according to facility protocol.
      (5) Maintain quiet environment.
      (6) Prevent injury: fall from stretcher, scratch corneas with random movements.
   d. Protracted delirium may resolve with physostigmine; consult anesthesia provider.
   e. Judiciously treat pain: chemical restraint
      (1) Prevent sudden somnolence.
      (2) Pain may be severe in patients who chronically use oral narcotics.
         (a) Did patient take scheduled narcotics preprocedure?
         (b) If not, likely reacting incoherently to severe pain
C. Recall of intraoperative or procedural events
   1. Rare and haunting occurrence for patient and anesthesia provider
      a. Alert, oriented patient, perhaps ready for discharge, relates details of intraoperative events.
         (1) Specifics of conversations, comments, or an occurrence
            (a) Pain and being "unable to tell anyone"
            (b) Interprets conversations he or she overheard to be about self, even if they were not
         (2) Most associated with "light" general anesthetic for
            (a) Cesarean section
            (b) Bypass cardiac surgery
      b. Allow to talk.
         (1) May feel scared, angry, sad, confused
         (2) Listen closely; *document* all communication.
         (3) Acknowledge that awareness does occur.
         (4) Consult and inform anesthesia provider, who should visit patient.
D. Local anesthetic toxicity
   1. Central nervous system effects: cross blood-brain barrier
      a. Tinnitus
      b. Light-headedness and/or confusion
      c. Circumoral numbness
      d. Unresponsiveness, seizures
   2. Cardiovascular and respiratory effects
      a. Peripheral vasodilatation: relaxation of vascular smooth muscle
      b. Hypotension, circulatory collapse at extremely high doses
      c. Arrhythmias: bradycardia, AV block, intraventricular conduction delay
      d. Respiratory arrest

      3. Cause: large intravascular bolus of local anesthetic
         a. Sudden release or failure of tourniquet during Bier Block
         b. Inadvertent injection when placing regional blocks
         c. Improperly set infusion rate of IV lidocaine
      4. Intervention: largely supportive to resuscitate
         a. Oxygenation, airway maintenance
         b. Generous IV fluid volume
         c. Symptomatic treatment of seizures, hypotension, apnea

VII. Thermal balance

  A. Hypothermia: iatrogenic complication

      1. Perianesthesia origins

         a. Vasodilating anesthetic medications and techniques
           (1) General anesthetics: alter thermoregulation at the hypothalamus.
             (a) Patient cools to temperature of room (poikilothermia).
           (2) Spinal blockade: lose heat through dilated peripheral vessels
             (a) Heat loss continues until spinal resolved, even in PACU.
         b. Open body cavities, room temperature tissue irrigants during procedure
         c. Cold room temperatures in procedure rooms

      2. Heat loss physics

         a. *Radiation:* heat transfer between two surfaces of different temperatures
         b. *Convection:* surface loss of heat when fluid flows across at a lower temperature
         c. *Conduction:* heat transfer between two touching objects of different temperatures as when warm human body in direct contact with cooler OR table
         d. *Evaporation:* heat loss through insensible water loss from skin, the respiratory tract, open incisions, and wet drapes

      3. Potential consequences: vary with significance of heat loss

         a. Increased oxygen consumption as a result of shivering
           (1) Normal autonomic response to generate heat
           (2) Heat production by muscular contractions
           (3) Potential cardiac or pulmonary failure for compromised patient
             (a) Oxygen consumption increases 400% to 500%.
             (b) Tachycardia and hypertension
             (c) Pain and thermal discomfort: *feels* cold
                (1) Temperature may actually meet discharge criteria.
                (2) Patients describe as "thought I'd freeze to death."
         b. Wound infection: studies indicate hypothermia delays wound healing.
         c. Cardiac disturbance: marked increase in cardiac output, breathing
         d. Delayed emergence from anesthesia: prolonged medication effect and delayed elimination, especially if temperature below 95° F (35° C)
         e. Coagulopathy
         f. Assessment interference
           (1) Vasoconstriction and shivering movements impede measurement of oxygen saturation.

      4. Interventions: *Preventing* unplanned heat loss recommended

         a. Rewarming measures: gradual to prevent sudden hypotension
           (1) Active methods for warmth and comfort
             (a) Forced-air warming system: billowy blankets filled with warmed air
           (2) Passive insulation
             (a) Warmed cotton blankets
             (b) Thermal drapes
             (c) Fluid and blood warmers
             (d) Heated humidifiers for oxygen delivery
             (e) Infrared lights
           (3) Increasing the thermostat to warm the procedure area

    b. Supplemental oxygen, particularly if shivering

    c. Regularly measure temperature, every 30 minutes if hypothermic

        (1) Discharge *only* after attaining facility's discharge temperature.

        (2) Discharge criteria per ASPAN discharge criteria: 96.8° F (36° C)

        (3) ASPAN clinical practice guideline, established at a multispecialty consensus conference on hypothermia, defines normothermia as 36° to 96.8° to 100.4° F (38° C).

    d. Meperidine, as little as 10 mg IV, effectively suppresses shivering.

B. Hyperthermia

    1. *Fever*: normal physiologic response to infection

      a. May arrive for surgery, perhaps for wound debridement or appendectomy: less febrile postoperatively

      b. May be indication for surgery cancellation of elective spine, joint replacement involving implanted hardware

        (1) Evaluate for pulmonary infection.

        (2) Urinary tract infection

      c. Prelude to sepsis?

        (1) Heighten vigilance and assessment.

        (2) Anticipate hypotension, hypoxia.

    2. *Malignant hyperthermia*: a true anesthesia crisis

      a. Causes

        (1) Rare, genetically determined skeletal muscle response

           (a) Calcium prevented from reentering cell

        (2) Specific triggers

           (a) Succinylcholine

           (b) Volatile inhalation agents, including desflurane, isoflurane, enflurane, halothane, and sevoflurane

        (3) Most likely in the young and healthy

      b. Goal: *prevention*

        (1) Identify susceptibility: ask *all* preoperative patients if a

           (a) Personal or family history of anesthetic-related death?

           (b) Muscle disorder?

           (c) Develop fever or dark urine after previous surgery?

      c. Observations

        (1) Sudden unexplained tachycardia may be initial signal.

        (2) Unexpected surge of end-tidal CO_2 in anesthetized patient

        (3) Profound muscle rigidity: often first noted at masseter muscle

        (4) Extreme metabolic acidosis

        (5) Cyanosis, tachypnea, hemodynamic instability

        (6) Fever a final sign

      d. Interventions: aggressive, intensive to ward off terminal acidosis

        (1) Immediate *cooling*: pack in ice, chill IVs required

        (2) Massive doses of dantrolene sodium (Dantrium), a skeletal muscle relaxant

        (3) Find personnel *help*: a crisis with multiple tasks.

        (4) Oxygenate: hyperventilate at 100%.

        (5) Work to correct severe metabolic acidosis.

        (6) Monitor hemodynamics, urine, laboratory measures.

BIBLIOGRAPHY

1. American Society of PeriAnesthesia Nursing: *2002 Standards of perianesthesia nursing practice.* Cherry Hill, New Jersey: American Society of PeriAnesthesia Nursing, 2002.

2. Anthony D, Jasinski DM: Postoperative pain management: Morphine versus ketorolac. *J PeriAnesth Nurs* 17:30-42, 2002.

3. Ard JL, Prough DS: Perioperative electrolyte and acid-base abnormalities. In Benumof JL, Saidman LJ, editors: *Anesthesia and perioperative complications,* ed 2. St Louis: Mosby, 1999, pp 503-535.

4. Barnes S, O'Brien D: Considering bypass of phase I PACU? *J PeriAnesth Nurs* 17: 193-195, 2002.

5. Bennett J, Wren KR, Haas R: Opioid use during the perianesthesia period. *J PeriAnesth Nurs* 16:255-259, 2001.

6. Benumof JL: Obstructive sleep apnea in the adult obese patients: Implications for airway management. *Anesthesiol Clin North America* 20:789-811, 2002.

7. Bogetz MS: Using the laryngeal mask airway to manage the difficult airway. *Anesthesiol Clin North America* 20:863-780, 2002.

8. Burns SM: Safely caring for patients with a laryngeal mask airway. *Crit Care Nurse* 21:72-74, 2001.

9. Burns SM: Revisiting hypothermia: A critical concept. *Crit Care Nurse* 21:83-86, 2001.

10. Burns SM: Delirium during emergence from anesthesia: A case study. *Crit Care Nurse* 23:66-69, 2003.

11. Calswell JE: Rapid sequence intubation: Is rocuronium an alternative? *Sem Anesth Periop Med Pain* 21:99-103, 2002.

12. Childs SG: Tension pneumothorax: A pulmonary complication secondary to regional anesthesia from brachial plexus interscalene nerve block. *J PeriAnesth Nurs* 17:404-412, 2002.

13. Connor EL, Wren KR: Detrimental effects of hypothermia: A systems analysis. *J PeriAnesth Nurs* 15:151-155, 2000.

14. Cowling GE, Haas R: Hypotension in the PACU: An algorithmic approach. *J PeriAnesth Nurs* 17:159-163, 2002.

15. Erickson LI: Acquired neuromuscular disorders in the critically ill patient. *Sem Anesth Periop Med Pain* 21:135-139, 2002.

16. Floyd PT: Latex allergy update. *J PeriAnesth Nurs* 15:26-30, 2000.

17. Golembiewski JA, Obrien D: A systematic approach to the management of postoperative nausea and vomiting. *J PeriAnesth Nurs* 17:364-376, 2002.

18. Gray JR: Steering clear of sepsis skid: Interventions in sepsis, organ, and renal failure. Lecture on April 21, 2003. North Memorial Center, Robbinsdale, MN.

19. Irvin SM: Sensorineural hearing loss after select procedures. *J PeriAnesth Nurs* 17: 89-101, 2002.

20. Harris SN: Hypotension, hypertension, perioperative myocardial ischemia, and infarction. In Benumof JL, Saidman LJ, editors: *Anesthesia and perioperative complications*, ed 2. St Louis: Mosby, 1999, pp 286-307.

21. Kervin MW: Residual neuromuscular blockade in the immediate postoperative period. *J PeriAnesth Nurs* 17:152-158, 2002.

22. Knoerl DV, McNulty P, Estes C, et al: Evaluation of orthostatic blood pressure testing as a discharge criterion from PACU after spinal anesthesia. *J PeriAnesth Nurs* 16:11-18, 2001.

23. Krau SD: Selecting and managing fluid therapy. *Crit Care Nurs Clin North America* 10:401-410, 1998.

24. Learman JB: The challenging role of the perianesthesia nurse in the office-based surgical suite. *J PeriAnesth Nurs* 15:31-52, 2000.

25. Lui ACP, Thompson GE: Perioperative nerve injury. In Benumof JL, Saidman LJ, editors: *Anesthesia and perioperative complications*, ed 2. St Louis: Mosby, 1999, pp 192-206.

26. Moline BM: Pain management in the ambulatory surgical population. *J PeriAnesth Nurs* 16:388-398, 2001.

27. Nunnelee JD, Spaner DS: Assessment and nursing management of hypertension in the perioperative period. *J PeriAnesth Nurs* 15:163-168, 2000.

28. O'Brien D: Acute postoperative delirium: Definition, incidence, recognition and interventions. *J PeriAnesth Nurs* 17:384-392, 2002.

29. Prielipp RC, Young CC: Current drugs for sedation of critically ill patients. *Sem Anesth Periop Med Pain* 20:85-94, 2001.

30. Redmond MC: Malignant hyperthermia: Perianesthesia recognition, treatment, and care. *J PeriAnesth Nurs* 16:259-269, 2001.

31. Rose JB, Watcha MF: Postoperative nausea and vomiting. In Benumof JL, Saidman LJ, editors: *Anesthesia and perioperative complications*, ed 2. St Louis: Mosby, 1999, pp 425-440.

32. Sandlin D: Transderm scopolamine: A painless, noninvasive option for control of postoperative nausea and vomiting. *J PeriAnesth Nurs* 17:427-429, 2001.

33. Sommers MS: The cellular basis of septic shock. *Crit Care Nurs Clin North America* 15:13-26, 2003.

34. Spitellie PH, Holmes MA, Domino KB: Awareness during anesthesia. *Anesthesiol Clin North America* 20:317-332, 2002.

35. Watkins AC, White PF: Fast-Tracking after ambulatory surgery. *J PeriAnesth Nurs* 16:379-387, 2001.

36. Watson CB: Respiratory complications associated with anesthesia. *Anesthesiol Clin North America* 20:275-299, 2002.

37. Watche MF: Postoperative nausea and emesis. *Anesthesiol Clin North America* 20:471-484, 2002.

38. Williams EL: Postoperative blindness. *Anesthesiol Clin North America* 20:367-384, 2002.

39. Wilson M: Giving postanesthesia care in the critical care unit. *Dimens Crit Care Nurs* 19:38-43, 2000.

37 PACU Phase I Discharge Criteria

SUSAN JANE FETZER

OBJECTIVES
At the conclusion of this chapter the reader will be able to:

1. Define terminology describing discharge definitions.

2. Describe commonly used postanesthesia care unit (PACU) discharge criteria rankings.

3. Recognize purposes of discharge criteria.

■■ PACU nurses must assess and evaluate the patient's readiness for discharge. Using a criteria-based scoring system ensures patients are adequately prepared for transfer to PACU phase II or a nursing unit.

I. Overview
   A. Definitions
      1. Discharge ready (adj): a multifaceted concept that describes a patient's functional and cognitive state as sufficiently recovered from anesthesia with the ability to leave the PACU and be safely cared for in a less intensive nursing environment
      2. Discharge readiness (noun): the state of being ready to leave the PACU and be cared for in a less intensive nursing environment
      3. Discharge criterion (noun): a standard or test by which to judge or decide if a PACU patient is discharge ready
      4. Discharge score (noun): a quantitative measurement applied to one or more discharge criteria that have been assigned numerical values to categories of achievement; a discharge score is a summation of criteria ratings into a total score
      5. Ready for transfer (adj): a description of the patient who is discharge ready with consideration of patient and institutional characteristics
      6. Fast tracking (verb): bypassing PACU phase I recovery when phase I criteria have been met prior to leaving the operating room
      7. Functional and cognitive ability pertaining to discharge readiness is evidenced by
         a. An assessment by the attending anesthesia personnel
         b. Meeting established criterion or criteria
         c. Achieving an acceptable score on an established discharge scoring system
         d. Narrative nurses' notes that reflect that the patient is stable, responsive, free from complications and has adequately recovered from the major effects of anesthesia.
      8. *Ready for transfer* may include patient characteristics not included in a discharge criteria but considered as related factors in nursing decisions such as
         a. Acceptable level of pain
         b. Acceptable level of nausea
         c. Need for ongoing pharmacological or technological treatments
            (1) Blood transfusion complete
            (2) Chest x-ray

      d. Need for ongoing collaboration with other health care providers
        (1) Respiratory therapy
        (2) Surgeon
  9. *Ready for transfer* may include institutional characteristics that affect the patient's ability to leave the PACU environment such as
      a. Receiving unit able to accept transfer (i.e., bed available)
      b. Nursing personnel availability

B. Purpose of discharge criteria
  1. Ensure same standard of care for all patients.
  2. Guides practice decisions but does not make practice decisions
  3. Promotes efficient use of fiscal and personnel resources
  4. Allows nurses to act on behalf of anesthesia personnel: American Society of Anesthesiologists (ASA) (1988) "In the absence of the physician responsible for the discharge, the PACU nurse shall determine that the patient meets the discharge criteria."[6]
  5. Meets Joint Commission on Accreditation of Healthcare Organizations (JCAHO) requirements
      a. Relevant discharge criteria are rigorously applied to determine the readiness of the patient for discharge.
      b. The discharge criteria are approved by the medical staff.
  6. Meets American Society of PeriAnesthesia Nurses (ASPAN) Standards: determining discharge assessment is included in ASPAN Practice Standards.
  7. Nurse Practice Act: determining discharge readiness is a delegated act (refer to specific practice act of each state).

C. Requirements for determining discharge readiness
  1. ASA Standards for Post Anesthesia Care (1988)
      a. Standard V: Physician is responsible for the discharge of the patient from the post anesthesia care unit.
      b. Standard V. 1. When discharge criteria are used, they must be approved by the Department of Anesthesiology and the medical staff.
      c. Standard V. 1. [Discharge criteria] may vary depending upon whether the patient is discharged to a hospital room, to the ICU, to a short stay unit, or home.
  2. Discharge criteria must be applied consistently.
  3. Discharge criteria must be enforced.
  4. Compliance to discharge criteria must be monitored.

D. Application of discharge criterion
  1. Applied when patient is admitted to PACU as part of nursing assessment
  2. Applied routinely (every 15 or 30 minutes depending on institutional policy) as part of nursing assessment
  3. Applied when patient is about to leave the operating room (OR) to determine eligibility for fast tracking
  4. Used to monitor intraoperative and postanesthesia interventions for effectiveness during quality assurance activities
  5. Used in nursing research to monitor the effect of interventions on patient outcomes
  6. Gives support for physician and nursing critical judgment of discharge readiness

E. Variations of discharge readiness
  1. PACU to intensive care unit (ICU)
      a. Achievement of discharge criteria reflects need for ongoing critical care nursing to monitor and intervene.
      b. All discharge criteria may not be met.
      c. Discharge score may not be attained.
      d. Physician evaluation is used in place of discharge criteria or discharge score.
      e. Discharge readiness and ready to transfer should occur concurrently.

   2. PACU to acute care
      a. Achievement of most discharge criteria, which reflects need for continuing nursing care to monitor patient's status.
      b. Discharge criteria are met, with one or two exceptions.
      c. Discharge score is attained within acceptable range set by policy.
      d. Reasons for exceptions are documented in nurses' notes.
      e. Institutional policy refers to exceptions that must be reported to the physician prior to transfer.
      f. Discharge readiness may be attained before ready to transfer.
   3. PACU to phase II
      a. Achievement of most discharge criteria with the belief that all discharge criteria will be attained within short period of time.
      b. Discharge criteria are met; occasionally other patient characteristics (e.g., pain control, nausea) restrict the patient from discharge to home.
      c. Discharge score is attained within acceptable range set by policy.
      d. Discharge readiness may be attained before ready to transfer.
   4. PACU to home
      a. Achievement of all PACU discharge criteria and all phase II discharge criteria are met.
      b. Any exceptions are documented, are reported to the physician, and an order to discharge home is noted.
II. Standards for discharge criteria
   A. Objective
      1. Be measurable
      2. Be understandable
      3. Be able to be applied by knowledgeable health care providers
   B. Validity
      1. Is judged by determining if the criteria reflects the concept being measured (e.g., Sao_2 is a more valid measurement of oxygenation than patient color)
      2. Has been acknowledged as appropriate by content experts
      3. Can be established by comparing two criteria that evaluate the same concept (e.g., level of sensory block and extremity movement)
      4. Reflect the ability of the criterion to be sensitive to changes in patient status and able to measure change in patient status appropriately
      5. Can be supported by testing the criterion against future predictions
      6. Validity is evaluated on a continuum.
      7. A discharge criterion may be valid for one population of patients but not for another (e.g., O_2 saturation >92% for chronic obstructive pulmonary disease (COPD) patient who has baseline O_2 saturation of 89)
   C. Reliability
      1. Concerned with the ability of the criterion to be ranked the same way regardless of health care provider applying the criterion (inter-rater reliability)
      2. Documented by statistical analysis from research performed with the criterion
III. Commonly used PACU discharge criteria rankings
   A. Respiratory criteria
      1. Respiratory stability
         a. Able to breathe deeply[18]
         b. Able to breathe deeply and cough freely[1,3]
         c. Coughs on commands or cries[13,14]
         d. Tachypnea with a good cough[18]
         e. Maintains good airway[13,14]
         f. Dyspnea or limited breathing[1,3]
         g. Dyspnea, limited breathing or tachypnea
         h. Dyspnea with a weak cough[18]
         i. Apneic[1,3]
         j. Apneic or on mechanical ventilator[1]
         k. Requires airway maintenance[13,14]

   2. Oxygen saturation
      a. Maintains value >92% on room air[12,18]
      b. Needs O_2 inhalation to maintain saturation >90%[1]
      c. Requires supplemental oxygen[18]
      d. Saturation <92% with supplemental oxygen[18]
      e. O_2 saturation <90% with supplemental oxygen[1]
   3. Color
      a. Pink[3,13]
      b. Pink and warm[15]
      c. Pale, dusky, blotchy, jaundice, others[3,13]
      d. Cyanotic[3,13,14]
B. Cardiovascular criteria—hemodynamic stability
   1. Blood pressure +/− 15%, 30%, 50%[18]
   2. Blood pressure >90 mm systolic and +/− 30 mm Hg preoperative baseline[15]
   3. Blood pressure +/− 20%, 20% to 50%, 50% preanesthetic level[3,13]
   4. Blood pressure +/− 20%, 20% to 49%, 50% preanesthetic level[1]
   5. Exception: Children who are crying[14]
C. Musculoskeletal—physical activity
   1. Able to stand up and walk straight[1]
   2. Able to move all extremities on command[18]
   3. Able to move all extremities voluntarily or on command[1,3]
   4. Active motion, voluntary or on command[13]
   5. Head lift with closed mouth for 5 seconds[15]
   6. Moving limbs purposefully[14]
   7. Vertigo when erect[1]
   8. Some weakness in movement of extremities[12]
   9. Dizziness when supine[1]
   10. Weak motion, voluntary or on command[13]
   11. Able to move two extremities on command
   12. Able to move two extremities voluntarily or on command[1,3]
   13. Nonpurposeful movements[12]; unable to move extremities voluntarily[18]
   14. Unable to move extremities voluntarily or on command[1,3]
   15. No motion[13,14]
D. Neurological: Level of consciousness
   1. Fully awake[1,3,14]
   2. Awake and oriented[18]
   3. Fully awake or easily aroused when called[13]
   4. Verbal response to spoken command[15]
   5. Arousable with minimal stimulation[18]
   6. Responding to stimuli[14]
   7. Responds to stimuli and exhibits presence of protective reflexes[13]
   8. Arousable on calling[1,3]
   9. Responsive to only tactile stimulation[18]
   10. Not responding[1,3,14]
   11. No response or absence of protective reflexes[13]
E. Temperature
   1. Core temperature at least 36° C (96.8° F)[5]
   2. Patient described feeling acceptable level of warmth.[5]
   3. No signs and symptoms of hypothermia
   4. Exception: Can be discharged to critical care with hypothermia[5]
F. Pain assessment
   1. Pain free[1]
   2. No pain or mild
   3. Moderate to severe, controlled with analgesics
   4. Mild pain handled by oral medication[1]
   5. Persistent severe pain
   6. Severe pain requiring parenteral medication[1]
   7. Comfortable with regard to pain[15]

G. Patient characteristics considered concurrently with discharge criteria prior to determining whether ready to transfer
  1. Emetic symptoms
    a. Able to drink fluids[1]
    b. None or mild nausea with no vomiting
    c. Nauseated[1]
    d. Transient vomiting or retching
    e. Nausea and vomiting[1]
    f. Persistent moderate or severe nausea and vomiting
  2. Urinary symptoms
    a. Has voided[1]
    b. Unable to void but comfortable[1]
    c. Unable to void and uncomfortable[1]
  3. Surgical site
    a. Dry and clean[1]
    b. Wet but stationary or marked[1]
    c. Growing area of wetness[1]
H. Regional anesthesia (epidural/spinal) discharge criteria
  1. Orthostatic blood pressure challenges[12]
    a. Intervals of 30 minutes
    b. Less than 10% decrease in mean arterial pressure (MAP)
  2. Sensory level
    a. Less than or equal to T10[12,13]
  3. Block has started and continuing to recede[7]
  4. Two segment regression of sensory block[7]
  5. Receding to L1 or lower[12]
I. Regional anesthesia (shoulder/ankle) discharge criteria
  1. No sensory or motor criteria required for discharge from PACU
J. Minimum mandatory stay as a discharge requirement
  1. Insufficient research literature to support minimum 1 hour stay in PACU
  2. Length of stay should be determined on case-by-case basis
K. Sources of discharge criteria rankings noted in preceding sections A-H
  1. Postanesthesia recovery score (PARS)—Aldrete (1970)[3]
  2. Steward (1975)[14]
  3. Thomas and Davis (1984)[15]
  4. Soliman et al (1988)[13]
  5. Alexander et al (1989)[4]
  6. Postanesthesia Recovery Score for Ambulatory Patients (PARSAP)—modified Aldrete (1995)[1]
  7. Marley and Moline (1996)[12]
  8. White (1999)[18]
  9. Cohen et al (1998)[7]
  10. ASPAN (2001)[5]

IV. Overview of discharge criteria scoring systems
  A. Quantitatively summarizes clinical observations and judgments
  B. Composed of discharge criteria that best reflect the patient's overall status
  C. Discharge criteria for a scoring system may be patient specific (e.g., criteria and scoring system for general anesthesia patient, criteria and scoring system for obstetrical patient, criteria and scoring system for regional anesthesia patient).
  D. Each criteria has two or more levels on which to be ranked.
    1. Point for each level of criterion attained
    2. Greater total score reflects increased patient stability and lower risk of complications upon transfer and progress toward discharge readiness
  E. Requirements for scoring systems
    1. Simple
    2. Easy to remember
    3. Applicable to all situations
    4. Able to discriminate among patients at different levels of recovery (validity)

      5. Able to be scored similarly by two different providers simultaneously (reliability)

V. Examples of discharge criteria scoring systems

  A. Aldrete (also known as PARS)

    1. Developed in 1970

    2. Five criteria rated from 0 to 2

      a. Activity

      b. Respiration

      c. Circulation

      d. Consciousness

      e. Color

    3. Maximum score of 10

    4. Scores 8 and 9 reflect discharge readiness.

    5. Scores less than 7 are dangerous.

    6. Recommended assessment every 30 minutes

    7. Research support

      a. Aldrete (1970)[3]

        (1) Studied 352 patients undergoing general anesthesia

        (2) Seventy-eight percent of patients scored 8 or greater upon PACU admission.

      b. Figueroa (1972)[9]

        (1) Studied 500 cases with 89% having general anesthesia

        (2) Fifty-six percent of patients scored under 7 upon PACU admission.

        (3) Eleven percent of patients score 10 upon PACU arrival.

        (4) Age, sex and surgical procedure did not influence scores.

      c. Holzgrafe (1972)[10]

        (1) Studied 456 patients

        (2) Twenty-four percent of patients scored 8 or greater upon PACU admission.

        (3) Circulation criteria were likely to have higher score on admission.

        (4) Level of consciousness and activity had lowest scores on admission to PACU.

      d. Soliman et al (1988)[13]

        (1) Studied 81 children undergoing general anesthesia

        (2) Used PARS with oxygen saturation criterion

        (3) No significant association with PARS score and oxygen saturation was identified.

        (4) Twelve children had PARS scores >8 with SaO_2 less than 95%.

  B. Steward[14]

    1. Proposed in 1975

    2. Three criteria rated from 0 to 2

      a. Consciousness

      b. Airway

      c. Movement

    3. Maximum score of 6

    4. Excluded color because deemed color was difficult to interpret (not objective)

    5. Excluded blood pressure because of little constant relation to recovery from general anesthesia

    6. Minimum score for discharge not addressed

    7. Research support not published

  C. Thomas and Davis[15]

    1. Proposed in 1984

    2. Five criteria rated either 0 or 1

      a. Systolic blood pressure above 90 mm Hg but not 30 mm Hg above or below the preoperative reading

      b. Pink and warm

      c. Verbal response to spoken command

      d. Head lift with closed mouth for 5 seconds

      e. Comfortable with regard to pain

   3. Minimum score of 5 is required for discharge.

   4. Research support not published

D. Modified Aldrete (also known as PARSAP)

   1. Reported in 1995 in response to trends in ambulatory surgery for ambulatory surgery patients

   2. Modified one criteria of original PARS by replacing color index with SaO_2

   3. Ten criteria rated from 0 to 2

      a. Activity

      b. Respiration

      c. Circulation

      d. Consciousness

      e. Oxygenation

      f. Dressing

      g. Pain

      h. Ambulation

      i. Fast feeding

      j. Urine output

   4. Maximum score of 20

      a. PACU phase I discharge requires minimum score of 8 to 10 on original PARS criteria.

      b. Home discharge requires minimum score of 18.

   5. Addition of five criteria to original PARS when determining discharge from Phase II

      a. Dressing appearance

      b. Pain severity

      c. Ability to ambulate

      d. Tolerance of oral fluids

      e. Ability to urinate

   6. Useful for combined PACU phase I and phase II units

   7. Research support

      a. Aldrete (1998)[2]

      b. Studied 740 adult patients

      c. Sixty-two percent of patients scored 18 and above within an hour of arrival in PACU.

E. White[18]

   1. Developed in 1999

   2. Used for fast tracking

   3. More sensitive and selective than modified Aldrete

   4. Seven criterion rated from 0 to 2

      a. Level of consciousness

      b. Physical activity

      c. Hemodynamic stability

      d. Respiratory stability

      e. Oxygen saturation status.

      f. Postoperative pain assessment

      g. Postoperative emetic symptoms

   5. Maximum score of 14

   6. Requirements for discharge to phase II

      a. Minimum score of 12

      b. All scores 1 or above

F. Cohen et al[7]

   1. Reported in 1998

   2. Proposed specific discharge criteria for obstetrical PACUs after regional anesthesia

   3. Retrospective review of 6-month data on 358 patients

   4. All patients kept 1 hour in PACU and monitored for events

5. Criteria
   a. Stable cardiorespiratory status
   b. Block has started to recede.
   c. Block is continuing to recede.
6. Research found that patients who received epidurals were discharged sooner than those who received spinals.

BIBLIOGRAPHY

1. Aldrete JA: The post anesthesia recovery score revisited. *J Clin Anesth* 7:89-91, 1995.
2. Aldrete JA: Modifications to the postanesthesia score for use in ambulatory surgery. *J PeriAnesth Nurs* 13(3):148-155, 1998.
3. Aldrete JA, Kroulik D: A postanesthetic recovery score. *Anesth Analg* 49:924-933, 1970.
4. Alexander CM, Teller LE, Gross JB, et al: New discharge criteria decrease recovery room time after subarachnoid block. *Anesthesiology* 70:649-653, 1989.
5. American Society of PeriAnesthesia Nurses: Clinical guidelines for the prevention of unplanned perioperative hypothermia. *J PeriAnesth Nurs* 16:305-314, 2001.
6. ASPAN: *2002 Standards of perianesthesia nursing practice*, Resource 7. Cherry Hill, NJ: Author, 2002.
7. Cohen SE, Hamilton CL, Riley ET, et al: Obstetric postanesthesia care unit stays. *Anesthesiology* 89:1559-1565, 1998.
8. Fetzer S: Letter to the editor: Factors used to determine discharge readiness. *J PeriAnesth Nurs* 13:337-339, 1998.
9. Figueroa M Jr: The postanesthesia recovery score: a second look. *South Med J* 65(7):791-795, 1972.
10. Holzgrafe RE: A postanesthesia recovery score. *Wisc Med J* 71:239-241, 1972.
11. Kuc JA, Pietro J: Safe discharge from the PACU and ambulatory care setting. *J Nurs Law* 6(2):7-14, 1999.
12. Marley RA, Moline BM: Patient discharge from the ambulatory setting. *J PeriAnesth Nurs* 11:39-49, 1996.
13. Soliman IE, Patel RI, Ehrenpreis MB, et al: Recovery scores do not correlate with postoperative hypoxemia in children. *Anesth Analg* 67:53-56, 1988.
14. Steward DJ: A simplified scoring system for the post-operative recovery room. *Can Anaesth Soc J* 22:111-112, 1975.
15. Thomas D, Davis AC: A post-anesthetic scoring system. *Anaesth Intensive Care* 12:125-126, 1984.
16. Wetchler BV: Postanesthesia scoring system. *AORN J* 41:362-364, 1985.
17. White PF: Criteria for fast-tracking outpatients after ambulatory surgery. *J Clin Anesth* 11:78-79, 1999.
18. White PF, Song D: New criteria for fast-tracking after outpatient anesthesia: A comparison with the modified Aldrete scoring system. *Anesth Analg* 88:1069-1072, 1999.

SURGICAL SPECIALTIES

38 Respiratory Surgery

REX A. MARLEY

OBJECTIVES

At the conclusion of this chapter the reader will be able to:

1. Describe the anatomy and physiology relevant to the care of the pulmonary surgical patient.

2. Recognize essential components of the medical history and physical assessment.

3. Describe signs and symptoms of specific pulmonary pathologic conditions.

4. Describe components of preoperative assessment in the evaluation of a patient presenting for pulmonary surgery.

5. Explain surgical procedures used in the diagnosis and treatment of the pulmonary patient.

6. Identify special intraoperative considerations in the care of the pulmonary patient.

7. State the major complications seen postoperatively in the patient undergoing thoracic surgery.

8. Describe the key nursing assessments and interventions in the immediate postoperative phase of the patient undergoing thoracic surgery.

RESPIRATORY ANATOMY AND PHYSIOLOGY

The respiratory system, consisting of the upper and lower airways, promotes the interchange of gases between the atmosphere and the bloodstream.

I. Gross anatomy of the respiratory system
   A. Nose: during nasal breathing the nose serves to humidify, filter, heat, or cool the inspired air better than oral breathing
      1. The olfactory region senses whether the inspired gas has noxious qualities.
      2. If the inspired air is sufficiently noxious, a sneeze may result in an attempt to cleanse the nose of the noxious gas.
   B. Pharynx: stems from Greek word meaning "throat"
      1. Nasopharynx: pharynx above the soft palate
         a. Lymphatic tissue, known as the pharyngeal tonsils are located here.
            (1) When these tonsils hypertrophy, they are known as adenoids.
         b. Eustachian tubes allow for equalization of air pressure between the middle ear and the atmosphere.
      2. Oropharynx: region below the nasopharynx, above the laryngopharynx and posterior to the oral cavity
         a. Palatine tonsils, located in the posterior oropharyngeal wall
            (1) Similar to the pharyngeal tonsils
            (2) Located to interact with foreign material taken into the pharynx
         b. Tongue: the posterior portion of the tongue is located in the oropharynx.
            (1) It is highly innervated which accounts for the strong gag reflex when stimulated.
      3. Laryngopharynx: airway below base of tongue to larynx
   C. Larynx: complex series of cartilages connected to bones by muscles, which serves as the distinction between the upper and lower airways
      1. Functions include
         a. Gas conduction

    b. Prevention of food entry into the lower respiratory tract

    c. Facilitation of cough and phonation

  2. Consists of

    a. Three paired cartilages

      (1) Arytenoids

      (2) Corniculate

      (3) Cuneiform

    b. Epiglottis: chief guardian of the laryngeal opening by preventing pulmonary aspiration during swallowing

    c. Vocal cords: Altering positions of the vocal cords allows for phonation and the basis for speech.

    d. Glottic opening (glottis): opening between the vocal cords upon entry into the trachea

      (1) Narrowest portion of the adult's airway when factoring endotracheal tube size

    e. Thyroid cartilage: largest of all the laryngeal cartilages, the Adam's apple is the anterior prominence of the thyroid cartilage.

    f. Cricoid cartilage: located immediately caudal to the thyroid cartilage; it is the only completely ringed cartilage surrounding the trachea.

      (1) Narrowest portion of the child's airway when factoring endotracheal tube size

    g. Cricothyroid membrane: small space separating the thyroid and cricoid cartilages anteriorly

      (1) Cricothyroidotomy, consisting of a small incision into the cricothyroid membrane

      (2) May be made via a small incision to establish an emergency airway into the trachea

D. Trachea: the lower airway starts at the trachea and includes the tracheobronchial tree and parenchyma of the lungs (Figure 38-1).

  1. Composed of 16 to 20 horseshoe-shaped cartilages with the posterior wall composed of nonstriated trachealis muscle

    a. Differences between infants and adults are illustrated in Table 38-1.

  2. Carina: bifurcation point of trachea into right and left main-stem bronchi

    a. Important marker in endotracheal tube placement

    b. Anatomic landmark is the angle of Louis.

E. Lungs

  1. Primary bronchi: right and left bifurcate from trachea at the carina.

    a. Right is slightly larger in diameter than the left.

    b. Left angles more sharply (45° to 55° from midline) toward its lung than the right (20° to 30° from midline).

    c. Most common site of pulmonary aspiration is the right lung because it is wider and makes a smaller angle.

  2. Each primary bronchus further divides at least 20 times forming

    a. Lobar, segmental, subsegmental and small bronchi

    b. Primary, secondary, terminal, and respiratory bronchioles; a gradual transition begins at the respiratory bronchioles from conduction to gas exchange

    c. Alveolar ducts

    d. Alveoli (200 to 600 million in healthy lung)

F. Thoracic cavity: cone shaped; composed of bone and cartilage to protect the vital organs

  1. Bony structures

    a. Sternum (breastbone), which is composed of three parts in the adult

      (1) Manubrium (uppermost)

      (2) Body

      (3) Xiphoid process (lower end)

    b. Ribs

    c. Clavicle

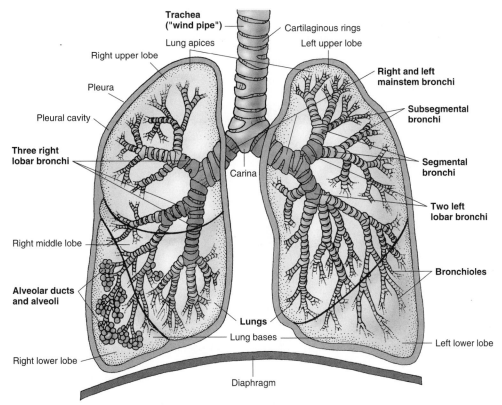

FIGURE 38-1 ■ Anatomy of lower respiratory tract. (From Ignatavicius DD, Bayne V: *Medical-surgical nursing: A nursing process approach*, 4th ed. Philadelphia: WB Saunders, 2002, p 469.)

d. Vertebrae

e. Scapulae

2. Muscles of breathing

   a. Inspiration (active phase)

   (1) Principle: diaphragm is the major muscle of inspiration, innervated by phrenic nerve from the cervical plexus (C3-C5).

   (2) Accessory: external intercostals, scalenes, sternocleidomastoids (silent during normal breathing)

   b. Expiration (normally proceeds passively to functional residual capacity; expiratory muscles become active when minute volume exceeds 40 L/minute)

   (1) Most important expiratory muscles are the abdominal.

   (a) Rectus abdominis

   (b) External and internal obliques

   (c) Transversalis

3. Pleurae: two layers that normally slide easily over each other during ventilation

   a. Visceral: lines the lungs; no sensory innervation

   b. Parietal: lines the chest wall; sensory innervation

   c. Pleural space: potential space containing thin residual film of fluid to provide lubrication for the sliding of the visceral pleura on the parietal pleura with each breath; pressure within is normally subatmospheric (-4 to -5 cm H_2O)

4. Mediastinum ("place in the middle"): located between the two lungs and contains portions or all of

   a. Aortic arch and branches

   b. Thymus

■ TABLE 38-1
■ ■ Comparative Mean Values for Normal Infant and Adult Airway Parameters

Parameter	Infant	Adult
ANATOMIC DIFFERENCES		
Narrowest portion of airway	Cricoid ring	Glottis
Epiglottis	Narrow, short, U-shaped	Broad
Tongue	Large	—
Glottis location	C3-4	C5-6
Tracheal length (mm)	57	120
Tracheal diameter (mm)	4	16
LUNG VOLUMES		
Tidal volume (V_T; ml/kg)	7	7
Anatomic dead space (V_D; ml/kg)	2-2.5	2.2
V_D/V_T ratio	0.3	0.3
Residual volume (ml/kg)	19	16
Closing volume (ml/kg)	12	7
Closing capacity (ml/kg)	35	23
Functional residual capacity (ml/kg)	27-30	34
Vital capacity (ml/kg)	35	70
Total lung capacity (ml/kg)	70	80
RESPIRATION		
Frequency (breaths/min)	30-50	12-16
Alveolar ventilation (ml/kg/min)	100-150	60
Airway resistance (cm H_2O/L/sec)	18-29	2-3
Oxygen consumption (ml/kg/min)	7-9	3

From Aker J, Marley RA, Manningham RJ: Anesthesia for pediatric patients with respiratory diseases. In Zaglaniczny K, Aker J, editors: *Clinical guide to pediatric anesthesia*. Philadelphia: WB Saunders, 1999, pp 241-264.

     c. Innominate veins
     d. Pulmonary artery and veins
     e. Vena cava
     f. Heart and pericardium
     g. Lymphatic tissue and thoracic ducts
     h. Trachea
     i. Hilum of each lung
     j. Azygos and hemizygous system
     k. Esophagus
     l. Vagus, cardiac, and phrenic nerves
    m. Sympathetic nerve chains
5. Lungs
    a. Right lung is shorter and wider than the left; right lung enjoys slightly greater ventilation than the left lung.
    b. Right lung has three lobes (upper, middle, lower), and the left has two (upper, lower).
    c. Apex of the lung extends upward into the base of the neck, about 4 cm above the midpoint of the clavicle.
    d. Base of the lungs is concave with the right lung base higher than the left.
    e. Hilum is the root portion of each lung, located medially containing
       (1) Pulmonary artery
       (2) Two pulmonary veins
       (3) Primary bronchus

                    (4) Bronchial vessels
                    (5) Lymphatics
                    (6) Lymph nodes
                    (7) Nerves
        G. Pulmonary circulation
            1. Purpose is to deliver deoxygenated blood to pulmonary capillaries where gas exchange occurs (oxygen taken on and carbon dioxide removed).
            2. Pulmonary circulation acts as reservoir for left ventricle; approximately 30% of pulmonary vessels are perfused at any given time.
            3. Low-pressure (one sixth of systemic arterial pressure), low-resistance system
                a. Arterioles perfuse each terminal bronchiole.
                b. Alveolar-capillary membrane is area for gas exchange.
                c. Bronchial circulation supplies bronchi and parenchymatous structures with oxygenated blood, main components of the anatomic shunt.
            4. Distribution of pulmonary ventilation and perfusion
                a. Distribution of blood flow affected by posture; in upright position, blood flow increases linearly from apex to base; in supine position, blood flow is greater to posterior (dependent) regions
                b. Zone I (upper): ventilation exceeds perfusion.
                c. Zone II (middle): ventilation equals perfusion.
                d. Zone III (lower): perfusion exceeds ventilation.
        H. Neural control of ventilation
            1. Respiratory center
                a. Medulla
                    (1) Inspiratory area: responsible for basic ventilatory rhythm
                    (2) Expiratory area: responsible for active expiration
                b. Pons
                    (1) Pneumotaxic center: located in upper pons; stimulates expiratory center, which turns off inspiratory area to cause inspiration to end and expiration to begin
                    (2) Apneustic center: located in lower pons; prolongs inspiration by stimulation of inspiratory area
            2. Chemical feedback mechanisms
                a. Central chemoreceptors
                    (1) Located on anterolateral surface of medulla
                    (2) Influenced by pH of cerebrospinal fluid (CSF); increase in hydrogen ion concentration stimulates ventilation to increase in depth and rate
                    (3) Responsible for normal control of ventilation
                    (4) In chronic situations of hypercapnia, chemoreceptors become less sensitive to changes in carbon dioxide levels as reflected in hydrogen ion concentration.
                b. Peripheral chemoreceptors
                    (1) Located in the aortic arch and bilaterally paired carotid bodies close to the bifurcation of the common carotid artery
                    (2) Have high metabolic rates so are sensitive to changes in oxygen supply
                    (3) A decrease in PaO_2 causes stimulation of respiratory center of the medulla, resulting in
                        (a) Increase in rate and depth of respiration
                        (b) Tachycardia
                        (c) Hypertension
                        (d) Increase in minute ventilation
                        (e) Increase in pulmonary resistance
                        (f) Increase in cardiac output
            3. Nerves
                a. Autonomic
                    (1) Parasympathetic: main neural influence over airways in normal conditions; cause smooth muscle contraction
                    (2) Sympathetic: cause smooth muscle dilation

      b. Phrenic: motor innervation for diaphragm

      c. Intercostals: motor innervation for intercostal muscles and muscles and skin of anterolateral thorax

    4. Receptors

      a. Pulmonary stretch receptors (Hering-Breuer reflex)

        (1) Located predominantly in the airways rather than in the alveoli

        (2) Stimulation causes slowing of ventilatory rate.

        (3) Minimal functional significance in healthy man

      b. Irritant receptors located between airway epithelial cells

        (1) Sensitive to foreign gases and materials

        (2) Stimulation initiates cough, bronchoconstriction, and increased respiratory rate.

      c. Juxtacapillary (J) receptors: located in alveolar walls adjacent to capillaries.

        (1) Increase respiratory rate in response to fluid or inflammation

      d. Extrapulmonary receptors

        (1) Upper airway: respond to mechanical and chemical stimuli

        (2) Joint and muscle: increase ventilation during exercise

        (3) Chest wall: probably instrumental in sensation of dyspnea

II. Components of gas exchange

  A. Ventilation: movement of gas between atmosphere and alveoli

    1. Pressure changes during ventilation

    2. Volumes (see Table 38-1)

      a. Tidal volume: volume of air inspired or expired during each respiratory cycle

      b. Minute ventilation: product of the tidal volume and respiratory frequency per minute; adult at rest approximates 6 L/minute

      c. Vital capacity: maximum volume of air that can be expelled from the lungs after the deepest possible inspiration

      d. Function residual capacity: volume of air present in the lungs after a normal expiration

      e. Alveolar ventilation: that part of ventilation that takes part in gas exchange

      f. Dead space ventilation: portion of ventilation that is not involved in gas exchange; two main components

        (1) Anatomic dead space (e.g., nose, mouth, pharynx, larynx, trachea, bronchi, bronchioles)

        (2) Alveolar dead space (e.g., ventilated but not perfused alveoli)

    3. Distribution of ventilation: dependent regions of lungs ventilate better than uppermost regions except at low lung volumes, where ventilation then becomes greater at apices of lung

    4. Work of breathing: energy required for ventilation can be divided into three components.

      a. Compliance work: work required to overcome elastic forces of lung

      b. Tissue resistance work: work required to overcome tissues of lung and thoracic cage

      c. Airway resistance work: work required to overcome resistance to air movement in and out of lungs

    5. Elastic recoil: tendency of lungs to collapse, tendency of chest wall to spring out

    6. Critical closing volume: volume of alveolar distension at which force of recoil becomes greater than force of distension; below this volume, alveolus collapses

    7. Compliance: a measurement of distensibility of chest and lung; how easily the elastic forces in the lung accept a volume of air; the volume change per unit of pressure change

      a. Conditions that increase compliance

        (1) Chronic obstructive pulmonary disease (COPD)

        (2) Aging process

    b. Conditions that decrease compliance (reduced compliance requires that patient do more muscular work to achieve same minute ventilation)

        (1) Adult respiratory distress syndrome (ARDS)

        (2) Bronchospasm

        (3) Pulmonary edema

        (4) Pulmonary fibrosis

        (5) Deformities of chest wall

        (6) Obesity, pregnancy, abdominal distension

        (7) Postoperative splinting, atelectasis, or pneumonia

  8. Resistance: pressure difference required for a unit of air flow; airway resistance can be modulated by physical, neuronal, or chemical factors; dynamic measurement of pressure flow relationship affected by both length and radius of area; major sites of resistance are medium-sized airways

    a. Conditions that can increase resistance (increased resistance requires that patient do more muscular work to achieve same minute volume)

        (1) Edema of airways

        (2) Bronchospasm

        (3) Obstruction: secretions, tumor, COPD

        (4) Endotracheal or tracheostomy tubes

B. Diffusion: movement of gas across alveolocapillary membrane

  1. Factors affecting diffusion

    a. Surface area of alveoli and capillaries available for diffusion

    b. Integrity of alveolocapillary wall, thickness of alveolocapillary membrane

    c. Hemoglobin level

    d. Difference of partial pressure of gas in alveolus versus blood

    e. Solubility of gas

  2. Disease processes that decrease diffusion

    a. Interstitial disease

    b. COPD

    c. Pulmonary edema

    d. Decrease in lung tissue: pneumonectomy

  3. Oxygen transport: oxygen is transported either dissolved or bound to hemoglobin.

    a. Dissolved: 3%

    b. Oxyhemoglobin: 97%

    c. Oxyhemoglobin dissociation curve graphically represents relationship of PaO_2 to percentage of oxygen saturation of hemoglobin.

        (1) Upper flat curve indicates a relatively unchanged hemoglobin affinity at PaO_2 levels greater than 70 mm Hg.

        (2) Steep slope of curve (less than 60 mm Hg) indicates small decreases in PaO_2 and results in massive unloading of oxygen from hemoglobin molecule

        (3) Factors favoring oxygen dissociation from hemoglobin (shift to right)

            (a) Acidosis

            (b) Hypercapnia

            (c) Hyperthermia

            (d) Increased levels of 2,3-diphosphoglycerate (2,3-DPG)

        (4) Factors that decrease oxygen dissociation (shift to left)

            (a) Alkalosis

            (b) Hypocapnia

            (c) Hypothermia

            (d) Decreased levels of 2,3-DPG

    d. Oxygen content: $CaO_2 = Hb \times 1.34 \times SaO_2 + (PaO_2 \times 0.003)$, where Hb = hemoglobin

    e. Oxygen transport: $CaO_2 \times 10 \times CO$

    f. Causes of hypoxemia

        (1) Hypoventilation

        (2) Diffusion abnormalities

        (3) Altered ventilation to perfusion ratios

        (4) Shunting

    4. Carbon dioxide transport

      a. Dissolved in plasma

      b. Carbaminohemoglobin

      c. Bicarbonate ion

C. Perfusion: movement of oxygenated blood to tissues

    1. Control of pulmonary circulation: hypoxic vasoconstriction

    2. Ventilation to perfusion ratios and abnormalities: normal ratio is 0.85.

      a. Changes in lung ventilation or pulmonary blood flow alter relationships.

      b. This results in abnormalities of gas exchange.

    3. Shunt: blood flow without alveolar ventilation

RESPIRATORY ASSESSMENT

  I. Medical history: four main objectives of the medical interview are to (1) collect information, (2) develop rapport, (3) respond to concerns, (4) educate the patient.

    A. Chief complaint and present illness

    B. Current health status

    C. Significant medical history

      1. Respiratory disease

      2. Acquired immune disease

      3. Cardiovascular disease

      4. Diabetes

      5. Renal or hepatic dysfunction

      6. Smoking history: smoking exposure is crudely derived by the number of "pack years" smoked, which is the number of years smoked multiplied by the number of packs per day smoked.

      7. Family history: for example, household exposure to tuberculosis, inherited diseases (cystic fibrosis, alpha1-antitrypsin deficiency, hereditary hemorrhagic telangiectasia, immotile cilia syndrome), familial intrinsic asthma, or passive smoke exposure

      8. Occupational or environmental exposure: for example, occupational asthma, asbestosis, silicosis, irritant inhalant injury, high-altitude pulmonary edema, berylliosis, Spanish toxic oil syndrome, occupational bronchitis, paraquat injury, acute silicosis, chronic cadmium exposure, hard metal disease, uranium mining, coke oven work

    D. Major pulmonary symptoms

      1. Cough: the most common symptom for which patients seek medical care and the second most common reason for a general medical examination

        a. Two main reasons for coughing are

          (1) To prevent pulmonary aspiration of foreign material

          (2) To clear foreign material and excessive secretions from the lower respiratory tract

        b. Acute (<3 weeks) or chronic (≥3 weeks) cough

          (1) Acute—most common causes are viral or bacterial upper respiratory tract infection (e.g., common cold, acute bacterial sinusitis, pertussis, exacerbations of chronic obstructive pulmonary disease), allergic rhinitis, and environmental irritant rhinitis.

            (a) Potentially life-threatening conditions such as asthma, congestive heart failure, pneumonia, pulmonary embolism, and pulmonary aspiration may also cause acute coughing.

          (2) Chronic—most common causes are postnasal drip syndrome secondary to rhinosinus conditions, asthma, gastroesophageal reflux disease, chronic bronchitis, or bronchiectasis.

      2. Sputum production

        a. Foul-smelling: indicative of anaerobic infection, for example, lung abscesses or necrotizing pneumonia

      b. Plentiful frothy salivalike: rare symptom of bronchoalveolar carcinoma

      c. Pink-tinged foamy: pulmonary edema

      d. Rust-colored or prune juice colored: pneumococcal pneumonia

      e. Copious purulent with intermittent blood streaking: bronchiectasis

3. Dyspnea

    a. Key areas to elicit

      (1) Persistence or variability of dyspnea

      (2) Intermittent dyspnea is probably caused by reversible events (e.g., bronchoconstriction, congestive heart failure, pleural effusion, acute pulmonary emboli, hyperventilation syndrome)

      (3) Continual or progressive dyspnea is more characteristic of chronic circumstances (e.g., COPD, interstitial fibrosis, chronic pulmonary emboli, dysfunction of the diaphragm or chest wall)

      (4) Aggravating or precipitating factors (e.g., activity, timing, position, exposures [cigarettes, allergens], eating)

      (5) Measures (e.g., positioning) or medications helpful in lessening dyspnea

    b. Physiologic conditions contributing to dyspnea

      (1) Mechanical interference with ventilation (e.g., obstruction to airflow, resistance to expansion of the lungs, or resistance to expansion of the chest wall or diaphragm)

      (2) Weakness of the respiratory pump (e.g., absolute [poliomyelitis, neuromuscular disease] or relative [hyperinflation, pleural effusion, pneumothorax])

      (3) Increased respiratory drive (e.g., hypoxemia, metabolic acidosis, or stimulation of intrapulmonary receptors)

      (4) Wasted ventilation (e.g., capillary destruction [emphysema, interstitial lung disease], large-vessel obstruction [pulmonary emboli, pulmonary vasculitis])

      (5) Psychologic dysfunction (e.g., bodily preoccupation, anxiety, depression, litigation)

4. Wheezing: Expiratory sound produced by turbulent gas flow through narrowed airways; be aware of the adage that "all that wheezes is not bronchospasm."

5. Hemoptysis: The expectoration of any blood is indicative of hemoptysis.

    a. Any newfound or substantial hemoptysis merits a complete diagnostic evaluation.

    b. The more common causes of hemoptysis include chronic bronchitis, bronchiectasis, neoplasm, and tuberculosis becoming less important.

6. Chest pain: sources, types, and most common causes include

    a. Pleuropulmonary disorders (e.g., pleuritic pain, pain of pulmonary hypertension, or tracheobronchial pain)

    b. Musculoskeletal disorders (e.g., costochondral pain, neuritis-radiculitis, shoulder-upper extremity pain, or chest wall pain)

    c. Cardiovascular disorders (e.g., myocardial ischemia, pericardial pain, or substernal and back pain)

    d. Gastrointestinal disorders (e.g., esophageal pain, or epigastric-substernal pain)

    e. Psychiatric disorders (e.g., atypical anginal pain)

    f. Others (e.g., substernal pain)

7. Voice changes or hoarseness may indicate recurrent laryngeal nerve damage or compression associated with tumor.

8. Dysphagia may indicate esophageal involvement.

9. Constitutional signs

    a. Weakness or decreased exercise tolerance

    b. Weight loss, anorexia

    c. Night sweats

    d. Fever

    10. Abnormal chest radiograph

    11. Superior vena cava syndrome: dyspnea; cough; dilation of veins on head, neck, and arms; and edema of face, arms, and upper body associated with compression of vena cava)

II. Physical examination

  A. Inspection: visual skill utilized to gather patient information during the patient interview

    1. General appearance (e.g., sex, age, size, posture)

    2. State of sensorium

    3. Temperature, turgor, moisture of skin

    4. Skin color

      a. Peripheral cyanosis

      b. Central cyanosis

    5. Nutritional status

    6. Speech

    7. Chest configuration: pectus excavatum, pectus carinatum, lordosis, kyphoscoliosis, scoliosis, ankylosing spondylitis

    8. Ventilatory effort (e.g., rate, rhythm, depth of respirations)

    9. Breathing abnormalities

      a. Tachypnea: rapid shallow breathing

      b. Kussmaul's breathing: relentless, rapid, deep breathing (air hunger)

      c. Cheyne-Stokes breathing: rhythmic waxing and waning of the depth of breathing with regularly recurring periods of apnea

      d. Biot's breathing: irregular breaths interspersed with variable periods of apnea, sometime prolonged

      e. Cough

      f. Stridor

      g. Wheezing

      h. Hoarseness

      i. Prolonged expiratory time

    10. Chest wall movement

      a. Excursion

      b. Symmetry

    11. Fingers for clubbing or nicotine stains

    12. Use of accessory muscles of ventilation

  B. Palpation: placing the palms of the hands on the chest to assess the degree of chest movement; least productive and thus not routinely performed by many

    1. Chest excursion and symmetry

    2. Tracheal position in the suprasternal notch may detect shifts of the mediastinum.

    3. Subcutaneous air

    4. Vocal fremitus: patient speaks "one, two, three" while examiner positions both palms horizontally from top to bottom on each side.

      a. Increased fremitus in areas of increased sound transmission (e.g., pneumonia)

      b. Decreased fremitus in areas of impaired sound transmission (e.g., pleural effusion)

  C. Percussion: tissue vibrations will produce different sounds with varying tissue density.

    1. Dullness: percussion note heard and felt over areas of lung consolidation or fluid accumulation

    2. Tympany: percussion note heard and felt in regions of increased air in the lung

  D. Auscultation: procedure utilized to deduce the quality and quantity of breath sounds

    1. Vesicular breath sounds: soft, low-pitched sounds heard over most of the normal chest

      a. Sound may originate in the periphery of the lung at the area of the terminal respiratory units.

   b. Inspiratory phase longer than expiratory phase (often softer or inaudible)
   2. Bronchial breath sounds: loud, high-pitched sounds usually of a "tubular" quality
      a. Normal sound if heard over the manubrium
      b. Pathologic if heard over the periphery
   3. Rales: most common abnormal sound
      a. Sound of air entry into small airways or alveoli containing fluid
      b. Usually heard during inspiration
   4. Rhonchi: low-pitched continuous sounds of increased air turbulence from an accumulation of fluid
      a. Will often clear with coughing
   5. Wheezes: High-pitched continuous sound of musical quality
      a. May be heard on inspiration and expiration
      b. Most commonly associated with a combination of bronchoconstriction and retained secretions
III. Diagnostic testing
   A. Laboratory
      1. Standard hematologic: routine laboratory screening is not cost-effective or predictive of complications.
         a. Various tests will be ordered based on the presenting symptoms and the likelihood that these symptoms will yield abnormal laboratory tests.
      2. Arterial blood gases: cornerstone in the diagnosis and management of clinical oxygenation and acid-base disturbances
      3. Cultures and serologic testing: the laboratory diagnosis of lower respiratory infection includes obtaining specimens for microbiologic examination.
   B. Radiographic techniques: play an essential role in the detection, diagnosis, and follow-up care of patients with pulmonary disease
      1. Chest radiography: provides instant and inexpensive imaging of the cardiopulmonary system and plays a primary role in screening, emergency medicine, and intensive care setting
         a. Routine examination consists of posteroanterior view and sometimes a left lateral projection with suspected chest disease.
      2. Pulmonary angiography: primarily used for the detection or exclusion of pulmonary embolism
      3. Computed tomography (CT)
         a. Has become the major imaging modality of choice for the evaluation of patients with lung carcinoma and entities such as arteriovenous fistulas, rounded atelectasis, fungus balls, mucoid impaction, and infarcts
         b. CT is useful for staging and as a guide to surgical management and in the determination of appropriate methods for surgical staging.
      4. Magnetic resonance imaging (MRI) techniques: valuable for specific problem solving of issues in the thorax, which include evaluation of mediastinal masses, superior sulcus tumors, and the thoracic aorta
         a. Advantages include multiplanar imaging, high tissue contrast, flow sensitivity, and use of gadolinium contrast agents.
      5. Positron emission tomography (PET) imaging in the thorax: emerging powerful tool that complements conventional radiologic assessment with most research focusing on tumor imaging
   C. Cardiac: certain electrocardiogram (ECG) changes might occur under various presenting pulmonary conditions.
      1. Severe asthma: sinus tachycardia, right axis deviation, clockwise rotation, partial right bundle branch block, ST-T abnormalities, P pulmonale (associated with hypercapnia and acidemia), and right ventricular strain
      2. COPD: 75% of these patients have abnormal ECGs; multifocal atrial tachycardia, right axis deviation, clockwise rotation, diminished QRS amplitude, incomplete to complete right bundle branch block.

3. Pulmonary embolism: sinus tachycardia, T-wave inversion, ST segment depression, low voltage in frontal plane, left axis deviation, ST segment elevation, right bundle branch block, and premature ventricular contractions
D. Pulmonary function tests: a multitude of tests designed to evaluate lung function; these tests may evaluate airway function, lung volumes and ventilation, diffusing capacity, or metabolic requirements

RESPIRATORY PATHOPHYSIOLOGY

I. Obstructive diseases
  A. Chronic diseases characterized by obstruction to airflow in lung parenchyma or airways; includes patients with
    1. Chronic airflow obstruction (bronchitis and emphysema)
    2. Destruction of alveolar tissue (emphysema)
    3. Potentially reversible airway disease (asthma)
    4. These diseases are seen commonly as secondary medical conditions in patients undergoing thoracic surgery.
  B. COPD: distinguished by the progressive development of airflow obstruction that is not fully reversible
    1. Primary diseases of COPD
      a. Emphysema
        (1) Condition of the lung characterized by abnormal permanent enlargement of the air spaces distal to the terminal bronchioles accompanied by destruction of their walls and without obvious fibrosis
        (2) The loss of elastic recoil allows collapse of distal, poorly supported airways leading to premature airway closure and chronic air trapping.
        (3) This leads to increased compliance and impairment of gas exchange.
        (4) Frequently found in association with chronic bronchitis
      b. Chronic bronchitis: chronic inflammation results in hypertrophy and hyperplasia of mucus-secreting glands resulting in
        (1) Increased sputum production
        (2) Narrowing of bronchioles and small bronchi by edema and mucous gland enlargement, and chronic cough
        (3) Definition: the presence of chronic productive cough for 3 or more months in each of 2 successive years in the absence of persistent cough-producing disorders (e.g., tuberculosis, neoplasm, bronchiectasis, cystic fibrosis, or chronic congestive heart failure have been ruled out)
    2. Etiology of COPD: chronic exposure to tobacco smoke is the major predisposing factor leading to the development of COPD.
    3. Clinical manifestations of COPD
      a. Chronic productive cough: most common symptom
      b. Dyspnea: reason for seeking medical attention
      c. Sputum production: mucoid but purulent during infections; greater in smokers
      d. Hemoptysis: chronic bronchitis is most common cause.
      e. Barrel-shaped chest, increased anteroposterior diameter of chest
      f. Tachypnea
      g. Prolonged expiratory time, indicative of significant obstruction when it exceeds 4 seconds
      h. Pursed lip breathing
      i. Decreased excursion
      j. Crackles (inspiratory), rhonchi (inspiratory and expiratory), and wheezing (not consistent finding)
      k. Diminished breath sounds
      l. Emaciation

   4. Laboratory findings
      a. Chest radiograph and computed tomography
         (1) Chronic bronchitis: "dirty chest" appearance, including increased bronchial wall thickness and prominent lung markings
         (2) Emphysema
            (a) Hyperlucency of the lungs secondary to arterial vascular deficiency (oligemia), attenuation of pulmonary vascular shadows
            (b) Hyperinflation: flattening of the diaphragm, increase in the width of the retrosternal air space
            (c) Bullae
      b. Pulmonary function test
         (1) Forced expiratory flow: tests, for example, FEV_1 (volume expired in the first second), FEV_1/FVC (forced vital capacity) ratio, FEF_{0-25}, PEF (peak expiratory flow) are decreased; typically minimal improvement in these tests in response to a bronchodilator
         (2) Lung volumes: total lung capacity, residual volume, and functional residual capacity are increased in emphysema; vital capacity is decreased secondary to the increased residual volume
         (3) Diffusing capacity: single-breath diffusing capacity is decreased with severe emphysema.
      c. Arterial blood gases
         (1) Early stage COPD: mild to moderate hypoxemia without hypercapnia
         (2) Late stage COPD: moderate to severe hypoxemia with hypercapnia and increased serum bicarbonate levels
   5. Complications
      a. Pneumothorax
      b. Cor pulmonale
      c. Pneumonia
      d. Sleep abnormalities
   6. Treatment
      a. Influenza and pneumococcal vaccinations
      b. Smoking cessation
      c. Improve airway clearance of secretions
      d. Chest physiotherapy
      e. Adequate hydration; diuresis if cor pulmonale present
      f. Mucolytic or expectorant medications
      g. Oxygen therapy: assess arterial blood gases for PaO_2 <55 mm Hg or hematocrit >55%; keep PaO_2 at 60-80 mm Hg.
      h. Minimize airflow obstruction with beta 2–agonists or anticholinergics (most effective in COPD).
      i. Reduce inflammation.
         (1) Corticosteroids
         (2) Antibiotics if infection present
         (3) Avoidance of smoking and other irritants
      j. Noninvasive nasal mask ventilation during acute exacerbations
      k. Lung volume reduction surgery in select emphysematous patients
      l. Emotional support
C. Asthma: a chronic disease characterized by chronic airway inflammation, airway hyperresponsiveness, and at least partially reversible airflow obstruction
   1. Etiology: see Box 38-1.
   2. Clinical manifestations: recurrent episodes of wheezing, dyspnea, chest tightness, and coughing, predominantly at nighttime or in the early morning
   3. Laboratory findings
      a. Chest radiograph: lung hyperinflation with flattened diaphragms
      b. Pulmonary function testing
         (1) Asthmatics are bronchodilator responsive, such that the airway obstruction is reversible.

■ BOX 38-1

■ **ETIOLOGIC FORMS OF ASTHMA ALLERGEN-INDUCED (IMMUNOLOGIC ASTHMA, MOST COMMON FORM OF REVERSIBLE EXPIRATORY AIRFLOW OBSTRUCTION)**

- Exercise-induced asthma
- Nocturnal asthma
- Aspirin-induced asthma (includes nonsteroidal antiinflammatory drugs; patients with asthma may be sensitive to bisulfite and food-processing and certain drugs)
- Occupational asthma (latex sensitivity in health care personnel may manifest as increasing expiratory obstruction to airflow during the normal workday in the operating room)
- Infectious asthma

From Stoelting RK, Dierdorf SF: Asthma. In *Handbook for anesthesia and co-existing disease,* ed 2, New York: Churchill Livingstone, 2002, p 151.

    (2) FEV_1 and maximum midexpiratory flow rates are diminished; during an asthmatic attack they may be <35% and <20% of normal respectively.

    (3) Periodic peak inspiratory flow measurements should be performed to evaluate the effectiveness of inhaled pharmacologic agents.

  c. Electrocardiogram: during an acute asthmatic attack, acute right heart failure and ventricular irritability may be present.

  d. Arterial blood gases

    (1) With mild asthma, PaO_2 and $PaCO_2$ typically are normal values.

    (2) With severe asthma (FEV_1 <25% of predicted), arterial hypoxemia may be present along with increasing $PaCO_2$ as the patient fatigues.

  4. Treatment

    a. Prevent and control bronchial inflammation with corticosteroids as a first line of therapy.

      (1) Cromolyn, a mast cell stabilizer, is effective in reducing inflammation and may be part of the treatment protocol.

    b. Beta 2–agonist bronchodilators are recommended for symptomatic relief of acute occurrences whenever corticosteroids are inadequate and for the prevention of exercise-induced asthma.

    c. Control of environmental factors (i.e., cigarette smoke, dust) to minimize acute exacerbations

    d. Figure 38-2 provides a therapeutic algorithm for the treatment of infrequent, frequent, and persistent asthma.

 D. Bronchiectasis: localized, irreversible dilation of proximal bronchi (>2 mm in diameter) caused primarily by chronic bacterial infections; inflammatory response may erode arteries, leading to hemoptysis

  1. Clinical manifestations

    a. Cough: chronic, productive

    b. Large quantities of purulent sputum production

    c. Hemoptysis

    d. Signs of recurrent infection

  2. Treatment

    a. Antibiotics as dictated by sputum or bronchoalveolar lavage fluid culture for aerobes, anaerobes, and mycobacteria

    b. Chest physical therapy, including chest percussion and vibration along with postural drainage

    c. Mucolytics and methods to increase mucociliary clearance

    d. Surgical resection may be considered in patients with localized disease that has not responded to medical management.

 E. Cystic fibrosis: inherited autosomal recessive disorder characterized by chronic airway obstruction and infection and by exocrine pancreatic insufficiency

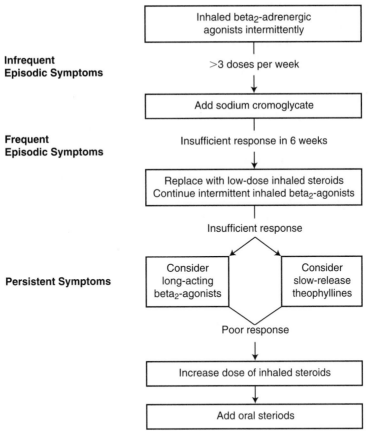

FIGURE 38-2 ■ Asthma treatment algorithm. (From Warner JO, Naspitz CK: Third international consensus statement on the management of childhood asthma. *Pediatr Pulmonol* 25:1-17, 1998.)

1. Clinical manifestations: very salty-tasting skin; persistent coughing, wheezing or pneumonia; excessive appetite but poor weight gain; and bulky stools
2. Laboratory findings
   a. The sweat test is the accepted diagnostic examination for cystic fibrosis by measuring the amount of salt in the sweat.
   b. A high salt level indicates that a person has cystic fibrosis.
3. Treatment: similar to that of bronchiectasis (infection control, airway clearance) plus the correction of organ dysfunction (pancreatic enzyme replacement) as well as bronchodilator therapy if the patient exhibits bronchial hyperreactivity

II. Restrictive diseases
   A. Pulmonary disorders resulting in impaired respiratory function characterized by decreases in total lung capacity
      1. Principally an intrinsic process that alters the elastic properties of the lungs, causing the lungs to stiffen
      2. As compared with obstructive lung diseases, in restrictive diseases the expiratory flow rates remain normal.
   B. Acute intrinsic restrictive lung disease: typically presenting clinical symptoms of pulmonary edema (i.e., intravascular fluid leakage into the lung interstitium and alveoli)
      1. Acute hypoxemic respiratory failure: arises from collapse or filling of alveoli leading to adverse consequences on gas exchange; interstitial and alveolar fluid accumulation causes an increase in lung stiffness

2. Aspiration pneumonitis: secondary to pulmonary aspiration of acidic gastric contents
3. Neurogenic pulmonary edema: develops secondary to acute brain injury; secondary massive expression of sympathetic nervous system impulses lead to widespread vasoconstriction and a shift of blood volume into the pulmonary circulation
4. Drug-induced pulmonary edema: principally heroin and cocaine, which may cause noncardiogenic pulmonary edema
5. High-altitude pulmonary edema: secondary to hypoxic pulmonary vasoconstriction and increased pulmonary vascular pressure that leads to high permeability pulmonary edema
6. Reexpansion of collapsed lung: unilateral pulmonary edema may occur in patients whose lung has been rapidly reinflated after a varied period of collapse
7. Postobstructive pulmonary edema: complication of upper airway obstruction (i.e., postextubation laryngospasm, epiglottitis) where subambient intrapleural pressures generated with inspiratory efforts against a closed glottis create increased pulmonary venous pressure and leakage of fluid and blood into the alveoli
8. Congestive heart failure

C. Chronic intrinsic restrictive lung disease: attributable to inflammatory response and diffuse scarring of alveolar walls leading to pulmonary fibrosis
   1. Sarcoidosis: systemic granulomatous disease resulting in inflammation, scarring, and occasionally hypercalcemia that interferes with organ function
   2. Hypersensitivity pneumonitis
      a. Diffuse granulomatous response to the breathing of dust containing fungi, spores, or animal or vegetable material
      b. Recurring period of hypersensitivity pneumonitis leads to pulmonary fibrosis.
   3. Eosinophilic granuloma
   4. Alveolar proteinosis: deposition of lipid-rich proteinaceous material in the alveoli
   5. Lymphangiomyomatosis
      a. Proliferation of smooth muscle in abdominal and thoracic lymphatics, veins, and bronchioles
      b. Occurs in females of reproductive age
   6. Drug-induced pulmonary fibrosis

D. Chronic extrinsic lung disease: secondary to disorders affecting the thoracic cage that interfere with lung expansion
   1. Obesity
   2. Ascites
   3. Pregnancy
   4. Deformities of the chest wall
      a. Kyphoscoliosis
      b. Ankylosing spondylitis
   5. Deformities of the sternum
   6. Chest trauma
      a. Flail chest: multiple rib fractures (typically double fractures of three or more contiguous ribs or combined sternal and rib fractures) produce a segment of the rib cage that is disconnected from the rest of the chest wall and deforms markedly with breathing (paradoxical).
      b. Pulmonary contusion: blunt injury to lung parenchyma, airways, and alveoli, which may result in ventilation and perfusion mismatches
   7. Neuromuscular disorders
      a. Spinal cord transection
      b. Guillain-Barré syndrome
      c. Myasthenia gravis
      d. Eaton-Lambert syndrome
      e. Muscular dystrophies

E. Disorders of the pleura and mediastinum
   1. Pleural thickening
   2. Pleural effusion: fluid in pleural space; may be exudative (high-protein content) or transudative (low-protein content)
      a. Etiology
         (1) Infection
         (2) Tumor
         (3) Congestive heart failure
         (4) Hepatic cirrhosis
         (5) Pancreatic abscess
      b. Signs and symptoms
         (1) Hypoxemia
         (2) Tachypnea, dyspnea
         (3) Dullness to percussion
         (4) Decreased or absent fremitus
         (5) Diminished breath sounds
      c. Treatment
         (1) Thoracentesis
         (2) Chest tube with water seal drainage
   3. Empyema: pus in pleural space; may be acute or chronic
      a. Etiology
         (1) Pneumonia
         (2) Following thoracic surgery
      b. Signs and symptoms: malaise, febrile, pleuritic pain, and leukocytosis
      c. Diagnosis: lateral chest radiograph
      d. Treatment
         (1) Appropriate antibiotic therapy based on pleural fluid cultures
         (2) Thoracentesis; consider closed or open drainage
         (3) Thoracoscopy with decortication
   4. Pneumothorax: air in pleural space as result of traumatic, iatrogenic, or spontaneous causes
      a. Etiology: trauma, surgical procedure or central venous line insertion, nerve block (i.e., intercostal, supraclavicular, interscalene), positive-pressure ventilation, spontaneous subpleural emphysematous bleb rupture
      b. Diagnosis: suggested by the clinical history and physical examination; chest radiograph and demonstrating a pleural line or chest CT
      c. Signs and symptoms: depend on the size
         (1) Dyspnea
         (2) Tachypnea
         (3) Chest pain
         (4) Increased work of breathing
         (5) Decreased fremitus
         (6) Decreased excursion
         (7) Tracheal deviation to contralateral side
         (8) Decreased or absent breath sounds
      d. Treatment
         (1) Supplemental oxygen therapy: increases rate of pleural absorption
         (2) If pneumothorax >15-20%, reexpand lung with chest tube to underwater seal drainage; Heimlich valve (one-way valve attached to pleural tube that allows exit of fluid and air but prevents entry of atmospheric air)
      e. Tension: life-threatening disorder in which air enters pleural space but cannot escape; as intrapleural volume of air increases, lungs and mediastinal structures are compressed and shifted to contralateral side, impairing respiratory and cardiac function
      f. Hemothorax: presence of blood in pleural space
         (1) Etiology: trauma, surgical procedure, neoplasm, pulmonary infarction
         (2) Treatment: depends on rate and volume of bleeding, thoracostomy and tube drainage, thoracoscopy or thoracotomy and exploration

     5. Mediastinal mass

     6. Pneumomediastinum

III. Vascular diseases

     A. Pulmonary edema: a pathologic state of abnormal accumulation of extravascular liquid in the lungs; acute pulmonary edema may be caused by increased capillary pressure (hydrostatic or cardiogenic edema) or by increased capillary permeability

          1. Signs and symptoms: dyspnea, cough, and tachypnea are early signs.

               a. Increased pressure edema: may complain of vague fatigue, mild pedal edema during the day, or exertional or paroxysmal nocturnal dyspnea.

                    (1) With severe alveolar edema, cough with frothy, pink sputum may be a presenting symptom.

               b. Increased permeability edema

                    (1) Do not have symptoms of underlying cardiac disease

                    (2) May offer history of exposure

                        (a) Toxic gases or chemicals

                        (b) Near drowning

                        (c) Drug ingestion

                        (d) Trauma

                    (3) Risk factors

                        (a) Sepsis

                        (b) Pancreatitis

                        (c) Pneumonia

                        (d) Emesis

                        (e) Seizures

                        (f) Burns

                        (g) High altitude

           2. Treatment

               a. Increased pressure edema (usually caused by cardiac failure): goal is to reduce the hydrostatic pressure.

               b. Treatment measures may include

                    (1) Upright position

                    (2) Antianxiety (morphine [also a vasodilator])

                    (3) Maintenance of satisfactory oxygenation

                        (a) Supplemental oxygen therapy

                        (b) Continuous positive airway pressure (CPAP) and positive end-expiratory pressure (PEEP)

                    (4) Decrease venous return (vasodilators).

                    (5) Improve cardiac output (positive inotropics).

                    (6) Diuresis

               c. Increased permeability edema

                    (1) Decrease edema accumulation.

                        (a) Ensure lowest possible pulmonary microvascular pressure.

                        (b) Reduce vascular volume.

                    (2) Identify infection and treat.

                    (3) Supportive therapy: administer oxygen; lung protection ventilation strategy; optimize blood pressure and cardiac output

                    (4) Avoid hypotension; avoid volume overload; avoid infection.

     B. Pulmonary embolism: an obstruction of the pulmonary artery or one of its branches; may be secondary to amniotic fluid, long bone fractures, or more commonly a result of venous thrombosis

          1. Signs and symptoms

                a. Dyspnea—acute onset

                b. Reflex bronchoconstriction

                c. Pulmonary edema

                d. Pleuritic pain

                e. Hemoptysis

                f. Rapid, shallow breathing

g. Right ventricular dysfunction: bulging neck veins; increased central venous pressure; right ventricular hypokinesis, accentuated pulmonic component of the second heart sound

h. Circulatory collapse

2. Treatment

a. Heparin: administered initially via continuous infusion to maintain activated partial thromboplastin time (APTT) between 1.5 and 2.5 times the control value

b. Inotropes (e.g., dopamine, dobutamine) to manage low cardiac output states

c. Supplemental oxygen therapy to alleviate the hypoxic pulmonary vasoconstriction

d. Endotracheal intubation and mechanical ventilation with PEEP as needed for oxygenation

e. Analgesics may be required to treat pleuritic pain.

f. Emergent pulmonary artery embolectomy with cardiopulmonary bypass for massive emboli may be required.

IV. Malignant diseases: ninety percent of cases are symptomatic and advanced when diagnosed; obstruction or compression of structures such as bronchi, blood vessels, and nerves are responsible for symptoms.

A. Symptoms include

1. Cough

2. Hoarseness

3. Hemoptysis

4. Chest pain

5. Dyspnea

B. Systemic symptoms are

1. Fatigue

2. Fever

3. Anorexia

4. Weight loss

5. Malaise

C. Lung cancer

1. Leading cause of cancer death worldwide (28% of all cancer deaths) with most patients who develop lung cancer dying of it (5-year survival <15%)

2. Cigarette smoking is the primary cause of lung cancer (90% of total deaths).

3. Squamous cell carcinoma

a. Approximately 30% of all lung cancers

b. Characteristic development in major segmental bronchi with extension to lobar and mainstem bronchus

c. Associated with the most favorable prognosis since this tumor is more amenable to resection

d. The lymph nodes should be examined, either by mediastinoscopy or by dissecting and sampling during the operation to stage the disease.

e. Lobectomy and pneumonectomy, as indicated, are recommended whenever possible.

f. Limited lung resection may be more appropriate in the patient with compromised pulmonary status.

4. Adenocarcinoma

a. Greater than 30% of all lung cancers

b. Characteristic development in peripheral parenchyma and is asymptomatic until mass becomes large; frequently metastasizes before becoming apparent

c. The lymph nodes should be examined, either by mediastinoscopy or by dissecting and sampling during the operation to stage the disease.

d. Lobectomy and pneumonectomy, as indicated, are recommended whenever possible; limited lung resection may be more appropriate in the patient with compromised pulmonary status.

    5. Large cell carcinoma
      a. Accounts for 9% of all lung carcinomas
      b. Characteristic rapid growth in lung periphery
      c. The lymph nodes should be examined, either by mediastinoscopy or by dissecting and sampling during the operation to stage the disease.
      d. Lobectomy and pneumonectomy, as indicated, are recommended whenever possible. Limited lung resection may be more appropriate in the patient with compromised pulmonary status.
    6. Small cell lung carcinoma (SCLC)
      a. Twenty percent of all lung cancers; incidence would be reduced 80% if exposure to tobacco smoke were eliminated
      b. Characteristic endobronchial lesion in chronic cigarette smokers with hilar enlargement and disseminated disease
      c. Two recognized subtypes
        (1) Pure SCLC: accounts for 90% of SCLC cases
        (2) Combined SCLC, with a mixture of any nonsmall cell type; occurs in fewer than 10% of cases
      d. Often metastases to brain, liver, bone, bone marrow, and adrenal gland at diagnosis
      e. Rarely amenable to surgical resection; early-stage solitary tumors without metastases may be treated with surgical resection
    7. Bronchial carcinoid tumor
      a. One to two percent of all invasive lung malignancies; frequently are invasive and metastasize
      b. Characteristic central tracheobronchial tree location
      c. Treatment is surgical resection. Typical carcinoid has excellent prognosis with the 5-year survival between 60% and 80%.
    8. Metastatic tumor
      a. Malignant tumors with pulmonary metastases are common and occur in 30% to 40% of patients with cancer.
      b. The majority of adults presenting with pulmonary metastases do not have curable cancers, and palliative therapy is suitable.
      c. Medical management for selected cancers may consist of chemotherapy, radiation therapy, hormonal therapy, or immunologic therapies.
      d. Surgical resection of the pulmonary metastases may be indicated if
        (1) The tumor's primary site has been controlled.
        (2) The patient's physical status is such that he or she can tolerate the surgery.
        (3) No metastases to other sites
        (4) No radiologic proof that the tumor is unresectable
  D. Pleural tumors
    1. Main primary tumors involving the pleura are malignant mesotheliomas.
    2. Asbestos exposure accounts for most cases of malignant mesothelioma.
    3. Primary attempts at curing malignant mesothelioma involve surgery (extrapleural pneumonectomy) along with chemotherapy and radiotherapy.
  E. Esophageal (see Chapter 42)
    1. Squamous cell
    2. Adenocarcinoma
  F. Mediastinal: common nonthoracic cancers that metastasize to the mediastinum include tumors arising from the skin (malignant melanoma), breast, genitourinary tract, and the head and neck.
    1. Tissue sampling techniques may include transbronchial needle aspiration, suprasternal mediastinoscopy, or anterior mediastinotomy.
    2. The majority of mediastinal tumors must be surgically removed whether they are benign or malignant.
    3. Neurogenic tumors (20% of adults; 40% of children) are mostly benign and asymptomatic in adults, but in children, most are malignant and symptomatic.

4. Thymoma: the most common mediastinal neoplasm is managed by surgical resection.
5. Germ cell tumors account for 10% to 12% of mediastinal tumors and are classified as either teratoma and teratocarcinoma, seminoma, embryonal cell carcinoma, and choriocarcinoma.
6. Lymphoma: 10% to 20% of mediastinal masses are lymphomas occurring from
   a. Hodgkin's disease
   b. Non-Hodgkin's lymphoma
   c. HIV-infected patients
   d. Anterior thoracotomy or mediastinoscopy are indicted to make the diagnosis, but surgical resection is typically not part of the therapy.

SURGICAL PROCEDURES

I. Diagnostic
   A. Bronchoscopy
      1. Indications include
         a. Visualizing the airways
         b. Assessing airway patency
         c. Removing abnormal tissue
         d. Retained secretions
         e. Mucous plugs
         f. Foreign bodies
         g. Evaluating lung lesions of unknown etiology by obtaining samples for
            (1) Culture
            (2) Cytologic study
            (3) Histologic examination
         h. Staging lung cancers
         i. Bronchoalveolar lavage
         j. Application of medication or radiopaque medium
         k. Performance of difficult intubations
      2. Complications
         a. Airway obstruction
            (1) Laryngospasm
            (2) Bronchospasm
            (3) Glottic or subglottic edema
         b. Hypoxemia
         c. Pneumothorax occurs in 5% to 10% of patients following transbronchial lung biopsies.
         d. Hemorrhage: <50 ml blood loss considered normal
         e. Local anesthetic toxicity (e.g., agitation, hypotension, seizure activity)
         f. Hemodynamic alterations (e.g., bradycardia, tachycardia, hypotension, asystole; 40% of patients experience atrial ectopy)
   B. Mediastinoscopy: a small, transverse incision just above the suprasternal notch for visualization or biopsy of tumors or lymph nodes at tracheobronchial junction, subcarina, or upper lobe bronchi
      1. Complications
         a. Hemorrhage
         b. Venous air embolism
         c. Airway, esophageal injury
            (1) Subcutaneous emphysema
            (2) Chest pain
            (3) Pneumothorax
         d. Recurrent laryngeal nerve injury; hoarseness, vocal cord paralysis
   C. Laryngoscopy: visualization and/or biopsy of oropharynx, laryngopharynx, larynx, and proximal trachea
      1. Complications: trauma to
         a. Upper lip

  b. Mucous membranes of oropharynx
  c. Teeth
  d. Eyes
  e. Rupture of esophagus
  f. Hypoxemia
  g. Laryngospasm

 D. Thoracoscopy
  1. Visualization within pleural cavity to allow diagnosis of variety of pulmonary diseases and conditions
  2. Able to perform variety of procedures
   a. Decortication of hemothorax and empyema
   b. Blebectomy and bullectomy for spontaneous or secondary pneumothorax with persistent air leak
   c. Lung volume reduction
   d. Pleurectomy and pleurodesis
   e. Biopsy and excision of mediastinal lesions
   f. Pulmonary resection for bronchogenic carcinoma
   g. Drainage of pleural effusion and pericardial effusion
   h. Sympathectomies
   i. Vagotomies
   j. Thymectomies
  3. Advantage of thoracoscopic surgery is minimization of incision pain and loss of muscle function.

 E. Percutaneous needle aspiration: used for the diagnosis of infectious and malignant diseases, often under the guidance of CT scanning or ultrasonography
  1. Complications: tension pneumothorax, endobronchial hemorrhage, air embolism

 F. Scalene node biopsy: positive biopsy indicates extramediastinal tumor involvement
  1. Complications: injury to the great vessels (internal jugular and subclavian veins), phrenic nerve, and thoracic duct (on left) or lymphatic structure (on right)

II. Therapeutic
 A. Repair of pectus excavatum (funnel chest) or carinatum (pigeon breast): principally a cosmetic procedure to improve contour and body image of the sternum and lower costal cartilages
 B. Chest wall reconstruction: removal of portions of the thoracic cage may be required, most commonly for lung cancer that has invaded the chest wall or radiation necrosis; wide skin flaps may be required to achieve adequate closure
  1. Complication: flap ischemia—assessment of tissue perfusion every hour, including color, temperature, flap turgor
 C. Thoracoplasty: removal of several ribs or portions of ribs to obliterate an existing pleural space (i.e., empyema) or to collapse a portion of diseased lung
 D. Decortication with pleurodesis: thoracoscopy is primarily performed to remove all fibrous tissue and pus from the pleural space; pleural sepsis is eliminated and the underlying lung is allowed to expand; this pleural thickening may develop secondary to empyema, blood, or fluid in pleural space
 E. Open window thoracostomy: surgical creation of an opening in the chest; involves resection of ribs to allow for drainage and irrigation of postpneumonectomy empyema; opening may be closed surgically at completion of empyema treatment
 F. Wedge resection of lung lesion: removal of a lung mass including 1 cm margins in a manner that does not remove an entire anatomic pulmonary segment
 G. Segmentectomy: excision of individual bronchoalveolar segments of a lobe of lung; can be done if peripheral lesion is present without chest wall involvement

H. Lobectomy: excision of a lobe of lung

I. Pneumonectomy: excision of either right or left lung

    1. Right pneumonectomy removes 55% of vascular bed and breathing capacity so it is tolerated less well than left pneumonectomy.

    2. Chest tube may be clamped after surgery to allow serosanguineous effusion to fill hemithorax.

        a. If bleeding suspected, chest film obtained to ascertain fluid level in chest

        b. Assess for tracheal deviation to ascertain excessive pressure in hemithorax.

    3. Dysrhythmias: may be digitalized preoperatively.

    4. Volume overload: extremely sensitive to volume administration

        a. Monitor for signs and symptoms of congestive heart failure (e.g., crackles, tachypnea, dyspnea, hypoxemia, or increased filling pressure).

    5. Phrenic nerve may be severed on operative side to elevate hemidiaphragm.

    6. Pericardium may be opened during procedure.

        a. Ascertain whether pericardial closure was performed.

        b. Check with surgeon regarding positioning restrictions.

        c. Monitor for signs of cardiac herniation (acute cardiovascular compromise).

J. Sleeve resection: removal of tracheobronchial tree and associated lung segment or lobe and reattachment of remaining lung tissue; sleeve pneumonectomy may also be performed

K. Lung volume reduction surgery: removal of emphysematous lung tissue; procedure relieves pressure and increases expansion of functional lung tissue, increases thoracic expansion and improves respiratory mechanics and gas exchange; unilateral or bilateral and usually requires multiple chest tubes

L. Lung transplant: removal of recipient lung and replacement with donor lung; most common reason for single lung transplant is end-stage emphysema

M. Thymectomy: performed via a median sternotomy; treatment of choice for myasthenia gravis

    1. Preoperative pulmonary function testing may be done.

    2. Will try to avoid or limit muscle relaxant during surgery

    3. Drugs that potentiate neuromuscular blockade are avoided.

    4. Neurologist may help to determine time to restart anticholinesterase drugs.

    5. Complications

        a. Ineffective breathing pattern

        b. Ineffective airway clearance

        c. Myasthenic, cholinergic crisis

        d. Phrenic nerve injury

        e. Bleeding: Innominate, internal mammary artery

CARE OF THE PATIENT UNDERGOING PULMONARY SURGERY

I. Preoperative preparation: the goal is to properly evaluate and optimize the patient's condition and thus decrease postanesthetic complications that may further compromise patient's status.

    A. The best evaluation of the patient's respiratory function comes from a comprehensive medical history of the patient's quality of life.

    B. Certain measures can be implemented prior to the patient's surgery in an attempt to optimize their condition (see Box 38-2).

    C. Laboratory testing may be expected to include

        1. Electrocardiogram

        2. Chest radiograph

        3. Complete blood count

        4. Prothrombin time

        5. Partial thromboplastin time

■ BOX 38-2

■ **RISK REDUCTION STRATEGIES TO DECREASE THE INCIDENCE OF POSTOPERATIVE COMPLICATIONS IN PATIENTS WITH COPD**

Preoperative
- Encourage cessation of smoking for at least 8 weeks.
- Treat evidence of expiratory airflow obstruction, e.g., bronchodilator therapy.
- Treat respiratory infection with antibiotics.
- Initiate patient education regarding lung volume expansion maneuvers.

Intraoperative
- Use minimally invasive surgical (laparoscopic) techniques when possible.
- Consider use of regional anesthesia.
- Avoid use of long-acting neuromuscular blocking drugs.
- Avoid surgical procedures >3 hours.

Postoperative
- Continue tracheal intubation and mechanical ventilation (likely after abdominal or intrathoracic surgery and a preoperative $Paco_2$ >50 mm Hg and FEV_1/FVC <0.5; maintain Pao_2 at 60-100 mm Hg and $Paco_2$ in a range that maintains the pH at 7.35-7.45).
- Institute lung-volume expansion maneuvers (voluntary deep breathing, incentive spirometry, continuous positive airway pressure).
- Chest physiotherapy
- Maximize analgesia (neuraxial opioids, intercostal nerve blocks, patient-controlled analgesia).

From Stoelting RK, Dierdoff SF: Chronic obstructive pulmonary disease. In *Handbook for anesthesia and co-existing disease,* ed 2, New York: Churchill Livingstone, 2002, p 142. Data from Smetana GW: Preoperative pulmonary evalution. *N Engl J Med* 340:937-944, 1999.

6. Electrolytes
7. Blood urea nitrogen
8. Creatinine
D. Pulmonary function tests: obtained in patients scheduled for major lung resection or if patients have severe pulmonary dysfunction.
   1. Arterial blood gases: increased postoperative risk with Pao_2 <50 mm Hg or $Paco_2$ >45 mm Hg
   2. Spirometry, including forced vital capacity (FVC), forced expiratory volume in the first second (FEV_1), and maximum breathing capacity (MBC)
      a. Increased postoperative risk with: FVC <50% of predicted, FEV_1 <50% of FVC or 2 liters, or MBC <50% of predicted or 50 L/minute
   3. Diffusion capacity: increased postoperative risk with diffusion capacity <50% of predicted
   4. Residual volume and total lung volume. increased postoperative risk with residual volume/total lung volume >50%
   5. Xenon scanning
   6. Pulmonary artery pressure with unilateral balloon occlusion (if pneumonectomy considered): increased postoperative risk if pulmonary artery pressure during unilateral occlusion >30 mm Hg
E. Premedication
   1. Sedation: given as needed to allay anxiety
      a. Diazepam, 5 mg orally in the adult, may be supplemented with incremental intravenous midazolam once the patient is under anesthesia provider care
      b. Opioids are typically avoided as they may impair ventilatory reflexes and spontaneous deep breathing.
   2. Antisialagogue: glycopyrrolate, 0.2 mg intravenously, adult, may be given to decrease oral secretions.

II. Intraoperative care
  A. Monitoring
    1. Circulatory
      a. Electrocardiogram to monitor heart rate, rhythm, and ischemia, using simultaneous leads II and V5
      b. Blood pressure cuff
      c. Arterial line, if frequent determinations of blood gases, one-lung ventilation, or serious cardiac problems are anticipated
      d. Central venous pressure, to evaluate circulatory volume and cardiac performance
      e. Pulmonary artery pressure monitoring, only when there is documented left ventricular dysfunction, severe pulmonary hypertension, or cor pulmonale
      f. Intake and output
      g. Capillary refill
    2. Respiratory
      a. Esophageal stethoscope or precordial stethoscope over the dependant lung
      b. Inspired oxygen concentration
      c. End-tidal CO_2
      d. Arterial blood gases, when indicated
      e. Airway pressure
      f. Pulse oximeter
    3. Temperature
    4. Urine output: to evaluate circulatory and renal function
    5. Neuromuscular blockade by peripheral nerve stimulator
  B. Anesthesia: general anesthesia in combination with epidural anesthesia is the preferred technique for major thoracic surgery.
    1. The thoracic epidural catheter is typically placed preoperatively.
    2. Induction of general anesthesia is usually with propofol.
    3. Maintenance is achieved with a potent volatile agent (e.g., sevoflurane or desflurane)
    4. The epidural catheter may be used for postthoracotomy pain management.
    5. Additional techniques for pain management may include
      a. Intercostal nerve block
      b. Parenteral opioids (e.g., patient-controlled analgesia)
      c. Nonsteroidal antiinflammatory agents
  C. Positioning: supine for mediastinoscopy; typically lateral decubitus for thoracotomy or thoracoscopy
    1. Circulatory effects of lateral decubitus
      a. Pooling of blood can produce decreased venous return and fall in cardiac output.
      b. Hyperabduction of the up-side arm, as might occur when the arm is suspended from the armrest, has resulted in peripheral gangrene.
      c. Extreme head rotation, especially in the elderly, may occlude the vertebral artery.
    2. Respiratory effects of lateral decubitus: mechanical interference with chest movement and thus limitation of lung expansion; most common long-term respiratory complication of lateral decubitus position is atelectasis
    3. Neurological effects of lateral decubitus: care must be exercised while positioning the patient to prevent injury to the brachial plexus and its peripheral branches, the long thoracic nerve, and nerves of the lower extremity (common peroneal nerve, sciatic nerve)
  D. One-lung ventilation: placement of a double-lumen endobronchial tube or bronchial blocker endotracheal tube is indicated for lung isolation.
    1. Absolute indications for lung isolation
      a. Isolation from spillage or contamination (e.g., infection or massive hemorrhage)

        b. Control the distribution of ventilation (e.g., bronchopleural fistula, giant unilateral lung cyst or bulla, tracheobronchial tree disruption, surgical opening of major conducting airway, unilateral bronchopulmonary lavage, pulmonary alveolar proteinosis)

    2. Relative indication for lung isolation

        a. Facilitation of surgical exposure (high priority) for thoracic aortic aneurysm, pneumonectomy, upper lobectomy, mediastinal exposure, thoracoscopy, or pulmonary resection via median sternotomy

        b. Facilitation of surgical exposure (low priority) for esophageal resection, middle and lower lobectomies and segmental resection, or procedures on the thoracic spine

    3. Special considerations

        a. Hypoxemia is a common occurrence when one-lung ventilation is employed; thus patients are ventilated with 100% oxygen during this time.

        b. If the patient cannot be extubated at the end of the surgery, the double lumen tube will be exchanged for a conventional endotracheal tube.

  E. Special intraoperative considerations

    1. Chest cavity may be filled with saline while the suture site is subjected to a sustained positive airway pressure of 30 cm H_2O to check for air leak from the site of resection. This maneuver is also beneficial for reexpanding atelectatic regions.

    2. Chest tube to water seal drainage (typically to −20 cm H_2O suction) to drain the pleural cavity and promote lung expansion

    3. Endotracheal extubation is the goal at the end of the surgery, depending on the surgery and patient condition; patient should be awake, warm, and comfortable.

III. Postoperative care

  A. Admission assessment: prior to the postanesthesia care unit (PACU) nurse accepting responsibility for the nursing care of the patient, the patient's condition will be reevaluated and a report will be given per the anesthesia care provider. The initial assessment and report will include

    1. Intraoperative vital sign trends

    2. Pertinent surgical and medical history

    3. Anesthetic medications administered

    4. Special intraoperative events

    5. Airway support measures

    6. Supplemental oxygen therapy requirements

    7. Vital signs, cardiac rhythm

    8. Pulse oximetry continually (arterial blood gases obtained as needed)

    9. Conditions of dressings, tubes

    10. Intravenous infusions and invasive monitoring

    11. Chest radiograph to verify chest tube positioning, resolution of pneumothorax, presence of hemothorax, and position of endotracheal tube or central intravenous line if present

  B. Physical assessment

    1. Inspection

        a. Airway patency and presence of artificial airways

        b. General condition

            (1) Level of consciousness

            (2) Confusion, restlessness, anxiety

                (a) Hypoxemia

                (b) Hypercapnia

                (c) Medication

                (d) Hemodynamic

        c. Respiratory rate

            (1) Tachypnea

                (a) Hypoxemia

                (b) Hypercapnia

         (c) Acidosis

         (d) Fever

         (e) Pain

      (2) Bradypnea

         (a) Hypercapnia

         (b) Residual anesthetic effect

         (c) Opioid effect

  d. Ventilatory rhythm

  e. Prolonged expiratory time?

  f. Depth: hypoventilation (with respiratory acidosis) common in early postoperative phase

  g. Chest wall movement

      (1) Decreased: hypoventilation

      (2) Asymmetric

         (a) Atelectasis

         (b) Pleural effusion

         (c) Diaphragmatic paralysis

         (d) Mainstem bronchus endotracheal intubation

         (e) Splinting

         (f) Hemothorax, pneumothorax

  h. Cyanosis: the blue color of skin and mucous membranes associated with deoxyhemoglobin

      (1) Cyanosis is not a reliable sign of hypoxemia; thus if cyanosis is present, PaO_2 should be determined.

      (2) At least 5 g% of deoxyhemoglobin must be present in the blood before cyanosis will appear; therefore

      (3) It may be marked in patients with polycythemia, yet difficult to detect in the anemic patient.

  i. Use of accessory muscles: indicative of increased work of breathing

  j. Retractions secondary to patient's effort to generate more negative pressure to improve ventilation

  k. Nasal flaring

  l. Sputum production

  m. Thoracoabdominal dyscoordination: retraction of abdomen during inspiration; indicates diaphragmatic fatigue and ventilatory failure

2. Palpation

  a. Chest expansion

  b. Trachea will deviate toward hemithorax with lowest intrathoracic pressure.

  c. Trachea deviates away from pathologic conditions: space-occupying disorders

      (1) Tension pneumothorax

      (2) Hemothorax

      (3) Pleural effusion

  d. Trachea deviates toward pathologic condition (e.g., atelectasis, phrenic nerve paralysis, pneumonia, and pneumonectomy)

  e. Subcutaneous emphysema

      (1) Palpable crackling sensation that results from air that has escaped from lungs into subcutaneous tissue.

      (2) Sources of air leak postoperatively include

         (a) Pneumothorax

         (b) Tracheostomy wound

         (c) Alveolar rupture from barotraumas

         (d) Tracheobronchial or esophageal injury

  f. Fremitus

      (1) Increased

         (a) Consolidation

         (b) Mucus in airways

(2) Decreased
    (a) Atelectasis
    (b) Pneumothorax
    (c) Pneumonectomy
    (d) COPD
    (e) Pleural effusion

3. Auscultation
  a. Absence of breath sounds, possibly from
    (1) Obstruction
      (a) Upper airway (e.g., tongue or soft tissue)
      (b) Kink in endotracheal tube
      (c) Laryngospasm
    (2) Secretions
    (3) Pneumonectomy
    (4) Pleural effusion
    (5) Pneumothorax
    (6) Mainstem endobronchial intubation
    (7) Atelectasis
  b. Diminished vesicular sounds from
    (1) Obesity
    (2) Hypoventilation
    (3) COPD
    (4) Mainstem endobronchial intubation
  c. Bronchial sounds in peripheral fields from increased tissue density (e.g., consolidation)
  d. Crackles
    (1) Atelectasis
    (2) Airway fluid
  e. Wheezes
    (1) High pitched: bronchospasm
    (2) Low pitched (rhonchus): mucus in airways
  f. Rhonchi: mucus in airways
  g. Rub
    (1) Grating or scraping sound of inflamed parietal visceral surfaces as they approximate at end inspiration
    (2) Normal sound postthoracotomy
  h. Voice sounds: amplified transmission of voice through thorax as a result of increased lung density of areas of atelectasis
    (1) Bronchophony: increased transmission of spoken words "ninety nine"
    (2) Egophony: spoken "ee" is auscultated "aa."
    (3) Whispered pectoriloquy: auscultation of whispered voice is enhanced.

C. Chest tube with closed water seal drainage
  1. Purpose
    a. Remove air and fluid from pleural space
    b. Reexpand a collapsed lung by restoring negative intrapleural pressure
  2. Components
    a. Chest tube; two tubes routinely placed; dressing changes may be required to keep tubes secured
      (1) Positioning
        (a) Apex, anterior for air removal
        (b) Base, posterior for fluid removal
      (2) Never clamp chest tubes unless
        (a) Changing drainage chamber
        (b) Assessing system leak
        (c) Evaluating readiness for chest tube removal
    b. Collection chamber: where the chest tube connects to the water-seal drainage system; maintain upright and below level of lungs

(1) Allows for collection and documentation of fluid drainage in a calibrated column

(2) Anticipate dumping of collected fluid into collection chamber with body position changes

c. Water seal chamber: acts as one-way valve and does not permit atmospheric pressure to equilibrate with the lung; air can exit but not reenter the lung; filled to 2 cm water without air leak

d. Suction chamber: provides negative pressure to facilitate removal of air or fluid

(1) Suction pressure is determined by the height of the sterile water.

(2) Wall suction should be adjusted to where a gentle bubbling is observed.

(3) Suction can be turned off with water seal intact, for ambulation, transfer, or weaning.

3. Care of patients with chest tube

a. Check for intactness of unit (i.e., all connections taped)

b. Position to facilitate drainage (i.e., no dependent loops)

c. Observe for "tidaling" or fluctuation of water seal column with respiration.

d. Monitor volume, color, and consistency of drainage. Over time, the volume of drainage should decrease, and the color of fluid should lighten.

e. Gently milk tubes as needed to maintain patency.

f. Maintain desired suction level; −20 cm H_2O is normal for adult patient.

(1) Following lung volume reduction surgery, suction may be omitted unless a >30% pneumothorax is present or if the patient demonstrates persistent hypoxemia or significant subcutaneous emphysema.

(2) Lower than normal (−10 cm H_2O) suction to the chest tubes may be applied.

g. Maintain suction so there is constant bubbling in suction chamber.

h. Assess for bubbling in water seal column, signaling air leak.

i. Assess for sudden cessation of drainage indicating clogged tube.

j. Assess for development or progression of subcutaneous emphysema indicating air leak.

POSTOPERATIVE NURSING CONCERNS

I. Oxygenation: alterations in the ability of the patient to normally oxygenate are impaired for several days following pulmonary surgery.

A. Etiology of postoperative hypoxemia

1. Alveolar hypoventilation as a result of impaired breathing or increased in dead space

2. Preexisting pulmonary dysfunction

3. Pain with splinting can make the patient prone to atelectasis.

4. Loss of lung parenchyma as a result of the surgery

5. Atelectasis

6. Decreased wall compliance secondary to surgery

7. ARDS

8. Mainstem endobronchial intubation

B. Signs and symptoms

1. Shallow, rapid respirations or normal, infrequent respirations depending upon the etiology

2. Dyspnea, increased work of breathing

3. Hypoxemia: oxyhemoglobin saturation <90%

4. Anxiety, restlessness, inattentiveness

5. Mental confusion

6. Altered mental status

7. Dimmed peripheral vision
8. Diaphoresis
9. Seizures, unconsciousness
10. Cyanosis
11. Increased cardiac output
12. Increased stroke volume
13. Hypertension—early sign
14. Hypotension—late sign
15. Tachypnea from carotid body chemoreceptor stimulation and lactic acidosis
16. Dysrhythmias
17. Tachycardia—early sign
18. Bradycardia—late sign

C. Interventions
1. Continually monitor oxyhemoglobin saturation.
    a. Adjust supplemental oxygen therapy to maintain sufficient oxyhemoglobin saturation; ABG as indicated.
2. Positioning: head of bed elevated 30° to 45° or, if needed, to an upright sitting position to facilitate diaphragmatic excursion
    a. Following pneumonectomy, the patient will be positioned supine or with the operative side in the dependent position.
    b. The nonoperative side should not be placed down in the lateral decubitus position.
3. Ensure sufficient alveolar ventilation.
    a. The residual anesthetic agents will depress ventilation and make the patient prone to hypoxemia.
    b. Judicious use of opioids and patient stimulation are effective management measures.
4. Periodic alveolar expansion and lung hyperinflation: measures designed to maintain terminal airway and alveolar patency to minimize the occurrence of microatelectasis
    a. Encourage the cooperative patient to take in a maximal breath and hold for several seconds; this can be repeated four times consecutively, then periodically while in the PACU.
    b. Incentive spirometry every hour
5. Appropriate pain management to promote effective ventilation
6. Chest physiotherapy, which incorporates postural drainage, breathing exercises, percussion, and chest compressions, is designed to improve the mobilization of secretions thus improving the matching of ventilation and perfusion; use pillow support to the appropriate rib cage location prior to coughing.
7. Nasal CPAP approximating 10 cm H_2O may be considered when derangements in oxygenation are severe yet the patient is adequately ventilating.
8. Encourage turning, coughing, and deep breathing.
9. Early ambulation as appropriate
10. Supplemental oxygen therapy can be anticipated for several days following thoracic surgery.

II. Ventilation: early extubation is goal to minimize barotrauma, which has disruptive influence on fresh suture lines, and development of bronchopleural fistula; most common causes of delayed extubation are concomitant pulmonary disease, cardiac dysfunction, multiorgan dysfunction, and hemodynamic instability.

A. Etiology: effective minute ventilation may be impacted by several factors occurring in the immediate postoperative phase.
1. Residual anesthetic effects (e.g., potent inhalational agents and opioids decrease the sensitivity of the respiratory center to carbon dioxide); residual neuromuscular relaxants will leave the patient with inadequate respiratory muscular function

    2. Epidural anesthesia with high block may impair intercostals muscle function.

    3. Preexisting pulmonary dysfunction

    4. Pain with splinting

  B. Signs and symptoms

    1. Shallow, rapid respirations (i.e., secondary to residual neuromuscular relaxants or bradypnea secondary to the effects of opioids or potent inhalational agents)

    2. Hypoventilation

    3. Hypercapnia

    4. Decreased breath sounds

  C. Interventions

    1. Assess level of consciousness, level of fatigue, work of breathing.

    2. Monitor rate, quality, and depth of respiration.

    3. Auscultate breath sounds.

    4. Pulmonary stir-up regimen

    5. Positioning: head of bed elevated 30° to 45° or, if needed, to an upright sitting position to facilitate diaphragmatic excursion

    6. Appropriate pain management to promote effective ventilation

    7. CPAP with mask-applied pressure support ventilation may be sufficient to temporarily mange the lethargic patient with respiratory acidosis in the PACU.

    8. ABG analysis to monitor and trend Pa_{CO_2}

    9. If adequate ventilation and oxygenation cannot be achieved with noninvasive measures, prepare for reintubation.

III. Pain: appropriate pain management is integral to patient care following pulmonary surgery; the degree of therapy is influenced by the patient, the surgical procedure, and preexisting conditions.

  A. Thoracic epidural analgesia: a dilute concentration of long-acting local anesthetic in conjunction with fentanyl may be continuously infused to improve postthoracotomy pain.

  B. Paravertebral or intercostal nerve blocks

    1. Usually done by the surgeon intraoperatively under direct vision

    2. May be administered as a bolus or continuous infusion with long-acting local anesthetic agents

    3. Preservation of pulmonary function and oxygenation are better following thoracotomy plus fewer side effects (e.g., nausea and vomiting, hypotension) when compared with thoracic epidural anesthesia.

  C. Intrathecal opioid: morphine when administered prior to thoracotomy has been shown to be effective in reducing postoperative pain; provides pain relief for 18 to 24 hours.

  D. Intermittent opioid administration: judicious use of opioids either intermittent intravenous or via patient controlled analgesia if required

  E. Interpleural local anesthesia: single or multiple catheters are positioned percutaneously into the pleural space, and a long-acting local anesthetic is injected; results in marginal efficacy secondary to drug dilution with blood and tissue fluid and drug evacuation with chest tube drainage.

  F. Cryoanalgesia: long-lasting (3-4 weeks) intercostal nerve block is obtained by intercostal nerve freezing with a cryoprobe.

  G. Nonsteroidal antiinflammatory drugs: ketorolac, 15 to 30 mg every 6 hours, over the first 24 to 48 hours, with supplemental opioid for breakthrough pain may be all that is required for thoracoscopy pain; used with caution in the elderly patient, patient with renal insufficiency, or patient with history of gastric bleeding

IV. Bleeding

  A. Etiology

    1. Inadequate perioperative hemostasis

    2. Postoperative coagulopathy

    3. Pulmonary artery rupture

    B. Signs and symptoms
        1. Chest tube drainage >100 ml/hour should be reported.
        2. Hypotension
        3. Decreased filling pressures
        4. Tachycardia
        5. Restlessness
        6. Decreased cardiac output
    C. Interventions
        1. Monitor chest tube output upon admission and at frequent intervals.
        2. Inspect dressing for excessive drainage.
        3. Frequent vital sign assessment
        4. Notify physician of
            a. Chest tube drainage as noted previously
            b. Sudden increase in wound or chest tube drainage
            c. Abrupt decrease in chest tube drainage
            d. Falling hematocrit

V. Cardiac dysrhythmias: occur >20%, usually supraventricular
    A. Predisposing factors
        1. Advanced age
        2. Preexisting cardiac disease
        3. Extensive resection (e.g., pneumonectomy)
        4. Intrapericardiac disease or dissection
    B. Etiology
        1. Mediastinal shifts
        2. Hypoxia, hypercapnia
        3. Vagal stimulation
        4. Atrial stretching, inflammation
        5. Alterations in pulmonary blood flow
        6. Increased sympathetic tone
        7. Acid-base disturbances
        8. Tachycardia
    C. Interventions
        1. Assess hemodynamic stability.
        2. Assess for precipitating factors.
            a. Acid-base disturbances
            b. Alteration in oxygenation and ventilation
            c. Electrolyte imbalance
            d. Adverse effect of bronchodilators
        3. Treatment
            a. Monitor and treat acid-base and electrolyte imbalances.
            b. Ensure adequate oxygenation and ventilation.
            c. Electrocardiographic evaluation
            d. Pharmacologic therapy for stable rhythms
            e. Cardioversion, pacing for unstable rhythms

VI. Cardiac herniation
    A. Etiology
        1. Displacement of heart through pericardial defect
        2. Twisting of great vessels obstructs inflow and outflow tracts of heart.
        3. May be precipitated by
            a. Change in position
            b. Coughing
            c. Positive-pressure ventilation
    B. Signs and symptoms
        1. Cardiovascular collapse
        2. Jugular venous distension, upper body cyanosis
        3. Tachycardia, myocardial ischemia
        4. Displaced point of maximum intensity
        5. Cyanosis

C. Interventions
   1. Check for positioning restrictions, especially with pneumonectomy patient or anytime that pericardium has been opened.
   2. Alert physician of precipitating factors of cardiovascular collapse.
   3. Reposition patient if turning causes symptoms.
   4. Prepare patient for emergent surgical reduction.

BIBLIOGRAPHY

1. Aker J., Marley RA, Manningham RJ: Anesthesia for pediatric patients with respiratory diseases. In Zaglaniczny K, Aker J, editors: *Clinical guide to pediatric anesthesia*. Philadelphia: WB Saunders, 1999, pp 241-264.
2. Conacher ID: Post-thoracotomy analgesia. *Anesthesiol Clin North America* 19:611-625, 2001.
3. Flick MR, Matthay MA: Pulmonary edema and acute lung injury. In Murray JF, Nadel JA, editors: *Textbook of respiratory medicine*, ed 3. Philadelphia: WB Saunders, 2000, pp 1575-1629.
4. Osann KE, Ernster VL, Mustacchi P: Epidemiology of lung cancer. In Murray JF, Nadel JA, editors: *Textbook of respiratory medicine*, ed 3. Philadelphia: WB Saunders, 2000, pp 1395-1414.
5. Slinger PD, Johnston MR: Preoperative assessment for pulmonary resection. *Anesthesiol Clin North America* 19:411-433, 2001.
6. Smetana GW: Preoperative pulmonary evaluation. *N Engl J Med* 340:937-944, 1999.
7. Stoelting RK, Dierdorf SF: Asthma. In *Anesthesia and co-existing disease*, ed 4. New York: Churchill Livingstone, 2002, pp 193-204.
8. Stoelting RK, Dierdorf SF: Chronic obstructive pulmonary disease. In *Anesthesia and co-existing disease*, ed 4. New York: Churchill Livingstone, 2002, pp 177-191.
9. Stoelting RK, Dierdorf SF: Restrictive lung disease. In *Anesthesia and co-existing disease*, ed 4. New York: Churchill Livingstone, 2002, pp 205-216.
10. Tagliavia AA, Cowan GA: Anesthesia for thoracic surgery. In Hurford WE, Bailin MT, Davison JK, et al, editors: *Clinical anesthesia procedures of the Massachusetts General Hospital*. Philadelphia: Lippincott-Raven, 1998, pp 347-368.
11. Travis WD: Pathology of lung cancer. *Clin Chest Med* 23:65-81, 2002.
12. Yao F-SF: Bronchoscopy and thoracotomy. In *Yao and Artusio's anesthesiology: Problem-oriented patient management*, ed 4. Philadelphia: Lippincott-Raven, 1998, pp 30-52.

Cardiovascular Surgery

SHERRIE L. SMARTT

OBJECTIVES
At the conclusion of this chapter the reader will be able to:

1. Explain the interrelationship of preload, afterload, contractility, and heart rate in the determination of cardiac output.
2. Describe the effects of congenital heart defects on the hemodynamics of the cardiovascular system.
3. Explain the effects of atherosclerosis on the coronary arteries.
4. Identify risk factors associated with coronary artery disease.
5. Identify complications that may result from coronary artery disease.
6. Discuss the diagnostic studies used to examine the cardiovascular system.
7. Identify psychosocial concepts that are applied to the nursing care plan for the cardiovascular surgical patient.
8. Explain the goals of preoperative teaching for the cardiovascular surgical patient.
9. Describe the preoperative assessment of the cardiovascular surgical patient.
10. Relate assessment findings to the selection of anesthetics to be used during the surgical procedure.
11. Compare the intraoperative management of the adult cardiac patient versus the pediatric cardiac patient.
12. Implement the nursing process for a postoperative cardiovascular patient in the postanesthesia care unit (PACU).
13. Identify basic cardiac dysrhythmias that may occur after cardiac surgery, and identify possible causes and treatments.
14. Identify the use of a pacemaker and management of a patient with a pacemaker in the PACU after cardiac surgery.
15. Identify the use of an intraaortic balloon pump (IABP) and management of a patient with an IABP.
16. Identify the use of a ventricular assist device (VAD) and management of a patient with VAD.

■
■■ Care of the postoperative cardiovascular patient depends on a thorough understanding of the concepts of oxygenation. The primary concern when caring for a patient in the early postoperative phase is to maximize oxygen delivery to body tissues and to minimize oxygen consumption (i.e., work load) of the heart. This requires a sound understanding of normal cardiac physiology, pathophysiology, pharmacology, and psychosocial aspects of postoperative nursing care. Although much progress has been made with respect to the care of cardiovascular surgery patients, the knowledge base and assessment skills of the nurse are the primary determinants of positive outcomes after surgery.

    I. Foundations of tissue oxygenation
        A. Effective postoperative care and positive outcomes for the cardiovascular surgical patient depend on a thorough understanding of oxygenation.
        B. Every assessment and intervention done in the immediate recovery phase (and thereafter) is focused toward optimizing tissue perfusion.
        C. Tissue perfusion is optimized by maximizing oxygen delivery (DaO_2) and minimizing oxygen consumption (VO_2)

   D. Key ingredients of oxygen delivery (Dao_2)
   1. Cardiac output (CO)
   2. Hemoglobin (HGB)
   3. Arterial oxygen saturation (Sao_2)
   E. Key ingredients of CO
   1. CO = Stroke volume (SV) × Heart rate (HR)
   2. CO is the biggest contributor (or detractor) from Dao_2.
   3. Control factors for HR
      a. Sympathetic nervous system (epinephrine): increases rate.
         (1) HR greater than 130 beats per minute (bpm) decreases diastolic filling time and myocardial perfusion.
      b. Parasympathetic nervous system (acetylcholine): decreases rate
         (1) HR less than 50 bpm may decrease cardiac output.
   4. Control factors for SV
      a. Preload: end-diastolic ventricular volume; measured by pressure; controls "stretch" of the myocardial fibers
         (1) An increase in preload stretches the myocardial fibers and improves contractility (Frank-Starling's law).
         (2) Excessive preload overstretches the fibers and results in decreased contractility.
         (3) Preload is affected by the volume returning to the ventricle and the volume leaving the ventricle.
      b. Afterload: The resistance to ejection of blood from the ventricle
         (1) Increased from
            (a) Peripheral vasoconstriction
            (b) Obstruction of flow (i.e., valvular stenosis, pulmonary embolus)
            (c) Ventricular diameter (i.e., congestive heart failure [CHF])
            (d) Blood viscosity (i.e., increased hematocrit)
         (2) Decreased from
            (a) Vasodilation
            (b) Incompetent valves
            (c) Hemodilution
      c. Contractility: inherent ability of the myocardial muscle fibers to shorten and contract
         (1) Decreased by
            (a) Hypothermia
            (b) Imbalances (i.e., hypocalcemia, hypomagnesemia, hypokalemia)
            (c) Acidosis
            (d) Cellular changes (i.e., CHF, cardiomyopathy)
 II. Congenital heart disease (CHD)
   A. Malformation of the heart or its associated blood vessels during fetal life
   1. Incidence: about 1% of live births
   2. Defects are categorized as
      a. Acyanotic: Increased pulmonary blood flow
      b. Cyanotic: Increased or decreased pulmonary blood flow
   3. Three major types
      a. Stenosis: results in obstruction to blood flow
      b. Left-to-right shunt: blood flows directly from the left side of the heart, or aorta, to the right side of the heart, or pulmonary artery, bypassing the systemic circulation (generally acyanotic).
      c. Right-to-left shunt: blood flows from the right side of the heart, or pulmonary artery, directly into the left side of the heart, or aorta, bypassing the lungs (generally cyanotic).
   4. Special considerations in CHD
      a. Surgical patient is usually pediatric with unique considerations.
      b. Effective care and positive outcomes mandate a thorough understanding of the unique physiology of each type of defect.

      c. Preoperative concerns

         (1) Preoperative teaching and preparation must be centered on the cognitive and social perception of the child's health.

         (2) It is important for the child and family to meet the staff before surgery.

         (3) Include the Child Life Specialist for assessment and teaching.

         (4) Understand the child's unique words or expressions for pain, thirst, fear, voiding, and identify the people or objects that comfort the child.

         (5) Surgical and anesthetic planning requires knowledge of the weight and body surface area, cardiac status, general health, and laboratory data, chest radiograph findings, and electrocardiogram (ECG) results (measure and weigh the child on the admitting unit's scale the night before surgery if possible).

         (6) Awareness of other significant congenital defects may influence surgical and postoperative course (e.g., hypoplastic lungs).

      d. Operative and postoperative concerns

         (1) Phases of postoperative recovery

            (a) Support of the myocardium to prevent secondary injury to the heart and other organs

            (b) Weaning of external support as the heart and other organs recover from the stress of surgery and cardiopulmonary bypass (CPB)

         (2) Body temperature (pediatric patients have a larger body surface area, and care must be taken to control heat loss) (e.g., hypothermia blanket, intravenous [IV] solution warmers)

         (3) Patients with severe CHF and little cardiac reserve require narcotic anesthetics.

         (4) Patients with severe outflow obstruction may benefit from Ketamine.

            (a) May utilize a prostaglandin E infusion to decrease pulmonary vascular vasoconstriction

         (5) Heart must be carefully purged of air to prevent embolism.

         (6) Complications include those associated with thoracotomy: bleeding, atelectasis, hemothorax, and pneumothorax.

         (7) For optimal postoperative care, personnel must have training in nursing care of the critically ill child.

  B. Left-to-right shunts

    1. Patent ductus arteriosus (PDA)—acyanotic (Figure 39-1)

      a. Definition: failure of ductus arteriosus to close during early months of life

      b. In the U.S. accounts for about 5% to 10% of all types of CHD: 1 in 1000-2000 full-term live births

      c. Signs and symptoms result from increased cardiac workload on the left side of the heart and increased pulmonary blood flow; may be decreased systemic blood flow if the PDA is large

         (1) May be asymptomatic or experience tachypnea, poor feeding and weight gain, frequent respiratory tract infections, fatigue, and diaphoresis

      d. Assessment and diagnostics

         (1) Diastolic murmur present (machinery murmur)

            (a) Best heard over pulmonic area (left second intercostal space close to sternum)

         (2) Arterial blood gas analysis (ABG) and mixed venous oxygen saturation (SVo_2)

         (3) Echocardiography

         (4) Pulmonary catheterization

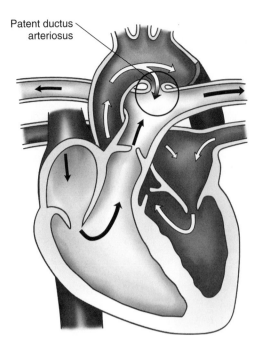

Patent ductus arteriosus

FIGURE 39-1 ■ Patent ductus arteriosus: Acyanotic. (From Kenner C, Lott JW: *Comprehensive neonatal nursing: a physiologic perspective*, 3rd ed. St. Louis: WB Saunders, 2003.)

  e. Effects on hemodynamics
    (1) Backward flow of blood from aorta (high pressure) to pulmonary artery (low pressure) through open ductus arteriosus
    (2) High pulmonary pressures caused by pulmonary congestion lead to increased right ventricular afterload, resulting in right ventricular hypertrophy.
    (3) Left ventricular hypertrophy results from increased pumping requirements of the left ventricle (two or more times cardiac output).
  f. Corrective surgical procedures: ligation or ligation and division of ductus arteriosus
 2. Ventricular septal defect (VSD)—acyanotic (Figure 39-2)
  a. Accounts for about 25% of CHD: Most common congenital cardiac lesion; often accompanied by other cardiac defects
  b. Definition: Hole in the ventricular septum (may vary in size)
  c. Type is based on location.
    (1) Conoventricular
    (2) Atrioventricular (AV) canal type
    (3) Muscular
  d. Signs and symptoms (same as PDA—infants; are asymptotic until 4 to 12 weeks when the pulmonary vascular resistance [PVR] begins to fall)
  e. Assessment
    (1) Physical
      (a) Right ventricular hypertrophy
      (b) Systolic murmur of VSD shunt
      (c) Presternal thrill
    (2) Chest film
      (a) Right ventricle (RV) hypertrophy
      (b) Pulmonary artery enlargement
      (c) Left atrial and left ventricular (LV) enlargement

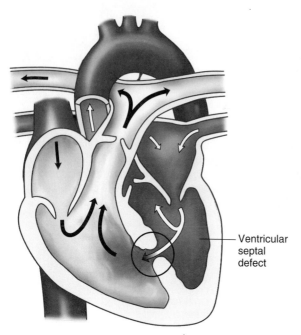

FIGURE 39-2 ■ Ventricular septal defect: Acyanotic. (From Kenner C, Lott JW: *Comprehensive neonatal nursing: a physiologic perspective*, 3rd ed. St. Louis: WB Saunders, 2003.)

Ventricular septal defect

   (3) Diagnostic assessment
       (a) Echocardiography (color Doppler)
       (b) Cardiac catheterization
       (c) ABG and SVo_2 analysis
   f. Effects on hemodynamics (depends on size of defect)
       (1) Blood flow from left to right ventricle
       (2) Increase in RV volume (increased preload) and pressure results in hypertrophy.
       (3) May develop aortic insufficiency (2% to 7%)
   g. Corrective surgical procedure
       (1) Timing is based on the location, symptoms, and the incidence of spontaneous closing (generally in the first year of life).
       (2) Antibiotic prophylaxis indicated for all VSDs
       (3) Patch closure of defect: Requires a median sternotomy, CPB, and hypothermia
       (4) Pulmonary artery banding: Palliative
3. Atrial septal defect (ASD) (Figure 39-3)
   a. Three to four percent of congenital heart defects
   b. Definition: communicating hole between the left and right atria, which results in blood flow from the left to right atrium
   c. Defects classified by location
       (1) Partial or incomplete (ostium primum ASD): two AV valves with a cleft in the mitral
       (2) Intermediate or transitional (ostium secundum ASD): AV valve configuration is between two AV valves and a common AV valve; ASD and no significant VSD (most common)
       (3) Complete (sinus venosus ASD): marked by a single common AV valve orifice as well as an ASD and VSD (least common)
   d. Signs and symptoms
       (1) Usually asymptomatic
       (2) Surgery done to prevent development of pulmonary hypertension that could lead to RV failure

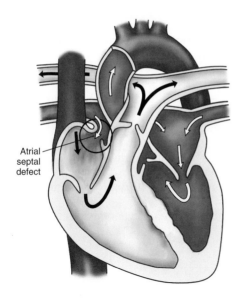

Atrial
septal
defect

FIGURE 39-3 ■ Atrial septal defect: Acyanotic. (From Kenner C, Lott JW: *Comprehensive neonatal nursing: a physiologic perspective*, 3rd ed. St. Louis: WB Saunders, 2003.)

    e. Assessment and diagnostics
      (1) Cardiac catheterization: demonstrates increased oxygen content in right atrium
      (2) Chest film: RV enlargement and prominent main pulmonary artery
    f. Effects on hemodynamics: increased RV volume (preload)
    g. Corrective surgical procedure: suture or patch closure of defect
      (1) Asymptomatic: Older than 3 months to early childhood but before pulmonary vascular disease develops
      (2) Symptomatic: Preferably 3-4 months of age
      (3) Requires median sternotomy and usually CPB
      (4) Complications: Dysrhythmias—heart block and sick sinus syndrome (usually transient)—and CHF (2%)
C. Right-to-left shunts
  1. Tetralogy of Fallot—cyanotic with decreased pulmonary blood flow (Figure 39-4)
    a. Eight to ten percent of CHD
    b. Definition: Composed of four anatomic defects
      (1) VSD
      (2) Aorta overriding VSD
      (3) RV outflow obstruction: pulmonary stenosis
      (4) RV hypertrophy (develops secondary to pulmonary stenosis)
    c. Presence of cyanosis depends on degree of RV obstruction and shunting caused by obstruction.
    d. If cyanosis is present, systemic and venous blood are mixing with pulmonary venous blood.
      (1) *It is imperative to eliminate any air in IV tubing as it may proceed to the cerebral circulation and result in stroke.*
    e. Corrective surgical procedure
      (1) Asymptomatic scheduled at 2-4 months of age and sooner for symptomatic
      (2) Requires CPB
      (3) Aortopulmonary shunt for palliation
      (4) Patch closure of VSD
      (5) Right ventricular outflow reconstruction

  (6) Complications include narrow complex tachycardia, varying degrees of heart block, residual ventricular septal defect, low cardiac output, residual ventricular outflow obstruction, and branch pulmonary artery stenosis.

  (7) Mortality for uncomplicated repair: 2% to 5%

 2. Complete transposition of great vessels—cyanotic mixing lesion (Figure 39-5)

  a. Five to seven percent of CHD

  b. Definition: Aorta arises from right ventricle and pulmonary artery arises from left ventricle.

  c. Forty-five percent have a co-existing VSD. Without mixing of oxygenated and venous blood, the patient will die.

  d. Produces chronic arterial desaturation, compensatory polycythemia, and cyanosis

  e. Diagnosis is frequently made by ruling out other cyanotic defects.

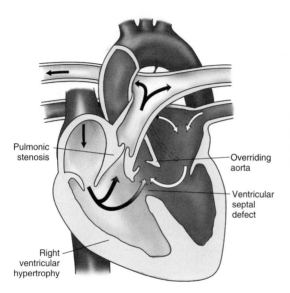

FIGURE 39-4 ■ Tetralogy of Fallot. (From Kenner C, Lott JW: *Comprehensive neonatal nursing: a physiologic perspective*, 3rd ed. St. Louis: WB Saunders, 2003.)

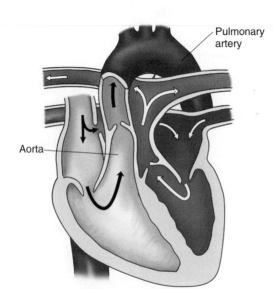

FIGURE 39-5 ■ Transposition of the great vessels: Cyanotic. (From Kenner C, Lott JW: *Comprehensive neonatal nursing: a physiologic perspective*, 3rd ed. St. Louis: WB Saunders, 2003.)

    f. Corrective surgical procedure
      (1) Balloon atrial septectomy for palliation
      (2) Arterial switch procedure: Places the pulmonary artery and aorta in their proper anatomic positions over the right and left ventricles
        (a) Requires CPB
        (b) Reimplantation of the coronary arteries is a critical component.
      (3) Mortality for arterial switch with uncomplicated lesions: 5% to 10%.
      (4) Complications: low cardiac output related to poor LV function and dysrhythmias related to decreased coronary artery perfusion and myocardial ischemia

  3. Total anomalous pulmonary venous return—cyanotic (Figure 39-6)
    a. Definition (1% of CHD)
      (1) No pulmonary veins enter the left atrium (pulmonary veins join the systemic venous circulation and mixed venous blood returns to the heart).
      (2) Anomalous common pulmonary venous channel formed
      (3) ASD (one half have a PDA or patent foramen ovale)
    b. Signs and symptoms
      (1) One half are cyanotic in the first month.
      (2) Two thirds exhibit CHF by 3 months.
      (3) Ninety percent have CHF and cyanosis by first year.
    c. Corrective surgical procedure
      (1) Anastomosis of collecting vein and enlargement of left atrium—requires median sternotomy, CPB, and profound hypothermia (20° C; 68° F)
      (2) Requires vigorous management of CHF and endocarditis (perioperative mortality is 90%)

D. Obstruction to blood flow—cyanotic
  1. Valvular pulmonic stenosis (Figure 39-7)
    a. Ten percent of CHD
    b. Definition: Thickening of valve with fusion of leaflets at their commissure, resulting in narrowing pulmonary outflow tract and poststenotic dilation of the pulmonary artery

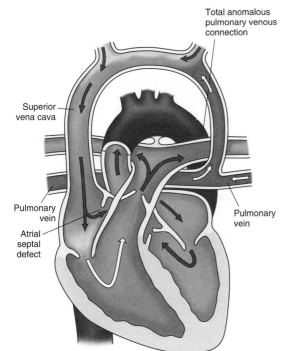

FIGURE 39-6 ■ Anomalous pulmonary venous return: Cyanotic. (From Kenner C, Lott JW: *Comprehensive neonatal nursing: a physiologic perspective*, 3rd ed. St. Louis: WB Saunders, 2003.)

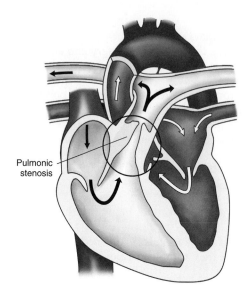

Pulmonic
stenosis

FIGURE 39-7 ■ Pulmonic stenosis: Cyanotic. (From Kenner C, Lott JW: *Comprehensive neonatal nursing: a physiologic perspective*, 3rd ed. St. Louis: WB Saunders, 2003.)

    c. VSD or ASD may also be present.
    d. Assessment: Cardiac catheterization defines the level of obstruction and identifies other lesions.
    e. Effects on hemodynamics: increased RV afterload and RV hypertrophy
        (1) Increased pressure gradient between the RV and pulmonary artery (PA)
           (a) Mild: 25-49 mm Hg
           (b) Moderate: 50-70 mm Hg
           (c) Severe: ≥80 mm Hg
    f. Corrective surgical procedure: pulmonary valvotomy—requires CPB
2. Valvular aortic stenosis (Figure 39-8)
    a. Five to ten percent of CHD
    b. Definition: thickened aortic valve, which is generally bicuspid instead of tricuspid, resulting in narrowing of aortic outflow
    c. May be present with PDA, coarctation of aorta, or both
    d. Physical assessment
        (1) Different blood pressure between two arms
        (2) Systolic thrill
        (3) Systolic ejection murmur
        (4) Tachypnea
        (5) Tachycardia
        (6) Cyanosis with severe stenosis
    e. Effects on hemodynamics: Increase in LV volume (preload) and pressure (afterload), results in hypertrophy
    f. Corrective surgical procedure: aortic valvotomy—requires CPB
3. Coarctation of aorta (Figure 39-9)
    a. Five to ten percent of CHD with male to female ratio of 2:1
    b. Definition: Localized narrowing of aortic lumen (usually at ligamentum arteriosum), two types are
        (1) Preductal (infantile): upper body supplied by LV and lower body supplied by RV through ductus arteriosus
        (2) Postductal (adult): LV supplies upper body and collaterals develop in utero through intercostal and internal mammary arteries to supply lower body.

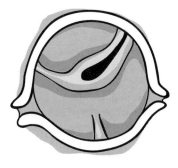

Bicuspid valve

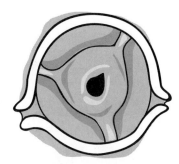

Conical valve

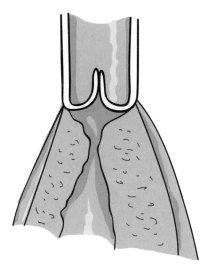

Diffuse hypertrophic
sub aortic stenosis

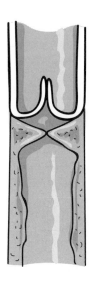

Sub aortic
stenosis

FIGURE 39-8 ■ Aortic stenosis: Cyanotic. (From Sanderson RG: Congenital heart disease. In Sanderson RG, Kurth CL, editors: *The cardiac patient: A comprehensive approach,* ed 2. Philadelphia: WB Saunders, 1983, p 33.)

    c. May present with PDA, valvular aortic stenosis, VSD, and other left-sided lesions

    d. Physical assessment

      (1) Classic finding

        (a) Disparity in impulses and blood pressures between the upper and lower extremities

      (2) Right upper extremity is the preferred location for blood pressure checks for accuracy.

      (3) Preductal coarctation: CHF (may occur early in infancy), cyanosis, diminished pulses in lower body

      (4) Postductal coarctation: Acyanotic, upper extremity hypertension, diminished pulses in lower body, midsystolic ejection murmur, leg pain with exercise, fatigability, and headaches

    e. Effects on hemodynamics

      (1) Increased LV afterload from obstruction to flow and increased arteriolar resistance

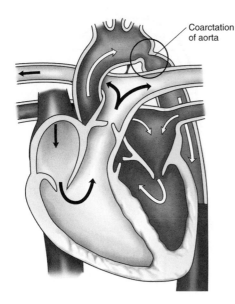

Coarctation
of aorta

FIGURE 39-9 ■ Coarctation of the aorta: Cyanotic. (From Kenner C, Lott JW: *Comprehensive neonatal nursing: a physiologic perspective*, 3rd ed. St. Louis: WB Saunders, 2003.)

      f. Corrective surgical procedure
          (1) Patch angioplasty or resection with end-to-end anastomosis
  E. Generalized signs and symptoms of CHD
    1. Cyanosis, results from
      a. Shunting of unoxygenated blood into the left side of the heart: right-to-left shunt (i.e., Tetralogy of Fallot)
      b. Poor oxygen uptake: CHF, pulmonary edema
    2. Tachypnea
      a. Physiologic chemical compensation to low oxygen content in blood
      b. Precipitated by mild exercise
    3. Effort intolerance
      a. Inability of infant to tolerate feedings; respiratory distress
      b. Fatigue with activity, inability to keep up with other children
    4. Failure to thrive
      a. Usually indicates left-to-right shunt or CHF
      b. Growth retardation, inability to gain weight
    5. Miscellaneous findings
      a. Frequent upper respiratory infections with ASD or PDA
      b. Headaches and leg pains with activity; coarctation of aorta
      c. Chest pain on exertion, fainting; aortic stenosis
      d. Clubbing of fingers, hypoxic episodes: Tetralogy of Fallot
III. Coronary artery disease (CAD)
  A. Definition: Progressive narrowing or total occlusion of the arterial lumen characterized by accumulation of lipids, fibrous tissue, and calcium deposits in the arterial wall
  B. Angina pectoris
    1. The sensory response (chest pain) to a transient lack of oxygen in the myocardium
    2. A symptom of CAD, not a disease
    3. Exhibited late in the disease process
    4. Results from an imbalance between oxygen supply and oxygen demand to myocardium
      a. Factors increasing demand
          (1) Increased afterload (i.e., hypertension)

(2) Increased preload (i.e., sodium and water retention)

(3) Dysrhythmias (i.e., tachydysrhythmias)

(4) Increased contractility

(5) Increased metabolism (i.e., fever, pain)

    (a) Factors decreasing oxygen supply

        (i) Hypotension

        (ii) Decreased afterload (i.e., peripheral vasodilation)

        (iii) Increased LV preload (i.e., CHF) (increases resistance to coronary artery filling)

5. Stress of surgery and postoperative pain are two of many precipitants of angina.

6. Characteristics

    a. Typically lasts 1 to 5 minutes and subsides when precipitating factor is removed

    b. May be described as heaviness in chest, squeezing, burning, aching, or tightness

    c. Location is usually precordial, middle or lower sternum; may radiate to jaw, neck, shoulder, arm or hand, usually on left side

    d. May be accompanied by dyspnea, diaphoresis, nausea, vomiting, and general fatigue

    e. Usually subsides with rest or is relieved with nitroglycerin within 30 to 90 seconds

7. Classification

    a. Stable

        (1) Predictable in onset, duration, location, radiation, and quality of pain

        (2) Typically subsides with rest

    b. Unstable (preinfarction)

        (1) Unpredictable with increased frequency

        (2) May require nitrates for relief

        (3) May signify impending infarction

    c. Vasospastic (Prinzmetal's)

        (1) Results from coronary artery spasm

        (2) Anginal pain at rest that is cyclic and unrelated to exertion

        (3) Pain may persist for longer duration and is difficult to relieve.

8. Diagnostic assessment

    a. Electrocardiogram (ECG)

    b. Treadmill or nonexercise (drug-induced) stress test (may include echocardiogram)

    c. Coronary catheterization

9. Noninvasive management

    a. Identify and reduce modifiable risk factors (e.g., diet, smoking, obesity).

    b. Decrease myocardial oxygen demand.

        (1) Preload reduction (i.e., diuretics)

        (2) Afterload reduction (i.e., antihypertensives)

        (3) Reduction of contractility (i.e., beta-blockers) (in the absence of CHF) and angiotensin-converting enzyme (ACE) inhibitors

    c. Improve coronary blood flow (i.e., nitrates and anticoagulation)

10. Invasive management

    a. Interventional cardiology

        (1) Percutaneous coronary transluminal angioplasty (PCTA)

        (2) Laser angioplasty

        (3) Stent placement

        (4) Atherectomy

    b. Surgical management

        (1) Coronary artery bypass grafting (CABG)

IV. Myocardial infarction (MI)

    A. Definition: Sustained myocardial ischemia resulting in death of myocardial tissue from sustained oxygen deprivation

    B. Causes

        1. Atherosclerosis of the coronary arteries (most common cause)

            a. Atherosclerotic lesions occlude the vessel lumen and restrict flow under resting conditions while making the vessel stiff and unable to dilate.

        2. Coronary artery thrombosis

            a. Thought to be present in almost all acute occlusions

        3. Plaque fissure or hemorrhage

            a. Considered a predisposing factor, this initiates the platelet aggregation, clotting cascade, and inflammatory response to injury.

        4. Coronary artery spasm

        5. Imbalance of myocardial oxygen demand versus supply (i.e., cocaine abuse, anemia, thyrotoxicosis)

            a. *Regardless of cause, the result is decreased driving pressure beyond the site of the lesion and less oxygenated blood available to the myocardial cells perfused by that vessel.*

    C. Description

        1. Location is described by the affected wall of the heart (i.e., inferior).

        2. Necrosis may extend through the full myocardial wall (transmural) or affect only the heart's inner lining (subendocardial or non-Q-wave MI).

        3. Signs and symptoms

            a. Chest pain is generally described as more severe (crushing) in quality than anginal pain and unrelieved after 20 to 30 minutes from either nitrates or rest.

            b. Pain may be accompanied by symptoms of nausea and vomiting, diaphoresis, intense anxiety, apprehension, and a feeling of doom.

            c. Some patients do not experience chest pain (e.g., diabetics and elderly may exhibit associated symptoms such as fatigue or syncope).

    D. Assessment

        1. Physical

            a. Inspection may include any of the previously mentioned symptoms (e.g., dyspnea, diaphoresis).

            b. Palpation may reveal a thrill over valvular areas, chest wall heaves, and a shift of the point of maximal impulse (PMI).

            c. Auscultation may reveal crackles, gallop rhythms, murmurs, and precordial friction rubs.

        2. ECG should be obtained within 10 minutes from onset of symptoms.

            a. ST segment depression and T-wave inversion indicate possible ischemia and unstable angina.

            b. ST segment elevation indicates pattern of injury.

            c. Q-wave appearance (more than 0.03 second width) indicates pattern of necrosis and is a definitive diagnosis of infarction.

        3. Laboratory findings (see Chapter 32 for discussion on laboratory assessment for the cardiac patient).

            a. Elevations in cardiac markers (i.e., creatine kinase MB isoenzyme [CK-MB] and troponin-I)

        4. Effects on hemodynamics

            a. Hemodynamic effects are a direct result of decreased pumping ability of the ventricle, which results in a backup of pressure and volume from the affected ventricle and decreased forward flow of blood

            b. Severe LV dysfunction results in cardiogenic shock and pulmonary edema.

            c. Severe RV dysfunction results in LV dysfunction (from decreased volume to the LV) and systemic congestion.

            d. Dysrhythmia is the number one complication and cause of death.

                (1) Other complications requiring surgical intervention include papillary muscle rupture, septal defect, and ventricular aneurysm.

E. Treatment
   1. The goal of treatment is to revascularize the ischemic myocardium and limit the size of the MI while supporting the patient and attempting to prevent complications.
   2. Treatment is categorized between ST elevation and new or presumed new left bundle branch block and ST depression or T-wave inversion.
      a. Revascularization
         (1) Fibrinolytics
         (2) Antithrombin agents
         (3) Antiplatelet agents
            (a) Aspirin
            (b) Glycoprotein (GP) IIb/IIIa inhibitors
         (4) Percutaneous coronary interventions (PCI)
            (a) PTCA
            (b) Coronary stents
         (5) CABG
      b. Inotropic support
         (1) Drugs (i.e., dobutamine, dopamine, digoxin, epinephrine, norepinephrine)
         (2) Mechanical
            (a) Intraaortic balloon pump (IABP)
            (b) Ventricular assist device (VAD)
      c. Pain control
         (1) Nitrates and morphine
      d. Prevention and treatment of symptoms depends on the manifestations but may include diuretics, antidysrhythmic agents, magnesium sulfate, beta-blockers, calcium channel blockers and ACE inhibitors.
V. Valvular heart disease
   A. Rheumatic heart disease (RHD)
      1. Characterized by scarring and deformity of heart valves resulting from rheumatic fever
      2. Rheumatic fever is a diffuse inflammatory disease affecting joints, heart, skin, and the nervous system.
         a. It is probably the result of an autoimmune process induced by streptococcal antigens.
      3. Valves commonly involved
         a. Mitral and aortic (most common)
         b. Tricuspid
         c. Pulmonary (rare)
      4. The extent of the cardiac disease depends on several factors.
         a. Duration and severity of inflammation
         b. Location of the valvular insufficiency and/or stenosis and the severity of hemodynamic effect
         c. Frequent recurrences of carditis
         d. Degree of valvular and myocardial scarring after resolution of the inflammation
         e. Presence of valvular disease unrelated to the underlying rheumatic inflammation
      5. Signs and symptoms
         a. Will depend on the degree of disease and the valve affected
      6. Diagnostic evaluation
         a. Echocardiography
         b. Cardiac catheterization
      7. Effects on hemodynamics
         a. Dependent on amount of regurgitation or stenosis and which valve(s) are affected
      8. Treatment
         a. Antibiotic therapy: penicillin (vancomycin if allergy to penicillin)

      b. Antiinflammatory agents: salicylates, corticosteroids

      c. Prevention of recurrence of streptococcal infections with prophylactic penicillin

      d. Valve surgery indicated if significant hemodynamic effects

B. Special considerations for valve replacement

  1. Categories

    a. Mechanical (i.e., ball-and-cage [Starr-Edwards®], tilting disc [Bjork-Shiley®, Lillehei-Caster®, Medtronic Hall®], and the central flow disc [St. Jude®])

      (1) Suitable for larger orifices (i.e., aortic and mitral)

      (2) Durable, but thrombogenic and require long-term anticoagulation

      (3) Suitable for patients with a life expectancy >10 years

      (4) Unsuitable for patients with a questionable ability for compliance with anticoagulation, liver dysfunction, or a stated desire to bear children

    b. Bioprosthetic

      (1) Porcine or bovine

      (2) Low risk of thromboembolic complications without coagulation

      (3) Low durability—8 to 10 years

      (4) Human allografts (homografts)

        (a) Removed and prepared from cadavers

        (b) Stored in a cryopreservation process

        (c) Technically difficult to implant

        (d) Contraindicated with history of an adverse immunological response to human allogenic tissue

        (e) Does not require anticoagulation

C. Nonrheumatic causes of valvular disease

  1. Atherosclerotic heart disease

  2. Congenital abnormalities

  3. Cardiothoracic trauma

  4. Calcification caused by aging

  5. Systemic infections

  6. Tumors

  7. Syphilis

  8. Marfan's syndrome

D. Pathophysiology of valvular disease

  1. Stenosis: narrowing of the valve orifice; obstructs blood flow

  2. Insufficiency: incompetent valve that results in regurgitation through the valve orifice

  3. Mixed lesion: stenosis and insufficiency

E. Specific valvular abnormalities

  1. Mitral stenosis (MS) (Figure 39-10)

    a. Principal cause is rheumatic fever.

    b. Most common valvular defect, especially in women in their third decades

    c. Pathologic findings

      (1) Progressive narrowing of the mitral valve (MV) from 4-6 cm to 1.5 cm

      (2) Fusion of commissures

      (3) Scarring of anterior and posterior leaflets' free margins

      (4) Shortening, fusion, and nodularity of chordae tendineae

    d. Signs and symptoms

      (1) Most common: dyspnea, fatigue, palpitations, cough, and hemoptysis

      (2) Less common: dysphasia, hoarseness, chest pain, embolic events, seizure, and cerebrovascular accident

      (3) Atrial fibrillation

        (a) Occurs in 40% to 50% of patients with MS

        (b) May decrease CO by as much as 15% to 20% and increases likelihood of clot formation caused by incomplete emptying of the atria

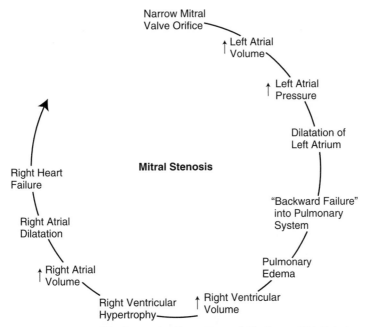

Narrow Mitral
Valve Orifice

↑ Left Atrial
Volume

↑ Left Atrial
Pressure

Dilatation of
Left Atrium

Mitral Stenosis

"Backward Failure"
into Pulmonary
System

Right Heart
Failure

Right Atrial
Dilatation

Pulmonary
Edema

↑ Right Atrial
Volume

Right Ventricular
Hypertrophy

↑ Right Ventricular
Volume

FIGURE 39-10 ■ Mitral stenosis. (From Abranczk EL, Brown MM: Valvular heart disease. In Kinney MR, Packa DR, Andreoli KG, et al, editors: *Comprehensive cardiac care,* ed 7 Philadelphia: Mosby, 1991, p 335.)

   (4) Thromboembolism: 80% of patients who develop systemic emboli are in atrial fibrillation
   (5) Murmur is early diastolic to middiastolic; low-pitched, rumbling sound heard best at the apex.
 e. Diagnostic studies
   (1) ECG (wide, notched P waves)
   (2) Echocardiogram
      (a) Most useful
      (b) Valve appears thick and shows diminished motion and posterior leaflet movement.
   (3) Cardiac catheterization (obtains valvular gradient data)
 f. Effects on hemodynamics
   (1) Increased left atrial (LA) pressures and volumes resulting in atrial strain and dysrhythmias
   (2) Progresses to low CO states, increased pulmonary artery pressures (PAP), and increased pulmonary artery occlusion (wedge) pressures (PAOP, PCWP)
 g. Treatment
   (1) Noninvasive: sodium restriction, diuretics, antidysrhythmics, anticoagulation
   (2) Surgical intervention
      (a) Indicated when the patient develops symptoms of atrial fibrillation, pulmonary edema, pulmonary hypertension, orthopnea, and fatigue
      (b) Commissurotomy: performed if valve is only stenotic with fusion of uncalcified commissures, chordae tendineae are not severely deformed, leaflets are mobile, and there is no associated insufficiency
      (c) Balloon mitral valvotomy

(d) Performed on an outpatient basis: Risk of damage to the MV, which would require mitral valve replacement (MVR)

(e) Mitral valve replacement

(f) Performed if preoperative catheterization, angiography, and echocardiography indicate valvular or subvalvular calcification and thickening.

h. Preoperative considerations

(1) It is extremely important to have a thorough evaluation of the cardiac disease, including exertional tolerance, history of CHF, and response to drug therapy.

(2) Review of all diagnostic testing, including cardiac catheterization, laboratory tests, ECG, and x-rays

(a) The cardiac catheterization data becomes immensely useful in patient management postoperatively.

(3) Baseline system evaluation with emphasis on neurologic, pulmonary, and renal.

(4) Patient teaching should include the criteria for selection of valve type (mechanical vs. porcine) and long-term considerations.

i. Intraoperative and postoperative considerations

(1) Pulmonary hypertension is common.

(2) Generally have insertion of PA catheter, possibly fiberoptic

(3) Preload management is important to maintain adequate CO and avoid pulmonary edema.

(a) Generally, use crystalloid or synthetic colloid fluid for volume replacement.

(b) It is very useful to know the preoperative PAP.

(4) Control of dysrhythmia is essential for CO (prone to atrial dysrhythmias)

2. Mitral insufficiency (Figure 39-11)

a. Second most common valvular defect

b. Causes

(1) Rheumatic fever

(2) Bacterial endocarditis

(3) Ruptured chordae tendineae

(4) Rupture or dysfunction of a papillary muscle

(5) Annular dilation (from dilated LV)

(6) Prolapse (prolapse and CAD most common causes)

(7) Trauma

(8) Calcification (common in elderly women)

c. Pathologic findings

(1) Backward leakage of blood from the LV into the LA during systole

(2) Scarring and calcification

(3) Bacterial destruction of uninvolved tissue

(4) Dilation of the annulus

d. Signs and symptoms

(1) Blowing, high-pitched, pansystolic murmur heard best at PMI, with radiation to the left axilla or infrascapular areas

(2) Atrial pulsation at the third left intercostal space

(3) Weakness and fatigue

(4) Atrial fibrillation

(5) Pulmonary edema

(6) CHF

(7) Chest pain (usually atypical)

e. Diagnostic studies (same as MS)

(1) ECG (altered P waves and QRS amplitude and nonspecific ST changes)

(2) Chest x-ray (LV and LA enlargement)

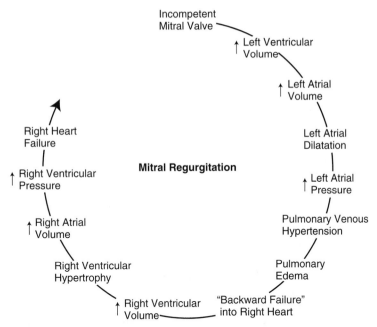

FIGURE 39-11 ■ Mitral regurgitation. (From Abranczk EL, Brown MM: Valvular heart disease. In Kinney MR, Packa DR, Andreoli KG, et al, editors: *Comprehensive cardiac care,* ed 7. Philadelphia: Mosby, 1991, p 336.)

    (3) Echocardiogram and echo Doppler (decreased ventricular wall motion and estimates severity of regurgitation)

    (4) Cardiac catheterization (LV end-diastolic pressure (LVEDP) and wall motion)

  f. Effects on hemodynamics

    (1) Backward flow of blood from the LV to the LA during ventricular systole increases LA and LV volumes (preload) and pressures causing a backup of pressure and volumes into the pulmonary vasculature (increased LVEDP [PAOP, PCWP] and PAP)

    (2) Increased pulmonary pressures result in pulmonary edema.

    (3) Over time, pulmonary edema and hypertension can result in failure of the right side of the heart (increased right arterial pressure).

  g. Treatment

    (1) Noninvasive (same as for MS)

    (2) Surgical interventions

      (a) Surgery should be timed to occur before irreversible LV dysfunction has developed.

      (b) Mitral valve replacement with removal of the mitral valve apparatus

      (c) Mitral valve replacement with preservation of at least part of the mitral valve apparatus

      (d) Mitral valve repair (valvuloplasty)

        (i) Preservation of the mitral valve apparatus helps to maintain LV performance and avoids the risks of prosthesis.

        (ii) Results of valvuloplasty are better in nonrheumatic valves.

  h. Preoperative consideration (same as MS)

  i. Intraoperative and postoperative considerations

    (1) Both the LA and LV are usually volume overloaded and dilated.

    (2) Goal of anesthesia is to maintain the heart rate at normal levels and control afterload with vasodilators.

(3) Generally have a PA catheter inserted after the initiation of anesthesia

(4) Requires heart-lung bypass and myocardial preservation techniques

(5) Usually performed via a medial sternotomy: Insertion of mediastinal chest drainage tubes and sometimes a left pleural drainage tube

(6) Patients are preload sensitive and require vigilant hemodynamic monitoring and fluid maintenance.

(7) Postoperative goal is rapid extubation and ambulation.

3. Aortic stenosis (Figure 39-12)

   a. A narrowing of the aortic valve orifice, which obstructs the ejection of blood from the LV

   b. Three times more common in men than women

   c. Causes

     (1) Congenital abnormalities (generally in patients less than 30 years of age)

     (2) Rheumatic fever (30 to 70 years of age)

     (3) Idiopathic calcification

       (a) Aging (>70 years of age)

       (b) Hypertrophic obstructive cardiomyopathy (HOCOM)

   d. Pathological findings

     (1) Narrowing of the normal valve orifice (2.6 to 3.5 cm^2)

       (a) A valve orifice of 0.5 cm^2 may still prove functional if it develops over several years with LV compensation.

       (b) A valve orifice of 0.4 cm^2 with peak systolic pressure gradients above 50 mm Hg results in a critical obstruction.

     (2) Congenital malformations may include unicuspid, bicuspid, multicuspid, or unequal aortic valve leaflets (1% of Americans are born with a bicuspid aortic valve).

   e. Signs and symptoms

     (1) Most patients with AS are initially asymptomatic.

       (a) There is a rapid increase in the risk of death with the development of symptoms.

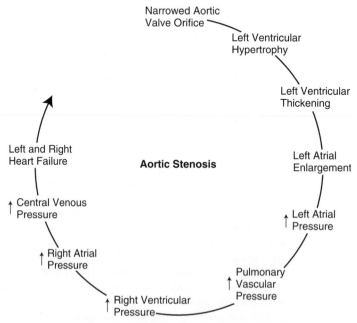

FIGURE 39-12 ■ Aortic stenosis. (From Abranczk EL, Brown MM: Valvular heart disease. In Kinney MR, Packa DR, Andreoli KG, et al, editors: *Comprehensive cardiac care,* ed 7. Philadelphia: Mosby, 1991, p 330.)

(2) Classic manifestations
  (a) Fatigue
  (b) Chest pain (approximately 50% experience exertional angina)
  (c) Syncope (15% to 30% as consequences of dysrhythmia or an abrupt fall in the systemic vascular resistance)
(3) Harsh, high-pitched systolic crescendo-decrescendo best heard at the right sternal border at the second intercostal space; may radiate to the neck or apex (the intensity of the murmur usually decreases as the disease progresses and the CO falls)
(4) Systolic thrill over the apex
(5) Narrowed pulse pressure

f. Diagnostic studies
  (1) ECG (LV hypertrophy, first degree atrioventricular block and left bundle branch block)
  (2) Chest x-ray (LV enlargement, a poststenotic dilation of the aorta, calcification of the valve cusps, pulmonary congestion)
  (3) Echocardiogram (LV thickening and reduced mobility and calcification of the cusps)
  (4) Nuclear scans (ventricular function and ejection fraction)
  (5) Cardiac catheterization (determines the gradient and evaluates LV function; also identifies the presence of other valvular lesions and CAD)

g. Effects on hemodynamics
  (1) Increase in afterload leads to LV hypertrophy and elevated LVEDP, resulting in elevated pulmonary vascular pressures, left heart failure, and eventual right heart failure.

h. Treatment
  (1) Symptomatic aortic stenosis is lethal if not treated.
  (2) Noninvasive
    (a) Patients must be asymptomatic or clearly nonsurgical candidates
    (b) Must always receive prophylactic antibiotics before and after dental and invasive medical procedures
    (c) Nitrates for chest pain should always be administered cautiously as the vasodilation may result in hypotension, syncope, and decreased CO.
  (3) Surgical intervention
    (a) Even patients with advanced heart failure and severe LV dysfunction may still benefit from aortic valve replacement, especially if the gradient exceeds 30 mm Hg.
    (b) Aortic valve replacement (most common procedure)
    (c) Indicated for patients who develop a gradient >50 mm Hg with CHF, angina, or exertional syncope; also for patients with a calculated aortic valve area index <0.8 cm^2/m^2
    (d) Requires use of extracorporeal circulation and the selection of a valvular prosthesis
    (e) Criteria for selection of mechanical or bioprosthesis is the same as for MS.
    (f) Approximately 20% of patients with a bioprosthetic aortic valve require a second valve replacement within 8 years.
  (4) Valvuloplasty
    (a) Indicated in patients who are severely symptomatic but are not candidates for aortic replacement to decrease the gradient and relieve symptoms
    (b) Does not decrease mortality

i. Preoperative considerations (same as MS)
j. Intraoperative and postoperative considerations
  (1) Most difficult to manage of all valvular diseases

   (2) *Extremely preload sensitive*
      (a) Replacement of the valve greatly decreases the afterload the ventricle must pump against to eject blood.
      (b) The decreased resistance allows the ventricle to easily eject, therefore decreasing the volume (preload) and stretch of the myocardium.
      (c) This can significantly impact ventricular filling and cardiac output by decreasing contractility.
   (3) Generally, have a PA catheter inserted; pay special attention to preload (right atrial [RA], PAOP [PCWP] and afterload SVR, pulmonary vascular resistance) parameters.
   (4) Prone to atrial fibrillation and tachycardia
4. Aortic insufficiency (AI) (Figure 39-13)
   a. Backward flow of blood from the aorta into the LV during ventricular diastole
   b. Causes
      (1) Cause can result from pathophysiology of the aortic root or the valve leaflet.
      (2) Most common valvular causes: endocarditis and rheumatic heart disease (endocarditis is the most common cause of acute AI)
      (3) Most common aortic root causes: Idiopathic dilation (annuloaortic ectasia) associated with hypertension and aging, Marfan's syndrome, aortic dissection, syphilis, collagen vascular disease, and trauma
   c. Signs and symptoms
      (1) Patients with normal LV function may be remarkably asymptomatic, even during strenuous exertion.
      (2) Symptoms are usually those of left-sided failure.
      (3) May develop angina because of the relative diastolic hypotension resulting in decreased coronary filling pressure; angina is usually associated with vasodilation and flushing

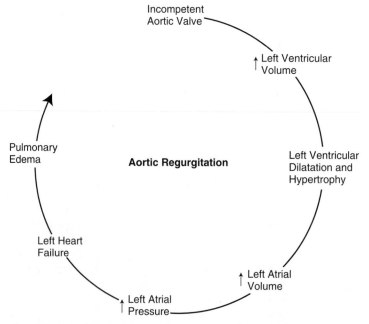

FIGURE 39-13 ■ Aortic regurgitation. (From Abranczk EL, Brown MM: Valvular heart disease. In Kinney MR, Packa DR, Andreoli KG, et al, editors: *Comprehensive cardiac care*, ed 7. Philadelphia: Mosby, 1991, p 332.)

    (4) *Acute AI's* presenting signs and symptoms are tachycardia, dyspnea, pulmonary edema and peripheral vasoconstriction, cyanosis, and a midpitched, short, diastolic murmur; a third heart sound may be audible.

    (5) *Chronic AI* generally has presenting signs and symptoms of exertional dyspnea, orthopnea and a high-pitched, blowing crescendo diastolic sound heard best at the second right intercostal space while patient is sitting; a third or fourth heart sound may be audible depending on the degree of regurgitation.

    (6) The patient may also have a rapid up stroke and down stroke of the carotid pulse (Corrigan's pulse).

d. Diagnostic studies

    (1) ECG

        (a) *Chronic*—LV hypertrophy (increased amplitude of the QRS and ST-T wave strain pattern); AV conduction is prolonged

        (b) *Acute*—ST-T wave changes are consistent with myocardial ischemia.

    (2) Chest x-ray

        (a) *Chronic*—dilation of the LV with elongation of the apex inferiorly and posteriorly; may see a prominent ascending aorta with Marfan's syndrome

        (b) *Acute*—normal sized heart, but may show pulmonary edema

    (3) Echocardiogram

        (a) May visualize vegetation formation on the valve leaflets from endocarditis

        (b) Quantifies the amount of regurgitation

        (c) Promptness of exam mandatory in acute AI

    (4) Cardiac catheterization

        (a) Estimates the severity of the regurgitation and evaluates the extent of the LV failure

        (b) Generally not indicated in young acute AI resulting from endocarditis

e. Effects on hemodynamics

    (1) Produces LV volume overload

    (2) With chronic AI, the increase in LVEDV results in a more forceful LV contraction; the force of contraction is maintained by LV hypertrophy and dilation.

    (3) Eventually, increased LVEDP is reflected backward to the LA, pulmonary vasculature, and right heart and results in pulmonary edema and right heart failure.

    (4) With acute AI, the LV does not have time to hypertrophy and increase the force of contraction; therefore, the increased LVEDP may actually exceed LA pressure and cause the mitral valve to close prematurely; this results in pulmonary venous hypertension and pulmonary edema.

f. Treatment

    (1) Noninvasive

        (a) Antibiotic prophylaxis

        (b) Treat CHF with diuretics, digoxin, vasodilators, and preload and afterload reducers.

        (c) Important to remember AI is a fluid *volume* overload problem, whereas AS is a *pressure* overload disturbance.

    (2) Surgical valve replacement

    (3) Must be performed before the development of irreversible LV dysfunction

    (4) Indications

        (a) Symptomatic chronic AI

        (b) Asymptomatic—"55 rule"

Good outcome can be expected if LV end-systolic diameter <55 and LV ejection fraction 55% or greater.

   (c) Acute

      (i) Seventy-five percent mortality if treated medically

      (ii) Twenty-five percent mortality if treated surgically

  (5) Prosthesis selection (same as mitral)

   (a) One to two percent incidence of prosthetic infective endocarditis regardless of the prosthesis selected

g. Preoperative considerations (same as MS)

  (1) Important to know degree of LV failure preoperatively to guide postoperative care

h. Intraoperative and postoperative considerations

  (1) Generally severely volume overloaded

  (2) Prevent bradycardias as they prolong filling time and result in volume overload.

  (3) Utilize afterload reduction: nitroglycerin and nitroprusside.

  (4) Mechanical valves carry a 2% to 5% incidence of thromboembolic and bleeding complications.

5. Tricuspid stenosis (TS) (Figure 39-14)

  a. Causes

   (1) Rheumatic heart disease

   (2) Frequently associated with MS also

   (3) Right atrial tumors

   (4) Congenital abnormalities

  b. Pathologic findings

   (1) A reduction of the normal tricuspid valve orifice of 7 cm² to 1.5 cm² or less

  c. Signs and symptoms

   (1) Major symptoms: dyspnea and fatigue

   (2) Peripheral edema and neck pulsation (especially when RA pressure is 10 mm Hg or greater)

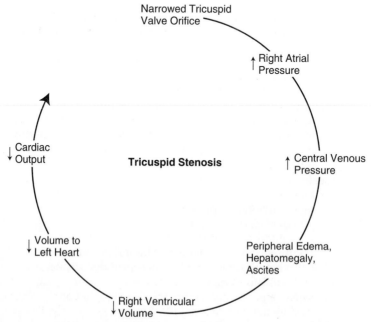

FIGURE 39-14 ■ Tricuspid stenosis. (From Abranczk EL, Brown MM: Valvular heart disease. In Kinney MR, Packa DR, Andreoli KG, et al, editors: *Comprehensive cardiac care,* ed 7. Philadelphia: Mosby, 1991, p 338.)

          (3) Murmur is a low-pitched diastolic rumble best heard at the fourth intercostal space to the left of the sternal border; increases in intensity with inspiration.

    d. Diagnostic studies

        (1) ECG: Large P waves

        (2) Chest x-ray: Prominent right atrium

        (3) Echocardiogram: Fibrosis, calcifications, and obstruction

        (4) Echo Doppler: Estimates the diastolic gradient

        (5) Cardiac catheterization: Confirms a gradient of greater than 1 mm Hg between the RA and the RV

    e. Effects on hemodynamics

        (1) Increased RA volume (preload) and pressure

        (2) Decreased CO because less blood fills the RV and therefore less blood reaches the left side of the heart

    f. Treatment

        (1) Noninvasive

            (a) Antibiotic prophylaxis

            (b) Peripheral edema may not respond to diuretics since the edema is a result of pressure overload and not volume overload.

        (2) Surgical intervention

            (a) Valve replacement

            (b) Long-term anticoagulation is warranted because of the high thrombogenic rate and therefore negates the benefit of a bioprosthesis.

    g. Preoperative considerations (same as MS)

    h. Intraoperative and postoperative considerations

        (1) Potential for valve infection is a persistent problem.

        (2) Will require extensive education regarding anticoagulation and signs and symptoms of endocarditis

        (3) May have considerations of other valvular diseases if have concomitant disease (e.g., mitral stenosis)

  6. Tricuspid insufficiency (TI) (Figure 39-15)

    a. Causes

        (1) Infective endocarditis

            (a) Occurs in 10% of the general endocarditis population, but increases to 50% among illicit intravenous drug users who develop endocarditis

            (b) RV dilation and failure secondary to LV failure and pulmonary hypertension

            (c) Congenital abnormality

    b. Signs and symptoms

        (1) Generally well tolerated by the RV

        (2) Presence worsens the symptoms of RV failure (i.e., fatigue, edema, and ascites)

        (3) Atrial fibrillation common

        (4) Murmur is high-pitched, blowing, and holosystolic; heard best at the fourth intercostal space at the left sternal border or xiphoid area; intensifies with inspiration.

    c. Diagnostic studies

        (1) ECG: atrial fibrillation or right bundle branch block

        (2) Chest x-ray: RA and RV enlargement

        (3) Echocardiogram: Recognition of vegetative lesions, ruptured chordae and papillary muscles, and the back-and-forth motion of the valve

        (4) Doppler: estimates severity of the regurgitation

        (5) Cardiac catheterization: Prominent V-wave in the RA

    d. Effects on hemodynamics

        (1) Backward flow of blood into the RA increases the RA volume (preload) and pressure.

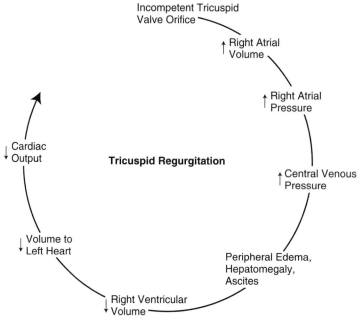

FIGURE 39-15 ■ Tricuspid regurgitation. (From Abranczk EL, Brown MM: Valvular heart disease. In Kinney MR, Packa DR, Andreoli KG, et al, editors: *Comprehensive cardiac care,* ed 7. Philadelphia: Mosby, 1991, p 339.)

      (2) Decreased CO resulting from a diminished amount of blood reaching the left side of the heart

   e. Treatment

      (1) Noninvasive

         (a) Alleviation of RV failure

         (b) Improvement of diseases responsible (e.g., endocarditis)

      (2) Surgical intervention (same as TS)

         (a) May have to replace a concurrent stenotic mitral valve

   f. Preoperative considerations (same as MS)

   g. Intraoperative and postoperative considerations

      (1) Will have right-sided volume overload

      (2) Will have long-term anticoagulation considerations

 7. Pulmonic valvular disease

   a. Stenosis: most common cause is congenital abnormality (Figure 39-16).

   b. Insufficiency: most common cause is dilation of the valve ring resulting from pulmonary hypertension (Figure 39-17).

   c. May be tolerated for years without difficulty unless it is complicated by pulmonary hypertension

   d. Signs and symptoms

      (1) Stenosis

         (a) Dyspnea, fatigue, and syncope proportional to the severity of the disease

         (b) Murmur is a sharp, systolic crescendo-decrescendo best heard at the left sternal border at the second or third intercostal space; the second heart sound may be widely split or absent.

      (2) Insufficiency

         (a) No symptoms except those of pulmonary hypertension

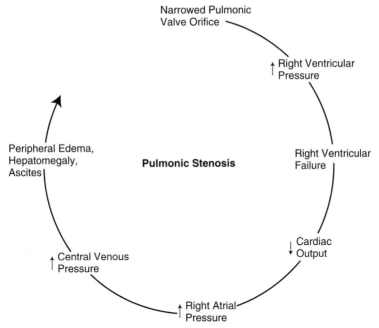

FIGURE 39-16 ■ Pulmonic stenosis. (From Abranczk EL, Brown MM: Valvular heart disease. In Kinney MR, Packa DR, Andreoli KG, et al, editors: *Comprehensive cardiac care,* ed 7. Philadelphia: Mosby, 1991, p 340.)

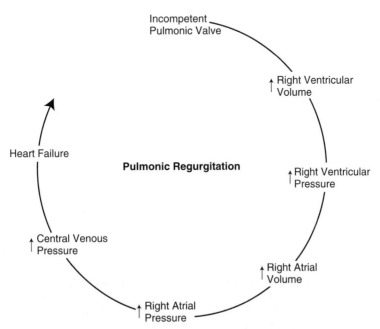

FIGURE 39-17 ■ Pulmonic regurgitation. (From Abranczk EL, Brown MM: Valvular heart disease. In Kinney MR, Packa DR, Andreoli KG, et al, editors: *Comprehensive cardiac care,* ed 7. Philadelphia: Mosby, 1991, p 341.)

       (b) Murmur is high-pitched with pulmonary hypertension and moderately pitched without pulmonary hypertension; it is a blowing sound most optimally auscultated at the fourth or fifth intercostal space to the left of the sternal border; hard to distinguish from aortic regurgitation.

  e. Diagnostic studies

    (1) Thorough history

    (2) Echocardiography is the most valuable noninvasive tool.

  f. Effects on hemodynamics

    (1) Stenosis is a right-sided pressure overload while insufficiency is a right-sided volume overload.

      (a) Both are evidenced by elevated RA pressures and eventual heart failure.

      (b) Stenosis will show evidence of diminished CO earlier than insufficiency.

  g. Treatment

    (1) Noninvasive intervention is aimed at alleviation of symptoms with insufficiency and preventing recurrent endocarditis and emboli with stenosis.

    (2) Surgical replacement of a stenotic valve is rare.

    (3) Replacement prosthesis will be a bioprosthesis because of the high incidence of emboli associated with the mechanical valves.

    (4) Valvotomy is the preferred invasive treatment for stenosis.

  h. Preoperative considerations (same as MS)

  i. Intraoperative and postoperative considerations

    (1) Hemodynamic monitoring and intervention will be focused on presence of pulmonary hypertension, decreased CO, and RV overload and failure.

    (2) Same considerations as any mechanical valve replacement

8. Multivalvular disease

  a. Common with rheumatic heart disease

  b. Should undergo right and left heart catheterizations for full assessment before surgery

  c. Common types

    (1) Mitral stenosis and aortic insufficiency

    (2) Mitral stenosis and aortic stenosis

    (3) Aortic stenosis and mitral insufficiency

    (4) Aortic and mitral insufficiency

  d. Management

    (1) Double valve replacement

      (a) Operative mortality 18.6%

      (b) Five year survival 47%

    (2) Triple valve replacement

      (a) Complicated with severe heart failure

      (b) Surgical correction generally the only option

      (c) Eighteen to forty percent operative mortality

    (3) Preoperative considerations

      (a) Patients and families have extensive educational, psychosocial, and physiologic needs.

      (b) Generally present with complex medical history and treatment regimens

    (4) Intraoperative and postoperative considerations

      (a) Effective postoperative care and outcome requires a thorough understanding of all the valvular pathologies and complications.

      (b) Hemodynamic measurements may be confounded by the multivalvular disease.

VI. Miscellaneous acquired lesions (unrelated to rheumatic or atherosclerotic heart disease)
- A. Primary myocardial diseases
  - 1. Cardiomyopathy
    - a. Heart muscle diseases that primarily affect the structural and/or functional capacity of the myocardium
    - b. Primary (no known cause—idiopathic)
    - c. Secondary (most common causes—ischemia, viral infections, alcohol, and pregnancy)
    - d. Functional classifications (Box 39-1)
      - (1) Dilated
        - (a) Characterized by systolic dysfunction
        - (b) Cardiomegaly with ventricular dilation
        - (c) Impairment of systolic function
        - (d) Atrial enlargement
        - (e) Stasis of blood in the LV
      - (2) Hypertrophic
        - (a) Characterized by diastolic dysfunction
        - (b) Ventricular hypertrophy (with normal or small ventricles and dilated atria)
        - (c) Rapid contraction of the LV, impaired relaxation
        - (d) Intracavity systolic pressure gradients
      - (3) Restrictive (least common)
        - (a) Diastolic dysfunction
        - (b) Principal characteristic is cardiac muscle stiffness caused by infiltrative changes in the heart muscle.
        - (c) Diminished CO
    - e. Signs and symptoms
      - (1) Dilated: CHF, fatigue, weakness, and pulmonary and systemic emboli
      - (2) Hypertrophic: dyspnea (most common), angina, fatigue and syncope
      - (3) Restrictive: similar to dilated; exercise intolerance the most common
    - f. Diagnostic studies: Echocardiogram is the most useful tool for diagnosis.
    - g. Effects on hemodynamics (see Table 39-1)
    - h. Treatment
      - (1) Noninvasive:
        - (a) The goal is to reduce the workload of the heart and improve the symptoms of CHF.
        - (b) May utilize beta-blocking agents and calcium-blocking agents for hypertrophic presentation
        - (c) Restrictive presentations may require pacemaker insertion for treatment of AV blocks.
      - (2) Surgical intervention
        - (a) Dilated: cardiac transplantation (last resort) or implantable LV assist devices (LVAD) (i.e., Novacor® and Heartmate®)

■ BOX 39-1
■ **FUNCTIONAL CLASSIFICATIONS OF CARDIOMYOPATHY**

Dilated	**Hypertrophic**	**Restrictive**
▪ Systolic dysfunction	▪ Diastolic dysfunction	▪ Diastolic dysfunction
▪ Cardiomegaly	▪ Ventricular hypertrophy	▪ Cardiac muscle stiffness
▪ Atrial enlargement	▪ Rapid LV contraction	▪ ↓ Cardiac output
▪ LV stasis	▪ Impaired relaxation	
	▪ Intracavity systolic pressure gradients	

■ TABLE 39-1
■ ■ **Cardiomyopathy Effects on Hemodynamics**

	Contractility	LV Filling Pressure
Dilated	↓↓↓	↑↑
Hypertrophic	↑↑→↓	Normal
Restrictive	Normal →↓	↑

From White-Williams C: Cardiomyopathy. In Kinney MR, Packa DR, Andreoli KG, et al, editors: *Comprehensive cardiac care*, ed 7. Philadelphia: Mosby, 1991, p 345.

      (b) Hypertrophic: Septal myotomy-myectomy (excision of a part of the hypertrophied septum)

      (c) Restrictive: Excision of the thickened endomyocardial plaque or mitral or tricuspid valve replacement

  i. Preoperative considerations

    (1) Cardiac transplantation

    (2) All patients present with advanced signs and symptoms of failure.

    (3) Will have to deal with the implications of end-stage cardiac disease

    (4) Imperative that patients and families understand risks, alternative and benefits, and the level of ongoing care required postoperatively (must assess willingness to comply with treatment regimen postoperatively)

  j. Intraoperative and postoperative considerations

    (1) Dependent on procedure preformed, but will have all the implications of any cardiac surgery performed on an extremely debilitated patient in end-stage cardiac failure

    (2) Likely to require complex and comprehensive hemodynamic monitoring and titration of vasoactive medications

    (3) Likely to require mechanical support postoperatively (i.e., IABP or LVAD)

2. Pericardial disease (pericarditis)

  a. Clinical syndrome caused by inflammation of the pericardial membrane

  b. Principle cause is viral infection; can also be caused by postpericardiectomy syndrome, trauma, or tumor.

  c. Signs and symptoms

    (1) Pleuritic, substernal chest pain

    (2) Dyspnea

    (3) Pericardial friction rub

  d. Diagnostic studies

    (1) Transthoracic echocardiography is the most sensitive and accurate tool for the detection and quantification of pericardial fluid.

    (2) ECG: Acute pericarditis—ST elevation is concave upward and usually present in all leads except V1 and aVR (diagnostic).

  e. Effects on hemodynamics

    (1) A build up of pericardial fluid or blood leads to constriction around the heart and results in tamponade.

      (a) Hypotension

      (b) Plateauing of all heart pressures

      (c) Decreased CO

  f. Treatment

    (1) Noninvasive: Antiinflammatory agents

    (2) Invasive intervention

      (a) Pericardiocentesis: Subxiphoid needle aspiration of pericardial fluid (may leave a catheter with stopcock in place)

          (b) Subxiphoid limited pericardiotomy
          (c) Pericardiectomy or pericardial window: Surgical resection of all or part of the pericardium

  g. Preoperative considerations
     (1) Dependent on cause

  h. Intraoperative and postoperative considerations
     (1) Pericardiectomy will require median sternotomy or thoracotomy (i.e., will have mediastinal tubes and/or pleural drainage tubes).
     (2) Pericardial window will require a small subxiphoid incision with mediastinal drain to vacuum initially, then gravity.
     (3) Pericardiotomy may have catheter left in for aspiration of fluid and infusion of antibiotics.
     (4) Tamponade remains the most worrisome complication.

3. Traumatic heart disease
  a. Types
     (1) Blunt
     (2) Penetrating

  b. Potential injuries
     (1) Lacerations to the heart muscle
     (2) Myocardial contusions
     (3) Aortic dissection

  c. Potential complications
     (1) Dysrhythmias
     (2) Hemorrhagic shock
     (3) Cardiogenic shock
     (4) Tamponade

  d. Presentation and effects on hemodynamics depend on extent of injuries acquired.

  e. Diagnostic studies: Same as other pathologies, but also includes computed tomography and magnetic resonance imaging (MRI) (emergent presentations may be self-obvious and be taken immediately to the operating room)

  f. Surgical intervention: Repair of injury, depends of type of injury

  g. Intraoperative and postoperative considerations
     (1) Dependent on type of surgical repair
     (2) Likely to require replacement of blood products (possibly uncrossmatched) and fluid resuscitation
     (3) May require CPB
     (4) Likely to have multiple injuries (initial surgical intervention will only address life-threatening injuries)

4. Cardiac tumors
  a. Primary or metastatic

  b. Complications
     (1) Pericardial effusion
     (2) Restrictive disease
     (3) Obstruction to blood flow
     (4) Impaired contractility

  c. Surgical intervention
     (1) Depends on the location of the tumor and the hemodynamic effects

  d. Preoperative considerations
     (1) Whether treatment is palliative or curative
     (2) May be dealing with psychosocial implications of cancer

  e. Intraoperative and postoperative considerations
     (1) Depends on the surgical intervention
     (2) May have experienced radiation and/or chemotherapy preoperatively (may be immunocompromised and have depressed cardiac function related to the cardiotoxic effects of chemotherapy agents)

5. Aneurysms
   a. Defined as lumen enlargement, which results in weakening of the aortic wall
   b. Sometimes confused with dissection (creation of a channel between the inner and outer portions of the wall of the aorta by the surging column of blood; dissection can occur in a previously aneurysmal segment, and dissection can lead to aneurysm formation if the false lumen continues to expand)
   c. Location
      (1) Thoracic (ascending, arch, or descending)
         (a) Ascending may involve the aortic valve.
      (2) Abdominal (suprarenal or infrarenal)
   d. Causes: Most common are atherosclerosis and trauma (common with Marfan's syndrome).
   e. Signs and symptoms: asymptomatic unless dissecting, which results in tearing abdominal pain and profound hypotension
   f. Diagnostic studies: Chest x-ray, transesophageal echocardiography, and MRI
   g. Treatment
      (1) Noninvasive: aimed at aggressive blood pressure (BP) control with beta-blocking agents
      (2) Aortic endoscopic grafting
      (3) Surgical intervention
         (a) Indications (see Table 39-2)
         (b) Risk of rupture
            (i) 10%: <4.0 cm
            (ii) 45%: 7.0 to 10.0 cm
            (iii) 60%: >10.0 cm
      (4) Mortality: 60% die before reaching the OR and 50% die intraoperatively or postoperatively.
   h. Preoperative considerations
      (1) Need a comprehensive assessment with emphasis on renal function (5% to 10% complication of renal failure)
   i. Intraoperative and postoperative considerations
      (1) Generally have insertion of arterial and/or central line; may have PA line
      (2) Will require vigorous BP control with nitroglycerin or nitroprusside
      (3) Typically, require large amounts of fluid resuscitation postoperatively to maintain preload

■ TABLE 39-2
■ ■ **Aortic Aneurysms: Criteria for Surgical Intervention**

Ascending Thoracic	Descending Thoracic	Thoraco-abdominal	Abdominal
Pain	Pain	As for descending thoracic or abdominal aorta	Pain, tenderness
Severe aortic regurgitation	Compression of adjacent structures		Athero-emboli
Size ≥6 cm	Size ≥6 cm		Size ≥5 cm
Marfan's ≥5 cm	Growth ≥1 cm/yr		Growth ≥1 cm/yr
Growth ≥1 cm/yr			

From Creager MA, Halperin JL: Aortic and arterial aneurysms. In Creager MA, volume editor: *Vascular disease*. Braumwald E, series editor: Atlas of Heart Diseases. Philadelphia: Current Medicine, 1996, pp 1.1-1.19.

(4) Important to maintain mean arterial pressure (MAP) of 60 to 70 mm Hg to maintain renal perfusion

(5) Aortic cross-clamp time may result in renal failure, paralysis, and neurologic injury.

    (a) May insert an intrathecal catheter with thoracic aneurysm repair and use to monitor and maintain intrathecal pressures ≤15 mm Hg by drainage of cerebral spinal fluid

    (b) May utilize spinal cord cooling

    (c) May utilize atrial-femoral bypass

VII. Classifications of cardiovascular disease

    A. New York Heart Association guidelines (see Chapter 32 for a detailed discussion of assessment of the cardiac patient)

    B. American Society of Anesthesiologists' Physical Status Classification

      1. Descriptive analysis of patient status

      2. Often used to classify patient's status relative to risks of operative intervention

      3. Classes

        a. Class 1: patient has no organic, physiologic, biochemical, or psychiatric disturbances; pathologic process for which operation is to be performed is localized and does not entail systemic disturbance.

        b. Class 2: mild to moderate systemic disturbance caused by either condition to be treated surgically or other pathophysiologic process

        c. Class 3: severe systemic disturbance or disease from whatever cause, even though it may not be possible to define degree of disability with finality

        d. Class 4: patient with severe systemic disorders that are already life threatening, not always correctable by operation

        e. Class 5: moribund patient who has little chance of survival but has submitted to operation in desperation

        f. Class 6: a declared brain death patient whose organs are being removed for donor purposes.

        g. Emergency operation (E): any patient in one of the classes listed previously who is operated on as an emergency is considered to be in less than optimal physical condition; the E is placed after the numeric classification

VIII. Postanesthesia unit admission (phase I)

    A. Major goals of patient care

      1. Maintain adequate cardiac function by minimizing oxygen demand of the myocardium and maximizing oxygen delivery to all body tissues

    B. What you want to know from operating room (OR)

      1. Type of surgical procedure

      2. Type of anesthesia and combinations of agents and reversal agents used

      3. Hemodynamic data and problems

      4. CPB (or cross-clamp) time

      5. Recent laboratory data (i.e., hemoglobin and hematocrit, K^+, activated clotting time [ACT])

      6. Estimated blood loss and fluids and blood products given

        a. Empty or mark all drainage devices, and ensure patency of tubes.

      7. Reversal of anticoagulation

      8. Pertinent medical history, especially pulmonary and cardiovascular

    C. Respiratory support

      1. Mechanical ventilator settings or high-flow humidified O_2 as ordered

      2. Monitor continuous SpO_2 and regular ABGs: acidosis increases myocardial oxygen demand and reduces contractility.

    D. Cardiac support

      1. Assess for and select best lead to detect dysrhythmias: adjust alarms for patient.

      2. Monitor measured and derived hemodynamic parameters: Ensure accuracy by leveling and zeroing transducer and record baseline data.

3. Assess for abnormal heart sounds.
4. Obtain baseline rhythm strips of all waveforms.
5. Be prepared to support heart rate with pacing (see Chapter 32 for a detailed discussion of care of the patient with temporary and permanent cardiac pacing).
   a. Type: transcutaneous, transvenous epicardial
   b. Mode: ventricular, atrial, AV sequential
   c. Sensitivity: Synchronous *(senses intrinsic cardiac rhythm)* versus asynchronous *(does not sense intrinsic cardiac rhythm)*

IX. Immediate patient management
  A. Dysrhythmias (see Chapter 32 for detailed discussion)
    1. Identify and treat cause if possible.
      a. Be alert for electrolyte imbalance related to diuresis, CPB, acidosis, and irritable myocardium; treat per Advanced Cardiac Life Support (ACLS) protocol.
      b. Be prepared to use pacing.
  B. Bleeding
    1. Be concerned for 100 ml/hour to 200 ml/hour for the first 3 to 4 hours or 1500 ml/4 hours.
    2. Causes of postoperative bleeding
      a. Clotting abnormalities: preexisting or after CPB
      b. Hypothermia
      c. Excessive hypertension
      d. Disrupted suture lines
      e. Protamine rebound
    3. Nursing interventions
      a. Stat laboratory tests as indicated (i.e., hemoglobin and hematocrit, partial thromboplastin time [PTT], prothrombin time [PT] or ACT and platelets)
        (1) Be concerned for
          (a) PTT >90, ACT >120 seconds
          (b) Platelets <50,000
          (c) Hemoglobin and hematocrit <8 (may be hemodiluted) (ideally hematocrit should be 28% to 30%.)
        (2) Replace blood products as ordered.
      b. Rewarm to 97° F (convection, warmed fluids, atmosphere).
      c. Treat hypertension: MAP <70 mm Hg (rewarming will also cause vasodilation which decreases MAP)
      d. Consider adding positive end-expiratory pressure (PEEP) up to 10 cm if hemodynamically stable.
      e. Give protamine (heparin reversal agent) and aminocaproic acid (Amicar®) as ordered (causes diffuse clotting).
    4. Tamponade
      a. Fluid accumulation within the pericardial space, which causes
        (1) Elevation and equilibration of intracardiac filling pressures
        (2) Progressive limitation of ventricular diastolic filling
        (3) Reduction of SV and CO
      b. Monitor for
        (1) Beck's triad (classic findings)
          (a) Increased central venous pressure (CVP)
          (b) Muffled heart tones
          (c) Pulsus paradoxus
        (2) Associated signs and symptoms may include
          (a) Tachycardia
          (b) ↓ Voltage of QRS complex
          (c) Narrow pulse pressure
          (d) Equalizing pressures (RA, PAP, PAOP [PCWP])
          (e) A sudden cessation of drainage from mediastinal tubes

(f) Decreased SVo$_2$ and CO

(g) Jugular venous distension

(3) Intervention

(a) *Cardiac tamponade in the cardiac surgery patient can be a true surgical emergency. Be prepared for possibility of open sternotomy at the bedside and/or emergent return to the OR.*

(b) Strip mediastinal tubes

(c) Supportive fluid and blood product replacement

C. Low cardiac output states

1. Be concerned for cardiac index (CI) <2.0 L/minute per m^2.

2. Assess for cause and treat accordingly (refer to Section I of this chapter).

   a. Assess and treat HR and rhythm disturbances.

   b. Assess and treat preload (most common cause and should be assessed for and treated first).

      (1) Be concerned for RA pressures <6 mm Hg and PAOP (PCWP) <10 mm Hg.

      (2) Lactated Ringer's or normal saline are usually the crystalloids of choice.

      (3) Hespan (hetastarch) is a frequent synthetic colloid used.

      (4) Blood products as indicated

      (5) Be sure to assess for tamponade.

   c. Afterload

      (1) Make sure patient is normothermic.

      (2) Strive to keep SVR 900-1200 dynes/second per cm-5 (keep low normal for dysfunctional myocardium).

      (3) Nitroglycerin and nitroprusside are the most common agents used.

   d. Contractility

      (1) Left ventricular stroke work index (LVSWI) is an indirect indicator of contractility (normal is 40-75 g/m^2/beat).

      (2) Medical interventions

         (a) Assess and treat electrolyte imbalance—especially hypokalemia, hypomagnesemia, hypocalcemia.

         (b) Assess and treat acidosis: respiratory and metabolic.

         (c) Assess and treat hypoxia.

         (d) May utilize dobutamine, milrinone, and possibly sympathomimetic agents such as dopamine, epinephrine and norepinephrine

3. IABP

   a. Temporary mechanical ventricular assist device, which augments systemic and coronary circulation and "unloads" the heart through the diastolic inflation and systolic deflation of a catheter mounted balloon placed in the descending thoracic aorta

   b. Inserted through the femoral artery (most common) or surgical transthoracic implantation

   c. Two major functions

      (1) Increase coronary artery perfusion

      (2) Decrease afterload

   d. Most common complications are

      (1) Ischemia to the extremity distal to insertion

      (2) Bleeding

      (3) Obstruction of blood flow to the kidneys

   e. Patient management (Box 39-2) should include

      (1) Frequent assessment of insertion site and extremity perfusion

      (2) Hourly urine output

      (3) Continuous hemodynamic monitoring

4. VAD

   a. Extracorporeal ventricular flow assist device that provides temporary circulatory support for single or biventricular failure

■ BOX 39-2
■ **CARE OF THE PATIENT ON AN INTRAAORTIC BALLOON PUMP (IABP)**

Rationale for use	↑ Coronary artery perfusion (balloon inflation)	↓ Afterload (balloon deflation)
Placement	Generally in the femoral artery Percutaneous or cutdown	
Timing	Inflate: On or near the dicrotic notch of the arterial waveform	Deflate: Slightly before systole
Troubleshooting	Increased afterload Decreased cardiac index	Adjust deflation point.
	Inadequate augmentation	Assess patient status. Adjust inflation point. Check trigger. Refill balloon. Check for balloon rupture.
	Balloon not pumping	Check augmentation setting. Check trigger. Check power source. Check connections. Look for kinks in tubing.

      b. May be a right or left VAD (RVAD or LVAD) or both (BIVAD)
      c. Requires surgical cannulation of the atria or ventricle and either pulmonary artery or aorta
      d. Blood is removed from the atria or ventricle and directed to the appropriate artery.
      e. The primary goals are (1) myocardial tissue recovery and (2) bridge to treatment (i.e., transplant).
      f. Most common types: (1) roller, (2) centrifugal (Bio-Medicus Bio-Pump®), (3) pneumatic (Abiomed 5000®), (4) electric (Hemopump®), (5) total artificial heart (AbioCor®)
      g. Most common complications: (1) bleeding and (2) embolus
      h. Patient management requires advanced training related to the specific device.
   D. Hypertension
     1. Goal: Maintenance of an adequate perfusion pressure for cellular oxygenation (MAP 65-75 mm Hg with an SVR of 900-1200 dynes)
     2. Excessive arterial pressures *(increased afterload)* *increases the work load on the heart and puts excessive pressure on suture lines.*
     3. Assessment and treatment
      a. Ideal assessment is continuous arterial pressure line monitoring of MAP.
      b. *Preload should always be assessed and treated first (use of vasodilators in a low preload situation will result in patient deterioration).*
      c. Vasodilators (see Chapter 32 for detailed discussion of cardioactive drugs)
        (1) Nitroglycerin
        (2) Nitroprusside
   E. Impaired oxygenation and ventilation
     1. Goal: Oxygen delivery sufficient to meet cellular oxygen demand needed to maintain aerobic metabolism
     2. Oxygen demand is specific to the individual and requires invasive and noninvasive monitoring: Respiratory rate, SpO_2, ABG analysis, urine output, skin color and temperature, pulses, for example.

   3. Treatment: Airway maintenance, administration of appropriate FiO_2 and mechanical support of ventilation
   F. Impaired renal functioning
   1. Kidneys are underperfused early in a low perfusion state.
   2. Intrarenal damage usually results from a prolonged MAP of <75 mm Hg.
      a. Mild reversible injury: ≤25 minutes of ischemia
      b. Severe damage: 40-60 minutes of ischemia
      c. Irreversible damage: 60-90 minutes of ischemia
   3. Most sensitive indicator of renal perfusion is urine output: Be concerned for urine outputs <0.5 ml/kg per hour.
   4. Treatment depends on whether decreased urine output is a result of a prerenal or intrarenal cause.
      a. Prerenal cause: Volume replacement and support of CO
      b. Intrarenal cause: Loop diuretics
      c. Renal failure may progress to the point of the need for hemofiltration.
   G. Impaired neurologic functioning
   1. Most common causes
      a. Air embolism
      b. Preexisting cerebrovascular disease
      c. Hypoxemia and hypercapnea
   2. Preoperative neurologic assessment is invaluable for postoperative assessment.
   3. Any change is significant and should be reported and investigated.
   4. Cornerstone of treatment is adequate oxygenation.
X. Special considerations for CABG
   A. Indications: Failure of medical management to control the pain and related sequelae of coronary heart disease
   B. Goal: Relief of symptoms and improved quality of life
   C. Selection criteria (controversial)
   1. Angina interfering with activity of daily living and/or evidence of severe ischemia
   2. Left main stenosis of at least 50% (least disputed)
   3. Proximal LAD stenosis of at least 70% with other major and significant coronary artery stenosis
   4. Proximal three-vessel disease of at least 50%
   5. Multivessel stenosis of at least 50% with moderate to severe LV dysfunction
   6. Failed PTCA or stent
   D. Conventional CABG
   1. Median sternotomy approach
   2. Utilizes vein grafts (saphenous), internal mammary artery (IMA), or other artery grafts (i.e., radial or gastroepiploic arteries [GEA])
   3. Cardiopulmonary bypass (CPB)
      a. Purpose: To provide a dry, quiet operative field while achieving myocardial preservation
      b. Blood is diverted from entering the heart by a single catheter placed in the RA or by catheters placed in the inferior and superior vena cava.
      c. Blood is directed back to the patient from the heart-lung machine through an arterial cannula placed in the ascending aorta.
      d. Main structures
         (1) Pump
         (2) Oxygenator with reservoir
         (3) Plastic circuitry
      e. Myocardial protection (incidence of intraoperative MI is 2% to 4%)
         (1) Hypothermia: Core cooling (28° to 32° C) is induced by the heart-lung machine via a heat exchanger and topical cooling to the myocardium (10° C).

(2) Cardioplegia
  (a) A cold (0° to 4° C) solution composed of a concentration of electrolytes, albumin, blood, and oxygenated crystalloid (some surgeons use warm cardioplegia, especially in patients with active ischemia).
  (b) Infused into the aortic root, coronary arteries, and myocardium, resulting in immediate electromechanical asystole
(3) Global ischemic arrest with topical cooling
  (a) Iced saline is instilled into the pericardial cavity.
  (b) The left side of the pericardium is protected to avoid phrenic nerve injury.
(4) Coronary perfusion
  (a) Antegrade: Injection of the cardioplegic solution into each new graft as the distal anastomosis is sutured
  (b) Retrograde: Injection of the cardioplegic solution into the coronary sinus and coronary veins
(5) Hemodilution: Decreases blood viscosity, SVR, hemolysis, use of blood products; and promotes postoperative diuresis
(6) Anticoagulation: Reduces the sludging of blood in the capillaries, blood cell trauma, and the incidence of thromboemboli; accomplished using heparin, which is reversed by protamine at the termination of CPB

E. Minimally invasive CABG
  1. Defined as either a small incisional field or absence of CPB
    a. Minimally invasive CABG (MimCAB or MiniCAB): Vein grafting is visualized and performed through laparoscopes inserted through the chest wall or a left thoracotomy approach. Heart continues to beat, but may be slowed with pharmacological agents (i.e., beta-blockers). Technically difficult. Limited to anterior anastomoses.
    b. Off-pump CABG (OPCAB) or beating heart bypass: Utilizes a median sternotomy, but does not rely on CPB or cardiac arrest. A stabilizing "foot" is used directly over the artery being sutured to stabilize the myocardium. Able to access more areas because of greater visibility.
  2. Benefit: Avoids complications associated with CPB, which may decrease recovery time and days of hospitalization
  3. Downside: Heart may be irritable postoperatively from manipulation without hypothermia, and intraoperative preload and contractility may be difficult to maintain.

F. Preoperative consideration
  1. Thorough history and physical exam with emphasis on medications and respiratory, neurologic, gastrointestinal, and renal status
    a. Include pulmonary function studies.
  2. Laboratory tests
    a. Complete blood count with differential
    b. Electrolytes
    c. Coagulation studies: PT, PTT, bleeding times
    d. Type and crossmatch
    e. ABGs (room air)
  3. Preoperative teaching is highly individualized and may be difficult as a result of an emergency presentation.
  4. Many cardiac medications may be continued up to the time of surgery, but warfarin must be discontinued several days before surgery and aspirin should be withheld for one week.
  5. Patients are generally given a bath or shower with a germicidal agent the evening before surgery.
  6. Broad spectrum prophylactic antibiotics are usually administered immediately before the incision and continued for up to 24 hours postoperatively.

G. Intraoperative and postoperative considerations
   1. Goal: first hour is stabilization—rewarm, stabilize vital signs and hemodynamics, and provide adequate oxygenation.
   2. Anesthesia utilizes a combination of inhalation and short-acting intravenous agents in the lowest possible doses to enhance a rapid emergence from anesthesia.
      a. Patients may be extubated in the OR (particularly minimally invasive).
      b. Pain must be anticipated and addressed quickly in the recovery phase.
   3. Fast track extubation (may vary with physician and facility)
      a. Goal: Extubation within 4-6 hours of arrival to the recovery area
         (1) Weaning criteria
             (a) Warm (37° C)
             (b) Able to lift head upon request
             (c) Spontaneous respirations
             (d) Negative inspiratory force (NIF) of at least 20 cm/20 seconds
             (e) ABGs and related parameters adequate
             (f) Hemodynamically stable
         (2) Acceptable extubation parameters
             (a) Alert and follows commands
             (b) Respiratory rate <30 breaths per minute
             (c) Tidal volume >50% of predicted (>5 ml/kg)
             (d) PEEP/CPAP <5 cm H_2O
             (e) SaO_2 >91%, FiO_2 <40%
             (f) Hemodynamically stable
         (3) Acceptable extubation gases
             (a) pH 7.33-7.46
             (b) PCO_2 ≥33-49 mm Hg
             (c) PO_2 ≥65 mm Hg
      b. Extubate to nasal cannula and stay with patient for 15-30 minutes to assess tolerance.
   4. Typical placement of intravenous and monitoring lines in the holding area or OR suite
      a. Two large bore (14 gauge) peripheral IV accesses
      b. Central line (usually subclavian)
      c. PA catheter (may be oximetric)
      d. Radial arterial line
      e. Foley urinary catheter (may have temperature probe)
   5. Median sternotomy incisions will have mediastinal tubes and possibly a pleural tube connected to −25 cm H_2O suction
      a. Assess drainage every 15 minutes until less than 200 ml an hour..
      b. Elevate head of bed 15° to 25° to promote drainage (may receive Amicar if had CPB).
   6. Monitor closely for electrolyte imbalances from massive diuresis postoperatively (be concerned with diuresis of 300 ml or greater for two consecutive hours).
   7. Address comfort as soon as possible; typical agents and routes are IV Fentanyl or morphine sulfate, IV ketorolac and oral analgesics after extubation.
   8. May receive Sulcrate per nasogastric tube until extubated
XI. Special considerations for transplant
   A. Potential therapy for patients experiencing end-stage disease refractory to medical and surgical therapy
   B. Recipient criteria (see Box 39-3)
      1. Fifty percent of potential recipients are disabled from dilated cardiomyopathy with the remainder from ischemic cardiomyopathy.
      2. United Network for Organ Sharing (UNOS) Status grouping for allocation of donor hearts (see Box 39-4)

■ BOX 39-3
■ **RECIPIENT CRITERIA FOR HEART TRANSPLANTATION**

Acceptance Criteria	Exclusion Criteria
New York Heart Association functional class III or IV despite optimal medical management	Refractory elevation of pulmonary vascular resistance
Maximal O_2 consumption <14 ml/kg/minute	Acute, unresolved malignancy
	Recent pulmonary infarction
	Active infection
Life expectancy 1 to 2 years	Active peptic ulcer disease
Age<65 years	Type I diabetes mellitus with significant end-organ damage
Stable family support system	Symptoms of cerebrovascular accident
Ability to adhere to complex medical regimen	
Normal renal and hepatic function	Irreversible end-organ failure
	Active substance abuse
	Psychological instability
	Morbid obesity

Compiled from the following publications: (1) McKellar SH: Cardiomyopathy/cardiac transplant donor and recipient selection. Available at http://www.ctsnet.org/doc/4499. (2) Inova Health System: Heart transplant: Treatment options. Available from http://www.inova.org/inovapublic.srt/transplant/heart/index.jsp. (3) Cardiac transplantation. Available from http://www.ctsnet.org/ doc/4475. Accessed on May 12, 2003.

C. Preoperative considerations
  1. Goal: Provide the patient and family with factual, realistic information
    a. Procedure, intensive care, recovery, change in diet, exercise, impact of immunosuppressive therapy, and risk of infection and rejection
    b. Emotional support is vital.

■ BOX 39-4
■ **UNITED NETWORK FOR ORGAN SHARING (UNOS) STATUS GROUPING FOR ALLOCATION OF DONOR HEARTS**

Status	Severity of Illness
1A	Candidate admitted to listing transplant center hospital with at least one of the following devices or therapies
	▪ VAD implanted for ≤30 days, TAH, IABC, or ECMO*
	▪ Mechanical ventilation*
	Continuous infusion of intravenous inotrope and continuous hemodynamic monitoring of left ventricular filling pressure†
1B	Candidate with at least one of the following devices or therapies
	▪ VAD implanted for >30 days
	▪ Continuous infusion of intravenous inotropes
2	Candidate does not meet criteria for status 1A or 1B listing.
7	Candidate is considered temporarily unsuitable to receive a thoracic organ transplant.

From UNOS, 2002 Amended UNOS Policy 3.7 (Allocation of Thoracic Organs). Effective November 15, 2002, Richmond, VA.
VAD, ventricular assist device; *TAH,* total artificial heart; *IABC,* intraaortic balloon counterpulsation; *ECMO,* extracorporeal membrane oxygenator.
*Must be recertified every 14 days.
†Valid for 7 days.

2. Operative procedure
    a. Donor heart is excised, preserving the sinoatrial node and passed through a series of cooled saline baths (if transported it is placed in iced saline solution (4° C).
    b. Ischemic time is <4 hours.
    c. Orthotopic (95%): Recipient's heart is removed, and the donor heart is implanted in its place in normal anatomic position in the chest.
    d. Utilizes cardiopulmonary bypass and a median sternotomy
    e. Transplanted heart is rewarmed, and epicardial pacing wires chest tubes and invasive lines are placed.
3. Postoperative considerations
    a. Early function affected by the length of the ischemic insult
    b. Neural control
        (1) There is no direct neural control of the conduction system.
        (2) The adrenal hormones exert primary stimulation of the heart by exciting the adrenergic receptors of the donor myocardium with circulating catecholamines.
        (3) The denervated donor heart may be less sensitive to drugs such as atropine and digoxin.
    c. Immediate postoperative care is similar to any open-heart surgery.
    d. Frequent use of inotropic and vasodilating drugs (i.e., dobutamine and Isuprel)
        (1) Common use is 3-5 days.
        (2) Transplanted heart has a relatively fixed stroke volume; therefore, CO is very dependent on rate.
        (3) Calcium channel blockers and beta-blockers should be used with caution because of negative inotropic activity.
    e. Rhythm disturbances: Uncommon in the initial postoperative period unless there has been significant ischemia
        (1) May have bradycardia 2-3 days postoperatively if the recipient received amiodarone preoperatively (accumulates rapidly in transplanted myocardium and peaks during the second postoperative week).
        (2) Adenosine for tachydysrhythmias should be used at one quarter to one half normal dose because of increased sinus node sensitivity.
    f. Immunosuppression: Immune response can occur by either humoral or cell-mediated mechanisms; *patient may be isolated;* infection is the leading cause of death in the first three months.
    g. Increased risk of tamponade
        (1) Preoperative warfarin for severe LV dysfunction
        (2) Previous cardiac operations
        (3) Diminished coagulation factors from chronic liver congestion
        (4) Donor heart may not fill the enlarged pericardial space.
    h. Intensive care unit 2-3 days and discharged in 7-10 days
    i. Require vigilant follow-up
    j. Morbidity: Three major types
        (1) Rejection
        (2) Infection
        (3) Coronary artery vasculopathy
    k. Classical signs of rejection:
        (1) Development of S3 and/or S4
        (2) Weakness, fatigue, malaise
        (3) Hypotension
        (4) Elevated atrial pressures
        (5) Decreased urine output
        (6) Weight gain
        (7) Dysrhythmias

     l. Mortality
       (1) Early operative (<30 days): 5% to 10%
       (2) One-year survival rate: 79%
 XII. Psychosocial factors
   A. Goal of nursing care: Provision of holistic nursing care
   B. Psychosocial concepts to consider when planning and implementing care for the cardiac surgery patient
     1. Body image and self-concept perception
     2. Self-esteem
     3. Stress
     4. Fear and anxiety
     5. Pain
     6. Sensory deprivation or overload
     7. Death
   C. Structured preoperative family and patient teaching enhances understanding.
     1. Surgical procedure information specific to the patient
     2. Tour of the postoperative unit and visiting hours
     3. Sequence of events of operative day: premedication, time of procedure, surgical waiting area for family
     4. Identification of equipment to be used postoperatively
     5. Procedure for coughing and deep breathing, stressing rationale for importance
     6. Review of expected postoperative course
     7. Adequate time for discussion to allow patient and family to ask questions and verbalize concerns
   D. Postoperative support of psychosocial factors
     1. Allow family to see patient as soon as appropriate in the recovery phase.
     2. Reinforce preoperative teaching.
     3. Utilize systems that allow for the family to get rest and nutrition: pagers, sleep rooms, for example.
     4. Utilize ancillary support services (e.g., social services, pastoral care, family liaisons)
     5. Utilize a Child Life Specialist if a child needs to be allowed into the critical care area to visit a family member.

BIBLIOGRAPHY

1. Accorda R, Kraus R, Casey PE: Advances in the surgical treatment of coronary artery disease. *Nurs Clin North America* 35(4): 913-931, 2000.
2. Ahrens TS, Martin NK, Powers C, et al: Angina pectoris and myocardial infarction. In Ahrens TS, Prentice D, editors: *Critical care certification: Preparation, review, and practice exams*, ed 4. Stamford, CT: Appleton & Lange, 1998, p 63.
3. Anderson AB , May OJ: *A notebook for the human heart valve patient*. Kennesaw, GA: Cryolife, 1998.
4. AneuRx™: Patient information booklet, *The AneuRx™ stent graft system: A new treatment for abdominal aortic aneurysms*. Minneapolis: Medtronic, 1999.
5. Barnason S, Rasmussen D: Comparison of clinical practice changes in a rapid recovery program for coronary artery bypass graft patients. *Nurs Clin North America* 35(2): 395-403, 2000.
6. Braunwald E: Acute myocardial infarction. In Goldman L, Braunwald E, editors: *Primary cardiology*. Philadelphia: WB Saunders, 1998, pp 257-283.
7. Burden N: The surgical specialties—part 2: Gynecologic and obstetric, urologic, orthopedic and podiatric, general, and cardiovascular surgical procedures. In Burden N, editor: *Ambulatory surgical nursing*. Philadelphia: WB Saunders, 1998, p 502.
8. Carabello BA: Valvular heart disease. In Goldman L, Braunwald E, editors: *Primary cardiology*. Philadelphia: WB Saunders, 1998, pp 370-389.
9. Carbone LM: An interdisciplinary approach to the rehabilitation of open-heart surgical patients. *Rehabil Nurs* 24(2):55-61, 1999.
10. Dec GW: Recognition and management of patients with cardiomyopathies. In Goldman L, Braunwald E, editors: *Primary cardiology*. Philadelphia: WB Saunders, 1998, pp 487-507.

11. Doering LV, Esmailian F, Imperial-Perez F, et al: Determinants of intensive care unit length of stay after coronary artery bypass graft surgery. *Heart Lung* 30(1):9-17, 2001.

12. Cambria RP, Davison JK, Zannetti S, et al: Clinical experience with epidural cooling for spinal cord protection during thoracic and thoracoabdominal aneurysm repair. *J Vasc Surg* 25:234-241, 1997.

13. Chan CB, Wright BP: Home care for the coronary artery bypass graft surgery patient. *Home Healthc Nurse* 16(8):563-566, 1998.

14. Clark JA, Kotyra LG, Brocious R: Rapid progression following cardiac surgery. *Critical Care Nurs Clin North America* 11(2):159-173, 1999.

15. Cummings CC, Byrum D: The beat goes on. *Am J Nurs* (Suppl Critical Care Nursing Update):9-12, 2001.

16. De Jong MJ, Morton PG: Predictors of atrial dysrhythmias for patients undergoing coronary artery bypass grafting. *Am J Crit Care* 9(6):388-395, 2000.

17. Griepp RB, Ergin MA, Galla JD, et al: Minimizing spinal cord injury during repair of descending thoracic and thoracoabdominal aneurysms: The Mount Sinai approach. *Semin Thorac Cardiovasc Surg* 10(1):25-28, 1998.

18. Finkelmeier BA: Coronary artery disease. In *Cardiothoracic surgical nursing.* Philadelphia: Lippincott, 2000, pp 5-22.

19. Finkelmeier BA: Valvular heart disease. In *Cardiothoracic surgical nursing.* Philadelphia: Lippincott, 2000, pp 23-36.

20. Finkelmeier BA: Disorders of the thoracic aorta. In *Cardiothoracic surgical nursing.* Philadelphia: Lippincott, 2000, pp 37-46.

21. Finkelmeier BA: Cardiomyopathies. In *Cardiothoracic surgical nursing.* Philadelphia: Lippincott, 2000, pp 59-64.

22. Finkelmeier BA: Congenital heart disease in adults. In *Cardiothoracic surgical nursing.* Philadelphia: Lippincott, 2000, pp 65-76.

23. Finkelmeier BA: Cardiopulmonary bypass. In *Cardiothoracic surgical nursing.* Philadelphia: Lippincott, 2000, pp 125-134.

24. Finkelmeier BA: Myocardial protection. In *Cardiothoracic surgical nursing.* Philadelphia: Lippincott, 2000, pp 134-140.

25. Finkelmeier BA: Blood conservation. In *Cardiothoracic surgical nursing.* Philadelphia: Lippincott, 2000, pp 141-148.

26. Finkelmeier BA: Surgical treatment of coronary artery disease . In *Cardiothoracic surgical nursing.* Philadelphia: Lippincott, 2000, pp 149-168.

27. Finkelmeier BA: Surgical treatment of valvular heart disease. In *Cardiothoracic surgical nursing.* Philadelphia: Lippincott, 2000, pp 169-188.

28. Finkelmeier BA: Surgery on the thoracic aorta. In *Cardiothoracic surgical nursing.* Philadelphia: Lippincott, 2000, pp 189-202.

29. Finkelmeier BA: Cardiovascular medications. In *Cardiothoracic surgical nursing.* Philadelphia: Lippincott, 2000, pp 327-340.

30. Finkelmeier BA: Complications of cardiac operations. In *Cardiothoracic surgical nursing.* Philadelphia: Lippincott, 2000, pp 341-356.

31. Finkelmeier BA: Heart, lung, and heart-lung transplantation. In *Cardiothoracic surgical nursing.* Philadelphia: Lippincott, 2000, pp 389-406.

32. Foster E, Cheitlin MD: Congenital heart disease. In Goldman L, Braunwald E, editors: *Primary cardiology.* Philadelphia: WB Saunders, 1998, pp 390-411.

33. George-Gay B, Hooper VD: Cardiovascular surgery. In Quinn DM, editor: *Ambulatory surgical nursing core curriculum.* Philadelphia: WB Saunders, 1999, pp 498-599.

34. Goldsborough MA, Miller MH, Gibson J, et al: Prevalence of leg wound complications after coronary artery bypass grafting: Determination of risk factors. *Am J Crit Care* 8(3):149-153,1999.

35. Goodwin JJ, Bissett L, Mason P, et al: Early extubation and early activity after open heart surgery. *Crit Care Nurse* 19(5):18-26.

36. Hayes EC, L'Ecuyer KM: A standard of care for radial artery grafting. *Am J Crit Care* 7(6):429-435, 1998.

37. Hicks FD: The cardiac surgical patient. In Litwack K, editor: *Core curriculum for perianesthesia nursing practice.* Philadelphia: WB Saunders, 1999, pp 271-305.

38. James S, Ashwill R, Droske S: The child with a cardiovascular alteration. In *Nursing care of children,* ed 2. Philadelphia: WB Saunders, 2002, pp 687-727.

39. Khan JH, McElhinney DB, Hall T, et al: Cardiac valve surgery in octogenarians: Improving quality of life and functional status. *Arch Surg* 133:887-893, 1998.

40. Koncsol K. DeVoogd K, Hravnak M, et al: Minimally invasive coronary artery bypass grafting: A kinder cut. *Dimens Crit Care Nurs* 18(2):21-23, 1999.

41. Maglish BL, Schwartz JL, Matheny RG: Outcomes improvement following minimally invasive direct coronary artery bypass surgery: The role of nursing in critical care and cardiovascular risk factor reduction. *Crit Care Nurs Clin North America* 11(2):177-188, 1999.

42. Marolda D, Finkelmeier BA: Postoperative patient management. In Finkelmeier BA: *Cardiothoracic surgical nursing.* Philadelphia: Lippincott, 2000, pp 255-276.

43. Maisel WH, Rawn J, Stenson W: Atrial fibrillation after cardiac surgery. *Ann Intern Med* 135(12):1061-1073, 2001.

44. Martich GD, Vega JD: Heart transplantation. In Shoemaker WC, Ayres S, Grenvik AN, et al, editors: *Textbook of critical care,* ed 4. Philadelphia: WB Saunders, 2000, pp 1958-1961.

45. Mason VF, Miller HH: Optimizing outcomes. *Am J Nurs* (Suppl Critical Care Nursing Update):13-15, 2001.

46. Michalopoulos A, Tzelepis G, Dafni U, et al: Determinants of hospital mortality after coronary artery bypass grafting. *Chest* 115(6):1598-1603, 1999.

47. Ockerman JC, Cronin SN: Day-of-surgery transfer after cardiac surgery. *Am J Nurs* (Suppl Critical Care Nursing Update): 33-37, 2000.

48. O'Gara PT: Diseases of the aorta: Aneurysms and dissection. In Goldman L, Braunwald E, editors: *Primary cardiology.* Philadelphia: WB Saunders, 1998, pp 413-426.

49. Ott RA, Gutfinger DE, Alimadadian H, et al: Simplified Parsonnet Risk Scale. *J Card Surg* 15(5):316-322, 2000.

50. Pottmeyer E, Stillman PC: Off-pump coronary artery bypass surgery. *Hosp Physician* 36(11):64-69, 2000.

51. Reger TB, Vargas G: The return of the radial artery in CABG. *Am J Nurs* 99(9):26-30, 1999.

52. Ryan TJ, Antman EM, Brooks NH, et al: The management of patients with acute myocardial infarction: American College of Cardiology/American Heart Association pocket guidelines. Vacaville, CA: Genentech, 2000.

53. Sakallaris BR, Halpin LS, Knapp M, et al: Same-day transfer of patients to the cardiac telemetry unit after surgery: The Rapid After Bypass Back into Telemetry (RABBIT) Program. *Crit Care Nurse* 20(2):50-68, 2000.

54. Savage LS, Grap M: Telephone monitoring after early discharge for cardiac surgery patients. *Am J Crit Care* 8(3):154-159, 1999.

55. Schmelz JO, Johnson D, Jorton JM, et al: Effects of position of chest drainage tube on volume drained and pressure. *Am J Crit Care* 8(5):319-323, 1999.

56. Schulze C, Conrad N, Schultz AE, et al: Reduced expression of systemic proinflammatory cytokines after off-pump versus conventional coronary artery bypass grafting. *Thorac Cardiovasc Surg* 364-369, 2000.

57. Shawgo R, York N: Preoperative versus postoperative weights: Which one should be used for cardiac surgery patients' drug and hemodynamic calculations? *Crit Care Nurse* 19(5):57-59, 1999.

58. Simpson K, Creehan PA: Congenital heart disease. In Simpson K, Creehan PA, editors: *Perinatal nursing.* Philadelphia: Williams & Wilkins, 2001, pp 579-582.

59. Sugimoto T, Masayoshi O, Nobuchika O, et al: Influence of functional tricuspid regurgitation on right ventricular function. *Ann Thorac Surg* 66:2044-2050, 1998.

60. Svensson LG, Hess KR, D'Agostino RS, et al: Reduction of neurologic injury after high-risk thoracoabdominal aortic operation. *Ann Thorac Surg* 66:132-138, 1998.

61. Young M, Bratina P, Hickenbottom S, et al: Neurologic complications after coronary artery bypass grafting. *J Cardiovasc Nurs* 13(1):26-33, 1998.

62. Zevola DR, Maier B: Improving the care of cardiothoracic surgery patients through advanced nursing skills. *Crit Care Nurse* 19(1):34-44, 1999.

Neurologic Surgery

PAMELA E. WINDLE

OBJECTIVES

At the conclusion of this chapter the reader will be able to:

1. Describe the anatomy and physiology of the nervous system as it relates to the patient undergoing neurologic surgery.

2. Discuss neurodiagnostic testing procedures.

3. Describe the pathophysiology, diagnosis, and treatment of the most common conditions requiring neurologic surgery.

Nursing care of the neurosurgical patient in the postanesthesia care unit (PACU) requires attention to all body systems and their interactions with the central nervous system (CNS). In particular, the PACU nurse must understand the pathophysiology, signs, and symptoms of increased intracranial pressure (ICP) and the appropriate medical and surgical interventions. Neurologic assessment and patient monitoring for potential complications are essential components of PACU nursing care.

ANATOMY AND PHYSIOLOGY OF THE CENTRAL NERVOUS SYSTEM

I. Cellular structure (Figure 40-1)
   A. Neuron: basic structural unit
      1. Nerve cell: receives and conducts impulses
      2. Functions
         a. Afferent, or sensory, neurons conduct impulses from receptors to CNS.
         b. Efferent, or motor, neurons conduct impulses to CNS to effector organs.
      3. Structure
         a. Cell body contains nucleus, cytoplasm, cell membrane.
         b. Nerve cell processes
            (1) Dendrites: short processes with multiple projects that conduct impulses to cell body; receive information
            (2) Axon: longest process of cell body; conducts impulses away from cell body; sends information
               (a) Myelinated (insulated)
               (b) Unmyelinated
      4. Functions (Figure 40-2)
         a. Sensory (afferent)
            (1) Special senses
               (a) Smell
               (b) Taste
               (c) Vision
               (d) Auditory
            (2) Pain and temperature
            (3) Proprioception (position sense and vibration)
            (4) Vibration
            (5) Touch (light and deep)
         b. Motor (efferent—to)
         c. Special (interneurons)

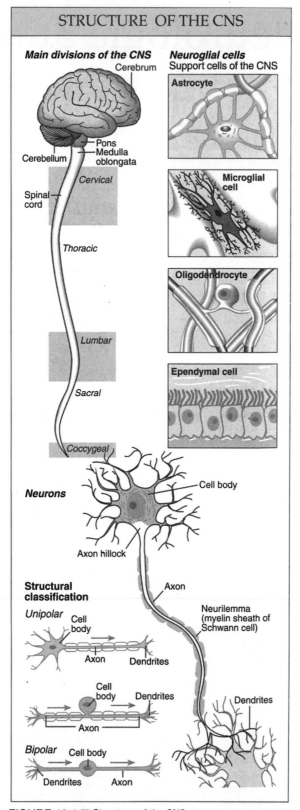

FIGURE 40-1 ■ Structure of the CNS. (From Luckmann J: *Saunders manual of nursing care.* Philadelphia: WB Saunders, 1997, p 652.)

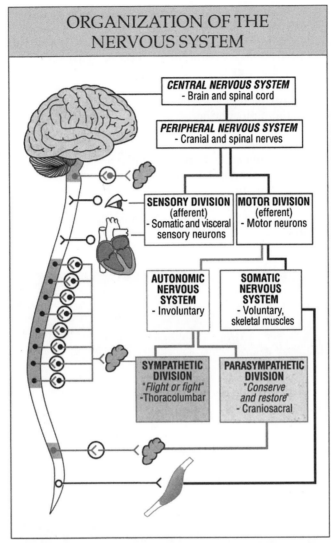

FIGURE 40-2 ■ Organization of the nervous system. (From Luckmann J: *Saunders manual of nursing care.* Philadelphia: WB Saunders, 1997, p 652.)

5. Transmission
   a. Electrical impulse
      (1) Depolarization—K+ ion influx, Na+ ion outflow
      (2) Repolarization—K+ ion pump, Na+ ion pump restore membrane potential
      (3) Axonal versus saltatory conduction
         (a) Axonal: entire axon must be depolarized, such as in unmyelinated fibers, making conduction slow.
         (b) Saltatory: sections of a myelinated axon are depolarized, impulse jumping from the node of Ranvier, leading to more rapid impulse conduction.
   b. Chemical transmission (Figure 40-3)
      (1) Synapse: vesicles release neurotransmitter (NT) from the presynaptic membrane into the synaptic cleft, which attaches to receptor sites on the postsynaptic membrane of the target organ (i.e., another neuron, muscle, other organs), resulting in the appropriate response (i.e., muscle

contraction or relaxation) or communication points between two neurons.

(2) Neurotransmitters (NT): protein substances that stimulate, facilitate, or inhibit impulse transmission across synapses
  (a) Adrenergic
    (i) Dopamine
    (ii) Norepinephrine
    (iii) Epinephrine
  (b) Cholinergic: acetylcholine
  (c) Serotonin
  (d) Gamma-aminobutyric acid (GABA)
  (e) Alpha-endorphins and beta-endorphins
  (f) Histamine
  (g) Substance P

B. Gray matter: cortex of brain; contains cell bodies and dendrites of CNS (Figure 40-4)

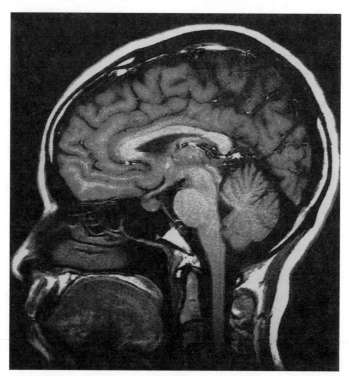

FIGURE 40-3 ■ Structure of a synapse. (From Luckmann J: *Saunders manual of nursing care.* Philadelphia: WB Saunders, 1997, p 653.)

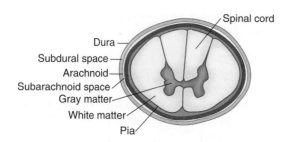

FIGURE 40-4 ■ Illustrations of the gray and white matter. Circulation of the CSF in the brain and spinal cord. (From Drain CB: *Perianesthesia nursing: A critical care approach*, ed 4. St Louis: WB Saunders, 2003, p 107.)

C. White matter: contains myelinated axons and neuroglia; supporting tissue
D. Neuroglia: support cells of CNS
  1. Nonexcitable
  2. More numerous than neurons
    a. Astrocytes
      (1) Small cell bodies with numerous projections
      (2) Projections end on blood vessels, ependyma, and pia mater.
      (3) Form the blood-brain barrier and provide structure
    b. Oligodendrocytes
      (1) Smaller and more delicate than astrocytes
      (2) Responsible for formation of myelin covering of axons
    c. Microglia
      (1) Smallest neurologic cells
      (2) Scavenger cells
    d. Ependymal cells
      (1) Line cerebrospinal fluid pathways (brain and spinal cord)
      (2) Single layer of cuboid cells with villi
      (3) Facilitate movement of cerebrospinal fluid (CSF)
II. Composition of the CNS
  A. Brain (Figure 40-5)
    1. Primary center for control
    2. Primary regulator for nervous system functions
    3. Three major structures
      a. Forebrain (prosencephalon) contains
        (1) Telencephalon (cerebrum) with its hemispheres
        (2) Diencephalon
      b. Midbrain (mesencephalon) contains
        (1) Cerebral peduncles
        (2) Corpora quadrigemina
        (3) Cerebral aqueduct
      c. Hindbrain (rhombencephalon) contains
        (1) Medulla oblongata
        (2) Pons
        (3) Cerebellum
        (4) Fourth ventricle
  B. Spinal cord
III. Extracerebral structures
  A. Scalp: protects integrity of skull
  B. Skull (Figure 40-6)
    1. Protects brain from external forces
    2. Composition
      a. Frontal bone (1)
      b. Parietal bones (2)
      c. Temporal bones (2)
      d. Occipital bone (1)
      e. Ethmoid bone (1)
      f. Sphenoid bone (1)
    3. Compartments (Figure 40-7)
      a. Anterior fossa: contains frontal lobes, olfactory nerves
      b. Middle fossa: contains temporal, parietal, occipital lobes
      c. Posterior fossa: contains cerebellum, brainstem (composed of midbrain, pons, and medulla)
  C. Meninges
    1. Function
      a. Protection for brain and spinal cord
      b. Support underlying structures

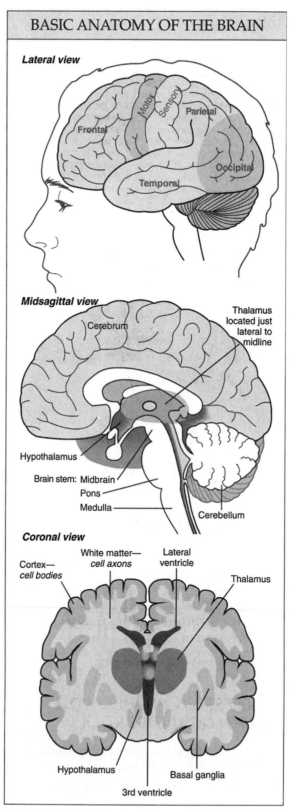

FIGURE 40-5 ■ Basic anatomy of the brain. (From Luckmann J: *Saunders manual of nursing care.* Philadelphia: WB Saunders, 1997, p 656.)

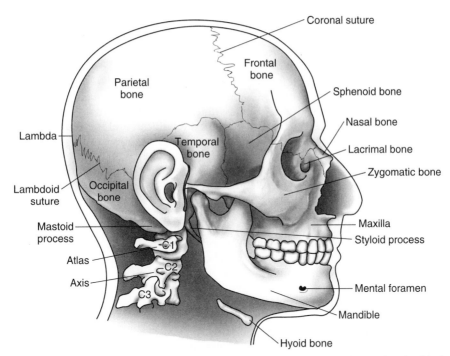

FIGURE 40-6 ■ Lateral view of the skull. (From Drain CB: *Perianesthesia nursing: A critical care approach,* ed 4. St Louis: WB Saunders, 2003, p 105.)

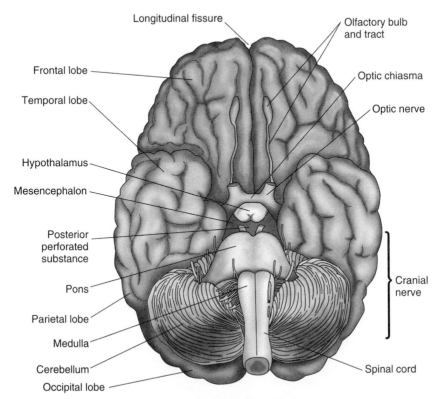

FIGURE 40-7 ■ Basal view of the brain. (From Drain CB: *Perianesthesia nursing: A critical care approach,* ed 4. St Louis: WB Saunders, 2003, p 95. Redrawn from Guyton AC: *Basic neuroscience: Anatomy and physiology,* ed 2. Philadelphia: WB Saunders, 1991.)

2. Layers from outermost layer inward; covering (Figure 40-12)
   a. Dura mater ("tough mother")
      (1) Skinny, dense, fibrous, inelastic membrane
      (2) Double layered, tough, fibrous covering
          (a) Outer layer (periosteal): periosteum of skull
          (b) Inner layer (meningeal): creates intracranial compartments
      (3) Dural folds: divide cranial vault into compartments
          (a) Falx cerebri: separates right and left cerebral hemispheres
          (b) Tentorium cerebelli: supports and separates the occipital and temporal lobes of cerebrum from cerebellum
          (c) Falx cerebelli: separates right and left cerebellar hemispheres
   b. Arachnoid membrane (weblike)
      (1) Fine, thin, delicate, elastic, fibrous
      (2) Closely adheres to dura mater
      (3) Separated from dura mater by subdural space
      (4) Contains blood vessels of varying sizes
      (5) Connects to pia mater by trabeculae
      (6) Arachnoid granulations and villi enable CSF to move from subarachnoid space to venous system.
      (7) CSF circulates through the "web."
   c. Pia mater ("soft mother") (Figure 40-8)
      (1) Innermost layer, one cell-layer thick, not visible
      (2) Rich in blood choroids plexuses and mesothelial cells
      (3) Meshlike, vascular membrane
      (4) Follows sulci and fissures
      (5) Inseparable from brain's surface, in direct contact with brain and spinal cord
3. Spaces
   a. Epidural
      (1) Potential space
      (2) Must be created by force (e.g., trauma, surgical dissection)
   b. Subdural
      (1) Potential space

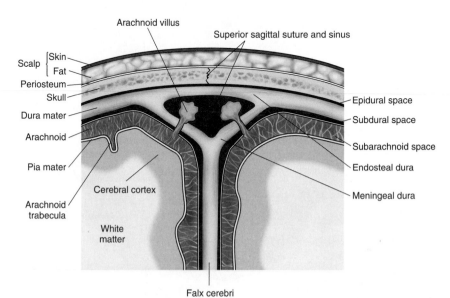

FIGURE 40-8 ■ Coronal section of the skull, brain, meninges, and superior sagittal sinus. (From Drain CB: *Perianesthesia nursing: A critical care approach*, ed 4. St Louis: WB Saunders, 2003, p 109.)

(2) Below dura, above arachnoid

(3) Subarachnoid: contains CSF, arteries, and veins

(4) Cisterns: pockets of arachnoid filled with CSF

IV. Cerebral vasculature

A. Arterial system: two paired systems of blood vessels (anterior and posterior) that combine to form circle of Willis (Figure 40-9, Figure 40-10)

1. Anterior arterial circulation

a. Common carotid: branches into external and internal carotid arteries

b. Internal carotid artery (ICA): enters cranial cavity at petrous portion of temporal bone; supplies most of hemispheres (except occipital lobe, basal ganglia) and upper two thirds of diencephalons

c. External carotid artery (ECA): supplies skin and muscles of face, scalp

d. Anterior cerebral artery (ACA): supplies medial surfaces of frontal and parietal lobes

e. Anterior communicating artery: connects anterior cerebral arteries

f. Middle cerebral artery (MCA)

(1) Largest branch of ICA

(2) Supplies two thirds of cerebral hemispheres (lateral surface)

2. Posterior arterial circulation

a. Vertebral arteries

(1) Paired arteries arising from subclavian artery

(2) Enter cranial vault through foramen magnum

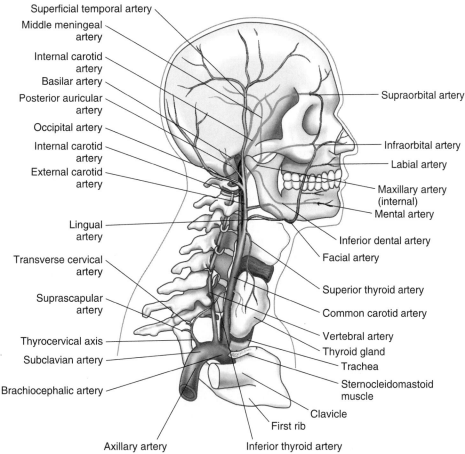

FIGURE 40-9 ■ Arterial supply to the neck and head. (From Drain CB: *Perianesthesia nursing: A critical care approach*, ed 4. St Louis: WB Saunders, 2003, p 113.)

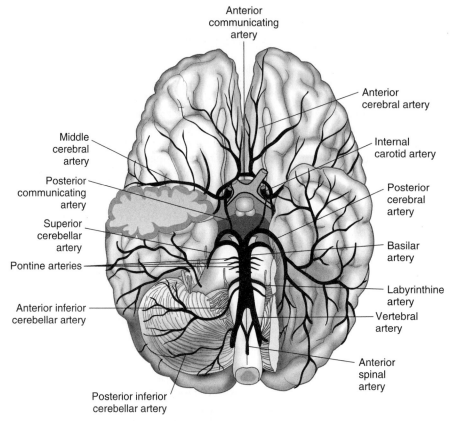

FIGURE 40-10 ■ Major arteries as seen on the base of the brain. (From Drain CB: *Perianesthesia nursing: A critical care approach,* ed 4. St Louis: WB Saunders, 2003, p 114.)

      (3) Branches supply spinal cord, underside of cerebellum, medulla, and choroid plexus of fourth ventricle.
      (4) Two arteries merge to form basilar artery.
   b. Basilar artery
      (1) Branches into posterior cerebral arteries and smaller vessels supplying posterior fossa
   c. Posterior cerebral artery (PCA): supplies brainstem, occipital lobe, inferior and medial surfaces of temporal lobe
B. Venous drainage: valveless, thin-walled system of superficial and deep veins and venous sinuses (Figure 40-11)
   1. Superficial veins: drain external surfaces of brain into superior sagittal, cavernous, sphenoparietal, and petrosal sinuses
     a. Superior cerebral veins
     b. Middle cerebral veins
     c. Inferior cerebral veins
   2. Deep veins: drain internal areas of brain
     a. Basal veins: connect superficial and deep cerebral veins
     b. Vein of Rosenthal
     c. Great cerebral vein (great vein of Galen)
   3. Venous sinuses: located between two layers of dura mater
     a. Posterior (superior) group
      (1) Superior sagittal
      (2) Inferior sagittal
      (3) Straight

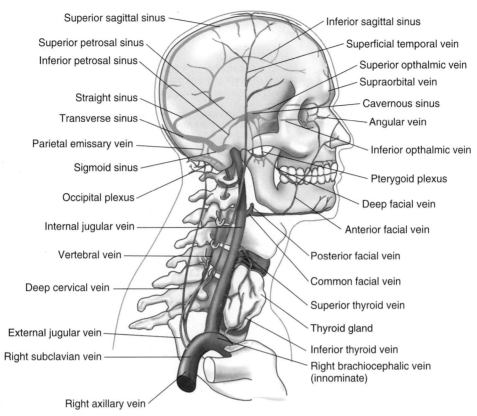

Superior sagittal sinus

Superior petrosal sinus

Inferior petrosal sinus

Straight sinus

Transverse sinus

Parietal emissary vein

Sigmoid sinus

Occipital plexus

Internal jugular vein

Vertebral vein

Deep cervical vein

External jugular vein

Right subclavian vein

Right axillary vein

Inferior sagittal sinus

Superficial temporal vein

Superior opthalmic vein

Supraorbital vein

Cavernous sinus

Angular vein

Inferior opthalmic vein

Pterygoid plexus

Deep facial vein

Anterior facial vein

Posterior facial vein

Common facial vein

Superior thyroid vein

Thyroid gland

Inferior thyroid vein

Right brachiocephalic vein (innominate)

FIGURE 40-11 ■ Venous drainage of the brain, head, and neck. (From Drain CB: *Perianesthesia nursing: A critical care approach,* ed 4. St Louis: WB Saunders, 2003, p 108.)

        (4) Transverse
        (5) Sigmoid
        (6) Occipital
    b. Anterior (interior) group
        (1) Cavernous
        (2) Superior petrosal (2)
        (3) Inferior petrosal (2)
        (4) Basilar plexus
V. Ventricular system (Figure 40-12)
  A. Formation of CSF
    1. Approximately 500 ml/day produced (0.37 ml/min)
    2. Volume of 150 ml in system at one time
    3. Secreted by choroid plexuses
    4. Choroid plexuses located in temporal horns of lateral ventricles, posterior portion of third ventricle, and roof of fourth ventricle
  B. Function
    1. Supports and cushions CNS
    2. Medium for exchange of nutrients and excretion pathways for cerebral metabolic waste products
    3. Maintains stable chemical environment
    4. Facilitates intercerebral transport
  C. CSF properties
    1. Appearance
      a. Clear
      b. Colorless
      c. Odorless

VENTRICLES OF THE BRAIN AND CEREBROSPINAL FLUID CIRCULATION

The ventricles are 4 fluid-filled cavities within the brain. They connect with one another and with the spinal canal, which descends down the center of the spinal cord.

These chambers and the spinal canal are filled with cerebrospinal fluid (CSF), a total volume of 135 ml.

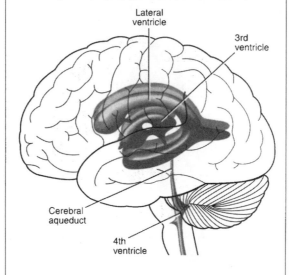

CSF circulates from the lateral ventricles, where most of it is formed, to the 3rd and 4th ventricles, down the spinal canal and throughout the subarachnoid space that surrounds the brain and spinal cord.
CSF provides cushioning for the central nervous system, allows fluid to shift from the cranial cavity to the spinal cavity, and carries nutrients to the brain. It returns to the general circulation primarily through the arachnoid villi, tiny projections of the subarachnoid space, which extend into the intradural venous sinuses. The venous sinuses collect venous blood as well as CSF and pass this mixture into the jugular veins.

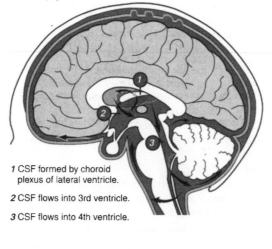

1 CSF formed by choroid plexus of lateral ventricle.

2 CSF flows into 3rd ventricle.

3 CSF flows into 4th ventricle.

FIGURE 40-12 ■ Ventricles of the brain and CSF circulation. (From Luckmann J: *Saunders manual of nursing care.* Philadelphia: WB Saunders, 1997, p 656.)

2. Protein: 15 to 45 mg/ml
3. Glucose
   a. 50 to 75 mg/dl
   b. Two thirds of serum glucose
4. White blood cells: 0 to 5/mm^3
5. Red blood cells: none
6. pH: 7.35 to 7.40
7. Specific gravity: 1.005 to 1.009
8. Pressure: 0 to 15 mm Hg or 50 to 150 mm H_2O (depending on the type of monitoring system used)

D. Blood-brain barrier (BBB)
   1. Composed of network of endothelial cells (cells of capillaries) and projections from astrocytes close to neurons
      a. Located throughout brain, except in hypothalamus, pineal gland area, and floor of fourth ventricle in upper medulla
      b. More permeable in newborn than adult
   2. Tight junctions between endothelial cells and astrocytes
   3. Functions
      a. Preserves homeostasis of CNS
      b. Selectively permeable to facilitate entry of needed metabolites and remove toxic or unnecessary metabolites
      c. Permeable to water, oxygen, carbon dioxide, other gases, glucose, and lipid soluble substances
      d. Breakdown of BBB by inflammation, tumors, and toxins allows large molecules to pass directly into CNS.

E. Cerebral hemispheres
   1. Cerebral cortex: outermost layer, composed of gray matter
      a. Gyri or convolution: raised projections
      b. Sulci: grooves between gyri
         (1) Shallow: Sulcus
         (2) Deeper: Fissure
      c. Left cortex: deals with symbols and symbolic material, including language, mathematics, abstractions, reasoning; analytic aspect
      d. Right cortex: deals with visual-spatial tasks, processing of whole sensory experiences such as dancing, art appreciation; creative aspect
   2. Lobes
      a. Frontal lobes (2)
         (1) Motor cortex: controls voluntary and fine motor movement
         (2) Sensory cortex: sensory association areas integrate and interpret sensory input
         (3) Memory, attention span
         (4) Personality and emotional behavior
         (5) Complex intellectual functioning, goal-directed behavior
         (6) Broca's area
             (a) Left hemisphere
             (b) Expressive speech (producing language)
      b. Parietal lobes (2): posterior to central sulcus of Rolando
         (1) Sensory discrimination
         (2) Tactile receptive area (i.e., soft, hard texture, smooth, etc.)
         (3) Body image, association area (allows body/self awareness/ orientation in space)
      c. Temporal lobes (2): located under fissure of Sylvius
         (1) Hearing
         (2) Olfaction
         (3) Sensory speech (Wernicke's area), left hemisphere
         (4) Short-term memory
         (5) Sound interpretation, right hemisphere
      d. Occipital lobe (1): integrates visual cortex reception

      3. Corpus callosum
        a. Bundle of nerve fibers
        b. Connects cerebral hemispheres
        c. Allows transfer of information from one hemisphere to the other
      4. Basal ganglia (cerebral nuclei) (Figure 40-13)
        a. Group of deep subcortical gray matter
        b. Buried deep in hemispheres near thalamus and lateral ventricle
        c. Group of neuron cell bodies lying within the CNS
        d. Important part of the extrapyramidal motor pathway
        e. Link cerebral cortex to certain thalamic nuclei
        f. Connect with hindbrain areas for coordination of muscle movements
        g. Modulate voluntary body movements, especially in hands and legs (as seen in Parkinson's syndrome)
      5. Internal capsule
        a. White matter pathways
        b. Carries ascending and descending motor and sensory fibers
  F. Limbic system (limbic lobe/rhinencephalon)
      1. Two rings of limbic cortex and other tissue surrounding ventricles
      2. "Visceral" or "emotional" brain and other behavioral response (anger, aggression)
      3. Interconnections with other cerebral structures and hemispheres
      4. Damage affects emotional responses, sexual behavior and drive, motivation, biologic rhythms.
  G. Diencephalon: Second major division of the forebrain, located within cerebrum and continuous with midbrain
      1. Epithalamus
        a. Narrow band forming roof of diencephalons
        b. Contains pineal body that secretes melatonin
        c. Associated with reproductive activity, inhibition or delay of gonadal development
      2. Thalamus (sensory relay station)
        a. Located on both sides of third ventricle
        b. Consist of right and left egg-shaped masses

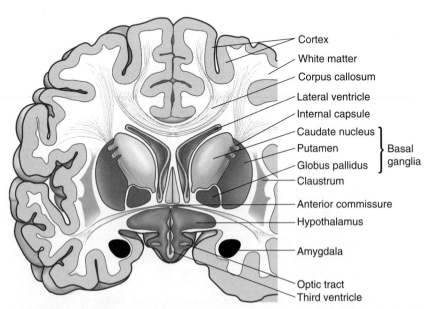

FIGURE 40-13 ■ Section of the cerebrum showing the basal ganglia. (From Drain CB: *Perianesthesia nursing: A critical care approach,* ed 4. St Louis: WB Saunders, 2003, p 96. Redrawn from Guyton AC: *Basic neuroscience: Anatomy and physiology,* ed 2. Philadelphia: WB Saunders, 1991.)

      c. Greatest bulk of diencephalon

      d. Acts as relay center for all incoming sensory (except for taste and smell) and motor tracts

      e. Perception of primary sensations of pain, touch, pressure, temperature

      f. Contributes to emotional activities, attentive processes, and behavioral expression

      g. Coordinates and regulates functional activity of cerebral cortex

   3. Subthalamus

      a. Located below the thalamus and above the midbrain

      b. Correlation center for the optic and vestibular impulses

      c. May cause violent involuntary movement on the opposite limb

   4. Hypothalamus

      a. Connected to pituitary gland by hypophyseal stalk (infundibulum)

      b. Forms base of diencephalons and part of the third ventricle

      c. Maintains internal body homeostasis and temperature control

         (1) Regulates body temperature, endocrine activities, water balance, carbohydrate and fat metabolism

         (2) Appestat: controls and regulates appetite

         (3) Has role in maintaining awake state

         (4) Hormonal feedback system (growth and sexual maturity)

         (5) Secretes neurohormones (hypothalamic releasing and inhibiting factors), oxytocin, vasopressin (antidiuretic hormone)

         (6) Sympathetic control (pulse rate, blood pressure)

      d. Influences behavior patterns

         (1) Helps control primitive responses such as fear, instinct, self-preservation

         (2) Physical expression of emotions and emotional behavior

         (3) Enhances CNS activity

      e. Cardiovascular regulation

      f. Uterine contractility and milk ejection

 H. Brainstem (Figure 40-14)

   1. Contains reticular activating system (RAS)

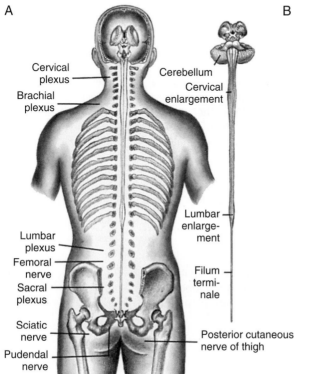

A

B

FIGURE 40-14 ■ **A,**Posterior view of brainstem; **B**, Anterior view of brainstem and spinal cord. (From Thompson J: *Mosby's clinical nursing,* ed 5. St Louis: Mosby, 2002, p 226. From Rudy EB: *Advanced neurological and neurosurgical nursing.* St. Louis: Mosby, 1984.)

Cervical plexus

Brachial plexus

Cerebellum

Cervical enlargement

Lumbar plexus

Femoral nerve

Sacral plexus

Sciatic nerve

Pudendal nerve

Lumbar enlargement

Filum terminale

Posterior cutaneous nerve of thigh

2. Relays messages between cerebral structures and spinal cord
3. Gives rise to cranial nerves third through twelfth (III to XII)
4. Composition
    a. Midbrain (mesencephalon)
        (1) Short narrow segment that connects the forebrain with the hindbrain
        (2) Conduction pathway and reflex control center
        (3) Connects to cerebrum through diencephalons
        (4) Control of various visual, auditory, postural, and righting reflexes
            (a) Third cranial nerve (oculomotor) dorsal or posterior portion
                (i) Moves eyes up, down, and medially
                (ii) Opens lid
                (iii) Parasympathetic outflow constricts pupil.
                (iv) Sympathetic outflow dilates pupil.
            (b) Fourth cranial nerve (trochlear)
                (i) Moves eye down and in
    b. Pons
        (1) Bridge between the midbrain and the medulla oblongata
        (2) Roof contains portion of reticular formation.
        (3) Lower pons regulates respiration.
        (4) Contains apneustic, pneumotaxic respiratory centers
            (a) Fifth cranial nerve (trigeminal)
                (i) Sensation of face (three branches)
                (ii) Sensation to cornea (corneal reflex)
                (iii) Muscles of mastication
            (b) Sixth cranial nerve (abducens)
                (i) Moves eye out laterally
            (c) Seventh cranial nerve (facial)
                (i) Movement of facial expression
            (d) Eighth cranial nerve (auditory or acoustic)
                (i) Auditory branch (hearing)
                (ii) Vestibular branch (balance)
    c. Medulla oblongata
        (1) Lower portion of brainstem
        (2) Located between the foramen magnum and pons
        (3) Connects to cervical spinal cord
        (4) Regulatory centers for cardiac, respiratory, vasomotor, rhythmicity functions
        (5) Center for protective reflexes: coughing, gagging, sneezing, swallowing, vomiting (respiratory and vomiting center)
            (a) Ninth cranial nerve (glossopharyngeal)
                (i) Taste—anterior two thirds of tongue
                (ii) Sensory to tongue and soft palate
            (b) Tenth cranial nerve (vagus)
                (i) Parasympathetic outflow
                (ii) Sensory to posterior pharynx
            (c) Eleventh cranial nerve (accessory)
                (i) Shoulder shrug
            (d) Twelfth cranial nerve (hypoglossal)
                (i) Extends tongue
I. Cerebellum
    1. Overlaps the pons and the medulla oblongata
    2. Located at base of brain, below occipital lobes
    3. No sensory function and does not initiate movement
    4. Right and left hemispheres connected at midline
    5. Connected to brainstem by three sets of cerebellar peduncles
        a. Superior
        b. Middle

        c. Inferior
6. Receives input from brainstem and spinal cord nuclei
7. Functions
        a. Coordinates muscle tone
        b. Coordinates voluntary movements
        c. Controls equilibrium posture and balance
        d. Motor gracefulness
8. Damage to a part of the cerebellum can result in nystagmus and a reeling gait.

J. The fourth ventricle
1. Diamond-shaped space
2. Located between cerebellum, pons, medulla oblongata
3. Contains CSF

K. Cranial nerves (Figure 40-15, Table 40-1)
1. Help in remembering names of cranial nerves (CN) (Table 40-2)
2. Help in remembering whether nerves are sensory, motor, or both (S, M, B) (Table 40-3)

L. Autonomic nervous system (Table 40-4)
1. Part of peripheral nervous system

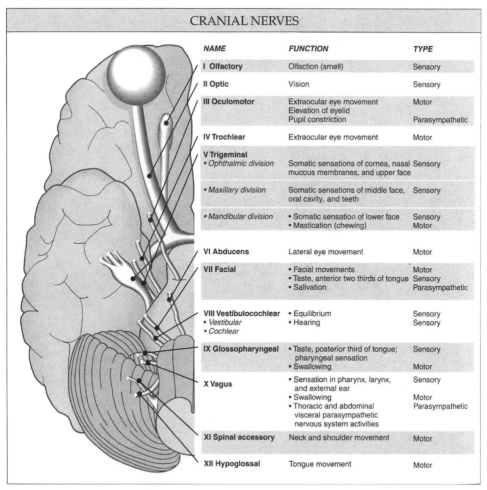

CRANIAL NERVES

NAME	FUNCTION	TYPE
I Olfactory	Olfaction (smell)	Sensory
II Optic	Vision	Sensory
III Oculomotor	Extraocular eye movement Elevation of eyelid Pupil constriction	Motor Parasympathetic
IV Trochlear	Extraocular eye movement	Motor
V Trigeminal • *Ophthalmic division*	Somatic sensations of cornea, nasal mucous membranes, and upper face	Sensory
• *Maxillary division*	Somatic sensations of middle face, oral cavity, and teeth	Sensory
• *Mandibular division*	• Somatic sensation of lower face • Mastication (chewing)	Sensory Motor
VI Abducens	Lateral eye movement	Motor
VII Facial	• Facial movements • Taste, anterior two thirds of tongue • Salivation	Motor Sensory Parasympathetic
VIII Vestibulocochlear • *Vestibular* • *Cochlear*	• Equilibrium • Hearing	Sensory Sensory
IX Glossopharyngeal	• Taste, posterior third of tongue; pharyngeal sensation • Swallowing	Sensory Motor
X Vagus	• Sensation in pharynx, larynx, and external ear • Swallowing • Thoracic and abdominal visceral parasympathetic nervous system activities	Sensory Motor Parasympathetic
XI Spinal accessory	Neck and shoulder movement	Motor
XII Hypoglossal	Tongue movement	Motor

FIGURE 40-15 ■ Cranial nerves. (From Luckmann J: *Saunders manual of nursing care.* Philadelphia: WB Saunders, 1997, p 658. Tabular material from Black JM, Matassarin-Jacobs E, editors: *Luckmann and Sorensen's medical-surgical nursing: A psychophysiologic approach,* ed 4. Philadelphia: WB Saunders, 1993, p 630.)

■ TABLE 40-1

■ ■ **Rapid Neurologic Evaluation of Cranial Nerve Function**

Nerve	Origin	Function	Method of Testing	Site of Involvement	Abnormal Findings	Frequency
I Olfactory	Olfactory bulb	Sensory—sense of smell	Identify odors, one nostril at a time	Fracture of cribriform plate or in ethmoid area	Anosmia	Uncommon
II Optic	Lateral geniculate body	Sensory—vision and circuit for light reflex	■ Acuity—Snellen chart or newspaper; test each eye separately ■ Visual fields—confrontation method, each eye separately; move finger from eight cardinal points and indicate when it is seen	Direct trauma to orbit or globe, or fracture involving optic foramen	Loss of both direct and consensual papillary constriction when light flashed in affected eye; unaffected eye has normal direct and consensual response	Common
III Oculomotor	Midbrain	Motor—papillary constriction, elevation of upper eyelid, extraocular movements conjointly with III, IV, and VI	■ Light flashed in affected eye ■ Light flashed in unaffected eye	Pressure on geniculate body; laceration or intracerebral clot in temporal, parietal, occipital lobes	Absence of blink when hand brought suddenly from side; indicates visual field defect (always homonymous)	Common
				Pressure of herniating uncus on nerve just before it enters cavernous sinus, or fracture involving cavernous sinus	■ Dilated pupil, ptosis; eye turns down and out ■ Direct pupil reflex absent; consensual reflux present ■ Direct pupil reflex absent; consensual reflux absent	Very frequent
IV Trochlear	Midbrain	Motor—extraocular movements of eye downward and inward (oblique muscles)	Follow fingers, using eight cardinal points	Course of nerve around brainstem	Eye fails to move down and out	Infrequent

Nerve	Location	Function	Assessment	Cause of Injury	Signs/Symptoms	Frequency
V Trigeminal	Pons	*Sensory* ■ Ophthalmic: cornea of eye and above ■ Maxillary: cheek and upper lips ■ Mandibular: lower lip and chin *Motor* ■ Masseter and temporal muscles: biting down and chewing, lateral movement of jaw	Touch cotton to both sides along divisions, corneal reflex	Direct injury to terminal branches, particularly second division in roof of maxillary sinus	■ Loss of sensation of pain and touch ■ Paresthesias	Uncommon (exception: trigeminal neuralgia)
VI Abducens	Pons	Motor—extraocular movements of eye laterally	Follow fingers using eight cardinal points; test III, IV, VI together	As with III, IV	Eyes fail to move laterally	Infrequent
VII Facial	Pons	Motor—facial muscles around eyes, mouth, and forehead	"Wrinkle your forehead"	Supranuclear: intracerebral clot	Forehead wrinkles because of bilateral innervation of frontalis; otherwise, paralysis of facial muscles as below	Frequent
				Peripheral: laceration or contusion in parotid area	Paralysis of facial muscles; eye remains open; angle of mouth droops; forehead fails to wrinkle	Frequent
		Sensory—taste receptors on anterior two thirds of tongue	Identify flavors—Does food taste the same?	Peripheral: fracture of temporal bone	As above, plus associated involvement of acoustic nerve (see below), dry cornea, and loss of taste on anterior two thirds of tongue	Frequent

Continued

TABLE 40-1 *Cont'd*

Rapid Neurologic Evaluation of Cranial Nerve Function

Nerve	Origin	Function	Method of Testing	Site of Involvement	Abnormal Findings	Frequency
VIII Acoustic	Pons	Sensory ■ Cochlear division: hearing ■ Vestibular division: maintenance of equilibrium and posturing of head	In children and unresponsive patients, clap hands close to ears ■ Weber's test: bone conduction with tuning fork ■ Rinne's test: air conduction using mastoid process Caloric test	Fracture of petrous portion of temporal bone; CN VII often involved Caloric test negative	Startle reflex Sound not heard by involved ear	Common
IX Glossopharyngeal	Medulla	Motor—constructors of pharynx used in swallowing Sensory—taste receptors on posterior one third of tongue	Touch walls of pharynx with tongue blade Identify tastes	Brainstem or deep laceration of neck	Loss of taste to posterior one third of tongue Loss of sensation on affected side of soft palate	Rare Rare
X Vagus	Medulla	Sensory—pharynx and larynx Motor—pharynx and larynx, movement of soft palate and uvula; conjointly with IX, ability to speak clearly	Touch with tongue blade to emit gag reflex Watch movement of uvula when patient says "ahhh"	Brainstem or deep laceration of neck Compression by herniation	Sagging of soft palate; deviation of uvula to normal side ■ Hoarseness from paralysis of vocal cords	Rare
XI Spinal accessory	Medulla	Motor—sternocleidomastoid, trapezius, and rhomboid muscles	Shrug shoulders against resistance, turn head against resistance, flex chin	Laceration of neck	Inability to shrug shoulders or turn head	Rare
XII Hypoglossal	Medulla	Motor—tongue	"Stick out tongue, wiggle tongue"	Neck laceration, usually associated with major vessel damage	Tongue protrudes toward affected side; dysarthria	Rare

■ TABLE 40-2
■ ■ **Help in Remembering Names of Cranial Nerves (CN)**

Mnemonic	CN Number Name
O (n)	I Olfactory
O (ld)	II Optic
O (lympus)	III Oculomotor
T (owering)	IV Trochlear
T (ops)	V Trigeminal
A	VI Abducens
F (inn)	VII Facial
A (nd)	VIII Auditory
G (erman)	IX Glossopharyngeal
V (iewed)	X Vagus
S (ome)	XI Spinal accessory
H (ops)	XII Hypoglossal

■ TABLE 40-3
■ ■ **Help in Remembering Whether Nerves Are Sensory, Motor, or Both (S, M, B)**

Mnemonic	CN Number Name
S (ome)	I Olfactory
S (ay)	II Optic
M (arry)	III Oculomotor
M (oney)	IV Trochlear
B (ut)	V Trigeminal
M (y)	VI Abducens
B (rother)	VII Facial
S (ays)	VIII Auditory
B (ad)	IX Glossopharyngeal
B (usiness)	X Vagus
M (arry)	XI Spinal accessory
M (en)	XII Hypoglossal

2. Implications for patient undergoing intracranial surgery should be considered.
3. Overall purpose: regulation of involuntary functions of internal organs
4. Sympathetic nervous system
   a. Originates in thoracic area of spine and upper lumbar segments of spinal cord
   b. Impulses travel from CNS to ganglia (relay stations outside spinal column), along postganglionic (adrenergic) fibers to effector organs where catecholamines are released (norepinephrine).
      (1) Regulates body's energy expenditures
      (2) Prepares body for stress (fight or flight)
5. Parasympathetic nervous system
   a. Cell bodies located in extreme ends of spinal cord (brainstem, sacrum)
   b. Transmits impulses from CNS along preganglionic fibers to ganglia located in or near effector organs
      (1) Nerves are cholinergic.
      (2) Acetylcholine released
   c. Helps in conservation of body's energy
   d. Affects localized, discrete areas rather than whole body

■ TABLE 40-4
■ ■ **Effects of Autonomic Nervous System**

Effector Organ	Sympathetic (Adrenergic Effect)	Parasympathetic (Cholinergic Effect)
Pupil	Dilates	Constricts
Salivary glands	Decreases secretion	Increases secretion
Bronchi	Dilates	Constricts
Respiratory rate	Increases	Decreases
Heart		
Pulse	Increases	Decreases
Contraction	Strengthens	Weakens
Blood pressure	Increases	Decreases
Stomach	Decreases contractions	Increases contractions
Adrenal glands	Stimulates secretion of epinephrine, norepinephrine	Decreases secretions
Digestive tract	Decreases motility	Increases motility
	Contracts sphincters	Relaxes sphincters
	Inhibits secretions	Stimulates secretions
Bladder	Relaxes	Contracts
	Relaxes sphincter	
Sweat glands	Increases activity	Decreases activity
Hair	Piloerection	Relaxes
Blood vessels		
Coronary	Dilates	No significant effect
Skeletal muscle	Dilates	Constricts
Skin	Constricts	No significant effect

DISORDERS POTENTIALLY REQUIRING SURGICAL INTERVENTION

I. Brain tumors
  A. Pathologic condition: damage to brain tissue through expansion, infiltration, or destruction
  B. Classification: no universally accepted system
    1. Benign versus malignant
      a. Malignancy depends on
        (1) Rate of growth
        (2) Infiltration
        (3) Location
        (4) Grading III to IV
          (a) Very poorly differentiated
          (b) Has lost characteristics of cell of origin
          (c) Poor prognosis
  C. Clinical findings: dependent on location of tumor and degree of increased ICP
    1. Headache
      a. Characteristically worse in morning
      b. Intensified by activity
    2. Seizures: adults with first-time seizure are considered to have brain tumor until proven otherwise.
    3. Papilledema
    4. Vomiting
    5. Sensory and motor dysfunctions
    6. Speech impairments
    7. Changes in personality or mental function

    D. Diagnostic tools
        1. History and physical assessment
        2. Skull films
        3. Computed tomography (CT) scan
        4. Magnetic resonance imaging (MRI)
        5. Angiography
    E. Treatment modalities
        1. Radiation therapy: often initially to shrink tumor
        2. Chemotherapy
        3. Craniotomy
        4. Radiosurgery: gamma knife
II. Brain abscess
    A. Pathologic condition: pocket(s) of exudates formed from infections of adjacent tissue or hematogenous spread
    B. Clinical findings
        1. Headache
        2. Focal signs
        3. Signs of increased ICP
    C. Diagnostic tools
        1. History and physical assessment
        2. Skull films
        3. CT scan
        4. MRI
        5. Culture of abscess exudates through stereotactic approach
        6. Routine laboratory studies
    D. Treatment modalities
        1. Aspiration or excision of abscess
        2. Intravenous antibiotic therapy
        3. Treatment of increased ICP
III. Trigeminal neuralgia
    A. Pathologic condition
        1. Cause unknown
        2. Most common in middle and later life
    B. Clinical findings
        1. Explosive, severe pain in distribution of CN V
        2. Pain may spontaneously remit and recur.
        3. Pain may cause patient to avoid activities that intensify it, such as eating, hygiene.
    C. Treatment modalities
        1. Pharmacologic
            a. Carbamazepine (Tegretol)
            b. Phenytoin (Dilantin)
        2. Alcohol block of one or more branches
        3. Surgical retrogasserian rhizotomy
        4. Sensory root decompression (Taarnhoj procedure)
        5. Microsurgical decompression of trigeminal root (Jannetta procedure)
        6. Radio frequency percutaneous electrocoagulation
        7. Vascular decompression of CN V through posterior fossa craniotomy
IV. Craniocerebral trauma
    A. Mechanism of injury
        1. Deceleration: head hits stationary object.
        2. Acceleration: head struck by moving object
        3. Acceleration-deceleration (coup-contrecoup): head hits object; brain rebounds inside cranium against opposite cranial bones.
        4. Shear strain: twisting, sliding motions of brainstem
    B. Types of injuries
        1. Primary (impact) injury: damage produced by blow
            a. Concussion: transient loss of consciousness lasting several minutes

     b. Contusion: actual bruising of brain tissue resulting in structural damage

     c. Laceration: actual tearing of brain tissue

     d. Fractures

        (1) Linear

        (2) Comminuted

        (3) Depressed

        (4) Basilar

  2. Intracranial secondary injury: damage that follows impact injury

     a. Hematomas

        (1) Epidural: bleeding, usually from middle meningeal artery; accumulates between skull and dura

        (2) Subdural: venous bleeding beneath dura mater; may be acute, subacute, or chronic

     b. ICP

     c. Brain swelling

     d. Cerebral edema

  3. Extracranial secondary injury

     a. Hypoxia

     b. Systemic hypotension

C. Clinical findings (variable) (Figure 40-16)

  1. Epidural hematoma

     a. Momentary loss of consciousness

     b. "Lucid interval"

     c. Rapid deterioration

     d. Signs of increased ICP

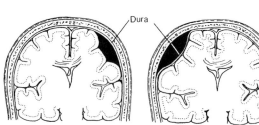

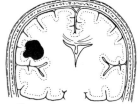

Part 1   **A.** Subdural hematoma   **B.** Epidural hematoma   **C.** Intracerebral hematoma

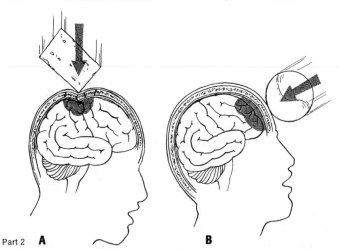

Part 2   **A**   **B**

FIGURE 40-16 ■ Types of hematomas. (In Drain CB: *Perianesthesia nursing: A critical care approach,* ed 4. St Louis: WB Saunders, 2003, p 522. From Clochesy J, Breu C, Cardin S, et al: (1996) *Critical care nursing,* ed 2. Philadelphia: WB Saunders, 1996; and Luckmann J, Sorensen KC: *Medical-surgical nursing: A psychophysiologic approach,* ed 3. Philadelphia: WB Saunders, 1987.)

2. Subdural hematoma
   a. Drowsiness
   b. Agitation
   c. Slow cerebration and confusion
   d. Signs of increased ICP
3. Intracerebral hematoma
   a. Immediate neurologic deficits
   b. Signs of increased ICP
   c. Loss of consciousness usually occurs from onset of injury.
4. Skull fractures (signs and symptoms depend on anterior or middle fossa)
   a. Basilar fracture most common
   b. Involves bones of floor of cranial vault
   c. Otorrhea, rhinorrhea
   d. Battle's sign: ecchymosis over mastoid process
   e. Raccoon's eyes: periorbital ecchymosis
   f. Otorrhagia
   g. Test ear or nasal drainage for glucose, and observe for concentric circles (halo or ring sign) on dressing or linens.
5. Open head injuries
   a. Gunshot and stab wounds
   b. Potential for infection is high.
D. Diagnostic tools
   1. History and physical assessment
   2. Skull films
   3. CT scan
   4. MRI (not for initial diagnosis; may be used for follow-up)
   5. Routine laboratory studies
      a. Alcohol and drug screen
      b. Arterial blood gases (ABGs)
   6. Cervical spine films
E. Treatment modalities
   1. Surgical evacuation of hematoma usually needed, depending on size and presence of signs of increased ICP
   2. Debridement
      a. Removal of bone fragments, foreign objects, infracted tissue
      b. Permits inspection of skull fractures and penetrating wound
V. Intracranial hemorrhage
   A. Pathologic condition
      1. Arterial aneurysm rupture: dilation of weakened arterial wall, causing blood-filled sac
      2. Arteriovenous malformation (AVM) rupture
         a. Congenital communication of arteries and veins without intervening capillaries
         b. Forms tangled, interwoven mass
         c. Occurs more often in younger patients
         d. Vessels rupture more easily than normal vessels.
      3. Hypertensive hemorrhage
   B. Clinical findings
      1. Subarachnoid hemorrhage
         a. Sudden, violent headache: "worst headache of my life"
         b. Altered level of consciousness (LOC)
         c. Signs of increased ICP
         d. Nausea and vomiting
         e. Meningeal irritation
            (1) Kernig's sign: resistance and pain when patient's leg is flexed at hip and knee
            (2) Brudzinski's sign: flexion of hips and knees in response to passive flexion of neck

        f. Focal signs depending on location of bleeding

        g. Bloody CSF

        h. Hunt and Hess classification of aneurysms (Table 40-5)

    2. Intracerebral hemorrhage

        a. Abrupt changes in LOC

        b. Signs of increased ICP

        c. Headache

        d. Nausea and vomiting

        e. Focal signs dependent on site of bleeding

C. Diagnostic tools

    1. History and physical assessment

    2. Lumbar puncture and CSF analysis

    3. Arteriogram, magnetic resonance angiography (MRA)

    4. CT scan

    5. Routine laboratory studies

D. Treatment modalities

    1. Medical

        a. Minimize increases in ICP.

        b. Promote cerebrovascular perfusion.

        c. Prevent complications.

    2. Surgical

        a. Craniotomy for evacuation of hematomas, clipping of aneurysm

        b. Carotid endarterectomy

        c. Extracranial-intracranial bypass

        d. Embolization of AVM, aneurysm

        e. Gamma knife radiosurgery

        f. Interventional neuroradiology

            (1) Insertion of balloons and coils

            (2) Angioplasty and stenting

VI. Hydrocephalus

A. Pathologic condition

    1. Noncommunicating hydrocephalus

        a. Obstruction of CSF flow within ventricular system, resulting in lack of communication within subarachnoid space

        b. Etiology

             (1) Congenital malformation of ventricular system

             (2) Adhesions caused by inflammatory processes (e.g., meningitis)

             (3) Obstructive, space-occupying lesions

    2. Communicating hydrocephalus

        a. Obstruction of CSF flow in subarachnoid space or basilar cisterns

        b. Too few or nonfunctioning arachnoid villi cannot reabsorb CSF sufficiently.

        c. Etiology

■ TABLE 40-5
■ ■ **Hunt and Hess Classification of Aneurysms**

Grade 0	Unruptured aneurysm
Grade I	Asymptomatic or minimal headache, slight nuchal rigidity
Grade I-A	Fixed neurologic deficit but not acute meningeal signs
Grade II	Moderate to severe headache; nuchal rigidity present; CN III palsy, but no other neurologic deficits
Grade III	Drowsy, confused, mild focal deficits
Grade IV	Stupor, moderate to severe hemiparesis, early decerebrate rigidity, vegetative disturbances
Grade V	Deep coma, decerebrate rigidity, moribund

(1) Congenital malformations

(2) Adhesions caused by inflammatory disorders

(3) Overproduction of CSF

(4) Occlusion of arachnoid villi by particulate matter (blood, pus)

B. Clinical findings: dependent on patient's age and type of hydrocephalus

1. Infants

a. Enlarged head

b. Thin, fragile, shiny-looking scalp

c. Weak, underdeveloped neck muscles

d. Poor sucking reflex

e. "Sunset" eyes

f. Signs of increased ICP

2. Older children and adults

a. Impaired mental function

b. Gait disturbances

c. Signs of increased ICP

d. Papilledema

e. Incontinence

f. Nausea and vomiting

C. Diagnostic tools

1. History and physical assessment

2. Skull series

3. CT scan

4. MRI

5. Isotope cisternogram (flow study)

6. Lumbar puncture

7. Transillumination of infant's skull

D. Treatment modalities

1. Removal of obstruction

2. Ventriculostomy with external ventricular drainage for temporary relief

3. Insertion of shunt

SELECTED OPERATIVE PROCEDURES

I. Burr hole (trephination)

A. Procedure: removal of isolated or multiple small, circular portions of cranium for purposes of clot removal or in preparation for a craniotomy where a series of burr holes are made and connected

B. Purpose

1. Evacuation of extracerebral clot

2. Removal of subdural fluid

3. Drainage of CSF

4. Aspiration of CSF

5. Instillation of medications

6. Instillation of air for ventriculography

II. Craniotomy

A. Procedure

1. Series of burr holes made into skull

2. Burr holes connected with saw

3. Bone flap created

4. Opening kept as small as possible without restricting surgical approach

5. Bone flap may or may not be replaced.

B. Purpose

1. Removal of tumor

2. Clipping of an aneurysm

3. Repair of a cerebral injury

4. Protection of cranial contents

     5. Improvement of cosmetic appearance

     6. Usually done only in supratentorial area because neck muscles protect infratentorial areas

III. Cranioplasty

    A. Procedure

       1. Repair of skull defects to reestablish the contour and integrity of the skull

    B. Purpose

       1. Protection of cranial contents

       2. Improvement of cosmetic appearance

       3. Usually done only in supratentorial area because neck muscles protect infratentorial areas

IV. Craniectomy

    A. Procedure

       1. Excision of a portion of the skull without replacement

    B. Purpose

       1. Surgical access

       2. Decompression after cerebral debulking

       3. Removal of bone fragments from skull fracture

V. Microsurgery

    A. Procedure

       1. Surgery performed with the assistance of an operating microscope

    B. Purpose

       1. Provides magnification of various intensities

VI. Transsphenoidal hypophysectomy

    A. Procedure

       1. Procedure

          a. Access to the pituitary gland by an incision inside the superior upper lip, in front of the hard palate

          b. Removal of pituitary gland through transnasal or sublabial approach

          c. Often requires collaboration of neurosurgeon and ENT specialist

    B. Purpose

       1. Removal of pituitary tumors, adenomas, or craniopharyngiomas

       2. Preservation of pituitary gland, infundibular stalk, and normal vital structures

       3. Palliation for breast cancer

       4. Identification of tumor tissue

       5. Decompression

       6. Control of bone pain in metastatic cancer

VII. Shunts

    A. Procedure

       1. Placement of primary catheter, one-way valve reservoir

       2. Connection of reservoir to tubing emptying into distal site

    B. Purpose

       1. Used to treat hydrocephalus

       2. Provide drainage of excessive CSF from the brain

       3. Improvement or preservation of neurologic status by providing alternative CSF pathway

       4. Emergency reduction of increased ICP

       5. Instillation of antibiotics, analgesics, omega reservoir

       6. Sampling of CSF

    C. Types

       1. Ventriculoperitoneal

       2. Ventriculoatrial

       3. Lumbar-peritoneal

       4. External lumbar drain

       5. Multiple shunt sites (ureter, pleura, etc.)

  D. Components of shunting system

   1. Primary catheter: into lateral ventricle through burr hole

   2. Reservoir: rests on mastoid bone to collect CSF

   3. One-way valve: at reservoir to prevent CSF reflux

   4. Terminal catheter: tunneled under skin to termination point and secured in position

VIII. Stereotactic procedures ("stereo" means three-dimensional; "tactic" means touch)

  A. Procedure

   1. Precise localization of lesion through use of three-dimensional coordinates, stereotactic frame, and instrumentation

   2. Involves intraoperative use of CT scans, radiographs

  B. Purpose

   1. Precise localization and treatment of deep brain lesions (thalamic lesions) for biopsy

   2. Evacuation of intracerebral hemorrhage

   3. Catheter placement for drainage of deep lesions, colloid cyst, or abscess

   4. Ventricular catheter shunt placement

   5. Placement of electrodes for epilepsy

   6. Implantation of radioactive seeds into brain tumor

   7. Ablative procedures for extrapyramidal diseases (Parkinson's disease)

   8. Especially useful with intractable, chronic pain with deep brain stimulator

 IX. Carotid endarterectomy

  A. Procedure

   1. Incision made in neck area

   2. Heparinization and clamping of artery above and below obstruction

   3. Small incision made into artery

   4. Obstruction removed

   5. End-to-end anastomosis, suturing of artery, or patching of artery with autologous vein or Gortex graft

  B. Purpose

   1. Removal of stenotic vessel area

   2. Removal of plaques in vessels

   3. Primarily involves carotid bifurcation and junction of carotid and vertebral vessels with aorta or subclavian and innominate arteries

   4. Bypass of occlusion by use of grafts

   5. Primary purpose is to restore flow to cerebral circulation and prevent stroke if vessel is more than 70% occluded.

 X. Microradiosurgery

  A. Procedure

   1. Gamma knife

    a. Precise destruction of deep and inaccessible lesions during single session using 201 radially distributed, sealed, radioactive, sharply focused sources of cobalt 60 radiation; surrounding healthy tissue not harmed

    b. Minute measurement and precise patient positioning

    c. Purpose

     (1) Excessive risk for conventional surgical procedure

     (2) Surgical inaccessibility of lesion (acoustic neuromas)

     (3) Prior surgical failure

     (4) Patient refusal to undergo conventional craniotomy

    d. Used for

     (1) Arteriovenous malformations (AVMs)

     (2) Tumors

     (3) Other intracranial lesions for which conventional surgery is inappropriate

    e. Time between treatment and results long

        f. Time required for treatment limits centers to one or two patients per day.

        g. Procedure can be done with local anesthesia, but patient needs to be cooperative.

     2. Cyberknife

        a. Used in conjunction with a frameless computerized guidance system

     3. Lasers

        a. Types

           (1) Carbon dioxide

           (2) Argon

           (3) Neodymium-doped yttrium aluminum garnet (Nd:YAG)

        b. Precise dissection without traumatizing surrounding tissues

        c. Formerly inaccessible anatomic areas can be reached

        d. Dissect tissue by vaporization, coagulate blood vessels, and shrink tumors

  B. Patient selection an important aspect

XI. Seizure surgery

  A. Procedure

     1. Phase 1: noninvasive scalp monitoring

     2. Phase 2: placement of depth electrodes

     3. Phase 3: placement of grids and resection of epileptogenic focus

  B. Purpose

     1. Localization of seizure focus

     2. Removal of epileptogenic focus without causing neurologic deficits

  C. Selection criteria

     1. Refractory to medical management

     2. Unilateral focus

     3. Significant alteration in quality of life

ANATOMY AND PHYSIOLOGY OF THE SPINAL CORD

I. Vertebral column

  A. Purpose

     1. Supports head and trunk

     2. Protection of spinal cord

     3. Flexibility for movement

  B. Unique aspects

     1. Atlas (C1): sits on odontoid process

     2. Axis (C2)

  C. Divisions (Figure 40-17)

     1. Cervical (7)

     2. Thoracic or dorsal (12): intermediate in size, becomes larger as descends

     3. Lumbar (5): largest segment

     4. Sacral (5): fused into one

     5. Coccygeal (4): fused as one

  D. Essential parts of vertebrae

     1. Body: Anterior solid segment separated by discs

     2. Arch: Posterior segment

        a. Pedicles (2): short, thick pieces of bone

        b. Laminae (2): broad plates of bone

        c. Articular processes (4): two on either side, provide spine stability

        d. Transverse processes (2): points of attachment for muscles and ligaments

        e. Spinous process (1): projects from rear of arch, serves as attachment for muscles and ligaments

     3. Foramen

        a. Opening where vertebral arch meets vertebral body

        b. Allows for passage of spinal cord

SPINAL CORD SEGMENTS

The spinal cord contains 31 pairs of spinal nerves (part of the peripheral nervous system), which innervate segments of the body, from the back of the head to the feet. It is divided into 8 cervical, 12 thoracic, 5 lumbar, 5 sacral segments, and 1 coccygeal segment.

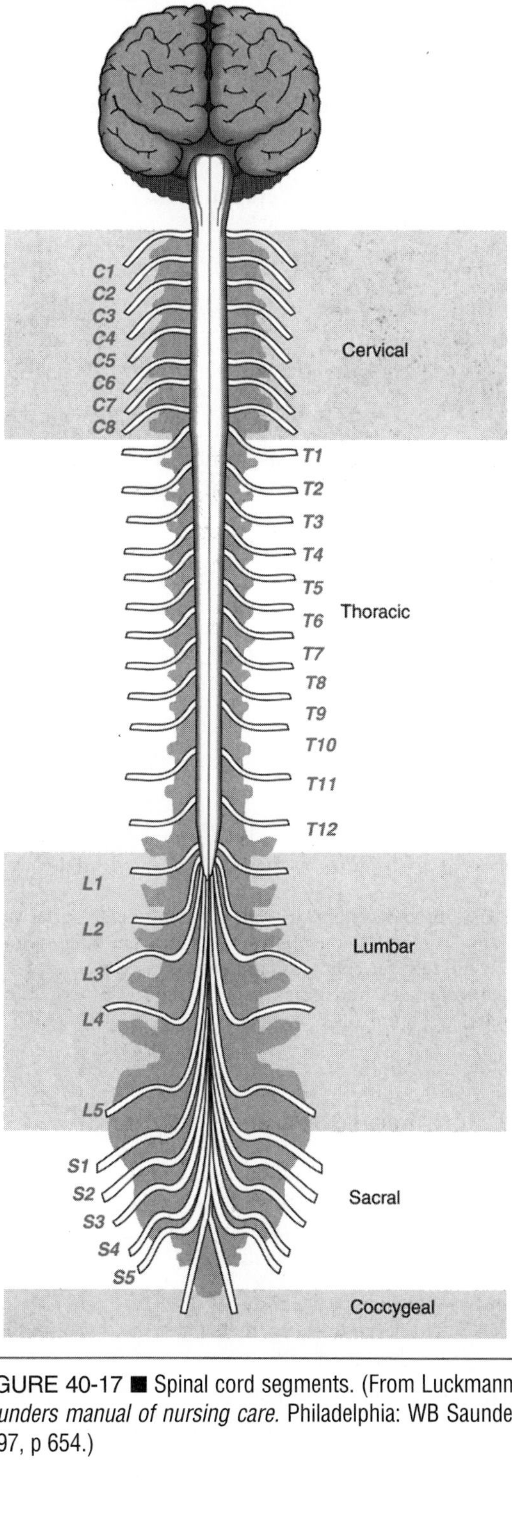

FIGURE 40-17 ■ Spinal cord segments. (From Luckmann J: *Saunders manual of nursing care.* Philadelphia: WB Saunders, 1997, p 654.)

E. Spinal ligaments
   1. Anterior longitudinal ligament
      a. Fibers attach to anterior surface of vertebral body and intervertebral disks.
      b. Broad, strong
      c. Extends from occipital bone and anterior tubercle of atlas to sacrum
   2. Posterior longitudinal ligament
      a. Attaches to posterior surface of vertebral bodies within spinal canal
      b. Thick, strong
      c. Extends from occipital bone to coccyx
   3. Ligamenta flava
      a. Yellow elastic fibers connecting lamina of adjacent vertebrae
      b. Extend from axis to first segment of sacrum
      c. Help hold body erect
      d. Thin, broad, and long in cervical area
      e. Thicker in thoracic area
      f. Thickest in lumbar region
   4. Supraspinous ligament
      a. Joins the spinous process tips from C7 to sacrum
   5. Interspinous ligament
      a. Connects adjacent spinous process from tips to roots
F. Intervertebral discs (Figure 40-18)
   1. Located between vertebral bodies from second cervical vertebra to sacrum
   2. Fibrocartilaginous, disc-shaped structures
   3. Vary in size, thickness, and shape at different spinal levels

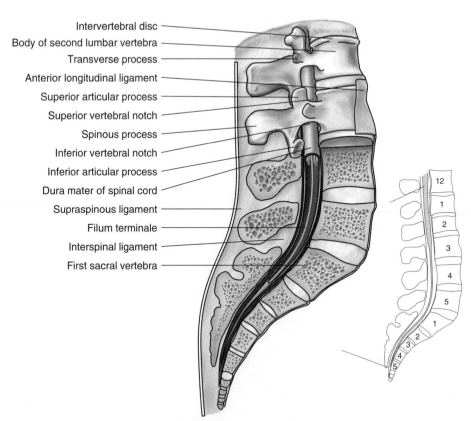

FIGURE 40-18 ■ Vertebral column showing structure. (From Drain CB: *Perianesthesia nursing: A critical care approach,* ed 4. St Louis: WB Saunders, 2003, p 118.)

        4. Serve as cushions between bony surfaces of vertebral bodies

        5. Parts

            a. Nucleus pulposus

                (1) Central, spongy core

                (2) Loses resiliency with age

            b. Anulus fibrosus

                (1) Fibrous capsule that surrounds nucleus pulposus

                (2) Degenerative changes can occur in middle and later life.

II. Spinal cord

    A. Characteristics

        1. Size: 1 cm in diameter; average length of 42-45 cm

        2. Originates at foramen magnum and ends at L2

        3. Elongated mass of nerve tissue that occupies upper two thirds of vertebral canal; is continuous with medulla oblongata

        4. Has 31 segments, each with a pair of spinal nerves

        5. Surrounded by meninges for protection

        6. Central canal contains CSF.

    B. Purposes

        1. Conducts sensory and motor impulses to and from brain

        2. Controls many reflexes

    C. Arterial blood supply

        1. From vertebral arteries

        2. Anterior spinal artery (1): runs full length of cord, midventrally

        3. Posterior spinal arteries: run full length of spinal cord along each row of dorsal roots

    D. Venous drainage

        1. Intradural vein: follows arterial pattern

        2. Extradural intravertebral veins: form plexus from cranium to pelvis with communication to veins of neck, thorax, abdomen

    E. Transverse section

        1. White matter

            a. Longitudinal myelinated fibers

            b. Comprises bulk of spinal cord

            c. Encases gray matter

            d. Each half divided into columns (funiculi) containing ascending (sensory), lateral and descending (motor) tracts

        2. Gray matter

            a. Unmyelinated fibers

            b. H-shaped appearance of inner core

            c. H divided into columns (horns) containing ascending (sensory) and descending (motor) tracts

                (1) Anterior (ventral) horns: motor, efferent

                (2) Posterior (dorsal) horns: sensory, afferent, axons from peripheral sensory neurons

                (3) Lateral horns

                      (a) Thoracic and upper lumbar segments only

                      (b) Sympathetic nervous system cell bodies

    F. Ascending tracts

        1. Spinothalamic

            a. Carry sensations of pain, temperature, light touch, pressure

            b. Originate in posterior gray column on opposite side and terminate in thalamus

        2. Spinocerebellar

            a. Carry impulses of proprioception (knowledge of position and body parts) or kinesthesia from lower body

            b. Originate in posterior gray horns and terminate in cerebellum

        3. Fasciculus gracilis and fasciculus cuneatus

        a. Carry impulses of proprioception from muscles, joints; light touch from skin, discrete localization, two-point discrimination, vibratory sense, stereognosis

        b. Originate in posterior white columns and terminate in medulla where they cross and continue to thalamus

  G. Descending tracts

    1. Lateral corticospinal (pyramidal)

        a. Voluntary motor movement, especially contraction of small muscle groups such as hands, fingers, feet, toes

        b. Originate in motor areas of cerebral cortex on opposite side and terminate in anterior gray columns

  H. Upper motor neurons

    1. Located entirely in CNS

    2. Neurons and their fibers

    3. Extend from cerebral centers to cells in spinal cord

    4. Facilitating and inhibitory descending pathways that modify lower motor neurons

    5. Paralysis

        a. Increased muscle tone and spasticity

        b. Little to no atrophy of muscles involved

        c. Hyperactive deep tendon reflexes

        d. Babinski's sign

  I. Lower motor neurons

    1. Located in anterior horn cells and spinal and peripheral nerves

    2. Receive impulses from different levels of CNS and channels to muscles

    3. Paralysis

        a. Total loss of voluntary muscle control with complete transection

        b. Decreased muscle tone and flaccidity

        c. Diminished or absent reflexes

        d. Absence of pathologic reflexes

        e. Local twitching of muscle groups

        f. Progressive atrophy of atonic muscles

  J. Spinal roots

    1. Dorsal (posterior) roots: convey afferent (sensory) impulses from skin segments (dermatomal areas) to dorsal root ganglia

    2. Ventral (anterior) roots: convey efferent (motor) impulses from spinal cord to body

    3. Dorsal and ventral roots meet and join to form spinal nerve.

  K. Spinal nerves

    1. Thirty-one pairs exit from spinal cord.

        a. Cervical (8): exit above corresponding vertebrae

        b. Thoracic (12): exit below corresponding vertebrae

        c. Lumbar (5): exit below corresponding vertebrae

        d. Sacrum (5): exit below corresponding vertebrae

        e. Coccyx (1): exits below corresponding vertebrae

    2. Formed by union of anterior and posterior roots attached to spinal cord

    3. Spinal segment made up of corresponding spinal cord segment plus spinal nerves

  L. Plexus

    1. Network of interlacing nerves formed by primary branch of nerves or by terminal funiculi

    2. Cervical

        a. Innervates muscles of neck and shoulders

        b. Gives rise to phrenic nerve, which supplies diaphragm

    3. Brachial: radial and ulnar nerves merge.

    4. Lumbar: gives rise to femoral nerve

    5. Sacral: gives rise to sciatic nerve

ASSESSMENT OF SPINAL CORD FUNCTION

I. Motor function
   A. Muscle size: inspect for atrophy, hypertrophy.
   B. Muscle strength: as described in neurologic assessment
   C. Muscle tone
   D. Coordination
      1. Rapid alternating movements
      2. Heel to shin
      3. Finger to nose
II. Sensory function
   A. Superficial sensation
      1. Light touch (cotton wisp)
      2. Pain (pinprick)
   B. Deep sensation
   C. Technique
      1. Have patient close eyes.
      2. Begin at feet and work upward systematically.
      3. Compare findings on both sides.
      4. Ask patient to tell you when sensation is felt.
      5. Note dermatome level.
III. Reflexes
   A. Superficial
      1. Abdominal
      2. Cremasteric
      3. Bulbocavernosus
      4. Perianal reflex (anal wink)
      5. Plantar
   B. Deep tendon reflexes (DTR)
      1. Biceps
      2. Triceps
      3. Brachioradial
      4. Patellar
   C. Pathologic
      1. Corticospinal tract involvement
         a. Babinski's reflex positive

DISORDERS REQUIRING SPINAL SURGERY

I. Herniated intervertebral disc (Figure 40-19)
   A. Major cause of severe and chronic back pain
      1. Disruption of anulus with leakage of nucleus pulposus
      2. May extrude into epidural space and compress nerve roots
   B. Often referred to as HNP (herniated nucleus pulposus)
   C. Cervical and lumbar regions most susceptible to injury and stress (especially lumbar disc disease)
   D. Patients often admitted with diagnosis of radiculopathy, disease of spinal nerve roots, complaining of arm and leg pain
   E. Occurs more in men
   F. Occurs most often in 30-year-old to 50-year-old age group
   G. Etiology
      1. Fifty percent: trauma (lifting, slipping, falling on buttocks or back, and suppressing a sneeze)
      2. Degenerative processes such as aging, osteoarthritis, or ankylosing spondylitis
      3. Congenital anomalies (scoliosis) can predispose to disc injury.
   H. Signs and symptoms
      1. Lumbar (90% to 95% at L4 to S1 level)

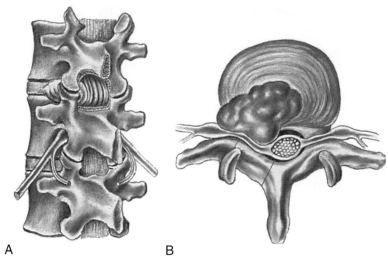

A   B

FIGURE 40-19 ■ Herniated nucleus pulposus (A) and laminectomy (B). (From Drain CB: *Perianesthesia nursing: A critical care approach*, ed 4. St Louis: WB Saunders, 2003, p 545. From Thompson J: *Mosby's clinical nursing*, ed 5. St Louis: Mosby, 2002.)

    a. Pain aggravated by sneezing, coughing, stooping, straining, standing, or by jarring movements while walking or riding
    b. Postural deformity
        (1) Lumbar lordosis absent (60%)
        (2) Restriction in lateral flexion
        (3) Limited lumbar spine movement
        (4) Painful when climbing stairs
    c. Motor changes
        (1) Hypotonia
        (2) Atrophy of affected muscles
        (3) Paresis
        (4) Footdrop
        (5) Difficult micturition and sexual activity
    d. Sensory deficits
        (1) Paresthesias
        (2) Numbness of leg and foot
        (3) Tenderness over L5 and S1
    e. Alteration in reflexes (diminished knee or ankle reflexes)
    f. Other diagnostic signs
        (1) Straight leg raising test (Lasegue's Sign)
        (2) Neri's sign (patient bends forward after knee flexion on affected side)
        (3) Naffziger's test (pain when both jugular veins simultaneously compressed while standing)
        (4) Kernig's sign (unable to extend knee to normal range while in dorsal recumbent position)
  2. Cervical (most commonly C6 to C7, then C5 to C6)
    a. Pain
    b. Paresthesias
    c. Reflex loss
    d. Motor weakness in hand, forearm
    e. Restricted neck movement
    f. Atrophy of affected muscles
    g. Tenderness when pressure exerted over cervical area of spine

I. Diagnostic tools
  1. History and physical assessment
  2. Spinal films
  3. Contrast myelography
  4. MRI
  5. CT scan
II. Spinal cord injury (Figure 40-20)
  A. Mechanisms of injury
    1. Hyperflexion (head-on collision and diving incident)
    2. Hyperextension (rear-end collision, elderly who fell and struck chin)
    3. Axial loading (falling from height and land on feet or buttocks)
    4. Rotational (extreme flexion or twisting of head and neck)
    5. Penetrating (bullets penetrate spinal column or soft tissue)
  B. Classifications of injury
    1. Concussion—jarring resulting in temporary loss of function
    2. Compression—distortion of normal curvatures
    3. Contusion—bruising, edema, and necrosis from compression
    4. Laceration—actual tear resulting in permanent injury
    5. Transection—severing of cord (complete or incomplete)
    6. Hemorrhage—blood in or around spinal cord

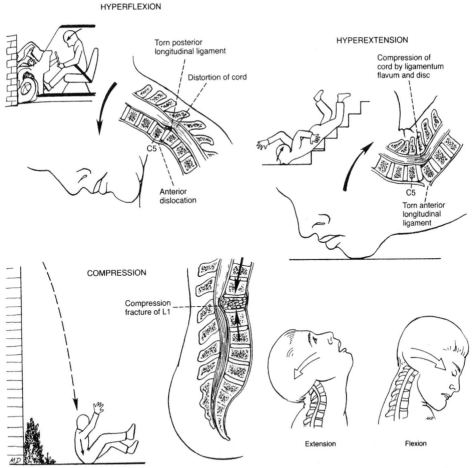

FIGURE 40-20 ■ Closed spinal injury mechanism. (In Drain CB: *Perianesthesia nursing: A critical care approach,* ed 4. St Louis: WB Saunders, 2003, p 538. From Clochesy J, Breu C, Cardin S, et al: (1996) *Critical care nursing,* ed 2. Philadelphia: WB Saunders, 1996; and Luckmann J, Sorensen KC: *Medical-surgical nursing: A psychophysiologic approach,* ed 3. Philadelphia: WB Saunders, 1987.)

7. Damage to blood vessel—results in ischemia and possible necrosis

C. Spinal cord injury syndromes

1. Quadriplegia
   a. Lesion involves one or more cervical segments.
   b. Loss of motor and sensory function below level of lesion, usually upper and lower extremities
   c. Bowel, bladder, and sexual dysfunction

2. Paraplegia
   a. Lesion involves one or more of thoracic, lumbar, or sacral regions.
   b. Loss of motor and sensory function below level of lesion, usually lower extremities
   c. Bowel, bladder, and sexual dysfunction

3. Complete lesion: implies total loss of motor and sensory function below the injury

4. Incomplete lesion
   a. Preservation of motor or sensory function or both below level of lesion
   b. Classified according to area of damage
   (1) Central cord syndrome
       (a) More motor deficits in upper extremities than lower extremities
       (b) Sensory loss varies
       (c) Bowel, bladder dysfunction variable or, function may be completely preserved.
       (d) Injury to central area of spinal cord, usually cervical area
   (2) Anterior cord syndrome
       (a) Loss of perception of pain, temperature, and motor function below level of lesion
       (b) Light touch, position, vibration intact
       (c) Injury to anterior spinal artery through trauma, hyperflexion
       (d) Injury in anterior part of spinal cord including spinothalamic tracts (pain), corticospinal tracts (temperature), anterior gray horn motor neurons
   (3) Brown-Séquard syndrome (lateral cord syndrome)
       (a) Ipsilateral paralysis or paresis
       (b) Ipsilateral loss of touch, pressure, and vibration
       (c) Contralateral loss of pain and temperature
       (d) Transverse hemisection of cord, usually as a result of knife or missile injury or acute ruptured disc
   (4) Posterior cord syndrome
       (a) Rare syndrome
       (b) Position and vibration senses of posterior columns are involved.
   (5) Root syndrome (peripheral syndrome)
       (a) Tingling, pain, motor weakness of selected muscles; absent or decreased reflexes in involved area
       (b) Sacral roots: bowel and bladder dysfunction
       (c) Cervical roots: tingling and weakness in arm; pain radiating down arm and into shoulder
       (d) Compression or vertebral subluxation with compression of nerve roots
   (6) Horner's syndrome
       (a) Seen with partial transection at T1 level or above
       (b) Associated with miosis, ptosis, loss of sweating on ipsilateral side
       (c) Lesions of preganglionic sympathetic trunk or cervical postganglionic sympathetic neurons

D. Treatment

1. Medical: dependent on patient's symptoms and severity of injury
   a. High dose steroid for acute cord injury
   b. Immobilization

       c. Bed rest
   2. Surgery
       a. May be delayed
          (1) Allow for decrease in cord edema.
          (2) Allow for immobilization and realignment of vertebral column.
          (3) Allow for reduction of fracture dislocation.
       b. May occur within 12 to 72 hours if any of following are present
          (1) Compression of spinal cord
          (2) Progressive neurologic deficits
          (3) Bony fragments with compound fractures (because they could penetrate cord)
          (4) Penetrating wounds
          (5) Bone fragments in spinal cord
       c. Purpose
          (1) Decompress spinal cord or spinal nerves to prevent the following
             (a) Pain
             (b) Loss of neurologic function
             (c) Ischemia or necrosis of neural tissue
          (2) Stabilization
       d. Procedures
          (1) Decompression laminectomies with fusion
          (2) Posterior laminectomy using acrylic wire mesh and fusion
          (3) Insertion of Harrington rods or instrumentation for stabilization
 E. Complications: affect all body systems
   1. Neurologic
       a. Spinal shock
       b. Autonomic dysreflexia
       c. Spinal instability
       d. Pain
       e. Spasticity
   2. Respiratory
       a. Hypoxia
       b. Aspiration
       c. Pulmonary embolus
       d. Pneumonia
       e. Atelectasis
   3. Cardiovascular
       a. Bradydysrhythmias
       b. Orthostatic hypotension
       c. Deep vein thrombosis
   4. Orthopedic, musculoskeletal, integumentary
       a. Contractures
       b. Osteoporosis
       c. Pressure ulcers
   5. Gastrointestinal
       a. Bleeding
       b. Fecal impaction or incontinence
       c. Paralytic ileus
   6. Genitourinary
       a. Urinary tract infections
       b. Urinary calculi
       c. Urinary retention or incontinence
       d. Sexual dysfunction
 F. Spinal shock
   1. Condition occurring immediately after injury; may last hours to months, depending on severity of injury
   2. Commonly lasts 1 to 6 weeks after injury
   3. Characteristics

   a. Loss of motor, sensory, reflex and autonomic activity below level of injury

   b. Flaccid paralysis of all skeletal muscle

   c. Loss of pain perception, light touch, temperature and pressure below level of injury

   d. Loss of ability to perspire

   e. Absence of somatic and visceral sensation

   f. Bowel and bladder dysfunction

   g. Hypotension, bradycardia

  4. Resolution of spinal shock

   a. Gradual process (4-6 weeks)

   b. Varies with patient and level of injury

 G. Autonomic dysreflexia

  1. Usually occurs after resolution of spinal shock and return of reflex activity

  2. Occurs most often with lesions at T6 or above

  3. Results from uninhibited sympathetic discharge

  4. Causes

   a. Bladder distension

   b. Fecal impaction

   c. Noxious stimuli (vary with individual patient)

  5. Symptoms

   a. Pounding headache

   b. Hypertension (can be dangerously high)

    (1) Changes in mental status

    (2) Seizures

    (3) Intracerebral hemorrhage

   c. Profuse sweating above level of lesion

   d. Nasal congestion

   e. Flushed skin above level of lesion

   f. Pallor below level of lesion

   g. Piloerection (goose pimples) below level of lesion

   h. Anxiety

   i. Visual disturbances

  6. Treatment

   a. Assess patient.

   b. Remove stimulus.

   c. Elevate head of bed.

   d. Notify physician immediately.

   e. Fast-acting antihypertensive medications may be ordered.

III. Spinal cord tumors (Figure 40-21)

 A. Less common than brain tumors

 B. Usually occur in young and middle-aged adults, with men and women equally affected

 C. Sites

  1. Cervical: 30%

  2. Thoracic: 50%

  3. Lumbosacral: 20%

 D. Classification

  1. Intramedullary

   a. Within spinal cord tissue

   b. May compress cord and nerve roots and destroy cord tissue

   c. Usually malignant

   d. Types

    (1) Astrocytoma

    (2) Ependymoma

    (3) Oligodendroglioma

    (4) Hemangioblastoma

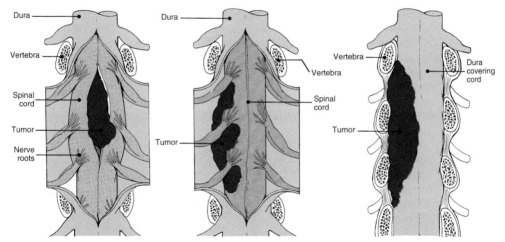

FIGURE 40-21 ■ Spinal cord tumors. (From Drain CB: *Perianesthesia nursing: A critical care approach,* ed 4. St Louis: WB Saunders, 2003, p 546. From Thompson J: *Mosby's clinical nursing,* ed 5. St Louis: Mosby, 2002.)

        e. Characteristics
            (1) Slow growing
            (2) May extend over more than one spinal segment
            (3) Loss of pain and temperature
            (4) Caudal area tumors may precipitate sexual, bladder, and bowel dysfunction.
        f. Compression is usually on central portion of spinal cord, rather than on nerve roots.
    2. Extramedullary
        a. Can occur inside or outside dura, but do not occur within spinal cord parenchyma
            (1) Extradural: occur outside the spinal dura, within the epidural space
                (a) Symptoms occur rapidly.
                (b) Mostly malignant
                (c) Pain is a common symptom and may occur before signs of spinal cord compression.
                (d) Metastatic tumors (from lungs, breast, prostate, kidneys, gastrointestinal tract)
                (e) Multiple myeloma
                (f) Lymphoma, chordomas, and sarcomas
            (2) Intradural: occur within the spinal dura but not within the spinal cord
                (a) Most common spinal cord tumor
                (b) Most frequently seen in thoracic area
                (c) Gradual onset of symptoms of cord compression
                (d) Pain may not always be present.
                (e) Meningioma
                (f) Neurofibroma
                (g) Congenital: dermoid, epidermoid
  E. Symptoms
    1. Etiology
        a. Destruction of spinal cord parenchyma
        b. Compression of spinal cord or spinal nerves
        c. Compression or occlusion of spinal blood vessels
        d. Obstruction of CSF flow

      2. Dependent on the following

         a. Level of lesion

         b. Tumor type

   F. Diagnostic tools

      1. History and physical assessment

      2. Spinal films

         a. Assess destruction of bony structures.

         b. Assess presence of vertebral column lesions.

      3. Contrast myelography

         a. Identifies obstruction of spinal CSF pathway (subarachnoid space)

         b. Identifies location, size, boundaries of lesion

         c. Considered hallmark of diagnostic armamentarium

         d. May be scheduled immediately before surgery, so patient may proceed directly from myelogram to operating room

      4. CT scan: identifies location, size, boundaries of lesion

      5. MRI

         a. Identifies location, size, boundaries of lesion

         b. Identifies destruction of bony structures

      6. CSF analysis

         a. Routine analysis as discussed with cranial space-occupying lesions

         b. CSF collected from below level of lesion may show increases in protein, absence of large amounts of cells, rapid coagulation.

      7. Spinal angiogram: assists in differentiating vascular lesions

      8. Electromyogram: used for differential diagnosis

      9. Other laboratory test or x-ray films as indicated by patient's symptoms and condition

OPERATIVE PROCEDURES

  I. Laminectomy

    A. Most frequent surgical procedure

    B. Procedure

      1. Removal of laminae, part of posterior arch of vertebrae, and attached ligamentum flavum

      2. Hemilaminectomy: excision of part of laminae

    C. Purpose

      1. Decompression of spinal cord or spinal nerves

      2. Allow for discectomy.

    D. Spinal fusion may be performed at the same time for stability of spinal column.

    E. Approaches

      1. Posterior (traditional): with cervical surgery, incision is made through back.

      2. Anterior: with cervical surgery, incision is made anteriorly through throat and neck area.

  II. Hemilaminectomy

    A. Removal of part of the lamina and posterior arch

 III. Discectomy

    A. Procedure

      1. Lumbar

         a. Posterior approach always used

         b. Entire disc and cartilaginous plate removed

      2. Cervical

         a. Posterior approach: only extruded disc fragments removed

         b. Anterior approach: total disc removed

    B. Purpose: removal of nuclear disc material with or without laminectomy

 IV. Microdiscectomy

A. Procedure and purpose: microscopic surgical technique
   1. Allows for easier identification of anatomic structures
   2. Improves precision in removing small fragments
   3. Decreases tissue trauma and pain: smaller incision
B. Patient able to ambulate sooner
C. Advantages
   1. Decreases risk of CSF leak through dural laceration
   2. Improved hemostasis: decreases vascular trauma and hematoma formation
   3. Decreases muscle spasms by decreasing traction on spinal nerve roots
   4. Less risk of stripping muscle from fascia
   5. Decreases risk of infection
V. Percutaneous discectomy
   A. Procedure and purpose: endoscopic lumbar surgical technique
      1. Posterolateral approach
      2. High-power suction shaver and cutter system
      3. Local anesthesia
   B. Alternative to microdiscectomy
   C. Indicated in disc-related root compression with minor deficits
VI. Spinal fusion—with or without instrumentation
   A. Procedure: insertion of bone chips, usually from iliac crest, between vertebrae; variety of surgical hardware (rods, screws, bolts) may also be used
   B. Purpose
      1. Immobilization of vertebral column
      2. Stabilization of weakened vertebral column
   C. Types
      1. Lumbar
         a. Motion increased above level of lesion
         b. Patient often unaware of permanent area of stiffness
      2. Cervical
         a. Increased limitation of movement
         b. Anterior approach: used when cervical area of spine is unstable
         c. Often performed with anterior laminectomy and discectomy
VII. Foraminotomy
   A. Procedure: surgical enlargement of intervertebral foramen to accommodate exit of spinal nerves
   B. Purpose
      1. Decrease pressure on spinal nerve
      2. Release entrapped spinal nerve
   C. Most often done in cervical area where foramen is smaller in diameter
VIII. Chemonucleolysis
   A. Procedure
      1. Injection of chymopapain, enzyme found in papaya plant, into nucleus pulposus
      2. Fluoroscopy and local anesthesia used
   B. Purpose
      1. Decreases size of disc by hydrolysis
      2. Decreases pain
   C. Fallen out of favor
      1. Increased incidence of pain recurrence
      2. Adverse reactions to chymopapain
IX. Rhizotomy
   A. Procedure: destruction of sensory nerve roots at entrance to spinal cord
   B. Purpose: interruption of transmission of pain
   C. Types
      1. Closed: percutaneous insertion of catheter to destroy nerve root through coagulation, injection of neurolytic chemicals, or cryodestruction

2. Open
   a. Requires laminectomy
   b. Nerve roots isolated and destroyed

X. Chordotomy
   A. Procedure: pain pathways transected at midline portion of spinal cord before impulse ascends through spinothalamic tract
   B. Purpose: interruption of transmission of pain

XI. Other procedures
   A. Carpal tunnel release (example of peripheral median nerve entrapment)
      1. Disorder
         a. Characteristics
            (1) Results from pressure on the median nerve
            (2) Associated health factors
                (a) Diabetes mellitus
                (b) Pregnancy
                (c) Premenstrual fluid retention
                (d) Obesity
                (e) Arthritis
            (3) Most common in females ages 40 to 60
         b. Symptoms
            (1) Pain, paresthesia ("pins and needles"), numbness in the hand that may radiate up the arm
            (2) Exacerbation of pain upon wrist flexion, often interrupting sleep from normal wrist flexion during sleep
            (3) Weakness in the thumb, first, second, and third fingers
      2. Procedure
         a. Anesthesia may be from local infiltration, Bier block, axillary block, or general.
         b. The carpal ligament is sectioned vertically over the median nerve.
         c. Incision
            (1) Along the ulnar or medial side of the thenar groove (most common)
            (2) Along the median groove
            (3) Endoscopically (one half inch incision)
      3. Postprocedure
         a. Assessment: check all fingers, but most particularly the thumb, index, and middle fingers every 15 minutes for 1 hour, then every 30 minutes for 1 hour, then every hour until discharged.
            (1) Sensation to touch
            (2) Sensation to pin prick or temperature; this is intact if patient is describing pain
            (3) Blanching of fingertips—compare with uninvolved fingertips
            (4) Assess dressing for drainage and increasing tightness.
         b. Care
            (1) Keep hand elevated at level of, or higher than, the heart.
            (2) If dressing becomes constrictive, request or have standing order to clip dressing one half to one and one half inches on back of hand.
            (3) Do not take blood pressure in affected arm.
            (4) Use sling for elevation and protection only when ambulating.
            (5) Keep elbow free of pressure.
            (6) Exercise the fingers throughout the day.
            (7) Check fingers for movement, sensation, and color (compare with uninvolved hand) several times a day (upon arising, at each meal, and at bedtime).
            (8) Avoid soiling dressing or hand; use unaffected hand or ask for assistance.

    B. Epidural patch
       1. Disorder
          a. Characteristics
             (1) Follows a lumbar puncture (LP)
                (a) Postmyelogram
                (b) Post-LP for diagnostic tests
                (c) Post–intrathecal catheter removal
                (d) Post–intrathecal injection of medication
             (2) Most often related to large-bore lumbar puncture needle >20 gauge
          b. Symptoms
             (1) Severe headache
                (a) Worsens when up
                (b) May extend into neck
                (c) Prevents activities
             (2) Nausea and vomiting
          c. Conservative treatment
             (1) Bed rest
             (2) Fluid challenge
             (3) Analgesics and antiemetics
             (4) Abdominal binder
       2. Procedure
          a. Have patient lie down in quiet, dark room with limited visitors.
          b. Patient may be too ill to listen to detailed instructions; limit information.
          c. Detailed explanations may be given to significant other.
          d. Establish at least one intravenous route (two sites may be needed if severely dehydrated).
          e. Prepare to obtain 15 to 20 ml of blood under careful aseptic technique for patch (physician may prefer to obtain blood).
            (1) Intermittent intravenous (IV) access for blood retrieval
            (2) Prepare site for phlebotomy.
              (a) Povidone preparation
          f. Place patient prone (pillow under abdomen).
            (1) May be done under fluoroscopy
          g. Epidural puncture is performed.
            (1) Anesthesia
              (a) Local infiltration
              (b) IV conscious sedation
          h. Assist with LP preparation.
          i. Obtain or assist with blood for patch.
          j. Blood is injected into epidural space.
          k. Band-Aid applied
       3. Postprocedure
          a. Assessment
            (1) Severity of headache (pain scale)
            (2) Description of headache (observe for changes)
            (3) Observe for nerve root irritation.
              (a) Symptoms worsen.
              (b) Pain in legs or groin area
              (c) Inability to void
          b. Care
            (1) Force fluid, caffeinated (IV fluid bolus, if nausea persists).
            (2) Caffeine
              (a) Beverages
              (b) Tables
              (c) IV (caffeine, sodium benzoate)
            (3) Bed rest, with head of bed flat

(4) Establish ability to void.

(5) At any point, if symptoms return, bed rest must be resumed (patch procedure may be repeated).

C. Excision of neuroma

1. Disorder

a. Characteristics

(1) Results from trauma to the nerve, particularly the axon

(a) Surgical or traumatic incision

(b) Amputation sites

(c) Repeated trauma

(i) Oral from dentures, for example

(ii) Wrist or hand from repetitive work injuries, for example

(iii) Morton's neuroma from trauma to the digital nerve

(iv) Any traumatized nerve

(2) Associated health factors

(a) Traumatic injuries

(b) Familial tendency

(c) Poorly fitted shoes

(3) Morton's neuroma more common in adult women

b. Symptoms

(1) Pain at neuroma site

(2) Numbness and tingling around neuroma and distally

c. Conservative treatment

(1) Injection with various medications and saline

(2) At operative and amputation sites, many methods have been and are currently being tried to prevent neuroma formation.

(3) Morton's neuroma

(a) Padding in shoes

(b) Limiting walking and standing

(c) Proper fitting footwear, avoiding heels >1 inch

2. Procedure

a. Anesthesia may be local infiltration, nerve block, epidural, spinal, or general.

b. The neuroma is excised, and the nerve ending may be buried into bone or muscle or other attempts made to prevent reoccurrence.

c. Morton's neuroma

(1) Incision

(a) Vertical plantar

(b) Dorsal

3. Postprocedure

a. Assessment: check extremity distal to surgical site every 15 minutes for 1 hour, every 30 minutes for 1 hour, and every hour until discharge.

(1) Sensation to touch distal to surgical site (consider type of anesthesia, document resolution)

(2) Sensation to pain and temperature distal to surgical site: compare preoperative pain score and description with postoperative pain score and description (consider type of anesthesia, document resolution).

(3) Capillary refill and warmth of digits compared with unaffected extremity (capillary refill <1 second)

(4) Assess dressing for drainage and increasing tightness.

b. Care

(1) Keep extremity elevated at level or above heart.

(2) If dressing becomes constricting, obtain order or have standing order to clip one half to one and one half inches on opposite surface of incision.

(3) If upper extremity, avoid taking blood pressure in affected arm.
  D. Microendoscopic discectomy (lumbar disc removal)
    1. Disorder
      a. Characteristics
        (1) Ruptured intravertebral disk with resulting pressure on a nerve
        (2) Associated health factors: no clear indication of a particular risk factor except age; disc rupture in most cases is thought to be caused by the weight loading of an erect posture
          (a) Misuse of back
          (b) Static positions at work
            (i) Sitting at a desk or work station
            (ii) Standing at a work station
            (iii) Sedentary lifestyle
          (c) Weight-loading phenomenon
            (i) Load that is too heavy
            (ii) Load that is too bulky
        (3) Age-related phenomenon
          (a) Greatest risk between 30 to 50 years of age
          (b) Peak occurrence in the 40s
      b. Symptoms
        (1) Pain
          (a) Sharp, stabbing, burning
          (b) Radiates into a dermatome and can be fairly accurately traced by the patient
          (c) Pain increases with any straining, Valsalva's maneuver, sneezing, coughing.
        (2) Paresthesia may exist anywhere along the affected dermatome.
        (3) Weakness and atrophy may become evident in the muscles innervated by the specific nerve root.
        (4) Decreased or loss of reflexes specific to the innervation of the involved nerve root
        (5) Specific nerve root involvement (disc rupture at one level may involve more than one root, and with individual anatomic variations symptoms may vary)
          (a) Pressure on L4, L5, or S1 nerve root (sciatica)
            (i) Pain radiating down one buttock, possibly into the ipsilateral posterior thigh, knee, calf, and may extend all the way into the foot
            (ii) Usually more comfortable with leg flexed
            (iii) Sitting may be particularly painful.
            (iv) Weakness
              [a] L5—unable to walk on heels because of weakness of dorsiflexion
              [b] S1—unable to walk on toes because of weakness of plantar flexion
            (v) L4 and L5—most common areas of disc herniation in the lumbar spine
          (b) Pressure on L2 or L3 nerve root (more rare)
            (i) Pain radiating into the groin, anterior thigh, and medial calf of affected leg
            (ii) Will usually assume a position of knee and hip flexion with lateral rotation of the hip
      c. Conservative treatment
        (1) Activity restrictions
          (a) Bed rest
          (b) Avoid sitting for >30 minutes at a time.

              (2) Steroid or antiinflammatory treatment
                 (a) Topical
                 (b) Oral medication
              (3) Traction
              (4) Exercise
              (5) Heat and massage
              (6) Ice massage or ice application
              (7) Sleeping position and mattress adjustments
              (8) Ergonomic evaluation of work environment

    2. Procedure
        a. A small 15-mm incision is made over the site (left or right of the midline).
        b. The endoscope is positioned and verified with x-ray.
        c. Part of the lamina is removed to allow access to the nerve root.
        d. The nerve root is identified and protected as the loose pieces of disc are removed.
        e. The nerve root is verified as being "free" without pressure.
        f. A foraminotomy may be performed (bone along the neural foramen can be drilled away, leaving a slightly larger area for the nerve to pass through).
        g. Benefits
            (1) Can be done under local or epidural anesthesia
            (2) Minimal tissue damage to skin, muscle, and other tissue at entry site
            (3) Minimal scarring, therefore less morbidity

    3. Postprocedure
        a. Assessment
            (1) Description of pain, paresthesia, numbness; compare with preoperative
            (2) Pain scale score; compare with preoperative
            (3) Weakness
               (a) Walk on heels
               (b) Walk on toes
               (c) Difficulty ambulating
            (4) Band-Aid intact without bleeding
            (5) Able to void
        b. Care
            (1) Remove Foley catheter.
            (2) Teach to get out of bed "statue style."
               (a) Turn to unaffected side.
               (b) Lower legs off bed, while pushing upper body up with upper extremities, keeping back straight.
            (3) Ambulate increasing distances and to bathroom, to ensure ambulation ability at home.

POSTANESTHESIA CARE

  I. Postoperative assessment
    A. Ongoing, frequent, and careful observation
    B. Specific spinal cord assessment form may assist in consistent documentation of improvement or deterioration.
    C. Assess for signs of meningeal irritation.
      1. Headache
      2. Photophobia
      3. Nuchal rigidity
      4. Kernig's sign: resistance and pain when patient's leg is flexed at hip and knee
      5. Brudzinski's sign: flexion of hips and knees in response to passive flexion of neck

  D. Hemodynamic monitoring: especially useful for patient with spinal cord injury who may be in spinal shock
    1. Swan-Ganz catheter
    2. Arterial lines
    3. Central venous pressure line
  E. Respiratory status
    1. Especially important with cervical lesions
    2. Assess rate, use of accessory muscles, nasal flaring.
    3. Breath sounds
    4. Ability to handle secretions
    5. For patients with anterior cervical approach (may have damage to laryngeal nerves, vocal cords, hematoma formation)
       a. Hoarseness
       b. Tracheal deviation (edema)
    6. Pulse oximetry
    7. ABGs
  F. Neurovascular checks
  G. Urinary elimination
    1. Voiding pattern
    2. Intake and output
    3. Palpate abdomen for distension.
  H. Auscultate bowel sounds, presence of distension.
 II. Postoperative complications
  A. Increase in existing deficits
  B. Motor loss: paralysis of upper or lower extremities
  C. Sensory loss
  D. Urinary retention
  E. Paralytic ileus
  F. Leakage of CSF fistula
  G. Nerve root injury
  H. Postural deformity
  I. Hematoma at operative site (will increase neurologic deficits)
  J. Arachnoiditis: Inflammation of arachnoid layer of meninges
  K. Infection
  L. Respiratory distress
  M. Spinal cord–injured patients may experience any of the complications indicated in discussion of spinal cord injury.
III. Signs of deterioration in status
  A. Increase in existing deficits
  B. Appearance of new deficits
  C. Spinal shock
  D. Autonomic dysreflexia
IV. Nursing interventions after spinal injury
  A. Maintain patent airway.
    1. Coughing and deep breathing
    2. Use of incentive spirometry
    3. Supplemental oxygen
    4. Assistance with mechanical ventilation may be needed with cervical lesions.
  B. Frequent assessment of neurologic status: not deviations from patient's baseline
  C. Positioning
    1. Factors
       a. Type of surgery
       b. Type of lesion
       c. Site of lesion
       d. Presence of complications

2. Reduce pressure on operative site.
3. Reposition every 2 hours once specified by surgeon.
4. Log rolling
   a. Maintains alignment
   b. Decreases pain
   c. Decreases muscle spasms
   d. Use of turning sheet decreases stress on caregiver and helps ensure alignment.
5. Avoid twisting.
6. Proper body alignment
7. Stryker frame
   a. May be used for a variety of spinal surgeries depending on patient condition and severity of injury
   b. May be used in conjunction with halo apparatus or Gardner-Wells tongs
      (1) Maintain traction.
      (2) Observe pin sites.
      (3) Assess stability of halo apparatus and security bolts.
   c. Physician must be present first time patient is turned down.
   d. Psychosocial and emotional support needed, because patients frequently are afraid and anxious on frame.
8. Cervical collar or Philadelphia collar
D. Maintain skin and mucous membrane integrity.
   1. Monitor incision site.
      a. Hematoma development
      b. Edema at surgical site
      c. CSF leakage
         (1) Test for glucose.
         (2) Look for halo or ring sign.
   2. Pad bony prominences.
   3. Frequent repositioning for paralyzed patients
E. Pain control
   1. Assess pain.
      a. Level, location, duration
      b. Use of pain scale
   2. Patient-controlled analgesia (PCA) often used with spinal surgery
   3. Frequent repositioning
   4. Maintenance of stabilizing devices
   5. Administration of pain medications if patient-controlled analgesia not used
   6. Alternative methods of pain relief
      a. Relaxation
      b. Imagery
F. Antiembolic stockings or sequential compression devices
G. Psychosocial and emotional support
   1. Reassure patient frequently.
   2. Inform patient when assessing, performing procedures.
   3. Keep family informed of patient's condition.
   4. Answer patient's and family's questions as honestly as possible.

BIBLIOGRAPHY

1. American Association of Neuroscience Nurses. *Clinical guidelines series: Intracranial pressure monitoring.* Chicago: American Association of Neuroscience Nurses, 1997.
2. American Heart Association. Available at http://www.americanheart.org. Accessed on December 21, 2003.
3. Back Bubble. Available at http://www.backpainrelief.com. Accessed on December 21, 2003.
4. Cammermeyer M, Appledorn C: *AANN's core curriculum for neuroscience nursing,* ed 3. Chicago: American Association of Neuroscience Nurses, 1996.

5. Chipps E, Clanin N, Campbell V: *Neurologic disorders*. St Louis: Mosby–Year Book, 1992.

6. Defazio Quinn D: *ASPAN's ambulatory surgical nursing core curriculum*. Philadelphia: WB Saunders, 1999.

7. Hickey J: *The clinical practice of neurological and neurosurgical nursing*. ed 4. Philadelphia: Lippincott, 2002.

8. Litwack K: *Core curriculum for post anesthesia nursing practice*. ed 3. Philadelphia: WB Saunders, 1995.

9. Luckmann J: *Saunders manual of nursing care*. Philadelphia: WB Saunders, 1997.

10. Marshall BA, Miller RH: *Essentials of neurosurgery: A guide to clinical practice*. New York: McGraw-Hill, 1995.

11. Medtronic Sofamor Danek. Available at http://www.sofamordanek.com. Accessed on December 20, 2003.

12. National Institute of Neurological Disorders and Stroke. Available at http://www.ninds.nih.gov/health_and_medical/disorders/brainandspinaltumors.htm. Accessed on December 20, 2003.

13. Neck Reference. Available at http://neckreference.com. Accessed on December 20, 2003.

14. Spinal Cord Injury Information Network. Available at http://www.spinalcord.uab.edu. Accessed on December 20, 2003.

41 Endocrine Surgery

LAURA F. MONETTE

OBJECTIVES

At the conclusion of this chapter the reader will be able to:

1. Describe the basic function of the endocrine system including the hormones produced by the thyroid, parathyroid, pituitary, and adrenal glands.

2. Identify the signs, symptoms, and diagnostic testing used to assess abnormal endocrine gland function.

3. Identify the surgical procedure and perioperative concerns of the patient having surgical treatment for hyperthyroidism, hypothyroidism, pheochromocytoma, hypersecretion of the pituitary gland, hyperaldosteronism, and hyperparathyroidism.

4. Identify postanesthesia nursing diagnosis, and develop a plan of care for the patient having subtotal thyroidectomy, bilateral adrenalectomy, hypophysectomy, and parathyroidectomy.

5. Discuss the postanesthesia concerns of the patient with Addison's disease.

6. Discuss the postanesthesia care of the patient with endocrine conditions, thyrotoxicosis, tetany, hypoglycemia in the insulin-dependent diabetic patient, diabetes insipidus, Addisonian crisis, and hyperparathyroid crisis.

7. Discuss the postanesthesia care of the diabetic patient.

■■ Endocrine dysfunction may be the primary reason for surgery, as with hyperthyroidism, or it may be a chronic condition coexisting with the patient's primary diagnosis, as with diabetes mellitus. Understanding endocrine dysfunction both as a primary reason for surgical intervention and as a complicating factor with other disorders is essential for the postanesthesia care unit (PACU) nurse to provide appropriate care.

THE THYROID GLAND

Hyperthyroidism

    I. Anatomy and physiology
      A. The thyroid gland
        1. Sits in the anterior portion of the neck
        2. Right lobe is below the larynx.
        3. Left lobe beside the trachea
        4. Middle portion called the isthmus lies at the base of the neck.
      B. Thyroid receives its blood supply from the external carotid arteries.
      C. Nerve supply from the cervical sympathetic trunk
      D. Function of the thyroid gland
        1. Regulates energy, metabolism and growth, and development
          a. Produces three hormones,
            (1) Thyroxine (T_4)
            (2) Triiodothyronine (T_3)
            (3) Thyroid-stimulating hormone (TSH), which is a combination of two iodine-producing hormones
          b. TSH is synthesized by the anterior pituitary, which stimulates the release of thyroid hormone (TH) and the uptake of iodide.

        c. As a result, the hypothalamus secretes thyrotropin-releasing hormone (TRH) to regulate the synthesis and release of the TSH on a negative-feedback cycle.

        d. When the TH levels decrease, TSH and TRH levels increase.

        e. Conversely, if the TH levels increase, the TSH and TRH levels decrease.

    2. T_3 has a short half-life, and T_4 has a half-life of 5 to 7 days.

    3. Peripheral tissue converts T_4 to T_3.

    4. T_3 is considered the true tissue thyroid hormone.

    5. T_4 is considered a plasma prohormone.

    6. Most patients seen in the PACU are in a euthyroid state.

        a. Patients who are hyperthyroid are usually those with large airway thyroid glands or pregnant women in their first trimester.

II. Description of hyperthyroidism

  A. Hypermetabolic condition

    1. Results in excessive secretion of thyroid hormone

III. Causes of hyperthyroidism

  A. Multinodular toxic diffuse enlargement; Graves' disease

  B. Adenomas

  C. Malignancy

  D. Thyroiditis

    1. Viral, autoimmune, or unknown etiology

    2. Immunoglobulins found in serum of hyperthyroid patients mimic thyrotropin (also called thyroid-stimulating hormone, or TSH).

IV. Signs and symptoms

  A. Cardiopulmonary

    1. Hypertension

    2. Tachycardia: 150 to 200 beats per minute (bpm) demonstrated as palpitations

    3. Increased cardiac output

    4. Systolic murmurs

    5. Tachypnea

    6. Atrial fibrillation

  B. Gastrointestinal

    1. Weight loss

    2. Increased peristalsis

    3. Diarrhea and abdominal pain

  C. Integumentary

    1. Fine, silky hair

    2. Hair loss

    3. Fever

  D. Musculoskeletal

    1. Body thinness

    2. Muscle atrophy

    3. Muscle weakness

  E. Nervous system

    1. Fine tremors

    2. Diaphoresis

    3. Hyperactive emotional state

  F. Miscellaneous

    1. Enlarged thyroid gland

    2. Exophthalmos

    3. Menstrual cycle changes

    4. Heat intolerance

V. Diagnostic laboratory values—see Table 41-1

  A. T_3 and T_4 levels; T_3 proportionately higher

  B. Radioactive iodine (RAI) uptake elevated in Graves' disease

  C. TSH level decreased in Graves' disease

■ TABLE 41-1
■ ■ **Tests to Determine Thyroid Dysfunction**

	Thyroxine T_4	Triiodothyronine T_3	TSH
Hyperthyroidism	Elevated	Elevated	Normal
Hypothyroidism Primary	Low	Low/normal	Elevated
Hypothyroidism	Low	Low	Low
Pregnancy	Elevated	Normal	Normal

   D. Thyroid scan: demonstrates iodide-concentrating capacity of the thyroid
      gland
   E. Ultrasonography: distinguishes between cystic and solid tumors
   F. Antibodies to thyroid gland distinguish left thyroiditis from cancer.
VI. Operative procedures
   A. Subtotal thyroid lobectomy: unilateral or bilateral excision of portion of
      lobe(s)
   B. Thyroid lobectomy: removal of one lobe
   C. Total thyroidectomy: removal of entire gland
VII. Preoperative objectives
   A. Promote euthyroid state with antithyroid drugs; several weeks required to
      promote euthyroid state.
      1. Propylthiouracil
         a. Dosage: 300 to 900 mg daily in divided doses given 6 to 12 weeks
            preoperatively
         b. Blocks peripheral conversion of T_4 and T_3
      2. Methimazole
         a. Dosage: 30 to 60 mg daily in divided doses
         b. May take 1 to 3 months to produce euthyroid state
         c. Blocks uptake of iodine
      3. Sodium iodide and potassium iodide (Lugol's solution)
         a. Emergently, iodide, 1 to 2 g of sodium salt intravenously (IV)
         b. Less acutely, SSKI, 2 to 10 drops per day, or 10 to 20 drops of Lugol's
            solution daily
         c. Decreases vascularity of gland
         d. Inhibits release of thyroxine
      4. Propranolol
         a. Dosage: 40 to 640 mg/day in divided doses
         b. Best single pharmacologic agent to control thyroid function
   B. Control hyperdynamic cardiovascular state.
      1. Sodium restriction
      2. Digitalization
      3. Diuretics
      4. Propranolol (Inderal)
         a. Drug of choice for severe tachycardia
         b. Does not reduce oxygen demand
         c. Blocks T_4 transformation to T_3
      5. Antihypertensive: reserpine; also causes bradycardia
   C. Increased preoperative sedation for already hyperactive patient
      1. Anticholinergics such as atropine may be omitted because of their
         tachycardic effect.
   D. Preoperative instruction: emphasis on head and neck support when turning

VIII. Intraoperative and anesthesia concerns
  A. Agents
    1. Thiopental: succinylcholine is paralyzing induction agent of choice because it does not induce a hyperdynamic cardiovascular effect.
    2. Propofol: short-acting without cardiotonic properties
    3. Ketamine: may cause cardiovascular problems in euthyroid patients with a history of thyrotoxicosis
      a. Increased cardiac output
      b. Hypertension
      c. Dysrhythmias
  B. Increased oxygen requirements because of
    1. Hypermetabolic state
    2. Increased temperature
    3. Tracheal deviation from retrosternal goiter compressing trachea
  C. Corneal drying or abrasions of exophthalmic eyes
  D. Vocal cord visualization for injury to recurrent laryngeal nerves
  E. Monitor for signs of thyroid storm: increased temperature, increased heart rate; esmolol 100 to 300 mcg/kg per minute to control tachydysrhythmia.
  F. Avoidance of bucking (coughing) on endotracheal tube, which may stimulate hemorrhage
  G. Avoidance or treatment of hypotension
IX. Postanesthesia nursing concerns
  A. Related nursing diagnostic categories
    1. Ineffective airway clearance related to edema of surgical area
    2. Impaired gas exchange or inability to move secretions
    3. Altered peripheral tissue perfusion
    4. Ineffective thermoregulation related to altered metabolic state
  B. Airway maintenance
    1. Supplementary humidified oxygen: aerosol or high-humidity face mask or tent
    2. Observation for respiratory distress
      a. Causes
        (1) Edema of glottis
        (2) Hematoma formation
      b. Signs
        (1) Dyspnea
        (2) Cyanosis
        (3) Crowing respirations or stridor
        (4) Retraction of neck muscles
        (5) Tracheal deviation
      c. Strategy
        (1) Immediate intubation if possible
        (2) Emergency tracheostomy
  C. Suture line observation
    1. Wound hemorrhaging: usually an early complication
    2. Hematoma formation: can create respiratory difficulty
    3. Drainage devices: Penrose or Jackson-Pratt drains
  D. Assessment of recurrent laryngeal nerve damage
    1. Assess and record quality of vocalization.
    2. Assess and record any difficulty in swallowing.
  E. Positioning
    1. Semi-Fowler's position after reaction
    2. Neck support
    3. Avoidance of extremes in head flexion or extension
  F. Avoidance of vigorous coughing; enhances hemorrhage
  G. Protection of exophthalmic eyes
    1. Sterile artificial tears
    2. Lubricating ophthalmic ointment

  H. Awareness of hormonal imbalances
   1. Tetany and hypocalcemia if parathyroid glands were removed
   2. Thyrotoxic crisis (storm)
     a. Caused by sudden increase in circulating thyroid hormone
     b. May be confused with malignant hyperthermia
     c. Seventy percent mortality if untreated
     d. Can occur up to 18 hours postoperatively
     e. Signs
       (1) Tachycardia
       (2) Profuse sweating
       (3) Hyperthermia
       (4) Severe dehydration
       (5) Delirium, agitation, psychosis, convulsions, coma
       (6) Pulmonary edema
       (7) Atrial fibrillation
       (8) Tachypnea
       (9) Hypertension followed by hypotension
       (10) Congestive heart failure
     f. Treatment
       (1) Adequate hydration with thiamine added because high output is causing this deficiency
       (2) Cooling; aspirin is *not* recommended for treatment because it displaces T_4 from its carrier protein
       (3) Sedation
       (4) Medication
         (a) Sodium potassium iodide, 1 to 5 g every 24 hours
         (b) Propylthiouracil, 200 mg every 4 to 6 hours
         (c) Cortisone: (100 to 200 mg) for persistent hypotension
       (5) Supplementary oxygen support
       (6) Control of tachycardia: beta-blockers to compete with catecholamines (propranolol)

Hypothyroidism

  I. Description of hypothyroidism
   A. A decrease in circulatory T_3 and T_4.
   B. Development of hypothyroidism is usually gradual and insidious.
   C. Incidence
    1. Subclinical presentation of hypothyroidism may be evident in as many as 8% to 10% of adult women and 1% to 2% of adult men.
    2. Incidence of diagnosed hypothyroidism is low (<1.5%) in the general population.
  II. Causes of hypothyroidism
   A. Chronic thyroiditis (Hashimoto's thyroiditis)
    1. Progressively destroys thyroid function
  III. Signs and symptoms
   A. Intolerance to cold
   B. Bradycardia
   C. Lethargy
   D. Peripheral vasoconstriction
   E. Decrease in cardiac output
   F. Hyponatremia
   G. Atrophy of adrenal cortex
   H. Reduced platelet adhesiveness
  IV. Diagnostic laboratory values (see Table 41-1)
  V. Anesthesia concerns
   A. Sensitivity to opioids

      1. No controlled studies exist to support the claim that hypothyroidism promotes sensitivity to inhaled anesthetic drugs or opioids.
      2. One should suspect sensitivity because exaggerated effects of depressants have been reported.

  B. Need for supplemental cortisone to correct adrenal insufficiency
  C. Slow metabolism of drugs
  D. Unresponsive baroreceptor reflexes
  E. Impaired ventilatory response to arterial hypoxemia or hypercapnia
  F. Hypovolemia
  G. Delayed gastric emptying
  H. Hyponatremia
  I. Hypothermia
  J. Anemia
  K. Hypoglycemia
  L. Adrenal insufficiency
  M. Induction and maintenance of anesthesia
      1. Ketamine is commonly used for induction because it supports the cardiovascular system.
      2. Succinylcholine used for paralysis of skeletal muscles
  N. Early recognition of a decrease in cardiac dysfunction resulting in congestive heart failure

VI. Postanesthesia nursing concerns
  A. Examples of related nursing diagnostic categories include
      1. Impaired cardiac output leading to congestive heart failure
      2. Decrease in circulating cortisone
      3. Fluid volume deficit
      4. Impaired thermoregulation related to metabolic rate
      5. Impaired fluid and electrolyte balance related to hyponatremia
      6. Potential alteration in comfort related to reduced sensitivity to opioids

THE PARATHYROID GLAND
Hyperparathyroidism

  I. Anatomy and physiology
  A. The parathyroid gland
      1. Consists of four small ovoid masses of tissue lying behind the thyroid gland
         a. Rarely, within the thyroid gland inside the pretracheal fascia
      2. The parathyroid gland secretes parathyroid hormone (PTH).
      3. PTH and vitamin D are responsible for the regulation of calcium and phosphorous.
      4. When the parathyroid is stimulated, the decrease in serum calcium levels results in bone reabsorption followed by increased renal reabsorption and gut uptake (with vitamin D).
      5. The release of PTH is inhibited by rising serum calcium.
      6. Magnesium is necessary for PTH release and for its bone effect.

  II. Description: Hyperparathyroidism
  A. Primary hyperparathyroidism characterized by hypercalcemia and hyperphosphatemia
  B. Disturbances in these two minerals result in major kidney and bone lesions.
  C. Secondary hyperparathyroidism results from parathyroid hyperplasia, producing decreased serum calcium levels.
  D. Bone lesions are primary outcomes.
  E. Overactivity of one or more parathyroid glands
  F. Excessive secretion of PTH

      G. Imbalance in calcium and phosphorus metabolism; increased calcium, 10.5 mg/dl (normal, 9 to 10.5 mg/dl)

III. Cause of disease process
  - A. Secondary hyperparathyroidism
    1. Adenomas: 80% to 90%
    2. Hyperplasias: 10% to 15%
    3. Malignancies: <5%
    4. Previous head or neck radiation: therapy of choice during 1950s and 1960s for benign conditions of face and neck

IV. Signs and symptoms
  - A. Cardiovascular
    1. Electrocardiogram (ECG) changes
      - a. Prolonged PR intervals (rare)
      - b. Shortened QT intervals (rare)
    2. Heart failure: tachydysrhythmias
  - B. Gastrointestinal: constipation
  - C. Musculoskeletal
    1. Muscle weakness
    2. Osteopenia
    3. Pathologic fractures
    4. Bone pain
  - D. Renal: chronic renal insufficiency, a late manifestation
    1. Polyuria
    2. Hypertension
      - a. Renal impairment
      - b. Calcium deposits in vessels
    3. Dehydration
  - E. Neurologic
    1. Somnolence
    2. Psychosis

V. Diagnostic laboratory values
  - A. Hypercalcemia
    1. Serum level greater than 10.5 mg/dl (normal range: 9.0-10.5 mg/dl)
    2. Excessive bone resorption
  - B. Hypercalciuria
    1. Urine level greater than 300 mg/24 hours
    2. Leads to renal calculi and kidney damage
  - C. Hyperphosphaturia
  - D. Hypophosphatemia: less than 2.5 mg/dl
  - E. Elevated serum PTH level (absolute values vary based on laboratory)
  - F. Radiographic identification of bone demineralization

VI. Preoperative objectives
  - A. Correct preexisting hypovolemia.
  - B. Reduce elevated calcium levels.
    1. Rehydration with normal saline, 6 to 10 L/24 hours
      - a. Not Ringer's lactate (contains calcium chloride)
    2. Furosemide (Lasix): 80 mg/24 hours to enhance diuresis
  - C. Control dysrhythmias secondary to hypercalcemia.

VII. Anesthesia concerns
  - A. Hypotension: usually caused by hypovolemia
  - B. Bradycardia: occurs with manipulation near carotid sinus
  - C. Impaired renal function
    1. Volume overload possibility
    2. Monitoring for hyperkalemia
  - D. Pneumothorax possible during mediastinal exploration

VIII. Operative procedures
  - A. Total parathyroidectomy
    1. Removal of all glands

    B. Partial parathyroidectomy

        1. Removal of up to three and one half of the four glands, leaving metal clip in place to identify remaining glandular tissue

IX. Postanesthesia nursing concerns

    A. Related nursing diagnostic categories

        1. Ineffective airway clearance related to edema of surgical area

        2. Impaired gas exchange or inability to move secretions

        3. Altered peripheral tissue perfusion

        4. Potential for impaired renal function

        5. Alteration in fluid and electrolyte status

    B. Airway maintenance

    C. Suture line observation (hematoma formation)

    D. Assessment of recurrent laryngeal nerve damage

    E. Positioning

    F. Awareness of hormonal imbalances

        1. Within immediate postoperative period, calcium concentration begins to fall.

        2. Uptake of calcium into bone may also deplete serum calcium.

        3. Tetany: Decreased PTH secretion and acute hypocalcemia

            a. Signs

                (1) Laryngeal spasm

                (2) Apprehension

                (3) Tingling in toes, fingers, mouth

                (4) Positive Chvostek's sign: twitching of facial muscles if cheek is tapped over facial nerve

                (5) Positive Trousseau's sign: carpopedal spasm if circulation in arm is impeded with blood pressure cuff

            b. Treatment

                (1) Calcium chloride administered slowly IV (so as not to irritate veins)

                (2) Vitamin D_2 (calciferol) replaces PTH, increases serum calcium.

                (3) Monitor for dysrhythmias, especially if patient is taking digitalis.

        4. Hyperparathyroid crisis: increased circulating parathyroid hormone, calcium greater than 11mg/dl up to 18 mg/dl

            a. Signs

                (1) Nausea and vomiting

                (2) Abdominal pain

                (3) Thirst, dehydration, hypovolemia

                (4) Dyspnea

            b. Treatment

                (1) Normal saline hydration

                (2) Calcitonin (parathormone antagonist)

                (3) Mithramycin for thrombocytopenia, renal problems

                (4) Prednisone to correct hypercalcemia

    G. Psychologic support and reassurance; elevated calcium levels produce altered psychologic states

    H. Hyperventilation: reduces calcium level

THE PITUITARY GLAND
Hyposecretion or Hypersecretion

  I. Anatomy and physiology

    A. Location: Pituitary gland is located at the base of the skull in the sphenoid bone.

        1. Lies within the sella turcica, near the hypothalamus and the optic chiasm

        2. Connected to the hypothalamus by the pituitary stalk, which links the endocrine and nervous systems

        3. Composed of anterior (75% of gland) and posterior lobes (25% of gland)

II. Pathophysiology
- A. Causes of glandular dysfunction
  1. Adenomas
  2. Malignancies
  3. Congenital abnormalities
  4. Traumatic injuries causing increase in intracranial pressure
  5. Infarction
  6. Hypothalamic dysfunction
- B. Hormonal influences
  1. Anterior pituitary hormones: normal physiology
     a. Growth hormone (GH)
        (1) Increases rate of protein synthesis
        (2) Increases lipolysis
        (3) Decreases carbohydrate use
        (4) Works with insulin, thyroid hormone, and sex steroids to promote growth
     b. Adrenocorticotropic hormone (ACTH)
        (1) Production and release of adrenocortical hormones
     c. Thyroid-stimulating hormone (TSH)
        (1) Increases synthesis of thyroid hormone
        (2) Releases stored thyroid hormone
     d. Luteinizing hormone (LH)
     e. Prolactin
     f. Follicle-stimulating hormone (FSH)
  2. Anterior pituitary hypersecretion caused by adenomas
     a. Increases (ACTH) (Cushing's disease)
     b. Increases GH (acromegaly)
     c. Increases prolactin
  3. Anterior pituitary hyposecretion caused by adenomas or hypothalamic dysfunction
     a. Decreases GH (dwarfism)
     b. Decreases TSH (hypothyroid)
     c. Decreases ACTH (chronic: adrenal insufficiency; acute: Addisonian crisis)
  4. Posterior pituitary hormones: normal physiology
     a. Antidiuretic hormone (ADH)
        (1) Increases water permeability in renal collecting duct, controlling extracellular fluid osmolality
        (2) Constricts arterioles to control blood pressure
     b. Oxytocin
  5. Posterior pituitary excess or deficiency caused by intracranial tumors or infarctions
     a. Excess: Syndrome of inappropriate ADH secretion (SIADH)
        (1) Characterized by high levels of ADH
        (2) Clinical signs include serum hypoosmolality and hyponatremia.
     b. Deficiency: Diabetes insipidus (DI)
        (1) Characterized by insufficiency in ADH
        (2) Clinical signs include polyuria, polydipsia, low urine specific gravity.

III. Signs and symptoms
- A. Anterior pituitary hypersecretion
  1. Acromegaly
     a. Bone overgrowth of mandible, hands, feet
     b. Soft tissue thickening
  2. Menstrual disturbances
  3. Headaches
  4. Visual disturbances
  5. Diagnostic tests
     a. Radiographs of skull, hands, feet
     b. Radioactive plasma human growth hormone (HGH) levels

    B. Anterior pituitary hyposecretion
       1. Hypothyroidism
       2. Obesity
       3. Decreased secondary sexual characteristics
       4. Dwarfism
       5. Headaches
       6. Diagnostic tests
          a. Radiographs of skull
          b. Decreased radioactive iodine (RAI) uptake
          c. Decreased T_4
          d. Decreased urine ACTH level
    C. Posterior pituitary hyposecretion: diabetes insipidus
       1. Polydipsia
       2. Polyuria
       3. Dehydration
       4. Diagnostic test
          a. Hypoosmolar polyuria
IV. Operative procedures
    A. Hypophysectomy (removal of pituitary gland)
       1. For primary pituitary disease, tumors
       2. Palliative measure for treatment of breast and prostate cancer
    B. Operative approaches
       1. Frontal craniotomy
       2. Transsphenoidal approach through nasal floor
V. Anesthesia concerns
    A. Anterior pituitary hypersecretion (increases ACTH, GH)
       1. Acromegaly
          a. Overgrown mandible
          b. Jaw protrusion
          c. Soft tissue thickness, which may cause recurrent laryngeal nerve entrapment leading to paralysis
       2. Intubation problems: airway
          a. Mask fit may be a problem.
          b. Long intubation blades may be indicated.
       3. Retention of sodium and potassium may lead to cardiac dysfunction.
       4. Inhibition of insulin leads to diabetes mellitus.
       5. Cushing's disease–like symptoms (see information on adrenal gland: Cushing's disease)
       6. If a recent air pneumoencephalogram was performed, nitrous oxide is avoided to decrease risk of increased intracranial pressure.
    B. Anterior pituitary hyposecretion (decreases TSH, ACTH)
       1. Decreased anesthesia requirements as result of hypometabolism
       2. Intolerance to hypothermia
       3. Bradycardia
    C. Posterior pituitary hyposecretion (decreases ADH): diabetes insipidus
       1. Tendency to dehydration with enormous urinary output
       2. Hypovolemia
       3. Hypotension
VI. Postanesthesia nursing concerns
    A. Related nursing diagnostic categories
       1. Potential for infection
       2. Potential ineffective airway clearance–related difficult intubation
       3. Impaired thermoregulation related to metabolic rate
       4. Impaired fluid and electrolyte balance related to fluid volume deficit or excess
       5. Altered cerebral tissue perfusion

B. Decreased ACTH of greatest concern (see information on Addisonian crisis)
   1. Requires lifelong cortisone replacement
      a. Surgical stress increases cortisone requirements.
      b. Persistent, unexplained hypotension; usually reversible with cortisone supplements
   2. Underlying diabetes mellitus (often unmasked with large doses of cortisone)
      a. Monitor blood sugar.
      b. Observe for acidosis and diabetic coma.
   3. Decreased resistance to infection should the following complications occur
      a. Wound contamination
      b. Respiratory infection
C. Decreased ADH results in diabetes insipidus; deficiency state causes inability to conserve water.
   1. Diabetes insipidus occurs immediately postoperatively (and for 24 hours after).
      a. Polyuria (6 to 24 L/day)
      b. Polydipsia
   2. Nursing intervention
      a. Observe for dehydration and hypotension.
         (1) Monitor increased urinary output.
         (2) Check specific gravity of urine.
         (3) Monitor serum electrolytes; Na^+ important
      b. Administer as ordered.
         (1) Vasopressin (Pitressin), 10 units subcutaneously every 6 hours
         (2) Fluids at prescribed rates
      c. Observe for signs of fluid overload.
         (1) Water intoxication: decreases serum sodium
         (2) Coma
         (3) Convulsions
D. Neurologic sequelae (because pituitary gland lies adjacent to hypothalamus)
   1. Hyperthermia
   2. Increased intracranial pressure
   3. Cerebrospinal fluid leakage
   4. Convulsions
E. Other concerns
   1. Temperature
      a. Hyperthermia from hypothalamic influence
      b. Hypothermia intolerance from decreased TSH, causing hypothyroid symptoms
   2. Suture line observation
      a. Hematoma formation
      b. Cerebrospinal fluid leakage

THE ADRENAL GLAND (CORTEX)

Hyperaldosteronism

I. Anatomy and physiology
   A. Adrenal glands
      1. Lie retroperitoneal beneath the diaphragm capping the medial aspect of the superior pole of each kidney
      2. The right adrenal is triangular and adjacent to the inferior vena cava.
      3. The left adrenal is round or crescent shaped and sits posterior to the stomach and the pancreas.
   B. Adrenal medulla
      1. Ten percent of the gland secretes catecholamines.

C. The adrenal cortex
   1. Ninety percent of the gland secretes steroids and hormones (i.e., aldosterone, glucocorticoids, and adrenal androgens).
II. Pathophysiology
   A. Cortical hormones (cortisol) normal physiology
      1. Glucocorticoids
         a. Carbohydrate metabolism
         b. Protein metabolism
         c. Promotes lipolysis
         d. Increases tissue responsiveness to other hormones
         e. Antiinflammatory effects
      2. Mineral corticoids (aldosterone)
         a. Increases sodium reabsorption
         b. Increases potassium secretion
   B. Medullary hormones
      1. Catecholamines (epinephrine and norepinephrine)
         a. Systemic responses to stress (fight or flight)
   C. Primary aldosteronism
      1. Definition
         a. Syndrome caused by inappropriate increase in adrenal gland production of the mineralocorticoid aldosterone
         b. Normally, aldosterone produced in response to hyperkalemia and hypovolemia through renin-angiotensin system
         c. Aldosterone acts with kidney to increase potassium wasting and sodium retention.
      2. Etiology
         a. Adenomas (Conn's syndrome): aldosterone producing
         b. Adrenocortical malignancies
         c. Adrenocortical hyperplasias
      3. Effects of increased aldosterone (most potent mineralocorticoid produced by adrenal glands)
         a. Sodium retention
         b. Water retention (hypervolemia)
         c. Hypertension
         d. Hypokalemia leads to alkalosis, dysrhythmias
         e. Generalized weakness
         f. Paresthesia
         g. Tetany
         h. Hyperglycemia
         i. Lowered plasma renins: renin-angiotensin system is primary regulator of aldosterone secretion.
   D. Secondary aldosteronism
      1. Definition: aldosteronism caused by high renin activity from pathologic edematous condition and hypertension
      2. Etiology
         a. Ascites
         b. Congestive heart failure
         c. Obstructive renal artery disease
      3. Resultant symptoms
         a. Hypovolemia
         b. Hyponatremia
         c. Hypokalemia
III. Diagnostic parameters
   A. Laboratory evaluation
      1. Hypernatremia
      2. Hypokalemia
      3. Increased urinary aldosterone excretion
      4. Hyperglycemia and glycosuria

B. Other diagnostic tests
   1. Computed tomography (CT) scan for tumors
   2. ECG changes reflecting hypokalemia
   3. Changes in personality (hyperglycemia)
   4. Adrenal vein serum aldosterone levels
      a. Elevated values on side of tumor
      b. Elevated values on both sides in secondary aldosteronism
IV. Operative procedures
   A. Unilateral adrenalectomy: removal of one adrenal gland
   B. Bilateral adrenalectomy: removal of both adrenal glands
V. Preoperative concerns
   A. Preoperative correction of hypokalemia and hypertension
      1. Spironolactone (Aldactone, Aldactazide): reverses physiologic effects of aldosterone
      2. Potassium chloride supplements
      3. Sodium restriction to promote potassium retention
      4. Diuretics and digitalis for heart failure
   B. Achieve highest possible state of stability before administration of anesthesia.
VI. Anesthesia concerns
   A. Maintain normotensive blood pressure.
      1. Control of hypertension
         a. Aggravated on induction and during tumor manipulation
         b. Antihypertensive agents
            (1) Vasodilators
               (a) Nitroglycerin
               (b) Sodium nitroprusside (Nipride)
            (2) Angiotensin-converting enzyme (ACE) inhibitors, calcium channel blockers, potassium-sparing agents
      2. Control of hypotension
         a. Most likely occurrence after tumor removal (with decreased circulating aldosterone)
         b. Management
            (1) Increased volume administration
            (2) Use of expanders (blood, albumin) may counter need for vasopressors
   B. Deep muscle relaxation and anesthesia level
      1. Necessary for adequate exposure and manipulation of retroperitoneal tumors
      2. Aggravates hypotension after tumor removal
   C. Maintain normal serum potassium.
   D. Monitor dysrhythmias.
      1. Causes: hypokalemia, decreases in catecholamine levels
      2. Counteracting agents: digitalis, calcium channel blockers
   E. Anesthetic agents and adjuncts
      1. Halothane: inhibits sympathetic responses but can sensitize myocardium to epinephrine, leading to dysrhythmias
      2. Enflurane: avoid if hyperaldosteronism is caused by renal disease.
      3. Droperidol and fentanyl citrate (Innovar)
         a. Droperidol raises epinephrine threshold, reducing dysrhythmias in those with low levels of circulating epinephrine.
         b. Fentanyl has fewer histamine effects than other narcotics.
      4. Nondepolarizing muscle relaxants increase histamine activity.

Cushing's Disease

I. Physiology of adrenal gland
   A. The anterior pituitary gland when stimulated by the hypothalamus will release ACTH.
      1. This release usually occurs early in the morning.

       2. In response to the ACTH, the adrenal cortex releases about 20 mg of cortisol daily.

       3. These hormones react on a negative-feedback basis.

       4. Cortisol has an anti-inflammatory effect, but its most important role is its response to stress.

  II. Etiology: Excess output of cortisol and androgens from adrenal cortex

     A. Hyperactivity of adrenal cortex resulting from adenoma or carcinoma

     B. Overstimulation of adrenal cortices by increased ACTH from pituitary gland

     C. Iatrogenic etiology: prolonged use of glucocorticoids

     D. Congenital disorders

 III. Signs and symptoms

     A. Plethoric facies

     B. Moon-shaped face

     C. Hypertension

     D. Ecchymosis and easy bruising

     E. Thin skin

     F. Buffalo hump

     G. Hirsutism

     H. Centripetal (truncal) obesity with muscle wasting

     I. Poor wound healing

     J. Osteoporosis

 IV. Diagnostic parameters

     A. Laboratory indicators

       1. Elevated cortisol levels

       2. Decreased eosinophil levels

       3. Increased plasma ACTH if cause is pituitary gland

       4. Hypokalemia

     B. Diagnostic indicators

       1. Skull films to identify pituitary tumors if increased ACTH level

       2. Adrenal scanning

         a. CT scan

         b. Radioactive cholesterol uptake

       3. Dexamethasone suppression test: failure to suppress cortisol secretion confirms diagnosis of Cushing's syndrome

  V. Operative procedures (dependent on etiology)

     A. Unilateral adrenalectomy: removal of one adrenal gland for localized adenoma

     B. Bilateral adrenalectomy: removal of both adrenal glands; may be performed for pituitary tumors to decrease ACTH influence on adrenal glands

     C. Hypophysectomy: removal of pituitary gland for microadenomas

 VI. Operative concerns

     A. Preoperative and intraoperative concerns

       1. Hypertension

       2. Hyperglycemia

       3. Hypokalemia

       4. Edema

     B. Intraoperative and anesthesia concerns

       1. Compromised lung expansion

         a. Truncal obesity

         b. Awkward positioning for flank approach

       2. Positioning for exposure

         a. Abdominal approach; increases chance of splenic or pancreatic injury

         b. Flank approach

           (1) Pneumothorax possible if twelfth rib resected

           (2) Vena caval injury (rare)

       3. Cortisone supplement for surgical stress

       4. Electrolyte monitoring, especially of potassium

       5. Avoid hyperglycemia greater than 200 mg/dl.

       6. Control hypertension resulting from blood volume increase.

7. Control hypotension resulting from loss of mineralocorticoids (aldosterone deficiency).

Addison's Disease

I. Pathophysiology
   A. Definition: adrenocortical insufficiency manifested by hyposecretion of cortisol and aldosterone
   B. Etiology
      1. Autoimmune reaction
      2. Influence from other glandular conditions
      3. Congenital disorder
      4. Malignancy
      5. Infection
      6. Most common: glandular atrophy resulting from steroid therapy for other conditions (iatrogenic)
II. Postanesthesia significance
   A. Failure to recognize patients taking cortisone (for rheumatoid arthritis, asthma, colitis, etc.) or inadequately replacing cortisone during and after surgical procedures can result in acute Addisonian crisis and death.
   B. Addisonian crisis is major complication after adrenal surgery.
III. Acute Addisonian crisis
   A. Signs and symptoms
      1. Prolonged hypotension and cardiac dysrhythmia (atrial fibrillation with rapid ventricular response)
         a. Decreased cardiac output
         b. Decreased vascular resistance
         c. Decreased wedge pressure
         d. Lack of response to vasopressors; vessels respond poorly to dopamine or volume expanders
      2. Fever
      3. Nausea and vomiting
      4. Electrolyte imbalance
         a. Hypoglycemia
         b. Hyponatremia
         c. Hyperkalemia
      5. Lethargy, somnolence lead to altered mental state and coma.
   B. Treatment
      1. Hydrocortisone: up to 300 mg/70 kg per day
      2. Symptomatic treatment of accompanying electrolyte imbalance

THE ADRENAL GLAND (MEDULLA)

Pheochromocytoma

I. Pathophysiology
   A. Preganglionic fibers of the sympathetic nervous system end in the medullary portions of both adrenal glands.
   B. They stimulate the release of catecholamines and have very short half-lives, usually less than 1 minute.
   C. Catecholamines have both inotropic and chronotropic effects on the heart and blood vessels, inhibit the release of insulin, but stimulate liver glycogenesis.
   D. These effects are commonly seen in the "fight or flight" situation.
   E. Pheochromocytomas are catecholamine-producing tumors that typically cause hypertension.
   F. These tumors are present in 0.1% to 1% of individuals with sustained hypertension.

II. Etiology
    A. Benign tumor of adrenal medulla: 90% of cases
    B. Tumors in other locations
        1. Thorax
        2. Bladder
        3. Brain
        4. Along sympathetic chain
        5. Aorta
        6. Ovaries
        7. Spleen
    C. Tumors secrete catecholamines (norepinephrine, epinephrine).
III. Effects of increased catecholamine secretion
    A. Severe hypertension (paroxysmal or sustained)
    B. Orthostatic hypotension
    C. Cardiomegaly
    D. Elevated blood sugar (from insulin suppression)
    E. Elevated white blood cell count
    F. Increased hematocrit (from decreased plasma volume)
    G. Hypermetabolism
IV. Diagnostic parameters
    A. Laboratory testing
        1. Twenty-four–hour urine collection for catecholamines
            a. Increase in both norepinephrine and epinephrine indicates adrenal pheochromocytoma.
            b. Increase in only norepinephrine indicates tumor may be of sympathetic origin.
        2. Vanillylmandelic acid (VMA), a by-product of catecholamine degradation, elevated in 80% of pheochromocytomas
        3. Radioenzymatic: costly but measures plasma level
        4. Clonidine: treat with single dose; decreases plasma norepinephrine
    B. CT scan
        1. Localizes tumor
        2. Ninety-eight percent accurate
    C. Signs and symptoms
        1. Cardiovascular (paroxysmal)
            a. Angina
            b. Palpitations
            c. Tachycardia
        2. Gastrointestinal
            a. Abdominal pain
            b. Nausea
            c. Weight loss
        3. Neuromuscular and vascular
            a. Headaches
            b. Diaphoresis
            c. Irritability
            d. Visual disturbances
V. Preoperative management
    A. Establish alpha-adrenergic blockage with phenoxybenzamine hydrochloride (Dibenzyline).
        1. Beginning doses: 20 to 30 mg daily, increasing to 60 to 250 mg daily until blood pressure controlled
        2. Volume repletion
        3. Control of tachycardia with beta-blockers
VI. Operative procedure
    A. Radical adrenalectomy performed with removal of affected gland and adjacent areolar tissue

VII. Operative concerns with alpha-blocker and beta-blocker drugs
   A. Avoidance of drugs causing histamine release or sympathetic stimulation
      1. Narcotics
         a. Substitution of barbiturates for preoperative narcotic medication
         b. Use of fentanyl because of its decreased histamine release
      2. Nondepolarizing muscle relaxants
      3. Adrenergic drugs
      4. Cholinergic blockers
   B. Avoid sympathetic response during
      1. Anesthesia induction
      2. Tracheal intubation
      3. Positioning
      4. Manipulation of tumor
      5. Ligation of venous drainage of tumor
   C. Need for adequate CO_2 absorption to reduce increased catecholamine production
   D. Continuous blood pressure monitoring
      1. Electronic apparatus
      2. Arterial monitoring
   E. Have drugs readily available.
      1. Before tumor excision
         a. Phentolamine mesylate (Regitine)
         b. Sodium nitroprusside (Nipride)
      2. After tumor excision, if rebound hypotension occurs
         a. Norepinephrine
         b. Blood and volume expanders
         c. Cortisone for replacement only if both adrenal glands excised

POSTANESTHESIA NURSING CARE FOR PATIENTS WITH ADRENAL GLAND CONDITIONS

   I. Related nursing diagnostic categories
      A. Potential for infection
      B. Decreased cardiac output
      C. Ineffective airway clearance
      D. Potential for impaired gas exchange
      E. Fluid volume excess or deficit
      F. Potential for electrolyte disturbances
  II. Hypotension
      A. More common than hypertension
      B. Bleeding: adrenocorticoid insufficiency
      C. Persistent, unexplained hypotension may precede adrenal crisis.
      D. Rebound epinephrine shock: complicated by receptors that have become insensitive and vascular reflexes that are slow to respond
 III. Hypertension
      A. Occasionally seen after excision of pheochromocytoma
      B. Antihypertensive agents often more effective than when administered before tumor excision
  IV. Electrolyte values (serum and urine)
      A. Monitor
         1. Decreases in serum Na^+
         2. Increases in urine Na^+
         3. Increases in serum K^+
            a. In unrecognized Addisonian patient
            b. Transient with primary hyperaldosteronism
            c. When hypokalemia overcorrected

4. Serum glucose
   a. Hypoglycemia: unrecognized Addisonian patient
   b. Hyperglycemia: after excision of pheochromocytoma from related preoperative insulin suppression

V. Fluid administration
   A. Hypertonic saline at prescribed rate
   B. Blood, plasma, albumin for decreased hemoglobin, hematocrit, and volume
   C. Sudden withdrawal of catecholamines postoperatively makes patient susceptible to rapid changes in blood pressure and fluid and electrolyte balance

VI. Wound observation
   A. Increased infection susceptibility
   B. Increased bleeding or hematoma formation
      1. Resulting from easy bruisability and/or hypertension
      2. Signal of internal hemorrhaging
      3. Meticulous care necessary for dressing changes

VII. Chest film confirmation
   A. Bilateral lung expansion after adrenalectomy (if twelfth rib resection necessary)
   B. Central venous pressure catheter placement

VIII. Complications
   A. Shock
      1. Causes
         a. Addisonian crisis caused by decreased cortisol and aldosterone levels
            (1) After bilateral adrenalectomy
            (2) After any surgery on patients taking cortisone for chronic medical conditions
         b. Decreased circulating catecholamines after excision of pheochromocytoma
         c. Inadequate blood volume
      2. Treatment (specific to underlying causes)
         a. Hydrocortisone for Addisonian-related problems
         b. Norepinephrine (Levophed) drip for decreased catecholamine effects
         c. Blood, plasma, albumin for hypovolemia
   B. Pneumothorax: atelectasis
      1. Occurs usually after rib resection
      2. Signaled by dyspnea, uneven chest expansion, chest pain, decreased to absent breath sounds
      3. Confirmed by chest film
      4. Treated with insertion of chest tube
   C. Cerebrovascular accident
      1. Risk increases intraoperatively.
         a. With inadequately controlled hypertension accompanying excision of pheochromocytoma
         b. With increased catecholamines and fluid overload
         c. With inappropriate aldosterone release, renal artery ligation
      2. Ascertained by postanesthesia evaluation
         a. Level of consciousness
         b. Ability to move all extremities
         c. Bilateral Babinski's sign present
         d. Pupillary changes
         e. Slurred speech
   D. Cardiac dysrhythmias
      1. Causes
         a. Tachydysrhythmias: increased catecholamine circulating after excision of pheochromocytoma
         b. Uncorrected hypokalemia after hyperaldosteronism and Cushing's disease

    2. Treatment (specific to underlying cause)

      a. Beta-blockers for tachydysrhythmias

      b. Potassium supplements if decreased serum potassium

      c. Amiodarone or lidocaine for ventricular tachycardia and fibrillation

  E. Infection

    1. Resulting from cortisone masking signs of infection

    2. Poor wound healing

  F. Hypoglycemia

    1. Occurs from rebound hyperinsulinemia

    2. Results from removal of anti-insulin factor in tumor, enhanced glucoreceptor reactivity to insulin, or both

DIABETES MELLITUS IN THE SURGICAL PATIENT

  I. Pathophysiology

    A. Etiology

      1. Syndrome characterized by glucose intolerance, large vessel disease, microvascular disease, and neuropathy

      2. Diabetic patient at higher risk for surgery and anesthetic complications than nondiabetic patient

      3. Cardiovascular complications responsible for 80% of diabetic deaths

      4. Amputation 20 times more likely in diabetic population

    B. Types of diabetes mellitus

      1. Type I: insulin dependent (ketosis prone)

        a. Characteristics

          (1) Little or no endogenous insulin

          (2) Children and young adults

          (3) Lower than average body weight

        b. Causes

          (1) Genetic: human leukocyte antigen (HLA) immune antigen

          (2) Body's immune system destroys pancreatic beta cells, the only cells in the body that make the hormone insulin that regulates blood glucose.

          (3) Environmental: viruses

          (4) Autoimmunity: circulating islet cell antibodies

      2. Type II: maturity onset (no longer referred to as non–insulin-dependent, NIDDM, as patients may require insulin as part of their disease management), nonketotic

        a. Characteristics

          (1) Overweight

          (2) Middle aged

          (3) Sometimes high levels of circulating insulin

          (4) Carbohydrate intolerance

        b. Causes

          (1) Problems at beta-cell level

          (2) Insulin resistance or decrease in receptor sites

      3. Type III: impaired glucose tolerance (chemical or borderline diabetes); causes: receptor sites decreased or not receptive to insulin

  II. Prevalence of diabetes

    A. Estimated 17 million people have diabetes—6.2% of the population

    B. Many surgical disorders such as cataracts, cholelithiasis, vascular disease have been identified in this group.

    C. Estimated that 50% of diabetic population experience at least one surgical intervention in their lifetimes

  III. Special effects of diabetes on surgical problems

    A. Increased prevalence of macrovascular disease affecting coronary and cerebral arteries as well as peripheral arterial supply

    B. Gastrointestinal and urinary bladder dysfunctions

C. Causes of occult infections
1. Lowered resistance during periods of stress-induced hyperglycemia; glucose levels greater than 200 inhibit white blood cell activity
2. Catabolic effect of insulin deficiency, which results in protein wastage and adversely affects wound healing
3. Electrolyte and hormone deficiencies
    a. Potassium depletion causing decreased stroke volume, dysrhythmias
    b. Hyperkalemia may be result of renal impairment causing bradycardia, ventricular fibrillation.
    c. Stress and trauma lead to hyperglycemia, may lead to ketoacidotic coma.

IV. General adaptation syndrome (GAS) described by Selye
A. Sympathetic nervous system (adrenal medulla) stimulates production of catecholamines.
1. Increases heart rate
2. Increases blood pressure
3. Dilates bronchi
B. Blood glucose increases.
1. Catecholamines cause glycogen stores in liver to release glucose into blood system.
2. Glucocorticoids (primary cortisol) secreted by adrenal cortex cause liver to produce additional carbohydrates from fats, proteins.
3. Gluconeogenesis may elevate blood glucose levels six to eight times normal.
C. Along with increasing glucose levels, catecholamines inhibit pancreas from releasing insulin.
D. Glucocorticoids decrease use of glucose in adipose tissue and stimulate formation of circulating insulin antagonist.
E. Proclivity for infection
1. Inadequate circulation to extremities
2. Hyperglycemia; excellent culture media

V. Operative concerns
A. Preoperative evaluation
1. Cardiovascular system
    a. One of most common causes of mortality in diabetic patients
    b. Painless angina occurs more often in diabetics than in general population.
    c. For diabetics who have experienced a myocardial infarction, risk of reinfarction within 4 to 6 months is 10%.
    d. Diagnostic tests
        (1) Serum lipid values
        (2) ECG
2. Renal function
    a. Serum creatinine
    b. Blood urea nitrogen (BUN)
    c. Urinary output
3. Serum values
    a. Glucose and acetone levels
    b. Glycosylated hemoglobin (hemoglobin A1C) to determine long-term (3 months) control of diabetes
    c. Electrolytes
        (1) Potassium
        (2) Sodium
        (3) Chloride
        (4) Bicarbonate
B. Drugs altering glucose levels
1. Thiazides and loop diuretics
    a. Contribute to hyperglycemia
    b. Hyperglycemic effect may be outweighed by antihypertensive value.
2. Phenytoin (Dilantin): may cause mild hyperglycemia.

       3. Propranolol

         a. Modified hypoglycemic reaction of insulin by blocking catecholamine release

         b. Possibly inhibits insulin release from pancreas

       4. Chlorpropamide (Diabinese): lengthy half-life necessitates discontinuance 24 to 36 hours preoperatively.

   C. Gastroparesis

       1. Caused by autonomic neuropathy

       2. Results in weak or absent esophageal motility

         a. When diabetic patients lie flat, food and liquids pool in esophagus.

         b. Delay in gastric emptying

         c. Risk of aspiration of gastric contents is intensified.

   D. Control of diabetes during surgery: both diabetic and nondiabetic patients are somewhat resistant to insulin during this stress period.

       1. Goal: prevent hyperosmolar coma (usually in type II) and ketoacidosis without inducing hypoglycemia.

         a. Maintain patient in well-hydrated anabolic state.

         b. Avoid hypoglycemia or hyperglycemia by adequate preoperative preparation.

         c. Frequent monitoring of blood glucose levels

       2. Operative strategy

         a. Schedule procedure as early in morning as possible.

         b. Discontinue oral agents before surgery.

            (1) Patients taking oral hypoglycemics may be given regular insulin before surgery.

            (2) Titrated according to glucose levels

         c. Assess preoperative fasting blood glucose levels.

         d. Begin IV fluids containing glucose at rate appropriate to keep patient well hydrated.

       3. Insulin regimens

         a. Common method of insulin administration on day of surgery: of patient's usual dose of intermediate-acting insulin subcutaneously on morning of surgery; absorption may be impeded if patient becomes too cold while exposed to low temperatures in operating suite

         b. More controlled method of insulin administration achieved with constant infusion of D_5W, 25 to 100 ml/hour piggyback with an insulin solution at 1 to 5 U/hour; most critical issue for maintaining insulin blood glucose levels is reliable blood glucose monitoring; rapid access crucial in monitoring these levels; many practitioners maintain intraarterial lines, a practical approach to access

         c. Glucose and insulin infusions may induce hypokalemia; potassium chloride may be added to infusion if renal function is satisfactory.

VI. Anesthesia concerns

   A. Type of anesthesia

       1. No "best" anesthetic for diabetic patients

       2. Inhalation agents cause less pronounced changes in blood glucose.

       3. Stress and practice of rapid administration of glucose-containing IV fluids have more profound effect on blood glucose.

       4. Regional blocks may be considered in some diabetic patients because they produce fewer metabolic disturbances.

   B. Avoidance of hypoglycemia and serious cerebral dysfunction

       1. Blood glucose level for diabetic patients commonly maintained between 120 and 220 mg/dl

         a. For protection against unexpected drop to hypoglycemia

         b. Elevations capable of causing significant glycosuria

       2. Subtle external signs

         a. Slight increase in pulse

         b. Decrease in urinary output

C. Avoidance of hyperglycemia
    1. Leads to glycosuria and significant polyuria, electrolyte imbalance, and dehydration of osmotic diuresis
    2. Diuresis and vasodilating drugs may render diabetic patient hemodynamically unstable during anesthesia.
    3. Less resistance to infection
        a. Impaired phagocytosis
        b. Decrease in tissue strength and healing of wounds
        c. Increase in free fatty acids
    4. Hypoglycemic agents (see Table 41-2)
D. Avoidance of hypoxemia, hypotension, impaired cardiac function
    1. Myocardial infarction
        a. Results from increased severity of large-vessel atherosclerosis
        b. One of leading causes of high mortality in diabetic patients
    2. Hypotension caused by persistent urinary losses will result in ketoacidosis.
    3. Hypoxemia
        a. Influenced by long-term control of diabetic patients
        b. Increase in glycosylated hemoglobin will influence tissue oxygenation.
        c. Increase in oxygen consumption in patient already borderline oxygenated as result of increased shunting (commonly seen in anesthetized patient) may result in pronounced hypoxemia.
E. Avoidance of injury during anesthesia
    1. Patients with peripheral neuropathy vulnerable to positioning injuries
    2. Impaired gastric emptying should be anticipated.
VII. Postanesthesia concerns
A. Related nursing diagnostic categories
    1. Potential for decreased cardiac output
    2. Potential for infection
    3. Potential for fluid volume deficit
    4. Potential for impaired gas exchange
    5. Potential for ineffective airway clearance
B. Assess levels of consciousness.
    1. Persistent disorientation, unconsciousness may portend hypoglycemia.
    2. Hyperglycemia (diabetic coma); occurs rarely immediately postoperatively.
C. Monitor serum glucose on admission to PACU.
    1. Serum levels are only accurate indication for insulin requirement.
    2. Urinary glucose and acetone values reflect serum level of preceding few hours and lead to erratic control of hyperglycemia.
D. Continue hydration.
    1. Monitor urinary output.
    2. Monitor vital signs.
E. Monitor cardiac dysrhythmias.
    1. Note hypokalemic change of ECG.
        a. Depressed T wave and ST segment
        b. Prolonged QT interval
        c. U waves

■ TABLE 41-2
■ ■ **Insulin Profiles**

Insulin Agent	Onset (hours)	Peak (hours)	Duration (hours)
Rapid acting (Lispro)	15 minutes	30-90 minutes	5
Short acting (regular)	30 minutes	2-4	4-8
Intermediate acting (NPH/Lente)	2-6	4-14	14-20
Long acting (Ultralente)	6-14	Little (10-16)	20-24

    2. Hypokalemia leads to increased premature ventricular contractions.

    3. Supplemental potassium for hypokalemia

    4. Tachydysrhythmias; propranolol helpful

    5. Persistent hypotension may require hydrocortisone.

  F. Prevention of infection: meticulous attention to sterile technique

    1. Surgical dressings

    2. Urinary catheter insertion

    3. Invasive monitoring lines

    4. Pulmonary hygiene

  G. Complications

    1. Sudden death from respiratory or cardiac arrest; respiratory arrests may be caused by severe autonomic neuropathy.

      a. Avoid dehydration and electrolyte deficits.

      b. Lactic acidosis

        (1) Associated with circulatory collapse, renal or hepatic failure, alcoholism

        (2) High mortality

    2. Diabetic coma or acidosis caused by decreased insulin and increased insulin-antagonistic hormones (cortisol)

      a. Rarely seen in PACU

      b. Confirmation

        (1) Serum electrolytes

        (2) Increased potassium

        (3) Increased BUN

        (4) Increased serum osmolarity

        (5) Increased serum glucose and acetone level

        (6) Arterial blood gas pH decreases to 7.30; decreased bicarbonate levels

        (7) Tachypnea

        (8) Tachycardia

        (9) Polyuria

        (10) Hypotension

      c. Treatment

        (1) Fluid and electrolyte correction

        (2) Insulin administration

        (3) Bicarbonate for pH less than 7.20 (1 mEq/kg)

    3. Hypoglycemic reaction

      a. Causes

        (1) Inadequate amount of glucose after insulin administration

        (2) Incorrect or overdosage of insulin

        (3) Hyperfunction of beta-cells in pancreatic tumors

        (4) Brittle and juvenile diabetics eliciting undue response to insulin action

      b. Symptoms (sudden onset)

        (1) Weakness, dizziness

        (2) Moist, pale skin

        (3) Shallow breathing pattern

        (4) Confusion, incoherence

        (5) Combativeness

      c. Treatment (initiated before laboratory confirmation)

        (1) Obtain serum glucose for future confirmation.

        (2) Immediate administration of dextrose 50% bolus (50 ml)

        (3) Observance of (often dramatic) return of orientation after dextrose bolus

PANCREAS TRANSPLANTATION

  I. Overview

    A. At present, transplantation of the pancreas is the only treatment that can render type I diabetic patients euglycemic.

B. In addition, secondary complications of diabetes are lessened and in some cases ameliorated.

C. The incidence of success in whole organ pancreas transplant is 77% with the new antirejection agents.

D. Higher morbidity exists with pancreas transplantation than in the more common simultaneous pancreas and kidney transplantation.

E. Islet cell transplants are less common.

F. Clinical trials for patients with diabetes and without kidney disease have not been performed in the number that would provide validity to the research.

G. Less than 10% of a small sample of patients have achieved insulin independence.

II. Preoperative assessment

A. Pancreas transplants are *elective* procedures: hence the patient should have attained

   1. Absence of infection: diabetic patients should be screened for remote infection (i.e., urinary tract infection, respiratory, dental).

   2. Tight control of blood sugar

   3. Balance of electrolytes

B. Systems review

   1. Nervous system: peripheral neuropathy and gastroparesis

   2. Cardiopulmonary hypervolemia, hyperkalemia, coronary artery disease (CAD)

   3. Musculoskeletal: joint immobilities or contracture osteopenia

III. Preoperative preparation

A. Medication

   1. Ranitidine, 50 mg, and metoclopramide, 10 mg

   2. Antibiotics: vancomycin or cefotaxime

B. Blood availability

C. Control hyperglycemia with regular insulin 25 U/250 ml in 0.9% normal saline solution.

D. Arterial lines

IV. Anesthesia concerns

A. Rapid induction because of gastroparesis

B. Muscle relaxants: succinylcholine used to induce if patient is eukalemic (3.5 to 5 mEq/L)

C. Atracurium for maintenance of blockade in patients with end-stage renal disease (ESRD)

   1. Glucose management: attempt to maintain serum glucose at 70 to 100 mg/dl

   2. After reperfusion of graft, slow the insulin infusion.

D. Control of K^+ levels: this is difficult to do because a high percentage of patients have wide fluctuations; treating variations in serum K^+ levels should be anticipated even with adequate glucose control.

E. Administration of immunosuppressive agents before graft reperfusion

V. Postanesthesia concerns

A. Pain management: incisional, joint, and neuropathic

B. Hypovolemia if recently dialyzed; hyperkalemia and hypervolemia if not dialyzed

C. Aspiration pneumonitis

D. Control of glucose levels

   1. Usually an insulin infusion with 25 units of regular insulin in 250 ml 0.9% normal saline solution is used to maintain blood sugar at 70 to 100 mg/dl.

   2. Hyperglycemia of 300 mg/dl is treated with boluses of regular insulin in addition to the insulin drip.

   3. Important to control serum glucose by changing infusion rate rather than by bolus in patients who have glucose levels less than 250 mg/dl

E. Noncardiogenic pulmonary edema associated with intraoperative immunosuppressives

F. Protection of hemodialysis access sites

G. Infection control: patients remain at high risk for infection.

H. Blood loss intraoperatively may require replacement in PACU.

BIBLIOGRAPHY

1. American Diabetes Organization: Diabetes statistics. Available at https://www.diabetes.org/about-diabetes.jsp. Accessed on December 22, 2003.

2. Clark OH, Duh QY, editors: *Textbook of endocrine surgery.* Philadelphia: WB Saunders, 1997.

3. Clement B: Parathyroid pathophysiology. *Semin Perioper Nurs* 7(3):186-192, 1998.

4. Davidson JK, editor: *Clinical diabetes mellitus: A problem oriented approach,* ed 3. New York: Thieme, 2000.

5. DeGroat LJ, Jamison JL, editors: *Endocrinology,* ed 4. Philadelphia: WB Saunders, 2001.

6. Dorn L, Cerrone P: Cognitive functioning on patients with Cushing's Syndrome: A longitudinal perspective. *Clin Nurs Res* 9(4):420-440, 2000.

7. Lawrence P, editor: *Essentials of surgical specialties.* Philadelphia: Lippincott Williams & Wilkins, 2000.

8. Meeker M, Rothrock JC, editors: *Alexander's care of the patient in surgery.* St Louis: Mosby, 2002.

9. Morwessel N: The genetic basis of diabetes mellitus. *AACN Clin Issues* 9(4):539-554, 1998.

10. Roizen MF, Fleisher LA, editors: *Essence of anesthesia practice.* Philadelphia: WB Saunders, 1997.

11. Selye H: *Stress without distress.* Philadelphia: Lippincott, 1974.

12. Sprung J, Kinney M, Warner M, et al: Anesthetic aspects of laparoscopic adrenalectomy. *Semin Anesth* 21(1):35-45, 2002.

13. Williams M: Disorders of the adrenal gland. *Semin Perioper Nurs* 7(3):179-185, 1998.

42 Gastrointestinal Surgery

DENISE O'BRIEN

■■ Acknowledgement: I thank Lisa Colletti, MD, for her assistance in preparing this chapter.

OBJECTIVES

At the conclusion of this chapter the reader will be able to:

1. Describe the fluid and electrolyte problems most frequently encountered in the patient with a gastrointestinal disorder.

2. Incorporate the care of the other body systems into the postoperative management of the gastrointestinal surgery patient.

3. Describe two specific system complications of the gastrointestinal surgery patient.

4. State the rationale for placement of tubes and drains in the gastrointestinal surgery patient.

5. State the rationale for observations necessary in postanesthesia care of the patient undergoing gastrointestinal surgery.

■■ The gastrointestinal system is one of the longest systems in the human body, offering many opportunities for pathology. Many operative procedures are performed on this system. The most frequently encountered procedures in the adult population will be discussed. A few references will be made to those pediatric gastrointestinal procedures performed primarily for congenital defects.

ANATOMY AND PHYSIOLOGY

Before using this review text, the reader will have independently reviewed the anatomy and physiology for this system (Figure 42-1) and be able to do the following:

1. Correctly name and locate the major anatomic components of the gastrointestinal tract and the accessory organs of digestion;

2. Identify the major functions of each of the divisions of the gastrointestinal system and the accessory organs of digestion.

PATHOPHYSIOLOGY

A list of causes of gastrointestinal pathophysiologic conditions follows. The causes are varied, and therefore this list is not inclusive. Examples of disease processes or operative procedures are included parenthetically for clarification.

    I. Neoplasms and growths
        A. Malignancies, either primary or metastatic
        B. Polyps: a benign proliferation of cells lining the gastrointestinal tract, some with potential for malignant transformation
        C. See also III.A, III.B.

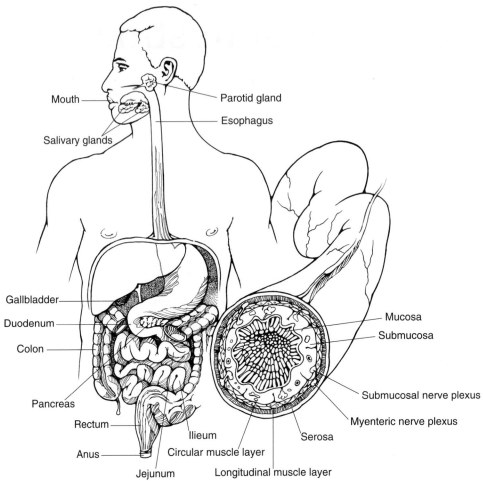

FIGURE 42-1 ■ The gastrointestinal system. (From Ignatavicius DD, Bayne MV: *Medical-surgical nursing*, 4th ed. Philadelphia: WB Saunders, 2002, p 1160.)

II. Calculi
   A. Calculi or stones (e.g., cholelithiasis), primarily resulting from supersaturation of bile with cholesterol
III. Strictures or obstructions
   A. Stricture: abnormal narrowing of gastrointestinal passage
      1. Neoplasms commonly cause strictures, for example, in the colon and biliary tree.
      2. Strictures can progress to obstruction (blockage of gastrointestinal passage) or be caused by adhesions.
   B. Adhesions: union of two normally separate surfaces or a fibrous band that connects them, occasionally producing obstruction or malfunction of an organ
      1. Adhesions are the result of the formation of scar tissue.
      2. Abdominal surgery always results in the formation of adhesions or scar tissue; the magnitude of these adhesions or scar tissue varies.
      3. Approximately 5% of cases associated with adhesions occur in persons who have had no previous abdominal surgery; however, this is virtually always the result of some other previous or ongoing pathologic process, such as pelvic inflammatory disease, appendicitis, or diverticulitis.

IV. Ulceration
  A. Ulcer disease
    1. Peptic ulcer disease
      a. *Helicobacter pylori (H. pylori)*
      b. Medications (e.g., aspirin, steroids, and especially nonsteroidal antiinflammatory agents [NSAIDs])
    2. Stress ulceration, resulting from the following
      a. Surgical stress
      b. Burns
      c. Cranial trauma
      d. Sepsis associated with multisystem failure
  B. Ulcerative colitis (also an inflammatory process)
V. Perforations
  A. Caused by ulceration
  B. Resulting from trauma
  C. Can also result from vascular compromise or strangulation obstruction
VI. Inflammations
  A. Regional enteritis (Crohn's disease)
  B. Cholecystitis
  C. Pancreatitis
  D. Appendicitis
  E. Diverticulitis
  F. Esophagitis
  G. Gastritis
VII. Altered innervation
  A. Achalasia
VIII. Congenital defects
  A. Hirschsprung's disease
  B. Tracheoesophageal fistula
  C. Imperforate anus
  D. Pyloric stenosis
  E. Arteriovenous malformation
IX. Ischemia: arterial or venous infarction
  A. Complication after abdominal aortic aneurysmectomy
  B. After repair of coarctation of aorta
  C. After coronary artery bypass
X. Gastroesophageal reflux disease (GERD)
  A. Symptomatic clinical condition or change in tissue structure
  B. Results from the reflux of stomach or duodenal contents into the esophagus
  C. Symptoms may include heartburn, gastric regurgitation, dysphagia, pulmonary manifestations (asthma, coughing, wheezing, laryngeal inflammation)

ASSESSMENT PARAMETERS AND PREOPERATIVE EVALUATION

I. Diagnostic tests or procedures: Tests ordered depend on gastrointestinal area thought to be involved.
  A. Laboratory tests
    1. Basic hematology and electrolyte studies
    2. Serum enzyme levels (amylase, lipase, and liver function tests [LFTs])
    3. Serum markers
      a. CA 19-9 for pancreatic cancer
      b. Alpha-fetoprotein (AFP) for hepatocellular cancer
    4. Carcinoembryonic antigen (CEA) for some types of cancer, especially cancers of the pancreas, large intestine (colon and rectum), breast, or lung

     5. Coagulation studies if liver involvement suspected or with malabsorption syndromes; these syndromes cause malabsorption of vitamins that can compromise metabolism of the coagulation factors produced by the liver

     6. Bilirubin studies, alkaline phosphatase

     7. Twenty-four hour pH monitoring with probe for reflux

B. Endoscopic procedures

     1. Motility studies (e.g., esophageal manometry)

     2. Esophagogastroduodenoscopy (EGD)

     3. Endoscopic retrograde cholangiopancreatography (ERCP), with or without stents, sphincterotomy

       a. Purpose: to remove retained common duct stones before or after biliary tract surgery, or as an emergency measure in patients with common bile duct obstruction (single or multiple stones) resulting in cholangitis; may be done preoperatively to explore common bile duct in patients needing laparoscopic cholecystectomies

       b. Description: by use of side-viewing fiber optic endoscope, pancreatic, biliary, and hepatic ducts are cannulated through ampulla of Vater and visualized fluoroscopically after retrograde injection of radiopaque contrast medium.

     4. Colonoscopy

     5. Sigmoidoscopy

C. Radiologic examinations

     1. Barium swallow

     2. Upper gastrointestinal series

     3. Cholangiogram (operative): typically done as part of an ERCP, percutaneous transhepatic cholangiography (PTC), or operatively

     4. PTC

     5. Barium enema

     6. Flat plate of abdomen

     7. Visceral angiography

       a. Angiography

       b. CO_2 digital subtraction angiography

D. Other modalities

     1. Endoscopic ultrasonography

       a. Endoscopic ultrasonography of esophagus, stomach, pancreas and biliary tree, and rectum

       b. Transanal ultrasonography

     2. Computed tomography (CT)

     3. Radionuclide

       a. Gastrointestinal

       b. Liver and spleen

       c. Hydroxyiminodiacetic acid (HIDA) scan for acute cholecystitis or to detect biliary leak

       d. Labeled red blood cells (RBCs) to check site of bleeding

     4. Magnetic resonance imaging (MRI)

     5. Magnetic resonance angiography (MRA): used to evaluate vasculature

     6. Magnetic resonance cholangiopancreatography

E. Tissue biopsies as indicated with cytologic or histologic studies

F. Laparoscopy

INTRAOPERATIVE CONCERNS

I. Proper positioning

  A. Maintain neurovascular integrity.

     1. Padding and support of all body parts with particular attention given to vulnerable areas (e.g., elbows, sacrum, heels, occiput)

     2. For comfort

      3. To maintain proper alignment in presence of arthritis, lumbar disorders, and contractures

      4. To preserve integrity of popliteal nerve and/or ulnar and brachial nerve plexi when lithotomy or exaggerated arm abduction is used

   B. Prevent complications.

      1. Proper application of electrosurgical grounding pads to prevent cautery burns; avoid contact with metal or hard surfaces

      2. Careful positioning changes of anesthetized patient (to and from Trendelenburg or lithotomy position) to prevent adverse alterations in tidal volume and cardiac output; position of padding and support rechecked after each change

      3. Protect skin from shearing while positioning and moving.

II. Cardiovascular stability

   A. Factors influencing altered fluid volume, electrolyte, and nutritional status

      1. Chronic bleeding

      2. Diarrhea

      3. Vomiting

      4. Increased secretions

      5. Fluid loss: nasogastric suctioning, fistula drainage, bowel preparation, and length of operative procedure

   B. Problems with preceding factors if not corrected preoperatively

      1. Hypotension: caused by deficits in circulating volume

         a. Poorly tolerated in pediatric, elderly, and debilitated patients vulnerable to adverse effects of hypotension as result of decreased body reserve necessary to handle crises

         b. Rapid fluid (blood) loss is potential problem as result of rich intestinal blood supply and its proximity to aorta and vena cava.

         c. Rapid fluid resuscitation with crystalloid or colloid solution can result in overhydration, leading to pulmonary edema and congestive heart failure in compromised patient.

      2. Altered electrolyte balance: cardiac dysrhythmias can occur with abnormal potassium or calcium levels.

      3. Clotting abnormalities caused by poor nutritional status or hemodilution or in presence of liver disease

         a. Decreased vitamin K, leading to decreased levels of factors V, VII, IX, and X

         b. Prolonged prothrombin times

III. Thermal regulation

   A. Hyperthermia

      1. Elevated temperature on arrival in the operating room, possibly as a result of infection, peritonitis, or other inflammatory process

      2. Anesthesia care provider must observe for signs and symptoms of possible adverse reaction to anesthetic agents and muscle relaxants, which may lead to malignant hyperthermia, either in operating room or in postanesthesia care unit (PACU) (see Chapter 28).

   B. Hypothermia

      1. Prolonged exposure of abdominal viscera causes loss of body heat leading to hypothermia.

         a. Procedures of 3 or more hours

         b. Extensive gastrointestinal resection

      2. Temperature control methods

         a. Room temperature control

         b. Use of warming mattresses, convective warming devices, and protective coverings

         c. Warming of intravenous (IV) and irrigating fluids

IV. Drug interactions and other concerns

   A. Nondepolarizing muscle relaxants (see Chapter 26)

      1. Antagonized by hypothermia

      2. Patients may reparalyze with postoperative warming.

    3. May have slowed return of neuromuscular function because of hypothermia and decreased elimination of some relaxants (those eliminated by Hoffman elimination [ester hydrolysis])

    4. Potentiated by broad-spectrum antibiotics (mycins, aminoglycosides)

  B. Metabolism and excretion of medications impaired in presence of liver dysfunction, renal failure, and obesity

  C. Avoidance of use of histamine-releasing agents such as morphine sulfate is important consideration in certain patients.

    1. Histamine release can cause hypotension in hypovolemic patient.

  D. All opioids increase biliary tract pressure that may cause spasm of sphincter of Oddi, producing severe right upper quadrant or substernal pain in the patient with biliary obstruction or disease.

    1. Severity of symptoms (pain, nausea, diaphoresis, hypotension) requires that myocardial infarction be ruled out.

    2. Symptoms usually abate with administration of naloxone (Narcan) or glucagon.

  E. Rapid sequence induction ("crash" induction): possible indications

    1. History of gastroesophageal reflux

    2. Stricture of gastroesophageal sphincter

    3. History of recent eating before emergency surgery

    4. Bowel obstruction

    5. History of gastroparesis

  F. Spillage of feces or bile into peritoneal cavity is potential cause of chemical or bacterial peritonitis and should be documented.

GENERAL POSTANESTHESIA CARE CONCERNS

  I. Routine immediate postanesthesia assessment following American Society of PeriAnesthesia Nurses (ASPAN) Standards of Perianesthesia Nursing Practice and American Society of Anesthesiologists (ASA) Standards for Postanesthetic Care

  II. General postanesthesia observation and care for gastrointestinal procedures

  A. Cardiovascular system

    1. Monitor vital signs per unit routine; check perfusion to extremities.

      a. Risk for radical shifts in body fluids as result of inadequate fluid replacement, excessive replacement, preoperative status, presence of fistula, vomiting, diarrhea, intestinal obstruction, third spacing, nasogastric drains and tubes

      b. Sequestered fluid in gastrointestinal tract (resulting from tumor, stricture, adhesions, paralytic ileus, or surgical manipulation) is lost to circulating volume of body; it is in a potential or "third" space; in general, third space fluid does not begin to mobilize until second or third postoperative day.

      c. Stress responses resulting in hormonal alterations can lead to retention of fluids and potential for fluid overload postoperatively.

    2. Observe for hemostasis; observe for and document coagulation deficiencies (oozing, bruising, and petechiae).

      a. In a patient with a history of coagulation problems or one who has received massive transfusions, coagulation difficulties can occur; malabsorption, impaired digestion, or altered liver function will affect clotting.

    3. Leg exercises, range of motion (ROM) at least every hour as part of "stir-up" regimen; antiembolism stockings, intermittent pneumatic or sequential compression devices, or low-dose anticoagulation as ordered

      a. Deep vein thrombosis (DVT) formation is potential complication of immobility; laparoscopic procedures increase risk of emboli as result of air insufflation and resultant increase in intraabdominal pressure, and decreasing venous return, particularly from the lower extremities.

      b. Active ROM exercises stimulate venous return from extremities.

B. Genitourinary system

1. Monitor intake and output every hour and specific gravity every 4 hours.
   a. Potential for decreased urine output as result of fluid shifts (see information on cardiovascular system)
2. Assess bladder distension if no indwelling catheter in place.
   a. Bladder distension is common postoperative problem.
   b. Palpation or bladder ultrasound may be used.
3. Note color of urine.
   a. Retraction or pressure placed on bladder or kidney during surgery can traumatize bladder or kidney.

C. Endocrine system

1. Document blood glucose levels, urine glucose, and ketones as appropriate.
   a. Surgical intervention and operative stress on body systems alter pancreatic enzymes and insulin production.
      (1) Patients with diabetes are observed for same reasons.
   b. Blood glucose can be monitored with blood glucose monitor at bedside.

D. Respiratory system

1. Document routine postanesthesia nursing interventions ("stir-up" or "wake-up" regimens) and their results concerning lung auscultation, deep breathing, incentive spirometry, coughing to mobilize and expectorate secretions, turning, and ROM exercises.
   a. Prevention of decreased lung expansion leading to atelectasis, congestion, and hypostatic pneumonia resulting from oversedation or lack of sedation, hypoxia, fluid overload, decreased ventilatory excursion
2. If central line (CVP or pulmonary artery catheter) is placed intraoperatively or in PACU, obtain chest film.
   a. Demonstration of correct catheter placement and confirmation of presence or absence of pneumothorax
3. Document chest drainage and chest tube function.
   a. Follow PACU routine for care of chest tubes for patients undergoing pulmonary approach for upper gastrointestinal surgery (esophageal resection, hiatal herniorrhaphy).

E. Gastrointestinal system

1. NPO (nothing by mouth)
   a. Nausea and vomiting may be present because of effects of anesthesia, decreased intestinal motility, malfunctioning nasogastric tube, and disease process.
2. Nasogastric tube assessment
   a. Check for proper tube placement by auscultating with stethoscope over gastric area while inserting 20 to 50 ml air into tube.
      (1) If nasogastric tube was placed intraoperatively under direct visualization, check with surgeon before irrigating or repositioning; if tube is properly placed, rush of air should be heard.
   b. Secure tube to nares with correct taping technique.
      (1) Taping or securing tube properly decreases risk of necrosis or damage of nares and inadvertent dislodgment of tube; alar necrosis is disfiguring and difficult to repair if it occurs.
3. Maintain patency of nasogastric or gastrostomy tube.
   a. To decrease tension on gastric suture line
   b. Notify surgeon of excessive drainage from tubes or drains so that IV fluid and rates can be adjusted.
   c. Initial 24-hour drainage may be bloody changing to dark serosanguineous to bile colored over the next 24 to 72 hours; color and consistency vary with location of surgery (if esophageal or gastric expect bloody drainage; if hepatic, biliary or intestinal surgery drainage should not be bloody).

    4. Irrigation or manipulation of nasogastric tubes
       a. Do not irrigate or manipulate nasogastric tube unless specifically ordered.
         (1) Nasogastric tube lies close to anastomosis (gastric resection, some pancreatic procedures involving stomach).
       b. Check, if nasogastric tube to dependent drainage, for proper securing of tube to eliminate manipulation.
         (1) Nasogastric tube may be used as stent anastomosis in esophageal procedures.
       c. Notify surgeon if nasogastric tube is accidentally removed or becomes displaced.
         (1) Attempts to replace tube can result in esophageal perforation.
    5. Assess abdominal girth (abdominal distension), and auscultate bowel sounds.
       a. Anastomotic leak, hemorrhage, malfunctioning nasogastric tube, ileus, and mechanical obstruction may cause abdominal distension, nausea, and vomiting.
    6. Observe and document status of stoma color and drainage from stoma and position of stoma to skin; notify surgeon of any sudden or progressive change in stoma color.
       a. Altered color may indicate increasing edema leading to decreased circulation or generalized poor circulation to bowel.
  F. Dressings and drains
    1. Document dressing status every hour or as needed.
       a. Keeping dressing dry promotes wound healing by minimizing potential breeding ground for bacterial contamination.
    2. Reinforce or change dressing per preferred routine or as ordered.
       a. Dry dressings are more comfortable for patient.
    3. Monitor amount of drainage on dressings and from drains; establish expected drainage amounts with surgeon when patient arrives in PACU; notify surgeon of excessive or questionable quantities of drainage.
       a. Significant blood or fluid losses can occur from incisions or drain sites that may require replacement or exploration of site.
    4. Document both abdominal and perineal dressings after abdominoperineal resection.
       a. Sump or Penrose (cigarette or tube) drains may be present in perineal incision, a likely area for copious serosanguineous drainage.
  G. Positioning
    1. Lateral recumbent position
       a. Side-lying position is usually more comfortable for patients who have had rectal or perineal procedures.
    2. Elevate head of the bed (reverse Trendelenburg, not head up and hips flexed).
       a. Elevating head decreases weight against diaphragm to promote improved respiratory excursion and facilitate gas exchange.
  H. Temperature (see information on hyperthermia and hypothermia under Intraoperative Concerns)
    1. Monitor temperature on admission to PACU; warm or cool patient as indicated with warming lights, hypothermia or hyperthermia blankets, and convective warming devices.
       a. Vital signs should include temperature monitoring on PACU admission and every 1 to 2 hours until discharge.
    2. Take axillary, oral, or tympanic temperatures (avoid rectal temperatures) on patients with permanent colostomies, ileostomies, or rectal or anal incisions or following pull-through or stapled low anterior resections.
       a. Perforation of suture or staple lines is possible if rectal or anal incision exists or if rectum has been totally removed.

I. Pain control
   1. Assess location, pattern, intensity, and duration of pain; if possible, use pain assessment tool, requiring patient to identify quality of pain or discomfort; initiate pain relief measures; medicate patients according to PACU routine and approved pain guidelines (see Chapter 29).
      a. Pain management practices will vary from institution to institution; pain is subjective; patient complaining of pain should be believed and comfort measures initiated.
   2. Observe for incisional splinting.
      a. Splinting can lead to increased Pco_2 level because of inadequate gas exchange.
   3. IV route preferred for opioid and analgesic administration
      a. Absorption time and onset of action are less predictable when intramuscular injections are administered in cold patient.
   4. Patient-controlled analgesia, epidural analgesia, incisional or field blocks may provide significant pain relief in selected patients.
      a. Adequate pain control may improve ventilation, promote deep breathing and coughing, and allow patient to move more easily, especially after procedures with large or upper abdominal incisions.
      b. Gastric surgical procedures are generally considered the most painful postoperatively; aggressive and appropriate pain management is desirable.
III. Phase II priorities
   A. Pain management
      1. Initiate oral analgesics to prepare for discharge.
      2. Instruct patients to call if pain unrelieved by oral medications, severe pain, or questions related to pain (amount, location, duration).
   B. Diet
      1. Encourage fluids if desired; do not force fluids.
      2. Instruct patients to begin with light foods and progress to full diet as tolerated.
      3. If nauseated or vomiting for more than 6 hours after discharge, instruct patients to call and report nausea and vomiting.
   C. Wound care
      1. Review basic wound care with patients, companions, and families.
      2. Provide written and verbal instructions, especially for specialized incisional and/or drain care.
      3. Instruct patients to call if incision shows signs of infection or a fever is present.
   D. Activity
      1. Generally, activities limited first day postoperatively
      2. Dependent on operative procedure, lifting and activity restrictions may be ordered.
   E. Complications
      1. Provide patient, companion, and family with information on expected outcomes and complications.
      2. Instruct in appropriate follow-up if needed for complications.
IV. Postoperative complications
   A. General complications (not in order of occurrence or severity)
      1. Paralytic (adynamic) ileus: although this is commonly listed as a complication, it is an expected part of any abdominal or intestinal procedure; *all* patients who have these procedures will experience ileus.
      2. Atelectasis and respiratory problems
      3. Bladder distension
      4. Hemorrhage or shock
      5. Wound infection
      6. Dehiscence or evisceration
      7. Peritonitis

8. Hiccups (singultus)
9. Anastomotic leak
10. Anastomotic or stomal obstruction
11. External fistulas
12. Electrolyte and fluid imbalances
13. Stress ulceration
14. DVT and possible pulmonary embolus
15. Pancreatitis
16. Toxic shock syndrome

B. Specific system complications
  1. Pulmonary
    a. Hypoventilation: most frequent and dangerous pulmonary complication after surgery; various causes
      (1) Preoperative medication
      (2) Anesthetic agents
      (3) Narcotic administration preoperatively, intraoperatively, and postoperatively
      (4) Pain
      (5) Patient position
    b. Atelectasis constitutes 90% of all pulmonary complications.
      (1) Acute gastric dilation or ascites in advanced cancer can cause elevation of diaphragm, leading to decreased size of chest cavity and atelectasis (can also lead to shock).
  2. Cardiovascular
    a. Venous thrombosis
    b. Hypotension
    c. Shock
      (1) Hypovolemic
      (2) Septic
    d. Myocardial infarction
    e. Cerebrovascular accident

GASTROINTESTINAL OPERATIVE PROCEDURES

Surgical intervention is usually indicated when a medical regimen or conservative therapy is no longer sufficient to alleviate or control the underlying gastrointestinal pathophysiologic condition. At other times, emergent surgery is required, as when the patient experiences perforation, uncontrolled hemorrhage, or significant vascular compromise. Some of the more frequently encountered surgical procedures will be briefly defined.

For procedures requiring no additional assessment or concerns, refer to the above general information. The reader is advised to review chapters related to immediate postoperative assessment, perianesthesia complications, and PACU phase I discharge criteria for additional information.

I. Esophageal procedures
  A. Cervical esophagostomy
    1. Purpose: often done as part of first-stage repair for tracheoesophageal fistula or esophageal atresia repair in infants
    2. Description: surgical formation of opening into esophagus at cervical level
    3. Preoperative assessment and concerns
      a. At risk for aspiration; gastrostomy tube placed as soon as atresia or fistula identified
      b. May have multiple anomalies of cardiovascular, gastrointestinal systems
    4. Postanesthesia priorities
      a. Phase I
        (1) Maintain normothermia.

        (2) Tracheal leak may be present.

        (3) Pain management

    5. Complications

      a. Pulmonary aspiration

      b. Vocal cord paralysis

B. Esophagectomy with colon or gastric interposition

    1. Purpose: used in presence of esophageal atresia or for esophageal damage anywhere, except very proximal cervical esophagus

    2. Description: usually a piece of colon or stomach (more common) is used to establish continuity between esophagus and stomach.

    3. Preoperative assessment and concerns

      a. May have recurrent aspiration pneumonia from gastric reflux

      b. Malnutrition related to dysphagia or anorexia

      c. Evaluation of cardiovascular and respiratory status

    4. Intraoperative concerns

      a. Hypothermia

      b. Positioning to avoid neural injuries or soft tissue damage

    5. Postanesthesia priorities

      a. Phase I

        (1) At risk for aspiration and atelectasis; head of bed elevated

        (2) Pain management; thoracic epidural continuous analgesia for postoperative pain

        (3) Assess for hypoventilation, pneumothorax, anastomotic leak.

        (4) Patient may be hoarse.

    6. Complications

      a. Aspiration

      b. Atelectasis, hypoventilation

      c. Hemorrhage

      d. Pneumothorax

      e. Esophageal anastomotic leak

      f. Recurrent laryngeal nerve injury

C. Esophageal dilation

    1. Purpose: to allow freer passage of food and fluids into stomach; used to correct achalasia, esophageal spasms, and strictures

    2. Description: dilating instruments (bougies or balloons) passed in increasingly larger sizes or inflated to enlarge lumen of esophagus

    3. Preoperative assessment and concerns

      a. NPO prior to procedure

    4. Intraoperative concerns

      a. Procedure may be done with sedation and analgesia or general anesthesia.

    5. Postanesthesia priorities

      a. Phase I

        (1) Minimal postprocedure pain expected

        (2) Observe for subcutaneous emphysema, severe pain, aspiration.

        (3) Monitor temperature.

      b. Phase II

        (1) Assess gag reflex prior to giving fluids.

        (2) Review appropriate instructions for postsedation or postanesthesia care with patient, companion, and family.

    6. Psychosocial concerns

      a. Patient may require frequent dilations.

      b. Patient may prefer particular type of sedation or anesthesia for procedure based on past experience.

    7. Complications

      a. Esophageal perforation

      b. Pain

      c. Hemorrhage

      d. Bacteremia or sepsis

D. Esophagomyotomy (Heller procedure)

    1. Purpose: to allow food to pass from esophagus to stomach when a segment of esophagus is narrowed, causing functional obstruction

    2. Description: surgical division or anatomic dissection of muscles at distal esophagogastric junction, leaving mucosa intact

    3. See preceding sections B.3 to B.6 for perianesthesia care and concerns.

E. Herniations (see Chapter 43 for additional information)

    1. Surgical repair of hiatal or diaphragmatic hernias accomplished through either an abdominal or a thoracic approach

    2. Herniation is part of stomach protruding through an opening, or hiatus, in diaphragm.

    3. Hiatal hernias are not true hernias, while diaphragmatic hernias are.

      a. Hiatal hernia occurs when the gastroesophageal (GE) junction slides up and down between the chest and abdomen.

      b. Tend to be associated with GERD

      c. There is really no indication to fix them unless the patient also has GERD.

    4. Diaphragmatic hernia is a true hernia and should always be fixed.

    5. Purposes

      a. To restore herniated part below diaphragm for diaphragmatic hernias (the following sections 2.b, 2.c, and 2.d pertain only to GERD and hiatal hernias)

      b. For patients with GERD and hiatal hernias

        (1) To narrow esophageal hiatus

        (2) To recreate esophagogastric angle to enhance lower esophageal sphincter (LES) function

        (3) To stop reflux of gastric contents

    6. Description (these procedures are done for GERD and not specifically for a hiatal hernia)

      a. Collis-Belsey and Collis-Nissen repairs: esophageal lengthening with antireflux wrap of distal esophagus

      b. Hill repair: abdominal approach that narrows esophageal orifice and fixes esophagogastric junction in intraabdominal position; includes 180° wrap of stomach around esophagus

      c. Belsey Mark IV repair: performed through incision in left side of chest; consists of 240° wrap of distal portion of esophagus with fundus of stomach; this partial fundoplication is technically difficult, and risk of leakage or diverticulum developing in esophagus is higher because sutures are required in esophageal wall; newer procedure: modified thoracoscopic Belsey repair

      d. Nissen fundoplication: transabdominal or laparoscopic (similar to open approach and most common procedure for this condition) treatment for sliding esophageal hiatal hernia; a portion of fundus of stomach is mobilized and completely wrapped around (360°) distal portion of esophagus to prevent stomach displacement into posterior portion of mediastinum through diaphragmatic defect

      e. Toupet partial fundoplication: alternative antireflux procedure; the fundal wrap is reduced to 180° to 200°

    7. Preoperative assessment and concerns

      a. Possible recurrent aspiration pneumonia

      b. Antacid and antireflux prophylaxis recommended

      c. Laparoscopic approach may be contraindicated in patients with severe cardiovascular and respiratory disease.

    8. Intraoperative concerns

      a. Aspiration risk during induction and emergence

      b. Pneumoperitoneum

      c. Hemorrhage

        d. Visceral injury

        e. Hypothermia

    9. Postanesthesia priorities

        a. Phase I

           (1) Nausea and vomiting

           (2) Shoulder pain (if laparoscopic approach)

           (3) Pain management

           (4) Hypoventilation

        b. Phase II

           (1) Patients may go home in 2 to 4 hours after laparoscopic Nissen fundoplication in some settings.

           (2) Patients need to swallow fluids without vomiting and have pain controlled prior to discharge.

   10. Complications

        a. Gastric perforation

        b. Bleeding, hemorrhage

        c. Pneumothorax

        d. Aspiration

        e. Hypoventilation

F. Esophageal band ligation

    1. Purpose: to obliterate esophageal varices to reduce risk of bleeding or hemorrhage

    2. Description: endoscopic procedure involves placing a band around (ligation) varices in esophagus.

    3. Preoperative assessment and concerns

        a. NPO prior to procedure

    4. Intraoperative concerns

        a. Procedure may be done with sedation and analgesia or general anesthesia.

    5. Postanesthesia priorities

        a. Phase I

           (1) Minimal postprocedure pain expected

           (2) Observe for subcutaneous emphysema, severe pain, aspiration.

           (3) Monitor temperature.

        b. Phase II

           (1) Assess gag reflex prior to giving fluids.

           (2) Review appropriate instructions for postsedation or postanesthesia care with patient, companion, and family.

    6. Psychosocial concerns

        a. Patient may require repeat procedures.

        b. Patient may prefer particular type of sedation or anesthesia for procedure based on past experience.

    7. Complications

        a. Esophageal perforation

        b. Aspiration pneumonitis

        c. Hemorrhage

        d. Bacteremia and sepsis

II. Gastric procedures

  A. Gastrectomy

    1. Purpose: to remove all or a portion of diseased organ

    2. Description: surgical removal of whole or a part of stomach

        a. Antrectomy: involves almost a 50% distal gastrectomy; antral mucosa (site of gastrin formation) is removed, usually in conjunction with truncal vagotomy; remaining portion of stomach is anastomosed to duodenum.

        b. Billroth I (gastroduodenostomy): one type of reconstructions used with an antrectomy; the first portion of the duodenum is sewn to the remaining portion of the stomach (see Figure 42-2)

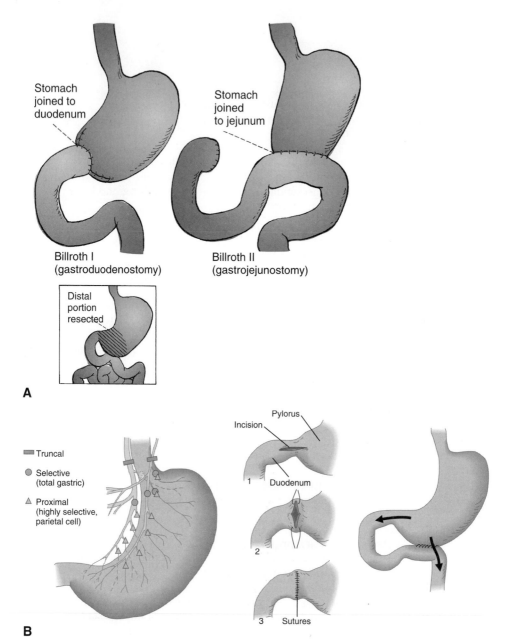

FIGURE 42-2 ■ **A,** Gastric surgical procedures: Billroth I, Billroth II. **B,** Gastric surgical procedures: *left,* vagotomy; *middle,* pyloroplasty; *right,* gastroenterostomy. (From Black JM, Hawks JH, Keene AM: *Medical-surgical nursing: Clinical management for positive outcomes,* ed 6. Philadelphia: WB Saunders, 2001.)

    c. Billroth II (gastrojejunostomy): another type of reconstruction used with an antrectomy; in this case, the first portion of the duodenum is unable to reach the remaining portion of the stomach; the first portion of the duodenum is sewn shut, and a loop of jejunum just distal to the ligament of Treitz is brought up and sewn to the remaining stomach remnant (see Figure 42-2)

    d. Total gastrectomy: usually done for cancer of stomach or abdominal esophagus; reconstruction after total gastrectomy is usually by esophagojejunostomy

    e. Near total gastrectomy: may be done for treatment of gastroparesis

f. Roux-en-Y gastrojejunostomy: reconstruction procedure for the stomach; may be used for reconstruction after an antrectomy or after a total gastrectomy; it can be used as a bypass procedure for unresectable pancreatic cancer, but more commonly a loop gastrojejunostomy is used in this situation (a loop of jejunum is sewn to the stomach to bypass an obstructed distal stomach or duodenum)

3. Preoperative assessment and concerns
   a. Rehydration
   b. Possible transfusion because of bleeding
   c. Possible hyperalimentation for nutritional deficits
   d. Electrolyte abnormalities
4. Intraoperative concerns
   a. Volume status
   b. Anticipate significant third space losses.
   c. Acute hemorrhage
5. Postanesthesia priorities
   a. Phase I
      (1) Low thoracic epidural for pain management; patient-controlled analgesia also an option
      (2) Maintain nasogastric tube patency and position.

B. Gastric bypass (usually done with a Roux-en-Y limb; sometimes called a Roux-en-Y gastric bypass)
   1. Purpose: performed for morbid obesity (defined as 100 pounds above ideal body weight or 100% over ideal body weight)
   2. Description: lower 90% to 95% of stomach is stapled off, allowing only upper 5% to 10% of stomach to receive food; upper stomach is anastomosed by an approximately 1 cm opening to jejunum to allow intestinal absorption and elimination of food.
   3. Preoperative assessment and concerns
      a. As a result of excessive weight, patients may suffer from multiple respiratory, cardiovascular, endocrine, and musculoskeletal system issues.
      b. Obstructive sleep apnea common in morbidly obese patient
   4. Intraoperative concerns
      a. Patients at risk for aspiration; may be an awake intubation or rapid sequence induction with cricoid pressure
      b. May be done laparoscopically
   5. Postanesthesia priorities
      a. Phase I
         (1) Position for optimal respiratory effort.
         (2) Provide appropriate equipment for safe patient care.
   6. Complications
      a. Open procedures increase risk of cardiopulmonary complications, wound infection, and late incisional hernia.
      b. Leaks, obstructions, sepsis
      c. Venous thromboembolism

C. Gastroenterostomy (see Figure 42-2)
   1. Purpose: to create an artificial passage between stomach and small intestine
   2. Description: surgical anastomosis between stomach and small intestine, usually jejunum, for unresectable pancreatic cancer with gastric outlet obstruction

D. Gastrostomy
   1. Purpose: used for long-term stomach decompression or to introduce food into gastrointestinal system
   2. Description: creation of gastric fistula or opening through abdominal wall, usually with a tube in place
      a. May be done operatively or endoscopically (insertion of gastrostomy tube through incision made at point where anterior portion of stomach wall is tented with endoscope, making contact with parietal peritoneum)
      b. Traction on tube maintains contact between stomach and abdominal wall.

      3. Percutaneous endoscopic gastrostomy (PEG): endoscopic procedure
        a. Performed with local anesthesia
        b. Relative and/or absolute contraindications to PEG: prior gastric surgery, portal hypertension with varices and/or ascites, ascites from other causes, prior abdominal surgery

  E. Pyloromyotomy
    1. Purpose: to widen pyloric opening
    2. Description: muscle fibers of outlet of stomach are cut without severing mucosa.

  F. Pyloroplasty (see Figure 42-2)
    1. Purpose: to increase size of pyloric opening in presence of pyloric stenosis or scarring caused by ulcer disease; usually performed in conjunction with vagotomy when done for latter
    2. Description: repair of pylorus used to establish opening in presence of pyloric or prepyloric obstruction

  G. Vagotomy (see Figure 42-2)
    1. Purpose: to reduce amount of gastric acid secreted and lessen chance of recurrence of gastric ulcer
    2. Description: sectioning of vagus nerve or its branches; choices of vagotomy include truncal, selective, proximal (highly selective, parietal cell); may be accomplished by laparoscopic approach

III. Biliary, hepatic, and pancreatic procedures
  A. Surgical correction of biliary atresia (condition in which extrahepatic bile ducts are nonpatent, seen primarily in infants)
    1. Roux-en-Y procedure
      a. Purpose: used when proximal extrahepatic bile ducts are patent and distal ducts are occluded; for bypass in cancer of bile duct and pancreatitis
      b. Description: distal end of divided jejunum is anastomosed to patent remnant of proximal bile duct.
    2. Hepatic portoenterostomy (Kasai procedure)
      a. Purpose: used when proximal extrahepatic ducts are totally occluded
      b. Description: removal of entire extrahepatic biliary tree; bile drainage is established by anastomosis of intestinal conduit to transected ducts at liver hilus
    3. Preoperative assessment and concerns
      a. May have impaired elimination of drugs because of hepatic dysfunction
      b. Coagulation values need to be evaluated.
    4. Intraoperative concerns
      a. Potential for large third space losses
    5. Postanesthesia priorities
      a. Phase I
        (1) Monitor volume status.
    6. Complications
      a. Cholangitis

  B. Cholecystectomy (see Chapter 43 for additional information)
    1. Purpose: to treat cholelithiasis and cholecystitis
    2. Description: removal of gallbladder and its cystic duct
      a. May be through traditional "open" approach or by laparoscopy
      b. Laparoscopic approach may use laser, electrosurgical cautery, or harmonic scalpel to remove gallbladder from liver bed and ligate vessels and ducts.
    3. Intraoperative concerns
      a. High incidence of postoperative nausea and vomiting; prophylactic antiemetics recommended prior to end of case
      b. Pneumoperitoneum if laparoscopic; risk of gas embolism

   4. Postanesthesia priorities
      a. Phase I
         (1) Postoperative nausea and vomiting management
         (2) Shoulder pain (both open and laparoscopic approaches)
      b. Phase II
         (1) Minimal nausea and vomiting for discharge home
         (2) Oral analgesics initiated as needed for pain management prior to discharge
         (3) Instruct patient and companion regarding diet, incision sites, and care of incisions.
C. Cholecystostomy
   1. Purpose: to decompress gallbladder of debilitated patient with acute cholecystitis or cholelithiasis unable to tolerate cholecystectomy at that time
   2. Description: formation of opening into gallbladder through abdominal wall; if stones are present, approach may be by angiography with lithotripsy to break up stones
   3. Preoperative assessment and concerns
      a. Dehydration from fever, vomiting, decreased oral intake; may require fluid resuscitation prior to operative procedure
      b. Peritonitis
D. Choledochotomy
   1. Purpose: usually for removal of stones
   2. Description: incision of common bile duct
   3. Preoperative assessment and concerns
      a. As in preceding section C.3
E. Common bile duct exploration
   1. Purpose: to check for stones and/or strictures; frequently performed at time of cholecystectomy
   2. Description: exploration of common bile duct; T-tube drain is left in place for a period of time postoperatively to ensure patency of common bile duct; can use laparoscopic approach
F. Hepaticojejunostomy
   1. Purpose: to repair stricture of common bile duct after laparoscopic or open cholecystectomy; may also be done for patients with bile duct cancer
   2. Description: creation of anastomosis between hepatic duct and jejunum
G. Portal systemic shunt
   1. Purpose: primarily used for treatment of portal hypertension and decompression of esophagogastric varices
      a. Increasing use of transjugular intrahepatic portosystemic shunt (TIPS) procedures reducing the number of older shunt procedures
      b. Since liver transplantation is now much more commonly performed, these patients are also treated with hepatic transplantation, rather than shunting.
   2. Description: shunts divert, either partially or totally, venous blood flow to liver; types of shunts include
      a. End-to-side, side-to-side, interposition, Sarfeh portacaval; interposition (adult) or direct (pediatric) mesocaval; distal splenorenal, mesoatrial (Budd-Chiari syndrome management)
      b. Sugiura procedures (combines esophageal transection, extensive esophagogastric devascularization, and splenectomy, while paraesophageal collateral vessels are preserved) are done for varices in patients who are not candidates for other types of shunt procedures.
      c. Transjugular intrahepatic portosystemic shunt (TIPS)
         (1) Purpose: definitive treatment for patients who bleed from portal hypertension; major limitation is that up to 50% have shunt stenosis or shunt thrombosis within the first year; may be ideal therapy for patients needing short-term portal decompression (those awaiting liver transplantation who fail sclerotherapy)

        (2) Description
            (a) Nonoperative; functions similarly to a side-to-side portosystemic shunt (effective in treating ascites); adverse side effects include total portal diversion and encephalopathy
            (b) Procedure: a needle is advanced from a hepatic vein to a major portal branch, and a guide wire is placed; a hepatic parenchymal tract is created by balloon dilation and an expandable metal stent is placed, creating the shunt

    3. Preoperative assessment and concerns
      a. Hypoxemia secondary to ascites
      b. Portal hypertension
      c. Risk for bleeding from esophageal and gastric varices
      d. Renal failure
      e. Anemia
      f. Altered drug elimination
      g. Electrolyte disturbances
    4. Intraoperative concerns
      a. Anticipate large blood loss for open procedures.
      b. Pulmonary artery catheter for monitoring
    5. Postanesthesia priorities
      a. Phase I
        (1) Intensive care monitoring usual following these procedures
    6. Complications
      a. Coagulopathy
      b. Encephalopathy
      c. Renal failure

H. Hepatectomy: excision of all or part of liver
    1. Increasing use of segmentectomies and wedge resections for patients with liver metastases
    2. Cryotherapy or radiofrequency ablation also used to treat primary liver cancer or hepatic metastases

I. Hepatic lobectomy: surgical removal of one of the two (right, left) lobes of liver; each lobe is then divided into several segments (eight total)—if a segment is removed, segmentectomy; may be accomplished with total vascular occlusion intraoperatively
    1. Intraoperative concerns (for hepatectomy and hepatic lobectomy)
      a. Potential for large blood loss
    2. Postanesthesia priorities
      a. Phase I
        (1) Epidural analgesia for pain management
        (2) May remain intubated and ventilated; anticipate intensive care monitoring
    3. Complications
      a. Massive hemorrhage
      b. Disseminated intravascular coagulopathy
      c. Hypoglycemia
      d. Electrolyte imbalance
      e. Pulmonary insufficiency

J. Peritoneovenous shunts (e.g., LeVeen or Denver)
    1. Purpose: used in an attempt to control ascites by reinfusing peritoneal fluid into venous system; patients with limited hepatic reserve who may not tolerate blood being shunted away from liver are candidates; also used to palliate patients with malignant ascites
    2. Description: unidirectional silicone elastomer valve and catheter are inserted into peritoneum; other end is tunneled subcutaneously up to neck and inserted into internal jugular vein and then threaded into superior vena cava or right atrium

K. Liver transplant
  1. Purpose: replacement of diseased liver with donor liver; may use cadaveric, living related, and split-liver organs
  2. Description: native liver is removed and replaced with whole liver, split liver, or liver segment; effective approach for treatment of liver failure of various causes because of development of improved surgical techniques, venous bypass method, and newer antirejection agents
  3. Preoperative assessment and concerns
    a. Fifteen percent of all liver transplant recipients in the United States are children.
    b. Premedications used with care
    c. Avoid intramuscular injections.
  4. Intraoperative concerns
    a. Monitoring includes arterial line, central venous pressure, or pulmonary artery catheter; transesophageal echocardiogram
    b. Warming essential
    c. Massive blood loss and subsequent transfusion
    d. Volume management
  5. Postanesthesia priorities
    a. Phase I
      (1) Remain intubated and mechanically ventilated
      (2) Monitored in intensive care setting
      (3) Pain can be severe.
  6. Psychosocial concerns
    a. Psychological preparation essential
    b. If donor is living related (relative), provide family support.
  7. Complications
    a. Bleeding and neurologic deficits
    b. Hepatic artery and/or portal vein thrombosis
    c. Bile leaks
    d. Rejection: primary or delayed
    e. Renal failure
    f. Electrolyte abnormalities
    g. Pulmonary complications
L. Pancreatectomy
  1. Purpose: to treat necrosis, abscess, pseudocysts, or intractable pain from injury or pancreatitis; most commonly used to treat pancreatic cancer
  2. Description: partial resection or total removal of pancreas; total removal results in diabetes and other metabolic difficulties; may use jejunal loop to drain
M. Pancreaticoduodenectomy (Whipple's procedure)
  1. Purpose: to treat cancer of head of pancreas and for resectable localized cancers of ampulla, distal common bile duct, or duodenum; also used to treat chronic pancreatitis
  2. Description: removal of proximal portion of pancreas, adjoining duodenum, lower portion of stomach, gallbladder, and common bile duct
N. Cystogastrostomy, cystoduodenostomy, cystojejunostomy
  1. Purpose: to treat pancreatic pseudocysts that do not disappear spontaneously
  2. Description: decompressive procedures for internally draining pseudocysts that are fixed to retrogastric area or duodenum or not in proximity to either stomach or duodenum
  3. Preoperative assessment and concerns (for pancreatectomy, pancreaticoduodenectomy, and cystogastrostomy)
    a. Jaundice and abdominal pain may be present.
    b. Electrolyte abnormalities
    c. Glucose monitoring

      4. Intraoperative concerns

        a. Anticipate large fluid loss.

        b. Invasive monitoring usually required

      5. Postanesthesia priorities

        a. Phase I

          (1) Epidural analgesia for pain management

          (2) Glucose monitoring; prone to hyperglycemia

      6. Complications

        a. Hypovolemia

        b. Hyperglycemia

        c. Hypocalcemia

   O. Pancreas transplant

      1. Purpose: to treat diabetes mellitus; establishes an insulin-independent euglycemic state

      2. Description: donor pancreatic tissue transplanted into recipient, achieved through various techniques: whole organ or segmental graft, with duct management occluded or drained into a hollow viscus; usually combined with a renal transplant procedure

      3. Preoperative assessment and concerns

        a. Absence of infection, dental evaluation completed

        b. Blood glucose assessment and monitoring

        c. If on dialysis, may need dialysis prior to procedure

      4. Intraoperative concerns

        a. Increased risk for aspiration

        b. Blood glucose monitoring

      5. Postanesthesia priorities

        a. Phase I

          (1) Pain management; use caution with opioids if renal failure or nonfunctioning renal transplant

          (2) Blood glucose monitoring; early return to euglycemic state possible after surgery

      6. Complications

        a. Rejection

        b. Graft thrombosis

   P. Splenectomy or splenorrhaphy

      1. Purpose: to treat traumatic injuries to spleen; thrombocytopenic purpura refractory to other treatment, anemias, and myeloproliferative disorders (e.g., leukemia); splenorrhaphy is *only* used for traumatic injuries; all other listed disorders (including trauma) are treated with total splenectomy

      2. Description: excision or repair of spleen, either by open or by laparoscopic approach; the laparoscopic approached is generally *not* used for trauma

IV. Small intestine

   A. Duodenojejunostomy

      1. Purpose: relieve duodenal obstruction

      2. Description: creation of opening or passage from obstructed or stenosed duodenum into jejunum

   B. Feeding jejunostomy

      1. Purpose: to allow access for alimentation in presence of functioning gastrointestinal tract

      2. Description: permanent opening or fistula into jejunum through abdominal wall, usually with placement of a tube

   C. Ileostomy

      1. Purpose: created after total proctocolectomy for Crohn's disease or ulcerative colitis or less frequently for multiple colorectal carcinomas, familial polyposis coli, ischemia, trauma, and congenital anomalies in which colon remains intact

      2. Description: creation of passage through abdominal wall into ileum

   3. Psychosocial concerns
      a. Acceptance of stoma and stoma care
      b. Concerns related to social and physical activities
D. Continent ileostomy (Kock pouch or Barnett continent intestinal reservoir)
   1. Purpose: to create a reservoir for feces after total proctocolectomy
   2. Description: construction of an intestinal reservoir created by joining a loop of terminal ileum and forming a nipple valve; after healing is complete, patient controls expulsion of feces and gas by emptying reservoir or pouch with catheter
   3. Postanesthesia priorities
      a. Phase I
         (1) Maintain patency of decompression tube after creation of continent ileostomy; gently irrigate pouch with normal saline solution (30 ml every 3 hours is commonly ordered).
         (2) Surgically created pouch is fragile until healed and matured because of many anastomoses.
E. Small bowel resection
   1. Purpose: to treat trauma, mesenteric thrombosis, regional enteritis, radiation enteropathy, strangulated small bowel obstruction, neoplasm, congenital atresia, or enterocutaneous fistulas
   2. Description: excision of varying lengths of small intestine; profound consequences with resection of more than 75% of small intestine (e.g., "short-gut" syndrome)
      a. In general, patients need 150 cm of small intestine without their ileocecal valve or 100 cm of small intestine with their ileocecal valve.
      b. Less small intestine than this generally results in "short-gut" syndrome and the need for supplemental total parenteral nutrition.
V. Colon or large intestine
   A. Abdominoperineal resection
      1. Purpose: generally performed for cancer of rectum; occasionally for severe Crohn's, especially in the presence of severe perianal disease
      2. Description: surgical procedure in which anus, rectum, and sigmoid colon are removed en bloc; through incision extending from pubis to above umbilicus
         a. A segment of lower bowel is mobilized and divided.
         b. Proximal end is exteriorized through separate stab wound as a single-barreled colostomy or ileostomy.
         c. Distal end is pushed into hollow of sacrum, and rectum is removed through perianal route.
      3. Preoperative assessment and concerns
         a. Patients may experience significant dehydration subsequent to extensive bowel preparation.
      4. Complications
         a. Ureter or bladder injury
         b. Wound dehiscence or infection
   B. Cecostomy
      1. Purpose: temporary measure to relieve obstruction distal to cecum
      2. Description: construction of opening into cecum, generally by placing a tube
   C. Colectomy
      1. Purpose: to treat tumors, bleeding, inflammation, or trauma of large intestine
      2. Description: surgical removal of all or part of colon
   D. Restorative proctocolectomy (total proctocolectomy with ileal reservoir and anal anastomosis)
      1. Purpose: to maintain the anal sphincter muscles and allow the patient to avoid a permanent ileostomy (a patient with a good to excellent result has 4-12 bowel movements per day); used for selected patients with ulcerative colitis or familial polyposis coli

   2. Description: pouch made from terminal ileum is created and then anastomosed to rectum at or just above dentate line; J-shaped ileoanal or larger W-shaped reservoir is most common; also S shaped

E. Colostomy
   1. Purpose: incision of colon to create fistula between bowel and abdominal wall
   2. Description: either temporary or permanent; placement of ostomy site is individualized; location depends on pathologic condition involved (e.g., transverse colostomy, sigmoid colostomy) and patient's anatomy and lifestyle; mucous fistula may also be created for decompression of cancer-caused obstruction of lower colon

F. Low anterior resection
   1. Purpose: to treat malignancies of rectosigmoid area or diverticulitis
   2. Description: rectum-containing tumor is excised; rectal stump and proximal bowel are anastomosed either with suture or with staples

G. Omphalocele (excision): rare defect of periumbilical abdominal wall seen primarily in premature infants; omphalocele sac may contain small and/or large bowel, liver, or spleen
   1. Primary closure
      a. Purpose: used for omphaloceles with small abdominal defects
      b. Description: omphalocele sac is excised, and abdominal wall muscles and skin edges are reapproximated.
   2. Staged repair
      a. Purpose: used for large omphaloceles
      b. Description: omphalocele is encased in silicone elastomer mesh sack that is sutured in place around defect; viscera are gradually moved into abdominal cavity in stages.
   3. Preoperative assessment and concerns
      a. Often associated with other anomalies
      b. Decompression of stomach to prevent regurgitation or aspiration
   4. Intraoperative concerns
      a. Closure may be primary or staged depending on size of defect, abdominal tension.
   5. Postanesthesia priorities
      a. Phase I
         (1) Patients with large defects may remain intubated and mechanically ventilated.
         (2) Fluid management
   6. Psychosocial concerns
      a. Parental support
   7. Complications
      a. Circulatory and renal dysfunction
      b. Infection

H. Polypectomy
   1. Purpose: to remove isolated gastrointestinal polyps
   2. Description: using snare and electrocautery, polyps are removed endoscopically; large polyps may require open colectomy.

VI. Rectal and anal procedures
A. Transanal excision of polyps or masses
   1. Purpose: to remove polyps or masses from the anal or rectal areas
   2. Description: excision of polyps or masses using an anal approach
B. Lateral internal sphincterotomy
   1. Purpose: to treat chronic anal fissures
   2. Description: cutting of anal sphincter; anoplasty normally is required to reestablish anal tissue and mucosal integrity
C. Anal fistulotomy or fistulectomy
   1. Purpose: to treat, by either incision or excision, fistulous tracts in anal canal

    2. Description: infection of anal duct gland creates fistula in ano, which may be incised and drained or excised and packed to heal by granulation.
        a. Usually has presenting condition of a perianal abscess, which is incised and drained
        b. A chronic draining tract may develop, which communicates with the anal canal.
        c. Treated with fistulotomy (opening the fistula) if not deep and crossing the sphincters
        d. If deep and cross multiple sphincters, more complicated anorectal procedures are required repair the defect.

  D. Duhamel and Soave operations
    1. Purpose: to treat congenital megacolon (Hirschsprung's disease) in children
    2. Description: in both Duhamel and Soave procedures, aganglionic bowel is resected, and proximal, healthy colon is pulled through and anastomosed to rectum.
    3. Preoperative assessment and concerns
        a. Present with prior colostomy
        b. Mildly malnourished with associated malabsorption state
        c. Diarrhea may be present.
    4. Intraoperative concerns
        a. Potential for large third space losses
    5. Postanesthesia priorities
        a. Phase I
           (1) Continuous epidural analgesia for pain management

BIBLIOGRAPHY

1. Alspach JG, editor: *Core curriculum for critical care nursing,* ed 5. Philadelphia: WB Saunders, 1998.
2. American Society for Gastrointestinal Endoscopy: Complications of upper GI endoscopy. *Gastrointest Endosc* 55(7):784-793, 2002.
3. Ball KA: *Endoscopic surgery.* Mosby's Perioperative Nursing Series. St Louis: Mosby–Year Book, 1997.
4. Black JM, Hawks JH, Keene AM: *Medical-surgical nursing: Clinical management for positive outcomes,* ed 6. Philadelphia: WB Saunders, 2001.
5. Gray H, Pick TP, Howden R, editors: *Gray's anatomy: Descriptive and surgical.* Philadelphia: Running Press, 1991.
6. Guyton AC: *Human physiology and mechanisms of disease,* ed 5. Philadelphia: WB Saunders, 1996.
7. Hulka JF, Reich H: *Textbook of laparoscopy,* ed 3. Philadelphia: WB Saunders, 1998.
8. Jaffe RA, Samuels SI, editors: *Anesthesiologist's manual of surgical procedures,* ed 2. Philadelphia: Lippincott, Williams & Wilkins, 1999.
9. Lynn-McHale DJ, Carlson KK, editors: *AACN procedure manual for critical care,* ed 4. Philadelphia: WB Saunders, 2001.
10. Moody FG, Carey LC, Jones RS, et al, editors: *Surgical treatment of digestive disease,* ed 2. Chicago: Year Book Medical Publishers, 1990.
11. O'Brien D: Care of the gastrointestinal, abdominal, and anorectal surgical patient. In Drain CB: *Perianesthesia nursing: A critical care approach,* ed 4. Philadelphia: WB Saunders, pp 551-565, 2003.
12. O'Brien D, Walters VA, Burden N: Special procedures in the ambulatory setting. In Burden N, Quinn DMD, O'Brien D, et al, editors: *Ambulatory surgical nursing,* ed 2. Philadelphia: WB Saunders, 2000.
13. O'Hanlon-Nichols T: Book assessment series: Gastrointestinal system. *Am J Nurs* 98(4):48-52, 1998.
14. Ray S: Result of 310 consecutive patients undergoing laparoscopic Nissen fundoplication as hospital outpatients or at a freestanding surgery center. *Surg Endosc* 17: 378-380, 2003
15. Roizen MF, Fleisher LA: *Essence of anesthesia practice,* ed 2. Philadelphia: WB Saunders, 2002.
16. Suter M, Giusti V, Heraief E, et al: Laparoscopic roux-en-Y gastric bypass. *Surg Endosc* 17:603-609, 2003.

17. Thibodeau GA, Patton KT: *Anthony's textbook of anatomy and physiology,* ed 17. St Louis: Mosby, 2002.

18. Thompson J, McFarland G, Hirsch J, et al: *Mosby's clinical nursing,* ed 5. St Louis: Mosby, 2002.

19. Tilkian SM, Conover MH, Tilkian AG: *Clinical nursing implications of laboratory tests,* ed 5. St Louis: Mosby, 1996.

20. Townsend CM, Beauchamp RD, Mattox KL, et al: *Sabiston's textbook of surgery,* ed 16. Philadelphia: WB Saunders, 2000.

21. Widmaier E, Raff H, Strang K: *Vander's human physiology,* ed 9. New York: McGraw-Hill, 2003.

43 General Surgery

MARY C. REDMOND

OBJECTIVES

At the conclusion of this chapter the reader will be able to:

1. Identify common laparoscopic and open general surgical procedures.
2. Describe anatomy and physiology relative to selected surgical procedures.
3. Review assessment considerations prior to selected surgical procedures.
4. Describe selected laparoscopic and open surgical procedures.
5. Describe PACU phase I and II care and key educational elements specific to selected surgical procedures.
6. Describe the advantages of minimally invasive procedures.
7. Describe equipment used in minimally invasive procedures.
8. Identify perioperative and perianesthesia issues concerned with minimally invasive procedures.
9. Identify potential perioperative complications associated with some procedures.

GENERAL SURGERY

General surgery refers to a variety of surgical procedures. This chapter covers some of the more common general surgery procedures. Many procedures can be done either using open or using minimally invasive techniques.

I. Anatomy and physiology
   A. Breast: Refer to Figure 43-1.
      1. Bilateral mammary glands
         a. Lie on pectoralis major fascia of anterior chest wall
         b. Surrounded by layers of fat enclosed in envelope of skin
      2. Muscle
         a. Fixed to overlying skin and underlying pectoral fascia with fibrous bands
      3. Lobes
         a. Twelve to twenty lobes subdivided into lobules, composed of acini
         b. Arranged in spiral fashion around nipple
         c. Each lobe drained by duct (12-20) opening on nipple
      4. Nipple
         a. In adult women it is center of fully developed breast with pigmented areola.
         b. Located in fourth intercostal space
         c. Bundles of smooth muscle fibers have erectile properties.
         d. Fifteen to twenty lactiferous ducts arranged radially under areola
         e. Areolar epithelium contains small hairs and glands.
            (1) Sebaceous glands (Montgomery's glands)
            (2) Sweat glands
            (3) Accessory mammary glands
      5. Blood supply
         a. Arteries
            (1) Internal mammary
            (2) Lateral branches of anterior aortic intercostal arteries

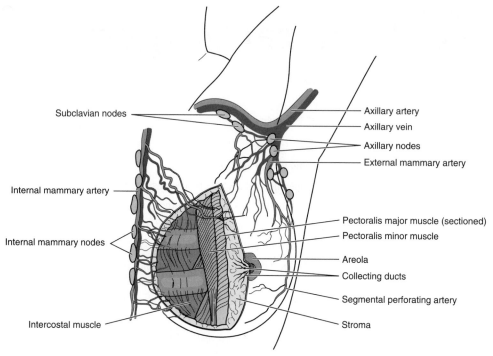

Subclavian nodes

Axillary artery
Axillary vein
Axillary nodes
External mammary artery

Internal mammary artery

Internal mammary nodes

Pectoralis major muscle (sectioned)
Pectoralis minor muscle

Areola
Collecting ducts

Segmental perforating artery

Intercostal muscle

Stroma

FIGURE 43-1 ■ Female breast. (From Phillips NF: *Berry & Kohn's operating room technique,* ed 10. St Louis: Mosby, 2004.)

      b. Veins
         (1) Main veins follow arterial pattern.
         (2) Superficial veins frequently dilated during pregnancy or over areas of disease
    6. Lymph system
      a. Generally follows course of blood vessels
      b. Drains into axillary nodes (approximately 53) and into internal mammary nodes (few in number)
    7. Nerve supply
      a. Anterior cutaneous branches of upper intercostal nerves
      b. Third and fourth branches of cervical plexus
      c. Lateral cutaneous branches of intercostal nerves
  B. Gallbladder: Refer to Figure 43-2.
    1. Location
      a. Lies in sulcus on undersurface of right lobe of liver
      b. Terminates in cystic duct
    2. Bile
      a. Becomes concentrated in gallbladder during storage period
      b. Consists of water, salts of bile acids, pigments, inorganic salts, cholesterol, and phospholipids
      c. Presence of certain food stuffs, especially fat in duodenum, cause release of cholecystokinin-pancreozymin, resulting in gallbladder contraction.
      d. As sphincter of Oddi in ampulla of Vater relaxes, bile pours forth into duodenum to aid digestion.
    3. Blood supply
      a. From cystic artery, a branch of the hepatic artery
  C. Spleen: Refer to Figure 43-3.
    1. Location
      a. Lies in upper left abdominal cavity beneath dome of diaphragm

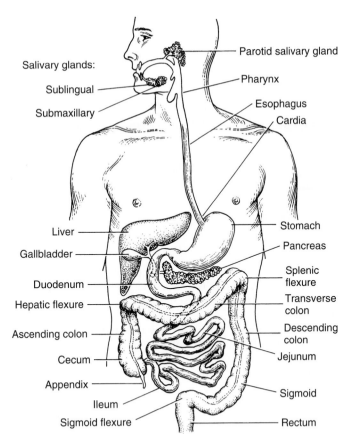

FIGURE 43-2 ■ Alimentary canal.

   b. Covered with peritoneum and held in place by numerous suspensory
      ligaments
 2. Blood supply
   a. Splenic artery furnishes arterial blood supply.
   b. Splenic vein drains into portal system.
 3. Function
   a. Largest lymphatic organ of body, having intimate role in immunologic
      defenses of body
   b. Involved in formation of blood elements
   c. Acts as a blood reservoir
   d. Site of red blood cell destruction
D. Esophagus-stomach: Refer to Figure 43-2.
 1. Location
   a. Esophagus
      (1) Musculocutaneous canal between pharynx in the throat and the
         stomach in the abdomen
      (2) Passes through thoracic cavity and enters abdominal cavity through
         esophageal hiatus of diaphragm
      (3) Lies between liver and aorta and between right and left branches of
         vagus nerve
   b. Stomach
      (1) Hollow muscular organ situated in upper left abdomen between
         esophagus and duodenum

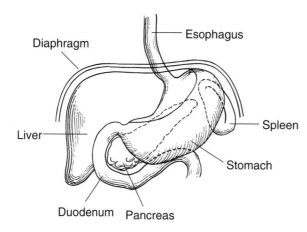

FIGURE 43-3 ■ Organs in upper abdominal cavity. (From Phillips NF: *Berry & Kohn's operating room technique*, ed 10. St Louis: Mosby, 2004.)

      (2) Divided into fundus, body, and pyloric antrum
      (3) Omentum, attached to lesser and greater curvatures, covers stomach and small intestine
  2. Nerve supply
    a. Autonomic nervous supply from vagus nerve
      (1) Controls reflex activities of movement and secretions of alimentary canal
      (2) Significant in rhythmic relaxation of pyloric sphincter
 E. Appendix: Refer to Figure 43-2.
  1. Location
    a. Blind, narrow tube that extends from inferior portion of cecum
    b. Some appendices are retrocecal.
  2. Has no known useful function
 F. Intestine: Refer to Figure 43-2.
  1. Location
    a. Continuous muscular tube of bowel extending from lower end of stomach to rectum
    b. Intestines divided into
      (1) Small intestine extends from pylorus to ileocecal valve.
        (a) Duodenum (proximal portion)
        (b) Jejunum (middle section)
        (c) Ileum (distal portion joining large intestine)
      (2) Large intestine (colon) extends from ileum to rectum.
        (a) Ascending
        (b) Transverse
        (c) Descending
        (d) Sigmoid
    c. Mesentery
      (1) A peritoneal fold attaching small and large intestines to posterior abdominal wall
      (2) Contains arteries, veins, lymph nodes that supply the intestines
  2. Purpose: Food and digestive products pass through alimentary canal during
    a. Digestion
    b. Absorption
    c. Elimination of waste products
 G. Hemorrhoids
  1. Location
    a. Masses of vascular tissue found in anal canal
    b. Internal hemorrhoid
      (1) Found above internal sphincter
      (2) Covered with columnar mucosa

   c. External hemorrhoids
    (1) Found outside external sphincter
    (2) Covered by anoderm and perianal skin
   d. May have combination of internal and external hemorrhoids
  2. Classification
   a. First degree: project slightly into anal canal
   b. Second degree: prolapse with defecation and reduce spontaneously
   c. Third degree: prolapse with defecation and reduce manually
   d. Fourth degree: irreducible
 H. Anal fissure
  1. Small tear in lining of anus resembling slitlike crack
  2. May extend from anal verge to pectinate line
 I. Anorectal fistula
  1. Location
   a. Hollow, fibrous tunnel or tract with two openings
   b. Primary, or internal, opening usually at a crypt near pectinate line
  2. May have single or multiple fistulas
 J. Pilonidal cyst
  1. Midline of upper portion of gluteal fold
  2. Rarely symptomatic until adulthood
 K. Hernias: Refer to Figure 43-4.
  1. Sac lined by peritoneum that protrudes through defect in layers of abdominal wall
  2. Type
   a. Acquired
   b. Congenital
  3. Weak places or intervals in abdominal aponeurosis
   a. Inguinal canals
   b. Femoral rings
   c. Umbilicus
  4. Contributing factors
   a. Age
   b. Sex
   c. Previous surgery
   d. Obesity
   e. Nutritional status

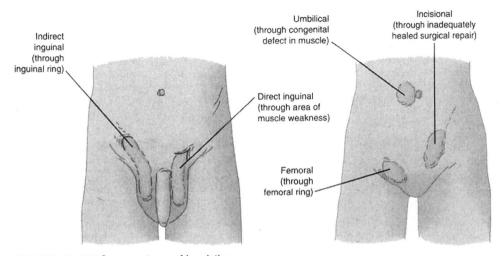

FIGURE 43-4 ■ Common types of herniation.

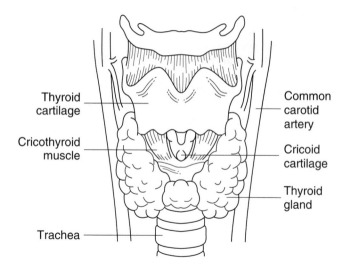

FIGURE 43-5 ■ Thyroid gland. (From Phillips NF: *Berry & Kohn's operating room technique,* ed 10. St Louis: Mosby, 2004.)

      f. Pulmonary and cardiac disease
      g. Loss of skin turgor
         (1) Aging
         (2) Chronic debilitating diseases
  L. Thyroid: Refer to Figure 43-5.
    1. Location
      a. Butterfly-shaped gland composed of two lobes
         (1) Positioned on either side of trachea
         (2) Joined by isthmus
      b. Isthmus situated near base of neck
      c. Posterior surface of isthmus adherent to anterior surface of tracheal ring
      d. Upper pole of gland beneath upper end of sternothyroid muscle
      e. Lower pole extends to sixth tracheal ring.
      f. Enclosed by pretracheal fascia
    2. Blood supply
      a. Arteries
         (1) External carotid arteries via superior thyroid artery
         (2) Subclavian artery via inferior thyroid arteries
      b. Veins
         (1) Three pairs
         (2) Extend from a plexus formed on surface of gland and on front of trachea
    3. Nerve supply
      a. Superior laryngeal nerve lies bilateral in proximity to superior thyroid artery.
      b. Recurrent laryngeal nerve that supplies vocal cord
         (1) Ascends from mediastinum
         (2) In close association with tracheoesophageal sulcus and interior thyroid artery
      c. Sympathetic and parasympathetic nerves enter gland, probably exerting influence primarily on blood supply.
    4. Physiology
      a. In response to thyroid-stimulating hormone (TSH, released by pituitary in response to thyrotropin-releasing hormone)
      b. Produces thyroxine (T_4) and triiodothyronine (T_3) each day
         (1) T_3 has short half-life.
         (2) T_4 has half-life of 5-7 days.
         (3) Peripheral tissue converts T_4 to T_3.

(4) T_3 considered as true tissue thyroid hormone, whereas T_4 considered a plasma prohormone

(5) Control of hormones exists in hypothalamus and pituitary on negative feedback cycle.

M. Parathyroid: Refer to Figure 43-6.

1. Consists of four small masses of tissue lying behind or within thyroid gland, inside pretracheal fascia
   a. Upper pair lies behind superior pole of thyroid.
   b. Lower pair lies near pole of thyroid.
2. Aberrant nodules of parathyroid tissue may be found outside pretracheal fascia as low as superior mediastinum, especially within thymus.
3. Normally measure 3-4 mm in diameter
4. Blood supply
   a. Superior thyroid arteries
   b. Inferior thyroid arteries
5. Physiology
   a. Parathyroid hormone (PTH) regulates and maintains.
      (1) Metabolism
      (2) Hemostasis of blood calcium concentration
   b. Regulation of parathyroid hormone secretion

N. Lymph nodes: Refer to Figure 43-7.

1. Lymphatic system closely related anatomically and physiologically to circulatory system
2. Lymphatic system consists of lymphatic vessels and lymph nodes.
3. Lymph nodes are small oval bodies enclosed within fibrous connective tissue capsules.
   a. Trap foreign matter
   b. May become enlarged, infected, or the focus of metastatic cancer
4. Lymphatic vessels
   a. Transport lymph fluid from interstitial spaces to venous bloodstream
   b. Help protect body from disease

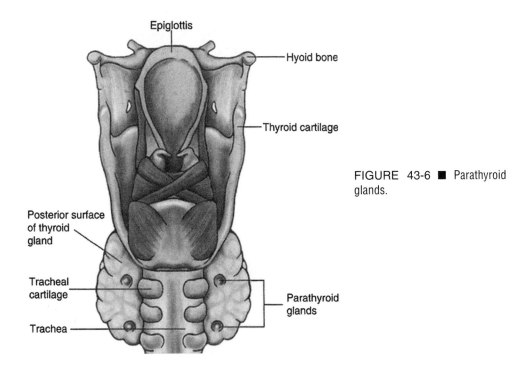

FIGURE 43-6 ■ Parathyroid glands.

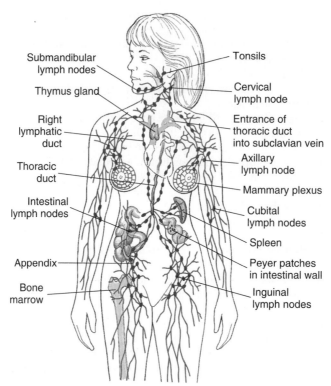

FIGURE 43-7 ■ Schematic representation of lymphatic system. (From Huether SE, McCance KL, editors: *Understanding pathophysiology,* 2nd ed. St. Louis: Mosby, 2000.)

5. Nodes occur in clusters in specific regions of body.
   a. Popliteal, inguinal nodes of lower extremity
   b. Lumbar nodes of pelvic region
   c. Cubital, axillary nodes of upper extremity
   d. Thoracic nodes of chest
   e. Cervical nodes of neck
   f. Peyer's patches of mesentery
O. Skin: Refer to Figure 43-8.
   1. Largest organ of body
   2. Integumentary system composed of
      a. Skin
         (1) Epidermis
            (a) Basal layer
            (b) Spiny layer
            (c) Granular layer
            (d) Clear layer
            (e) Hornlike layer
         (2) Dermis
            (a) Papillary layer
            (b) Reticular layer
         (3) Hypodermis (subcutaneous tissue)
            (a) Connects skin to underlying organs
      b. Epidermal modifications
         (1) Hair
         (2) Glands
         (3) Nails

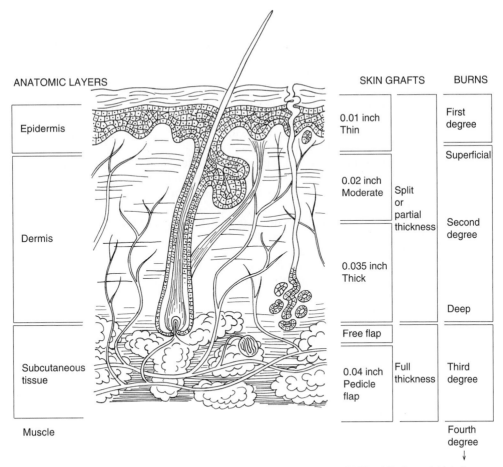

ANATOMIC LAYERS   SKIN GRAFTS   BURNS

Epidermis

0.01 inch
Thin

First
degree

Superficial

0.02 inch
Moderate   Split
or
partial
thickness

Dermis

Second
degree

0.035 inch
Thick

Deep

Free flap

Subcutaneous
tissue

0.04 inch   Full
Pedicle   thickness
flap

Third
degree

Muscle

Fourth
degree
↓

FIGURE 43-8 ■ Cross-section of skin and subcutaneous tissue. (From Phillips NF: *Berry & Kohn's operating room technique,* ed 10. St Louis: Mosby, 2004.)

3. Physiology
   (1) Functions as protective barrier against physical, chemical, bacterial agents
   (2) Maintains body temperature
   (3) Functions as sensory organ for pressure, touch, temperature, pain
   (4) Prevents loss of body fluid
   (5) Excretes waste from sweat glands
   (6) Contributes to self-concept and body image

II. Pathophysiology
  A. Breast
    1. Affected by three types of physiologic changes related to
      a. Growth and development
      b. Menstrual cycle
      c. Pregnancy and lactation
    2. Benign breast tumors
      a. Fibrocystic disease
        (1) Accounts for 45% of all biopsied female breast lesions
      b. Adenofibroses
        (1) Disease of youth, mean age 21
      c. Papilloma (intraductal papillomas)
        (1) Grows in terminal portion of duct or throughout duct

  d. Duct ectasia (comedomastitis)
   (1) Disease of ducts in subareolar zone
   (2) Disease of aging breast, most commonly in or near menopause
   (3) No demonstrated association with carcinoma
 3. Malignant breast tumors
  a. Early: solitary, unilateral, hard, painless, solid, irregular, poorly outlined, nonmobile lump, usually located in upper, outer quadrant of breast; opaque to translumination
  b. Moderately advanced locally: axillary nodes, nipple retraction or elevation, skin dimpling, nipple discharge
  c. Far advanced locally: supraclavicular nodes, fixation of axillary nodes, fixation of tumor to chest wall, edema (peau d'orange or redness over more than one third of breast), edema of arm, ulceration of skin, satellite nodules
  d. Distant metastasis: inoperable, partial, osseous or visceral
B. Gallbladder
 1. Cholelithiasis
  a. Precipitating factors for stone formation
   (1) Disturbances in metabolism
   (2) Biliary stasis
   (3) Obstruction
   (4) Infection
  b. Especially prevalent in women who are
   (1) Multiparous
   (2) Taking estrogen therapy
   (3) Using oral contraceptives
  c. Other risk factors
   (1) Obesity
   (2) Dietary intake of fats
   (3) Sedentary lifestyle
   (4) Familial tendencies
  d. Frequently seen in disease states such as
   (1) Diabetes mellitus
   (2) Regional enteritis
   (3) Certain blood dyscrasias
  e. Classification
   (1) Cholesterol
    (a) More common in the United States
   (2) Pigment stones
    (a) Black-pigment stones associated with cirrhosis and chronic hemolysis
    (b) Brown-pigment stones predominant in native Asians and associated with bacterial infection of the bile
 2. Cholecystitis
  a. Frequently associated with
   (1) Cystic duct obstruction caused by impacted gallstones
   (2) Stasis
   (3) Bacterial infection
   (4) Ischemia of the gallbladder due to trauma, massive burns, or surgery
C. Spleen
 1. Hypersplenism
  a. Causes a reduction in circulating quantity of red cells, white cells, platelets, or a combination of them
 2. Splenomegaly
  a. Congestive
  b. Hemolytic

   3. Hematologic disorders
      a. Hemolytic anemia
      b. Thrombocytopenia
   4. Tumors or cysts
   5. Accessory spleen
   6. Trauma
D. Esophagus-stomach
   1. Hiatal or diaphragmatic hernia
      a. Esophagitis
      b. Gastritis
      c. Aspiration of reflux contents
      d. Ulceration
      e. Bleeding
      f. Stenosis
      g. Chest and back symptoms
   2. Barrett's esophagus
      a. Ulcerations at distal esophagus
      b. May be precancerous
   3. Obesity
      a. Most common nutritional disorder in United States
      b. Causes
         (1) Social
         (2) Metabolic
         (3) Physiologic
         (4) Psychological
E. Appendix
   1. Appendicitis
      a. Most common in adolescents and young adults, especially
         males
      b. Can imitate other condition
         (1) Ruptured ovarian cyst
         (2) Ureteral calculus
      c. Usually caused by obstruction of appendiceal lumen
      d. Inflammation and infection result from normal bacteria invading
         devitalized wall.
   2. Peritonitis
      a. Result of severely inflamed and ruptured appendix
      b. Local or generalized
F. Intestine
   1. Inflammation
      a. Diverticulitis
      b. Ulcerative colitis
   2. Intestinal obstruction
      a. Neoplasms
      b. Strangulation from adhesions
      c. Volvulus
G. Hemorrhoids
   1. Bleeding: if severe can cause iron-deficiency anemia
   2. Strangulation: prolapsed hemorrhoid in which blood supply is cut off by
      anal sphincter
   3. Thrombosis: clotting of blood within hemorrhoid
H. Anal fissure
   1. Loss of elasticity of anal canal may predispose; caused by
      a. Laxative abuse
      b. Scarring from anal surgery
      c. Chronic diarrhea disease
      d. Frequent anal intercourse

I. Anorectal fistula
   1. Infection in crypt progresses to form abscess that drains spontaneously or surgically.
   2. Tract preserved as abscess heals
   3. Associated with
      a. Traumatic injury
      b. Crohn's disease
      c. Cancer
      d. Radiation therapy
J. Pilonidal cyst
   1. Sinus channel develops; lined with epithelium and hair
   2. Occurs during embryonic development when small amount of endothelial tissue is included beneath skin
K. Hernias
   1. Internal hernias
      a. Congenital
      b. Associated with failure of intestine to rotate in usual sequence in fetus
   2. External hernias
      a. Inguinal hernia
         (1) Most common
         (2) Types
            (a) Indirect: herniation protrudes through inguinal ring and follows round ligament or spermatic cord.
            (b) Direct: herniation goes through posterior inguinal wall.
            (c) Reducible: hernia contents can be returned to the normal cavity by manipulation.
            (d) Irreducible or incarcerated
               (i) Hernia contents cannot be returned to the normal cavity by manipulation.
               (ii) Bowel may lack adequate blood supply.
               (iii) Bowel may become obstructed or strangulated.
      b. Femoral
         (1) More frequent in women
         (2) Protrusion through femoral ring into femoral canal
         (3) Seen as bulge below inguinal ligament
         (4) Can easily strangulate
      c. Ventral
         (1) Associated with muscle weakness from abdominal incisions
         (2) Types
            (a) Epigastric
               (i) Protrusion of fat through defects in abdominal wall
               (ii) Between xiphoid process and umbilicus
            (b) Umbilical
               (i) Children
                  [a] More common
                  [b] Frequently disappears spontaneously by age two years
               (ii) Adult
                  [a] Acquired
                  [b] More common in females
                  [c] Increased abdominal pressure
                  [d] Obesity
                  [e] Multiparity
            (c) Incisional
               (i) Muscle weakness from prior surgeries
               (ii) Poor nutritional state
               (iii) Faulty surgical technique
               (iv) Obesity associated with ascites

(v) Wound infection

(vi) Wounds healed by secondary intention

L. Thyroid

    1. Multinodular toxic diffuse enlargement (Graves' disease)

    2. Adenomas

    3. Malignancy

    4. Thyroiditis

        a. Viral, autoimmune, or unknown etiology

        b. Immunoglobulins found in serum of hyperthyroid patients mimic thyrotropin (also called thyroid-stimulating hormone, or TSH).

M. Parathyroid

    1. Primary hyperparathyroidism

        a. Characterized by hypercalcemia and hypophosphatemia

        b. Results in major kidney and bone lesions

    2. Secondary hyperparathyroidism

        a. Results from parathyroid hyperplasia

        b. Produces decreased serum calcium levels

    3. Results in

        a. Bone lesions

        b. Overactivity of one or more parathyroid glands

        c. Excessive secretion of PTH

        d. Imbalance in calcium and phosphate metabolism

N. Lymph nodes

    1. Infectious mononucleosis

    2. Lymphadenopathy

    3. Malignant lymphomas

        a. Hodgkin disease

        b. Non-Hodgkin lymphoma

    4. Metastasis

O. Skin

    1. Cuts and punctures

    2. Burns and frostbite

    3. Abrasions

    4. Inflammation and infections

    5. Ulceration

    6. Disease conditions

    7. Neoplasms

        a. Malignant

            (1) Basal cell carcinoma

                (a) Most common skin cancer

                (b) Nodular with ulcerated center or crusted, dermatitis-like

            (2) Squamous cell carcinoma

                (a) Begins as red papule

                (b) Progresses to area that ulcerates, then crusts

                (c) Invades underlying tissue

            (3) Malignant melanoma

                (a) Changes size

                (b) Changes color (brown to black)

                (c) Changes smooth to rough

                (d) Borders become irregular.

                (e) Satellite lesions may be present.

        b. Nonmalignant

            (1) Nevus

                (a) Most common skin lesion

                (b) Round shape

                (c) Brown or black color

                (d) Flat or raised

                (e) With or without hair

III. Assessment
  A. General
    1. Test requirements are individualized according to institutional policy.
    2. History and physical
    3. Laboratory tests
      a. Basic hematology and electrolyte studies
      b. Urinalysis
    4. Chest x-ray
    5. Electrocardiogram with follow-up evaluation as dictated by medical history and/or physical findings
    6. Psychological assessment
  B. Breast
    1. Clinical manifestations
      a. Benign breast tumor may include
        (1) Breast pain and tenderness
        (2) Change in mass size with menstrual cycle
        (3) Palpable masses: firm, round, freely movable
      b. Conditions affecting nipple include
        (1) Bloody nipple discharge (intraductal papilloma)
        (2) Eczematous or ulcerated nipple (Paget's disease)
        (3) Usually minimal pain
      c. Malignant breast tumor may include
        (1) Nontender lump, usually in upper, outer quadrant
        (2) Axillary lymphadenopathy (late)
        (3) Fixed, nodular, nodular breast mass (late)
    2. Diagnostic studies
      a. Monthly breast self-examination
      b. Annual breast examination by physician
      c. Annual mammography for women 40 years and older
      d. Annual or periodic mammography for younger women if
        (1) Familial history of breast cancer
        (2) Early menarche
        (3) Multiparous or birth of first child after 34 years of age
        (4) High-fat diet
        (5) Oral contraceptive use
        (6) Radiation exposure
        (7) Presence of other cancer
    3. Laboratory studies
      a. Estrogen receptor protein
      b. Carcinoembryonic antigen (CEA)
      c. Gross cystic disease protein
      d. Liver function studies
    4. Scans
      a. Bone scan
      b. Brain or computed tomography (CT) scan
      c. Chest x-ray
      d. Ultrasonography
      e. Thermography
  C. Gallbladder
    1. Clinical manifestations
      a. Episodic, cramping pain in right upper abdomen quadrant or epigastrium, possibly radiating to back near right scapular tip (biliary colic)
      b. Nausea and/or vomiting
      c. Fat intolerance
      d. Fever and leukocytosis
      e. Signs and symptoms of jaundice
      f. Heartburn
      g. Flatulence

2. Laboratory studies
   a. Serum liver enzyme levels
   b. Bilirubin studies, liver function tests, alkaline phosphate
3. Radiologic studies
   a. Flat plate of abdomen
   b. Ultrasonography
   c. Oral cholecystogram
   d. Intravenous (IV) cholangiogram
   e. Upper gastrointestinal series
4. Other studies
   a. Endoscopic retrograde cholangiopancreatography (ERCP)
   b. CT scan

D. Spleen
1. History of
   a. Fatigue
   b. Lassitude
   c. Easy bruising
   d. Frequent nosebleed
   e. Hematuria
   f. Blood in stools
   g. Excessive bleeding after minor injuries or dental extractions
2. Physical examination
   a. Petechiae or bruising
   b. Pallor or cyanosis of skin and mucous membranes
   c. Hepatomegaly
   d. Splenomegaly
   e. Evidence of rupture
      (1) Increased abdominal girth
      (2) Abdominal pain
      (3) Signs and symptoms of shock
3. Laboratory studies as indicated
   a. Lactate dehydrogenase
   b. Bilirubin
   c. Sickle cell test
   d. Bone marrow aspiration
4. Radionuclide scanning
5. Other radiographic studies

E. Esophagus-stomach
1. Clinical manifestations of esophageal reflux
   a. Reflex esophagitis
      (1) After eating
      (2) While sleeping or reclining
      (3) With stress
      (4) With increased intraabdominal pressure
   b. Heartburn
   c. Belching
   d. Regurgitation
   e. Vomiting
   f. Retrosternal or substernal chest pain (dull, full, heavy)
   g. Hiccups
   h. Mild or occult bleeding and mild anemia
   i. Dysphagia
   j. Pneumonitis caused by aspiration
   k. Peptic stricture
2. Physical assessment
   a. Not diagnostic
   b. Not usually helpful in making a diagnosis
3. Diagnostic tests

    a. Barium swallow

    b. Chest x-ray

    c. Upper endoscopy and biopsy

    d. Esophageal motility studies

    e. Gastric analysis

    f. Stool occult blood test

    g. Electrocardiogram

4. Clinical manifestations of morbid obesity

    a. Weight more than 100 pounds (45.4 kg) more than ideal weight

    b. Failure to lose weight despite years of medical treatment

    c. Comorbid conditions possibly also present

        (1) Hypertension

        (2) Peripheral vascular disease

        (3) Cardiac disease

        (4) Degenerative arthritis or joint disorders

        (5) Gallbladder disease

        (6) Hiatal hernia

        (7) Diabetes mellitus

        (8) Obstructive sleep apnea

5. Diagnostic tests

    a. Diagnostic tests for comorbid conditions

        (1) Blood pressure (BP) checks

        (2) Doppler studies for circulatory status

        (3) Cardiac dysfunction studies

        (4) Motion analysis

        (5) Gastrointestinal (GI) studies

        (6) Nutritional studies

        (7) Electrolyte studies

        (8) Glucose studies

        (9) Pulmonary function studies

        (10) Psychological studies

F. Appendix

1. Assessment

    a. Early stage

        (1) Epigastric or umbilical pain

        (2) Vague and diffuse pain or mild cramping

        (3) Fever

        (4) Nausea and vomiting

    b. Acute stage

        (1) Rebound tenderness in right lower quadrant at McBurney's point

        (2) Pain aggravated by walking, coughing, movement

        (3) Sensation of constipation

        (4) Anorexia

        (5) Malaise

        (6) Diarrhea

        (7) Diminished peristalsis

    c. Acute appendicitis with perforation

        (1) Increasing, generalized pain

        (2) Recurrent vomiting

2. Physical examination

    a. Temperature increases

    b. Generalized abdominal rigidity

    c. Rigid position with flexed knees

    d. Tender, palpable mass in the presence of abscess

    e. Possible abdominal distension

3. Diagnostic tests

    a. Complete blood count (CBC) with differential (elevated white blood cell count)

       b. Urinalysis

       c. Abdominal x-ray

       d. Intravenous pyelogram

       e. Abdominal ultrasound

       f. Abdominal CT scan

G. Intestine

  1. Assessment

     a. Signs and symptoms

       (1) Severe, cramping abdominal pain

       (2) Back pain

       (3) Restlessness

       (4) Hiccups

       (5) Belching

       (6) Inability to pass stool or flatus with feeling of fullness

     b. Physical assessment

       (1) Abdominal distention

       (2) Abdominal tenderness

       (3) High pitched and intermittent bowel sounds above point of obstruction

       (4) Absent bowel sounds with paralytic ileus

       (5) Signs of intravascular volume depletion

         (a) Decreased urinary output

         (b) Poor skin turgor

         (c) Dry skin and mucous membranes

       (6) Bleeding on rectal examination

     c. History of

       (1) Abdominal hernia

       (2) Recent or past abdominal surgery

       (3) GI inflammation or perforation secondary to various disease processes

  2. Diagnostic tests

     a. CBC

     b. Abdominal x-ray

     c. Contrast studies

     d. CT scan of abdomen

     e. Endoscopy (sigmoidoscopy, colonoscopy)

H. Hemorrhoids

  1. Clinical manifestations

     a. External hemorrhoids

       (1) Pruritus

       (2) Pain

     b. Internal hemorrhoids

       (1) Bleeding

       (2) Thrombosis

       (3) Edema

  2. Diagnostic tests

     a. Anoscopy

       (1) Visualization of hemorrhoids as instrument is removed

     b. Sigmoidoscopy

     c. Barium enema

I. Anal fissure

  1. Clinical manifestation

     a. Inflammation

     b. Bleeding

     c. Burning

     d. Pain on defecation

  2. Diagnostic tests

     a. Digital rectal exam

       (1) Induration

       (2) Sphincter spasm

    b. Anoscopy (proctoscopy)

       (1) Visualization of anorectal fissure

       (2) Superficial tear

         (a) Bleeds easily

         (b) Has a reddish base

  3. Differential diagnosis

    a. If fissure not found in midline, rule out

       (1) Inflammatory disease

       (2) Bowel disease

       (3) Carcinoma

       (4) Tuberculosis

       (5) Syphilis

       (6) Herpes or other venereal disease

J. Anorectal fistula

  1. Physical examination

    a. Digital rectal examination

    b. Palpate tract direction internally.

  2. Diagnostic tests

    a. Anoscopy (proctoscopy)

       (1) May reveal primary opening in a cyst

    b. Sigmoidoscopy

       (1) Used to rule out other sources of fistula formation

    c. Fistulography

       (1) Used if tract is of questionable origin

       (2) Rule out colonic, small bowel, or urethral fistulas.

K. Pilonidal cyst

  1. Physical examination

    a. Hairy dimple in gluteal fold

    b. Open, draining lesion in sacral region with hair protruding from sinus opening

L. Hernias

  1. Physical examination of abdomen

    a. Examine supine and sitting.

    b. Can often see hernia protrude when

       (1) Changing position

       (2) Coughing

       (3) Laughing or crying

    c. Palpate weakened muscle area.

  2. Signs of intestinal obstruction

    a. Abdominal distention

    b. Nausea

    c. Vomiting

  3. Signs of strangulation

    a. Pain of increasing severity

    b. Fever

    c. Tachycardia

    d. Abdominal rigidity

M. Thyroid (hyperthyroidism)

  1. Clinical manifestations

    a. Nervousness, irritability, hyperactivity, emotional lability, and decreased attention span

    b. Weakness, easy fatigability, exercise intolerance

    c. Heat intolerance

    d. Weight change (loss or gain), increased appetite

    e. Insomnia, interrupted sleep

    f. Frequent stools, diarrhea

      g. Menstrual irregularities, decreased libido

      h. Warm, sweaty, flushed skin with a velvety-smooth texture; spider telangiectasis

      i. Exophthalmos, retracted eyelids, staring gaze

      j. Tremor, hyperkinesia, hyperreflexia

      k. Hair loss

      l. Goiter

      m. Bruits over thyroid gland

      n. Elevated systolic blood pressure, widened pulse pressure, S3 heart sound

    2. Diagnostic laboratory tests

      a. Thyrotropin-releasing hormone (TRH) stimulation test

      b. Serum T_4 and T_3

      c. Serum free T_4 and T_3

      d. Radioactive T_3 uptake (RT_3U)

      e. Radioactive iodine uptake (RAIU)

      f. TSH

      g. Thyroid-stimulating immunoglobulins (TSI)

N. Parathyroid

    1. Clinical manifestations

      a. Fatigue, muscular weakness, listlessness

      b. Loss of height, frequent fractures

      c. Renal calculi

      d. Anorexia, nausea, abdominal discomfort

      e. Memory impairment

      f. Polyuria, polydipsia

      g. Back and joint pain

      h. Hypertension

    2. Diagnostic laboratory tests

      a. Serum calcium levels

      b. Serum Po_4

      c. Urinary calcium levels

      d. Urinary PO_4

      e. Creatine clearance

      f. Hydroxyproline

      g. Urinary cyclic adenosine monophosphate (cAMP)

O. Lymph nodes

    1. Clinical manifestations

      a. Enlarged, painless lump or swelling

      b. Fever, sometimes intermittent

      c. Weakness, malaise

      d. Weight loss

      e. Anemia

      f. Local symptoms caused by pressure or obstruction

        (1) Pain, nerve irritation

        (2) Obliteration of pulse

    2. Diagnostic tests

      a. Chest x-ray

      b. Lymphangiography

      c. Biopsy

P. Skin

    1. Physical examination

      a. Color

      b. Texture

      c. Temperature

      d. Moisture or dryness

      e. Turgor

      f. Aging

  g. Sensory reception

  h. Condition of

   (1) Hair

   (2) Nails

   (3) Glands

 2. Diagnostic tests

  a. Biopsy

  b. Culture and sensitivity

IV. Operative procedures

 A. Breast

  1. Preoperative concerns

   a. Possible malignancy

   b. Losing a body part

   c. Facing negative reaction from spouse and family

   d. Change in self-image

   e. Life expectancy and ability to raise family

  2. Intraoperative concerns

   a. Mammogram films available

   b. Correct side verified

   c. Specimen properly prepared and labeled for pathology

  3. Procedures

   a. Needle biopsy

    (1) Purpose: Remove tissue sample for biopsy via needle aspiration

    (2) Vim-Silverman or disposable cutting-type needle introduced and advanced into breast mass to entrap a core of tissue

    (3) Needle withdrawn and tissue specimen sent for diagnostic examination

    (4) Definitive surgical treatment should only follow formal biopsy.

   b. Incisional biopsy

    (1) Purpose: Remove a sample of involved tissue for biopsy

    (2) Portion of mass is surgically excised using a curved incisional line.

    (3) Tissue sent for diagnostic examination

   c. Excisional biopsy

    (1) Purpose: Remove entire tumor mass for biopsy

    (2) Needle localization may be done preoperatively to locate mass.

    (3) Specimen sent for diagnostic examination

    (4) Usually done under local anesthesia or IV sedation

    (5) Short delay between biopsy and further treatment does not adversely affect survival.

   d. Sentinel node or primary lymph node biopsy

    (1) Purpose: Identify first lymph nodes along lymphatic channel from primary tumor site to determine need for additional or more extensive surgeries and treatments.

    (2) Small amount of radioisotope injected and sentinel node identified during a nuclear medicine scan

    (3) Node excised in addition to the malignant breast mass

    (4) Less extensive than axillary lymph node dissection

   e. Incision and drainage of abscess

    (1) Purpose: Incise inflamed and suppurative area of breast to drain abscess

    (2) Abscesses occur most frequently in infected lactating breast; chronic abscesses rare

    (3) Free drainage required with abscesses around nipple or in breast tissue

   f. Partial mastectomy (lumpectomy, segmental resection, quadrant resection, wedge resection)

    (1) Purpose: Remove tumor mass with at least one inch of surrounding tissue

    (2) Appears to provide results equal to more radical procedure when combined with axillary node or sentinel node dissection and irradiation in stages I and II

  g. Subcutaneous mastectomy

    (1) Procedure: Removal of all breast tissue with overlying skin and nipple left intact

    (2) Purpose: Remove benign subcutaneous involved tissue

    (3) Recommended for patients who have

     (a) Central tumors of noninvasive origin

     (b) Chronic cystic mastitis

     (c) Hyperplastic duct changes

     (d) Multiple fibroadenomas

     (e) Undergone several previous biopsies

  h. Simple mastectomy

    (1) Procedure: Removal of entire breast without lymph node dissection

    (2) Purpose: Performed

     (a) To remove extensive benign disease

     (b) If malignancy is believed to be confined only to breast tissue

     (c) As a palliative measure to remove an ulcerated advanced malignancy

  i. Procedure: Reduction of the male breast

    (1) Purpose: Performed to relieve gynecomastia

     (a) Occurs primarily after 40 years or during puberty

     (b) Usually related to alterations in normal hormonal balance

     (c) All subareolar fibroglandular tissue removed with reconstruction of resultant defect

     (d) Liposuction may be used to debulk male breast.

B. Gallbladder

 1. Cholecystectomy: Removal of the gallbladder

 2. Purpose: Treatment of cholelithiasis or cholecystitis

 3. Preoperative concerns

  a. Anxiety related to impending surgical procedure and knowledge deficit

  b. Self-consciousness about body image if obese

  c. Concern about ability to resume normal activity and work

 4. Intraoperative concerns

  a. Fluid volume deficit related to hemorrhage

  b. Altered body temperature

  c. Infection related to invasive GI procedure

  d. Perforation of bladder, bowel, vascular organs

  e. Injury related to positioning

  f. Long instruments for obese or tall patient

 5. Procedures

  a. Laparoscopic cholecystectomy

    (1) Accomplished through three or four incisions made in abdominal wall

    (2) Rigid fiberoptic laparoscope inserted into peritoneal cavity

    (3) Specialized, long-handled instruments used to resect gallbladder with electrocautery or laser cautery

    (4) Advantages

     (a) Less postoperative pain

     (b) Fewer complications

     (c) More rapid postoperative recovery

    (5) Disadvantages

     (a) Longer surgery time

     (b) Longer exposure to anesthesia

     (c) More costly than open abdominal cholecystectomy

    b. Open abdominal cholecystectomy
- (1) Performed through right subcostal incision that may be extended over the midline
- (2) Performed if laparoscopic cholecystectomy is unsuccessful or contraindicated
- (3) Common duct exploration done if stones suspected

    c. Cholelithotripsy: High-energy shock waves used to fragment cholesterol gallstones
- (1) Performed under IV sedation or general anesthesia
- (2) Pulverized stone fragments pass through bile duct.

C. Spleen
1. Splenectomy: Removal of spleen
2. Purpose: Provide symptomatic relief, depending on cause of anemia or hemorrhage, or prophylactically to reduce potential for rupture and massive blood loss
3. Preoperative concern
   - **a.** Anxiety related to impending surgical procedure and knowledge deficit
   - **b.** Concern about ability to resume normal activity and work
   - **c.** Scheduled splenectomy patients may require preoperative
     - (1) Whole blood immediately prior to procedure
     - (2) Corticosteroids to stabilize cell membranes and decrease inflammatory response
4. Intraoperative concerns
   - **a.** Fluid volume deficit related to hemorrhage
   - **b.** Altered body temperature
   - **c.** Infection related to invasive GI procedure
   - **d.** Perforation of bladder, bowel, vascular organs
   - **e.** Injury related to positioning
   - **f.** Inflammatory response
5. Procedures
   - **a.** Laparoscopic splenectomy
     - (1) Accomplished through three or four incisions made in abdominal wall
     - (2) Rigid fiberoptic laparoscope inserted into peritoneal cavity
     - (3) Performed in patients with benign disease
     - (4) Advantages
       - (a) Less postoperative pain
       - (b) Fewer complications
       - (c) More rapid postoperative recovery
     - (5) Disadvantages
       - (a) Longer surgery time
       - (b) Longer exposure to anesthesia
       - (c) More costly than open abdominal splenectomy
   - **b.** Open abdominal splenectomy
     - (1) Left rectus paramedian, midline, or subcostal incision
     - (2) Splenic artery and vein often friable

D. Esophagus-stomach
1. Preoperative concerns
   - **a.** Anxiety related to impending surgical procedure and knowledge deficit
   - **b.** Self-consciousness about body image if obese
   - **c.** Concern about ability to resume normal activity and work
2. Intraoperative concerns
   - **a.** Adequately sized cart, table, procedural instruments, and equipment
   - **b.** Adequate moving help and mechanical aids
   - **c.** Difficult IV access
   - **d.** Difficult intubation
   - **e.** Respiratory problems, especially during intubation or laryngospasm

f. Aspiration

g. Thromboembolism

h. Fluid volume deficit related to loss of blood and electrolyte-rich gastric and intestinal juices

i. Altered body temperature

j. Infection related to invasive GI procedure

k. Perforation of bladder, bowel, vascular organs

l. Injury related to positioning

3. Procedures

  a. Esophageal hiatal herniorrhaphy: Repair hiatal hernia

  b. Purpose: Prevent reflux of gastric contents into esophagus

    (1) Laparoscopic Nissen fundoplication (one of several common procedures)

      (a) Performed on selected patients

      (b) Performed through five stab wounds in abdomen

      (c) Portion of upper stomach is wrapped around distal esophagus and sutured to itself to prevent reflux.

      (d) Advantages

        (i) Less postoperative pain

        (ii) Fewer complications

        (iii) More rapid postoperative recovery

      (e) Disadvantages

        (i) Longer surgery time

        (ii) Longer exposure to anesthesia

        (iii) More costly than open abdominal fundoplication

    (2) Open abdominal approach

      (a) Accomplished through midline or left subcostal incision, possibly extending over lower rib cage

      (b) Hiatus narrowed and fundus of stomach anchored against diaphragm

  c. Bariatric surgery: Gastric restriction in the morbidly obese patient

  d. Purpose: Reduce the size of the stomach to facilitate weight loss

    (1) Laparoscopic gastric banding

      (a) Stomach capacity reduced to approximately 50 ml to restrict food absorption or intake

      (b) Silicone tubing or silastic rings applied to stomach

      (c) Advantages

        (i) Less postoperative pain

        (ii) Fewer complications

        (iii) More rapid postoperative recovery

      (d) Disadvantages

        (i) Longer surgery time

        (ii) Longer exposure to anesthesia

        (iii) More costly than open abdominal fundoplication

    (2) Open abdominal approach (gastric bypass)

      (a) Performed through a transabdominal incision

      (b) Stomach size reduced by creating small pouch in fundus

      (c) Gastrojejunostomy is constructed between the pouch and the jejunum.

      (d) Gastric, biliary, and pancreatic fluids feed into jejunum.

E. Appendix

  1. Appendectomy: Removal of appendix

  2. Purpose: Prevent a progression to gangrene and the perforation of friable tissue with subsequent peritonitis

  3. Preoperative concerns

    a. Anxiety related to impending surgical procedure and knowledge deficit

    b. Concern about ability to resume normal activity and work

4. Intraoperative concerns
    a. Potential or actual rupture
    b. Potential peritonitis
    c. Potential bladder or bowel perforation
5. Procedures
    a. Laparoscopic appendectomy
        (1) Performed through periumbilical incision with additional stab wounds at suprapubic area and left lower quadrant
        (2) May be done incidental to gynecologic procedures or for acute or chronic appendicitis
        (3) Advantages
            (a) Earlier ambulation and hospital discharge
            (b) Decreased risk of wound infection
            (c) More aesthetically appealing appearance
            (d) Less pain
        (4) Disadvantages
            (a) Longer surgical time
            (b) Increased general anesthesia exposure time
            (c) Increased cost
    b. Open appendectomy
        (1) Involves a muscle-splitting incision over McBurney's point in right lower quadrant
        (2) Following amputation of appendix, stump may be cauterized with phenol and alcohol or wiped with Betadine to reduce contamination.
        (3) Drainage indicated in presence of
            (a) Abscess
            (b) Appendix rupture
            (c) Gross contamination of wound
F. Intestine
    1. Bowel resection: Remove a portion of intestine
    2. Purpose: Relieve an obstruction or remove a portion of diseased intestine or adhesions
    3. Preoperative concerns
        a. Anxiety related to impending surgical procedure and knowledge deficit
        b. Concern about ability to resume normal activity and work
    4. Intraoperative concerns
        a. Fluid volume deficit related to hemorrhage
        b. Altered body temperature
        c. Infection related to invasive GI procedure
        d. Perforation of bladder, vascular organs
        e. Injury related to positioning
        f. Long instruments for obese or tall patient
    5. Procedures
        a. Laparoscopic intestinal resection
            (1) Performed through minimal access incision made in abdominal wall
            (2) Large or small bowel mobilized and resected through scope
            (3) Stomas can also be created with this technique.
            (4) Advantages
                (a) Less postoperative pain
                (b) Fewer complications
                (c) More rapid postoperative recovery
            (5) Disadvantages
                (a) Longer surgery time
                (b) Longer exposure to anesthesia
                (c) More costly than open intestinal resection procedure
            (6) Performed through midline abdominal incision
            (7) Peritoneal cavity walled off with intestine incised and clamped
            (8) Continuity reestablished by anastomosis

G. Hemorrhoids
1. Hemorrhoidectomy: Remove varicosities of veins or prolapsed mucosa of the anus and rectum
2. Purpose: Relieve discomfort and control bleeding
3. Preoperative concerns
   a. Embarrassment because of private nature of site
   b. Concern about excessive pain
   c. Concern about fecal incontinence
   d. Concern about painful suture removal
   e. Concern about ability to resume normal activity and work
4. Intraoperative concerns
   a. Maintaining privacy
   b. If used, laser safety
   c. Contamination of vagina with bloody anal fluid
5. Procedures
   a. Usual procedure
      (1) Sphincter dilated
      (2) Hemorrhoidal pedicle ligated with suture ligatures
      (3) Mass excised with dissection, laser, cautery or cryosurgical unit
      (4) Petrolatum gauze packed into anal canal
   b. Alternative procedure
      (1) Rubber band ligation placed around base of each hemorrhoid
      (2) Sloughing of avascularized hemorrhoid occurs in 7-10 days
      (3) Can be done as an office procedure under local anesthesia
      (4) Advantages
         (a) Less postprocedure pain
         (b) Fewer complications
         (c) More rapid postprocedure recovery
      (5) Disadvantage
         (a) Local pain and potential for hemorrhage
H. Anal fissure
1. Anal fissurectomy: Dilatation of anal sphincter and removal of lesion
2. Purpose: Relieve discomfort
3. Preoperative concerns
   a. Embarrassment because of private nature of site
   b. Concern about excessive pain
   c. Concern about fecal incontinence
   d. Concern about painful suture removal
   e. Concern about ability to resume normal activity and work
4. Intraoperative concerns
   a. Maintaining privacy
   b. If used, laser safety
5. Procedure
   a. Anal sphincter dilation may be only surgical treatment necessary.
   b. Scarred tissue removed for chronic conditions
I. Anorectal fistula
1. Anal fistulotomy: Incision and drainage of a fistulous tract
2. Anal fistulectomy: Excision of fistula
3. Purpose: Prevent spread of infection
4. Preoperative concerns
   a. Embarrassment because of private nature of site
   b. Concern about excessive pain
   c. Concern about fecal incontinence
   d. Concern about painful suture removal
   e. Concern about ability to resume normal activity and work
5. Intraoperative concerns
   a. Maintaining privacy
   b. If used, laser safety

6. Procedure
   a. In a fistulotomy the tract is opened, packed, and allowed to drain and heal by granulation.
   b. In a fistulectomy the tract is excised and sometimes partially closed with suture.
J. Pilonidal cyst
   1. Pilonidal cystectomy: Remove cyst with sinus tract
   2. Purpose: Prevent recurrence of infection and abscess formation in pilonidal sinus
   3. Preoperative concerns
      a. Embarrassment because of private nature of site
      b. Concern about excessive pain
      c. Concern about painful suture removal
      d. Concern about ability to resume normal activity and work
   4. Intraoperative concerns
      a. Maintaining privacy
      b. Contamination of vagina with bloody fluid
   5. Procedure
      a. Cyst with sinus tracts removed from intergluteal fold on posterior surface of lower sacrum to prevent recurrence of infection and abcess formation in pilonidal sinus
      b. Wound may be packed open, closed, or closed with tissue flaps.
K. Hernia
   1. Herniorrhaphy: Repair of weakened abdominal wall
   2. Hernioplasty: Reinforcement of weakened area with wire, fascia, or mesh
   3. Purpose: Reduce or repair hernia; may be inguinal, femoral, ventral, umbilical, or incisional in origin
   4. Preoperative concerns
      a. Anxiety related to impending surgical procedure and knowledge deficit
      b. Concern about ability to resume normal activity and work
   5. Intraoperative concerns
      a. Fluid volume deficit related to hemorrhage
      b. Altered body temperature
      c. Infection related to invasive GI procedure
      d. Perforation of bladder, bowel, vascular organs
      e. Injury related to positioning
      f. Long instruments for obese or tall patient
   6. Procedures
      a. Laparoscopic hernia repair
         (1) Transabdominal preperitoneal (TAPP) approach uses intraperitoneal trocars and the creation of a peritoneal flap over posterior inguinal region.
         (2) Totally extraperitoneal approach (TEPA) provides access to the preperitoneal space without entering peritoneal cavity.
         (3) Advantages
            (a) Less oral analgesics required
            (b) Recovery period shorter
            (c) Wound infection rate lower
            (d) Tension-free application of mesh enabled
            (e) Bilateral herniorrhaphy can be performed using same port sites.
            (f) Postoperative adhesions reduced
         (4) Disadvantages
            (a) Surgical time longer
            (b) General anesthesia exposure time increased
            (c) Potential for nerve injury greater
            (d) Cost increased

      b. Open hernia repair
        (1) Incision depends on hernia location and type.
        (2) Principle is same regardless of hernia location and type.
          (a) Free tightly bound hernias.
          (b) Examine contents of hernia for ischemic change.
          (c) Repair hernia defect with or without reinforcement.

L. Thyroid
  1. Thyroidectomy: Removal of all or part of thyroid gland
  2. Purpose: Relates to the patient's medical diagnosis
    a. To relieve tracheal obstruction
      (1) Graves' disease (hyperthyroidism)
      (2) Hashimoto's thyroiditis (autoimmune disease)
    b. To relieve tracheal or esophageal obstruction
      (1) Nontoxic nodular goiter
      (2) Rule out a malignant nodule of thyroid gland.
    c. To remove malignant tumors
  3. Preoperative concerns
    a. Anxiety related to disease state and impending surgical procedure with knowledge deficit
    b. Success of surgery
    c. Cosmetic results of surgery
    d. Concern about ability to resume normal activity and work
  4. Intraoperative concerns
    a. Edema resulting in impaired swallowing, ineffective airway clearance, or ineffective gas exchange postoperatively
    b. Ineffective thermoregulation
    c. Laryngeal nerve damage
    d. Positioning to prevent distorted body contour in neck region
  5. Procedures
    a. Unilateral thyroid lobectomy: removal of one thyroid lobe with division at isthmus
    b. Subtotal lobectomy: lobectomy that spares posterior capsule and possibly a portion of adjacent thyroid tissue
    c. Bilateral subtotal thyroidectomy: removal of both lobes of thyroid
    d. Near-total thyroidectomy: total lobectomy with contralateral subtotal thyroidectomy
    e. Total thyroidectomy: removal of both lobes of thyroid and attempted removal of all thyroid tissue present
    f. All procedures performed through a transverse incision parallel to normal skin lines

M. Parathyroid
  1. Parathyroidectomy: Excision of one or more parathyroid glands
  2. Purpose: Relates to the patient's medical diagnosis
    a. Presence of adenomas (hypersecreting neoplasms)
    b. Hyperplasia
    c. Carcinomas
      (1) Require surgical excision
      (2) Resection of lymphatics is essential
    d. Inability to locate glands
    e. Underlying medical conditions
      (1) Renal failure
      (2) Severe cardiac disorders
      (3) Hypercalcemia of nonparathyroid etiology
  3. Preoperative concerns
    a. Anxiety related to disease state and impending surgical procedure and knowledge deficit
    b. Success of surgery

        c. Cosmetic results of surgery

        d. Concern about ability to resume normal activity and work

    4. Intraoperative concerns

        a. Edema resulting in impaired swallowing, ineffective airway clearance, or ineffective gas exchange postoperatively

        b. Ineffective thermoregulation

        c. Laryngeal nerve damage

        d. Positioning to prevent distorted body contour in neck region

    5. Procedures

        a. Total parathyroidectomy: removal of all glands

        b. Partial parathyroidectomy: removal of three and one half to four glands

           (1) Metal clips left in place to identify remaining glandular tissue

        c. Procedures performed through a transverse incision parallel to normal skin lines

  N. Lymph node

    1. Lymph node biopsy: Excision of one or more lymph nodes and possibly some surrounding tissue

    2. Purpose: Relates to the patient's medical diagnosis

    3. Preoperative concerns

        a. Cosmetic appearance of surgical site

        b. Possible malignancy

        c. Life expectancy and ability to raise family

    4. Intraoperative concerns

        a. Lymphangiogram reports available

        b. Correct side verified

        c. Specimen properly prepared and labeled for pathology

    5. Procedure

        a. Depends on site of procedure

        b. Removal of nodes done through small incision

        c. Identification and microscopic examination of nodes determines

           (1) Diagnosis

           (2) Staging of malignancy

           (3) Need for additional or more extensive surgeries and adjunct treatment

  O. Skin

    1. Skin biopsy and excision of lesion: Excision of involved layers of tissue

    2. Purpose: Relates to the patient's medical diagnosis

    3. Preoperative concerns

        a. Cosmetic appearance of surgical site

        b. Possible malignancy

        c. Life expectancy and ability to raise family

    4. Intraoperative concerns

        a. Correct side verified

        b. Specimen properly prepared and labeled for pathology

    5. Procedure

        a. Excision of involved tissue to

           (1) Depth of involvement

           (2) Clean margins

        b. Graft may be required depending on

           (1) Size of lesion

           (2) Depth of lesion

V. Postanesthesia priorities: Phase I

  A. General immediate care: Refer to Chapter 35.

  B. Breast surgery

    1. Monitor and document drainage output.

        a. Monitor competency of drainage system.

        b. Monitor dressing for hemorrhage or oozing.

   2. Assess comfort level.
      a. Pain may increase anxiety and feeling of powerlessness.
      b. If severe, may limit chest expansion
      c. Assess effectiveness of any analgesics given.
   3. Position for comfort
      a. Usually supine or semi-Fowler's
      b. Affected arm may be elevated on pillow to decrease swelling and enhance circulation.
   4. Psychological support
      a. Respond appropriately to patient's verbalized questions and responses.
      b. Avoid making unfounded promises or encouraging false or unreasonable hopes.
      c. Respect patient's privacy.
C. Gallbladder surgery: Laparoscopic or open cholecystectomy
   1. Monitor intake and output.
      a. Assess nasogastric tube for proper placement; if ordered, discontinue.
      b. Note patency of catheter, color and amount of urine; if ordered, discontinue.
   2. Assess comfort level.
      a. Note location of discomfort, and position for comfort.
      b. Administer prescribed medications, and evaluate relief.
D. Spleen surgery: Laparoscopic or open splenectomy
   1. Monitor intake and output.
      a. Assess nasogastric tube for proper placement; if ordered, discontinue.
      b. Note patency of catheter, color and amount of urine; if ordered, discontinue.
   2. Assess comfort level.
      a. Note location of discomfort, and position for comfort.
      b. Administer prescribed medications, and evaluate relief.
   3. Maintain preoperative corticosteroid treatment if ordered.
   4. Monitor for internal bleeding.
      a. Abdominal girth and distension
      b. Abdominal firmness
      c. Signs and symptoms of shock
E. Esophagus-stomach surgery
   1. Laparoscopic or open Nissen fundoplication
      a. Initiate chest physiotherapy.
         (1) Coughing and deep breathing
         (2) Observe for indications of pneumothorax.
            (a) Dyspnea
            (b) Cyanosis
            (c) Sharp chest pain
      b. Initiate care of chest tubes if present for open procedure.
      c. Monitor intake and output.
         (1) NPO until
            (a) Absence of nausea and vomiting
            (b) Bowel sounds present
         (2) Assess nasogastric tube for proper placement; if ordered, discontinue.
         (3) Administer IV fluids and electrolytes as ordered.
         (4) Note patency of catheter, color and amount of urine; if ordered, discontinue.
      d. Monitor for internal bleeding.
         (1) Abdominal girth and distension
         (2) Abdominal firmness
         (3) Signs and symptoms of shock
      e. Assess comfort level.
         (1) Note location of discomfort, and position for comfort.
         (2) Administer prescribed medications, and evaluate relief.

    2. Laparoscopic or open bariatric procedures
      a. Protect airway
        (1) Elevate head.
          (a) Prevent aspiration.
          (b) Improve ventilation.
        (2) Lateral positioning
        (3) Oxygen
        (4) Cough, deep breathing
        (5) Vigilant observation
      b. Monitor intake and output.
        (1) NPO until
          (a) Absence of nausea and vomiting
          (b) Bowel sounds present
        (2) Administer IV fluids and electrolytes as ordered.
          (a) Avoid overhydration.
        (3) Note patency of catheter, color and amount of urine.
      c. Provide nasogastric (NG) tube care if tube present.
        (1) Ensure patency.
        (2) Anchor tube securely.
      d. Wound care
        (1) Observe for excessive drainage.
        (2) Splint incision when coughing.
        (3) Apply binders as ordered.
      e. Prevent thromboemboli.
        (1) Continue antiembolism stockings and sequential pneumatic devices as ordered.
        (2) Encourage leg movement.
        (3) Avoid groin and popliteal pressure.
      f. Assess comfort level.
        (1) Note location of discomfort, and position for comfort.
        (2) Administer prescribed medications, and evaluate relief.
        (3) Beware of prolonged somnolence caused by drugs stored in adipose tissue (e.g., barbiturates, fentanyl, sufentanil, meperidine diazepam, etc.).
      g. Provide psychological support.
        (1) Provide privacy.
        (2) Respect dignity.
F. Appendix surgery: Laparoscopic or open procedure
    1. Monitor intake and output.
      a. NPO until
        (1) Absence of nausea and vomiting
        (2) Bowel sounds present
      b. Administer IV fluids and electrolytes as ordered.
      c. Note patency of catheter if present, color and amount of urine.
      d. Provide NG tube care if tube present.
        (1) Ensure patency.
        (2) Anchor tube securely.
    2. Administer antibiotics as ordered.
    3. Assess comfort level.
      a. Note location of discomfort, and position for comfort.
      b. Administer prescribed medications, and evaluate relief.
G. Intestine surgery: Laparoscopic or open procedure
    1. Monitor intake and output.
      a. NPO until
        (1) Absence of nausea and vomiting
        (2) Bowel sounds present
      b. Assess nasogastric tube for proper placement.
      c. Administer IV fluids and electrolytes as ordered.
      d. Note patency of catheter, color and amount of urine.

    2. Monitor for internal bleeding.
      a. Abdominal girth and distension.
      b. Abdominal firmness
      c. Signs and symptoms of shock
    3. Assess comfort level.
      a. Note location of discomfort, and position for comfort.
      b. Administer prescribed medications, and evaluate relief.

H. Anorectal surgery
    1. Monitor for urinary retention.
    2. Monitor for bleeding.
    3. Assess comfort level.
      a. Note location of discomfort, and position for comfort.
      b. Administer prescribed medications, and evaluate relief.
    4. Monitor for hypotension secondary to vasodilation of pelvic blood vessels.

I. Hernia surgery: Laparoscopic or open procedure
    1. Monitor for hematoma formation in laparoscopic procedure.
      a. Perforation of bowel
      b. Perforation of epigastric vessels
      c. Perforation or damage of ilioinguinal vessels
    2. Monitor for scrotal edema and ecchymosis.
      a. Ice packs for scrotal edema as ordered
    3. Monitor for sensory and motor alterations.
      a. Damage of ilioinguinal nerves during manipulation and dissection of various anatomical structures
      b. Infiltration of incisional area with local anesthesia
    4. Assess for bladder distention.
      a. Urinary retention
      b. Perforation of urinary bladder during dissection
    5. Monitor for internal bleeding.
      a. Abdominal girth and distension
      b. Abdominal firmness
      c. Signs and symptoms of shock
    6. Assess comfort level.
      a. Note location of discomfort, and position for comfort.
      b. Administer prescribed medications, and evaluate relief.

J. Thyroid-parathyroid surgery
    1. Assess surgical site.
      a. Assess neck dressings for signs of hemorrhaging.
      b. Assess and document presence of drain and drainage.
      c. Assess neck for swelling.
        (1) Nerve damage; have patient say "e."
        (2) Obstructed airway
        (3) Vascularity of neck
      d. Encourage patient to remain calm, and prevent neck thrashing.
    2. In thyroidectomy instruct patient in importance of remaining silent to rest vocal cords.
    3. In parathyroidectomy assess for neurologic sequelae.
      a. Hyperthermia
      b. Increased intracranial pressure
      c. Cerebrospinal fluid leakage
      d. Convulsions

K. Node biopsy
    1. Assess surgical site for drainage.
    2. Assess comfort level.
      a. Pain may increase anxiety and feeling of powerlessness.
      b. Assess effectiveness of any analgesics given.
    3. Assess circulation in affected extremity.

      4. Psychological support

        a. Respond appropriately to patient's verbalized questions and responses.

        b. Avoid making unfounded promises or encouraging false or unreasonable hopes.

VI. Postanesthesia priorities: Phase II

    A. General immediate care: Refer to Chapter 56.

    B. Breast surgery

      1. Assess dressing and bra firmness.

      2. Assess security of drain.

      3. Assess emotional feelings.

      4. Key educational components

        a. Depends on extent of the procedure and diagnosis

        b. Reinforce need for firm-fitting bra without underwire to provide support.

        c. Provide information on range-of-motion exercises as directed by the physician.

        d. Provide information about resources and support systems as appropriate.

      5. Provide written and verbal instructions; assess and ensure patient and family understanding.

      6. Psychosocial concerns

        a. Possible malignancy

        b. Depression

          (1) Loss of a body part

          (2) Change in self-image

          (3) Possible negative reaction from spouse and family

          (4) Possible distancing of friends who "don't know what to say"

          (5) Life expectancy and ability to raise family

      7. Complications

        a. Detached or occluded drain

        b. Hematoma

        c. Hemorrhage or shock

        d. Wound infection

    C. Gallbladder surgery

      1. Laparoscopic cholecystectomy

        a. Assess dressings.

        b. Assess abdominal girth and firmness.

        c. Key educational components

          (1) Instruct patient and family about routine care following abdominal surgery.

            (a) Ambulate regularly.

            (b) Rest frequently.

            (c) Gradually increase activity as tolerated.

            (d) Keep incisions dry.

            (e) Report redness, increasing pain, or incision drainage.

            (f) Avoid heavy lifting as ordered.

            (g) Splint abdomen when coughing.

          (2) Stress importance of follow-up care with surgeon.

          (3) Instruct regarding pneumoperitoneum (retained CO_2 under diaphragm).

          (4) Stress adequate nutrition; low-to-moderate-fat diet.

        d. Provide written and verbal instructions; assess and ensure patient and family understanding.

        e. Psychosocial concerns

          (1) Fear of not being able to eat a normal diet without pain

          (2) Body image related to possible obesity

          (3) How soon will the patient be able to resume normal activity and work?

        f. Complications

          (1) Atelectasis and respiratory problems

          (2) Bladder distention

      (3) Hemorrhage or shock

      (4) Wound infection

      (5) Hiccups, especially in laparoscopic procedure

      (6) Pneumoperitoneum in laparoscopic procedure

      (7) Electrolyte and fluid imbalance

  2. Cholelithotripsy

    a. Assess for comfort.

      (1) Position for comfort.

      (2) Medicate for comfort.

    b. Key educational components

      (1) Instruct patient and family about routine care following abdominal procedure.

        (a) Ambulate regularly.

        (b) Rest frequently.

        (c) Gradually increase activity as tolerated.

        (d) Avoid heavy lifting as ordered.

        (e) Splint abdomen when coughing.

      (2) Stress importance of follow-up care with physician.

      (3) Take deoxycholic acid daily as ordered to dissolve stone fragments.

    c. Provide written and verbal instructions; assess and ensure patient and family understanding.

    d. Psychosocial concerns

      (1) All stones may not be eliminated or may recur.

      (2) Surgery may be necessary.

      (3) How soon will the patient be able to resume normal activity and work?

    e. Complications

      (1) Retained fragments

D. Spleen surgery: Laparoscopic splenectomy

  1. Usually stay for extended observation

  2. Key educational components

    a. Instruct patient and family about routine care following abdominal surgery.

      (1) Ambulate regularly.

      (2) Rest frequently.

      (3) Gradually increase activity as tolerated.

      (4) Keep incisions dry.

      (5) Report redness, increasing pain, or incision drainage.

      (6) Avoid heavy lifting as ordered.

      (7) Splint abdomen when coughing.

    b. Stress importance of follow-up care with surgeon.

    c. Stress adequate nutrition.

    d. Stress awareness of susceptibility to infection.

      (1) Prevention is best defense.

      (2) Need for medical care at earliest possible signs and symptoms of infection

    e. Follow-up as ordered

  3. Provide written and verbal instructions; assess and ensure patient and family understanding.

  4. Psychosocial concerns

    a. Susceptibility to infection

    b. Fear of germs, obsessive concern about cleanliness

    c. Social isolation and avoidance of social gatherings

    d. Concern about ability to return to normal activity

    e. Concern about ability to return to same line of work or need to change jobs

  5. Complications

    a. Atelectasis and respiratory problems

    b. Hemorrhage or shock

  c. Wound infection
  d. Generalized infection
  e. Inflammatory response
  f. Electrolyte and fluid imbalance
 E. Esophagus-stomach surgery
  1. Laparoscopic Nissen fundoplication
   a. Stay for extended observation
   b. Key educational components
    (1) Instruct patient and family about routine care following abdominal surgery.
     (a) Ambulate regularly.
     (b) Rest frequently.
     (c) Gradually increase activity as tolerated.
     (d) Keep incisions dry.
     (e) Report redness, increasing pain, or incision drainage.
     (f) Avoid heavy lifting as ordered.
    (2) Splint abdomen when coughing.
    (3) Instruct in indicators of reflux recurrence.
     (a) Dysphagia
     (b) Hematemesis
     (c) Increased pain
    (4) Instruct in occasional, temporary side effects.
     (a) Inability to vomit
     (b) Gas bloat
     (c) Early satiety
   c. Provide written and verbal instructions; assess and ensure patient and family understanding.
   d. Psychosocial concerns
    (1) Persistent GI disorders (bloating, nausea, diarrhea)
    (2) Recurrence of reflux
    (3) Inability to enjoy eating
    (4) Concern about ability to resume normal activity and work
   e. Complications
    (1) Pneumothorax
    (2) Perforation
    (3) Hemorrhage
    (4) Pneumonia
    (5) Dysphagia
    (6) Reflux, although less severe than preoperative
    (7) Gas bloat
    (8) Inability to vomit
    (9) Early satiety
    (10) Diarrhea
    (11) Nausea
  2. Open bariatric procedures
   a. Stay for extended observation
   b. Key educational components
    (1) Good nutrition to support wound healing
    (2) Pulmonary toilet for optimal respiratory function
    (3) Thrombosis prevention
     (a) Hydration
     (b) Activity
     (c) Positioning to avoid groin and popliteal pressure
    (4) Ambulation
    (5) Wound care and reportable symptoms
    (6) Maintenance of medication protocols for comorbid conditions
    (7) Expectations and rights regarding dignity and privacy

    c. Provide written and verbal instructions; assess and ensure patient and family understanding.

    d. Psychosocial concerns

        (1) Fear of being hungry

        (2) Fear of not being able to lose "enough" weight

        (3) Body image related to morbid obesity

        (4) Possible negative reaction from spouse, family, and friends over "new image"

        (5) Concern about ability to resume normal activity and work

    e. Complications

        (1) Pulmonary complications

        (2) Fluid and electrolyte imbalance

        (3) Nutritional deficiencies

        (4) Anemia

        (5) Wound infection

        (6) Failure of staple lines

        (7) Incisional hernia

        (8) Adhesions

        (9) Thromboembolism

F. Appendix surgery

  1. Stay for extended observation

  2. Key educational components

    a. Instruct patient and family about routine care following abdominal surgery.

        (1) Ambulate regularly.

        (2) Rest frequently.

        (3) Gradually increase activity as tolerated.

        (4) Wound care, dressing changes, bathing restrictions if appropriate

        (5) Report redness, increasing pain, or incision drainage.

        (6) Avoid heavy lifting as ordered.

        (7) Splint abdomen when coughing.

    b. Bowel management: if needed for constipation, laxatives or stool softeners may be used only as prescribed. Avoid enema unless or until approved by physician.

    c. Stress importance of follow-up care with surgeon.

  3. Provide written and verbal instructions; assess and ensure patient and family understanding.

  4. Psychosocial concerns

    a. Concern about how soon patient will be able to resume eating

    b. Concern about cosmetic appearance of scar (especially in young females)

    c. Concern about ability to resume normal activity and work

  5. Complications

    a. Wound infection

    b. Peritonitis

G. Intestine surgery

  1. Stay for extended observation

  2. Key educational components

    a. Instruct patient and family about routine care following abdominal surgery.

        (1) Ambulate regularly.

        (2) Rest frequently.

        (3) Gradually increase activity as tolerated.

        (4) Wound care, dressing changes, bathing restrictions if appropriate

        (5) Report redness, increasing pain, or incision drainage.

        (6) Avoid heavy lifting as ordered.

        (7) Splint abdomen when coughing.

b. Bowel management: if needed for constipation, laxatives or stool softeners may be used only as prescribed. Avoid enema unless or until approved by physician.

c. Stress importance of follow-up care with surgeon.

3. Provide written and verbal instructions; assess and ensure patient and family understanding.

4. Psychosocial concerns

a. Bowel movements

(1) Will it hurt?

(2) Possibility of constipation

b. Concern about eating normal diet

c. Concern about bloating or flatus

d. Concern about ability to resume normal activity and work

e. Concern about resuming sexual activity

5. Complications

a. Wound contamination

b. Peritonitis

H. Anorectal surgery

1. Assess dressings.

2. Key educational components

a. Pain control

(1) Analgesics

(2) Position for comfort.

(a) Side-lying

(b) Recumbent

b. Observe for adequate output.

c. Wound care

(1) Packing removal

(2) Sitz baths as ordered

(3) Perianal cleansing after each stool

(4) Dressing changes

d. Bowel management to avoid constipation

(1) Adequate hydration

(2) Exercise

(3) Fiber intake

(4) Stool softener

(5) Mild laxative if ordered

3. Provide written and verbal instructions; assess and ensure patient and family understanding.

4. Psychosocial concerns

a. Bowel movements

(1) Will it hurt?

(2) Not eating to postpone the first bowel movement

(3) Fecal incontinence

b. Concern about ability to resume normal activity and work

c. Concern about resuming sexual activity

5. Complications

a. Hemorrhage or shock

b. Urinary retention

c. Constipation

d. Diarrhea

e. External fistulas

f. Nonhealing wound

g. Fluid and electrolyte imbalance

I. Hernia surgery

1. Key educational components

a. Instruct patient and family about routine care following abdominal surgery.

       (1) Activity
         (a) Ambulate regularly.
         (b) Rest frequently.
         (c) Gradually increase activity as tolerated.
         (d) Avoid coughing, straining, stretching, heavy lifting until approved by physician.
         (e) Splint incision while coughing, sneezing.
         (f) Use proper body mechanics for moving and lifting.
         (g) Avoid sexual activity until approved by physician.
       (2) Wound care
         (a) Dressing changes
         (b) Binder or scrotal support
         (c) Ice to incision or scrotum if ordered
         (d) Bathing restrictions if appropriate
         (e) Signs of infection
           (i) Redness
           (ii) Fever
           (iii) Tenderness
           (iv) Incisional drainage
       (3) Pain control
       (4) Assess adequate intake and output.
       (5) Bowel management to avoid constipation
         (a) Hydration
         (b) Fiber
         (c) Exercise
         (d) Stool softener
         (e) Mild laxative if ordered
    b. Stress importance of follow-up care with surgeon.
  2. Provide written and verbal instructions; assess and ensure patient and family understanding.
  3. Psychosocial concerns
    a. Concern about resuming normal diet
    b. Concern about ability to urinate
    c. Concern about constipation and bowel movements
    d. Concern about ability to resume normal activity and work
    e. Concern about resuming sexual activity
  4. Complications
    a. Pneumoperitoneum in laparoscopic procedure
    b. Atelectasis and respiratory problems
    c. Bladder distention
    d. Paralytic ileus
    e. Hemorrhage or shock
    f. Wound infection
    g. Dehiscence or evisceration
    h. Electrolyte and fluid imbalance
    i. Pulmonary embolus
J. Thyroid
  1. Usually stay for extended observation
  2. Key educational components
    a. Instruct patient in signs and symptoms of
      (1) Hyperthyroidism
        (a) Nervousness, irritability, hyperactivity, emotional lability, decreased attention span
        (b) Weakness, easy fatigability, exercise intolerance
        (c) Heat intolerance
        (d) Weight change (loss or gain), increased appetite
        (e) Insomnia, interrupted sleep
        (f) Menstrual irregularities, decreased libido

            (g) Tremor, hyperkinesia, hyperreflexia

            (h) Exophthalmos, retracted eyelids, staring gaze

            (i) Hair loss

        (2) Hypothyroidism

            (a) Physical and mental sluggishness

            (b) Slow, clumsy movements

            (c) Dry, flaky skin, dry, brittle head and body hair, reduced nail and hair growth

            (d) Obesity

            (e) Cool skin and cold tolerance

            (f) Dyspnea

            (g) Fluid retention

            (h) Decreased appetite, constipation, weight gain

            (i) Muscle aching, stiffness

        (3) Hypocalcemia

            (a) Nervousness

            (b) Muscle cramps

            (c) Paresthesias

            (d) Tingling and numbness of feet

            (e) Positive Chvostek's sign: abnormal spasm of facial muscles when facial nerve is tapped

            (f) Carpopedal spasms

            (g) Laryngeal stridor

            (h) Convulsions

    b. Wound care

        (1) Report incisional pain.

        (2) Report redness, swelling, drainage, fever.

    c. Teach patient to support head and neck.

        (1) When turning or lifting head

        (2) When rising from a lying position

    d. Establish alternate means of communication (writing, sign language).

    e. Stress importance of follow-up care with physician.

3. Provide written and verbal instructions; assess and ensure patient and family understanding.

4. Psychosocial concerns

    a. Quality of voice

    b. Cosmetic appearance of surgical scar

    c. Concern about ability to resume normal activity and work

5. Complications

    a. Incisional bleeding

    b. Recurrent laryngeal nerve damage with resultant vocal cord impairment or paralysis

    c. Pneumothorax

    d. Tracheal compression from bleeding or edema

    e. Hypothyroidism

    f. Thyroid storm

        (1) Cause

            (a) Severe hyperthyroidism

            (b) Excessive stress

        (2) Symptoms

            (a) Hyperthermia

            (b) Tachycardia, especially atrial tachydysrhythmias

            (c) High-output heart failure

            (d) Agitation or delirium

            (e) Nausea, vomiting, or diarrhea contributing to fluid volume depletion

K. Parathyroid

    1. Usually stay for extended observation

2. Key educational components
   a. Instruct patient in signs and symptoms of hypocalcemia.
      (1) Nervousness
      (2) Muscle cramps
      (3) Paresthesias
      (4) Tingling and numbness of feet
      (5) Positive Chvostek's sign: abnormal spasm of facial muscles when facial nerve is tapped
      (6) Carpopedal spasms
      (7) Laryngeal stridor
      (8) Convulsions
   b. Wound care
      (1) Report incisional pain.
      (2) Report redness, swelling, drainage, fever.
   c. Activity
      (1) Importance of mobility, especially with irreversible skeletal impairment
   d. Nutrition
      (1) Monitor weight.
      (2) Take dietary supplements containing calcium.
      (3) Take calcium replacement medication.
3. Provide written and verbal instructions; assess and ensure patient and family understanding.
4. Psychosocial concerns
   a. Cosmetic appearance of surgical scar
   b. Concern about ability to resume normal activity and work
5. Complications
   a. Incisional bleeding
   b. Tracheal compression from bleeding or edema
   c. Tetany
   d. Hyperparathyroid crisis
      (1) Polyuria, polydipsia, kidney stones
      (2) Abdominal pain, constipation, nausea, anorexia
      (3) Joint or back pain
      (4) Muscle weakness and atrophy
      (5) Depression, paranoia, mood swings

L. Nodes
   1. Assess emotional feelings.
   2. Key educational components
      a. Depends on extent of the procedure and diagnosis
      b. Provide information on wound care.
      c. Provide information on range-of-motion exercises as directed by the physician.
      d. Provide information about resources and support systems as appropriate.
      e. Stress importance of follow-up with physician.
   3. Provide written and verbal instructions; assess and ensure patient and family understanding.
   4. Psychosocial concerns
      a. Possible malignancy
      b. Depression
         (1) Change in self-image
         (2) Possible negative reaction from spouse and family
         (3) Possible distancing of friends who "don't know what to say"
         (4) Life expectancy and ability to raise family
      c. Concern about ability to resume normal activity and work
   5. Complications
      a. Hematoma
      b. Wound infection

M. Skin
  1. Assess dressings.
    a. Note location and amount of drainage.
    b. Note hematoma formation.
  2. Assess circulation and sensation.
    a. Impaired circulation
    b. Sensation deficit
  3. Assess comfort level.
    a. Note location of discomfort and position for comfort.
    b. Administer prescribed medications and evaluate relief.
  4. Key educational components
    a. Depends of extent of the procedure and diagnosis
    b. Wound care
      (1) Dressings
      (2) Signs and symptoms of infection
    c. Impaired circulation or sensation
    d. Medications
      (1) Analgesics
      (2) Antibiotics
    e. Activity limitations or restrictions
  5. Provide written and verbal instructions; assess and ensure patient and family understanding.
  6. Psychosocial concerns
    a. Cosmetic appearance of surgical site and possible skin graft
    b. Possible malignancy
    c. Depression
      (1) Change in self-image
      (2) Possible negative reaction from spouse and family
      (3) Possible distancing of friends who "don't know what to say"
      (4) Life expectancy and ability to raise family
    d. Concern about ability to resume normal activity and work
  7. Complications
    a. Hematoma
    b. Wound infection

MINIMALLY INVASIVE SURGERY CONSIDERATIONS

Virtually any area of the body can be examined and treated via endoscopic procedures. General information about minimally invasive surgery follows.

  I. General information
    A. Definitions
      1. Endoscopy: visual examination of interior of a body cavity, hollow organ, or structure with an endoscope
      2. Endoscope: instrument designed for examination with an optical system in a tubular structure; named for anatomic area it is designed to visualize
      3. Minimally invasive surgery: a variety of surgical modalities, including endoscopy, video technology, and energies, or a combination of these technologies, used during least disruptive surgical interventions
    B. Types of endoscopic procedures
      1. Through natural orifice (e.g., mouth, anus, cervix, urethra)
      2. Through small skin incision and/or trocar puncture (e.g., through a joint space or the abdominal wall)
    C. Advantages of minimally invasive surgery
      1. Shorter postoperative stay
      2. Decreased postoperative pain
      3. Small incisions enable faster healing.
      4. Decreased infection rate

       5. Shorter rehabilitation time

       6. Quicker return to activities of daily living

    D. Disadvantages of minimally invasive surgery

       1. May take longer than open procedures

       2. Longer procedures mean longer exposure to anesthesia.

       3. May be more expensive than open procedures

II. Technology

    A. Endoscopes

       1. Rigid scope

          a. Hollow tube that permits viewing in a forward direction only

       2. Flexible scope

          a. Hollow tube that contours the lensed tip into and around anatomic curvatures to permit visualization of all surfaces of the wall of a hollow structure

    B. Laparoscopy equipment: See Figure 43-9.

       1. Veress needle or other pneumoperitoneal needle

          a. Used to penetrate abdomen

          b. Has outer sharp tip to penetrate abdomen and inner blunt tip to protect underlying tissue

       2. Carbon dioxide insufflator

          a. Machine that delivers metered flow of CO_2 into peritoneal cavity through disposable tubing connected to needle

          b. Creates a pneumoperitoneum before laparoscope inserted through abdominal wall

          c. Pneumoperitoneum expands abdomen and allows for visualization of organs and structures within peritoneal cavity

       3. Trocar and cannula

          a. Sharp inner obturator penetrates abdomen.

          b. Or cannula inserted via open laparoscopy technique

          c. Trocar has valve to maintain pneumoperitoneum.

       4. Laparoscope

          a. Consists of lenses and channels for fiber optics and viewing

          b. Available in various angles for viewing straight ahead or around intraabdominal tissue

          c. Position maintained by assistant or scope holder

       5. Light source

          a. Provides illumination through fiber optic cables to laparoscope

       6. Camera and video

          a. Permit real-time video imaging

          b. Videocassette recorder can document procedure.

       7. Instruments

          a. Disposable or reusable

          b. Classification

             (1) Grasping

             (2) Retracting

             (3) Cutting

          c. Insulated for use with electrocautery devices

          d. Nonreflective for use with lasers

       8. Devices being developed for laparoscopy visualization without risk of pneumoperitoneum

          a. Slings, wires, T-shaped, L-shaped, or fan-shaped devices

          b. Require additional puncture sites for retractors

          c. Enable use of ordinary surgical instruments

       9. Staples and clips

          a. Used to

             (1) Ligate vessels

             (2) Close abdominal structures with lumens

             (3) Approximate tissue

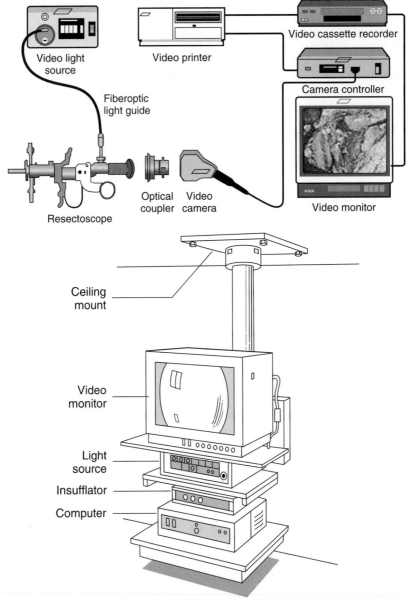

FIGURE 43-9 ■ Endoscopic machinery. Two examples of video system setups. (From Phillips NF: *Berry & Kohn's operating room technique,* ed 10. St Louis: Mosby, 2004.)

      b. Forms of clips
         (1) Occlusive
         (2) Tacking
      c. Staples pushed into tissue and closed
      d. Advantages
         (1) Save time
         (2) Less difficult than laparoscopic knot tying
 10. Association of periOperative Registered Nurses (AORN) resources
      a. Teaching videos for endoscopic surgery
         (1) Equipment
         (2) Handling, cleaning, care of equipment

      b. Published information: Recommended Practices for Endoscopic Minimally Invasive Surgery

        (1) Practices that reduce risk of injuries and complications

        (2) Endoscopic instruments and equipment performance and safety criteria

C. Electrosurgical unit (ESU) commonly called Bovie

   1. Adapted for use in laparoscopic procedures

   2. Modes

      a. Monopolar

        (1) Grounding pad placement

          (a) On same side or close to surgical site

          (b) Over muscle mass

          (c) Avoid

            (i) Bony prominences

            (ii) Metal implant areas

            (iii) Hairy areas

            (iv) Pooled prep solution areas

      b. Bipolar

   3. Action

      a. Coagulate

      b. Cut

   4. Risk of leakage current

D. Plane expander

   1. Balloon device inserted between tissue layers

   2. Expanded with saline to separate and bluntly open preperitoneal plane of dissection

   3. Balloon then deflated and withdrawn as space then insufflated

E. Laser

   1. Acronym for light amplification by stimulated emission of radiation

   2. Laser-tissue interaction

      a. Reflection

      b. Scattering

      c. Transmission

      d. Absorption

   3. Laser action

      a. Cuts

      b. Vaporizes

      c. Coagulates

   4. Types

      a. Argon laser: Used on cutaneous lesions, in GI procedures, ophthalmology, otolaryngology, gynecology, urology, neurosurgery, dermatology

      b. Carbon dioxide (CO_2) laser: Used primarily in otolaryngology, gynecology, plastic surgery, dermatology, neurosurgery, orthopedic, cardiovascular, general surgery

      c. Excimer laser: Used in ophthalmology, peripheral and coronary angioplasty, orthopedics, neurosurgery

      d. Diode laser: Used in ophthalmology, pain management

      e. Free electron laser: Used to fragment calculi, precisely cut tissue

      f. Holmium:YAG laser: Used in orthopedics

      g. Krypton laser: Used in ophthalmology

      h. Neodymium:YAG (Nd:YAG) laser: Used in rhinolaryngology, urology, gynecology, neurosurgery, orthopedics, ophthalmology, thoracic surgery, general surgery

      i. Potassium triphosphate (KTP) laser: Used in all surgical specialties for good cutting properties

      j. Ruby laser: Used to eradicate port wine stain lesions and tattoos.

      k. Tunable dye laser: Used for photodynamic therapy

    5. Laser safety
        a. Regulatory controls of Health and Human Services (DHHS)
            (1) National Center for Devices and Radiological Health (NCDRH) is the regulatory section of the Food and Drug Administration (FDA) in the Department.
            (2) American National Standards Institute (ANSI) provides for
                (a) Laser safety officer
                (b) Education of users
                (c) Protective measures
                (d) Management of accidents
            (3) Occupational Safety and Health Administration (OSHA)
            (4) State and local agencies
            (5) Facility policy and procedures include but not limited to
                (a) Credentialing and clinical practice privileges of medical staff
                (b) Initial and ongoing educational laser use and safety programs for perioperative personnel
                (c) Continuous quality improvement
                (d) Documentation
        b. Protective measures
            (1) Eye safety measures
                (a) Protective eyewear of appropriate optical density for anyone entering area
                (b) Protection (eyewear or moist gauze pads) for patient's eyes
            (2) Environmental controls
                (a) Mark laser-use area with laser safety symbol.
                (b) Limit traffic.
                (c) Cover glass windows.
                (d) Leave laser key with authorized personnel, not with laser.
            (3) Fire safety
                (a) Sources of ignition
                    (i) Surgical drapes
                    (ii) Anesthesia tubing
                    (iii) Surgical sponges
                (b) Contributors to flammability
                    (i) Oxygen
                    (ii) Anesthetic gases
                    (iii) Vapors from alcohol-based preparation solutions
                (c) Safety measures
                    (i) Use special drapes and endotracheal tubes.
                    (ii) Keep sponges wet.
                    (iii) Keep oxygen concentrations low.
                    (iv) Prevent preparation solutions from pooling.
                    (v) Locate laser foot pedal for safe activation by surgeon.
                    (vi) Laser plume
                        [a] Smoke produced by laser may contain particles of tissue, toxins, steam.
                      [b] Smoke evacuators remove smoke and particles.
                      [c] High-filtration masks filter plume not captured by evacuator.
    6. Advantages of laser surgery
        a. Precise control for accurate incision, excision, ablation of tissue
        b. Access to areas inaccessible to other surgical instruments through minimally invasive techniques
        c. Unobstructed view of surgical site
        d. Minimal handling of and trauma to tissues
        e. Dry, bloodless surgical field
        f. Minimal thermal effect on surrounding tissue

g. Reduced risk of contamination or infection
h. Prompt healing with minimal postoperative edema, sloughing of tissue, pain, scarring
i. Reduced operating time
7. Disadvantages of laser surgery
a. High program start-up expenses
b. Decide on disposable versus reusable supplies and impact on patient care.
c. Increased medical liability; need for credentialing medical practitioners, and need for continuing education to maintain staff competence
F. Ultrasound
1. Sound waves are mechanical energy.
2. Used to remove or reduce tumors in highly vascular, delicate tissue
a. Ultrasonic aspirator fragments, irrigates, and aspirates tissue.
b. Harmonic scalpel cuts and coagulates.
3. Used in open or laparoscopic procedures
G. Robotics and telemedicine
1. Combination of mechanical manipulators and a computer
a. Computer controls complex movements of joints and arms of manipulators
b. Surgeon verbally controls other computer-generated information during surgical procedure.
(1) Can see diagnostic reports
(2) Operative report generated by electronic media
c. Surgeon sits at console to command verbally multiple robotic arms while many miles away.
2. Virtual reality training for surgeons
a. Surgeon practices procedure without touching real patient.
b. Allows for evaluation of surgeon's skill and dexterity
III. Perioperative and perianesthesia issues
A. Preoperative considerations
1. Patient selection
a. Not all patients appropriate candidates for laparoscopic procedures
b. Relative contraindications
(1) Prior abdominal or pelvic surgery
(2) Previous peritonitis or pelvic fibrosis
(3) Obesity
(4) Umbilical abnormality
(5) Abdominal or iliac artery aneurysm
(6) Severe pulmonary disease
(7) Acute and chronic inflammation
(8) Uncontrolled coagulopathy
(9) Pregnancy
c. Absolute contraindications
(1) Hypovolemic shock
(2) Large pelvic or abdominal mass
(3) Severe cardiac decompensation
(4) Congestive heart failure
(5) Increased intracranial pressure
(6) Ventricular or peritoneal shunts
2. Patient education
a. Usual preparatory activities
b. Method depends on patient's ability and readiness to learn.
c. Patients and families tend to trivialize minimally invasive and ambulatory procedures.
d. Prepare patients and families for
(1) Nature of procedure
(2) Potential complications
(3) Aftercare required

    B. Intraoperative considerations

       1. Efficient and accessible room layout

       2. Video monitors on either side of patient or at foot of operating room table

       3. Insufflation equipment and ESU or laser easily accessible and observable by surgical team

    C. Anesthesia considerations

       1. Types of anesthesia

         a. Local

           (1) For brief, simple procedures

           (2) Injection of local anesthetic with epinephrine at each trocar site

         b. Monitored anesthesia care (MAC)

           (1) In conjunction with local anesthetic

           (2) Advantages

              (a) Avoids general anesthesia risks

              (b) Less postoperative nausea and vomiting

              (c) Rapid postoperative recovery

           (3) Disadvantages

              (a) Intraoperative anxiety

              (b) Respiratory compromise and shoulder and abdominal pain from insufflation

         c. Epidural

           (1) Rarely used in abdominal procedures

              (a) Viable alternative in selected cases to avoid risks of general anesthesia

           (2) Appropriate for procedures on extremities

         d. General anesthesia

           (1) Most common technique

           (2) Endotracheal intubation

              (a) Decreases risk of regurgitation and aspiration

              (b) Allows control of ventilation to compensate for compromised intraoperative pulmonary status

           (3) Gastric considerations

              (a) NPO status confirmed

              (b) Administration of metoclopramide or an H_2 blocker preoperatively

              (c) Placement of NG tube to decrease risk of injury to stomach

           (4) Placement of catheter (unless patient has voided preoperatively) to reduce risk of injury to bladder

           (5) Goals

              (a) Maintain end-tidal CO_2 <40 mm Hg

              (b) Maintain oxygen saturation at least 93%

       2. Physiologic effects of pneumoperitoneum

         a. Increased pressure in abdominal cavity

           (1) Causes circulatory impairment by decreasing venous return

           (2) Decreases central venous pressure, which is managed with fluids

           (3) Can lead to acute pulmonary edema in patients with cardiac compromise

         b. CO_2 is absorbed from abdomen into circulation.

           (1) Leads to hypercarbia and dysrhythmias

           (2) Tidal volume must be increased to compensate.

         c. Increased tidal volume

           (1) Results in increased wedge pressures

           (2) Decreased stroke volume

           (3) Decreased cardiac output

         d. Cardiovascular collapse can occur from

           (1) CO_2 embolus

           (2) Vagal effects of manipulation of abdominal organs

     e. Pulmonary effects include
       (1) Atelectasis
       (2) Decreased functional residual capacity
       (3) High peak airway pressures
     f. Kidneys effects include
       (1) Renal cortical perfusion diminished with pressure of 15 mm Hg, resulting in oliguria
       (2) Perfusion rapidly restored when pressure released
       (3) Urinary output may not promptly return because of abdominal compartment syndrome.

D. Complications of endoscopy
  1. Perforation of major organ
     a. Cause
       (1) Sharp trocars and rigid scopes
       (2) Trendelenburg position shifts intraabdominal anatomy, causing elevation of major organs of lower abdomen.
     b. Signs and symptoms
       (1) Usually seen at time of occurrence
     c. Treatment
       (1) Minor injury controlled with suturing or staples
       (2) Major injury requires suturing, clips, or open repair.
       (3) Thorough irrigation
       (4) Postoperative antibiotics
  2. Bleeding
     a. Cause
       (1) Perforation of vessel by sharp object
       (2) From biopsy site, pedicle of polyp, or other area where tissue cut
       (3) From dislodged endoscopic sutures or clips
     b. Signs and symptoms
       (1) Blood apparent at site
       (2) Decrease in BP
     c. Treatment
       (1) Minor vascular injury controlled with pressure
       (2) Major vascular injury requires clips, suturing, or open vascular repair.
  3. Thermal injury
     a. Cause
       (1) ESU burns
       (2) Laser injury
     b. Signs and symptoms
       (1) Not always readily apparent until 2-3 days postoperatively
         (a) Abdominal pain
         (b) Nausea
         (c) Fever
       (2) Slowed healing process
     c. Treatment
       (1) Antiemetics
       (2) Antibiotics
  4. Hypothermia
     a. Cause
       (1) CO_2 gas colder than body temperature
       (2) Exposed skin
       (3) Cold infusion fluids
     b. Signs and symptoms
       (1) Decreased temperature
       (2) Altered effects of drugs
       (3) Increased incidence of hypothermic coagulopathy

    c. Treatment
       (1) Forced air warming blankets
       (2) Warmed IV fluids
5. Electrical
    a. Cause
       (1) Improperly grounded electrical equipment
       (2) Unsuspected current leaks
          (a) Insulation failure
          (b) Direct coupling
          (c) Capacitive coupling
    b. Signs and symptoms
       (1) Not always readily apparent until 2-3 days postoperatively
          (a) Abdominal pain
          (b) Nausea
          (c) Fever
       (2) Slowed healing process
    c. Treatment
       (1) Antiemetics
       (2) Antibiotics
6. Complications related to pneumoperitoneum
    a. Pneumothorax and pneumomediastinum
       (1) Cause
          (a) Air accumulates in pleural space.
       (2) Signs and symptoms
          (a) Unilateral breath sounds
          (b) Confirmed by chest x-ray
       (3) Treatment
          (a) Decompress pneumoperitoneum.
          (b) Terminate procedure.
          (c) Reverse muscle relaxants.
          (d) Ventilate with oxygen.
    b. Subcutaneous emphysema
       (1) Cause
          (a) Improper positioning of Veress needle
          (b) In conjunction with pneumothorax, pneumomediastinum, or both
          (c) Weak areas in diaphragm allow CO_2 to leak through and enter mediastinum
       (2) Signs and symptoms
          (a) Increase in end-tidal CO_2
          (b) Cannot be lowered by
             (i) Increasing tidal volume
             (ii) Increasing rate of ventilation
          (c) Crepitus upon palpation of head and neck
          (d) Facial and conjunctival subcutaneous emphysema
       (3) Treatment
          (a) Observe for compromised airway.
    c. Gastric reflux
       (1) Cause
          (a) Increased risk with history of
             (i) Obesity
             (ii) Hiatal hernia
             (iii) Gastric outlet obstruction
          (b) Increased abdominal pressure associated with pneumoperitoneum
       (2) Signs and symptoms
          (a) Reflex esophagitis
          (b) Heartburn
          (c) Belching

(d) Regurgitation

(e) Vomiting

(f) Retrosternal or substernal chest pain

(g) Hiccups

(h) Mild or occult bleeding and mild anemia

(i) Dysphagia

(j) Pneumonitis caused by aspiration

(3) Treatment

(a) Nasogastric or orogastric tube insertion

(b) Stomach decompression

(i) Decreases risk of visceral puncture

(ii) Improves visualization

(iii) Decreases risk of aspiration

(iv) Decreases risk of postoperative nausea and vomiting

(c) Pharmacological interventions

(i) Metoclopramide, 10 mg IV, preoperatively to promote gastric emptying

(ii) Metoclopramide, 10 mg IV, at end of procedure to decrease potential for nausea and vomiting

d. CO_2 embolus

(1) Cause

(a) Large amount CO_2 enters central venous circulation through opening in venous channels.

(2) Signs and symptoms

(a) Sudden decrease in BP

(b) Cardiac dysrhythmias

(c) Heart murmur

(d) Cyanosis

(e) Pulmonary edema

(f) Increase in end-tidal CO_2

(3) Treatment

(a) Deflate peritoneum immediately.

(b) Place patient in left lateral decubitus position.

(c) Position head below level of right atrium.

(d) Establish IV access to central circulation to aspirate gas from heart.

e. Abdominal wall hematoma

(1) Cause

(a) Injury

(2) Signs and symptoms

(a) Depends on size

(b) Pressure on adjacent organs or vessels

(3) Treatment

(a) Evacuation

f. Cardiovascular collapse

(1) Possible causes include

(a) Hemorrhage

(b) Pulmonary embolus

(c) Myocardial infarction

E. Postoperative considerations

1. Immediate postoperative assessment: See Chapter 35.

2. Postoperative care associated with surgical specialties

3. Postoperative complications

a. Observe for any signs and symptoms as noted previously.

b. Notify anesthesiologist and surgeon.

c. Treat accordingly.

4. Patient and family teaching

a. Regarding signs and symptoms of potential complications

b. Specific to procedure

5. Minimally invasive surgery affects length of stay.
   a. Some are ambulatory patients.
   b. Some are fast-track patients.
   c. Some become phase III short-stay patients.

BIBLIOGRAPHY

1. Association of periOperative Registered Nurses: Standards, recommended practices and guidelines. Denver: Association of periOperative Registered Nurses, 2002.
2. Baker CL Jr, Jones GL: Current concepts: Arthroscopy of the elbow. *Am J Sports Med* 27:251-264, 1999.
3. Ball KA: Surgical modalities. In Meeker MH, Rothrock JC, editors: *Alexander's care of the patient in surgery*, ed 11. St Louis: Mosby, 1999, pp 49-63.
4. Baravarian B: Soft-tissue disorders of the ankle: A comprehensive approach. *Clin Podiatr Med Surg* 19:271-283, 2002.
5. Beaulac BN: Gastrointestinal disorders: Disorders of the mouth and esophagus. In Swearingen PL, Ross DG, editors: *Manual of medical-surgical nursing care: Nursing interventions and collaborative management*, ed 4. St Louis: Mosby, 1999, pp 405-409.
6. Beaulac BN: Gastrointestinal disorders: Obstructive processes. In Swearingen PL, Ross DG, editors: *Manual of medical-surgical nursing care: Nursing interventions and collaborative management*, ed 4. St Louis: Mosby, 1999, pp 420-424.
7. Beaulac BN: Gastrointestinal disorders: Peritonitis. In Swearingen PL, Ross DG, editors: *Manual of medical-surgical nursing care: Nursing interventions and collaborative management*, ed 4. St Louis: Mosby, 1999, pp 424-428.
8. Beaulac BN: Gastrointestinal disorders: Appendicitis. In Swearingen PL, Ross DG, editors: *Manual of medical-surgical nursing care: Nursing interventions and collaborative management*, ed 4. St Louis: Mosby, 1999, pp 428-432.
9. Burns AH: Thyroid and parathyroid surgery. In Meeker MH, Rothrock JC, editors: *Alexander's care of the patient in surgery*, ed 11. St Louis: Mosby, 1999, pp 600-615.
10. Carlson MA, Frantzides CT: Complications and results of primary minimally invasive antireflux procedures: A review of 10,735 reported cases. *J Am Coll Surg* 193:428-439, 2001.
11. Castell DO, Brunton SA, Earnest DL, et al: GERD: Management algorithms for the primary care physician and specialist. *Pract Gastroenterol* 22:18-46, 1998.
12. Earnhart SW: What's the best mix of procedures for ASC? *OR Manager* 18:26-27, 2002.
13. Fischer CP, Castaneda A, Moore F: Laparoscopic appendectomy: Indications and controversies. *Semin Laparosc Surg* 9:32-39, 2002.
14. Fleisher LA, Yee K, Lillemoe KD, et al: Is outpatient laparoscopic cholecystectomy safe and cost-effective? A model to study transition of care. *Anesthesiology* 90:1746-1755, 1999.
15. Fortunato NH: General surgery. In Berry EC, Kohn ML, editors: *Operating room technique*, ed 9. St Louis: Mosby, 2000, pp 313-345, pp 629-651.
16. Fuchs KH: Minimally invasive surgery. *Endoscopy* 34:154-159, 2002.
17. Gervasio BA: The endocrine surgical patient. In Litwack K, editor: *Core curriculum for perianesthesia nursing practice*, ed 4. Philadelphia: WB Saunders, 1999, pp 569-594.
18. Gordon SA, Ardila SC: Robotic doctors: Virtual laparoscopic surgery. *Surg Serv Manage* 7:18-21:2001.
19. Gregory Dawes BS: Otorhinolaryngology and head and neck surgery. In Burden N, DeFazio Quinn DM, O'Brien D, et al, editors: *Ambulatory surgical nursing*, ed 2. Philadelphia: WB Saunders, 2000, p 710.
20. Jones SB, Jones DB: Surgical aspects and future developments of laparoscopy. *Anesthesiol Clin North America* 19:107-124, 2001.
21. Joshi GP: Complications of laparoscopy. *Anesthesiol Clin North America* 19:89-105, 2001.
22. Keen JH: Gastrointestinal disorders: Disorders of the mouth and esophagus. In Swearingen PL, Ross DG, editors: *Manual of medical-surgical nursing care: Nursing interventions and collaborative management*, ed 4. St Louis: Mosby, 1999, pp 405-409.
23. Keen JH: Gastrointestinal disorders: Malabsorption/maldigestion. In Swearingen PL, Ross DG, editors: *Manual of medical-surgical nursing care: Nursing interventions and collaborative management*, ed 4. St Louis: Mosby, 1999, pp 415-420.
24. Keen JH: Hepatic and biliary disorders: Cholelithiasis and cholecystitis. In Swearingen PL, Ross DG, editors: *Manual of medical-surgical nursing care: Nursing interventions and collaborative management*, ed 4. St Louis: Mosby, 1999, pp 494-499.
25. Khaitan L, Holzman MD: Laparoscopic advances in general surgery. *J Am Med Assoc* 287:1502-1505, 2002.
26. Lo V, Newman B: Exemplar: Patient education and the prevention of incisional hernia. *Contemp Nurse* 11:50-54, 2001.
27. Ludwig-Beymer P, Huether SE, Zekauskus SB: Alterations of hormonal regulation. In

Huether SE, McCance KL, editors: *Understanding pathophysiology.* St Louis: Mosby, 1996, pp 480-483.

28. Mansen TJ, McCance KL: Alterations of hematologic function. In Huether SE, McCance KL, editors: *Understanding pathophysiology.* St Louis: Mosby, 1996, pp 549-553.

29. Nedeff DD, Back BR Jr: Arthroscopic anterior cruciate ligament reconstruction using patellar tendon autografts. *Orthopedics* 25:343-359, 2002.

30. O'Brien D: The gastrointestinal surgical patient. In Litwack K, editor: *Core curriculum for perianesthesia nursing practice,* ed 4. Philadelphia: WB Saunders, 1999, pp 467-485.

31. Pavlak L: General surgery. In Burden N, DeFazio Quinn DM, O'Brien D, et al, editors: *Ambulatory surgical nursing,* ed 2. Philadelphia: WB Saunders, 2000, pp 741-748.

32. Petty LR: Gastrointestinal surgery. In Meeker MH, Rothrock JC, editors: *Alexander's care of the patient in surgery,* ed 11. St Louis: Mosby, 1999, pp 335-370.

33. Petty LR: Surgery of the liver, biliary tract, pancreas, and spleen. In Meeker MH, Rothrock JC, editors: *Alexander's care of the patient in surgery,* ed 11. St Louis: Mosby, 1999, pp 382-416.

34. Roth RA: Breast surgery. In Meeker MH, Rothrock JC, editors: *Alexander's care of the patient in surgery,* ed 11. St Louis: Mosby, pp 617-621, 625-632.

35. Smith DA: Repair of hernias. In Meeker MH, Rothrock JC, editors: *Alexander's care of the patient in surgery,* ed 11. St Louis: Mosby, 1999, pp 424-438.

36. Smith I: Anesthesia for laparoscopy with emphasis on outpatient laparoscopy. *Anesthesiol Clin North America* 19:21-41, 2001.

37. Williams GM Jr, Kelly M: Management of rotator cuff and impingement injuries in the athlete. *J Athl Train* 35:300-315, 2000.

44 Renal/Genitourinary Surgery

GRATIA M. NAGLE

OBJECTIVES

At the conclusion of this chapter the reader will be able to:

1. Identify the structure and function of the genitourinary system.
2. Understand the pathophysiologic implications of each urologic disorder reviewed.
3. Discuss indications for common urologic surgical procedures.
4. Synthesize principles of physical assessment with the principles of the nursing process.
5. Identify the specific postanesthesia care unit (PACU) considerations in patient care after each urologic procedure discussed in the chapter.
6. Incorporate biologic, psychologic, social, and cultural assessment of the patient.

The genitourinary system includes two adrenal glands, two kidneys, two ureters, one urinary bladder, a single urethra, and the genital organs (Figure 44-1). The most important structure, the nephron, lies within the kidney (Figure 44-2). The nephron is responsible for removing wastes from the blood and regulating fluid and electrolyte content, thereby contributing to urine formation and homeostasis (Figure 44-3).

The entire system and its related anatomy are capable of succumbing to a host of disorders. It is essential to possess adequate knowledge of how these units function in interrelationships under normal circumstances. This chapter addresses many of the genitourinary disorders commonly encountered in the PACU. The treatment of acute renal failure is beyond the scope of this chapter's objectives. The reader is urged to consult the Bibliography for more information.

ANATOMY AND PHYSIOLOGY OF THE GENITOURINARY SYSTEM

I. Adrenal gland(s)
   A. Cap each kidney superiorly
      1. Right is triangular, between liver and vena cava.
      2. Left is rounded and crescent shaped, close to aorta, and partially covered by pancreas.
   B. Composed of cortex and medulla
   C. Secretions influenced by pituitary gland
      1. Cortex secretes steroids, hormones.
      2. Medulla secretes adrenaline and noradrenaline (epinephrine and norepinephrine).
   D. Arterial blood supply
      1. Inferior phrenic artery
      2. Renal (and suprarenal) artery
      3. Aorta
   E. Venous blood supply
      1. Right has short vein that empties into inferior vena cava.
      2. Left terminates in left renal vein.

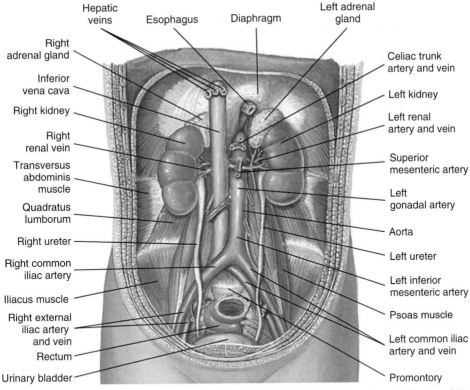

FIGURE 44-1 ■ Location of urinary system organs. (From Rothrock JC: *Alexander's care of the patient in surgery,* 12th ed. St Louis: Mosby, 2003, p 520.)

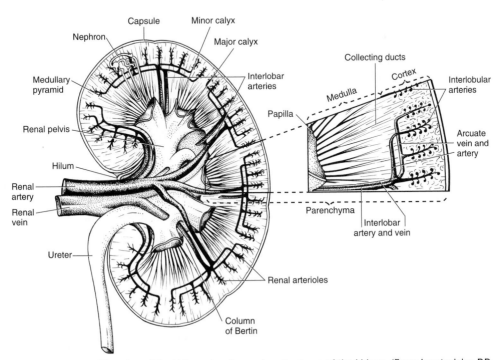

FIGURE 44-2 ■ Bisection of the kidney showing major structures of the kidney. (From Ignatavicius DD, Workman ML, editors: *Medical-surgical nursing: Critical thinking for collaborative care*, ed 4. Philadelphia: WB Saunders, 2002, p 1590.)

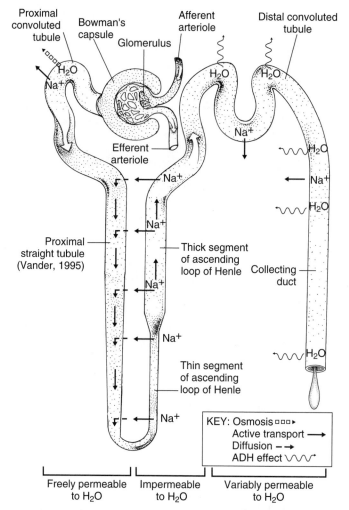

FIGURE 44-3 ■ Sodium and water reabsorption by the tubules of a cortical nephron. (From Ignatavicius DD, Workman ML, editors: *Medical-surgical nursing: Critical thinking for collaborative care*, ed 4. Philadelphia: WB Saunders, 2002, p 1594.)

   F. Lymphatics
      1. Accompany suprarenal vein
      2. Drain into lumbar lymph nodes
   G. Adrenal disease often directly affects renal function (refer to pathophysiology section of this chapter).
      1. Alport's syndrome
      2. Cushing's disease
      3. Pheochromocytoma
      4. Adenoma
      5. Carcinoma
II. Kidney
   A. Comprises hilum; parenchyma containing medulla, cortex, calices, and nephrons; and renal pelvis
      1. Hilum
         a. Concave, on medial aspect of kidney
         b. Pelvis, artery, vein, nerves, and lymphatics enter and exit parenchyma.

2. Parenchyma is functional tissue of kidney.
    a. Medulla
        (1) Five to eighteen cone-shaped pyramids that drain into 4-13 minor calices
        (2) Base of pyramids face hilum of kidney, and apices face renal pelvis.
    b. Cortex
        (1) Extends inward between two pyramids
        (2) Forms renal columns that contain nephrons
    c. Calices
        (1) Minor calices drain into two or three major calices.
        (2) Major calices join in center of medulla, forming and opening directly into renal pelvis.
    d. Nephron(s)
        (1) Approximately 1 million tiny nephrons comprise functional unit of kidney.
        (2) Each is composed of secretory or excretory tubules lined with thin epithelial cells.
            (a) Secretory tubule within renal cortex consists of renal corpuscle (Bowman's capsule and glomerulus) and secretory portion of renal tubule.
            (b) Excretory tubule within medulla is collecting tubule continuous with ascending limb of proximal convoluted tubule.
            (c) Excretory tubule empties into minor calyx.
        (3) Contains the glomerulus, Bowman's capsule, proximal tubule, loop of Henle, distal tubule, and collecting ducts
    e. Renal pelvis
        (1) May be intrarenal and extrarenal
        (2) Cone-shaped structure extending from center of medulla, exiting through the hilum, and curving downward to form the ureters
        (3) Left lies at level of first or second lumbar vertebra.
        (4) Right is lower than left because of the presence of the liver.
3. Glomerulus
    a. Segment of proximal nephron enclosed in Bowman's capsule
    b. Tuft of capillaries is site of blood filtration for selective secretion or reabsorption.
    c. Blood enters via afferent arterioles and exits via efferent arterioles.
4. Bowman's capsule (glomerular capsule)
    a. Membrane surrounding glomerulus
    b. Tubular system of nephron begins here.
5. Renal corpuscle
    a. Vascular glomerulus projects into Bowman's capsule.
        (1) Selectively permeable membrane
        (2) Permeable to water and solutes (crystalloids)
        (3) Impermeable to large molecules and plasma proteins
    b. Continuous with epithelium of proximal convoluted tubule
6. Secretory renal tubule
    a. Proximal convoluted tubule, extension of Bowman's capsule where 65% of glomerular filtrate is reabsorbed
    b. Loop of Henle
        (1) Ascending limb, impermeable to water, actively reabsorbs electrolytes (especially chloride, sodium, potassium) and generates medullary hypertonicity by forming hypotonic tubular fluid
        (2) Reabsorbs 25% of glomerular filtrate
        (3) Descending limb permeable to water and salts, diffuses NaCl from ascending limb across interstitial space
        (4) NaCl recycles through Loop of Henle multiple times.
        (5) Essential for water conservation with dehydration and hemorrhage

7. Distal convoluted tubule
   a. Tiny collecting ducts form larger duct that empties into renal pelvis.
   b. In the presence of ADH (anti-diuretic hormone), water is reabsorbed.
   c. Urine flows from renal pelvis to ureters to bladder.
B. Retroperitoneal location
   1. Parallel to vertebrae and psoas muscle
   2. Covered with a thin fibrous capsule (Gerota's fascia or fascia renalis) and perirenal fat
      a. Length: 12-14 cm
      b. Width: 5-7 cm
      c. Thickness: 3 cm
      d. Weight: 150 g
C. One kidney can provide adequate renal function.
D. Autonomic innervation with intraperitoneal organs accounts for gastrointestinal symptoms that accompany genitourinary disease, including nausea, vomiting, and pain.
E. Arterial blood supply
   1. End arteries (absence of collateral connections)
   2. Renal artery
      a. Arises from abdominal aorta and enters hilum between pelvis and renal vein
      b. Receives 25% of cardiac output
      c. Divides into anterior and posterior branches
      d. Anterior supplies upper and lower poles and anterior surface.
      e. Posterior supplies posterior surface.
      f. Divides again into interlobar arteries to glomeruli
F. Venous blood supply
   1. Renal veins paired with renal arteries
   2. Left renal vein is three times longer than right.
   3. Empties into inferior vena cava
G. Accessory renal vessels
   1. Common, although renal artery and vein are usually sole blood supply
   2. May compress ureter to cause hydronephrosis
H. Lymphatics drain into lumbar lymph nodes.
I. Nerve supply
   1. Sympathetic and parasympathetic innervation
   2. Supplied by splanchnic nerves
III. Ureter(s)
   A. Paired cylindrical fibromuscular tubes that follow smooth S curve
   B. Lies on psoas muscle, passes medial to sacroiliac joints and lateral near ischial spines
   C. Penetrates base of bladder medially at oblique angle
      1. Posteroinferior to bladder dome
      2. Distance apart: 5 cm
   D. Areas of narrowing
      1. At ureteropelvic junction
      2. As it crosses over external iliac vessels
      3. As it passes through bladder wall
   E. Averages 26 to 30 cm long and 1 mm to 6 mm wide in adult
   F. Peristaltic action of small muscle fibers in middle layer of ureter transports urine from renal pelvis to urinary bladder.
   G. Tunneling of the ureter prevents reflux (backflow) of urine from bladder to kidney
IV. Bladder
   A. Hollow, muscular, pelvic organ
      1. Inner lining composed of transitional epithelium
      2. Submucosal layer composed of lamina propria (fibroelastic connective tissue) and contains smooth muscle
      3. Muscular layer and detrusor muscle lie outside of submucosal layer.

    B. Reservoir for urine

        1. Adult capacity: 350 to 700 ml

        2. Urge to urinate common at 400 to 450 ml

    C. Lies behind symphysis pubis in adult, slightly higher in child

        1. When full, rises above symphysis pubis, especially in children

        2. Easily palpated, especially when full

        3. If overdistended, may cause visible lower abdominal bulge

        4. Postponing urination strains bladder capacity and weakens musculature.

    D. Ureteral orifices are on proximal trigone at extremities of interureteric ridge.

        1. Distance apart: 2.5 cm

        2. Trigone located between ridge and bladder neck

    E. Bladder neck (internal sphincter) formed of interlaced muscle fibers of detrusor on bladder floor

        1. Muscle fibers converge.

        2. Pass distally to form smooth musculature of urethra

    F. Dome and posterior surface covered by peritoneum

    G. Arterial blood supply comprised of superior, middle, inferior vesical arteries

        1. From trunk of internal iliac (hypogastric) artery

        2. From obturator and inferior gluteal arteries

        3. In females, also has branches from uterine and vaginal arteries

    H. Venous blood supply rich and empties into internal iliac (hypogastric) veins

    I. Lymphatics drain into vesical, external and internal iliac, and common iliac lymph nodes.

    J. Urine storage

        1. Highly coordinated two-phased process of filling and emptying

        2. Controlled by sympathetic, parasympathetic, and central nervous system

    K. Micturition

        1. Increase in volume of urine in bladder causes slow rise in intravesical pressure.

        2. Stretch receptors in bladder wall convey afferent impulses through pelvic nerve to spinal cord.

            a. Stimulates sympathetic efferent nerves

            b. Impulses conveyed back to bladder through hypogastric nerves

            c. Activates internal sphincter to maintain continence

            d. Allows for complete bladder filling

        3. When bladder sufficiently distended, nerve impulses transmitted to brain

        4. Brain stem activates micturition.

            a. Efferent pelvic nerve stimulates bladder to contract.

            b. Bladder neck and urethra open.

            c. External urethral sphincter and perineal muscles relax with opening of bladder neck.

        5. Normal micturition dependent on certain factors

            a. Appropriate bladder sensation during filling stage

            b. Closed bladder neck at rest

            c. Absence of involuntary contractions

V. Urethra

    A. Mucosal tubular structure

        1. Adult male

            a. Length: 15 to 30 cm with "S" shaped curve

            b. Posterior urethra

                (1) Membranous

                (2) Prostatic

            c. Anterior urethra

                (1) Bulbous

                (2) Penile

                (3) Glandular

            d. Surrounded by internal and external sphincter

      e. Curves at strong right angle where bulbous urethra joins prostatic urethra (urogenital diaphragm)

      f. Empties by contraction of bulbocavernous muscle

  2. Adult female

    a. Length: 4 cm and slightly curved

      (1) Lies anterior to vagina and beneath symphysis pubis

      (2) Urethral orifice (meatus) lies between clitoris and vaginal introitus (opening).

      (3) Short length common cause of cystitis and urinary tract infection (UTI)

    b. Voluntary external sphincter surrounds middle third.

    c. Composed of submucosa of connective and elastic tissue

      (1) Filled with spongy venous spaces

      (2) Contains many periurethral glands that secrete mucus

    d. Empties by gravity

  B. Transports urine from bladder to meatus for excretion

VI. Adult male anatomy

  A. Prostate gland

    1. Encapsulated, glandular, fibromuscular organ lying below and behind bladder in front of the rectum

      a. Contributes to seminal fluid

      b. Muscular fibers contract during ejaculation.

      c. Transports spermatozoa to ejaculate

      d. Posterosuperior surface adjacent to vas deferens and seminal vesicles

    2. Doughnut configuration around bladder outlet

      a. Walnut size

      b. Chestnut shape

    3. Contains 2.5 cm posterior urethra and prostatic urethra

    4. Supported by puboprostatic ligaments and urogenital diaphragm

    5. Ejaculatory ducts pierce prostate posteriorly and empty through verumontanum.

      a. On floor of prostatic urethra

      b. Proximal to striated external urinary sphincter

    6. Consists of five lobes or zones

      a. Anterior, posterior, median, right lateral, and left lateral lobes

      b. Peripheral, central, transitional, anterior, and preprostatic sphincteric zones

    7. Periurethral glands at median and lateral lobes are usual site of prostatic adenoma.

    8. Posterior lobe prone to malignancy

    9. Prostatic fluid alkaline with high fructose content

      a. Component of semen nourishes sperm cells.

      b. Activates sperm cell motility

      c. Protects sperm from acidic vaginal secretions

    10. Blood supply

      a. Arterial blood supply from inferior vesical, internal pudendal, and middle rectal arteries

      b. Venous blood supply drains into periprostatic plexus.

      (1) Connects to deep dorsal vein of penis

      (2) Connects to internal iliac (hypogastric) veins

    11. Nerve supply derived from sympathetic and parasympathetic nerve systems

    12. Lymphatics drain into internal iliac, sacral, vesical, and external iliac lymph nodes.

  B. Cowper's glands (bulbourethral glands)

    1. Pea-sized glands on each side of posterior urethra

    2. Secrete mucus (component of seminal fluid) into ejaculatory ducts and out urethra during ejaculation

C. Seminal vesicles
   1. Convoluted membranous pouches
   2. Lie under base of bladder and above prostate gland
   3. Each joins corresponding vas deferens to form ejaculatory duct.
   4. Nerve supply is mainly from sympathetic system.
   5. Lymphatics supply prostate gland.
D. Spermatic cord
   1. Extends from internal inguinal ring through inguinal canal to testis bilaterally
   2. Contents of each cord
      a. Vas deferens
         (1) Firm cylindrical tubular structure
         (2) Connects epididymis with ejaculatory duct
         (3) Peristaltic contraction of thick muscular walls helps propel sperm through duct.
         (4) Capable of storing sperm cells for as long as 42 days
      b. Internal and external spermatic arteries
      c. Artery of vas (deferential artery)
      d. Venous pampiniform plexus (forms spermatic vein superiorly)
      e. Lymph vessels that empty into external iliac lymph nodes
      f. Autonomic nerves
   3. Enclosed in layers of thin fascia
   4. Serves to suspend testis
   5. Some cremaster nerve fibers penetrate cords in inguinal canal.
E. Epididymis
   1. Comma-shaped coiled duct that is continuous with vas deferens at its lower pole
   2. Consists of head (upper pole), central body, and tail (lower pole)
   3. Connected to posterolateral surface of testis at upper pole
   4. Appendix often found on upper pole
   5. Efferent ductules in head carry spermatozoa from testis to vas deferens.
   6. Stored sperm mature during transportation to vas.
F. Testis
   1. Essential for male reproductive system
      a. Produces spermatozoa (spermatogenesis)
      b. Secretes testosterone
      c. Housed in scrotal sac to provide lower temperature for sperm viability
   2. Testes are two oval-shaped organs covered by thick fascial layer of tunica albuginea.
      a. Posteriorly forms mediastinum testis
      b. Fibrous septa separate testis into approximately 250 lobules.
      c. Each lobule contains one to three tightly coiled seminiferous tubules.
   3. Covered with and separated from scrotal wall by tunica vaginalis
   4. Appendix testis, similar to epididymis testis, located at upper pole
   5. Seminiferous tubules lie adjacent to interstitial Leydig's cells (essential for testosterone production).
      a. Densely packed within testis
      b. Long convoluted threadlike tubules converge into rete testis.
      c. Rete testis leads to epididymis.
      d. Epididymis leads to vas deferens, which converges into ejaculatory ducts.
   6. Shares common embryologic origin with kidney and closely associated blood supply
      a. Internal spermatic artery originates in aorta just below renal artery.
      b. Internal spermatic artery joins deferential artery.
      c. Right spermatic vein enters vena cava just below right renal vein.
      d. Left spermatic vein empties into left renal vein.

       7. Lymphatics drain into paraaortic lymph nodes, which are connected to mediastinal nodes.

    G. Scrotum

       1. Relaxation and contraction of muscular layer regulate internal temperature.

         a. Temperature generally 1° to 2° F lower than body temperature

         b. Temperature regulation necessary for fertility

       2. Septum of connective tissue divides internal sac into two pouches.

         a. Dartos (internal septum) consists of superficial fascia and connective tissue.

         b. Median raphe is external central scrotal ridge formed by dartos.

       3. Provides support to testes

       4. Arterial blood supply from femoral, internal pudendal, and inferior epigastric arteries.

       5. Veins are paired with arteries.

       6. Lymphatics drain into subinguinal and superficial inguinal lymph nodes.

    H. Penis

       1. Organ of excretion and reproduction

         a. Glans or tip

           (1) Before circumcision, prepuce forms hood over glans (foreskin).

           (2) Prepuce may be smoothed back to expose glans and urethral meatus.

           (3) Contains nerve endings

           (4) Glans formed by distal, expanded end of bulbospongiosus muscle

         b. Shaft or body

           (1) Suspensory ligament from pubic symphysis

           (2) Ligament inserts into fascia of corpus cavernosa.

         c. Two corpus cavernosa and corpus spongiosum underlie.

           (1) Corpus cavernosa run along either side of corpus spongiosum along major portion of penile shaft.

           (2) Urethra surrounded by corpus spongiosum

           (3) All contain vascular cavities.

           (4) Corpus cavernosa fills with blood during sexual arousal and produces erection.

       2. Arterial blood supply from internal pudendal arteries

         a. Deep artery of penis supplies corpus cavernosa.

         b. Dorsal artery of penis

         c. Bulbourethral artery supplies corpus spongiosum, glans, and urethra.

       3. Venous blood supply

         a. Superficial dorsal vein

         b. Deep dorsal vein

         c. Drains into internal pudendal vein

       4. Lymphatic system

         a. Lymphatics from penile skin drain into deep and superficial inguinal lymph nodes.

         b. Lymphatics from glans, corpora, and urethra drain into deep inguinal external iliac lymph nodes.

   I. Organs of reproduction

       1. Prostate gland

       2. Seminal vesicles

       3. Testes

       4. Penis

VII. Adult female anatomy

    A. Glands of Skene

       1. Open on floor of urethra inside meatus

       2. Stimulate mucus secretion during sexual arousal to lubricate vagina

       3. Inflammation may contribute to urethritis or cystitis.

    B. Bartholin's gland

       1. Small mucus gland opening on each inner aspect of labia minora within vagina (homologue of bulbourethral gland in male)

    2. Supplements lubrication during sexual intercourse
    3. Inflammation may contribute to chronic urethritis or cystitis.
  C. Arterial blood supply
    1. Inferior vesical artery
    2. Vaginal artery
    3. Internal pudendal artery
  D. Venous blood supply empties into internal pudendal veins.
  E. Lymphatic system
    1. Lymphatics from external urethra drain into subinguinal and inguinal lymph nodes.
    2. Lymphatics from deep urethra drain into internal iliac lymph nodes.
  F. Organs of reproduction
    1. Uterus
    2. Fallopian tubes
    3. Ovaries
    4. Vagina

RENAL PHYSIOLOGY

Fluid and electrolyte balance (homeostasis) within the kidney is maintained through a complex, and not fully understood, interaction of hormonal systems, electrolyte balance, renal blood flow, glomerular filtration, red blood cell formation, and calcium formation. Tubular reabsorption, secretion, and excretion ultimately provide long-term regulation of acid-base balance by controlling the concentration of body fluid constituents.

The kidney filters approximately 180 L of plasma in 25 hours; 1 L becomes urine and the balance is reabsorbed. This process is affected by the composition, pressure, and volume of blood flowing through the kidney. Renal shutdown may quickly ensue with hypovolemia, because the nephrons become unable to adequately manufacture urine as a result of decreased blood supply to the kidney. When this occurs, measures must be taken to reverse the situation.

  I. Endocrine function (hormonal interactions)
    A. Renin-angiotensin-aldosterone system (RAAS) cascade is major renal hormonal regulator for
      1. Systemic blood pressure
      2. Regional blood flow
      3. Sodium and potassium balance
    B. Renin
      1. Enzyme-catalyzing agent
      2. Manufactured in specialized lining of afferent renal arterioles
        a. Volume receptors
        b. Response to reduced arterial blood pressure or renal perfusion as a result of
          (1) Hemorrhage
          (2) Sodium depletion
          (3) Heart failure
          (4) Dehydration
        c. Responsible for initiating conversion of angiotensinogen to angiotensin I and II
    C. Angiotensin II
      1. Powerful vasoconstrictor
      2. Raises blood pressure
      3. Stimulates aldosterone release
      4. Feedback mechanisms have limited compensatory ability to affect alterations in volume.
      5. Medical management directed toward external efforts
        a. Replacement of blood, fluids, electrolytes
        b. Drug therapies

    D. Aldosterone
        1. Release from adrenal cortex stimulated by
            a. Decreased sodium levels
            b. Increased potassium levels
        2. Prompts kidney to
            a. Absorb more sodium
            b. Excrete more potassium
        3. Net effect of release
            a. Conserve sodium and water
            b. Raise blood volume
            c. Prevents acidosis
        4. Potential adverse effects
            a. Systemic vasoconstriction
            b. Decreased organ perfusion
    E. Prostaglandin
        1. Produced, metabolized, and acted on in renal medulla
        2. Maintains renal function by effect on afferent and efferent arterioles of glomerular capillary
        3. Modulates renin release
        4. Affects urine concentration through synergistic activity with AVP (arginine vasopressin, an antidiuretic hormone)
        5. Nonsteroidal antiinflammatory agents must be cautiously used.
            a. Cause salt and water retention
            b. Acute renal failure can occur in states of dehydration.
    F. Erythropoietin
        1. Secreted by kidney in response to decrease in tissue oxygen tension
        2. Stimulates production of new red blood cells
        3. Exerts effect directly on bone marrow
        4. Insufficient levels often found in patients with impaired renal function
    G. ADH (antidiuretic hormone or vasopressin)
        1. Exerts effect on distal tubules of nephrons
        2. Acts as messenger in tubules, informing of body's need for water
        3. Secreted by posterior pituitary gland when significant loss of body water occurs
        4. Results in increased reabsorption of water and decrease in urine output
        5. Causes constriction of arterioles thereby raising blood pressure
    H. Vitamin D
        1. Activated in kidney
        2. Deficiency plays major role in chronic renal failure.
            a. Losses in urine with nephrotic syndrome
            b. Defective enzyme activity in kidney caused by
                (1) Renal disease
                (2) Diminished parenchymal function
        3. Decreased levels with hypocalcemia
        4. Stimulates intestinal absorption of calcium and phosphate
        5. Increases reabsorption of calcium and phosphorus by kidney
  II. Fluid-electrolyte balance (electrolyte interactions)
    A. Sodium
        1. Kidney regulates total body sodium by varying urinary excretion in relation to intake.
        2. Secretion adjusted in response to alterations in blood volume
        3. Reabsorption accounts for most of energy consumed by kidney.
    B. Potassium
        1. Filtration and excretion are independent of one another.
            a. Once filtered, is almost totally reabsorbed in proximal tubules and loop of Henle
            b. Excreted is derived from tubular secretions in distal nephron.
        2. Secretion enhanced by tubular fluid flow rate and increases in sodium reabsorption

C. Calcium
  1. Renal excretions and net intestinal absorption must be equal for proper calcium balance.
  2. Calcium phosphates crystallize in alkaline urine (hereditary distal tubular acidosis).
  3. Ionized in plasma
  4. Two thirds reabsorbed in proximal tubules by bulk flow with sodium and fluids
  5. Direct relation to sodium balance
D. Phosphates
  1. Ninety percent reabsorbed in proximal tubule through sodium-dependent process
  2. Balance reabsorbed in distal tubule
  3. Plasma level constant when renal function is normal
    a. Excess concentrations of saline decrease proximal reabsorption.
    b. Phosphate depletion raises reabsorption.
    c. Excretion depressed with hyperparathyroidism and vitamin D deficiencies
  4. At saturation point, excess load is excreted in urine.
E. Glucose in glomerular filtrate completely reabsorbed at normal blood concentrations
III. Glomerular filtration
  A. Nephrons operate in highly sophisticated pressure system.
  B. Pressure gradients affect filtration.
    1. Blood reaches glomerulus through renal artery at forward pressure of about 90 mm Hg.
    2. Fluid in Bowman's capsule creates hydrostatic pressure at about 15 mm Hg, resisting filtration.
    3. Presence of protein in plasma and not in capsule creates opposing force.
      a. Uneven distribution of protein causes water concentration of plasma to be lower than capsule's.
      b. Difference in water concentration induces osmotic flow of fluid from capsule into capillary.
        (1) Water
        (2) Crystalloids
    4. Osmotic gradient creates difference in hydrostatic pressure of about 30 mm Hg.
    5. When opposing forces are subtracted from original renal artery pressure, forward pressure is decreased to 45 mm Hg.
    6. Net filtration pressure
      a. Protein-free filtrate forced through glomerulus into Bowman's capsule
      b. Filtrate passes down into tubules
      c. Urine production initiated
IV. Urine production
  A. Originates in glomerulus (filtering agent)
    1. Selectively permeable membrane leaves filtrate virtually protein free.
    2. Composed basically of water and solutes (crystalloids)
  B. Filtrate passes through proximal convoluted tubule.
    1. Water and crystalloids reabsorbed according to body's need
    2. Loop of Henle concentrates urine.
    3. Distal convoluted tubule can reabsorb or excrete water and solutes.
      a. Reabsorbs only what body requires
      b. Excretes remainder
V. Key points
  A. Kidneys depend on minimum blood flow and on pressure regulated by renal arteries.
  B. Net filtration pressure can be affected by change in renal artery pressure.
  C. Pressure has direct effect on urine production.
  D. Sustained changes in pressure cause compromise in system function.

    E. Kidneys maintain electrolyte balance.
    F. End products of metabolism excreted in urine

PATHOPHYSIOLOGY

  I. Upper genitourinary system
    A. Adrenal gland
      1. Alport's syndrome
        a. Hereditary nephritis accompanied by deafness
        b. Managed with diet and medication
        c. Generally progresses to require dialysis and subsequent renal transplantation
      2. Cushing's disease
        a. Caused by overproduction of cortisol (hydrocortisone) as a result of
          (1) Bilateral adrenocortical hyperplasia from overproduction of adrenocorticotropic hormone (ACTH) in pituitary gland (85%)
          (2) Adrenal adenoma (10%)
          (3) Adenocarcinoma of adrenal gland (5%)
        b. Signs and symptoms
          (1) Marked muscle weakness, especially in quadriceps
          (2) Obesity with abnormal fat distribution
            (a) Extremities unaffected
            (b) Moon face with facial flushing
            (c) Cervical vertebral hump ("buffalo hump")
            (d) Clavicular fat pads
            (e) Pendulous abdomen
            (f) "Skinny" legs
          (3) Striae
            (a) Thighs and abdomen
          (4) Skin ulcerations
          (5) Hypertension
          (6) Calcium loss
            (a) Osteoporosis
            (b) Compression fractures of lumbar spine and ribs
            (c) Renal calculi
          (7) Sleep disturbances
            (a) Irritability
            (b) Psychosis
          (8) Diabetic glucose tolerance curve
          (9) Vascular fragility (bruises easily)
          (10) Slow wound healing
        c. Surgical intervention usually alleviates symptoms with exception of osteoporosis.
          (1) Total bilateral adrenalectomy
          (2) Transsphenoidal hypophysectomy
      3. Pheochromocytoma
        a. Tumor of the chromaffin cells of adrenal medulla, may be
          (1) Bilateral
          (2) Extraadrenal
        b. Surgically curable hypertensive syndrome
          (1) Systolic and diastolic hypertension
          (2) Hypertension may be sustained, or more commonly, paroxysmal.
          (3) Other frequent symptoms
            (a) Headache (severity directly related to degree of hypertension)
            (b) Unprovoked diaphoresis with flushing or blanching
            (c) Tachycardia with palpitations from epinephrine excess
            (d) Postural hypotension
              (i) Diminished plasma volume

(ii) Ganglionic blockage

(iii) May result in profound weakness

(e) Weight loss

(i) Anorexia resulting from elevated blood glucose and fatty acid levels

(ii) Decreased gastrointestinal motility: nausea, vomiting, constipation

c. Often occurs in combination with other glandular diseases

d. Laboratory analysis

(1) Elevated hematocrit (HCT), white blood cells (WBCs), serum protein

(2) Few lymphocytes

(3) Elevated fasting glucose level with diabetic glucose tolerance curve

(4) Urine hormonal analysis reveals elevated epinephrine and sometimes norepinephrine.

e. Administration of 1 mg intravenous (IV) glucagon will raise blood pressure and catecholamine in 2 minutes.

B. Kidney

1. Agenesis

a. Absence of one kidney

b. Presence of atrophic kidney (not fully developed)

2. Hypoplasia

a. Presence of small kidney with small renal artery

b. Contributes to renal hypertension

3. Polycystic kidneys (hereditary)

a. Occurs in renal cortex from defective collecting system

b. Bilateral cystic disease leading to progressive functional impairment as cysts enlarge

c. Symptoms

(1) Bilateral flank pain, often with colic

(2) Hematuria

(3) Hypertension

(4) Nodular, palpable kidneys, often tender

d. Usually results in need for dialysis and possible transplantation

4. Congenital ureteropelvic junction obstruction

5. Glomerulonephritis (Bright's disease)

a. Inflammatory process that attacks glomerulus

b. Possible immune reaction

c. Contributing causes

(1) Infectious organisms

(a) Streptococci

(b) Staphylococci

(2) Systemic diseases

(a) Lupus erythematosus

(b) Polyarteritis nodosa

(i) Result of trauma, anticoagulants, or tumor

(ii) Cause of spontaneous subcapsular hematoma

(c) Diabetic glomerulosclerosis

(d) Amyloidosis

(e) Alport's syndrome

6. Nephrotic syndrome (combination of symptoms)

a. Massive edema

b. Proteinuria

c. Hypoalbuminemia

d. Hyperlipidemia

e. Lipiduria

7. Renal artery stenosis

a. Plaque formation

b. Embolism

    c. Thrombosis

    d. Contributes to renal hypertension

8. Simple (solitary) renal cyst

9. Pyelonephritis (often a complication of *Escherichia coli* infection elsewhere in the body)

10. Perinephric abscess

11. High-output renal failure (oliguria)

    a. Urine output volume insufficient relative to body's excretory need

        (1) Occurs with urine volumes less than 400 ml/day if kidney can concentrate to normal specific gravity (1.010 to 1.025)

        (2) Occurs with urine volumes of 1000 to 1500 ml/day when concentrating ability impaired causing low specific gravity

    b. Metabolites retained

    c. High loss of body water

    d. Etiology

        (1) Inadequate plasma volume with vasodilation and substantially decreased protein levels

        (2) Normal kidney function compromised by poor perfusion

            (a) Decreased plasma volume results in decreased perfusion.

            (b) Poor perfusion accompanies decrease in cardiac contractility.

        (3) Prerenal azotemia (rising serum urea blood levels)

12. Acute renal failure

    a. Substantial decrease in glomerular filtration rate results in decrease in clearance of metabolites excreted by kidneys: urea, potassium, phosphate, creatinine.

    b. Body retains metabolites in bloodstream.

        (1) Abnormally high creatinine level in bloodstream (best indicator of renal failure)

        (2) Retention produces state known as azotemia (excess of urea in blood).

        (3) Azotemia can be tolerated until treatment interventions are instituted.

        (4) Uremia characterized by progressively higher levels of circulating metabolites

        (5) Uremia (intoxication) seen in advanced nephritis and anuria, incompatible with life

    c. Causes

        (1) Prerenal

            (a) Dehydration (volume depletion)

                (i) Hemorrhage

                (ii) Gastrointestinal losses (vomiting, diarrhea)

                (iii) Renal losses (excessive diuretic therapy)

                (iv) Burns

                (v) Heat prostration

            (b) Volume shifts

                (i) "Third space" losses

                (ii) Vasodilating drugs

                (iii) Gram-negative sepsis

            (c) Volume expansion

                (i) Congestive heart failure

                (ii) Nephrotic syndrome

                (iii) Cirrhosis with ascites

            (d) Vascular anomalies

                (i) Dissecting arterial aneurysms

                (ii) Malignant hyperthermia

                (iii) Atheroembolism

        (2) Intrarenal (parenchymal) conditions

            (a) Glomerulonephritis

                (b) Ischemic reaction to vascular compromise

                (c) Acute tubular necrosis

                (d) Acute cortical necrosis

                (e) Antibiotic nephrotoxicity

           (3) Postrenal conditions

                (a) Calculus in patients with solitary kidney

                (b) Bilateral ureteral obstruction: stricture

                (c) Bladder outlet obstruction: benign prostatic hypertrophy

                (d) Postrenal trauma

13. Chronic renal failure

    a. Irreversible destruction of renal tissue

    b. Reduced metabolite clearance requiring peritoneal dialysis or hemodialysis

    c. Chief parameters indicative of renal failure

        (1) Elevated blood urea nitrogen (BUN)

        (2) Elevated serum creatinine

        (3) Decreased creatinine clearance

    d. Lengthy disease course

        (1) Azotemia

        (2) End-stage renal disease

    e. Etiology

        (1) Primary causes

             (a) Glomerulonephritis

             (b) Pyelonephritis

             (c) Congenital hypoplasia

             (d) Polycystic kidney disease

        (2) Secondary causes

             (a) Diabetes

             (b) Hypertension

             (c) Systemic lupus erythematosus

             (d) Alport's syndrome

             (e) Amyloidosis

                (i) Idiopathic, often malignant condition

                (ii) Increased protein levels

                (iii) May also involve bladder and prostate

    f. Treatment modalities

        (1) Maintenance hemodialysis

        (2) Peritoneal dialysis

        (3) Renal transplantation

C. Ureter

    1. Congenital abnormalities

        a. Incomplete ureter

        b. Duplication of ureter

            (1) Y formation

            (2) Double ureter on one or both sides

        c. Ureterocele

        d. Ureteral stricture

        e. Ureterovesical reflux

        f. Ureteral stenosis

    2. Acquired condition

        a. Stenosis

            (1) Surgical trauma

            (2) External trauma

         b. Metastatic lymph node enlargement

        c. Endometriosis

        d. Tumors

        e. Calculi

II. Lower genitourinary system
   A. Bladder
      1. Exstrophy
         a. Congenital fusion of bladder wall
         b. Bladder eversion
      2. Interstitial cystitis
         a. Multifactorial syndrome of pelvic and/or perineal pain with urinary urgency and frequency
         b. Loss of normal bladder capacity develops.
         c. Biopsy of bladder wall may reveal presence of Mast cells, thought to be an integral cause of this syndrome.
      3. Stress incontinence
         a. Leakage of urine with sneezing, coughing, laughing, straining
         b. Common in older females and after multiple pregnancies
      4. Bladder diverticulum
      5. Bladder tumors
   B. Prostate gland
      1. Benign prostatic hypertrophy (BPH)
         a. Gland enlarges.
         b. Evident bladder outlet obstruction necessitates surgical intervention.
      2. Carcinoma
         a. Nonsurgical treatments
            (1) Androgen therapy
            (2) Radiation
         b. Surgical modalities
            (1) Orchiectomy
               (a) Testosterone production dramatically reduced
                  (i) Adrenal production of testosterone not altered
                  (ii) Antiandrogen therapy may be required.
               (b) Alternative to "medical" hormonal therapies
            (2) Prostatectomy
            (3) Cryoablation
            (4) Radioactive seed implantation
   C. Penis and male urethra
      1. Phimosis
         a. Foreskin unretractable over glans
         b. Tendency for infection and fibrosis
         c. Circumcision indicated
      2. Paraphimosis
         a. Retracted phimotic foreskin
         b. Painful swelling of glans occurs.
         c. Dry gangrene can result if severe.
         d. Circumcision indicated
      3. Balanoposthitis
         a. Inflamed glans and mucous membrane
         b. Purulent discharge
         c. Circumcision indicated
      4. Urethral stricture (stenosis)
         a. Congenital or acquired condition
         b. Surgical interventions
            (1) Urethral dilation
            (2) Meatotomy
            (3) Urethroplasty
      5. Hypospadias
         a. Congenital anomaly
         b. Opening of meatus proximal to its normal glandular position at tip of penis
         c. Requires surgical reconstruction of urethra

6. Epispadias
    a. Congenital anomaly (often associated with bladder exstrophy)
    b. Absence of dorsal urethral wall
    c. Requires surgical correction
7. Carcinoma of penis and/or urethra
8. Trauma (e.g., fractured urethra)
D. Testis, spermatic cord, and scrotum
    1. Cryptorchidism (undescended testis)
        a. Evident at birth
        b. Absence of one or both testis in scrotum
        c. Requires surgical intervention by the age of 1 to 2 years
            (1) Sterility ensues when left untreated much beyond this time.
            (2) Maturation will not occur.
            (3) Tendency for cancerous development increases over time if left
                untreated.
    2. Testicular tumors
        a. Usually malignant
        b. Common in 18-year to 35-year age group
        c. Enlargement of testis occurs, usually painless.
        d. Requires metastatic workup, orchiectomy, and chemotherapy
    3. Spermatocele
        a. Intrascrotal cystic mass
        b. Attached to superior head of epididymis
        c. Caused by obstruction of sperm-carrying tubular system
        d. Most commonly occurs after vasectomy
    4. Varicocele
        a. Most often seen on left side
        b. Veins of spermatic cord become engorged because of venous
           backflow.
        c. Often painful
        d. Uncorrected can affect fertility.
    5. Hydrocele
        a. Collection of fluid within scrotal sac
        b. May compromise testicular blood supply
    6. Torsion of testis or spermatic cord
        a. Strangulation of testicular blood supply
        b. Usually of traumatic origin
        c. Patient has presenting symptom of extreme pain.
        d. Requires immediate surgery
E. Female urethra
    1. Urethrovaginal fistula (vesicovaginal fistula)
        a. Abnormal passageway between urethra and vagina
        b. Develops after trauma
            (1) Pelvic fracture
            (2) Surgery
            (3) Radiotherapy
        c. Vaginal urethroplasty performed to correct condition
    2. Urethral diverticulum
        a. Urethral pouch develops.
        b. Can be a congenital abnormality
        c. Traumatic causes
            (1) Cystitis
            (2) Urethritis
            (3) Obstetric
        d. Requires excision and plastic repair
    3. Urethral carcinoma
    4. Urethral caruncle

III. Voiding dysfunctions
- A. Frequency
  1. Perception of urge to urinate at more frequent intervals
  2. Causes
     a. Residual urine
     b. Inflamed bladder mucosa or submucosa
     c. Bladder capacity inadequate
     d. Bladder instability
     e. Interstitial cystitis
     f. Bladder infection
- B. Urgency
  1. Strong sensation of having to void immediately
  2. Causes
     a. Cystitis
     b. Bladder instability
- C. Nocturia
  1. Need to urinate often during normal sleep time
  2. Often symptom of renal or prostate disease
  3. Causes
     a. Fluid retention (shift of circulating fluids to kidneys during rest)
     b. Excess fluid intake before bedtime
     c. BPH
     d. Renal calculi
     e. Cystitis
- D. Dysuria
  1. Painful urination
  2. Causes
     a. Prostatitis
     b. Cystitis
     c. Urethritis
     d. Pyelonephritis
- E. Enuresis
  1. Involuntary urination, often during sleep
  2. Normal in first 2 to 3 years of life
  3. Causes
     a. Delayed neuromuscular maturation
     b. Organic disease: infection, urethral stenosis, neurogenic bladder, pituitary malfunction
     c. Emotional or behavioral problems
- F. Incontinence (includes stress, urge, mixed, and paradoxic or overflow types)
  1. Inability to control urination
  2. Causes
     a. Exstrophy of bladder
     b. Epispadias
     c. Vesicovaginal fistula
     d. Trauma: childbirth, prostatectomy
     e. Bladder instability: detrusor, sphincter
- G. Hematuria
  1. Presence of gross or microscopic blood in urine
  2. Causes
     a. Tumors or cysts
     b. Calculi
     c. Infection
     d. Sickle cell disease
     e. Glomerulonephritis
- H. Obstruction and stasis
  1. Backflow of urine may occur, leading to hydronephrosis.

    2. Normal urinary flow blocked or arrested
       a. Prostatic obstruction
       b. Urethral obstruction
       c. Vesicoureteral reflux
       d. Pyelonephritis
       e. Calculi
    3. Contributing causes
       a. Hypercalciuria
          (1) Increased calcium intake
          (2) Increased vitamin D intake
       b. Hyperphosphatemia
       c. Hyperparathyroidism
       d. Gout
       e. Cushing's disease
          (1) Increased cortisol production
          (2) Protein loss in urine
I. Infection
    1. Specific (organisms capable of causing clinical disease)
       a. Tuberculosis
       b. Gonorrhea
       c. Actinomycosis
    2. Nonspecific (similar manifestations among several conditions)
       a. Gram-negative rods
       b. Gram-positive cocci
    3. Venereal diseases
       a. Gonorrhea
       b. Syphilis
       c. Lymphogranuloma venereum
       d. Granuloma inguinale
       e. Herpes genitalis
       f. Condylomata acuminata

THE NURSING PROCESS

I. Assessment
  A. Inspect (consistent with observation).
    1. Observe for visible signs of pathologic conditions.
       a. Abdomen (kidneys, bladder, lungs)
          (1) Costovertebral fullness
          (2) Distension
          (3) Oxygen perfusion
       b. Penis
          (1) Edema
          (2) Discharge
          (3) Inflammation, rash
          (4) Ulcerations, lesions
       c. Scrotum
          (1) Edema, crepitus
          (2) Discoloration
          (3) Alteration in testicular shape, size, or position
       d. Operative wounds
          (1) Bleeding
          (2) Drainage
          (3) Assess frequently.
    2. Interview patient for presence of postoperative sequelae.
       a. Collaborate with other perioperative caregivers to promote optimum follow-through.

     b. Compare findings with preoperative psychosocial assessment.
       (1) All patients
         (a) Use comprehensive assessment tools.
         (b) Establish presence of preexisting physical impairments and disease processes.
         (c) Note allergies and need for ancillary drug therapies.
       (2) Pediatric patient
         (a) Age crucial to proper assessment and intervention
         (b) Establish cognitive level of child; note phobias, peculiarities, emotional maturity.
         (c) Allow treasured toy or other "security blanket" to be nearby.
         (d) Evaluate merit of parental comfort.
    c. Expand on preoperative and intraoperative teaching.
       (1) Initiate deep breathing, coughing, mobilization.
       (2) Explain presence of any invasive devices resulting from operative experience.
         (a) Urinary catheters: urge to void, application of traction
         (b) Wound drains
         (c) IV and arterial lines
       (3) Offer medications to control discomfort or agitation frequently.
       (4) Alleviate fears of embarrassment because of altered body image.
         (a) Promote calming environment.
         (b) Provide privacy.
         (c) Provide warmth.
       (5) Communicate as care is being given to patient.
         (a) Wound and drain inspections
         (b) Frequent vital signs
         (c) O_2 therapy

B. Auscultate (first step after inspection of urologic patient).
   1. Abdomen
    a. Palpation alters normal peristalsis.
    b. Evaluation of bowel sounds important after abdominal and flank surgeries
   2. Lungs
    a. Evaluate presence and character of breath sounds.
    b. Absence of sounds may infer blockage of airway or abnormal screening in pleural cavity.
   3. Heart
    a. Detection of murmurs or bruits associated with aneurysms and renal artery stenosis
    b. Note rate and character of apical beats.
    c. Palpate (not part of routine nursing assessment).
   4. Kidneys
    a. Realistic only in thin adult
    b. Normal kidney is firm and smooth.
      (1) Tenderness should be expected after renal surgery.
      (2) Tenderness or pain may also indicate renal abnormality.
    c. Palpate deeply anteriorly as supine patient inhales deeply.
      (1) Use left hand for left kidney.
      (2) Use right hand for right kidney.
    d. Place palm of hand over costovertebral angle posteriorly, and deliver light blow.
      (1) Necessary for patient to be sitting
      (2) Angle formed by lower thoracic vertebrae and eleventh and twelfth ribs
      (3) Lower poles of kidneys below rib cage bilaterally
        (a) Should be perceived by patient as dull thud
        (b) Sharp tenderness or pain may require further evaluation.

5. Abdomen
   a. Patient should be in supine position.
   b. Note any resistance to light palpation over lower abdomen and suprapubic region.
      (1) May indicate bladder distension
      (2) May indicate bladder infection
      (3) Pelvic mass may elicit similar reaction.
6. Penis
   a. Palpate shaft with patient in supine position.
   b. Note tenderness or nodules.
7. Testes
   a. Determine presence of testis in each hemiscrotum.
   b. Testis is oval with C-shaped tube dorsally.
   c. Should be sensitive to pressure
      (1) Tenderness to light palpation may indicate need for further evaluation.
      (2) Distinct hard nodules should not be present.
8. Prostate gland
   a. Rectal examination with patient in lateral recumbent position
   b. Establish symmetry, smooth consistency, size, contour, and mobility.
      (1) Normal size 30 ml, 4 cm
      (2) BPH: symmetric enlargement common
      (3) Adenocarcinoma: asymmetric enlargement; discrete nodule or lobular induration often
      (4) Inflammation and prostatitis: boggy, symmetric enlargement and moderate to extreme tenderness
      (5) Neurologic impairment: inability to tighten anal sphincter common
   c. Urethral secretions may be obtained and analyzed for bacterial infection.
C. Percuss
   1. Kidneys
      a. Rarely achievable
      b. May be possible on child
   2. Bladder
      a. Tympany normal over bladder because of proximity of bowel
      b. Dullness occurs with distension.
   3. Lungs
      a. Anterior aspects and apices should be resonant.
      b. Posterior aspect resonant to ninth rib
      c. Bases reveal gradual transition from resonance to dullness over borders.
      d. Bases should move downward 5 to 6 cm on inspiration.
D. Review pertinent preoperative diagnostic data.
   1. Laboratory studies
      a. Urinalysis
         (1) Most fundamental and valuable of all screening methods
         (2) Value dependent on
            (a) Proper specimen collection
            (b) Prompt delivery of specimens
         (3) Components
            (a) pH (4.6 to 8)
            (b) Appearance (color, clarity)
               (i) Normal clarity is clear.
               (ii) Normal color is straw to amber.
            (c) Odor (aromatic)
            (d) Specific gravity (1.010 to 1.025)
               (i) Infant (1.001 to 1.020)
               (ii) Elderly (values decrease with age)
            (e) Protein (albumin, 0 to 8 mg/dl)
            (f) Glucose (sugar, 0)

(g) Ketones (0)

(h) Blood (red blood cells [RBCs], 0 to 2; casts, 0)

(i) Leukocytes (WBCs, 0)

(j) Microscopic evaluation

  (i) Casts, crystals, bacteria

  (ii) RBCs, WBCs

  b. Creatinine clearance

  (1) Urine collected for 24 hours

  (2) First A.M. voiding discarded and first voiding of following morning collected

  (3) Requires refrigeration

  c. Urine culture and sensitivities

  d. BUN, 10 to 20 mg/dl

  (1) Infant or child, 5 to 18 mg/dl

  (2) Above 100 mg may infer renal function impairment.

  e. Urine osmolality

  (1) Monitors electrolyte and water balance

  (2) Evaluate dehydration.

  f. Serum creatinine (0.5 to 1.2 mg/dl)

  (1) Range for females slightly lower

  (2) Above 1.5 mg/dl indicates impairment of renal function.

  g. Complete blood count (CBC) and differential

  h. Serum electrolytes

  i. Cholesterol (120 to 200 mg/dl)

  j. Coagulation studies (prothrombin time [PT], partial thromboplastin time [PTT], platelets, bleeding time)

2. Diagnostic procedures

  a. Ultrasonography

  (1) Able to focus on particular organ

  (2) Picture of organ displayed on screen

    (a) Measure shape and size.

    (b) High-frequency sound waves

  (3) Affected areas alter image by response to sound waves.

  b. Intravenous pyelogram (IVP)

  (1) Visualizes entire urinary system through IV administration of contrast dye

  (2) Isolates abnormalities

  (3) Mortality has decreased with use of nonionic dyes.

  (4) Dye may prove nephrotoxic when certain abnormalities are present.

  c. Renal scan (renal isotope studies)

  (1) Evaluates renal flow and function

  (2) Displays space-occupying lesions

  d. Computed tomography (CT scan)

  (1) Retroperitoneal lymph nodes can be evaluated.

  (2) Intraabdominal and prostate abnormalities revealed

  e. Magnetic resonance imaging (MRI)

  (1) Better contrast between normal and pathologic tissue

  (2) Avoids obscuring bone artifacts

  (3) Allows direct imaging of transverse, sagittal, and coronal planes

  (4) Valuable in evaluating renal and prostate abnormalities

  (5) Useful tool in assessing cancer response to radiotherapy and chemotherapy

  f. Cystogram

  (1) Radiopaque dye instilled into bladder through cystoscopy or catheterization

  (2) Usually performed when reflux is suspected

  g. Retrograde pyelogram, ureteroscopy

  (1) Done with cystoscopy using radiopaque dye

       (2) Ureters catheterized

       (3) Direct vision and fluoroscopic views of ureters and kidneys

    h. Angiogram

       (1) Renal arteries catheterized under fluoroscopy

       (2) Demonstrates integrity of renal circulation and great vessels

       (3) Renal artery stenosis and pheochromocytoma may be identified.

    i. Chest x-ray

    j. Flat plate x-ray (KUB)

    k. Electrocardiogram (ECG)

  E. Establish nursing diagnosis based on data retrieval.

  F. Develop care plan according to findings.

  G. Implement care using criteria of nursing process.

  H. Evaluate patient outcomes.

II. Nursing diagnosis (examples of related categories)

  A. Fluid volume imbalance

  B. Altered tissue perfusion

  C. Alteration in urinary elimination

  D. Potential for infection

  E. Electrolyte imbalance

  F. Disturbance of self-esteem

  G. Pain

  H. Impaired pulmonary exchange

  I. Anxiety

  J. Potential for positional injury

OPERATIVE PROCEDURES

I. Renal surgery

  A. Adrenalectomy

    1. Purpose or procedure

      a. Correct hypersecretion of adrenal hormones.

      b. Remove neoplasms.

      c. Secondary treatment of hormonal-dependent carcinomas

       (1) Breast

       (2) Prostate

      d. Surgical approaches

       (1) Transthoracic

       (2) Thoracolumbar

       (3) Upper abdominal

       (4) Flank

       (5) Laparoscopic

    2. Intraoperative concerns

      a. Damage to liver, pancreas, spleen, or pleura

      b. Maintenance of appropriate cortisone levels

      c. Fluid volume imbalance

      d. Inadequate pulmonary perfusion

      e. Hypotension with pheochromocytoma

    3. Postanesthesia priorities

      a. Cortisone administration may be indicated if bilateral.

      b. Counteract preoperative antihypertensive agents.

      c. IV fluids to maintain blood volume

      d. Alertness to signs of hemorrhage and shock

      e. Maintain adequate pulmonary perfusion.

      f. Closely monitor cardiovascular status.

      g. Hourly urine and electrolyte values

      h. Increased susceptibility to infection requires strict dressing and drain techniques.

        i. Judicious use of narcotics (heightened effect with decreased adrenal function)

   4. Psychosocial concerns
      a. Change in lifestyle
      b. Threat of cancer

   5. Complications
      a. Hypovolemic and hyponatremic shock
      b. Hemorrhage
      c. Dehydration
      d. Infection

B. Renal transplantation
   1. Purpose or procedure
      a. Reverse end-stage renal disease
      b. Transplantation from cadaver or living donor
      c. Includes anastomosis of renal artery of donor organ to hypogastric or common iliac artery of recipient
      d. Kidney placed in pelvic fossa
      e. Continuity of urinary tract established by implanting donor ureter into recipient bladder
      f. Midline abdominal incision, xiphoid to pubis, with bilateral supraumbilical transverse extensions

   2. Intraoperative concerns
      a. Preoperative elimination of potential sources of infection
        (1) Dialysis cannulas
        (2) Bladder infection
        (3) Dental abscesses
        (4) Upper respiratory infection
        (5) Skin conditions
      b. Minimize shock that adversely affects new kidney's function.
      c. Control hypertension.
      d. Avoid agents metabolized by kidney.
      e. Monitor and control electrolyte balance.

   3. Postanesthesia priorities
      a. Preparation and assembly of patient care supplies
        (1) Blood collection tubes
          (a) CBC
          (b) Clotting factors
          (c) Electrolytes
          (d) BUN
          (e) Creatinine
          (f) Liver enzymes
          (g) Glucose
          (h) Arterial blood gases (ABGs)
        (2) Urine collection containers
        (3) Sterile specimen tubes
        (4) Hemodynamic monitoring equipment
        (5) Intravenous solutions
          (a) D_5 one half normal saline
          (b) D_5 one quarter normal saline
          (c) Ringer's lactate
          (d) Plasmanate
          (e) D_5W
        (6) Medications
          (a) Furosemide (Lasix)
          (b) Sodium bicarbonate
          (c) Methylprednisolone (hydrocortisone)
          (d) Antihypertensive agents

        (e) Immunosuppressive drugs as per hospital protocol
           (e.g., cyclosporin A)
    (7) Sterile irrigating solutions and syringes
    (8) Protective isolation measures as per hospital protocol (patient immunosuppressed)

  b. Data retrieval
    (1) Establish presence of hepatitis or serum-positive antigens.
    (2) Note times of last steroids and antibiotics.

  c. Monitor all vital signs frequently.
    (1) Patients generally hypertensive
    (2) Temperature may fluctuate.

  d. Monitor central venous pressure lines frequently.
    (1) Assess blood volume.
    (2) Ensure adequate kidney perfusion.

  e. Replace crystalloids and colloids.
    (1) Urinary output may be massive (especially with living donor kidney).
    (2) Measure urinary output scrupulously and at specified intervals.
    (3) Insensible body fluid loss

  f. Maintain patency of catheters.

  g. Initiate pulmonary toilet to combat upper respiratory complications.

  h. Collect ordered laboratory specimens.
    (1) Blood
    (2) Urine

  i. Administer medications as indicated.
    (1) Steroids
    (2) Antibiotics
    (3) Immunosuppressants
    (4) Antihypertensive agents

4. Psychosocial and interfamily concerns
  a. Patient has undergone extreme physical, mental, and psychologic strain.
    (1) Hemodialysis
    (2) Transplant seen as last chance for health
    (3) Fear of rejection
    (4) May display excessive concern about renal function
  b. Nurse will need to maintain inner calm and tolerance.

5. Complications
  a. Early onset
    (1) Anuria or oliguria from hypovolemia
      (a) Acute tubular necrosis
      (b) Thrombosis (especially renal artery)
      (c) Operative difficulties
    (2) Hyperacute rejection (immediate nephrectomy mandated)
  b. Delayed onset
    (1) Acute or chronic rejection
    (2) Ureteral obstruction
    (3) Infection
      (a) Constant threat to success of transplant
      (b) Nonpathogenic bacteria and viruses may become opportunistic organisms.
    (4) Steroid reaction
      (a) Gastric bleeding or perforation
      (b) Emotional disturbances or altered body image
      (c) Aseptic bone necrosis
        (1) Position and turn patient gently.
        (2) Minimal use of tape on tissue-fine skin
      (d) Nephrotoxicity to cyclosporin A

C. Nephrectomy (radical nephrectomy, nephroureterectomy)
1. Purpose or procedure
   a. Reasons for removal of kidney
      (1) Malignancy
      (2) Extensive renal calculi
      (3) Trauma
      (4) Renal vascular disease
      (5) Infection
      (6) Polycystic disease
         (a) Medical management and eventual transplant are preferred methods.
         (b) Carcinoma may develop from long-term dialysis, requiring organ removal.
   b. May include excision of ureter or adrenal gland or both
   c. Surgical approaches
      (1) Flank or lumbar incision
      (2) Transabdominal
      (3) Thoracoabdominal
      (4) Laparoscopic (also includes "partial nephrectomy")
         (a) Renal cyst decortication
         (b) Cryoablation of renal neoplasm
         (c) Refer to laparoscopic procedures.
2. Intraoperative concerns
   a. Flank and lumbar approaches
      (1) Position causes compression of dependent side.
         (a) Altered pulmonary perfusion
         (b) Pressure points on bony prominences
         (c) Brachial plexus injuries
         (d) Compromise of arterial and venous circulation
         (e) Pneumothorax
      (2) Potential injury to peritoneum
   b. Transabdominal (not commonly used)
      (1) Potential injury to liver, pancreas, or spleen
      (2) Proximity to aorta and vena cava
      (3) Fluid volume and electrolyte depletion
         (a) Increased incidence of third space losses with this approach
         (b) Altered tissue perfusion
   c. Thoracoabdominal approach
      (1) Same concerns as flank approach
      (2) Dependent lung deflated intraoperatively; postoperative chest tube may be indicated
   d. Laparoscopic
      (1) Potential injury to liver, spleen, or pleura
      (2) Hemorrhage
      (3) Concerns related to flank approach
3. Postanesthesia priorities
   a. Accurate intake and output records
   b. Skin integrity
   c. Adequate pulmonary perfusion
   d. Fluid volume and electrolyte replacement
   e. Maintain comfort level.
      (1) Position on affected side to limit stress on suture line.
      (2) Pain medication
4. Psychosocial concerns
   a. Threat of disease to remaining kidney
   b. Anxiety over potential metastases

      5. Complications

         a. Hemorrhage

         b. Atelectasis

  D. Extracorporeal shock wave lithotripsy (ESWL)

      1. Purpose or procedure

         a. Noninvasive treatment modality for obstructive renal stone disease

            (1) Patient placed over water-filled cushions

            (2) External shock waves directed at renal and ureteral calculi

            (3) Calculi selectively disintegrated

         b. Remnants pass in urine through forced diuresis.

         c. Ureteral stent placed to maintain patency of ureter (not always required)

      2. Intraoperative concerns

         a. Hemorrhage

         b. Ureteroscopy or percutaneous nephroscopy may be necessary.

         c. Maintenance of pulmonary exchange and heart rate

            (1) Monitored intravenous sedation, general or spinal anesthesia

            (2) ECG is monitored to assess for arrhythmias as result of shock waves.

      3. Postanesthesia priorities

         a. Maintain adequate fluid replacement.

         b. Management of postoperative pain

         c. Strain all urine for stone debris (patient to go home with strainer).

      4. Psychosocial concerns

         a. Altered body image if nephrostomy tube present

         b. Bruising over areas of shock entry

         c. Anxiety over potential postoperative hematuria

         d. Anxiety about safety of procedure

      5. Complications

         a. Hemorrhage

         b. Subcapsular hematoma

         c. Steinstrasse ("street of stones," often resulting in obstruction)

         d. Renal colic

         e. Sepsis

         f. Hypertension

         g. Skin bruising

  E. Ureterolithotomy, pyelolithotomy, or nephrolithotomy

      1. Purpose or procedure

         a. Surgical removal of large and adherent renal and ureteral calculi

         b. Flank, supine, prone, or laparoscopic approach

         c. Ureteral stent placed to maintain patency of ureter

      2. Intraoperative concerns

         a. Compression of dependent side (see information on nephrectomy in section C above)

         b. Hemorrhage

         c. Renal ischemia and parenchymal damage

         d. Hypertension

      3. Postanesthesia priorities

         a. Meticulous maintenance of ureteral stents and catheters

         b. Pain management

         c. Adequate pulmonary ventilation

         d. Fluid volume replacement

         e. Intake and output

      4. Psychosocial concerns

         a. Fear of developing more stones necessitating further surgery

         b. Fear of pain postoperatively

      5. Complications

         a. Hemorrhage

         b. Occlusion of ureteral and urethral catheters

         c. Paralytic ileus

 F. Ureteral reimplantation or dismembered pyeloplasty
  1. Purpose or procedure
   a. Repair of ureteral pelvic junction obstructions or reflux
   b. Ureter repositioned at newly created hiatus in bladder or renal pelvis
    (1) Abdominal approach for reimplantation
    (2) Flank or laparoscopic approach for pyeloplasty
  2. Intraoperative concerns
   a. Minimize trauma to involved ureter.
   b. Avoid injury to renal vessels.
   c. Maintenance of pulmonary and circulatory perfusion in flank position
   d. Strong fixation of ureter
   e. Integrity of ureteral blood supply
  3. Postanesthesia priorities
   a. Management of catheters, drains, and ureteral stents
    (1) Collection bags labeled
    (2) All drainage devices properly secured
   b. Monitor urinary output.
    (1) Separate record for each catheter
    (2) Assess for blood and sediment.
    (3) All drainage may not equal 30 ml/hour.
    (4) Report any significant drops in output volume.
   c. Administer antibiotics as ordered.
  4. Psychosocial concerns
   a. Patients are frequently children.
   b. Concern over long-term prognosis of repair
   c. Potential for infection high in early stages of recovery
  5. Complications
   a. Infection
   b. Hemorrhage
   c. Hydronephrosis
   d. Hypertension
   e. Ureteral leak or stricture
 G. Ureteroscopy and electrohydraulic lithotripsy (EHL) or laser disintegration of calculi
  1. Purpose and procedure
   a. Diagnose and evaluate patency of ureter
   b. Removal of obstructing calculi
   c. Involves rigid or flexible instrumentation
   d. Saline irrigation used
  2. Intraoperative concerns
   a. Extravasation of irrigating fluids
   b. Peripheral vascular circulation
   c. Ureteral spasm and perforation
   d. Radiation exposure
  3. Postanesthesia priorities
   a. Monitor electrolyte balance.
   b. Maintenance of stents and catheters
   c. Pain management
  4. Psychosocial concerns
   a. Recurrence of calculi
   b. Threat of long-term treatment for retained stone fragments
  5. Complications
   a. Avulsion or perforation of ureter
   b. Ileus
   c. Urinoma
   d. Ureteral stricture
   e. Alteration in vascular supply to ureter

II. Genitourinary surgery
  A. Cystoscopy
     1. Purpose or procedure
        a. Evaluation of bladder, urethra, trigone, prostate, and ureteral orifices
        b. Involves flexible or rigid instrumentation
        c. Biopsies may be accomplished.
        d. Method to instill bladder medications
        e. Possible to crush or laser fragment bladder calculi (litholapaxy)
        f. Commonly an outpatient procedure
     2. Intraoperative concerns
        a. Anesthetic may be local, general, or spinal.
        b. Bladder perforation, urethral trauma
     3. Postanesthesia priorities
        a. Catheter patency and output
        b. Observe for hemorrhage.
        c. Monitor for dysuria.
        d. Unaltered urinary elimination after procedure or catheter removal
     4. Psychosocial concerns
        a. Fear of cancer
        b. Concern about process of urination
     5. Complications
        a. Incontinence
        b. Hemorrhage
        c. Bladder perforation
        d. Infection
  B. Transurethral resection of bladder tumor or bladder neck (TURB)
     1. Purpose or procedure
        a. Resection of lesions and contractures
        b. Cystoscopy approach
     2. Intraoperative concerns
        a. Electrocautery safety
        b. Peripheral vascular integrity
        c. Bladder perforation may lead to extravasation of irrigating fluids (very low incidence).
        d. Blood volume and electrolyte balance
        e. If laser is used, implementation of appropriate precautions
        f. Hypothermia (irrigation warming units)
     3. Postanesthesia priorities
        a. Catheter patency
        b. Continuous irrigation may be indicated.
        c. Monitor urinary output and character.
        d. Infection
        e. Hypothermia
     4. Psychosocial concerns
        a. Fear of cancer
        b. Fear of recurrence
     5. Complications
        a. Urinary retention
        b. Hemorrhage
        c. Electrolyte imbalance
  C. Cystectomy (partial/radical)
     1. Purpose or procedure
        a. Removal of malignancy
        b. Radical required when widespread
           (1) Involves urinary diversion techniques
           (2) Entire bladder removed with lymphadenectomy
           (3) Lengthy surgery

2. Intraoperative concerns
   a. Abdominal or laparoscopic approach
   b. Pulmonary and renal function
   c. Fluid and electrolyte balance
   d. Control of body temperature
3. Postanesthesia priorities
   a. Fluid and electrolyte replacement
   b. Pulmonary perfusion
   c. Catheter maintenance
   d. Nasogastric tube or gastrostomy tube may be present.
   e. Maintenance of wound drains and ureteral stents
4. Psychosocial concerns
   a. Altered body image
   b. Change in lifestyle
   c. Fear of metastases
5. Complications
   a. Shock
   b. Hemorrhage
D. Urinary diversion
   1. Purpose or procedure
      a. Divert ureters before or following radical cystectomy, for neuropathic bladder, or noncompliant interstitial cystitis
         (1) Diverted to abdominal stoma generally
         (2) Newer techniques create neobladder with internal ureteral diversion and urethral anastomosis.
         (3) Ureteral stents placed to maintain ureteral patency
         (4) Midline abdominal or laparoscopic approach
      b. Segment of ileum generally used
      c. Various types of diversion
         (1) Ileal conduit
         (2) Bladder replacement with section of colon, sigmoid, or ileum
         (3) Continent diversion (Kock pouch, Indiana pouch)
   2. Intraoperative concerns
      a. Fluid and electrolyte balance
      b. Gastric control
      c. Pulmonary and renal function
      d. Patient's body temperature
      e. Peripheral vascular integrity
   3. Postanesthesia priorities
      a. Nasogastric or gastrostomy tube
      b. Stomal care
      c. Maintenance of ureteral stents and catheters
      d. Measure intake and output hourly.
      e. Pulmonary perfusion and peripheral circulation
      f. Fluid and electrolyte balance (metabolic acidosis or alkalosis)
      g. Pain management
      h. Central venous pressure and arterial lines
   4. Psychosocial concerns
      a. Depression caused by poor body image
      b. Prognosis may be poor.
   5. Complications
      a. Distension
      b. Mucous plugs
      c. Hemorrhage
      d. Intestinal leaks, ulcers
      e. Infection
      f. Stomal necrosis, obstruction, herniation, or fistula
      g. Vitamins B_{12}, A, and D and iron deficiencies

E. Bladder augmentation
  1. Purpose or procedure
     a. Increase bladder capacity
     b. Neuropathic bladder
     c. Segment of small or large bowel or stomach anastomosed to bladder at dome
  2. Intraoperative concerns
     a. Fecal spills
     b. Fluid and electrolyte balance
     c. Gastric control
  3. Postanesthesia priorities
     a. Nasogastric or gastrostomy tube
     b. Hourly urinary output measurements
     c. Pulmonary perfusion
     d. Peripheral vascular circulation
     e. Fluid and electrolyte imbalance
     f. Urinary catheters and irrigations
  4. Psychosocial concerns
     a. Need for intermittent catheterization
     b. Copious mucous discharge
  5. Complications
     a. Metabolic disorders
     b. Hyperchloremic acidosis
     c. Vitamin B_{12} deficiency
     d. Bladder rupture
     e. Urinary retention
F. Bladder neck suspensions
  1. Purpose or procedure
     a. To correct urinary stress incontinence
     b. Various endoscopic techniques require lithotomy position.
        (1) Raz sling
        (2) Stamey or Pereyra endoscopic suspension procedure
        (3) Pubovaginal or tension-free vaginal tape (TVT) sling
        (4) Laparoscopic modified Burch procedure
        (5) Male sling
     c. Traditional abdominal approach: supine frog-legged or modified lithotomy position
        (1) Marshall-Marchetti-Krantz
        (2) Endoscopy not performed
  2. Intraoperative concerns
     a. Pressure on bony prominences
     b. Peripheral vascular circulation
     c. Bladder perforation
  3. Postanesthesia priorities
     a. Maintenance of urinary catheters
     b. Urinary output
  4. Psychosocial concerns
     a. Fear that procedure will be ineffective
     b. Body image
  5. Complications
     a. Urinary retention
     b. Wound infection
     c. Urinary tract infection
     d. Continued incontinence
     e. Retroperitoneal hemorrhage
     f. Organ perforation
G. Artificial urinary sphincter implantation
  1. Purpose or procedure

      a. To correct persistent incontinence and urinary leakage

      b. Most often performed on postprostatectomy patient

      c. Mechanical device placed around bladder neck or bulbous urethra

         (1) Inflation pump in scrotal sac or labia majora

         (2) Reservoir placed behind rectus abdominis muscle

  2. Intraoperative concerns

      a. Maintain body temperature

      b. Strict adherence to aseptic technique

      c. Prevent urethral damage

  3. Postanesthesia priorities

      a. Catheter care and maintenance

      b. Wound and skin care (skin often raw from persistent leakage of urine)

      c. Fluid and electrolyte balance

      d. Administration of antibiotics as required

  4. Psychosocial concerns

      a. Embarrassment

      b. Low self-esteem

  5. Complications

      a. Infection

      b. Recurrence of persistent stress incontinence

      c. Urinary retention

      d. Cuff erosion

      e. Urethral atrophy

      f. Fluid leaks

      g. Tubing obstruction (kinks)

H. Neuromodulation of voiding dysfunction (InterStim)

  1. Purpose or procedure

      a. Treatment of urinary frequency, urgency, urge incontinence, or nonobstructive urinary retention

      b. Pacemaker type stimulation of sacral nerves ("bladder pacemaker")

      c. Pocket created for pacemaker below waist and adjacent to the pelvic bone

      d. Thin wires are tunneled from sacral foramen to pacemaker.

      e. MRI is contraindicated with implant.

  2. Intraoperative concerns

      a. Patient prone

      b. Monitored intravenous sedation and local injection

      c. Avoid muscle relaxants intraoperatively.

      d. Bipolar cautery is preferred.

  3. Postanesthesia priorities

      a. Pain management

      b. Edema (ice)

  4. Psychosocial concerns

      a. Fear of injury to device

      b. Fear of dislodging leads

      c. Inability to operate device

  5. Complications

      a. Infection

      b. Persistent pain at pacemaker site

      c. Blunt trauma damage to pacemaker

I. Pelvic lymph node dissection (lymphadenectomy)

  1. Purpose or procedure

      a. Histologic staging of prostatic and bladder carcinomas

      b. Abdominal approach through laparotomy or laparoscopy

      c. Nodes along external iliac, obturator, and hypogastric veins removed

      d. May include removal of nodes along aorta and vena cava (retroperitoneal lymph node dissection) in testicular cancer

      e. Midline abdominal or laparoscopic approach

2. Intraoperative concerns
   a. Bowel perforation or herniation with laparoscope
   b. Damage to arteries, veins, nerves
   c. Pulmonary perfusion, especially with laparoscopy
   d. Increased intraabdominal pressure with laparoscopy (pneumoperitoneum)
   e. Hemorrhage
   f. Adequate tissue retrieval
3. Postanesthesia priorities
   a. Adequate pulmonary perfusion
   b. Intraabdominal hemorrhage
4. Psychosocial concerns
   a. Fear of cancer and metastases
   b. Altered body image related to possible future surgery
   c. Anticipation of impotence and sterility
5. Complications
   a. Lymphocele
   b. Lymph obstruction
   c. Ileus
   d. Wound infection
   e. Pneumonia
   f. Retrograde ejaculation
   g. Infertility and impotence
   h. Scrotal hematoma or pneumoscrotum
J. Prostatectomies
   1. Purpose or procedure
      a. Transurethral resection of prostate (TURP)
         (1) For BPH
         (2) Done endoscopically with resectoscope
         (3) Laser may be incorporated into procedure for ablation of bleeders.
      b. Retropubic
         (1) Lower abdominal approach to expose and open bladder at urethral juncture with prostate
         (2) Avoids incision into bladder
         (3) Radical procedure for carcinoma of prostate
            (a) Entire gland and seminal vesicles removed, penile vessels ligated
            (b) Nerve-sparing approach has become more common.
            (c) Significant blood loss may occur.
         (4) Simple retropubic may be done for BPH.
            (a) Seminal vesicles are not removed.
            (b) Reserved for extremely large glands
      c. Perineal (simple and radical)
         (1) For BPH and carcinoma respectively
         (2) Patient in lithotomy position
         (3) Incision made behind scrotum between ischial fossae
         (4) Blood loss more easily controlled
      d. Suprapubic (seldom used)
         (1) For BPH when prostate too large to remove endoscopically
         (2) Low abdominal incision to expose and enter bladder
         (3) Enucleation of lateral and medial lobes
      e. Laparoscopic
         (1) For carcinoma of prostate
         (2) Lengthy surgery, 6 to 8 hours
         (3) Requires magnification of laparoscopic image
         (4) Procedure still evolving
   2. Intraoperative concerns
      a. TURP
         (1) Fluid and electrolyte balance

          (a) Extravasation, extraperitoneal or intraperitoneal absorption of irrigants (sorbitol, glycine)

            (i) Transurethral resection syndrome

            (ii) Newer irrigants have decreased risk.

            (iii) Abdominal pain, restlessness, pallor, and diaphoresis

          (b) Blood loss

       (2) Cardiac and pulmonary status

          (a) Hypertension or hypotension

          (b) Bradycardia or tachycardia

          (c) Dyspnea

       (3) Pressure on bony prominences because of lithotomy position

       (4) Peripheral vascular circulation

       (5) Perforation of bladder neck, prostatic capsule, or bladder wall

    b. Suprapubic

       (1) Suture line integrity

       (2) Bleeding because of vascular nature of gland

    c. Retropubic (radical and simple)

       (1) Bleeding

       (2) Fluid volume depletion

       (3) Hypothermia

       (4) Cardiac status

       (5) Integrity of urethral anastomosis

       (6) Damage to nerves

    d. Perineal (radical and simple)

       (1) Pressure on bony prominences

       (2) Peripheral vascular perfusion

       (3) Integrity of urethral anastomosis

       (4) Pulmonary and cardiac status altered by extreme position

       (5) Bleeding

    e. Laparoscopic

       (1) Perforation of viscera, bowel or bladder

       (2) Pulmonary and cardiac perfusion

       (3) Integrity of vascular ties or clips

       (4) Bleeding

       (5) Security of urethral anastomosis

       (6) CO_2 embolus

3. Postanesthesia priorities (consistent for all; radical and TURP patient at increased risk)

    a. Catheter maintenance and irrigation

       (1) Traction on catheter may be indicated to promote hemostasis of prostatic fossa.

       (2) Observe for occlusion from clots.

       (3) Sudden, excessive bleeding could indicate balloon has slipped into prostatic fossa.

    b. Urinary output

       (1) Alertness to signs of hemorrhage (pink to frank blood)

       (2) Record hourly output volumes.

       (3) Observe for massive diuresis with TURP patient.

    c. Fluid or electrolyte replacement

       (1) Evaluate serum osmolality and other pertinent laboratory data.

          (a) Hemoglobin and hematocrit

          (b) Potassium

          (c) Sodium hyponatremia (transurethral resection syndrome)

       (2) Decreased sodium values may indicate dilutional syndrome and water intoxication; TURP patient at increased risk

          (a) Other hyponatremic signs

             (i) Shortness of breath, hypoxemia

            (ii) Mental disorientation (confusion)

(iii) Nausea and vomiting

(iv) Muscle twitch, apprehension

(v) Tachycardia

(vi) Hypotension

(b) Treatment

(i) Furosemide to mobilize edema and diurese excess fluid combined with saline drip

(ii) Infuse hypertonic saline (3% to 5%) in 100 ml/hr increments for 2 to 4 hours if serum osmolality is low.

(iii) Untreated, transurethral resection syndrome has led to seizures and vascular collapse.

d. Monitor cardiac and pulmonary status.

(1) Sedate to combat restlessness.

(2) Evaluate for hypoxemia.

e. May have nasogastric tube

f. May have epidural catheter for postoperative pain control

4. Psychosocial concerns

a. Impotence

b. Infertility

c. Fear of metastases

5. Complications

a. Urinary retention

b. Incontinence

c. Fistula formation

d. Urethral calculi formation

e. Congestive heart failure or pulmonary edema

f. Dilutional hyponatremia

g. Delayed wound healing or infection

h. Hemorrhage

i. Transurethral resection syndrome (often manifested in PACU)

j. Erectile dysfunction

k. Bladder neck contracture

l. Epididymitis

m. Osteitis pubis

K. Minimally invasive surgery for prostate cancer

1. Cryosurgical ablation of the prostate

a. Purpose or procedure

(1) Percutaneous transperineal approach

(2) Utilizes ultrasound with transrectal transducer

(3) Multiple small probes are placed into prostate gland.

(4) Freezes gland using helium and argon gas (Joules Thompson effect)

(a) Argon gas creates freeze.

(b) Helium causes thaw.

b. Intraoperative concerns

(1) Damage to urethra, sigmoid, rectum and bladder

(2) Peripheral vascular injury

(3) Urethral warming catheter to prevent urethral freeze

c. Postanesthesia priorities

(1) Maintain catheter patency.

(2) Monitor urinary output.

d. Psychosocial concerns

(1) Fear of impotence

(2) Fear of incontinence

(3) Concern about recurrence

e. Complications

(1) Urinary retention secondary to edema

(2) Sloughing of urethra

2. Brachytherapy (transperineal implantation of radioactive seeds)
   a. Purpose or procedure
      (1) Percutaneous transperineal approach
      (2) Iodine-125 or palladium-123 seeds
      (3) Utilizes ultrasound with transrectal transducer and fluoroscopy
   b. Intraoperative concerns
      (1) Risk for seed migration into urethra, bladder, perineum, neurovascular bundles, and rectum
      (2) Peripheral vascular compromise (alternating compression stockings)
   c. Postanesthesia priorities
      (1) Pain management
      (2) Maintain catheter patency.
      (3) Monitor urinary output.
      (4) Alpha-blockers may be used to assist voiding.
      (5) Perineal bruising and swelling (ice)
   d. Psychosocial concerns
      (1) Concern over radiation exposure to others
      (2) Fear of recurrence
   e. Complications
      (1) Voiding dysfunction secondary to edema
      (2) Rectal complications
      (3) Urethral stricture
L. Minimally invasive surgery for BPH
   1. Interstitial laser coagulation of the prostate (Indigo)
      a. Purpose or procedure
         (1) Treatment of urinary outflow obstruction secondary to BPH
         (2) May be combined with transurethral incision of the prostate (TUIP) and/or suprapubic cystostomy
         (3) Intended for men over 50 with prostate glands of 20 to 85 cc
            (a) Minimizes risk for impotence and incontinence
            (b) Prostate shrinks over time; no tissue is sloughed.
      b. Intraoperative concerns
         (1) Peripheral vascular injury
         (2) Ultrasound guidance with transrectal transducer
         (3) Monitored intravenous sedation with local instillation, general or spinal anesthesia
      c. Postanesthesia priorities
         (1) Maintain catheter patency.
         (2) Observe for dysuria.
         (3) Increase intake to minimize bleeding.
      d. Psychosocial concerns
         (1) Fear of cancer
         (2) Fear of recurrence
      e. Complications
         (1) Urinary retention
         (2) Dysuria
   2. Transurethral microwave therapy (TUMT) (Prostatron)
      a. Purpose or procedure
         (1) Microwave therapy applies heat to prostate.
         (2) Able to treat deep transitional zone of gland
      b. Intraoperative concerns
         (1) Cooling catheter in urethra
         (2) Rectal temperature probe
         (3) Monitored intravenous sedation with local instillation

        c. Postanesthesia priorities

           (1) Maintain catheter patency.

           (2) Observe for signs of discomfort.

           (3) Catheter commonly removed before discharge from hospital

           (4) Patient should demonstrate ability to void.

        d. Psychosocial concerns

           (1) Fear of cancer

           (2) Fear of continued urinary symptoms

        e. Complications

           (1) Urethral burn

           (2) Rectal burn

           (3) Urinary retention secondary to edema

M. Penile implant or penile vein ligation

    1. Purpose or procedure

        a. Correct erectile dysfunction through implant or venous diversion

        b. Techniques for arterial revascularization also being accomplished but less common

    2. Intraoperative concerns

        a. Infection

        b. Hemorrhage

    3. Postanesthesia priorities

        a. Frequent dressing assessment for hemorrhage

        b. Maintenance of urinary catheter

        c. Compression dressings with venous ligations

    4. Psychosocial concerns

        a. Impotence anxiety

        b. Loss of self-esteem

    5. Complications

        a. Wound infection

        b. Erosion of implant

        c. Mechanical failure of implant

        d. Hemorrhage

        e. Persistent pain

N. Circumcision

    1. Purpose or procedure

        a. Correction of constricting foreskin

        b. Surgical excision of redundant foreskin

    2. Intraoperative concerns

        a. Bleeding

        b. Suture line integrity

    3. Postanesthesia priorities

        a. Frequent dressing assessment

           (1) Edema

           (2) Hemorrhage

        b. Ice applications as needed

        c. Pain management

    4. Psychosocial concerns

        a. Embarrassment

        b. Loss

    5. Complications

        a. Excessive scarring

        b. Hemorrhage

O. Hypospadias repair or urethroplasty

    1. Purpose or procedure

        a. Urethral or meatal reconstruction and repositioning

        b. Often a staged procedure

        c. High percentage is children.

    2. Intraoperative concerns

    a. Urethral damage

    b. Infection

    c. Peripheral circulation or body temperature

  3. Postanesthesia priorities

    a. Catheter care and maintenance

    b. Monitor urinary output.

    c. Fluid and electrolyte balance

    d. Body temperature

    e. Frequent dressing assessment or changes

  4. Psychosocial concerns

    a. Anxiety (most are children)

    b. Parental separation in PACU

  5. Complications

    a. Infection

    b. Urethral stricture

    c. Excessive scarring

    d. Urinary retention

P. Orchiectomy (radical, simple)

  1. Purpose or procedure

    a. Removal of diseased testis

    b. Scrotal or inguinal approach

    c. Adjunct therapy for prostatic carcinoma

    d. Radical may include retroperitoneal lymphadenectomy.

  2. Intraoperative concerns

    a. Cardiac dysrhythmias from traction on spermatic cord

    b. Hypothermia

    c. Hemorrhage

  3. Postanesthesia priorities

    a. Compression dressings

    b. Ice packs

    c. Catheter and drain care

    d. Fluid and electrolyte balance

    e. ECG changes

  4. Psychosocial concerns

    a. Altered body image (loss of manhood)

    b. Concern over fertility

    c. Concern over sexual ability

  5. Complications

    a. Hemorrhage

    b. Shock

    c. Infection

Q. Penectomy (partial or total)

  1. Purpose or procedure

    a. Carcinoma of the penis

    b. Extent of resection dependent on location and stage of tumor

    c. Prognosis dependent on lymph nodes and metastasis

    d. Inguinal dissection may be necessary.

  2. Intraoperative concerns

    a. Hemostasis

    b. Urinary function

  3. Postanesthesia priorities

    a. Edema (compression and ice)

    b. Pain management

    c. Hemorrhage

    d. Urinary output

  4. Psychosocial concerns

    a. Altered body image (disfigurement)

    b. Fear of metastasis

     5. Complications
       a. Sloughing of tissue
       b. Inability to urinate
       c. Bleeding
       d. Infection
 R. Orchidopexy (orchiopexy)
     1. Purpose or procedure
       a. Placement of undescended testis in normal anatomic position within scrotum
       b. Inguinal approach usually includes hernia repair.
       c. Performed for torsion of the testis to prevent recurrence
     2. Intraoperative concerns
       a. Body temperature (many are small children)
       b. Burns
         (1) Warming blankets
         (2) Preparation solutions
         (3) Electrocautery
       c. Bleeding
     3. Postanesthesia priorities
       a. Traction on testis usually afforded by subdartos pouch
         (1) Older methods used external fixation with rubber band to inner upper thigh or dental roll to scrotum
         (2) Older methods increase risk of testicular necrosis.
       b. Titrate small doses of pain remedies as ordered.
       c. Examine frequently for edema and hemorrhage.
       d. Ice packs to scrotum
     4. Psychosocial concerns
       a. Anxiety separation from parents
       b. Fear of surroundings
       c. Promote calm environment to limit activity of child.
     5. Complications
       a. Compromise of testicular blood supply
       b. Torsion of spermatic cord
       c. Hemorrhage
       d. Dislodgment of traction device
 S. Varicocelectomy
     1. Purpose or procedure
       a. Collection of large dilated veins ligated
       b. Commonly in left scrotum
       c. Varicosities affect fertility.
       d. Necessary for pain relief
       e. Scrotal or low inguinal incision
       f. May be performed laparoscopically
     2. Intraoperative concerns
       a. Damage to companion arteries
       b. Bleeding
       c. Injury to vas deferens
     3. Postanesthesia priorities
       a. Edema (ice)
       b. Pain (medication)
       c. Hemorrhage (compressive dressings)
     4. Psychosocial concerns
       a. Infertility
       b. Concern about long-term pain relief
     5. Complications
       a. Scrotal hematoma
       b. Hemorrhage
       c. Continued persistent pain
       d. Injury to vas deferens

   T. Spermatocelectomy
1. Purpose or procedure
   a. Removal of cystic mass at head of epididymis
   b. Not uncommon complication following vasectomy
2. Intraoperative concerns
   a. Injury to vas deferens
   b. Hemorrhage
   c. Compromise to spermatic vessels
3. Postanesthesia priorities
   a. Edema (ice)
   b. Hemorrhage (compressive dressings)
   c. Pain (medication, ice)
4. Psychosocial concerns
   a. Infertility
   b. Pain
5. Complications
   a. Injury to vas deferens
   b. Scrotal hematoma

   U. Hydrocelectomy
1. Purpose or procedure
   a. Excision of tunica vaginalis
   b. Expression of excessive accumulation of normal fluid between testis and tunica
   c. Generally scrotal incision
2. Intraoperative concerns
   a. Testicular damage
   b. Drain insertion
3. Postanesthesia priorities
   a. Pressure dressings
   b. Assess character and amount of drainage.
   c. Scrotal support
   d. Ice to area
      (1) Edema
      (2) Pain
      (3) Hemorrhage
4. Psychosocial concerns
   a. Embarrassment
   b. Concern about sexual function
5. Complications
   a. Hematoma
   b. Compromise of testicular blood supply

   V. Detorsion of spermatic cord/testis
1. Purpose or procedure
   a. Spermatic cord brought into proper position and sutured to scrotal wall
   b. Highest incidence in teenage boys
   c. Bilateral often done to avoid same occurrence in unaffected testis
2. Intraoperative concerns
   a. Compromise of blood supply to testis
   b. Testicular hypertrophy
3. Postanesthesia priorities
   a. Observe for sudden severe pain.
   b. Maintain compressive dressings.
4. Psychosocial concerns
   a. Anxiety about testicular integrity
   b. Embarrassment
5. Complications
   a. Hemorrhage (orchiectomy could result if strangulation ensues)

      b. Persistent pain

      c. Sterility

  W. Vasectomy

    1. Purpose or procedure

      a. Elective sterilization

      b. Scrotal approach with patient under any type of anesthesia

    2. Intraoperative concerns

      a. Adequate ligation of bilateral vas deferens

      b. Too high a ligation could result in chronic pain

    3. Postanesthesia priorities (see information on hydrocelectomy in section U above)

    4. Psychosocial concerns

      a. Ambivalence over decision

      b. Fear of impotence

      c. Association with prostate cancer has been disproved; many patients still express concerns, however.

      d. Concern about continued presence of viable sperm

    5. Complications

      a. Varicocele

      b. Spermatocele

      c. Chronic pain

      d. Migration of vas causing reconnection and resumption of fertility

  X. Vasovasostomy or epididymovasostomy

    1. Purpose or procedure

      a. To reverse previous vasectomy

      b. To correct stenosis of vas deferens or epididymis

      c. Involves microscopic techniques

    2. Intraoperative concerns

      a. Presence of live sperm cells

      b. Stress on anastomosis because of inadequate length

    3. Postanesthesia priorities

      a. Compression dressings

      b. Assess for bleeding.

      c. Ice to control edema

    4. Psychosocial concerns

      a. Desire for fertility

      b. Fear that procedure will not help

    5. Complications

      a. Infection

      b. Fibrosis at anastomosis site

III. Laparoscopy

  A. Recent surgical modality used as alternate operative approach

  B. Purpose or procedures

    1. Large incisions are avoided.

    2. Postoperative course tends to be shorter.

    3. Procedures currently being performed

      a. Adrenalectomy

      b. Nephrectomy, nephroureterectomy

      c. Ureteropelvic junction (UPJ) repair (pyeloplasty)

      d. Ureteral reimplantation

      e. Ureterolithotomy, pyelolithotomy

      f. Renal cyst decortication

      g. Cryoablation of renal neoplasms

      h. Pelvic lymph node dissection

      i. Retroperitoneal lymph node dissection

      j. Bladder neck suspension

      k. Radical prostatectomy

      l. Radical cystectomy

      m. Ileal conduit, Indiana pouch, and orthotopic neobladder

    n. Varicocelectomy (uncommon presently)

    o. Lymphocele excision

C. Intraoperative concerns

    1. Improper trocar placement

      a. Subcutaneous emphysema

      b. Preperitoneal insufflation

      c. Vascular injury

      d. Organ perforation

    2. Incorrect positioning can lead to peripheral nerve damage.

      a. Well-padded bony prominences

      b. Pronated hands

      c. Shoulder braces placed over bony aspects, not soft tissue

      d. Extreme hip or sacral positions done cautiously

    3. Cardiac dysrhythmias (bradycardia, premature ventricular contractions, sinus tachycardia)

    4. Blood pressure fluctuations (hypotension, hypertension)

    5. Central venous pressure irregularities

    6. Venous gas embolus

    7. Hypoxemia from restricted movement of diaphragm or pulmonary blood pooling

    8. Aspiration from increased abdominal pressure

    9. Pneumothorax if CO_2 enters pleural space

    10. Pneumoscrotum—most common postoperative complaint

D. Postanesthesia priorities

    1. O_2 to assist pulmonary exchange

    2. Pain management to lessen effects of abdominal distension and muscular soreness from position (patient may experience referred shoulder pain from CO_2 mobilization)

    3. Frequent vital signs with attention to blood pressure and respiration

    4. Monitor urinary output.

    5. ECG monitor to assess cardiac status

E. Psychosocial concerns

    1. Fear of cancer

    2. Anxiety over potential internal injury resulting from surgery

F. Complications

    1. Fever or peritonitis from bowel perforation

    2. Hemorrhage from vessel injury intraoperatively

    3. Incisional hernias

    4. Ascites, hyponatremia, or azotemia from unrecognized bladder perforation

    5. Abdominal adhesions caused by excessive manipulation

    6. Pneumoscrotum, pneumothorax, lymphocele, or lymph obstruction

BIBLIOGRAPHY

1. Appell R, Boone T, et al: *Guidelines: Treatment options for patients with overactive bladder; 2000-version 1.0.* Baltimore, MD: National Association for Continence/American MECCA, 2000.

2. Cancer Treatment Centers of America at Tulsa: Hormone therapy for prostate cancer. Available at http://www.brachytherapy.com/hormone.html. Accessed on August 27, 2001.

3. Donnelly BJ, Saliken JC: Management of radiation failure in prostate cancer: Salvage cryosurgery—how I do it. *Rev Urol* 4(2): 25-29, 2002.

4. Ellsworth P, Heaney JA, Gill O: *100 Questions and answers about prostate cancer.* Sudbury, MA: Jones & Bartlett, 2003.

5. Gill IS, Ulchaker JC: World's first laparoscopic orthotopic neobladder: The final frontier? *Urology news*: Laparoscopy, 2001. Available at http://www.clevelandclinic.org/urology/news/laparo/vol8d.htm. Accessed on December 29, 2002.

6. Gillenwater JY, Howards SS, Grayhack JT, et al, editors: *Adult and pediatric urology*, ed 4. St Louis: Mosby, 2002.

7. Kirby RS: *An atlas of uro-oncology.* New York: Parthenon/CRC, 2002.

8. Kirby R, Carson C, Goldstein I: *Erectile dysfunction: A clinical guide.* Oxford, UK: Isis Medical Media, 1999.

9. Krane RJ, Siroky MB, Fitzpatrick JM: *Surgical skills: Operative urology,* Philadelphia: Churchill Livingstone, 2000.

10. Marks S: *Prostate and cancer,* Cambridge: Fisher Books/Perseus, 1999.

11. Miller RD, Miller ED, Reves, JG, et al: *Anesthesia,* ed 5. Philadelphia: Churchill-Livingstone-Harcourt, 2000.

12. Nagle GM: Genitourinary surgery. In Rothrock JC, editor: *Alexander's care of the patient in surgery,* ed 12. St Louis: Mosby, 2003, pp 519-618.

13. Pagana KD, Pagana TJ: *Diagnostic testing and nursing implications: A case study approach,* ed 5. St Louis: Mosby, 1999.

14. Pagana KD, Pagana TJ: *Mosby's diagnostic and laboratory test reference,* ed 6. St Louis: Elsevier Science, 2002.

15. Partin AW, Schell PJ: *eMediguides.com— urology and nephrology: 05/02-04/03,* Princeton, NJ: Thomson Medical Economics, 2002.

16. Perry K, Zisman A, Pantuck AJ, et al: Ablative techniques in the treatment of renal cell carcinoma. *Rev Urol* 4(3):103-111, 2002.

17. Prostate cancer (early stage). Available at LifeExtension Foundation Web site: http://www.lef.org/protocols/prtcl-093a.shtml. Accessed on August 27, 2001.

18. *Prostate cancer: What it is and how it is treated,* Wilmington, DE: AZ Pharmaceuticals, 2002.

19. Ragde H, Grado GL, Nadir B, et al: Modern prostate brachytherapy. *CA Cancer J Clin* 50(6):380-393, 2000.

20. Schultz RE, Oliver AW: *Humanizing prostate cancer: A physician-patient perspective,* White Stone, VA: Brandylane, 2000.

21. Tanagho EA, McAninch JW: *Smith's general urology,* ed 15. East Norwalk, CN: Lange Medical Books/McGraw-Hill, 2000.

22. Tanga SS, Smith RB, Ehrlich RM: *Complications of urologic surgery: Prevention and management,* ed 3. Philadelphia: WB Saunders, 2001.

23. Testicular cancer and self-exam. Available at http://www.mcare.org/healthathome/testicul.htm. Accessed on December 24, 2003.

24. Walsh P, Retick AB, Darracott VE Jr, et al: *Campbell's urology,* ed 8. Philadelphia: WB Saunders, 2002.

25. Walsh P, Worthington JF: *Dr. Patrick Walsh's guide to surviving prostate cancer,* New York: Warner, 2001.

26. Winkelman C: Assessment of the renal/urinary system. In Ignatavicius DD, Workman ML, editors: *Medical-surgical nursing: Critical thinking for collaborative care,* ed 4. Philadelphia: WB Saunders, 2002, pp 1589-1597.

45 Gynecologic and Reproductive Surgery

DENISE O'BRIEN

OBJECTIVES

At the conclusion of this chapter the reader will be able to:

1. Describe anatomy and physiology of female reproductive organs and structures pertinent to the patient undergoing gynecologic and reproductive procedures.

2. Identify assessment parameters for patients undergoing gynecologic and reproductive operative procedures.

3. Define nursing care priorities in each postanesthesia phase.

4. Describe patient education following gynecologic and reproductive procedures related to diet, pain management, wound care, activity, and follow-up.

Patients undergo gynecologic surgery for acute or chronic, elective or emergent reasons. Surgical intervention may be required for a variety of indications ranging from simple diagnostic procedures to radical excisions for malignancy.

This chapter defines and discusses major and minor gynecologic procedures and perioperative concerns. Nursing management strategies are discussed as they relate to specific complications.

I. Anatomy and physiology
    A. External genitalia collectively known as vulva (see Figure 45-1)
        1. Mons: rounded fleshy prominence over the symphysis pubis
        2. Labia
            a. Majora: larger outer skin folds surrounding the vaginal orifice
            b. Minora: inner folds surrounding the vaginal orifice
        3. Clitoris: small projection of erectile tissue located at the upper ends of the labia minora
        4. Hymen: thin membrane partially covering the vaginal orifice (may be absent)
        5. Vestibule: space between the labia minora into which the urethra and vagina open
        6. Skene's ducts: paraurethral ducts that drain a group of urethral glands into the vestibule
        7. Bartholin's glands: two small mucoid-secreting glands on either side of and posterior to the vaginal orifice
        8. Urinary meatus: opening of urethra, located between clitoris and vaginal orifice
        9. Perineum: between the vulva and anus
    B. Internal genital structures (see Figure 45-2)
        1. Vagina
            a. Canal, extending from vulva to cervix uteri, between the bladder and rectum
            b. Lined with mucous membrane; muscles and fibrous tissue form the walls
            c. Coital organ, passage for menstrual discharge, functions as the birth canal
        2. Uterus
            a. Hollow muscular organ, normally pear sized; muscular walls, lined with mucous membrane

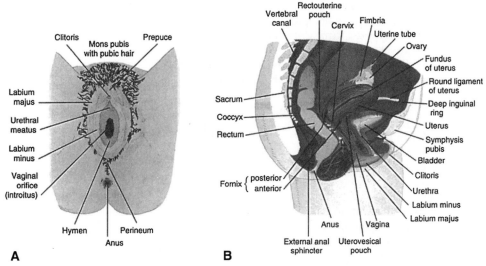

FIGURE 45-1 ■ **A,** Anatomic landmarks of external female genitalia. **B,** Midsagittal section of the female pelvis. (From Black JM, Matassarin-JE: *Medical-surgical nursing, Clinical management for continuity of care,* ed 5. Philadelphia: WB Saunders, 1997.)

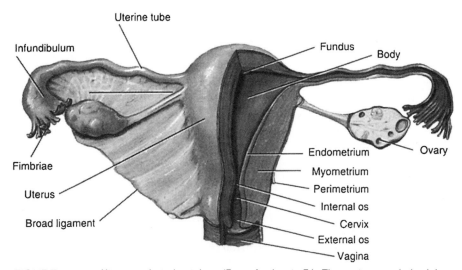

FIGURE 45-2 ■ Uterus and uterine tubes. (From Applegate EJ: *The anatomy and physiology learning system.* Philadelphia: WB Saunders, 1995.)

    b. Consists of corpus and cervix
        (1) Corpus includes fundus (dome)
        (2) Cervix (neck): lower, narrow part of uterus, extending into vagina
    c. Myometrium: muscular substance of uterus
    d. Endometrium: inner lining composed of mucous membrane
    e. Functions
        (1) Contain products of conception until time of delivery
        (2) Lining shed (menstruation) in monthly cycle in the absence of
            fertilization and implantation of embryo
  3. Fallopian tube
    a. One of two tubes, attached on each side of uterus, extending to ovary
    b. Conveys ova to uterus, spermatozoa in opposite direction

        c. Fertilization usually occurs in the tube.

        d. Typical site of ectopic pregnancy

        e. Interrupted during sterilization procedures

    4. Ovary

        a. Paired oval organs one on either side of uterus

        b. Attached to the posterior surface of the broad ligament

        c. Functions

            (1) Production of ovum

            (2) Hormone production: estrogen, progesterone

    5. Ligaments

        a. Broad

        b. Round

        c. Cardinal

        d. Uterosacral

        e. Utero-ovarian

        f. Infundibulopelvic

    6. Vasculature

        a. Internal and external iliac artery and vein after common iliac artery and common iliac vein bifurcate

        b. Hypogastric (same as internal iliac)

        c. Branches

            (1) Pudendal

            (2) Uterine artery: superior, inferior

    7. Nerves

        a. Femoral

        b. Obturator

        c. Genitofemoral

        d. Pudendal

        e. Superior and inferior hypogastric plexus

  C. Associated structures

    1. Bladder, ureters, urethra

    2. Sigmoid colon and rectum

    3. Pelvic floor muscles

    4. Lymph nodes

II. Pathophysiology

  A. Congenital and anatomic abnormalities

    1. Imperforate hymen

    2. Herniations

        a. Cystocele: herniation of bladder that causes anterior vaginal wall to bulge downward

        b. Rectocele: formed by protrusion of anterior rectal wall (posterior vaginal wall) into vagina

        c. Enterocele: herniation of cul-de-sac of Douglas, which almost always contains loops of small intestine

        d. Urethrocele: pouchlike protrusion of urethral wall and thickening of connective tissue around urethra

    3. Uterine displacement

    4. Prolapsed uterus

    5. Bicornuate uterus

    6. Septate uterus

    7. Tubal incompetency

  B. Endocrine (hormonal) dysfunction

    1. Endometriosis

    2. Dysfunctional uterine bleeding

    3. Stein-Leventhal syndrome (polycystic ovary syndrome)

  C. Growths and neoplasms

    1. Cysts: closed sack or pouch with definite wall that contains fluid, semifluid, or solid material

        a. Bartholin's (gland)

        b. Ovarian

    2. Uterine fibroids or myomatas: tumor containing muscle tissue

    3. Carcinomas: malignant tumor growth in epithelial tissue

        a. Vulvar

        b. Cervical

        c. Uterine

        d. Ovarian

    4. Polyps: benign tumor with pedicle; usually removed if there is a possibility that it will become malignant; prone to bleed

        a. Cervical

        b. Uterine

    5. Condylomata: wartlike growths of the skin; usually seen on external genitalia or in anal region

  D. Infections and inflammatory processes

    1. Pelvic inflammatory disease (PID)

        a. Affects abdominal organs

        b. May result in infertility

    2. Abscesses

        a. Perineal region

        b. Abdominal organs

    3. Fistulas

        a. Urethrovaginal

        b. Rectovaginal

  E. Pregnancy related

    1. Abortion

        a. Incomplete: abortion in which parts of products of conception have been retained in uterus

        b. Missed: abortion in which fetus has died before twentieth completed week of gestation, but products of conception are retained in uterus for 8 weeks or longer

        c. Therapeutic: abortion performed when mental or physical health of mother is endangered by continuation of pregnancy

    2. Incompetent cervix

    3. Ectopic pregnancy: pregnancy occurring outside uterine cavity

        a. Commonly occurs in fallopian tube

        b. Life threatening if ruptured; may result in hemorrhage or loss of tube or ovary

    4. Hydatidiform mole: degenerative process in chorionic villi that gives rise to multiple cysts and rapid growth of uterus with possible hemorrhage; usually surgically removed by laparotomy

III. Preanesthesia assessment priorities

  A. Examination

    1. Pelvic

        a. Inspection of external genitalia

        b. Speculum exam of vagina and cervix

        c. Palpation of any visible abnormalities to determine consistency, mobility, and relation to adjacent structures

        d. Papanicolaou's test (Pap smear): for detection and diagnosis of malignant and premalignant conditions of the vagina, cervix, endometrium

        e. Obtain wet preparation (yeast infection, bacterial infection, and trichomonas) and cultures for sexually transmitted diseases (gonorrhea and chlamydia).

        f. Bimanual: the abdominal hand presses the pelvic organs to be palpated toward the intravaginal hand.

    2. Menstrual history

        a. Onset of menses, length of cycles, regularity of cycles

        b. Duration, amount, and content of flow

      c. Date of last menstrual period

      d. Contraceptive use or absence

      e. Definitions

         (1) Menarche: beginning of menstrual function

         (2) Amenorrhea: absence or abnormal stoppage of menses

         (3) Oligomenorrhea: infrequent menstrual flow occurring at intervals of 35 days to 6 months

         (4) Menorrhagia: hypermenorrhea

         (5) Menometrorrhagia: excessive uterine bleeding occurring both during menses and at irregular intervals

3. Gravidity

  a. Number of pregnancies

  b. Number of deliveries, terminations (spontaneous, elective)

4. Virilizing features: hair growth, irregular absent periods

5. Emotional state

  a. Psychosocial: family and partner support or lack of support

  b. Need sympathetic and understanding approach

  c. Infertility

     (1) May be associated with specific psychological problems, ranging from anxiety and stress disorders to compulsive-obsessive neurosis

  d. Loss of desired pregnancy

  e. Surgically induced hormonal changes

  f. Concerns or fears for invasion of privacy

  g. History of sexual abuse and violence

6. Other assessment factors

  a. Neurovascular assessment of lower extremities

  b. Laboratory values

     (1) Hematology values: complete blood cell count, type, and screen

     (2) Chemistry values: serum electrolytes, glucose, beta HCG (pregnancy)

     (3) Urinalysis: bacteria, glucose, protein, ketones, red blood cells, pregnancy

     (4) Cytologic studies: Papanicolaou (Pap) smears, previous cryotherapy, biopsy reports

  c. Radiologic studies

     (1) Chest film: as indicated by history of cardiopulmonary problems

  d. Ultrasonography

  e. Electrocardiogram and stress test: as indicated by history of cardiopulmonary problems

  f. Physical limitations relating to

     (1) Arthritis

     (2) Musculoskeletal disorders

     (3) Implanted joints

  g. Resulting in potential alteration of anesthetic choice or positioning of patient (e.g., lithotomy)

  h. Allergies to dyes (injected during procedure)

B. Increased risk associated with history or need to alter perioperative management

  1. Deep vein thrombosis (DVT)

  2. Obesity

  3. Tobacco use

  4. Pregnancy

  5. Chronic pain

    a. Pain tolerance alterations

    b. Chronic analgesic use may alter postoperative analgesic management.

  6. Developmentally challenged

    a. Potential behavioral problems (combative, disruptive, abusive)

    b. Legal authorization appropriately obtained before treatment commences

    C. Determine the educational needs of patient, caregiver.
        1. Analgesia, preoperative anxiety
        2. Projected effect (if any) on sexual activity, fertility
        3. Discharge planning
            a. Comfortable loose clothing to wear home, especially following laparoscopy
            b. Supply of dressings or supplies needed (perineal pads, tampons)
            c. Possible need for catheters and drains
            d. Caregiver available for first 24 hours postoperatively (for outpatients)
IV. Intraoperative priorities
    A. Anesthesia choice
        1. General
            a. Endotracheal tube (ETT), laryngeal mask airway (LMA), or mask depending on operative procedure, patient needs and physical habitus
            b. Use of total intravenous technique (propofol and an opioid analgesic) can reduce the incidence of postoperative nausea and vomiting (PONV).
        2. Regional: spinal or epidural
        3. Monitored anesthesia care (MAC)
        4. Sedation and analgesia with local anesthesia
        5. Local anesthesia used alone for minor or office procedures
            a. Paracervical block
            b. Pudendal block
    B. Intraoperative concerns
        1. Lithotomy position
            a. Elevate and lower legs together to avoid strain of back and leg muscles.
            b. Avoid any abnormal movement of the knee or pressure on the knee.
            c. Avoid extreme flexion of hips or popliteal pressure.
            d. Pad lumbar region to prevent pressure.
            e. After positioning, assess neuromuscular status and reposition if compromised.
        2. Arms and hands are safely positioned and shoulders are padded during Trendelenburg position.
        3. Fingers need protection from impingement, especially when positioning and at end of procedure when repositioning for transfer.
        4. Maintain patient's dignity.
        5. Skin integrity can be compromised if iodine-based preparation solutions are allowed to pool under the patient; can lead to burns of the skin.
    C. Procedural techniques: Special cautions and care are required with each technique. Refer to equipment training and maintenance literature for specific information on precautions, hazards, and safe use of the equipment in the operating room (OR) environment.
        1. Microsurgical
        2. Endoscopic
            a. Laparoscope
                (1) Usually use CO_2 gas as insufflating medium for creation of pneumoperitoneum
                (2) Gasless: uses a mechanical lift method
            b. Hysteroscope
                (1) Rigid scope most commonly used
                (2) Flexible scopes available, not widely used
        3. Laser, cautery, cryotherapy
        4. Transvaginal ultrasonography
        5. Transvaginal fluoroscopy: used infrequently because of risk of radiation exposure to reproductive organs
    D. Intraoperative complications
        1. Gas embolism
        2. Fluid overload, dilutional hyponatremia
        3. Hemorrhage

    4. Perforation of hollow organs or vessels

    5. Thermal injuries

    6. Aspiration

    7. Perioperative neuropathy

V. Postanesthesia priorities (see Box 45-1)

    A. Phase I priorities

        1. Airway

            a. Spontaneous, unassisted breathing

            b. Adjunct or endotracheal tube in place

            c. Observe for respiratory complications.

                (1) Risk for pulmonary edema following hysteroscopy if excessive irrigant or distending media used

                (2) If intubated, assess location of tube by auscultating chest (dislocation of tube can occur from pneumoperitoneum).

        2. Hemodynamic stability

            a. Vital signs stable, consistent with baseline

            b. Observe for cardiovascular complications.

        3. Bleeding

            a. Vaginal

                (1) Cervical

                (2) Uterine

                    (a) Assess uterine firmness following dilation and extraction (D & E).

                        (i) Oxytocin (Pitocin®) may be needed in advanced pregnancy termination to produce control bleeding.

                    (b) Methylergonovine (Methergine®) for prevention and treatment of postpartum and postabortion hemorrhage.

                    (c) Rh factor identified for Rh-negative patients to receive Rh immune globulin injection

                    (d) Observe for passage of clots.

■ BOX 45-1
■ **KEY PATIENT EDUCATIONAL OUTCOMES**

Phase I
Patient will express feelings of lessened anxiety.
Patient will describe minimal to tolerable pain.
Patient will request analgesic to manage pain.

Phase II
Patient will tolerate discomfort following administration of oral analgesics.
Patient, family, and partner will describe wound care following instruction.
Patient will progress to upright position with minimal orthostatic effects: dizziness, lightheadedness, nausea.

Phase III
Patient, family, and partner will describe follow-up required.
Patient, family, and partner will identify risks associated with operative procedure: infection, hemorrhage, pain, vomiting.
Patient, family, and partner will describe wound observation, hand washing, how to change dressing and pads, how to cleanse wounds, and expected drainage.
Patient, family, and partner will describe at-home activity, restrictions, diet, and pain management.
Patient, family, and partner will demonstrate knowledge of medications (analgesics, antibiotics, antiemetics, etc.) by describing purpose and administration of each medication prescribed.
Patient, family, and partner will express understanding of necessity to report uncontrolled bleeding or pain.

      b. Incisional

        (1) Oozing or frank bleeding

        (2) Hematoma beneath incision

      c. Internal

        (1) Perforation of organ or vessel

        (2) Operative hemostasis not achieved or oozing

4. Report from anesthesia, surgeon, perioperative nurse

    a. Positioning of patient intraoperatively

    b. Estimated blood loss

    c. Complications

      (1) Perforation

      (2) Burn

      (3) Excessive fluid administration

5. Discomfort

    a. Incisional

    b. Cramping

    c. Significant pain following procedure: suspect perforation, hematoma formation, intraabdominal trauma

    d. Cervical and intrauterine manipulation may result in prostaglandin release, which can result in continued postoperative pain.

6. Dressing and drains

    a. Abdominal incisions

      (1) Adhesive bandages or no dressing over trocar insertion sites following laparoscopic procedures

      (2) Gauze and tape dressing over longer incisions

    b. Perineal pad in place following cervical, uterine procedures

      (1) Assess on arrival and regularly for type and amount of bleeding.

      (2) Notify surgeon of bleeding saturating more than a pad an hour.

    c. Vaginal packing: removable, absorbable, hemostatic material

      (1) Observe minimal perineal bleeding.

      (2) Patient may have urge to defecate from pressure of packing.

    d. Drains

      (1) Bartholin cyst incision and drainage or marsupialization

      (2) Vaginal drains include T tube, Malecot.

      (3) Grenade (Jackson-Pratt)

      (4) Maintain patency of drains.

7. Edema

    a. May observe subcutaneous edema from laparoscopic CO_2 insufflation

    b. External vulvar lesions: swelling may be reduced with application of ice or cold therapy.

8. Fluids and nutrition

    a. Do not force fluids, especially when nausea and vomiting present.

    b. Causes of nausea and vomiting

      (1) Opioid analgesics, neuromuscular reversal (neostigmine and pyridostigmine have been associated with increased PONV)

      (2) Pain also major cause of nausea after gynecologic surgery

      (3) Starvation leading to weakness, low blood sugar levels

      (4) Controversy exists regarding effect of menstrual cycle and timing of operative procedure on PONV.

    c. Hydrate with intravenous (IV) fluids (replacement and maintenance).

      (1) Usual lactated Ringer's (Hartmann's) or dextrose-containing solutions

      (2) Long laparoscopic procedures with dry insufflating gases may increase patient's fluid replacement needs.

    d. When nausea or vomiting are present

      (1) Administer antiemetics as ordered; determine if antiemetic prophylaxis given.

> (2) Commonly use promethazine, 5HT3 serotonin antagonists (e.g., ondansetron, dolasetron)

   9. Postlithotomy and postlaparoscopy neurovascular checks

     a. Nerve damage secondary to positioning or retractor injuries or surgical transection

     b. Pain, numbness, tingling of extremities, and loss of motor function in a given muscle group should be reported.

   10. Urinary distention

     a. Risk following gynecologic procedures, which either results in edema surrounding the urethra or injury to urethra and related structures (e.g., vaginal hysterectomy)

     b. Overdistention can cause temporary paralysis of the detrusor muscle, taking several days to resolve.

     c. May require indwelling catheter or intermittent catheterization

   11. Emotional support needed; may express anger, fear, depression

     a. Adolescents and young adults embarrassed

     b. Pregnancy loss

     c. Negative findings and outcomes

B. Phase II priorities

   1. Operative site

     a. Observe for bleeding, superficial hematoma formation around trocar insertion sites.

     b. Change or reinforce dressing as necessary.

     c. Monitor perineal pad drainage every hour and when patient ambulates first time.

       (1) Note amount and type of drainage.

       (2) Notify surgeon of significant bleeding or passage of clots, excessive cramping.

   2. Discomfort

     a. Gently palpate abdomen.

       (1) Expect soft, slightly tender to touch, slightly distended.

       (2) Notify surgeon of excessive tenderness, firmness, swelling, or suspected hematoma formation.

     b. Oral analgesic medications initiated in preparation for discharge home

       (1) May have started in postanesthesia care unit (PACU) phase I

       (2) Combination of opioid medication and nonsteroidal antiinflammatory drugs (NSAIDs) can provide effective analgesia following gynecologic procedures.

       (3) Determine effectiveness of medication before patient discharged home on same analgesic(s).

       (4) Patient with history of chronic pain or analgesia use may require greater support and alteration of usual pain-management protocols.

       (5) If ineffective, may need prescription changed or other follow-up

     c. Comfort measures

       (1) Positioning and repositioning to relieve or diminish discomfort

       (2) Back rub or massage may be comforting.

       (3) Continue ice therapy as ordered.

       (4) Promote relaxation techniques.

   3. Urinary retention

     a. Assess bladder status.

     b. Avoid overdistention.

     c. Determine adequate fluid replacement.

     d. May need intermittent catheterization until able to void

   4. Fluids and nutrition

     a. Avoid forced fluid intake if nausea and/or vomiting present.

     b. Dry crackers may help ease nausea.

     c. Maintain intravenous fluids to ensure adequate hydration.

5. Education
   a. Includes patient, family, responsible adult
   b. Instructions
      (1) Infections—signs and symptoms
      (2) Persistent pain or bleeding
      (3) Be alert for complications.
      (4) Pain-relief alternatives
C. After discharge—phase III
   1. Nutrition and diet
      a. Eat lightly following the procedure.
      b. If foods do not sound good, avoid and continue to drink fluids.
      c. Usually can begin regular diet after 24 hours, if not earlier
      d. Encourage fluid intake especially during hot weather.
      e. Avoid constipation through increased dietary fiber, bulking agents.
   2. Nausea and vomiting
      a. Prepare patient, family, and partner for possibility of nausea and vomiting.
      b. Caution patient, family, and partner to call surgeon or facility if nausea and/or vomiting persists for >6 hours.
   3. Pain
      a. Oral analgesics
         (1) Suggest contacting surgeon if pain is not relieved by prescribed analgesics or is intolerable or increasing.
         (2) Unrelieved or increasing pain may indicate
            (a) Infection
            (b) Peritonitis
            (c) Perforation
            (d) Hematoma
      b. Postoperative deep vein thrombosis can develop following hysterectomy or lengthy lithotomy procedures.
         (1) The following may indicate deep vein thrombosis
            (a) Lower extremity pain
            (b) Edema
            (c) Erythema
            (d) Prominent vascular pattern of the superficial veins
         (2) The following are diagnostic of pulmonary embolism
            (a) Pleuritic chest pain
            (b) Hemoptysis
            (c) Shortness of breath
            (d) Tachycardia
            (e) Tachypnea
         (3) Patient should call surgeon immediately and proceed to the nearest medical facility for diagnosis and treatment.
      c. Alternatives
         (1) Intermittent ice for external lesions to help reduce swelling, hematoma development, and pain
         (2) Sitz baths for easing discomfort of external lesion
         (3) Explore with patient, family, or partner other potential pain management techniques.
   4. Medications: instruct on administration and how to apply.
      a. Antibiotics
      b. Analgesics
      c. Vaginal applications
      d. Topical sprays and creams
   5. Wound care
      a. Instruct the patient to wash hands before and after changing pads, dressings, applying medications.
      b. Perineal care

   (1) Change pads every 4 hours or as needed.
   (2) Note drainage: type, amount, and color.
   (3) Gently wash the perineum with mild soap and warm water, rinse, and pat dry.
   (4) Sitz baths or perineal wash as prescribed
   c. Incisional care
   (1) Keep wound clean and dry for minimum of 24 to 48 hours.
   (2) May be instructed to remove dressing after 24 to 48 hours
   (3) Observe incision for signs of infection.
      (a) Redness
      (b) Swelling
      (c) Drainage
   (4) Replace original dressing with fresh gauze or adhesive bandage as needed or as ordered.
   (5) Report signs and symptoms of infection to surgeon or nurse practitioner.
   d. Vaginal bleeding
   (1) Heavier than a menstrual period must be reported to surgeon.
   (2) Seven to ten days after cone biopsy and cervical conization bleeding may increase.

6. Urinary care
   a. Indwelling catheter (e.g., Foley) left in for continued urinary drainage
   b. Wash carefully around the urinary meatus with gentle soap and warm water, and pat dry.
   c. Keep drainage bag below level of bladder to prevent back flow.
   d. Remove at home if ordered by surgeon (send with 10 ml syringe and instructions on how to aspirate balloon and pull catheter), or arrange return appointment for catheter removal.

7. Activity
   a. Rest
   (1) Limit activity until pain, nausea, and dizziness subside.
   (2) While taking opioid analgesics, avoid operating machinery, automobiles, using sharp or potentially injurious articles, or drinking alcohol.
   b. Exercise
   (1) For first 24 hours, exercise is discouraged.
   (2) Defer vigorous activity, heavy lifting.
      (a) Restrict until surgeon allows; may be up to 4 weeks after surgery
      (b) Aerobic activity may increase heart rate and blood pressure, leading to increased bleeding.
   c. Sexual activity
   (1) Depending on location of incision, operative procedure
   (2) May be advised to avoid douching and coitus for up to 6 weeks

8. Follow-up care
   a. Arrange for return visit with surgeon in specified time interval.
   b. Return to work dependent on procedure, patient work: usually next day for minor procedures; following hysterectomy: return in 1 to 2 weeks or when capable
   c. Home visit by a registered nurse may be arranged by the surgeon following certain procedures.
   d. Fever: contact surgeon if temperature over 100.4° F (38° C) or as ordered by surgeon; check temperature every 4 hours for 2 days following procedures such as hysterectomy, twice a day following laparoscopic procedures (risk for development of peritonitis).
   e. Particularly with endoscopic procedures, patient should continue to get better every day; if not, an injury should be suspected.
   f. Keep surgeon's and surgery facility's telephone number available when questions or concerns arise.

VI. Operative procedures

Common operative procedures and techniques are included. The reader is referred to a comprehensive text on gynecologic and reproductive surgery for additional procedures and techniques.

A. External
    1. Hymenectomy
      a. Purpose: to enlarge the vaginal orifice
      b. Description: surgical excision of hymen membrane
    2. Hymenotomy
      a. Purpose: to open the vaginal orifice; used to drain hematocolpos
      b. Description: surgical incision of the hymen membrane
    3. Excision and drainage of Bartholin's cysts
      a. Purpose: surgical drainage of Bartholin's gland for relief of pain and/or infection
      b. Description: removal by cutting or systematic withdrawal of fluids or discharges with placement of Word catheter
      c. Bartholinectomy: excision of Bartholin's gland
        (1) Marsupialization of Bartholin's cyst
          (a) Creation of open pouch around excised Bartholin's gland and cyst
          (b) Facilitates drainage and healing
    4. Excision external lesion
      a. Purpose: removal of lesions (warts [condylomata], papilloma, malignant growths)
      b. Description: lesions removed by cutting, laser, electrocautery methods
        (1) Laser therapy (carbon dioxide, Nd:YAG, argon)
    5. Vulvectomy
      a. Purpose: treatment for premalignant or malignant lesions of the vulva
      b. Description: excision of labia majora, labia minora, and surrounding structures; usually requires skin graft
    6. Postanesthesia priorities
      a. Perineal care
      b. Sitz baths may be ordered.
      c. Pain management
B. Transvaginal
    1. Cervical conization and colposcopy
      a. Purpose: diagnosis or treatment of cervical infection or carcinoma in situ removal of a cone of cervical tissue (partial excision)
      b. Description: removal of a cone of cervical tissue (partial excision)
    2. Loop electrosurgical excision procedure (LEEP)
      a. Purpose: Allows entire specimen to be sectioned for diagnosis
      b. Description: removes intact tissue
        (1) Advantage over CO_2 laser for diagnostic excision, small biopsies, or ablations of human papillomavirus (HPV)–related lesions of anogenital tract
        (2) Primarily used for cervical lesions, but may also be used for external warts, or flat lesions of the vagina, vulva, or anus
    3. Laser therapy (carbon dioxide, Nd:YAG, argon)
      a. Cervical cancer in situ
    4. Dilatation and curettage (D & C)
      a. Purpose: removal of growths and other materials from the uterine cavity
      b. Description: stretching the cervix beyond normal dimensions and removal of contents from the walls of the uterine cavity with a curet (spoon-shaped sharp-edged instrument)
      c. Often performed in conjunction with hysteroscopy
    5. D & E
      a. Purpose: uterine aspiration and emptying

    b. Description: stretching the cervix beyond normal dimensions and removing the contents of the uterus by curettage, suction
6. Endometrial ablation and resection
    a. Purpose: treatment of dysfunctional uterine bleeding
    b. Description: Nd:YAG laser with a hysteroscope; roller ball or loop electrode with a modified resectoscope most commonly used
7. Fertility procedures
    a. Cerclage
        (1) Purpose: preservation of uterine contents
        (2) Description: encircling an incompetent cervix uteri with a ring or loop (or a stitch into the cervix)
    b. In vitro fertilization (IVF)
        (1) Purpose: pregnancy
        (2) Description: Using transvaginal ultrasound-guided follicle aspiration, healthy mature oocytes are retrieved; oocytes and sperm are mixed; the resultant embryo is transferred to the uterine fundus after two days
    c. Transcervical balloon tuboplasty
        (1) Purpose: open obstructed fallopian tubes
        (2) Description: Performed under fluoroscopy, sonography, or via hysteroscopy; a catheter is passed through the cervix and, after injection of dye to detect obstruction, the balloon attached to the catheter is inflated inside the fallopian tube to dilate the interior of the tube until recanalization is achieved
8. Tension-free vaginal tape (TVT)
    a. Purpose: correction of stress incontinence
    b. Description: placement of a synthetic mesh tape under the midurethra
        (1) Local anesthesia most commonly used; general or regional anesthesia if additional procedures needed
    c. Preanesthesia assessment and concerns
        (1) Patient taught self-catheterization; may need to self-catheterize postoperatively
    d. Postanesthesia priorities
        (1) Phase II—standard voiding trial before discharge
            (a) May be discharged with indwelling (e.g., Foley) catheter in place
            (b) Patient education: catheter care and removal
    e. Complications
        (1) Bladder perforation
        (2) Hematoma
        (3) Postoperative voiding dysfunction
            (a) Incomplete bladder emptying
            (b) Persistent urgency and urge incontinence
        (4) Urinary tract infection
9. Vaginal hysterectomy
    a. Purpose: removal of uterus
    b. Description: excision of the uterus through the vagina
    c. Postanesthesia priorities
        (1) May require 23-hour stay (extended recovery) following procedure
10. Anterior colporrhaphy
    a. Purpose: Tightens vaginal wall; prevents or corrects bladder herniation into vagina
    b. Description: Removal of excess anterior vaginal tissue
11. Posterior colporrhaphy
    a. Purpose: tightens vaginal wall; prevents or corrects rectal herniation into vagina
    b. Description: removal of excess posterior vaginal tissue

12. Culdoscopy: direct visualization of uterus and adnexa through endoscope passed through posterior vaginal wall
13. Culdocentesis
    a. Purpose: Used to detect intraperitoneal bleeding or cul-de-sac hematoma
    b. Description: aspiration through vaginal wall of blood or pus through cul-de-sac; good diagnostic tool to rule out ruptured ectopic pregnancy
C. Endoscopic procedures—laparoscopy
    1. Laparoscopy
       a. Purpose: diagnostic or therapeutic procedures may be performed (biopsies, lysis of adhesions, sterilization, treatment of endometriosis, nerve ablative procedures, hysterectomy, myomectomy, cystectomy, pelvic reconstructive procedures).
       b. Description: examination of the interior of the abdomen (abdominal and pelvic organs) by means of a lighted endoscope (laparoscope) through small incision(s) in the abdominal wall
          (1) Pneumoperitoneum is created using CO_2 to enhance visualization by lifting the abdominal wall
    2. Tubal ligation
       a. Purpose: obliteration of the fallopian tubes to cause infertility (sterilization)
       b. Description: rings, clips, ligation (ties), cauterization commonly used
    3. Tubal lavage (chromopertubation)
       a. Purpose: ascertains fallopian tube patency
       b. Description: dye is injected through the fallopian tubes; spillage of dye indicates patent tubes.
    4. Fertility procedures
       a. Gamete intrafallopian transfer (GIFT)
          (1) Purpose: pregnancy
          (2) Description: follicle stimulation and oocyte retrieval same as for IVF; gametes (oocytes and sperm) replaced through the distal fallopian tube, via laparoscopy or sonographically guided tubal cannulation
       b. Zygote intrafallopian transfer (ZIFT)—also known as tubal embryo transfer (TET)
          (1) Purpose: pregnancy
          (2) Description: follicle stimulation and oocyte retrieval same as for IVF; zygote replaced through the distal fallopian tube, via laparoscopy or sonographically guided tubal cannulation
    5. Laparoscopic-assisted vaginal hysterectomy (LAVH)
       a. Purpose
          (1) Removal of uterus for myomata
          (2) Abnormal uterine bleeding
          (3) Adenomyosis
          (4) Malignancy
          (5) Pelvic pain
          (6) Endometriosis
       b. Description: hysterectomy begun by laparoscopy and completed vaginally
    6. Myomectomy
       a. Purpose: surgical removal of a myoma (leiomyoma, "fibroids") to preserve uterine integrity and fertility
       b. Description: accomplished by laparoscopic or hysteroscopic technique
    7. Oophorectomy: removal of an ovary or ovaries
    8. Ovarian cystectomy: excision of ovarian cyst, leaving functioning ovary
    9. Salpingectomy: removal of fallopian tube
    10. Neosalpingostomy: surgical restoration of the patency of the fallopian tube
    11. Salpingoplasty (tuboplasty)
        a. Purpose: to restore patency of fallopian tube

    b. Description: microscopic reconstructive surgery of the fallopian tube; obstructed portion of fallopian tube may be removed and the tube reconstructed to create patency to promote fertilization
      (1) Reversal of tubal ligation
      (2) Pelvic inflammatory disease (PID)
      (3) Adhesions

12. Intraoperative concerns
    a. Considerations unique to laparoscopic procedures
      (1) Pulmonary and cardiovascular changes
        (a) Pneumoperitoneum creates increased intraabdominal pressures.
        (b) Pulmonary inspiratory pressure increases, compliance decreases, atelectasis develops, and functional residual capacity decreases.
      (2) CO_2 absorption from peritoneal cavity into the blood can cause hypercarbia and respiratory acidosis.
      (3) Trendelenburg positioning can lead to increased mean arterial pressure, pulmonary artery pressure, aortic compression, and systemic vascular resistance accompanied by a drop in cardiac output.
      (4) Marked hemodynamic changes may be brought about by a significant release of catecholamines, prostaglandins, and vasopressin during the procedure.
      (5) Stretching of the peritoneum and manipulation of viscera can lead to bradycardia, which responds to atropine.
      (6) Pulmonary aspiration is a risk with abdominal insufflation.

13. Postanesthesia priorities—phase I
    a. Pain
      (1) Shoulder pain common following laparoscopy; referred pain caused by diaphragmatic irritation from residual CO_2 in abdomen
      (2) Peritoneal surface inflammation following laparoscopy may be caused by the formation of carbonic acid (reaction between CO_2 and intraperitoneal fluid) and persist for 2 to 3 days postoperatively.
      (3) NSAIDs effective in managing postlaparoscopic pain

D. Endoscopic procedures—hysteroscopy
  1. Hysteroscopy
    a. Purpose:
      (1) To examine the endometrium
      (2) Secure specimens for biopsy
      (3) Remove foreign bodies (e.g., intrauterine device [IUD])
      (4) Remove polyps
      (5) Intrauterine adhesions or submucous fibroids
      (6) Ablation
      (7) Diagnose uterine abnormalities
    b. Description: inspection of the interior of the uterus with an endoscope, using either a liquid or a gaseous distending medium
    c. Intraoperative concerns
      (1) Considerations unique to hysteroscopic procedures
        (a) Fluid (saline, glycine, dextran) used as distending media
        (b) Absorption and resultant circulatory overload
        (c) Dilution can lead to hyponatremia, hypoproteinemia, transurethral resection (TUR) syndrome (glycine)
        (d) Disseminated intravascular coagulation (DIC) (dextran)
        (e) Anaphylaxis (dextran)
      (2) Carbon dioxide used as distending medium
        (a) Abdominal distention from leak via fallopian tubes
        (b) CO_2 absorption leading to acidosis, arrhythmias
        (c) CO_2 embolism
      (3) Uterine perforation
      (4) Vaginal bleeding

(5) Careful attention should be paid to amount of fluid instilled and removed; excessive administration can lead to the preceding complications.

   d. Complications

      (1) Fluid overload may be result of significant absorption of irrigant through tissue and blood vessels; may lead to pulmonary edema, hyponatremia, with cerebral edema and subsequent seizures, respiratory arrest, coma and possibly death

         (a) Monitor respiratory status.

         (b) Check serum electrolytes.

         (c) Diuretics and IV fluid restriction may be needed.

E. Laparotomy (vertical, transverse)

  1. Laparotomy

    a. Purpose: allows for exploration of abdominal cavity

    b. Description: incision of abdominal wall; incision may be vertical or transverse

  2. Abdominal suspension procedures for stress urinary incontinence

    a. Purpose: surgical treatment for relief of stress incontinence

    b. Description: Marshall-Marchetti-Krantz (MMK) and Burch are the most common abdominal procedures; the Burch procedure is preferred; paravaginal fascia on each side of the urethra, near the bladder neck is sutured to the ligaments (Cooper's) attached to the pubic bone.

    c. Burch procedure may be performed with either a low transverse incision or laparoscopically.

  3. Metroplasty

    a. Purpose: repair of septate uterus

    b. Description: reconstructive surgery on the uterus

  4. Hysterectomy

    a. Purpose: excision of uterus

    b. Description: surgical approaches (vaginally, laparoscopic-assisted vaginal hysterectomy [LAVH]—see preceding; abdominally)

  5. Hysterosalpingo-oophorectomy: removal of uterus, fallopian tubes, and ovaries

  6. Radical hysterectomy and lymph node dissection

    a. Purpose: to remove uterus for cervical cancer, preserving the ovaries

    b. Description: laparotomy to remove uterus, tubes, upper vagina, supporting ligaments, and pelvic lymph nodes; extensive dissection of ureters and bladder also involved

    c. Portions of this procedure may be performed by laparoscopy (e.g., pelvic lymph node dissection).

  7. Radical vulvectomy

    a. Purpose: to treat invasive vulvar carcinoma

    b. Description: en bloc dissection of the inguinal-femoral region and the vulva; skin or myocutaneous graft may be needed for closure of wound

  8. Pelvic exenteration

    a. Purpose: curative, to remove all cancer tissue and reconstruction of diversions for urine and possibly colon

    b. Description: en bloc of all pelvic tissues, including uterus, cervix, vagina, bladder, and rectum

    c. Preanesthesia assessment and concerns

      (1) Full and thorough mechanical and antibiotic bowel preparation

      (2) Deep vein thrombosis prophylaxis initiated

    d. Postanesthesia priorities—phase I

      (1) Drain and stoma care

      (2) Potential for significant fluid loss and third spacing

      (3) Pain management

      (4) Psychosocial concerns

         (a) Prepare for altered body image.

         (b) Issues associated with cancer diagnosis and prognosis

    e. Complications
        (1) Fluid overload
        (2) Bleeding
        (3) Coagulopathy
        (4) Trauma to kidneys

BIBLIOGRAPHY

1. Azziz R, Murphy AA: *Practical manual of operative laparoscopy and hysteroscopy,* ed 2. New York: Springer-Verlag, 1997.
2. Black JM, Hawks JH, Keene AM: *Medical-surgical nursing: Clinical management for positive outcomes,* ed 6. Philadelphia: WB Saunders, 2001.
3. Darney PD, Horbach NS, Korn AP: *Protocols for office gynecologic surgery.* Cambridge, MA: Blackwell Science, 1996.
4. *Dorland's illustrated medical dictionary,* ed 29. Philadelphia: WB Saunders, 2000.
5. Evans MI, Johnson MP, Moghissi KS: *Invasive outpatient procedures in reproductive medicine.* Philadelphia: Lippincott-Raven, 1997.
6. Gershenson DM, DeCherney AH, Curry SL: *Operative gynecology.* Philadelphia: WB Saunders, 2000.
7. Jaffe RA, Samuels SI, editors: *Anesthesiologist's manual of surgical procedures*, ed 2. Philadelphia: Lippincott, Williams & Wilkins, 1999.
8. Karram MM, Segal JL, Vassallo BJ, et al: Complications and untoward effects of the tension-free vaginal tape procedure. *Obstet Gynecol* 101:929-932, 2003.
9. Mann WJ, Stovall TG: *Gynecologic surgery.* New York: Churchill Livingstone, 1996.
10. Miller-Keane, O'Toole MT: *Encyclopedia and dictionary of medicine, nursing, and allied health,* ed 7. Philadelphia: WB Saunders, 2003.
11. Penfield AJ: *Outpatient gynecologic surgery.* Baltimore: Williams & Wilkins, 1997.
12. Rock JA, Thompson JD: *TeLinde's operative gynecology,* ed 8. Philadelphia: Lippincott-Raven, 1997.
13. Thompson JM, McFarland GK, Hirsch JE, et al: (2002) *Mosby's clinical nursing,* ed 5. St Louis: Mosby, 2002.
14. Twersky RS: *The ambulatory anesthesia handbook.* St Louis: Mosby–Year Book, 1995.
15. White P: *Ambulatory anesthesia and surgery.* Philadelphia: WB Saunders, 1997.

46 Obstetric Surgery

DENISE O'BRIEN

OBJECTIVES

At the conclusion of this chapter the reader will be able to:

1. Describe the physiologic changes of pregnancy.

2. Describe the pathophysiology, potential problems, assessment parameters, and nursing implications for common complications of pregnancy.

3. Describe commonly used obstetric anesthesia techniques and their impact on pregnancy.

4. Identify various assessment techniques to ascertain fetal well-being.

5. List appropriate nursing interventions in the care of the postanesthesia obstetric patient after low-risk and high-risk vaginal and surgical delivery.

6. Describe the pathophysiology, potential problems, assessment parameters, and nursing implications for various postpartum complications.

7. Explain the pharmacology, indications for use, and potential complications of commonly used obstetric medications.

■
■ ■ Obstetrical surgery refers to female reproduction. This chapter covers the physiologic changes of pregnancy, potential complications, and surgical interventions. Obstetric anesthesia, cesarean birth (normal and high risk), and postpartum complications are also reviewed.

PHYSIOLOGIC CHANGES OF PREGNANCY

I. Cardiovascular system
   A. Maternal myocardial hypertrophy caused by increased circulatory volume load of pregnancy
   B. Enhanced myocardial contractility
   C. Third heart sound by 20 weeks' gestation (90% of women)
   D. Systolic ejection murmur (95% of women)
      1. Caused by systemic vasodilation and augmented cardiac ejection
   E. Cardiac output (CO) progressively increases 30% to 50% to 6 to 7 L/minute at rest.
      1. Before 20 weeks' gestation, increase is the result of
         a. Maternal tachycardia
         b. Increased blood volume
      2. After 20 weeks' gestation, increase is caused by:
         a. Significantly increased stroke volume
         b. Association with reversible myocardial hypertrophy
      3. Increases further with labor and certain disease states; highest immediately postpartum
      4. CO profoundly affected by maternal position
         a. Best in lateral or semi-Fowler's with uterine displacement
         b. Lowest in supine and standing position
   F. Heart rate increased 10% to 20% because of blood volume overload and hormonal changes
      1. Heart rate is positional: standing greater than sitting, sitting greater than supine.

G. Stroke volume increases 30% to 40%.
H. Exacerbation of preexisting cardiac disease with critical period for decompensation occurring between 24 to 32 weeks' gestation and in immediate postpartum period
I. Elevation of the diaphragm causes the heart to shift anteriorly and to the left.
J. Electrocardiography (ECG) changes during pregnancy.
   1. Sinus tachycardia with shortening of PR and uncorrected QT intervals
   2. QRS axis shifts
      a. To the right during the first trimester
      b. May shift left during the third trimester
   3. T-wave axis shifted left
   4. Depressed ST segments and isoelectric or low-voltage T waves in left-side precordial and limb leads
K. Circulatory blood volume progressively increases 40% to 50%.
   1. Women with preeclampsia do not expand their vascular volume to the extent that nonpreeclamptic women do; hemoconcentrated
   2. Pregnancy hypervolemia acts as protective mechanism against excessive peripartum blood loss.
   3. Pregnancy is a natural hypervolemic state with primary renal sodium and water retention.
L. Plasma volume progressively increases 45% to 50%.
   1. Responsible for
      a. Dilutional anemia during pregnancy
      b. Spontaneous autotransfusion at delivery
   2. Albumin binding of drugs and local anesthetic less in pregnant state
M. Red blood cell (RBC) volume increases 25% to 30%.
   1. Greater plasma volume than RBC mass results in physiologic anemia of pregnancy.
   2. Expansion related to increased hematopoiesis in bone marrow and liver
   3. Iron deficit of approximately 800 mg by midpregnancy created by
      a. Physiologic anemia
      b. Increased hematopoiesis
      c. Associated transfer of approximately 300 mg of maternal iron to fetus during gestation
   4. 2,3-diphosphoglycerate (2,3-DPG) concentration increased during pregnancy and affinity of maternal hemoglobin for oxygen decreased, enhancing oxygen transfer to fetus
N. White blood cell (WBC) volume increases 40% to 50%.
   1. Highest immediately postpartum
O. Coagulation
   1. Pregnancy is hypercoagulable state related to enhanced potential for coagulation and thrombosis; increases in late pregnancy and immediately postpartum
   2. Plasma fibrinolytic activity decreased as result of placental inhibitors but can return to normal within 1 hour after delivery
   3. Tissue thromboplastin released into circulation with placental separation; increases chance of thrombosis
   4. Platelet counts appear to remain in normal range.
P. Hemodynamic changes (Table 46-1)
II. Pulmonary system
A. Diaphragm elevated because of compression of enlarging uterus
B. Anteroposterior and transverse diameters increase, resulting in decreased residual volume.
C. Weight gain, edema, and mucosal hypervascularity may change anatomy significantly.
   1. Internal diameter of trachea reduced

■ TABLE 46-1
■ ■ **Normal Hemodynamics During Pregnancy**

Parameter	Normal value
Central venous pressure (CVP)	1-7 mm Hg
Pulmonary artery pressure (PAP)	Systolic, 18-30 mm Hg
	Diastolic, 6-10 mm Hg
	Mean, 11-15 mm Hg
Pulmonary artery occlusion pressure (PAOP)	6-10 mm Hg
Systemic vascular resistance (SVR)	1210 ± 266
Pulmonary vascular resistance (PVR)	78 ± 22
Cardiac output (CO)	6-7 L/min (at rest)
Cardiac index (CI)	3.2 ± 0.7
Left ventricular stroke work index (LVSWI)	45 ± 9

    2. If endotracheal intubation required, a small-caliber endotracheal tube should be used (e.g., a 6.5-mm endotracheal tube).
        a. Facilitates intubation
        b. Prevents mucosal trauma
    3. Should avoid nasotracheal intubation
  D. Nasal and respiratory tract mucosa become edematous and hyperemic.
  E. Nasal congestion and epistaxis common and may obstruct nasal airway.
  F. O_2 consumption increases to accommodate fetus and maternal hyperdynamic function.
    1. O_2 consumption increases progressively by 10% to 20% and may increase by 100% during labor.
  G. Respiratory rate increases 15%.
  H. Lung volumes
    1. Tidal volume increases 40%.
    2. Inspiratory reserve volume: no change or slight increase
    3. Expiratory reserve volume decreases 20%.
    4. Residual volume decreases 20%.
  I. Lung capacities
    1. Inspiratory capacity increases 5% to 10%.
    2. Vital capacity: no change
    3. Expiratory capacity decreases 20%.
    4. Functional residual capacity decreases 20%.
    5. Total lung capacity: no change or slight decrease
  J. Acid-base balance
    1. Maternal oxyhemoglobin dissociation curve shifted to right during pregnancy
    2. Arterial blood gas values (ABGs) (see Table 46–2)
    3. Pregnancy is state of compensatory respiratory alkalemia.
III. Gastrointestinal system
  A. Anatomic and physiologic changes in gastrointestinal tract predispose pregnant woman to
    1. Silent regurgitation
    2. Active vomiting
    3. Pulmonary aspiration, especially during impaired consciousness.[1]
        a. All pregnant women are considered a full stomach risk for anesthesia.
IV. Renal system
  A. Renal calyces, pelves, and ureters dilate progressively beginning at twelfth week because of mechanical compression at pelvic inlet.
    1. Increased risk of urinary tract infection (UTI) from urinary stasis

■ TABLE 46-2
■ ■ Arterial Blood Gas Values

S	Nonpregnant	Pregnant
pH	7.35-7.45	7.40-7.44
Pao_2	80-100	104-108
$Paco_2$	35-45	27-32
HCO_3^-	22-26	18-22

B. Glomerular filtration rate (GFR) and renal plasma flow (RPF) increase 40% to 50% by 20 weeks' gestation.
C. Blood urea nitrogen (BUN) and creatinine decrease 40% by midpregnancy because of increased GFR and RPF.
D. Renal tubular function
   1. Tubular reabsorption of electrolytes and water increases in proportion to GFR.
   2. Glycosuria common in pregnancy related to augmented GFR, which results in filtered load of glucose that exceeds tubular reabsorption capacity
      a. Increased concentrations of
         (1) Aldosterone
         (2) Estrogens
         (3) Cortisol
         (4) Human placental lactogen (HPL)
         (5) Prolactin
      b. Aortocaval compression by gravid uterus
   3. Renin-angiotensin-aldosterone system
      a. All components increase during pregnancy because of their increased regulatory roles in circulatory volume and sodium balance.
V. Hepatic system
   A. No change in hepatic size or blood flow; metabolism changes in pregnancy lead to liver storage and conversion changes
   B. See slight increase in
      1. Lactic dehydrogenase (LDH)
      2. Alkaline phosphatase
      3. Leukocyte alkaline phosphatase
   C. Unchanged are
      1. Aspartate aminotransferase (AST)
      2. Serum glutamic oxaloacetic transaminase (SGOT)
      3. Alanine aminotransferase (ALT)
      4. Serum glutamic pyruvic transaminase (SGPT)
   D. Serum albumin decreases.
   E. Cholesterol increases 40% to 50%, and free fatty acids increase 60%.
VI. Endocrine system
   A. Pituitary gland enlarges as result of its function as master of all glandular function.
   B. Thyroid gland enlarges in response to need for
      1. Increased basal metabolism rate (BMR)
      2. T_4 uptake increases.
      3. T_3 uptake decreases.
   C. Increased cortisol and catecholamine production raise maternal heart rate and BMR.
   D. Increased levels of human placental lactogen (HPL), an insulin antagonist, lead to diabetogenic state; insulin requirements increase in type I diabetic patients during pregnancy.

VII. Neurologic system
  A. During pregnancy, neurologic and sensory systems are influenced by altered hormonal levels and alterations in other systems.
  B. Eye shows mild corneal edema and thickening; intraocular pressure decreases; progressive decrease in blood flow to conjunctiva
  C. Edema and erythema of vocal cords accompanied by vascular dilation and small submucosal hemorrhage may occur.
  D. Pain response during intrapartum period
    1. Perception of pain influenced by the following factors
      a. Physiologic
      b. Psychologic
      c. Cultural
    2. Specific role of beta-endorphins in pregnancy is unknown.
      a. Pain during intrapartum period may be modulated by endorphins that alter release of neurotransmitters from afferent nerves and interfere with efferent pathways.
      b. Endorphins may increase pain threshold.
      c. Lower doses of analgesics and anesthetics during labor may be used because of increased endorphins.
  E. Musculoskeletal changes
    1. Mobility of sacroiliac joints and symphysis pubis increased from relaxin and progesterone effects.
    2. Distension of abdomen tilts pelvis forward, shifting center of gravity, changing posture and gait.
VIII. Reproductive system
  A. Changes in reproductive system are result of increased vascularity and hormone production.
  B. Vulva and vagina become more vascular and elastic because of increased estrogen levels.
  C. Cervix becomes softer and shorter and appears cyanotic (Goodell's sign) because of prostaglandins.
  D. Ovaries may be enlarged for up to 14 to 16 weeks because of corpus luteum production of progesterone and estrogen to maintain endometrium.
  E. Breast tissue becomes more vascular because of elevated progesterone and estrogen levels.

PREGNANCY COMPLICATIONS

  I. Ectopic pregnancy
    A. Definition
      1. Pregnancy implanted outside uterus
      2. Ninety percent occur in fallopian tube.
      3. Ultrasonography or laparoscopy for diagnosis
      4. Laparotomy may be performed after diagnosis; may remove pregnancy by laparoscopic procedure
    B. Potential problems
      1. Rupture
      2. Shock from preoperative or intraoperative hemorrhage
      3. Pain control
      4. Rh factor sensitization
      5. Aspiration during intubation and extubation
      6. Emotional crisis
    C. Nursing assessments and interventions
      1. Administer blood or blood products if indicated and as ordered.
      2. Assess for trauma to bladder, ureters.
      3. Assess and intervene for pain and discomfort.
      4. Assess for postoperative complications related to abdominal surgery or laparoscopy.

     5. Administer Rh immune globulin if woman is Rh negative.

     6. Give emotional support.

  II. Incompetent cervix

    A. Definition

      1. Painless dilation of cervix during second trimester

      2. Repeated second-trimester abortions in absence of uterine contractions

    B. Surgical intervention: cerclage

      1. McDonald's suture: Mersilene suture placed at cervicovaginal junction and removed for labor

      2. Shirodkar procedure: Mersilene tape encircles cervix, passed under mucosa

        a. May remove for labor

        b. If future childbearing desired, will remain intact and birth will be by elective cesarean

      3. Optimal timing for placement is after first trimester (~14 to 18 weeks' gestation completed)

    C. Potential postoperative complications

      1. Uterine contractions

      2. Rupture of membranes

      3. Hemorrhage

      4. Fetal compromise because of anesthesia

      5. Aspiration

      6. Urinary tract infection (UTI) related to indwelling (e.g., Foley) catheter

    D. Nursing assessments and intervention

      1. Maintain lateral position or uterine displacement to increase uterine perfusion.

      2. Administer O_2 through face mask at 8 to 12 L/minute.

      3. Maintain intravenous (IV) line for adequate hydration

      4. Assess Homan's sign (pain on dorsiflexion of foot).

      5. Monitor and interpret laboratory values, especially hemoglobin and hematocrit.

      6. Foley catheter care to prevent infection

      7. Reproductive

        a. Position in slight Trendelenburg position to decrease cervical pressure.

        b. Maintain perineal pad count, monitoring amount, color, and consistency of vaginal discharge.

        c. Assess fetal heart rate (FHR), which has a normal range of 120 to 160 beats per minute (bpm), through

          (1) Doppler ultrasonography

          (2) Fetoscope

          (3) Electronic fetal monitoring

        d. Palpate fundus for uterine resting tone and uterine activity.

        e. Assess for maternal perception of fetal movement if >20 to 22 completed weeks' gestation.

        f. Administer tocolytic agent as indicated (see Table 46-3).

      8. Assess for pain.

 III. Nonobstetric surgery during pregnancy

    A. Types of procedures

      1. Trauma most frequent indication for surgery in pregnant patient (see information on obstetric trauma in section VIII)

      2. Acute appendicitis and ovarian tumors second most common indications

      3. Cholecystectomy

      4. Orthopedic injuries

    B. Anesthesia

      1. Effects on altered maternal physiology must be considered.

        a. Goal is to provide maternal anesthesia without stimulating uterine activity or precipitating preterm labor.

        b. Surgical anesthesia designed to maintain uteroplacental perfusion and prevent preterm labor

■ TABLE 46-3
■ ■ **Commonly Used Obstetric Medications**

Class	Action	Indications	Potential Complications	Special Notes
Oxytocins	Increased uterine contractions	Stimulate labor Incomplete abortion	Transient dysrhythmias	Hypertensive crisis possible if Methergine given when patient is hypertensive
Pitocin Methylergo-novine maleate (Methergine)	Stimulate milk ejection	Postpartum bleeding	Uterine tetany Water intoxication	Undiluted IV oxytocin produces hypotension; administer as undiluted infusion.
Alprostadil (Prostin)	Increases uterine contractions	Second-trimester abortion Postpartum uterine atony unresponsive to oxytocin	Fever Chills Nausea and vomiting Diarrhea	Given IM or into myometrium
Magnesium sulfate (MgSO$_4$)	Decreases neuromuscular irritability and CNS irritability	Prevents seizures in preeclampsia-eclampsia Inhibits preterm contractions	Toxicity Loss of DTRs Respiratory depression Cardiovascular collapse	Toxicity reversible with calcium gluconate Careful administration of narcotics, CNS depressants, calcium channel blockers, beta-blockers
Tocolytics Terbutaline	Relaxes smooth muscle Beta-agonist	Bronchospasm Inhibits preterm labor	Tremors Anxiety Dysrhythmias Nausea and vomiting Pulmonary edema	May be given IV, subcutaneously, or orally
Ritodrine (Yutopar)	Decreased uterine contractions Beta-agonist	Preterm labor	Tachycardia Hypotension Dysrhythmias Restlessness and tremors Hyperglycemia or hypoglycemia Pulmonary edema	Contraindicated in abruptio placentae, intrauterine infection, severe preeclampsia, and diabetes
RhoGAM	Decreases immune response	Rh-negative woman after exposure to Rh-positive blood	Irritation at site Myalgias Lethargy	Must be given within 72 hours of delivery or abortion
Bromocriptine (Parlodel)	Inhibits prolactin	Prevents lactation Parkinson's disease Female infertility	Headache Nausea and vomiting Rash Orthostatic hypotension	With hypotensive agents, can produce significant hypotension May potentiate hypertension
Antihyperten-sives			Reflex tachycardia Headache Nausea and vomiting	

Continued

■ TABLE 46-3 *Cont'd*
■ ■ **Commonly Used Obstetric Medications**

Class	Action	Indications	Potential Complications	Special Notes
Hydralazine	Arteriolar dilator Decreases pulmonary vascular resistance	Essential hypertension, preeclampsia with diastolic BP >110 mm Hg	Bradycardia Dysrhythmias Nausea and vomiting	Alpha-blocker, beta-blocker
Labetalol	Adrenergic antagonist Increases BP	Essential hypertension Hypertensive crisis		

    c. Fetal oxygenation directly dependent on maternal oxygen and carbon dioxide tensions

  2. Effects on developing fetus must be considered in timing of surgery and anesthesia.

    a. Incidence of fetal loss increases during first and second trimesters.

    b. If elective, procedure should be deferred until at least 6 weeks' postpartum.

    c. Urgent surgical procedures that must be done but that can be delayed are best postponed until late second or early third trimester.

    d. Regional anesthesia decreases teratogenic drug exposure to fetus.

  C. Potential problems same as for cervical cerclage

  D. Nursing assessments and interventions same as for cervical cerclage

IV. Preterm labor

  A. Definition: labor that occurs between 20 and 37 completed weeks of pregnancy; exact cause usually unknown

  B. Risk factors

    1. Maternal

      a. Cardiopulmonary or renal disease

      b. Diabetes

      c. Hypertensive disease (preeclampsia-eclampsia, chronic hypertension)

      d. Abdominal surgery during pregnancy

      e. Abdominal trauma

      f. Uterine or cervical anomalies

      g. Maternal infection (systemic, intrauterine)

      h. Hypovolemia

    2. Fetal

      a. Multifetal gestation

      b. Polyhydramnios

      c. Fetal infection

      d. Placental abnormalities

  C. Nursing assessments

    1. Maternal

      a. History

      b. Uterine activity

        (1) Uterine contractions: ≥4/hour

        (2) Menstruation-like cramps, including thigh pain

        (3) Pelvic pressure

        (4) Low, dull backache

        (5) Change in vaginal discharge or leaking of fluid

        (6) Abdominal cramping with or without diarrhea

        (7) Thigh pain, cramping

        c. Cervical status
          (1) Effacement: ≥80%
          (2) Dilation: ≥2 cm
          (3) Soft consistency
        d. Membrane status
        e. Confirm gestational age of fetus or length of pregnancy.
     2. Laboratory test
        a. Complete blood count (CBC)
        b. Electrolytes
        c. Urinalysis or urine culture or both
        d. Cervical cultures
     3. Fetal
        a. Ultrasonography for fetal viability and to rule out anomalies incompatible with life
        b. Biophysical profile
        c. Nonstress test
        d. Electronic fetal monitor
  D. Interventions
     1. Initial supportive measures
        a. Bed rest
        b. Hydration
        c. Empty bladder
        d. Lateral position
     2. Pharmacologic interventions (see Table 46-3)
        a. Magnesium sulfate ($MgSO_4$)
        b. Beta-sympathomimetics
          (1) Terbutaline (Brethine)
          (2) Ritodrine (Yutopar)
        c. Calcium channel blockers
        d. Prostaglandin synthetase inhibitors
        e. Oxytocin antagonists (atosiban [Antocin])
     3. Implement management protocol specific to each patient.
        a. Baseline vital signs
          (1) Monitor for signs of intraamniotic infection (IAI).
          (2) Monitor for signs of pulmonary edema.
        b. Continuous fetal monitor
        c. Thorough systems assessment
        d. Strict measurement of intake and output (I&O)
        e. Maintain lateral decubitus position or uterine displacement.
     4. Assess for adverse effects of treatment.
     5. Provide psychosocial and emotional support.
     6. Administration of corticosteroids to enhance fetal lung maturation
V. Hypertensive disorders
  A. Definitions
     1. Chronic hypertension: hypertension present before pregnancy or elevations of blood pressure (BP) more than 6 weeks after delivery
     2. Preeclampsia: hypertension with proteinuria after 20 weeks' gestation
     3. Eclampsia: seizures or coma in woman with signs and symptoms of preeclampsia; no underlying neurologic history
     4. Chronic hypertension with superimposed preeclampsia-eclampsia
     5. Transient hypertension: development of hypertension during pregnancy or immediate postpartum period; no proteinuria
  B. Risk factors
     1. Young primigravida or older multipara
     2. Maternal age <18 years or >35 years
     3. Weight <100 pounds or morbid obesity
     4. Diabetes mellitus

     5. Hydatidiform mole

     6. Multifetal gestation, large fetus, fetal hydrops, polyhydramnios

     7. Preeclampsia in previous pregnancy

     8. Familial history of renal, hypertensive, or vascular disease

     9. Presence of chronic renal disease, hypertension, vascular, or autoimmune disease

C. Pathophysiology

     1. Early in disease process, increased CO or increased systemic vascular resistance (SVR) increases blood pressure (BP).

        a. Increased CO with decreased SVR causes turbulent blood flow through vessels; predisposes to endothelium damage.

        b. Endothelium damage activates hemostatic system.

        c. Kidneys respond to hemodynamic changes by inducing vasospasms as protective mechanism initially; later in process, vasospasms cause signs and symptoms seen.

     2. Multiorgan vasospasm

        a. Autoimmune or immune response occurs.

        b. Increased vascular tone

        c. Vasoconstriction caused by

           (1) Increased thromboxane levels

           (2) Decreased prostacyclin levels

     3. Disease process produces state of decreased uteroplacental perfusion.

        a. Decreased placental production of prostacyclin

        b. Activation of intravascular coagulation

        c. Decreased maternal vascular production of prostacyclin and other vasodilators causes vasoconstriction.

        d. Increased vascular permeability further decreases colloid oncotic pressure (COP).

D. Nursing assessments

     1. Signs and symptoms

        a. Hypertension

           (1) BP 140/90 after twentieth week

           (2) Mean arterial pressure >105 mm Hg; mean arterial pressure ≥85 in second trimester associated with increased risk of poor perinatal outcome

        b. Edema

           (1) Not necessary for diagnosis

           (2) Intracellular and extracellular edema may be present.

           (3) Window into organ integrity and oxygenation status

           (4) Significant finding when hypertension or proteinuria present

        c. Proteinuria

           (1) Ominous sign (doubles perinatal morbidity and mortality)

           (2) Late symptom caused by destruction of protein-sparing reticulum in kidney

           (3) Excretion of 1 g/L in random specimen or 0.3 g/L per 24 hours

     2. Clinical features of severe preeclampsia

        a. Systolic BP ≥160 mm Hg or diastolic BP ≥110 mm Hg

        b. Proteinuria >5 g/24 hours or 3+ or 4+ on dipstick

        c. Oliguria of <400 to 500 ml/24 hours (<30 ml/hour or 100 ml/4 hours)

        d. Cerebral or visual disturbances

        e. Hepatic, pulmonary, or cardiac involvement

        f. Thrombocytopenia

        g. Development of eclamptic seizures

        h. Development of HELLP (hemolysis, elevated liver enzymes, low platelets) syndrome (see section V.F)

     3. Laboratory studies

        a. CBC shows elevated hemoglobin and hematocrit and thrombocytopenia.

        b. Chemistries

        (1) Elevated serum creatinine, uric acid, and BUN

        (2) Reduced creatinine clearance, alkaline phosphatase

    c. Liver function

        (1) Increased LDH, ALT (SGPT), AST (SGOT)

        (2) Decreased serum glucose (severe hypoglycemia increases risk of maternal mortality)

    d. Coagulation studies

        (1) Decreased

           (a) Fibrinogen

           (b) Angiotensin (AT) III

           (c) Platelets

        (2) Increased fibrin degradation products, factor VIII activity, and platelet aggregability

4. Obtain thorough maternal health history to include medical and obstetric information.

5. Cardiovascular assessment

    a. Vital signs and BP; frequency of assessment dictated by condition of mother and fetus during the antepartum, intrapartum, and postpartum periods

    b. Edema increases or changes every shift.

    c. Daily weight at same time on same scale

    d. Assess skin color, temperature, turgor.

    e. Noninvasive assessments of cardiac output

    f. Capillary refill

    g. ECG and pulse oximetry as indicated by clinical condition

    h. Level of consciousness (LOC), behavior

6. Respiratory assessment

    a. Assess respiratory rate, quality, and pattern.

    b. Auscultate breath sounds at least every shift.

    c. Assess skin color and mucous membranes for cyanosis.

    d. Monitor oxygenation status with pulse oximetry as indicated.

    e. LOC, behavior

7. Renal assessment

    a. Assess urinary output every 1 to 4 hours.

    b. Evaluate urine for protein every 1 to 4 hours.

    c. Maintain 24-hour urine collection as indicated.

    d. *Strict I&O*

8. Central nervous system (CNS) assessment

    a. Assess deep tendon reflexes (DTRs) and clonus hourly (absence of DTRs is earliest sign of magnesium toxicity).

    b. Assess LOC and changes in behavior.

    c. Assess for headache or visual disturbances.

    d. Assess for signs of increasing intracranial pressure and cerebral edema.

9. Reproductive assessment

    a. Assess for uterine hypertonicity.

    b. Assess for postpartum hemorrhage.

    c. Fetal assessments for well-being or intolerance of intrauterine environment

10. Assess for signs of worsening disease.

    a. Headache

    b. Blurred vision

    c. Nausea and vomiting

    d. Change in LOC

    e. Epigastric pain

    f. Developing coagulopathy

11. Keep calcium gluconate at bedside (antidote for magnesium sulfate).

  E. Medical management
   1. Delivery only cure
   2. Magnesium sulfate for seizure prophylaxis (see Table 46-3); diazepam no longer used
   3. Antihypertensive therapy if diastolic BP ≥110 mm Hg
   4. Do not give diuretics.
     a. Will further deplete an already depleted intravascular bed
     b. Indicated for cardiogenic pulmonary edema
   5. Do not give heparin; will increase risk for intracranial hemorrhage
   6. Administration of colloid solutions will increase risk of pulmonary edema.
  F. HELLP syndrome
   1. Triad consists of hemolysis, elevated liver enzymes, and low platelets.
     a. Hemolysis
       (1) Vasospasms cause endothelial damage, leading to platelet aggregation and fibrin network formation.
       (2) RBCs forced through fibrin network at increased pressure, causing hemolysis
       (3) Hematocrit decreased; bilirubin and LDH levels increased
       (4) Burr cells and schistocytes may be present on red blood cell morphology.
     b. Elevated liver enzymes
       (1) Microemboli form in hepatic vasculature.
       (2) Hepatic blood flow decreases, resulting in ischemia.
       (3) Liver enzymes increase; LDH first to elevate
     c. Low platelets
       (1) Platelet consumption occurs.
       (2) Thrombocytopenia with platelets <50,000 associated with coagulopathies
       (3) Patient on low-dose aspirin therapy will have impaired platelet function irrespective of platelet number.
   2. Signs and symptoms
     a. Nausea and vomiting
     b. Epigastric tenderness
     c. Right upper quadrant pain or tenderness
     d. Significant hypertension and proteinuria may not be present initially.
     e. May be present as early as second trimester
   3. Is a form of severe preeclampsia; management same
  G. Eclampsia
   1. Complicates ~5% of all pregnancies
   2. Pathologic mechanisms implicated in development of eclampsia
     a. Cerebral vasospasm and ischemia
     b. Cerebral infarcts and hemorrhage
     c. Cerebral edema
     d. Disseminated intravascular coagulation (DIC)
     e. Hypertensive encephalopathy
     f. Metabolic encephalopathy
   3. Management
     a. Prevent maternal injury.
     b. Maintain adequate oxygenation.
       (1) Control airway and ventilation.
       (2) Mechanical ventilation may be required.
     c. Minimize risk of aspiration.
     d. Give adequate $MgSO_4$ (see Table 46-3).
       (1) Loading dose of 4 to 6 g IV over 20 minutes
       (2) Then 2 to 4 g/hour IV infusion
       (3) Always administer as secondary infusion.
     e. Assess for and control elevated increased intracranial pressure (ICP).

4. Goals of therapy
   a. Control of seizures
      (1) Magnesium sulfate as stated previously
      (2) If seizures persist, give additional 2 g IV bolus of MgSO$_4$ slowly at rate not to exceed 1 g/minute.
      (3) For seizures refractory to magnesium sulfate, give 250 mg IV sodium amobarbital slowly.
      (4) For rare case of status epilepticus, diazepam, 10 mg IV, may be administered slowly.
   b. Correction of hypoxia and acidosis
   c. Control of severe hypertension (diastolic BP >110 mm Hg)
      (1) Give antihypertensive agents cautiously because intravascular hypovolemia often accompanies preeclampsia-eclampsia; thus these patients are more sensitive to antihypertensive effects.
      (2) Not necessary to acutely normalize BP; overcorrection may result in uteroplacental hypoperfusion and fetal compromise
      (3) Maintain diastolic BP of 90 to 100 mm Hg.
      (4) Administer calcium channel blockers or beta-blockers with caution in patient receiving MgSO$_4$ therapy (can lead to cardiopulmonary collapse).
   d. Deliver products of conception.
      (1) During acute eclamptic episode, fetal bradycardia common
      (2) If fetal bradycardia persists beyond 10 minutes, preparation should be made for cesarean delivery, and abruption should be considered cause for bradycardia.
      (3) Often advantageous to fetus to allow intrauterine recovery from maternal seizure, hypoxia, and hypercapnia
   e. Monitor fluid I&O.
5. Nursing responsibilities
   a. Note onset of seizures, progress of seizure, body involvement, and length of convulsion.
   b. Maintain and protect airway.
   c. Administer oxygen by tight face mask at 10 to 12 L/minute.
   d. Administer anticonvulsant.
   e. Suction secretions.
   f. Evaluate lungs for aspiration.
   g. Evaluate cardiac status.
   h. Evaluate fetus.
   i. Evaluate uterine activity; placental abruption or precipitous birth possible
   j. Evaluation for timing and route of birth
6. Postpartum management
   a. Assessment and intervention continue with same intensity for minimum of 24 hours.
   b. Additional assessments done for
      (1) Recurrent eclampsia
      (2) Postpartum hemorrhage
      (3) Development of DIC
      (4) Development of HELLP syndrome
      (5) Development of acute renal failure
VI. Hemorrhage
   A. Hemorrhagic disorders in pregnancy are medical emergencies.
      1. Hemorrhage remains major cause of maternal death.
      2. Blood loss may reach 35% before hypovolemic shock occurs.
   B. Placenta previa
      1. Definition: improper implantation of placenta in lower uterine segment; either partial or complete
      2. Risk factors

a. Endometrial scarring
b. Early or late ovulation leading to immature or delayed development of decidua at time of implantation
c. Impeded endometrial vascularization
d. Increased placental mass

3. Pathophysiology
   a. Normally, blastocyst implants into upper portion of uterus, where blood supply is rich.
   b. With previa, blastocyst implants itself in lower uterine segment, over or near internal os.

4. Signs and symptoms and diagnosis
   a. Painless continuous or intermittent uterine bleeding, especially during third trimester
   b. Onset while woman at rest or in midst of activity without pain
   c. Normal uterine tone
   d. The earlier in gestation the bleeding, the worse the outcome; fetal effect depends on total blood loss, not number of bleeding episodes.
   e. Preterm labor develops in 30% of pregnancies complicated by placenta previa.

5. Management depends on gestational age, amount of bleeding, and placental location.
   a. Diagnosis by ultrasonography 95% to 99% accurate
   b. Gestational age <37 weeks: manage expectantly if bleeding stops, no labor, and fetal well-being established; home care appropriate for stable patient.
   c. Gestational age >37 weeks: deliver.
   d. Evidence of maternal or fetal compromise despite gestational age of fetus: deliver.

C. Abruptio placentae
   1. Definition: premature separation, either partial or total, of normally implanted placenta from decidual lining of uterus after 20 weeks' gestation
   2. Bleeding may be concealed or apparent with any classification of abruption.
   3. Risk factors
      a. Hypertensive disorders (chronic or preeclampsia-eclampsia)
      b. Multiparity
      c. Previous abruption
      d. Trauma, especially blunt abdominal
      e. Uterine anomaly
      f. Folic acid deficiency
      g. Smoking
      h. Cocaine use
      i. Premature rupture of membranes or sudden decompression of uterus
   4. Pathophysiology
      a. Degeneration of spiral arterioles that nourish endometrium and supply blood to placenta
      b. Process leads to rupture of blood vessels, and bleeding quickly occurs.
      c. Separation of placenta takes place in area of hemorrhage.
   5. Signs and symptoms and diagnosis
      a. Signs and symptoms related to amount of concealed blood trapped behind placenta and degree of separation
         (1) Sudden and stormy onset
         (2) External or concealed dark venous bleeding
         (3) Shock greater than apparent blood loss
         (4) Severe and steady pain
         (5) Uterine tenderness and hypertonicity (early finding)
         (6) Firm to boardlike uterine fundus (late finding)

(7) Uterus may enlarge and change shape.

(8) Fetal heart tones may or may not be present.

 b. Diagnosis made on basis of presenting symptoms and physical assessment

  (1) Severe and moderate abruptions are more easily diagnosed, whereas mild abruptions may be more difficult to diagnose because vaginal bleeding may be only presenting symptom.

  (2) Ultrasonographic examination ordered to rule out placenta previa; abruptio placentae may not be diagnosed by ultrasonography

 6. Management depends on degree of abruption suspected, fetal status, and maternal status.

  a. Expectant management: emphasis placed on maintaining cardiovascular status of mother and developing plan for birth of fetus

  b. Emergency management

   (1) Restore blood loss quickly.

   (2) Maintain vital organ function.

   (3) Continuous electronic fetal monitor

   (4) Correct coagulation defect or defects if present.

   (5) Expedite delivery.

  c. Vaginal delivery if woman hemodynamically stable, fetus stable, or fetal death

  d. Cesarean birth in presence of fetal distress, profuse bleeding, coagulopathy, or increasing uterine resting tone

D. Nursing assessments and interventions for placenta previa and abruptio placentae

 1. Fundamental areas of concern

  a. Mother's condition as primarily evidenced by degree of obstetric hemorrhage

  b. Fetal condition, including gestational age

 2. Nursing assessment plays vital role in this evaluation process.

 3. Intensive observation and monitoring

  a. Vital signs and noninvasive assessments of cardiovascular status and organ perfusion

  b. Strict I&O

  c. Record amount of bleeding.

 4. Fluid resuscitation

  a. Stable IV site with large-bore catheter (two IV lines possible)

  b. IV fluid replacement

  c. Blood replacement therapy

 5. Assessment of renal function

  a. Strict I&O

  b. Foley catheter

  c. Urinary output of at least 30 ml/hour

 6. Hemodynamic monitoring

  a. Pulmonary artery catheter more reflective of intravascular volume status

  b. Consider use of pulmonary artery catheter if aggressive fluid resuscitation required.

 7. Fetal evaluation as indicated

 8. Verify maternal Rh status; administer RhoGAM as indicated.

E. Adherent retained placenta

 1. Risks

  a. Associated with increased maternal morbidity and mortality because of hemorrhage leading to hypovolemic shock

  b. No sure signs of abnormally adherent placenta during pregnancy

 2. Types

  a. Placenta accreta: slight penetration of myometrium by placental trophoblast; most common; may be removed manually

      b. Placenta increta: deep penetration of myometrium by placental trophoblast; requires surgical intervention

      c. Placenta percreta: perforation of uterus by placenta; requires surgical intervention

   3. Unusual placental adherence may be partial or complete.

F. Uterine inversion

   1. Partial or complete inversion of uterus (turning inside out) after delivery is potentially life-threatening complication.

   2. Signs and symptoms

      a. Primary presenting sign is hemorrhage.

      b. Pelvic mass noted on vaginal examination

      c. No fundus palpable when attempting fundal massage

      d. Patient expresses feeling of fullness in vagina.

      e. Patient symptomatic for hypovolemic shock

   3. Management involves all of the following interventions.

      a. Combat shock.

      b. Replace uterus after woman has received tocolysis or deep anesthesia.

         (1) Give oxytocic as ordered, only after uterus has been replaced.

         (2) Uterus may be packed if inversion seems to recur.

      c. Abdominal or vaginal surgery may be necessary to reposition uterus if successful manual replacement fails.

      d. Give blood replacement therapy as indicated.

      e. Initiate broad-spectrum antibiotic therapy.

      f. Nasogastric tube to minimize paralytic ileus

   4. After replacement of uterus, do not massage fundus because inversion may recur.

G. Hydatidiform mole

   1. One of three types of gestational trophoblastic neoplasms

      a. Most often seen in women at both ends of reproductive age spectrum

      b. Increased risk for development of choriocarcinoma

   2. Signs and symptoms

      a. Vaginal bleeding may be dark brown (resembling prune juice) or bright red, either scant or profuse.

      b. Uterine size greater than expected gestational size

      c. Anemia from blood loss, excessive nausea and vomiting (hyperemesis gravidarum), and abdominal cramps caused by uterine distension relatively common findings

      d. Preeclampsia occurs in about 15% of cases, usually between 9 and 12 weeks' gestation.

   3. Management

      a. May abort spontaneously

      b. Suction curettage offers safe, rapid, and effective method of evacuation of hydatidiform mole in almost all women.

      c. If woman does not desire preservation of reproductive function, may benefit from primary hysterectomy as method of choice for evacuation of hydatidiform mole and concurrent sterilization

      d. Induction of labor with oxytocic agents or prostaglandins not recommended because of increased risk of hemorrhage

      e. Need to have negative beta human chorionic gonadotropin (HCG) for 6 months

VII. Multiple gestation

A. Perinatal morbidity and mortality increase with multifetal gestation because of

   1. Birth weight

   2. Gestational age

   3. Presentation of each fetus

   4. Mode of delivery

   5. Interval of time between deliveries

    B. Diagnosis

        1. Most important factor in successful outcome is early diagnosis

        2. Most important clinical finding suggestive of multifetal gestation is fundal height or uterine size disproportionately greater than date.

        3. Ultrasonography for confirmation of diagnosis

    C. Maternal complications

        1. Hypertension complicates 14% to 20% of twin pregnancies versus 6% to 8% of singleton pregnancies.

        2. Sepsis with premature rupture of membranes three times more frequent

        3. Postpartum hemorrhage occurs in approximately 20% of all multifetal pregnancies.

        4. Anemia occurs two times more frequently.

    D. Fetal and neonatal complications

        1. Preterm labor and birth

        2. Congenital anomalies

        3. Discordant growth

    E. Nursing implications

        1. Assess for

            a. Anemia

            b. Preeclampsia

            c. Polyhydramnios

            d. Preterm labor

        2. At risk for placenta previa

        3. After delivery, assess for postpartum hemorrhage.

VIII. Obstetric trauma

    A. Leading cause of nonobstetric maternal death in women of childbearing age

        1. Motor vehicle accidents currently leading cause of injury

        2. Physical abuse may become leading cause (~15% to 20% of all pregnant women are battered).

        3. Physiologic changes of pregnancy may contribute to injury severity and treatment.

        4. Maternal mortality most often from injuries sustained from motor vehicle accidents: head injuries; followed by multiple internal injuries, which lead to hypovolemic shock and exsanguination

    B. Abdominal trauma

        1. Significance

            a. First-trimester fetus protected by bony pelvis and amniotic fluid buffer

            b. Second-trimester pregnancy has become abdominal with minimum protection to fetus from pelvis

            c. Third trimester

                (1) With fetal engagement, increased risk for fetal skull fractures, intracranial bleeding

                (2) Increased risk for placental abruption; usually within first 48 hours

                (3) Complications unique to pregnancy

                    (a) Uterine trauma or rupture

                    (b) Bladder trauma or rupture

                    (c) Amniotic fluid embolus

                    (d) Placental abruption

            d. Significant trauma statistics in general population can be used to anticipate complications in pregnant trauma victim.

        2. Blunt abdominal trauma

            a. Motor vehicle accidents most common cause

            b. Head injury and exsanguination from vessel rupture most common cause of maternal death

            c. Leading cause of fetal death is maternal death.

            d. Leading cause of fetal death when mother survives is abruptio placentae.

3. Penetrating abdominal trauma
   a. Morbidity related to point of entry and number of organs penetrated
   b. As pregnancy advances, abdominal organs are displaced upward and laterally.
   c. Growing uterus may afford protection to abdominal organs located posterior to uterus, but fetus may be placed in position of greater risk.
   d. All penetrating abdominal wounds may require laparotomy for full surgical exploration.
   e. Gunshot wounds
      (1) Most common
      (2) Prognosis worse in that bullet path unpredictable and multiorgan involvement may occur
      (3) Greater damage to abdominal organs because of pregnancy displacement if bullet leaves uterine cavity
      (4) If bullet path limited to uterus, can have fetal, umbilical cord, or placenta damage
   f. Stab wounds
      (1) Second most common
      (2) Prognosis better than with gunshot wounds
      (3) Upper abdomen wounds may be complicated by damage to placenta, abdominal organs, lungs, heart; fetus usually protected
      (4) Lower abdomen wounds may be complicated by damage to fetus, bladder.
C. Thermal trauma
   1. Skin integrity affected—body systems compromised
   2. Prognosis depends on extent and depth of burn.
   3. Especially vulnerable to intravascular volume deficit and hypoxia
   4. Increased risk for preterm labor resulting from maternal hypoxemia (maternal Pao_2 <60 mm Hg increases fetal compromise)
   5. Fetal survival depends on maternal stabilization and survival.
D. Pelvic trauma
   1. Bony ring fracture may cause fetal skull fracture or maternal bladder trauma or rupture.
   2. Retroperitoneal bleeding risk increases because of engorgement of pelvic veins.
   3. Genitourinary trauma results in greater blood loss related to increased vascularity.
   4. Bowel (small and large) trauma possible
E. Modifications of care for pregnant trauma victim related to pregnancy physiology
   1. Cardiovascular system
      a. Blood volume increase means greater blood loss needed to show signs and symptoms of shock.
      b. Plasma volume expansion with greater red blood cell mass increase so there is physiologic anemia during pregnancy
      c. Resting heart rate increases by 15 to 20 bpm during pregnancy.
      d. Decreased SVR and increased CO may delay development of cool, clammy skin with hypovolemic shock.
   2. Respiratory system
      a. Normally in compensated respiratory alkalemia during pregnancy
      b. Decreased oxygen reserve and less tolerant of hypoxia as a result of increased metabolic rate and oxygen consumption
      c. Because chest wall is broadened and diaphragm elevated, thoracostomy will be performed above normal site.
      d. Peripheral edema, dyspnea, and third heart sound normal for pregnancy but may clinically mimic congestive ventricular failure

3. Gastrointestinal system
   a. Because abdominal viscera displaced and compressed, risk of liver or splenic rupture is increased; abdominal injury may be masked or mimicked; altered patterns for referred pain; rebound tenderness may be present or absent
   b. Decreased gastric motility, prolonged gastric emptying time, and incompetent esophageal sphincter: increased risk for aspiration
   c. Increased pelvic venous congestion: increased risk for hemorrhage
   d. Protruding uterus or bladder: increased risk for trauma
4. Hematologic system in hypercoagulable state: increased risk for thrombosis

F. Nursing assessments and implications
   1. Must remember that normal physiologic and anatomic changes of pregnancy will mask serious alterations in maternal status
   2. Primary survey assessment
      a. Airway
      b. Breathing
      c. Circulation
      d. Neurologic status
      e. Interventions
         (1) Establish and maintain airway; nasal airway inappropriate because of increased vascularity of pregnancy
         (2) Administer oxygen at 10 to 15 L/minute through tight nonrebreather mask.
         (3) Place nasogastric tube to decrease risk of aspiration.
         (4) Anticipate need for mechanical ventilation if respiratory rate <12 or >25; obtain ABGs and avoid exacerbation of acidosis by keeping Pco_2 to normal pregnancy values.
         (5) Initiate cardiopulmonary resuscitation (CPR) as indicated, maintaining uterine displacement.
         (6) Establish venous access.
         (7) Pneumatic antishock garment (MAST) may be indicated; abdominal compartment may be left uninflated once pregnancy becomes abdominal organ.
         (8) Control hemorrhage
   3. Secondary survey assessment
      a. Reassess neurologic status.
         (1) A: alert, oriented
         (2) V: responds to verbal stimulus
         (3) P: responds to pain only
         (4) U: unresponsive
      b. Examine for head injuries.
      c. Reassess chest and circulation.
      d. Anticipate laboratory and x-ray studies.
         (1) Kleihauer-Betke: maternal blood test to diagnose fetomaternal hemorrhage; indirect Coombs' test to detect maternal Rh sensitization
         (2) Alum-precipitated toxoid (APT) test: blood test to determine whether specimen is maternal or fetal blood
      e. Assess abdomen, noting pain, tenderness, distension.
      f. Assess musculoskeletal status.
      g. Reproductive assessment
         (1) Contraction frequency, duration, intensity, resting tone
         (2) Assess fundal height for approximate gestational age assessment.
         (3) Inspect perineum for bleeding, rupture of membranes.
         (4) If no bleeding, assess for cervical dilation.
         (5) Assess for signs and symptoms of abruptio placentae.
      h. Assess for fetal status.

    4. Circulatory support essential; however, vasopressors should not be routinely used

      a. Peripheral vasoconstrictors will increase maternal mean arterial pressure but decrease uterine blood flow.

      b. Central vasoconstrictors will concomitantly increase uterine blood flow and mean arterial pressure.

      c. Assessment and treatment priorities for pregnant burn victim same as any other

        (1) Airway patency

        (2) Maintain normal intravascular volume.

        (3) Provide maximum oxygenation.

IX. Cardiac disease

  A. Normal pregnancy physiology can have an impact on preexisting cardiac disease.

    1. Pregnancy is high-flow, low-resistance state.

    2. Increased CO causes patient to report signs and symptoms that mimic cardiac disease; diagnosis during pregnancy therefore complicated or missed

    3. Increased CO and blood volume in presence of decreased SVR and colloid oncotic pressure (COP) will predispose to peripheral edema, especially of lower extremities.

    4. Accentuated jugular pulse may be normal.

    5. Slight enlargement occurs because of upward and leftward displacement of heart; alters chest x-ray and ECG findings.

    6. Benign dysrhythmias occur.

    7. Hemodynamic values altered (see Table 46-1)

  B. Pregnancy counseling should be done before conception; pregnancy outcome depends on

    1. Functional capacity of heart

    2. Underlying lesion

    3. Likelihood of other complications that increase cardiac load during pregnancy and puerperium

    4. Quality of medical care available

    5. Psychosocial and economic capabilities of patient, her family, and community

  C. Significance of cardiac disease during pregnancy

    1. Maternal mortality based on New York Heart Association (NYHA) functional classification

      a. Class I: ≤1% mortality

      b. Class II: 5% to 15% mortality

      c. Class III: 25% to 50% mortality

      d. Class IV: >50% mortality

      e. Pregnancy increases NYHA class by at least one class; 40% of women with overt failure were class I early in pregnancy.

    2. Risk of maternal death by type of heart disease

      a. Group 1 consists of the following diagnoses:

        (1) Atrial septal defect

        (2) Ventricular septal defect

        (3) Patent ductus arteriosus

        (4) Pulmonic or tricuspid disease

        (5) Corrected tetralogy of Fallot

        (6) Bioprosthetic valve

        (7) NYHA class I and II mitral stenosis

        (8) Mortality risk <1%

      b. Group 2 consists of the following diagnoses:

        (1) NYHA class III and IV mitral stenosis

        (2) Aortic stenosis

        (3) Aortic coarctation without valvar involvement

        (4) Uncorrected tetralogy of Fallot

          (5) Previous myocardial infarction
          (6) Marfan syndrome with normal aorta
          (7) Mortality risk 5% to 15%
      c. Group 3 consists of the following diagnoses:
          (1) Pulmonary hypertension
          (2) Aortic coarctation with valvular involvement
          (3) Marfan syndrome with aortic involvement
          (4) Mortality risk 25% to 50%
D. General management of woman with cardiac disease during pregnancy
  1. Collaborative effort of obstetrician, cardiologist, anesthesiologist, nursing, and other needed disciplines
  2. Goals
    a. To prevent congestive heart failure (CHF)
    b. To react promptly to early signs of CHF
    c. To aggressively assess for and react to early signs of pregnancy complications
        (1) Preeclampsia
        (2) Diabetes
        (3) Infection
    d. To prevent recurrence of acute rheumatic fever
    e. To prevent infective endocarditis
  3. Avoid causes of tachycardia; treat when sustained heart rate >100 bpm.
E. Management principles
  1. Intrapartum
    a. First stage
        (1) Labor and deliver in same room
        (2) Monitor pulse, BP, respiratory status, lung bases, and I&O.
        (3) Keep heart rate <100 bpm.
        (4) Prophylactic antibiotics for ventricular septal defect, aortic and mitral disease
        (5) Examine and reevaluate cardiac status of patient in labor.
        (6) Semi-Fowler's position or best position as determined with invasive or noninvasive monitoring for CO and oxygenation status
        (7) Never place in lithotomy position, even for delivery.
        (8) Adequate analgesia (narcotic epidural appropriate)
        (9) Digitalis if needed
        (10) Drugs and equipment to treat pulmonary edema
        (11) Oxygen therapy and pulse oximetry
        (12) ECG monitoring as indicated
        (13) Cesarean birth for obstetric reasons only
        (14) Prevent fluid overload; use infusion pumps for all IVs and keep accurate I&O.
    b. Second stage of labor (delivery)
        (1) Recognize signs of decompensating heart.
        (2) Shorten second stage (episiotomy and forceps).
        (3) Avoid Valsalva's maneuver.
        (4) Cesarean birth for obstetric reasons only
        (5) Atraumatic delivery
        (6) Do not put patient in lithotomy position.
    c. Third stage of labor (delivery of placenta)
        (1) Avoid postpartum hemorrhage.
        (2) Strict I&O
        (3) Beware of antidiuretic effect and cardiovascular effects of oxytocin.
        (4) Beware of cardiovascular effects of prostaglandin preparations; avoid methylergonovine (Methergine).
  2. Fourth stage (postpartum)
    a. Observe in postanesthesia care unit (PACU) or labor and delivery (L&D) for at least 24 hours after delivery.

   b. Invasive hemodynamic monitoring as indicated

   c. At least one third of maternal deaths occur in first 24 hours after delivery.

 X. Pulmonary disease

  A. Pregnancy causes dramatic, predictable alterations in pulmonary function.

   1. Pao_2 must remain >60 mm Hg for adequate fetal oxygenation, providing all other factors influencing oxygen transfer across intervillous spaces remain optimum.

   2. Increased oxygen consumption associated with corresponding increase in CO_2 excretion

  B. Pulmonary edema

   1. Obstetric causes

    a. Noncardiogenic pulmonary edema

     (1) Aspiration of gastric contents

     (2) Sepsis

     (3) Blood transfusion reactions

     (4) DIC

     (5) Pregnancy-induced hypertension

     (6) Amniotic fluid embolism

    b. Cardiogenic pulmonary edema

     (1) Fluid overload

     (2) Magnesium sulfate or beta-mimetic tocolytic agents

     (3) Decreased contractility

   2. Predisposing conditions

    a. Frequent complication of preeclampsia-eclampsia

    b. Beta-mimetic therapy for preterm labor

    c. Preexisting cardiac disease

    d. Altered pulmonary capillary permeability

   3. Treatment same as any patient with pulmonary edema taking fetal status into consideration

  C. Pulmonary embolism

   1. Incidence

    a. Occurs in ~1:2000 pregnancies

    b. Untreated deep venous thrombosis (DVT) correlates with 15% to 24% incidence of pulmonary embolism.

    c. Mortality: 12% to 15%

   2. Predisposing conditions

    a. Pregnancy

    b. Prior history of DVT or pulmonary embolism

    c. Surgical procedures, immobility

    d. Obstetric complications

    e. Inherited coagulopathies

    f. Antiphospholipid antibody syndrome

    g. Age

    h. Race

    i. Greatest risk is in immediate postpartum period.

   3. Treatment

    a. Anticoagulation with heparin

    b. Antepartum management includes prophylactic anticoagulation.

    c. If anticoagulation given during antepartum period, maintain anticoagulation during labor.

    d. Low–molecular weight heparin preparations appropriate for use during pregnancy

  D. Pneumonia

   1. Associated with several maternal and fetal complications

   2. Pregnancy predisposes to aspiration; immune system altered during pregnancy

   3. Varicella very dangerous to mother and fetus

   4. *Mycoplasma* common in pregnancy and is difficult to diagnose

        5. Bacterial infection often occurs as a secondary infection.

        6. Treatment

           a. Prompt diagnosis

           b. Supportive therapy

           c. Oxygen

           d. Antibiotics

    E. Asthma

        1. Incidence

           a. Relatively common

           b. Prognosis during pregnancy depends on

              (1) Severity before pregnancy

              (2) Season of year

              (3) Presence of other respiratory infections

              (4) Patient's emotional state

        2. Effects of asthma during pregnancy

           a. No consistent effect

           b. Slightly higher risk for prematurity, intrauterine growth restriction (IUGR) because of decreased oxygenation

           c. Must consider fetal risks of drug therapy

           d. Exacerbations rare during labor

           e. If severe, may require pregnancy termination

           f. If prostaglandins used, should use prostaglandin E_2, a bronchodilator, instead of prostaglandin F_2-alpha, a bronchoconstrictor

        3. Treatment

           a. Supportive therapy

           b. Oxygen therapy

           c. Bronchodilators

           d. Antibiotics

    F. Amniotic fluid embolism

        1. Incidence

           a. Rare phenomenon, unique to pregnancy

           b. From National Registry, mortality >60%; of those women that survive insult, most sustain neurologic sequelae.

        2. Etiology; see Figure 46-1

        3. Presentation

           a. Acute onset of respiratory distress

           b. Shock out of proportion to blood loss

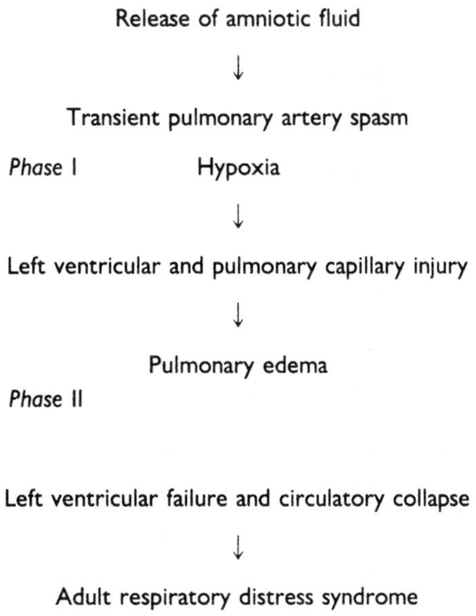

Release of amniotic fluid

↓

Transient pulmonary artery spasm

Phase I   Hypoxia

↓

Left ventricular and pulmonary capillary injury

↓

Pulmonary edema

Phase II

Left ventricular failure and circulatory collapse

↓

Adult respiratory distress syndrome

FIGURE 46-1 ■ Etiology of amniotic fluid embolism.

        c. Sudden, unexplained onset of DIC

        d. Seizures

        e. Acute-onset pulmonary edema

        f. Chest pain rare

        g. Acute cardiovascular collapse

    4. Treatment

        a. Maintain oxygenation.

        b. Maintain CO and BP.

        c. Treat coagulopathy.

        d. Initiate CPR.

  G. Nursing implications for pulmonary disease during pregnancy

    1. Multifaceted care

    2. Maintenance of adequate ventilatory function

    3. Optimize oxygen exchange.

    4. Arterial blood gas measurement

    5. Monitor patient's response to therapy.

    6. Emotional support

    7. Avoid hypoxemia during suctioning or ventilatory tubing changes.

    8. Hemodynamic monitoring as indicated

    9. Adjust mechanical ventilation setting to reflect normal pregnancy pulmonary parameters and arterial blood gas values.

XI. Maternal resuscitation

  A. Causes of cardiopulmonary arrest in pregnancy

    1. Maternal cardiac disease

    2. Severe preeclampsia, HELLP syndrome, eclampsia

    3. Preexisting medical conditions

    4. Acute complications

        a. Pulmonary embolism or amniotic fluid embolism

        b. Aspiration pneumonia

        c. Hypermagnesemia

        d. Anaphylaxis, laryngeal edema, bronchospasms

        e. Anesthesia

        f. Trauma

        g. Sepsis

  B. CPR during pregnancy

    1. Pregnancy is high-flow (CO), low-resistance (SVR) state.

    2. Thorax is less compliant, making mouth-to-mouth ventilation and chest compressions more difficult and less effective.

    3. Decreased chest compliance impedes success of standard closed-chest cardiopulmonary resuscitation.

    4. Before 24 weeks' gestation, objective is maternal conservation; after 24 weeks' gestation, fetal well-being may influence management decisions, but primary patient is the mother.

    5. Prompt emergent delivery increases maternal survival; if no maternal response within 4 minutes, bedside cesarean delivery or open-chest massage recommended

    6. After 12 weeks, uterus is abdominal organ.

        a. Decreased thoracic compliance

        b. Decreased venous return

        c. Causes aortic or vena caval compression

        d. Decreased forward flow of blood with compressions

        e. Causes respiratory impedance

    7. If fetus of viable gestational age (>24 weeks)

        a. Maternal hypoxia shunts blood from uteroplacental unit.

        b. Fetal $Paco_2$ increases as maternal $Paco_2$ increases, resulting in fetal metabolic acidosis.

  C. Modifications required during pregnancy when doing CPR

    1. Uterine displacement is essential.

   2. Correction of acidosis; rapid correction of maternal metabolic acidosis with sodium bicarbonate increases fetal $Paco_2$ levels
   3. Rapid initiation of endotracheal intubation for ventilation with 100% oxygen a must
   4. Defibrillation as indicated for appropriate cardiac dysrhythmias
   5. Resuscitation drug therapy as indicated
   6. Do not forget pulseless electrical activity, also known as electromechanical dissociation; common cause of pulseless rhythms during pregnancy is hypovolemia.
   7. Be prepared to initiate neonatal resuscitation.
   D. If delivery fails to facilitate successful maternal resuscitation
   1. Consider thoracotomy and open-chest cardiac massage.
   2. Consider use of cardiopulmonary bypass in the following situations.
      a. Method of rewarming hypothermic patients; especially if result of rapid, massive volume infusion
      b. Bupivacaine-induced cardiac toxicity (bupivacaine is slowly dissociated from the myocardial sodium channels)
      c. Pulmonary embolectomy in presence of massive pulmonary embolus
XII. Infectious diseases
   A. Significance
   1. Infections during pregnancy responsible for significant morbidity and mortality
   2. Pregnancy generally regarded as an immunosuppressed condition
   B. Sexually transmitted diseases
   1. *Chlamydia*
   2. Gonorrhea
   3. Syphilis
   4. Human immune deficiency virus (AIDS)
   5. Toxoplasmosis
   6. Hepatitis
   7. Cytomegalovirus
   8. Herpes simplex virus
   9. Human papillomavirus
   C. Treatment per identified infectious process

OBSTETRIC ANESTHESIA

I. General anesthesia
   A. Indications
   1. Rapid induction required for maternal or fetal compromise
   2. Failed regional anesthesia
   B. Anesthetic implications
   1. Decreased anesthesia required because of physiologic, anatomic, and hormonal changes of pregnancy
   2. More rapid loss of consciousness and protective airway reflexes at lower inspired concentrations of inhaled and IV anesthetics
   3. Airway changes may lead to difficulty in intubation.
   4. Magnesium sulfate therapy may cause prolonged neuromuscular blockade.
   C. Maternal effects
   1. Complications of endotracheal intubation and extubation
      a. Increased risk of gastric regurgitation and aspiration
      b. Failed intubation a leading cause of anesthesia-related maternal death
   2. Uterine activity
      a. Ketamine increases uterine resting tone and muscular activity.
      b. Nitrous oxide has no significant effect on uterine tone.
      c. Halogenated gases decrease uterine resting tone, uterine muscle tension, and spontaneous uterine activity.

3. Uterine blood flow
   a. Decreased with ultra–short-acting barbiturate induction agents
   b. Deep anesthesia leading to significant decrease in maternal CO and BP results in decreased uterine blood flow.
   c. Endogenous catecholamine release from inadequate general anesthesia or airway manipulation can decrease uterine blood flow.
D. Fetal effects
   1. Neonatal depression can result from placental transmission of depressant IV drugs or inhalation agents.
   2. Effects depend on length of time of exposure and agent used.
E. Nursing implications
   1. Premedicate obstetric patients with Bicitra or H_2-receptor antagonist to decrease gastric acidity.
   2. Judicious use of narcotic analgesia before delivery of fetus and during immediate PACU period
   3. Maintain uterine displacement with hip wedge at all times if undelivered.
      a. Aortocaval compression in supine position may cause profound hypotension.
   4. Hyperventilation should be avoided; hypocarbia and positive pressure ventilation decrease uterine blood flow.
   5. Be aware of potential for postpartum hemorrhage.

II. Regional anesthesia
A. Subarachnoid block (spinal)
   1. Anesthetic implications
      a. Increased blood volume and inferior vena caval compression by uterus during pregnancy lead to engorgement of epidural veins.
         (1) Increased risk of intravascular injections
         (2) Increased risk of catheter migration into epidural veins
      b. Epidural and subarachnoid spaces decrease in size and diameter.
      c. Higher levels of sensorimotor blockade achieved during spinal anesthesia in pregnancy
      d. Ability to generate expiratory airway pressure (cough) decreases by 50% with spinal; 10% with epidural.
      e. Contraindications same as general population
   2. Maternal effects
      a. Easier to perform than lumbar epidural
      b. Rapid onset of action
      c. Provides a solid sensory block and profound motor block
      d. Intense blockade of sympathetic fibers results in higher incidence of hypotension.
      e. Spinal headache may occur (<5%).
      f. Total spinal is rare but can lead to paralysis of respiratory muscles.
      g. Side effects may include
         (1) Nausea
         (2) Vomiting
         (3) Shivering
         (4) Urinary retention
      h. Uterine hypertonicity or hypercontractility and uterine artery vasoconstriction may occur from unintentional IV administration of the "caine" drug.
   3. Fetal effects
      a. Maternal hypotension may lead to decreased uteroplacental blood flow.
      b. Hypoxia can occur because of decreased uteroplacental perfusion.
      c. Fetal bradycardia (heart rate <100 bpm) may occur.
   4. Nursing implications
      a. Before administration, hydrate with minimum IV bolus of 500 to 1000 ml to compensate for vasodilation caused by sympathetic blockade.

      b. Assist with positioning and provide emotional support during procedure.

      c. Maintain uterine displacement intrapartum or intraoperatively.

      d. Monitor maternal vital signs frequently.

      e. Promptly treat hypotension (systolic BP <100 mm Hg) with lateral positioning, increase IV fluids, and/or administer IV ephedrine to maintain uteroplacental perfusion.

         (1) Slight Trendelenburg position with lateral tilt prevents cranial spread of intrathecal anesthesia.

         (2) Elevating legs increases preload.

         (3) Mean arterial pressure more reflective of hypotension status than systolic and diastolic BP

      f. Assess dermatome levels bilaterally.

      g. Assess for urinary retention.

      h. Monitor fetal heart tones; fetal bradycardia precedes maternal hypotension.

      i. Be alert for total spinal.

      j. Physician's order may include lying flat after administration to avoid headache; however, this is controversial.

B. Lumbar epidural and caudal anesthesia

    1. Epidural catheter frequently used as continuous technique to provide analgesia and anesthesia

    2. Anesthetic implications

      a. Epidural space decreased in diameter and size because of increased blood volume

      b. Pain relief is slower, and a higher volume of anesthetic agent is required than for spinal.

      c. Continuous infusion of low concentrations of local anesthetics into epidural space versus intermittent epidural injections offers the following advantages.

         (1) Total volume of anesthetic less

         (2) Degree of motor blockade minimized; pelvic muscle tone maintained

         (3) Fewer hypotensive episodes

      d. With continuous infusion a potential complication is intravascular or subarachnoid migration of catheter during infusion or progressively increasing levels of anesthesia with resulting hypotension and respiratory distress.

      e. Contraindications same as spinal

    3. Maternal effects

      a. Produces good analgesia, which alters maternal physiologic responses to pain and lowers maternal catecholamine levels

      b. Hypotension may occur because of sympathetic blockade.

      c. Woman awake and active participant in birth

      d. Systemic toxic reactions after epidural are rare but may be caused by

         (1) Unintentional placement of drug in subarachnoid space

         (2) Excessive amount of drug in epidural space

         (3) Accidental IV injection

    4. Fetal effects same as spinal

    5. Epidural opioids

      a. Use of intrathecal and epidural routes for opiate-type agents

      b. Common agents

         (1) Morphine (Duramorph)

         (2) Fentanyl (Sublimaze)

         (3) Hydromorphone (Dilaudid)

      c. Mechanism of action involves specific opiate receptors in spinal cord.

      d. Advantages

         (1) Decreased potential for toxic reaction

         (2) Long-lasting pain relief with minimal effects on voluntary muscle function or cardiovascular status

         (3) Minimal effects on fetus

  e. Disadvantages
    (1) Pruritus
    (2) Nausea and vomiting
    (3) Urinary retention
    (4) Respiratory depression
  6. Nursing implications
    a. Same as spinal
    b. With epidural opioids, pruritus most common side effect; can be treated with
      (1) Antihistamines
      (2) Naloxone
      (3) Opioid agonist–antagonist
    c. Sedation sometimes seen; not always accompanied by respiratory depression
    d. Respiratory depression can occur up to 24 hours after initial administration of opioid anesthesia.
    e. Platelet count <100,000 or bleeding times >10 minutes require anesthesia consultation before removing epidural catheter.
    f. Monitor for progression of profound block.
    g. Observe for intravascular infusion.
      (1) Tinnitus
      (2) Light-headedness
      (3) Circumoral tingling or numbness
      (4) Metallic taste in mouth
      (5) Convulsions
      (6) Urinary retention
III. Local anesthesia and nerve blocks
  A. Indications and actions
    1. Pudendal block
      a. Provides perineal anesthesia for second stage, delivery, episiotomy or laceration repair, forceps or vacuum extractor delivery
      b. Relatively simple procedure but requires thorough knowledge of pelvic anatomy
    2. Local infiltration
      a. Injection of anesthetic agent into intracutaneous, subcutaneous, and intramuscular area of perineum
      b. Used at time of delivery for episiotomy
    3. Paracervical block
      a. Anesthetizes inferior hypogastric plexus and ganglia to provide relief of pain from cervical dilation
      b. Given during active labor
      c. Does not give perineal pain relief
  B. Anesthetic implications
    1. Increased vascularity of perineal area, vagina, and cervix increases possibility of rapid absorption of agent, resulting in systemic toxic reactions.
    2. Relatively simple to administer
  C. Maternal effects
    1. Rapid onset of analgesia
    2. Hematomas may occur as result of vessel damage.
    3. Maternal hypotension rare
    4. No relief of uterine contractions
    5. Systemic toxic reaction can occur from IV injection.
  D. Fetal effects
    1. Fetal bradycardia frequently follows paracervical block because of systemic absorption of drug or accidental injection into fetal scalp.
    2. Usually few fetal effects with local infiltration
  E. Nursing implications
    1. Local anesthesia and nerve blocks usually do not alter maternal vital signs.

2. After paracervical block, carefully monitor FHR for bradycardia; if <110 bpm, increase IV infusion rate, displace uterus, administer supplemental oxygen.
3. Observe for vaginal hematoma.
IV. Psychologic and alternative techniques for pain relief
   A. Psychoprophylaxis
      1. Combines positive conditioning of mother with education on process of childbirth
      2. Basis is belief that pain of labor and birth can be suppressed by reorganization of cerebral cortical activity.
         a. Conditioned pain responses replaced by newly created "positive" conditioned reflexes
         b. Pain with purpose of delivering baby
   B. Hypnosis
      1. Hypnoidal trance provides maternal analgesia with no maternal or fetal compromise.
      2. Use not widespread
   C. Acupuncture or acupressure
   D. Therapeutic touch
   E. Water therapy
   F. Massage

ASSESSMENT OF FETAL WELL-BEING

I. Uterine activity
   A. Assessment of uterine activity
      1. Frequency
      2. Duration
      3. Intensity
   B. Resting tone (uterus at rest) is the time during which fetus receives most of its oxygen and nutrients and eliminates most of excess carbon dioxide.
II. FHR characteristics
   A. FHR tracing reflects complex physiologic processes that occur in fetus and mother.
   B. Mechanisms
      1. FHR is result of interaction between central and autonomic nervous systems and heart.
      2. Primary intrinsic factors
         a. Autonomic nervous system
            (1) Parasympathetic: cholinergic
            (2) Sympathetic: adrenergic
         b. Chemoreceptors
            (1) Respond to chemical changes in blood and compensate accordingly
            (2) Decreased O_2 results in increased heart rate.
         c. Baroreceptors
            (1) Maintain constant pressure
            (2) Increase heart rate with decreased BP to increase CO
      3. Secondary intrinsic factors
         a. Cerebral cortex
         b. Hypothalamus
         c. Medulla oblongata
         d. Adrenal medulla
         e. Adrenal cortex
      4. Extrinsic factors
         a. Placental physiology
         b. Umbilical blood flow
         c. Uterine blood flow
         d. Contractions

    e. Fetal reserve

    f. Maternal cardiopulmonary function

    g. Maternal environment

    h. Fetal-maternal response to drugs

C. Baseline FHR

  1. Approximate mean FHR during a 10-minute period excluding periodic or episodic changes, periods of increased FHR variability, or segments of the baseline that differ by 25 bpm or more; minimum baseline duration must be at least 2 minutes.

  2. Normal: 110 to 160 bpm

    a. Tachycardia

      (1) Rate: >160 bpm for >10 minutes

      (2) Causes

        (a) Fetal hypoxia (early sign)

        (b) Maternal fever

        (c) Drugs

        (d) Maternal hyperthyroidism

        (e) Fetal anemia

        (f) Fetal cardiac dysrhythmias

        (g) Maternal hypovolemia

    b. Bradycardia

      (1) Rate <110 bpm for >10 minutes

      (2) Causes

        (a) Hypoxia (late sign)

        (b) Fetal cardiac dysrhythmias

        (c) Drugs

        (d) Hypothermia

        (e) Reflex

D. Periodic FHR patterns

  1. Accelerations

    a. Sign of fetal well-being

    b. An abrupt (onset to peak in less than 30 seconds) increase in FHR over baseline of at least 15 bpm

      (1) Duration is at least 15 seconds from the onset to return to baseline and no longer than 2 minutes.

      (2) Before 32 weeks' gestation, acceleration will have a peak ~10 bpm above the baseline and will last ~10 seconds.

    c. Presence of accelerations rules out metabolic acidosis.

    d. No intervention required

  2. Early decelerations

    a. A visually apparent gradual decrease (onset of deceleration to nadir of at least 30 seconds) and return to baseline FHR associated with a uterine contraction

      (1) Coincident in timing; nadir of deceleration coincident with peak of contraction

      (2) In most cases the onset, nadir, and recovery are coincident with beginning, peak, and ending of contraction, respectively.

    b. Benign pattern

    c. Vagal response to head compression

    d. No intervention required

  3. Variable decelerations

    a. A visually apparent abrupt decrease (onset of deceleration to beginning of nadir <30 seconds) in FHR from baseline

      (1) Decrease below baseline is at least 15 bpm, lasting (from baseline to baseline) at least 15 seconds.

      (2) Onset, depth, and duration commonly vary with successive uterine contractions.

    b. Result of cord compression

      c. Reflects diminished blood flow to fetal heart and fetal hypoxia, hypotension, or hypertension

      d. Treat with maternal position change; obtain obstetric consultation.

    4. Late decelerations

      a. A visually apparent gradual decrease (onset of deceleration to nadir lasts 30 seconds or more) and return to baseline FHR associated with a uterine contraction

        (1) Delay in timing, with nadir of deceleration late in relation to peak of contraction

        (2) Onset, nadir, and recovery are late in relation to the beginning, peak, and ending of the contraction, respectively.

      b. Response to fetal hypoxia secondary to uteroplacental insufficiency

      c. In presence of abnormal baseline rate, may be ominous

      d. Treat with measures to improve uteroplacental perfusion; obtain obstetric consultation.

POSTPARTUM

  I. Vaginal birth without complications

    A. Anesthesia: see previous section.

    B. Postpartum observations

      1. Vital signs

        a. Blood pressure consistent with baseline during pregnancy

          (1) Orthostatic hypotension may be present for 24 hours.

          (2) Increased BP may be caused by

            (a) Preeclampsia

            (b) Anxiety

            (c) Essential hypertension

          (3) BP not reliable indicator of hypovolemia or shock

        b. Temperature >100.4° F (38° C) after 24 hours may indicate infection.

        c. Tachycardia (>100 bpm) may indicate

          (1) Hemorrhage

          (2) Pain

          (3) Fever

          (4) Dehydration

        d. Tachypnea (>24) may indicate respiratory disease.

        e. Lungs should be clear to auscultation.

      2. Condition of uterine fundus

        a. Firm, midline, at level of umbilicus first 24 hours

        b. Involution occurs at rate of 1 cm/day

        c. Boggy or higher than suggested normal level may indicate uterine atony related to overdistended uterus, structural anomalies, or overdistended bladder.

        d. Overdistended bladder may cause lateral deviation of uterus.

      3. Lochia

        a. Rubra

          (1) Bright red, bloody, may have small clots

          (2) Characteristic fleshy odor

          (3) Occurs 1 to 3 days postpartum

          (4) Heavy to moderate flow

        b. Serosa

          (1) Pink to pink brown, serous, no clots

          (2) Usually no odor

          (3) Occurs 5 to 7 days after delivery

          (4) Decrease in flow

        c. Alba

          (1) Cream to yellowish, may be brownish

          (2) Usually no odor

  (3) Occurs 1 to 3 weeks after delivery
  (4) Scant flow
  d. Excessive lochia may be caused by
   (1) Uterine atony
   (2) Laceration
   (3) Hematoma
   (4) Retained placental fragments
   (5) Infection
  e. Malodorous lochia indicative of infection
 4. Perineum
  a. Slight edema normal
  b. Assessment of episiotomy
   (1) Redness
   (2) Edema
   (3) Ecchymosis
   (4) Discharge
   (5) Approximation
  c. Rectal area free of hemorrhoids, hematoma
 5. Urinary system
  a. Output up to 3000 ml/day
  b. Distended bladder may cause uterine atony.
  c. Burning on urination or inability to void may suggest infection.
  d. Bladder atony may occur after instrument delivery or regional anesthesia.
 6. Intestinal elimination
  a. Bowel movement by day 2 or 3 after delivery
  b. Constipation may indicate sluggish bowel or pain (fear of pain also possible).
  c. Diarrhea may be from multiple factors.
 7. Breasts
  a. Assess feeding method.
  b. Soft to palpation
  c. Colostrum may be present; milk in 2 to 4 days.
  d. Nipples intact, erect
  e. Swollen, painful breasts may indicate infection.
 8. Rh status: is RhoGAM indicated?
 C. Personal care and comfort
  1. Ambulation
  2. Shower or bathing
  3. Perineal care
  4. Sitz bath
  5. Breast support and comfort
  6. Rest and exercise
  7. Nutrition
  8. Emotional adjustment
 D. Family relations
  1. Visitors
  2. Children at home
  3. Sexuality and birth control
  4. Role transitions
  5. Adaptation of family routines
 E. Infant care
II. Cesarean birth without complications
 A. Anesthesia: see previous section.
 B. Potential complications same as for any patient undergoing abdominal surgery
 C. Postoperative assessments same as for any patient undergoing abdominal surgery

    D. Postpartum assessments same as for vaginal delivery
III. High-risk versus critical care
    A. About 1% of obstetric population requires critical care management.
    B. Pregnant-specific diseases and medical complications of pregnancy that often require critical care management
        1. Preeclampsia
        2. Cardiac disease
        3. Septic shock
        4. Adult respiratory distress syndrome
        5. Diabetic ketoacidosis
        6. Thyroid storm
    C. Care multidisciplinary approach with collaboration between obstetric and critical care units
IV. Emergency hysterectomy
    A. Cesarean hysterectomy usually emergency procedure
        1. Emergency indications requiring hysterectomy
            a. Uterine atony (43%)
            b. Placenta accreta (30%)
            c. Uterine rupture (13%)
            d. Extension (unplanned) of low transverse incision (10%)
        2. Complications
            a. Increased blood loss
            b. Occasional injury to either bladder or ureters
            c. Increased anesthesia exposure
        3. Nursing assessments and interventions same as for nonobstetric abdominal hysterectomy

POSTPARTUM COMPLICATIONS

  I. Hemorrhage
    A. Remains major cause of maternal death
    B. Causes
        1. Early pregnancy
            a. Spontaneous abortion
               (1) Termination of pregnancy before viability of fetus
               (2) Of all clinically apparent pregnancies, ~15% end in spontaneous abortion
               (3) Caused by abnormal embryonic development, chromosomal defects, inheritable disorders; many early losses from unknown origin
               (4) Signs and symptoms depend on duration of pregnancy; bleeding, with varying degrees of pain.
            b. Incompetent cervix (see section on pregnancy complications)
            c. Ectopic pregnancy (see section on pregnancy complications)
            d. Hydatidiform mole (see section on pregnancy complications)
        2. Nursing implications for early pregnancy bleeding
            a. Obtain history of woman's
               (1) Chief complaint
               (2) Pain
               (3) Bleeding
               (4) Last menstrual period
            b. Initial database includes
               (1) Vital signs
               (2) Previous pregnancies
               (3) Previous pregnancy outcomes
               (4) Type and location of pain
               (5) Quantity and nature of bleeding

       (6) Allergies

       (7) Emotional status

   c. Possibility of ectopic pregnancy suspected in woman with history of

       (1) Missed menstrual period

       (2) Spotting

       (3) Pelvic pain

       (4) History of pelvic infection

       (5) Intrauterine device (IUD) use

       (6) Tubal surgery

   d. If internal bleeding present, assessment will reveal

       (1) Vertigo

       (2) Shoulder pain

       (3) Hypotension

       (4) Tachycardia

   e. Obtain ordered diagnostic and laboratory tests.

       (1) Pregnancy test

       (2) CBC

       (3) Blood typing for group

       (4) Rh factor

       (5) Crossmatching

       (6) Ultrasonography

       (7) Chest x-ray film

       (8) ECG if needed

   f. Immediate nursing care focuses on stabilization.

   g. Correct fluid and electrolyte imbalances.

   h. Analgesics as appropriate

   i. IV oxytocin, 10 IU in 500 ml of infusate, may be needed to induce or augment abortion; ergot products contraindicated until uterus is emptied

   j. Antibiotics as necessary

   k. Blood volume replacement; transfusion may be required

   l. RhoGAM should be given within 72 hours of pregnancy loss if patient is Rh negative.

   m. Prepare for surgical procedure if appropriate.

   n. Grief support and anticipatory guidance

3. Late pregnancy bleeding

   a. Placenta previa (see section on pregnancy complications)

   b. Abruptio placentae (see section on pregnancy complications)

4. Postpartum hemorrhage

   a. Most common and most serious type of excessive obstetric blood loss

       (1) Leading cause of maternal morbidity and mortality

       (2) Accounts for ~10% of nonabortive maternal deaths

       (3) Of all deliveries, ~8% complicated by postpartum hemorrhage

   b. Definition

       (1) Traditionally, loss of ~500 ml of blood after delivery

       (2) More meaningful definition is loss of 1% or more of body weight; 1 ml of blood weighs 1 g.

   c. Pathophysiology

       (1) Control of bleeding from placental site accomplished by prolonged contraction and retraction of interlacing strands of myometrium

       (2) Most common causes of postpartum hemorrhage, in approximate order of frequency, are

          (a) Mismanagement of third stage of labor

          (b) Uterine atony

          (c) Lacerations of birth canal

          (d) Hematologic disorders

          (e) Medical complications

          (f) Infection

        (3) Uterine atony is marked hypotonia of uterus.

          (a) Occurs with

            (i) Grand multipara

            (ii) Hydramnios

            (iii) Fetal macrosomia

            (iv) Multifetus gestation

          (b) Other causes include

            (i) Traumatic delivery

            (ii) Halogenated anesthesia

            (iii) Magnesium sulfate

            (iv) Rapid or prolonged labor

            (v) Chorioamnionitis

            (vi) Use of oxytocin for induction or augmentation of labor

            (vii) Postpartum filling of urinary bladder

          (c) Management goal is to

            (i) Eliminate cause

            (ii) Administer oxytoxic agent

            (iii) Maintain contraction of uterine muscle

       (4) Lacerations of birth canal

          (a) Second only to uterine atony as major cause of postpartum hemorrhage

          (b) Continued bleeding despite efficient postpartum uterine contractions demands inspection or reinspection of birth passage (labia, perineum, vagina, cervix).

          (c) Causative factors

            (i) Operative delivery (forceps or vacuum extraction)

            (ii) Aseptic or uncontrolled spontaneous delivery

            (iii) Congenital abnormalities of maternal soft tissue

            (iv) Contracted pelvis

            (v) Fetal size or position

            (vi) Prior scarring

            (vii) Varices

          (d) Management depends on identification of source of bleeding and repair of laceration.

5. Summary of diagnosis and management of hemorrhage

    a. Identify source of bleeding early.

    b. ORDER

      (1) O: oxygenation

      (2) R: replace intravascular volume.

      (3) D: drug therapy as needed to maintain hemodynamic status

      (4) E: evaluate patient status and effectiveness of treatment.

      (5) R: remedy underlying cause.

    c. REACT

      (1) Resuscitation: assessments, stabilization, venous access

      (2) Evaluate: did initial actions improve patient status?

      (3) Arrest hemorrhage: eliminate cause of hemorrhage, including traditional pharmacologic management or surgical intervention.

      (4) Consultation: care may require collaboration with medicine or anesthesia, transfer to critical care unit.

      (5) Treat complications: anticipate complications that occur because of hypovolemia, hypotension, and shock.

    d. Treat cause.

      (1) Atony

        (a) Fundal compression

        (b) IV solution of oxytocin; never given as undiluted IV push bolus

        (c) Methylergonovine (Methergine), 0.2 mg IM; *contraindicated in patient with history of hypertension*

           (d) Alprostadil (Prostin/15 M), 0.25 to 1.5 mg IM; use with caution in women with
              (i) History of reactive airway disease
              (ii) Asthma
              (iii) Cardiac disease
              (iv) Hepatic disease
              (v) Systemic lupus erythematosus
       (2) Hematoma
          (a) Evacuate.
          (b) Ligate areas of bleeding.
       (3) If patient is unresponsive
          (a) Arterial ligation or embolization
          (b) Hysterectomy
          (c) Umbrella pack
          (d) Military antishock trousers

II. Shock

  A. Because of expanded blood volume in pregnancy, early signs and symptoms of hemorrhagic shock may be masked.

    1. Earliest sign will be mild tachycardia with no change in blood pressure.

    2. COP reduced during pregnancy; will be further reduced with fluid resuscitation, increased risk for pulmonary edema

  B. Must be suspicious if excessive bleeding present; do not forget hidden sources of bleeding

    1. Placenta previa

    2. Abruptio placentae

    3. Placenta accreta

    4. Severe preeclampsia

    5. HELLP syndrome

    6. Eclampsia

    7. Coagulopathies (chronic DIC)

    8. Abdominal trauma

    9. Amniotic fluid embolism

  C. Shock is an emergency situation in which perfusion of body organs may become severely compromised and death may ensue.

  D. Aggressive treatment necessary to prevent adverse sequelae

    1. Initiate standing orders: start IV fluids and obtain CBC and coagulation studies, maintain airway.

    2. If patient is still pregnant, maintain uterine displacement.

    3. Trendelenburg position may interfere with cardiopulmonary functioning.

    4. Anticipate need for invasive hemodynamic monitoring.

  E. Nursing implications

    1. Assess and record respiratory rate, quality, and pattern.

    2. Assess and record pulse rate and quality.

      a. Rate increases and becomes irregular as shock progresses.

      b. Immediate postpartum period: physiologic bradycardia; may further mask mild tachycardia

    3. Assess and record blood pressure, capillary refill, pulse oximetry, skin color, and temperature.

    4. Assess and record LOC and mentation.

    5. Evaluate hemodynamic parameters if pulmonary artery catheter used.

III. Pulmonary embolism; deep vein thrombosis (DVT)

  A. Leading cause of maternal morbidity and mortality during pregnancy and puerperium is thromboembolic disease caused by hypercoagulable state.

  B. DVT

    1. Venous stasis in presence of hypercoagulability leads to development of DVT.

2. DVT predisposes to development of pulmonary embolism.
3. First sign of DVT may be pulmonary embolism.

C. Women with DVT or pulmonary embolism in association with pregnancy may have no significant medical risk factors or problems.

1. Conditions with increased associated risk include prior history of DVT or pulmonary embolism, surgical procedures, immobility, obstetric complications, and hereditary deficiency of antithrombin (AT) III, protein C, or protein S.
2. Time of greatest risk is immediate postpartum period, especially after cesarean birth.

D. Nursing implications

1. Primary goal is maintenance of pulmonary function.
2. Frequent assessments of respiratory status
3. Oxygen exchange should be facilitated by positioning and supplemental oxygen administration.
4. Pulse oximetry should be used to monitor oxygen saturation in conjunction with ABGs.
5. Administer heparin to maintain an activated partial prothrombin time (aPTT) of 1.5 to 2 times that of control levels or a plasma heparin level of 0.2 to 0.3 IU/ml antepartum (0.1 to 0.2 IU/ml intrapartum).
6. Anticipate need for protamine sulfate to reverse heparin effects (1 mg of protamine sulfate neutralizes 100 IU of heparin; maximal single dose, 50 mg).
7. Assess for signs of preterm labor if patient has not delivered (see information on preterm labor).

IV. DIC

A. Pathophysiology

1. Pathologic form of clotting that is diffuse and consumes large amounts of clotting factors
2. All aspects of coagulation system involved
3. Pregnancy predisposes to DIC because of changes in coagulation system.
4. Pregnancy conditions that increase risk for DIC
   a. Abruptio placentae
   b. Preeclampsia, HELLP syndrome, eclampsia
   c. Retained dead fetus syndrome
   d. Sepsis
   e. Amniotic fluid embolism
   f. Saline induction of abortions
   g. Excessive hemorrhage

B. Nursing implications

1. Be aware of maternal predisposing conditions.
2. Cardiovascular assessment
3. Respiratory assessment
4. Renal assessment
5. CNS assessment
6. Fetal assessment
   a. Assess whether FHR baseline is appropriate for gestational age.
   b. Assess for changes in baseline rate.
   c. Assess for late decelerations.
7. Monitor laboratory assessments for worsening condition or for signs of improvement.
8. Assess for preterm labor.
9. Institute supportive measures to correct acidosis, hypotension, and hypoperfusion.
10. Initiate vigorous volume replacement.
11. Initiate blood component replacement.

BIBLIOGRAPHY

1. American Academy of Pediatrics, American College of Obstetricians and Gynecologists: *Guidelines for perinatal care,* ed 5. Elk Grove, IL: American Academy of Pediatrics, 2002.

2. American College of Obstetricians and Gynecologists: ACOG Educational Bulletin No. 36: Obstetric analgesia and anesthesia. *Obstet Gynecol* 100:177-191, 2002.

3. Bader TJ: *OB/GYN secrets,* ed 3. Philadelphia: Hanley & Belfus, 2003.

4. Bonica JJ, McDonald JS, editors: *Principles and practice of obstetric analgesia and anesthesia,* ed 2. Baltimore: Williams & Wilkins, 1995.

5. Briggs GG, Freeman RK, Yaffee SJ: *Drugs in pregnancy and lactation,* ed 6. Baltimore: Williams & Wilkins, 2001.

6. Burke ME, Poole JH: Common perinatal complications. In Simpson KR, Creehan PA, editors: *AWHONN perinatal nursing.* Philadelphia: Lippincott-Raven, 1996.

7. Chestnut DH, editor: *Obstetric anesthesia: Principles and practice,* ed 2. St Louis: Mosby, 2000.

8. Clark SL, Cotton DB, Hankins GDV, et al: *Handbook of critical care obstetrics.* Boston: Blackwell Scientific, 1994.

9. Clark SL: New concepts of amniotic fluid embolism: A review. *Obstet Gynecol Surv* 45:360, 1990.

10. Clark SL, Hankins GDV, Dudley D, et al: Amniotic fluid embolus: Analysis of the National Registry. *Am J Obstet Gynecol* 172:1159, 1995.

11. Creasy RK, Resnik R, editors: *Maternal-fetal medicine,* ed 4. Philadelphia: WB Saunders, 1999.

12. Cunningham FG, MacDonald PC, Gant NF, editors: *Williams obstetrics,* ed 20. Stamford, CN: Appleton & Lange, 1997.

13. Daddario JB, Johnson G: Trauma in pregnancy. In Mandeville LK, Troiano NH, editors: *AWHONN's high-risk and critical care intrapartum nursing,* ed 2. Philadelphia: Lippincott, 1999.

14. Dantzker DR: Effects of pulmonary embolism on the lung. *Anesthesiol Clin North America* 10:781, 1992.

15. Datta S, editor: *Anesthetic and obstetric management of high-risk pregnancy,* ed 2. St Louis: Mosby, 1996.

16. Dehring DJ: Pulmonary thromboembolism. *Anesthesiol Clin North Am* 10:869, 1992.

17. Dunn PA, Poole JH: Critically-ill pregnant or postpartum woman: General principles for care. In Dunn PA, editor: *Maternal and newborn nursing.* Philadelphia: Little, Brown, 1996.

18. Gabbe SG, Niebyl JR, Simpson JL, editors: *Obstetrics: Normal and problem pregnancies,* ed 4. New York: Churchill Livingstone, 2002.

19. Gillie MH, Hughes SC: Amniotic fluid embolism. *Anesthesiol Clin North America* 10:55, 1993.

20. Hankins GDV, Synder R, Clark SL, et al: Acute hemodynamic and respiratory effects of amniotic fluid embolism in the pregnant goal model. *Am J Obstet Gynecol* 168:1113, 1993.

21. Harvey C, Hankins GDV, Clark SL: Amniotic fluid embolism and oxygen transport patterns. *Am J Obstet Gynecol* 174: 304, 1996.

22. Hayashi R: Obstetric hemorrhage and hypovolemic shock. In Clark SL, Cotton DB, Hankins GDV, et al, editors: *Critical Care Obstetrics.* Boston: Blackwell Scientific, 1991, pp 199-211.

23. Higby K, Xenakis E, Pauerstein C: Do tocolytic agents stop preterm labor? A critical and comprehensive review of efficacy and safety. *Am J Obstet Gynecol* 168:1247, 1993.

24. Hughes SG, Levinson G, Rosen MA: *Shnider and Levison's anesthesia for obstetrics,* ed 4. Philadelphia: Lippincott Williams & Wilkins, 2001.

25. James DK, Steer PJ, Weiner CP, et al, editors: *High risk pregnancy: Management options,* ed 2. Philadelphia: WB Saunders, 1999.

26. Johnson MD, Luppi CJ, Over D: Cardiopulmonary resuscitation in pregnancy. In Gambling, D, editor: *Obstetric anesthesia and uncommon disorders.* Philadelphia: WB Saunders, 1998.

27. Katz RL, editor: Obstetrical anesthesia. I. *Semin Anesth* 10:221, 1991.

28. Katz RL, editor: Obstetrical anesthesia. II. *Semin Anesth* 11:1, 1992.

29. Kaufmann BS, Young CC: Deep vein thrombosis. *Anesthesiol Clin North America* 10:823, 1992.

30. Knuppel RA, Drukker JE, editors: *High-risk pregnancy: A team approach,* ed 2. Philadelphia, WB Saunders, 1993.

31. Knuppel RA, Hatangadi SB: Acute hypotension related to hemorrhage in the obstetric patient. *Obstet Gynecol Clin North America* 22:111, 1995.

32. Mandeville LK, Troiano NH, editors: *AWHONN's high-risk and critical care intrapartum nursing,* ed 2. Philadelphia: Lippincott, 1999.

33. May KA, Mahlmeister LR: *Comprehensive maternity nursing: Nursing process and the childbearing family,* ed 3. Philadelphia: Lippincott, 1994.

34. Merkatz PD, Goldenberg RL: *New perspectives on prenatal care.* New York: Elsevier, 1990.

35. Parer JT: *Handbook of fetal heart rate monitoring,* ed 2. Philadelphia, WB Saunders, 1997.

36. Poole JH: Getting perspective on HELLP syndrome. *Am J Matern Child Nurs* 13:432, 1988.

37. Poole JH: Legal and professional issues in critical care obstetrics. *Crit Care Nurs Clin North America* 4:687, 1992.

38. Poole JH: Pulmonary embolism. *NAACOGS Clin Issu Perinat Womens Health Nurs* 3:461, 1992.

39. Poole JH: HELLP syndrome and coagulopathies of pregnancy. *Crit Care Nurs Clin North America* 5:475, 1993.

40. Poole JH: Hypertensive states, hemorrhagic disorders, and infectious disease. In Bobak IM, Lowdermilk D, editors: *Essentials of maternity nursing,* ed 4. St Louis: Mosby–Year Book, 1995.

41. Poole JH, White D, Hall SP: *Crisis OB: The video series, part I: Emergency and complicated deliveries.* St Louis: Mosby, 1995.

42. Poole JH, White D, Hall SP: *Crisis OB: The video series, Part II: Hypertension in pregnancy.* St Louis: Mosby, 1995.

43. Poole JH, White D, Hall SP: *Crisis OB: The video series, part III: Hemorrhagic disorders in pregnancy.* St Louis: Mosby, 1995.

44. Poole JH: Hematological/vascular disorders. In Dunn PA, editor: *Manual of maternal-newborn nursing.* Philadelphia: Little, Brown, 1996.

45. Poole JH: Hypertensive disease in pregnancy. In Dunn PA, editor: *Manual of maternal-newborn nursing.* Philadelphia: Little, Brown, 1996.

46. Poole JH: Sepsis. In Dunn PA, editor: *Manual of maternal-newborn nursing.* Philadelphia: Little, Brown, 1996.

47. Poole JH: Trauma. In Dunn PA, editor: *Manual of maternal-newborn nursing.* Philadelphia: Little, Brown, 1996.

48. Poole JH: Maternal hemorrhagic disorders. In Bobak IM, editor: *Maternity and gynecologic Care,* ed 6. St Louis: Mosby, 1997.

49. Poole JH: *Hypertensive disorders of pregnancy.* White Plains, NY: March of Dimes, Perinatal Nursing Education, 1997.

50. Poole JH: Aggressive management of HELLP syndrome and eclampsia. *AACN Clin Issues* 8(4):524-538, 1997.

51. Poole JH: Liver transplant and pregnancy. *J Perinatal Neonatal Nurs* 11(4):25-34, 1998.

52. Poole JH: Renal disease in pregnancy. *J Perinatal Neonatal Nurs* 15(4):13-26, 2002.

53. Repke JT: *Intrapartum obstetrics.* New York: Churchill Livingstone, 1996.

54. Scott JR, DiSaia PH, Hammond CB, et al, editors: *Danforth's obstetrics and gynecology,* ed 8. Philadelphia: Lippincott, 1999.

55. Simpson KR, Creehan PA, editors: *AWHONN Perinatal Nursing,* ed 2. Philadelphia: Lippincott Williams & Wilkins, 2001.

56. White D, Poole JH: *Obstetrical emergencies for the perinatal nurse.* White Plains, NY: March of Dimes, 1996.

47 Ophthalmologic Procedures

LINDA BOYUM

OBJECTIVES

At the conclusion of this chapter the reader will be able to:

1. Identify the important functions of the eye.

2. Describe the structure of the eye.

3. Discuss common ophthalmologic surgical procedures.

4. List drugs frequently used for ophthalmologic surgical procedures.

5. Identify possible complications of ophthalmologic surgery.

6. Discuss perianesthesia nursing care for the ophthalmologic surgery patient.

■
■■ This chapter covers surgical procedures performed on the eye. Surgical advances have revolutionized prevention of ocular disease as well as perfected operative interventions. Potential complications and perianesthesia nursing interventions are discussed.

I. Structure of the eye (see Figure 47-1)
   A. Orbit
      1. A pyramid-shaped bony cavity that functions as protection for the eye
      2. Consists of seven fused bones
         a. Ethmoid
         b. Sphenoid
         c. Frontal
         d. Lacrimal
         e. Zygomatic
         f. Palatine
         g. Maxilla
      3. The orbit contains the eyeball, six extraocular muscles, ophthalmic artery veins, the second (optic), third (oculomotor), fourth (trochlear), fifth (trigeminal), sixth (abducens), cranial nerves, lacrimal gland, lacrimal sac, orbital fascia, and fat and ligaments.
   B. Eyelids
      1. Act as protection for the anterior portion of the eyes, and the epithelium of the lids; is continuous with the conjunctiva lining the inner aspect of the lid.
      2. Spread lubricating solutions over globe
         a. Keep eyes moist
         b. Prevent evaporation of secretion
      3. Eyelashes are situated along the margins and act as protective fibers.
      4. Two muscle groups
         a. Sphincter called the orbicularis oculae—responsible for closing the eye
         b. Levator palpebrae—responsible for raising the lids
         c. Movements can be both involuntary and voluntary.
      5. Function of the eyelids
         a. Cover eyes during sleep
         b. Protect eyes from excessive light

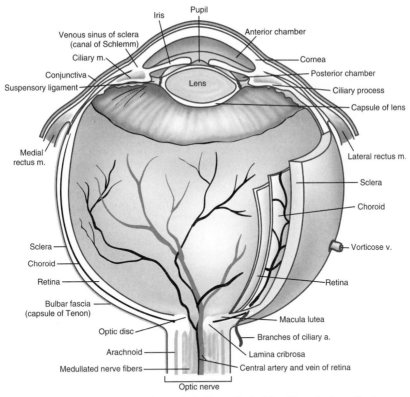

FIGURE 47-1 ■ Structure of the eyeball. (From Drain CB, editor: *Perianesthesia nursing: A critical care approach,* ed 4. St Louis: WB Saunders, 2003, p. 453.)

    c. Protect eye from injury
    d. Protect eye from foreign objects
    e. Lubricate the anterior surface of the eye
  6. Lined with mucous membrane called palpebral conjunctiva
C. Conjunctiva
  1. Thin transparent mucous membrane covering sclera and inner lids
  2. Lining upper and lower eyelids—palpebral conjunctiva
  3. Extends over sclera to corneal margin—bulbar conjunctiva
  4. Function of the conjuctiva
    a. Produces the mucin layer of the tear film, reducing the rate of tear evaporation
    b. Protects the eye against damage and infection
    c. Facilitates movement by moistening the surface of the eye and lids
D. Lacrimal apparatus: produces and drains tears
  1. Consists of
    a. Lacrimal gland—located in upper outer aspect of each orbit
      (1) Produces tears
      (2) Tears empty through lacrimal ducts onto conjunctiva of upper lid.
      (3) Tears are spread across eyeball by blinking.
      (4) Tears enter lacrimal puncta.
    b. Lacrimal puncta—two small openings located in the inner canthus of each upper and lower eyelid
      (1) Pass into lacrimal canals, lacrimal sac, nasolacrimal duct, and finally into inferior meatus of the turbinate bone of the nose
    c. Lacrimal sac—collects tears
    d. Nasolacrimal duct—Drains tears from lacrimal sac to nose

    2. Tears
       a. Contain water, protein, glucose, sodium, potassium, chloride, urea, and, lysozyme (bacterial enzyme)
       b. Purpose of tears
         (1) Aid refraction by providing an optically smooth corneal surface
         (2) Lubricate the anterior surface of the eye to aid movement
         (3) Clean dust particles from the eye
         (4) Protect against infection by the action of lysozymes
       c. Emotional stimulus of parasympathetic nervous system triggered
  E. Muscles controlling the eye (see Figure 47-2)
    1. Extraocular muscles (six)
       a. Attached to outside of eyeball and to bones of the orbit
       b. Consist of voluntary skeletal muscle
         (1) Four rectus
           (a) Superior—oculomotor nerve
           (b) Inferior—oculomotor nerve

Cardinal Directions of Gaze	Muscles Working for Each Direction
Eyes up, right	Right superior rectus and left inferior oblique
Eyes right	Right lateral rectus and left medial rectus
Eyes down, right	Right inferior rectus and left superior oblique
Eyes down, left	Right superior oblique and left inferior rectus
Eyes left	Right medial rectus and left lateral rectus
Eyes up, left	Right inferior oblique and left superior rectus

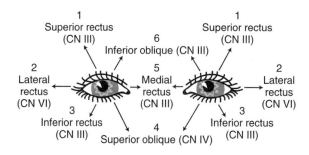

FIGURE 47-2 ■ The six cardinal directions of gaze and the muscles responsible for each. The six cardinal directions are (1) right, (2) left, (3) up and right, (4) up and left, (5) down and right, and (6) down and left. (From Black JM, Matassarin-Jacobs E: *Medical-surgical nursing clinical management for continuity of care*, ed 5. Philadelphia: WB Saunders, 1997, p 936.)

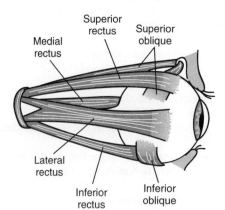

Muscles of Right Eye

(c) Medial—oculomotor nerve

(d) Lateral—abducens nerve

(2) Two oblique muscles

(a) Superior—trochlea nerve

(b) Inferior—oculomotor nerve

c. Action

(1) Muscles move eyeball through cranial nerves.

(a) Third (oculomotor)—moves eyeball and upper eyelid

(b) Size of iris (i.e., constriction and dilation of pupil to regulate amount of light admitted)

(c) Control of ciliary muscle to regulate degree of refraction by lens

(d) Fourth (trochlear)—movement of eyeball by superior oblique muscles

(e) Sixth (abducens)—movement of eyeball by lateral rectus muscle

(2) Muscles work in pairs

(3) Movement caused by

(a) Increase in tone of one set of muscles and a decrease in the tone of the antagonistic (opposite set) of muscles

2. Movement of upper eyelid

a. Raised (opened) by levator palpebrae superioris muscle

(1) Controlled by cranial nerve III and sympathetic nervous system

b. Closed by orbicularis oculi muscle

(1) Controlled by cranial nerve VII

3. Iris and ciliary muscles

a. Smooth, involuntary muscles

b. Work inside eyeball

(1) Regulate size of pupil

(2) Control shape of lens during accommodation

(3) Controlled through neural network

(a) Optic nerve (cranial nerve II)

(b) Oculomotor nerve (cranial nerve III)

F. Globe (eyeball): supported in orbital cavity on a cushion of fat and fascia; composed of three layers

1. External, corneal-scleral layer (fibrous, protects other two layers)

a. Cornea

(1) Anterior, transparent, avascular part of the external layer

(2) Serves as a window through which light rays pass to retina

(3) Supplied by branches of ophthalmic division of fifth cranial nerve

(4) Composed of five layers

(a) Epithelium

(i) Cell layers and nerve endings

(ii) Account for corneal sensitivity

(b) Bowman's membrane

(i) Composed of connective tissue fibers

(ii) Forms a barrier between trauma and infection

(iii) Does not regenerate if damaged

(iv) Will leave a permanent scar

(c) Stroma

(i) Accounts for 90% of corneal thickening

(ii) Composed of multiple lamellar fibers

(d) Descemet's membrane

(i) Thin layer between endothelial layer of cornea and substantia propria (fibrous, tough, and transparent main part of the cornea)

(ii) If inflamed, called descemetitis

(iii) If protrudes, called descemetocele

(e) Endothelium

(i) Single layer of hexagonal cells

(ii) Does not regenerate

(iii) Responsible for proper state of dehydration that keeps cornea clear

(iv) Damage causes corneal edema and loss of transparency.

   b. Sclera: posterior opaque part of the external layer; tough white outer coat of eyeball

     (1) Portion of sclera can be seen through the conjunctiva as the white of the eye

     (2) Made up of collagenous fibers loosely connected with fascia, which receives the tendons of the muscles of the globe

2. Middle layer: middle covering of the eye comprises the choroid, ciliary body, and iris (referred to as uveal tract).

   a. Choroid

     (1) Most posterior portion of middle coat

     (2) Contains many blood vessels; highly vascular

     (3) Deeply pigmented

     (4) Purpose

       (a) Absorbs light rays

       (b) Prevents reflection within eyeball

       (c) Main source of nourishment to retina (through its blood supply)

   b. Ciliary body

     (1) Consists of an extension of the choroidal blood vessels, a mass of muscle tissue, and an extension of the neuroepithelium of the retina

     (2) Composed of ciliary muscle and ciliary processes

     (3) Ciliary muscle

       (a) Affects accommodation

       (b) Alters shape of lens as needed to focus light rays from near or distant objects on retina

     (4) Ciliary processes

       (a) Produce aqueous humor

   c. Iris

     (1) Colored area of eye

     (2) Anterior portion of the middle layer

       (a) Thin membrane situated in front of the lens

     (3) Peripheral border attached to ciliary body

     (4) Central border is free.

     (5) Divides the space between the cornea and the lens

       (a) Anterior and posterior chambers

       (b) Chambers are filled with aqueous humor.

     (6) Regulates the amount of light entering the eye

       (a) Muscles contract and relax.

       (b) Changes size of opening in center (pupil)

       (c) Assists in obtaining clear images

3. Internal layer: innermost layer of neural coat (retina)

   a. Retina

     (1) A thin transparent membrane extending from the ora serrata to the optic disk

     (2) Consists of network of nerve cells and fibers

       (a) Receives images of external objects

       (b) Transfers the impressions via the optic nerve, optic tracts, lateral geniculate body, and optic radiations to the occipital lobe of cerebrum

       (c) Nerve fibers from retina converge to become optic nerve.

         (i) Point at which optic nerve enters eyeball is called optic disk (anatomic blind spot)

     (3) Covers choroid

     (4) Found only in back of eye

b. Retina is composed of layers.
  (1) Outer pigment
    (a) Stores vitamin A; needed to produce photopigment rhodopsin
  (2) Inner neural
    (a) Consists of photoreceptor cells (rods and cones)
      (i) Visual receptors that develop generator potentials
      (ii) Relays sensory information to ganglion cells of retina
    (b) Rods
      (i) Located in peripheral retina
      (ii) Allow for vision in dim light
      (iii) Responsible for perception of different shades of light and dark, shapes, and movement
    (c) Cones
      (i) Stimulated by bright light only
      (ii) Responsible for color vision and visual acuity
G. Refractive apparatus (cornea, aqueous humor, lens, and vitreous body)
  1. Cornea
    a. Has greatest refractive power of the ocular structures
    b. Variations in curvature of cornea change its refractive power
  2. Aqueous humor
    a. Fluid responsible for maintaining intraocular pressure
    b. Produced by ciliary processes
    c. Secreted by ciliary body into posterior chamber
    d. Flows from posterior chamber through pupil into anterior chamber
    e. Flows into anterior chamber angle and is filtered out through the trabecular meshwork into Schlemm's canal
    f. Channeled into capillary network and into episcleral veins
    g. Maintenance of normal intraocular pressure
      (1) Occurs as long as there is a balance between
        (a) Aqueous production and
        (b) Aqueous humor outflow
  3. Lens
    a. Suspended behind the iris
    b. Anterior and posterior surfaces are separated by rounded border.
    c. Does not shed cells; as it grows the cells compress and harden
    d. Lens expands and retracts through zonular fibers (accommodation).
    e. Accommodation power is lost with aging process.
    f. Hardening eventually causes opacity of lens (cataract).
  4. Vitreous body
    a. Glasslike transparent gelatinous mass (vitreous humor)
    b. Composed of 99% water and 1% collagen and hyaluronic acid
    c. Fills the posterior four fifths of the eyeball
    d. Supports the posterior cavity
    e. Keeps the retina in place
H. Nerve and blood supply
  1. Optic nerve (second cranial nerve)
    a. Extends between posterior eyeball and optic chiasma
    b. Carries visual impulses and sensations of pain, touch, temperature from eye to brain
  2. Muscle innervation
    a. Oculomotor (third cranial nerve): primary motor nerve to all rectus muscles (except lateral rectus)
    b. Abducens (sixth cranial nerve) innervates lateral rectus.
    c. Trochlear (fourth cranial nerve) innervates superior oblique muscle.
  3. Ophthalmic artery
    a. Main arterial supply to orbit and globe
    b. Branch of internal carotid artery

II. Common ophthalmic surgical procedures
   A. Blepharoplasty—repair of the upper or lower eyelids to remove redundant skin; may be cosmetic or therapeutic when the eyelid interferes with vision
      1. Types
         a. Upper blepharoplasty (upper eyelid only)
         b. Lower blepharoplasty (lower eyelid only)
         c. Quadrilateral blepharoplasty (involving all four eyelids)
      2. Preoperative considerations
         a. Patient may be examined by ophthalmologist prior to procedure to rule out ocular symptomatology.
      3. Surgical procedure
         a. Excess skin and muscle are resected; periorbital fat is trimmed.
         b. Requires meticulous hemostasis
         c. Closed using fine nonabsorbable suture
      4. Postoperative considerations
         a. Iced saline dressings applied immediately to control edema
   B. Removal of chalazion—granulomatous inflammation of a meibomian gland in eyelid, frequently caused by *Staphylococcus aureus*
      1. Surgical procedure
         a. Surgical incision and curettage
         b. Most commonly done under local anesthesia in physician's office
         c. Occasionally requires operating room (OR) setting
   C. Repair of entropion
      1. Entropion—eyelid margins turn in, especially the lower lid; caused by spasm of the orbicularis oculi muscle or scarring of the conjuctiva. Lashes scrape across cornea with each eye blink, which is painful and results in corneal abrasions, scarring, and ulcer.
      2. Surgical procedure
         a. Surgical removal of excision of skin and/or muscle and/or the tarsal plate; surgical correction of the muscular fibers of the lid, everting the lid margins and eyelashes
            (1) Performed under local or general anesthesia
         b. Cryotherapy—may be used to freeze and remove lashes, which destroys lash follicle and prevents regrowth of lashes
            (1) Preferred method of treatment
   D. Repair of ectropion
      1. Ectropion—outward turning or eversion of eyelid, usually bilateral
         a. Caused by
            (1) Relaxation of orbicularis oculi muscle
            (2) Scarring of the face near the eye
            (3) Normal aging process
            (4) Bell's palsy
            (5) Exposure of underlying conjunctiva
         b. Can lead to keratitis (inflammation or infection of the cornea)
      2. Surgical procedure
         a. Shortening of lower lid in a horizontal direction
         b. Mild case can be treated with deep electrocautery 4 to 5 mm from the lid margins.
            (1) Resulting scar formation will draw lid to its normal position.
   E. Ptosis
      1. Drooping of the upper eyelid; can affect one or both eyes; caused by weakness of levator muscle, or less frequently, Muller's muscle
      2. Three types of ptosis
         a. Congenital—caused by failure of levator muscle to develop, weakness of superior rectal muscles
         b. Acquired—associated with loss of superior visual field in primary gaze
            (1) Causes
               (a) Mechanical failure—weight of lid

       (b) Trauma—caused by laceration of third cranial nerve, the levator, or both

       (c) Myogenic, by disease—muscular dystrophy

       (d) Neurological disorders—myasthenia gravis

       (e) May be caused by a tumor

     (2) Treatment based on cause and severity

   c. Senile

  3. Surgical procedure

    a. Objective is to create a good upper lid fold with elevation of the lid.

    b. Surgical procedures based on advancement of levator muscle, frontalis muscles, or superior rectus muscle

F. Excision of pterygium

  1. Thick triangular growth of epithelial tissue that extends from corner of cornea to the canthus; appearances may be pale or white; may grow over the papillary opening.

    a. Cause thought to be exposure to constant irritant such as wind, dust, or ultraviolet light

  2. Surgical procedure

    a. Growth is dissected off the cornea and conjunctiva down to the sclera.

    b. Low-dose radiation on surgical wound may be used to prevent regrowth.

     (1) Regrowth rate is 20% to 40%.

G. Lacrimal duct disorders

  1. Dacryocystorhinostomy (DCR)—establishment of a new tear passageway for drainage directly into the nasal cavity

    a. Dacryocystitis is an infection in the lacrimal sac and its mucous membranes that extends to the surrounding connective tissue, resulting in localized cellulitis.

    b. Surgical procedure

     (1) Nasal cavity is anesthetized topically with cocaine preoperatively.

     (2) Usually performed under general anesthesia

     (3) Lacrimal sac is probed and opened.

     (4) A stent is placed through lacrimal duct drainage system to keep system open until epithelium forms around it and creates a new opening; stent, which is generally removed in 6 weeks.

  2. Conjunctivodacryocystorhinostomy

    a. Description

     (1) Variation of DCR

     (2) Necessary if lacrimal sac has been destroyed, must be recreated, or the canaliculi are absent

    b. Surgical procedure

     (1) After completion of DCR, conjunctiva taken from lower lid and sutured to nasal mucosa to form lacrimal sac

     (2) If canaliculus cannot be kept open or is absent

      (a) Permanent stent (Pyrex tube) is placed.

      (b) Patient teaching includes

        (i) How to place tube back in if it falls out

        (ii) How to clean tube

        (iii) How to hold tube in case of sneezing

  3. Endoscopic DCR

    a. Uses endonasal laser to open pathway into lacrimal sac

    b. Uses endoscopic equipment

    c. Benefits

     (1) Eliminates external incision and scar

     (2) Decreases amount of postoperative discomfort

     (3) Provides hemostasis

     (4) Increases healing time

     (5) Decreased cost

H. Surgery for strabismus
  1. Description
   a. The inability to direct the two eyes at the same object because of lack of coordination of extraocular muscles
   b. Misalignment of the axes of the eyes in which one or both eyes is turned inward or outward
   c. Often accompanied by amblyopia (normal vision fails to develop despite absence of disease or refractive error)
   d. Normally done on children less than 6 years of age
   e. May be done for cosmetic reasons for children older than 6 years of age
   f. Indications for performing procedure on adults
    (1) Bell's palsy
    (2) Muscular dystrophy
    (3) Traumatic injury
    (4) Untreated or unsatisfactory treatment of childhood strabismus
    (5) Muscular paralysis resulting from stroke
  2. Surgical procedure
   a. Corrective surgery is performed to change the relative strength of individual muscles and therefore improve coordination.
    (1) May require resection: the removal of a portion of muscle and attachment of cut ends
    (2) May require recession: severance of the muscle from its original insertion with reattachment more posteriorly on the sclera
    (3) May require transplanting a muscle to improve rotation of paralyzed muscle
   b. Intraoperative consideration
    (1) Manipulation of rectus muscle will cause transient bradycardia.
     (a) Treated with atropine
     (b) If severe, surgeon may have to stop manipulation of rectus muscle until heart rate returns to normal.
    (2) Bradycardia caused by innervation of branch of vagus nerve
I. Removal of globe
  1. Exenteration
   a. Entire contents of orbit are removed.
   b. Requires extensive plastic reconstruction
  2. Evisceration
   a. Removal of the contents of the globe
   b. Preserves sclera and muscular attachments
   c. Prosthesis inserted to maintain shape of eye
    (1) Sclera is closed over prosthesis.
    (2) Conjunctiva closed over sclera
    (3) Conformer placed under eyelids to maintain space until swelling subsides and artificial eye is created
   d. Advantages
    (1) Natural attachment of eye muscles
    (2) Normal eye movement
  3. Enucleation
   a. Removal of the diseased globe and a portion of the optic nerve
   b. General anesthesia usually administered
   c. Prosthesis may be inserted.
J. Corneal transplant (keratoplasty)
  1. Description
   a. Grafting of corneal tissue from one human eye to another
   b. Performed when patient's cornea is thickened and opacified
   c. Transparency of cornea may be impaired from infection, burns, or certain diseases.
   d. Corneal transplant performed to improve vision when basic visual structures of eye (optic nerve and retina) are functioning properly

      2. Types

         a. Penetrating keratoplasty (full-thickness)

            (1) Most common

            (2) Performed with microscope

         b. Lamellar keratoplasty (partial thickness)

            (1) More difficult than penetrating keratoplasty

            (2) Higher success rate

               (a) Success because of layered cellular arrangement of corneal tissue and avascularity

         c. Keratectomy (peeling of the cornea)

         d. Tattooing (simulation of a pupil)

            (1) Rarely done

      3. Postoperative considerations

         a. Eye patch and shield remain in place.

         b. Usually removed by surgeon day after surgery

         c. Diet and activity as tolerated

         d. Healing of cornea is very slow.

            (1) Recovery of vision longer than after cataract surgery

      4. Potential complications

         a. Rejection of corneal transplant

            (1) Cornea becomes opaque

            (2) Treated with steroids

            (3) May require repeated keratoplasty

K. Radial keratotomy

      1. Description

         a. Used to reduce myopia in adults

         b. Series of precise, partial-thickness radial incisions in the cornea

         c. Results in scar tissue that forms pulls and results in a flattening of the cornea, reducing refractive error

      2. Usually performed under local and topical anesthesia

      3. Potential complications

         a. Glaring from scars

         b. Permanent scarring

         c. Infection resulting in loss of vision

         d. Cataract formation caused by injury to lens

         e. Variations in the level of correction

      4. Correction with excimer laser

         a. Ablates top of cornea

         b. Fewer complications

            (1) Minimal glare sensitivity problems

            (2) No chance of perforation

         c. Performed with topical anesthesia

         d. Complications

            (1) Overcorrection

            (2) Undercorrection

            (3) Hazing

         e. Postprocedure treatment

            (1) Instillation of tobramycin dexamethasone suspension drops and 5% homatropine hydrobromide

            (2) Placement of disposable soft contact lens for first three weeks

               (a) Promotes epithelial growth

L. Cataract extraction

      1. Description

         a. Cataract: gradual developing opacity of the lens of the eye

            (1) Can occur at any time

               (a) Etiology in infants

                  (i) Heredity

                  (ii) Developmental abnormalities

   (iii) Infection

   (iv) Traumatic eye injury

   (v) Chemical imbalances (galactosemia and diabetes)

  (b) Etiology in adults

   (i) Same as infant

   (ii) Prolonged exposure to ultraviolet light

   (iii) Medications (those used to treat glaucoma)

   (iv) Normal part of aging process

 b. Cataract extraction is the removal of the opaque lens from the interior of the eye.

2. Types of procedures

 a. Intracapsular cataract extraction (ICCE)

  (1) Removal of lens, as well as the anterior and posterior capsule, the cortex, and nucleus

  (2) Method has largely been replaced by the extracapsular cataract extraction.

  (3) Risk of vitreous humor loss

 b. Extracapsular cataract extraction (ECCE)

  (1) Anterior portion of the capsule is first ruptured, then removed.

  (2) Lens cortex and nucleus are expressed from the eye, leaving the posterior capsule behind intact (posterior capsule is excellent support for intraocular lens implantation).

 c. Phacoemulsification

  (1) Removal of lens by fragmenting it with ultrasonic vibrations

  (2) Simultaneously there is irrigation and aspiration of the fragments without the loss of the lens capsule.

  (3) Very small incision needed

3. Correction of aphakia (absence of lens)

 a. Patient sees objects larger than normal.

 b. Objects appear blurred and without detail.

 c. Options available for correction

  (1) Glasses

   (a) Aphakia spectacles

   (b) Fitted 6 to 8 weeks after lens extraction

   (c) Acceptable only for binocular aphakia

   (d) Distorts peripheral vision

   (e) Produces change in image size

   (f) Clear image only in direct center of glasses

  (2) Contact lens

   (a) Excellent option for vision correction

   (b) Can be used for monocular aphakia

   (c) Patient has complete field of vision.

  (3) Epikeratophakia

   (a) Procedure considered for patients with low endothelial cell counts

   (b) Form of refractive keratoplasty

   (c) Description of procedure

    (i) Piece of donor corneal tissue is shaped to specific diopter on a cryolathe.

    (ii) Tissue sutured to recipient's cornea

    (iii) Changes corneal curvature

    (iv) Results in change of refractive power of cornea

  (4) Placement of intraocular lens (IOL)

   (a) Most commonly used procedure today

   (b) Description of lens

    (i) Made of Plexiglas or polymethyl methacrylate (PMMA)

    (ii) Center can be either biconvex or convexoplano and two haptics (spring-hook appendages).

[a] Polypropylene haptics break down over time.

[b] Should not be used on young patients

(iii) Lens cannot adjust anterior to posterior dimensions.

[a] Provides only myopic (nearsighted) or hyperopic (farsighted) vision

[b] Patient decides on need of glasses for distance or reading.

(5) Advantages of IOL

(a) Shorter rehabilitation period

(b) Lens used for monocular aphakic correction

(6) Lens placement

(a) Anterior chamber

(i) Used after ICCE

(ii) Used for secondary lens implantation

(b) Iris plane

(c) Posterior chamber

(i) Only when cataract removed by ECCE or phacoemulsification

(ii) Most physiologic position for artificial lens

(7) Sutureless cataract technique

(a) Increasingly popular

(b) Rapid visual rehabilitation

4. Preoperative considerations

a. Inquire as to patient's use of anticoagulants, nonsteroidal, and antiinflammatory drugs (Motrin or aspirin); can cause increase in bleeding intraoperatively

b. Identify adequate home support system; implement referrals if necessary.

c. Review preoperative instructions with patient; provide instructions in large type; use off-white paper to reduce glare.

d. Administer mydriatics and/or additional medications as ordered.

M. Procedures to treat glaucoma

1. Iridectomy

a. Description

(1) Removal of a section of iris tissue

(2) Peripheral iridectomy done in the treatment of acute, subacute, or chronic angle-closure glaucoma

(a) Extensive peripheral anterior synechiae not yet formed

(3) Reestablishes communication between posterior and anterior chambers

(4) Relieves pupillary block

(5) Facilitates movement of aqueous humor from posterior to anterior chamber

2. Trabeculectomy

a. Description

(1) Creation of a fistula between anterior chamber of eye and subconjunctival space

(2) Portion of the trabecular meshwork surgically excised

(3) Facilitates drainage of aqueous humor from the posterior chamber to the anterior chamber for treatment of glaucoma

b. Adjunctive medical therapy may be utilized to decrease postoperative fibrosis by applying 5-fluorouracil (5-FU) or mitomycin C under the conjunctival flap for 3 to 5 minutes.

N. Vitrectomy

1. Description

a. Removal of all or part of vitreous gel

2. Indications (anterior segment)

a. Vitreous loss during cataract extraction surgery

      b. Anterior segment opacities

      c. Miscellaneous causes

  3. Indications (posterior segment)

      a. Vitreous opacities

      b. Advanced diabetic eye disease

      c. Severe intraocular trauma

      d. Retained foreign bodies

      e. Endophthalmitis

  4. Procedural considerations

      a. Procedure varies according to location of pathologic condition.

         (1) Anterior

         (2) Posterior

      b. Requires use of operating microscope, illuminations system, and cutting-suction-infusion system

  5. Intraoperative considerations

      a. Procedure time varies from 1 hour to 6 hours.

      b. Protect pressure area on patient.

      c. May use elastic stockings

  6. Postoperative considerations

      a. May experience more postoperative pain than is generally associated with ophthalmologic surgeries

         (1) Strong analgesics may be necessary.

         (2) Ice packs may help reduce pain.

O. Retinal detachment

  1. Description

      a. Separation of a portion of the retina from the choroid

      b. Goal of treatment aimed at repairing tears and returning retina to normal anatomic position

  2. Causes

      a. Intraocular neoplasms

      b. Associated with injury (blow to head)

      c. Normal aging process

      d. Severe myopia

      e. Congenital

      f. Inflammatory process

  3. Signs and symptoms

      a. Patient may experience sudden onset of floaters (floating spots in front of eye).

      b. Loss of vision without pain

      c. Slow decrease in visual field (described as if someone were pulling a curtain in front of eye)

  4. Types

      a. Primary detachment—hole in retina permits fluid to enter space between retina and choroid.

      b. Secondary detachment—fluid or tissue builds up between choroid and retina with no hole in retina.

  5. Treatment

      a. Diathermy

         (1) Traditional method

            (a) Insertion of microneedles or needle tip of a probe into sclera

            (b) Shortwave radio frequency energy delivered through needles

            (c) Causes thermal changes in tissue

            (d) Results in scar formation and retinal reattachment at points of adhesion

            (e) Procedure rarely used anymore

      b. Cryotherapy

         (1) More popular method; less invasive than diathermy

         (2) Application of $-80°$ C cryoprobe to scleral area of detachment

           (3) Inflammation causes adhesion and reattaches retina.

           (4) Fewer complications than diathermy

      c. Pneumoretinopexy

           (1) Injection of air or expansile gases into vitreous cavity

           (2) Usually done in physician's office

           (3) Crymotherapy may be used to close and seal hole before gas is injected.

           (4) Patient may be instructed to hold head in certain position until retina reattaches (usually 2 weeks).

      d. Laser therapy

           (1) Used to "spot weld" retina

           (2) Done in physician's office

           (3) Can be done in OR in conjunction with vitrectomy

      e. Scleral buckling

           (1) Description

           (2) A procedure developed to create indentation in the retina so that adherence between the detached area and underlying tissues will result in permanent reattachment

      f. Posterior vitrectomy

           (1) Description

               (a) Objective is to remove vitreous humor without pulling on retina; permits surgeon to work directly on retina

              (b) Can be performed with all techniques for reattaching retina

  6. Preoperative considerations

      a. Instruct patient regarding activity limitations prior to surgery (reduces stress on area of detachment).

      b. Inform patient and family of potential for lengthy surgery (decrease anxiety level).

  7. Postoperative considerations

      a. Patient usually on cycloplegic agents (atropine or cyclopentolate) to dilate pupil and rest muscles of accommodation

      b. May be on antibiotic and steroid eyedrops

      c. Assess patient's ability to instill eyedrops.

  P. Laser therapy

    1. Description

      a. Noninvasive ambulatory procedures in which a slit lamp is used to deliver the laser beam

      b. May eliminate the need for more invasive procedures

      c. Argon or yttrium aluminum garnet (YAG) lasers are utilized in a procedure room.

      d. Topical anesthetic drops are instilled.

    2. Procedures

      a. Laser trabeculoplasty

           (1) Treatment for open-angle glaucoma

      b. Laser iridotomy

           (1) Treatment for acute or chronic angle-closure glaucoma

      c. Laser posterior capsulotomy

           (1) May be required when patients experience decreased vision within 2 years after ECCE

           (2) YAG laser used to create a window in the posterior capsule

           (3) Patients may have pupils dilated.

           (4) Iopidine may be used to prevent increased intraocular pressure.

III. Anesthetic considerations

  A. Types (overview)

    1. Topical

      a. Topical anesthetic eyedrops may be used.

      b. Rapid onset with moderate duration of action

    2. Local anesthesia block

      a. Used frequently

    b. Contraindications
        (1) Patients who have difficulty lying still
        (2) Children
        (3) Patients who have frequent cough
  3. Moderate sedation and analgesia used in conjunction with block
  4. General anesthesia
B. Topical anesthetic drops
  1. Used frequently
    a. Proparacaine hydrochloride 0.5%
    b. Tetracaine hydrochloride 0.5%
    c. Lidocaine hydrochloride 2%
C. Eye block
  1. Types
    a. Retrobulbar block
        (1) Injection of anesthetic solution into base of eyelids at level of orbital margins or behind the eyeball to block the ciliary ganglion and nerves
    b. Peribulbar block
        (1) Local anesthetic is deposited beside the globe instead of behind it.
  2. Performed in two stages
  3. Stage I—blocks eyelid
    a. Three methods
        (1) Van Lint method—blocks peripheral branches of cranial nerve VII in the orbicularis oculi muscle
        (2) Atkinson method—blocks temporal arborization of cranial nerve VII to the orbicularis muscle
        (3) O'Brien method—blocks the main trunk of cranial nerve VII near the temporomandibular joint
  4. Stage II—retrobulbar block
    a. Provides anesthesia to globe and muscular attachments
    b. Blocks branches of cranial nerves III, IV, V, and VI
    c. Common medications used
        (1) Lidocaine hydrochloride 2% or 4%; mixed with equal parts of 0.75% bupivacaine hydrochloride with hyaluronidase (used for diffusing local anesthetic to surrounding tissue)
        (2) May add epinephrine hydrochloride to prolong effectiveness of agents
        (3) May use as much as 6 ml for retrobulbar block and 10 ml for peripheral tissue
    d. Nursing considerations
        (1) Inform patient of possible burning sensation.
        (2) Inform patient of possible feeling of pressure behind eye during injection of medication.
        (3) Inform patient that physician may massage eye after injection of medication.
           (a) Decreases intraocular pressure
           (b) Aids in diffusing agents
        (4) Patient frequently given intravenous sedation to decrease discomfort during the injection; administer medications per protocol
        (5) Monitor vital signs per protocol.
        (6) Patient may be awake during procedure.
           (a) Monitor noise level.
    e. Nursing care following eye block
        (1) Patient will not have blink reflex; must keep eyelid closed to protect the cornea
           (a) Tape the eyelid closed.
           (b) Reassure patient that it is normal to be unable to open the eyelid.

        f. Effectiveness of eye block
          (1) Generally very effective
          (2) Occasionally a block may be incomplete, and patient will experience pain.
          (3) Instruct patient to use hand signal during surgery if he or she experiences pain or discomfort.
       g. Potential complications; cancellation of surgical procedure strongly advised for any of the following complications
          (1) Retinal detachment (caused by insertion of needle through globe)
          (2) Injection of anesthetic into optic nerve (irreparable damage)
          (3) Retrobulbar hemorrhage (most common)
            (a) Controlled by pressure to globe

D. General anesthesia
    1. Indications
      a. Children
      b. Patients unable to tolerate local anesthetic with sedation
      c. Extremely anxious patients
      d. Patients with certain systemic diseases
      e. Patients undergoing prolonged operations
    2. Postanesthesia care
      a. Same as any patient who has undergone general anesthesia

IV. Drugs frequently used for ophthalmologic surgery
  A. Mydriatics
    1. Action
      a. Blocks cholinergic stimulation of sphincter muscle of iris (dilation of pupil)
      b. Blocks accommodative ciliary muscle of lens (paralysis of accommodation)
    2. Types
      a. Phenylephrine hydrochloride (Alconefrin, Neo-Synephrine, Prefrin)
      b. Hydroxyamphetamine (Paredrine)
  B. Cycloplegics
    1. Action
      a. Dilate pupils and paralyze accommodation by acting on ciliary muscles (parasympatholytics)
    2. Types
      a. Atropine
      b. Homatropine (AK-Homatropine, Isopto Homatropine, Minims Homatropine)
      c. Cyclopentolate (Cyclogyl)
      d. Scopolamine (Isopto Hyoscine, Mydramide)
      e. Tropicamide (Mydriacyl)
  C. Miotics
    1. Action
      a. Used to constrict the pupil (parasympathomimetics)
    2. Types
      a. Cholinergics
        (1) Pilocarpine hydrochloride
        (2) Carbachol (Miostat, Carbacel)
        (3) Acetylcholine chloride (Miochol)
      b. Anticholinesterase
        (1) Physostigmine (Eserine)
        (2) Isoflurophate (Floropryl)
        (3) Echothiophate iodide (Phospholine Iodide)
  D. Osmotic agents
    1. Action
      a. Parenteral agents used to lower intraocular pressure through the blood-ocular gradient

       2. Types
         a. Mannitol (Osmitrol)
         b. Glycerin (glycerol, Glyrol, Osmoglyn)
   E. Viscoelastic agents
       1. Action
         a. Used to maintain the intraocular chamber during surgery
       2. Types
         a. Sodium hyaluronate (Healon, Amvisc)
   F. Carbonic anhydrase inhibitors
       1. Action
         a. Parenteral agent used to decrease intraocular pressure; used for glaucoma
       2. Types
         a. Acetazolamide (Diamox)
         b. Methazolamide (Neptazane)
   G. Corticosteroids
       1. Action
         a. Antiinflammatory agents
       2. Types
         a. Hydrocortisone (Solu-Cortef)
         b. Dexamethasone (Decadron)
         c. Prednisolone (Pred Forte)
   H. Topical antibiotics
       1. Action
         a. Used for prophylaxis of or treatment of infections; may be used in solutions or ointments
       2. Types
         a. Bacitracin, neomycin, erythromycin, tetracycline, Gantrisin, tobramycin, gentamycin
         b. Chloramphenicol
V. Preoperative considerations
   A. Assessment
       1. Patient and family's understanding of
         a. Eye disorder
         b. Goal of surgery
         c. What to expect before, during, and after surgery
       2. Assess in detail patient's understanding of intraoperative procedure, especially in cases where local anesthesia and sedation only is used.
       3. Identify patient's reaction to scheduled surgery.
         a. Unrealistic expectations regarding improved vision
         b. Anxiety over potential loss of vision
       4. Identify current visual status.
         a. May need additional safety precautions if severely impaired
         b. May need additional support postoperatively if visual status of unoperative eye is limited
   B. General health assessment per routine protocol
       1. Identify illnesses that can cause sneezing, coughing, or increase in intraocular pressure.
         a. Patient may not be a candidate for local anesthesia with sedation.
         b. May require general anesthesia
   C. Preoperative care
       1. Relieve anxiety related to impending surgery (the eyes are very sensitive to pain and pressure).
         a. Allow patient time to verbalize concerns.
            (1) Patient may have misconceptions regarding eye surgery.
            (2) Clarify misconceptions.
            (3) Some patients may think they will actually see the procedure through the operative eye.

  b. Involve the patient in the plan of care.
    (1) Provide clear written instructions in large type.
    (2) Reinforce physician's orders regarding preoperative and postoperative medications and eyedrop schedules.
  c. Provide emotional support.
    (1) Convey positive realistic attitude.
    (2) Acknowledge validity of patient concerns.
2. Verify correct surgical eye.
  a. Confirm with patient correct eye for surgery.
    (1) Document correct eye prior to preoperative sedation.
    (2) Keep in mind many patients may be unable to accurately identify the operative eye because of age or mental status.
  b. Document correct operative eye.
    (1) Verify the surgical consent and the history and physical with the scheduled procedure.
    (2) Investigate any discrepancy.
  c. Clearly identify surgical eye with skin marker (facility policy outlines process).
    (1) Visual marking should not be the sole way of identifying the correct surgical eye.
    (2) Every perianesthesia nurse caring for the patient should verify the patient's understanding, the consent, and the scheduled procedure before proceeding with care.
3. What to expect
  a. Length of time (preoperatively, intraoperatively, postoperatively)
  b. Eye patch (depending on surgical procedure)
  c. Reinforcement that improved vision may require a period of time
4. Demonstrate proper method of eyedrop instillation.
  a. Explain ways to avoid contamination of eye medications.
  b. Reinforce need to follow prescription instructions accurately.
  c. Teach proper technique for instillation of eyedrops.
    (1) Confirm on bottle that drops are for ophthalmic use.
    (2) Note the expiration date and discard if outdated.
    (3) Wash hands prior to using eyedrops.
    (4) Confirm proper eye.
    (5) Tilt head back for instillation.
    (6) Keep eyes open, and look upward.
    (7) Gently pull down tissue below the lower lid.
    (8) Place correct number of eyedrops into the conjunctival sac.
    (9) Close eyes, and try to avoid excessive blinking or squeezing for several minutes.
    (10) Gently blot any excess solution from beneath the eye.
    (11) Wait 5 minutes before instilling a different type of eyedrop.
    (12) Do not touch tip of eye medication dispenser to the eyelid or with hands.
D. Review postoperative routine.
  1. Include family and significant other as appropriate.
  2. Things to avoid postoperatively
    a. Quick movements
    b. Bending over from the waist
    c. Rubbing eyes
    d. Heavy lifting.
  3. Moderation in activity
  4. Proper hand washing before caring for the eye
E. Nursing considerations
  1. Visually impaired patient
    a. Approach from unaffected or least affected side.
    b. Identify self.

      c. Speak in normal tone.

      d. Provide method for patient to obtain immediate assistance (call bell in reach).

      e. Keep visual aids in close proximity.

      f. Allow patient to keep assistive devices as long as possible.

      g. Keep walking area clear of obstructions.

   2. Administer preoperative medications as ordered.

      a. Mydriatics to dilate pupil

      b. Notify physician if expected dilation does not occur.

   3. Allow patient to void prior to procedure.

      a. Patient will become restless in OR if he or she has a full bladder.

F. Overall assessment of patient's ability to tolerate anesthesia plan

   1. Procedure usually performed under local anesthesia with sedation (adults)

   2. Assess patient's ability to lie still under drapes for long period of time (1 to 3 hours).

   3. Factors influencing decision include

      a. Chronic cough

      b. Airway difficulties

      c. Claustrophobia

      d. Involuntary motions

VI. Postoperative considerations

A. Assessment

   1. Routine assessment per protocol

B. Positioning

   1. Assist patient to chair or recliner.

      a. Avoid bumping or jarring.

   2. Orient patient to surroundings.

   3. Certain operations (vitreoretinal surgery) may require special positioning.

      a. Surgeon should provide specific instructions as to positioning.

      b. Patient may need to be on side or back.

   4. Patient may have decreased pain with head of bed elevated.

C. Drainage

   1. Type and amount; document

   2. Notify physician per protocol.

D. Pain and discomfort level

   1. Varies with each procedure

      a. Usually uncommon after most eye surgeries

   2. Varies with type of anesthesia administered

   3. Patient may feel stiff and sore.

      a. Results from lying still and flat intraoperatively

   4. Pain usually relieved by acetaminophen, propoxyphene hydrochloride, or similar analgesics

   5. May experience significant pain after vitreoretinal surgery

      a. Administer narcotic analgesic as indicated.

      b. Apply ice pack.

      c. Notify ophthalmologist if pain not relieved by analgesics.

E. Nausea

   1. Caused by manipulation of eye and eye muscles during surgery

   2. May be caused by sedation

   3. Medicate immediately to prevent potential vomiting.

      a. Vomiting results in increased intraocular pressure.

      b. Instruct patient to notify nurse immediately if he or she begins to feel nauseous so that antiemetics may be given.

   4. To avoid potential for nausea and vomiting, oral fluids may be held for a while if patient underwent general anesthesia.

F. Visual impairment from surgery

   1. Ensure patient safety at all times.

        2. Requires assistance at home

        3. Verify arrangements prior to discharge.

  G. Eye shields and dressings

        1. Dressing or eye shields usually remain in place until the patient's first postoperative appointment at the physician's office.

            a. Instruct patient not to disturb or remove shield and dressing.

        2. Alteration in depth perception may be expected when one eye is bandaged.

            a. Evaluate patient for adequate balance before allowing him or her to ambulate unassisted.

        3. Provide clear written instructions for postoperative care at home.

            a. Wash hands before caring for eye.

            b. Do not rub eye.

            c. Surgeon will remove eye patch or shield during postoperative appointment.

            d. Wear glasses or shield at all times to protect the eye.

            e. Wear shield at night for sleeping.

            f. Do not bend at the waist.

            g. Avoid heavy lifting.

            h. Do not drive until after first postoperative appointment.

                (1) Do not drive at all if experiencing double vision.

            i. Take all eye medications as ordered.

            j. Notify physician if any of the following occur.

                (1) Pain not relieved by acetaminophen

                (2) Sudden loss of vision

                (3) Increasing double vision following surgery

                (4) Temperature greater than 100° F

                (5) Significant swelling or redness about the eye

                (6) Unexpected drainage from the eye

  H. Discharge instructions

        1. Inform patient to use strict aseptic technique when caring for eye and administering medications.

        2. Administer eye medications as directed by physician.

        3. Avoid activities that increase intraocular pressure.

            a. Bending

            b. Sneezing

            c. Sudden jarring or forceful movements

            d. Forceful nose blowing

            e. Sexual intercourse

            f. Straining during stools

         4. Wear sunglasses when outdoors.

        5. Avoid use of eye makeup.

        6. Notify physician if any increase in pain, vision changes, or signs and symptoms of infection (redness, increased swelling, purulent drainage).

VII. Possible complications of ophthalmic surgery

  A. Pain

        1. Minimal in most ophthalmic surgeries

        2. Causes: increased intraocular pressure, surgical manipulation, pressure from dressing

        3. Treatment: mild analgesic; be aware that need for stronger medication may indicate possible complications

  B. Bleeding

        1. Minimal for all ophthalmic surgeries

        2. Cause: dressing too loose

        3. Treatment: apply or reinforce dressing; notify physician.

  C. Nausea and vomiting

        1. Usually minimal following ophthalmic surgery

        2. Causes: oculocardiac reflex, surgical manipulation, general anesthesia

        3. Treatment: antiemetic; avoid potential vomiting

    D. Oculocardiac reflex (nervous response elicited by manipulation of extraocular muscles or surrounding ocular tissue)

        1. Causes: decreased heart rate, blood pressure, and level of consciousness

        2. Is seen immediately to 20 minutes postoperatively

        3. May be seen with all types of ophthalmic surgeries

            a. Risk increases with vitreoretinal and eye muscle surgeries.

            b. May be stimulated by retrobulbar block

        4. Treatment: IV atropine

BIBLIOGRAPHY

1. Burden N, editor: *Ambulatory surgical nursing,* ed 2. Philadelphia: WB Saunders, 2000.
2. Dirckx J, editor: *Stedman's concise medical dictionary for the health professions,* ed 4. Philadelphia: Lippincott Williams & Wilkins, 2001.
3. Drain C, editor: *Perianesthesia nursing: A critical care approach,* ed 4. St Louis: WB Saunders, 2003.
4. Karch A, editor: *2003 Lippincott's nursing drug guide.* Philadelphia: Lippincott Williams & Wilkins, 2003.
5. Meeker M; Rothrock J: *Alexander's care of the patient in surgery,* ed 11. St Louis: Mosby, 1999.
6. Nettina S, editor: *The Lippincott manual of nursing practice,* ed 7. Philadelphia: Lippincott, 2000.
7. Phippen M, Wells M, editors: *Patient care during operative and invasive procedures.* Philadelphia: WB Saunders, 2000.
8. Pudner R, editor: *Nursing the surgical patient.* London: Harcourt, 2000.
9. Maloney W: Beveled blades have simplified clear corneal technique. *Ocul Surg News* 15(18):11, 1997.

48 Oral/Maxillofacial/ Dental Surgery

DENISE O'BRIEN

OBJECTIVES

At the conclusion of this chapter the reader will be able to:

1. Describe anatomy and physiology of oral cavity pertinent to the patient undergoing oral and maxillofacial procedures.

2. Identify assessment parameters for patients undergoing oral and maxillofacial operative procedures.

3. Define nursing care priorities in each postanesthesia phase.

4. Describe patient education following oral and maxillofacial procedures related to diet, pain management, oral care, activity, and follow-up.

■■ Care of the oral or maxillofacial surgical patient in the postanesthesia care unit (PACU) presents many challenges to the perianesthesia nurse. Patients may experience feelings of suffocation as the surgical procedure may prevent normal breathing patterns (inability to breath through mouth or nose). Continuous reassurance and explanations from the nurse will assist the patients in understanding they are not in any danger. Astute assessment skills are necessary, because potential compromise of the airway can occur at any time, requiring immediate corrective actions.

I. Anatomy and physiology
   A. Mouth and oral cavity include the following structures:
      1. Lips, teeth, gums, buccal mucosa, tongue, palate (hard and soft), tonsils, pharynx, temporomandibular joint (see Figure 48-1)
   B. The oral cavity is bounded by the jawbones and associated structures (muscles and mucosa) (see Figures 48-2 and 48-3).
      1. Includes the cheek, palate, oral mucosa, the glands whose ducts open into the cavity, the teeth, and the tongue
      2. Except for the teeth, interior of mouth is covered with mucous membrane, lined with salivary glands.
         a. Secrete saliva
         b. Aid in the first step of digestion of food
   C. Oral cavity forms the beginning of the digestive system.
      1. This is where chewing occurs.
      2. The site of the organs of taste
      3. Mouth is entrance to the body for food, occasionally air.
      4. Major organ of speech and emotional expression
   D. Associated structures
      1. Buccal: pertaining to or directed toward the cheek
      2. Tooth: hard calcified structure set in the alveolar processes of the mandible and maxilla; for mastication of food
      3. Gingiva: mucous membrane (the gum) surrounding the teeth
         a. Covers the tooth-bearing border of the jaw
         b. Overlies crowns of unerupted teeth
         c. Encircles the necks of erupted teeth
         d. Supporting structure for subjacent tissues

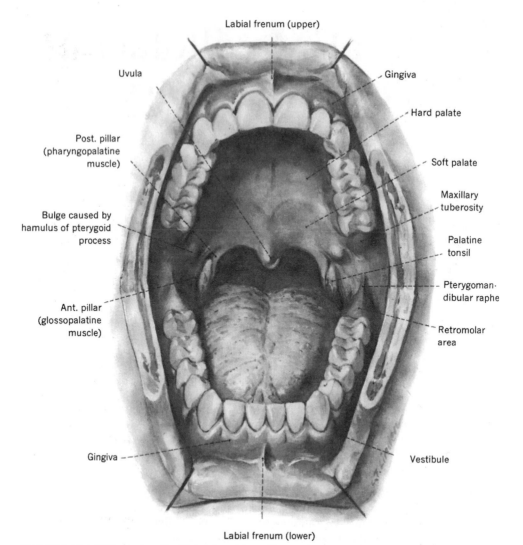

Labial frenum (upper)

Uvula

Gingiva

Post. pillar
(pharyngopalatine
muscle)

Hard palate

Soft palate

Maxillary
tuberosity

Bulge caused by
hamulus of pterygoid
process

Palatine
tonsil

Pterygoman-
dibular raphe

Ant. pillar
(glossopalatine
muscle)

Retromolar
area

Gingiva

Vestibule

Labial frenum (lower)

FIGURE 48-1 ■ The oral cavity. (Reproduced from Massler M, Schour I: *Atlas of the mouth in health and disease*, 1958, by permission of the American Dental Association, Chicago.)

4. Mandible: horseshoe-shaped bone forming the lower jaw; largest and strongest bone of the face; articulates with the skull at the temporomandibular joints
5. Maxilla: irregularly shaped bone that forms the upper jaw, actually two identically shaped bones that are considered one
   a. Assists in the formation of the floor of the orbits, part of the lateral walls and floor of the nasal cavity, and the palate; contains the maxillary sinuses and tear ducts, which drain into the nasal cavity
   b. Supports the upper teeth
   c. Described as the architectural key of the face, touches all facial bones except mandible
6. Palate: the roof of the mouth consists of
   a. Hard palate, the rigid anterior portion, formed by the maxillae and the palatine bones, covered by mucous membrane and forms a bony partition between the oral and nasal cavities; hinged to the soft palate

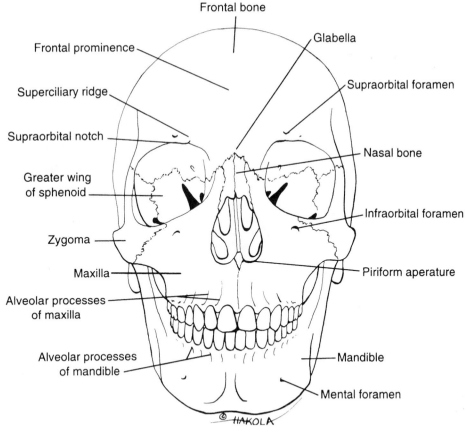

FIGURE 48-2 ■ The skull, anterior view. (Reproduced from Ferraro JW: *Fundamentals of maxillofacial surgery.* New York: Springer-Verlag, 1997, by permission.)

    b. Soft, the posterior, fleshy part of the palate; arch-shaped muscular partition between the oropharynx and nasopharynx, lined by mucous membrane, flanked by tonsils; in the middle of the soft palate is the uvula, a fleshy projection pointing down to the tongue; forms seal posteriorly with the pharynx to help direct food to the esophagus and air to the trachea; critical to the development of normal speech patterns

  7. Tongue: movable muscular organ on the floor of the mouth; accessory structure of the digestive system, composed of skeletal muscle covered with mucous membrane

    a. Location of organs of taste

    b. Aids in chewing, swallowing (deglutition), cleansing tooth surfaces, and the articulation of sound (phonetics)

  8. Nerves (see Figure 48-4)

    a. From the maxillary division of the trigeminal nerve (cranial nerve V), posterior, middle and anterior superior alveolar nerves supply sensation to the upper teeth.

    b. The mandibular division gives off the lingual nerve (sensation of anterior two thirds of tongue, the floor of mouth, gums), inferior alveolar nerve (sensation of premolar, molar teeth of mandible), and at its terminus, mental nerve (sensation of the lower lip and chin).

  9. Temporomandibular joint: bicondylar joint formed by the head of the mandible and the mandibular fossa and the articular tubercle of the temporal bone

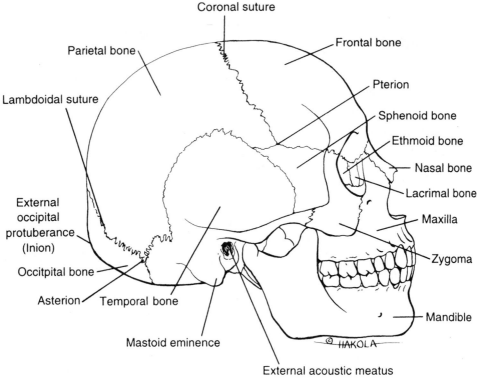

FIGURE 48-3 ■ Lateral view of the skull. (From Ferraro JW: *Fundamentals of maxillofacial surgery.* New York: Springer-Verlag, 1997.)

II. Preanesthesia assessment and parameters specific to procedures
   A. Examination
      1. Inspection and palpation of greatest use
         a. Head and neck
            (1) General appearance
            (2) Facial appearance
            (3) Trismus (limited degree of mouth opening)
            (4) Neck lumps
            (5) Gross facial swelling
            (6) Skin color and texture
         b. Intraoral
            (1) Tongue: size, mobility, color, and texture
            (2) Oral mucosa (palate, cheeks, labial mucosa, floor of mouth): examination for changes in color, texture, ulcers, lumps
            (3) Alveolar ridges and gingivae: color, texture, gingival recession, ulcers, and lumps
            (4) Teeth: number, position, restorations, crowns, caries, cracked and missing teeth, exposed structure
   B. Increased risk associated with history or need to alter perioperative management
      1. Cardiac: may require antibiotic prophylaxis
         a. Endocarditis
         b. Mitral valve prolapse with mitral regurgitation
         c. Valve implants
      2. Implants: antibiotic prophylaxis may be needed
         a. Joints (major replacements)
         b. Grafts of artificial materials

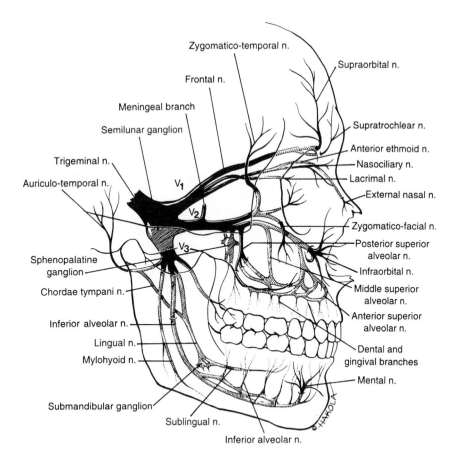

Zygomatico-temporal n.

Supraorbital n.

Frontal n.

Meningeal branch

Supratrochlear n.

Semilunar ganglion

Anterior ethmoid n.

Nasociliary n.

Trigeminal n.

Lacrimal n.

Auriculo-temporal n.

V_1

External nasal n.

V_2

Zygomatico-facial n.

V_3

Posterior superior alveolar n.

Sphenopalatine ganglion

Infraorbital n.

Chordae tympani n.

Middle superior alveolar n.

Anterior superior alveolar n.

Inferior alveolar n.

Lingual n.

Dental and gingival branches

Mylohyoid n.

Mental n.

Submandibular ganglion

Sublingual n.

Inferior alveolar n.

V_1 = ophthalmic division
V_2 = maxillary division
V_3 = mandibular division

FIGURE 48-4 ■ The trigeminal nerve (cranial nerve V). (From Ferraro JW: *Fundamentals of maxillofacial surgery.* New York: Springer-Verlag, 1997.)

3. Coagulation and bleeding disorders
   a. Factor VIII deficiency (hemophilia)
   b. Von Willebrand's disease
      (1) Factor VIII, synthetic factor VIII, aminocaproic acid (EACA or Amicar), or DDVAP (desmopressin acetate) may be given just before procedure begins.
   c. Anticoagulant therapy
      (1) Coagulation testing may be required (prothrombin, partial thromboplastin time, platelet count) to determine coagulation status before proceeding with elective surgery.
4. Immunocompromised patient or immune disorders
   a. Human immunodeficiency virus (HIV), acquired immunodeficiency syndrome (AIDS)
   b. Patient with history of organ transplant
   c. Universal precautions should be used with every patient.
   d. Immunocompromised patient may require special care (isolation, scheduling, altered medication regimen).

5. Patients with cancer receiving radiation therapy to the head and neck region
  a. Decreased salivary flow secondary to salivary gland atrophy require saliva substitutes and aggressive anticaries management with custom trays, topical fluoride applications, and immaculate oral hygiene.
  b. Hyperbaric oxygen treatment indicated for surgical procedures if radiation dose totals >6000 cGy.
6. Trauma
  a. Edema present
    (1) Recent injury
    (2) May delay operative repair until edema diminishes
  b. Disfigurement: may be significant and emotionally disturbing to patient and others
7. Chronic pain
  a. Pain tolerance alterations
  b. Chronic analgesic use may alter postoperative analgesic management.
8. Nutritional status changes
  a. Difficulty chewing, swallowing
  b. Pain may interfere with ability to eat and meet caloric demands and nutritional requirements.
9. Developmentally challenged
  a. Potential behavioral problems (combative, disruptive, abusive)
  b. Legal authorization appropriately obtained before treatment commences
C. Airway status evaluation
  1. Evaluation of airway for ease of intubation in oral or maxillofacial surgery
    a. Mobility of the neck—ability to touch chin to chest and each shoulder; flex and extend
    b. Position of the trachea relative to the mandible—distance from thyroid cartilage to anterior bony chin; at least 6.5 cm acceptable
    c. Ability of the patient to open the mouth—at least 3.6 cm in adults desirable
    d. Structures visualized when the patient opens the mouth and vocalizes "ahh..."—see the uvula and surrounding pharyngeal structures
D. Determine the educational needs of patient and caregiver.
  1. Oral care, analgesia, preoperative anxiety
  2. Discharge planning
III. Intraoperative priorities
  A. Anesthesia choice
    1. General: nasal intubation desired for unobstructed visualization of orofacial structures
    2. Sedation and analgesia with local anesthesia
      a. Midazolam, ketamine (glycopyrrolate to decrease oral secretions); less risk of respiratory depression; reduced emergence delirium after ketamine with midazolam
      b. Benzodiazepine with fentanyl: O_2 recommended when used with local anesthesia; may use methohexital or propofol for additional sedation
    3. Local anesthesia used alone for minor oral procedures or used as an adjunct during general anesthesia
      a. Minimize immediate postoperative pain.
      b. Minimize bleeding in operative field.
      c. Help separate tissue planes to ease dissection.
      d. Allow for less anesthetic agent because of reduced surgical stimulus.
  B. Intraoperative concerns
    1. Hemostasis and intraoral bleeding
      a. Hemostatic agent may be used.
      b. Gelfoam, Surgicel, Avitene, topical thrombin, bone wax (for bone bleeders), Tisseel (fibrin sealant)
    2. Airway
      a. Loss of reflexes with excessive sedation

      b. Positioning of endotracheal tube, potential displacement

      c. Foreign body aspiration

IV. Postanesthesia priorities

  A. Phase I

    1. Airway

      a. Spontaneous, unassisted breathing

      b. Adjunct in place: nasal trumpet, oropharyngeal airway

      c. Endotracheal tube: nasal insertion (most common)

      d. Observe for respiratory complications.

    2. Hemodynamic stability

      a. Vital signs stable, consistent with baseline

      b. Observe for cardiovascular complications.

    3. Bleeding

      a. Hemostasis may be difficult to obtain.

      b. Risk for hemorrhage

      c. Increases risk of nausea and vomiting: swallowed blood may precipitate nausea and vomiting from irritating effect of blood in stomach

    4. Report from anesthesia, oral surgeon, perioperative nurse (in addition to routine information)

      a. Implants and prostheses inserted

      b. Splints: location, type

      c. Oral packing: location, plan for removal

      d. Oral sutures: location, extreme care when suctioning

      e. MMF (wired jaws)

        (1) Wire cutters and scissors immediately available

        (2) Clear instructions from surgeon when appropriate to cut fixation wires and what wires to cut

        (3) Usually cut for vomit and for respiratory distress (in extreme cases only)

■ BOX 48-1
■ **KEY PATIENT EDUCATIONAL OUTCOMES**

Phase I
Patient will express feelings of lessened anxiety.
Patient will describe minimal to tolerable pain.
Patient will request analgesic to manage pain.
Patient will perform oral suctioning and handle oral secretions unassisted.
Patient will be able to communicate with nurse without using verbal skills.

Phase II
Patient will tolerate discomfort following administration of oral analgesics.
Patient and caregiver will describe oral hygiene following instruction.
Patient will demonstrate use of gauze sponge for tamponade of bleeding.
Patient will demonstrate safe, gentle, and effective oral suctioning.
Patient and caregiver will verbally describe wire cutting (patients with MMF).
Patient will progress to upright position with minimal orthostatic effects: dizziness, lightheadedness, nausea.

Phase III
Patient and caregiver will describe follow-up required.
Patient and caregiver will identify risks associated with operative procedure: infection, hemorrhage, pain, vomiting.
Patient and caregiver will describe oral care, activity, medications, and diet.
Patient and caregiver will demonstrate knowledge of medications (analgesics, antibiotics, antiemetics, etc.) by describing purpose and administration of each medication prescribed.

5. Discomfort
   a. Maximum pain intensity occurs about 3 hours after surgery; begin analgesics intraoperatively or immediately postoperatively.
   b. Long-acting local anesthetic infiltrated into operative site; usually bupivacaine with epinephrine to provide 8 to 12 hours of analgesia
   c. Opioids: decreasing use in ambulatory oral and maxillofacial surgery because increased use of NSAIDs (ketorolac)
   d. NSAIDs: ketorolac may provide superior analgesia following extractions.
6. Drainage from mouth
   a. Position to facilitate drainage of saliva, bloody secretions.
   b. Drooling or excessive salivation and unable to swallow (reflex absent or excessive pain)
   c. Suction as needed with soft catheter.
7. Dressing
   a. No dressing when incisions are intraoral
   b. Internal dressing may be moistened gauze sponge.
   c. External dressing
      (1) Pressure chin strap (Jobst® type)
      (2) Foam tape
      (3) Head wrap with fluffs and cling wrap generally for 24 hours
8. Edema
   a. Can be significant, especially in longer procedures
   b. Position with head of bed elevated 30°.
   c. Administer steroid if ordered; continued controversy regarding effectiveness in reducing inflammatory reaction
   d. Ice packs may help reduce blood flow to operative site and subsequent inflammatory response; check with surgeon before applying; may actually increase blood flow (rebound effect after ice pack removed)
9. Fluids and nutrition
   a. Clear to full liquid high-caloric diet as tolerated and ordered
   b. Do not force fluids, especially when nausea and vomiting present.
   c. Causes of nausea and vomiting
      (1) Opioid analgesics
      (2) Blood in stomach
      (3) Starvation leading to weakness, low blood sugar levels
   d. Hydrate with intravenous (IV) fluids (replacement and maintenance)
      (1) Lactated Ringer's (Hartmann's)
      (2) Dextrose-containing solutions
   e. When nausea and vomiting are present
      (1) Administer antiemetics as ordered; determine if antiemetic prophylaxis given.
      (2) Commonly use promethazine, 5HT3 serotonin antagonists (e.g., ondansetron, dolasetron), dexamethasone (see Chapter 36 for discussion on antiemetics)
10. Reaction to local anesthetics
    a. What appears to be an allergic reaction to local anesthetic (LA) may actually be a reaction to preservative methylparaben or sulfite.
    b. Allergy to LA is rare.
    c. Traumatic penetration of a nerve (prolonged numbness), vein (hematoma), or artery (systemic toxic effects)
    d. Systemic (cardiac) reactions to epinephrine (used to minimize bleeding) in LA, rather than LA itself
    e. Toxicity caused by overdose leads to excitation of central nervous system (CNS) followed by profound CNS depression, cardiovascular collapse, possible death.
11. Oral hygiene
    a. Take care to not disrupt clot; gently swab the oral cavity, hold saline rinse for 8 to 12 hours postprocedure.

        b. Lubricate lips with petroleum jelly or emollient cream, steroid (0.5% hydrocortisone) lip cream—for long procedures, expect significant edema of lips.
- **12.** Antibiotic as ordered: common following trauma, patients with cardiac valvular disease, history of rheumatic fever or implants
  - **a.** The oral cavity is laden with bacteria; bacteria enter the bloodstream through oral incisions, traumatic lacerations.
  - **b.** Infections can lead to loss of bone and teeth, distributive shock (septic), damage to heart valves, endocarditis, loss of implants, scarring, large vessel complications (carotid erosion or venous thrombosis).
- **13.** Provide patient with means of communication while in PACU.
  - **a.** Bell
  - **b.** Writing tools
    - (1) Pen or pencil, paper pad
    - (2) Magic slate and stylet
    - (3) Dry-erase board and marker
- **14.** Reasons for admission following outpatient operative procedure
  - **a.** Airway obstruction
  - **b.** Unanticipated maxillomandibular fixation (MMF)
  - **c.** Severe postoperative nausea and vomiting (PONV)
  - **d.** Excessive blood loss
  - **e.** Severe pain
  - **f.** Persistent bleeding from extraction sites
  - **g.** Slow recovery from anesthesia
- **B.** Phase II
  - **1.** Operative site
    - **a.** Continued bleeding: tamponade by biting saline-moistened gauze for approximately 30 minutes
    - **b.** Epinephrine-soaked gauze or packs not recommended; rebound vasodilation can occur when a vasoconstrictor is used, leading to increased bleeding
    - **c.** Pressure packs may need to be maintained for 2 hours or some specified time postprocedure—determine appropriate time for removal and discharge.
  - **2.** Discomfort
    - **a.** Oral analgesic medications initiated in preparation for discharge home
      - (1) May have started in phase I
      - (2) Determine effectiveness of medication before patient discharged home on same analgesic.
      - (3) If ineffective, may need prescription changed or other follow-up (see Chapter 29)
    - **b.** Continue ice pack as ordered.
  - **3.** Oral care
    - **a.** Oral suctioning initiated by patient when appropriate and patient capable
    - **b.** Begin oral fluids if desired and not already started in phase I; avoid extremes of heat.
  - **4.** Education
    - **a.** Includes patient, family, responsible adult companion
    - **b.** Instructions
      - (1) Oral hygiene
      - (2) Avoid temperature extremes in food and beverages.
      - (3) Avoid sucking motion (i.e., do not use a straw).
      - (4) Care of bands and wires
      - (5) For patient with MMF
        - (a) How and when to cut wires
          - (1) Airway distress
          - (2) Vomiting

        (6) Pain-relief alternatives
          (a) Dental wax may be used to protect oral mucosa and decrease irritation and discomfort from protruding wires or metal bands.

C. After discharge (phase III)
  1. Oral hygiene
    a. Brushing difficult if not impossible because of swelling and pain
      (1) Swelling reaches maximum in 2 to 3 days, subsides gradually.
      (2) Rinses may help in reducing swelling.
    b. Saline rinses (1 teaspoon table salt in one half glass hot water) for 2 minutes, three to six times a day, especially after meals)
      (1) No rinsing for at least 8 to 12 hours after procedure so as not to disturb clot (surgeon may order up to 24 hours before rinsing begins); disruption of the clot may lead to painful "dry socket" (localized osteitis)
        (a) Most often develops from second to fifth postoperative day
        (b) Chief complaint is pain; also may complain of odor or a bad taste
        (c) Treatment is conservative: gentle warm saline irrigation of site, sedative, dressing over site until patient no longer symptomatic.
      (2) Antiseptic mouthwashes may also be prescribed.
        (a) Most common is chlorhexidine 0.2%.
        (b) Held over surgical site for 1 minute, then expectorated
        (c) This should not be used for more than 1 week as it may stain the teeth.
    c. Continued bleeding
      (1) Instruct patient to replace gauze sponge over bleeding site and bite firmly for 20 to 30 minutes; if a bleeding tooth socket, a moist teabag over the socket may be helpful.
      (2) If bleeding persists, patient needs to be evaluated by surgeon.
  2. Nutrition
    a. Instruct patient regarding alcohol and smoking avoidance for first 48 hours.
    b. Diet and food preparation
      (1) Avoid hot foods and liquids for first 48 hours.
      (2) Instruct patient to advance to soft foods or pureed diet (nutritional supplement) as tolerated or ordered by surgeon.
    c. Encourage fluid intake especially during hot weather.
  3. Vomiting
    a. Prepare patient and family for possibility of vomiting swallowed blood; suggest adequately sized receptacle for ride home and at home in case of emesis.
    b. Caution patient and caregiver to call surgeon or facility
      (1) If vomiting persists for >6 hours
      (2) If continuing to swallow blood: may require evaluation to determine source of bleeding
  4. Pain
    a. Ice packs, heat application especially for temporomandibular joint (TMJ) procedures
    b. Oral analgesics
      (1) Suggest contacting surgeon if pain is not relieved by prescribed analgesics, intolerable, or increasing.
      (2) Unrelieved or increasing pain may indicate infection, retained root, bone, foreign body, maxillary sinus problems.
    c. Alternatives
      (1) Dental wax may be applied to wires and bands to reduce mucosal irritation.
      (2) Explore with patient and caregiver other potential pain-management techniques (see Chapter 29).

5. Wound care
   a. See oral hygiene instructions for intraoral incisions.
   b. For external incisions
      (1) Keep wound clean and dry for minimum of 24 to 48 hours.
      (2) May be instructed to remove dressing after 24 to 48 hours and clean incision with saline or half-strength hydrogen peroxide; cover with antibiotic ointment
      (3) Observe incision for signs of infection: redness, swelling, drainage.
6. Activity
   a. Rest
      (1) Limit activity until pain and swelling subside.
      (2) Sleep with head elevated on several pillows to reduce swelling and minimize bleeding.
      (3) While taking opioid analgesics, avoid operating machinery, driving automobiles, using sharp or potentially injurious articles, or drinking alcohol.
   b. Exercise
      (1) For first 24 hours, any exercise is discouraged.
      (2) Defer vigorous activity; restrict until surgeon allows; may be up to 4 weeks after surgery
         (a) Aerobic activity may increase heart rate and blood pressure, leading to increased bleeding from operative site(s).
7. Follow-up care
   a. Arrange for return visit with surgeon in specified time interval.
      (1) Patients with drains, MMF, extensive procedures may require return visit on first postoperative day.
      (2) Sutures removed in 5 to 7 days postoperatively
   b. Return to work dependent on procedure, patient work.
   c. Risk for secondary hemorrhage
      (1) Seven to 10 days after surgery
      (2) Often caused by an infected wound and poor oral hygiene
   d. Fever: contact surgeon if temperature over 100.4° F (38° C) or as ordered by surgeon.
V. Operative procedures

Common operative procedures and techniques are included. The reader is referred to a comprehensive text on oral and maxillofacial surgery for additional procedures and techniques. See also Chapter 50 and Chapter 52 for procedures that may also be done by oral and maxillofacial surgeons. The preceding preanesthesia, intraoperative, and postanesthesia care priorities apply to the following procedures with some additional notations.

A. Arch bars
   1. Purpose: Used for treatment of avulsed teeth, fractures of the mandible, or maxilla
   2. Description: Rigid metal bars used to splint and fix the teeth and/or maxilla or mandible; wire ligatures attach the bars to the teeth
B. Closed reduction of mandibular (jaw) fracture
   1. Purpose: Used for alignment and stabilization of fractures to allow proper healing
   2. Description: Erich-type arch bars ligated to teeth most common method of fixation; maxillomandibular fixation (MMF) using stainless steel loops or elastics for a minimum of 4 weeks considered best for providing reduction and fixation
   3. MMF acceptable for ambulatory surgery if there is no gross edema and/or bleeding
   4. Postanesthesia priorities
      a. Airway

  b. Nausea and vomiting

  c. Wire cutter at bedside, immediately available

 5. Psychosocial concerns

  a. Difficulty communicating

  b. Dietary modifications

 6. Complications

  a. Severe airway distress or emesis requiring wires to be cut

C. Dental examination

 1. Purpose: the oral cavity is inspected and the teeth and supporting structures are probed for defects, lesions, mobility, and infection.

 2. Description: visual and instrument methods are used for the examination.

D. Dental implant

 1. Purpose: replace a single missing tooth, lost to injury or other reasons

 2. Description: a prosthetic tooth with an anchoring structure surgically implanted beneath the mucosal or periosteal layer or in the bone

E. Dental prophylaxis

 1. Purpose: cleansing of teeth (stains, materia alba, calculus, removal of plaque)

 2. Description: dental instruments used to clean the teeth

F. Dental restoration

 1. Purpose: replacing tooth structure by artificial means

 2. Description: reforming lost tooth structure, missing, damaged, or diseased teeth with alloy of silver, gold, or acrylic resin

G. Genioplasty

 1. Purpose: operative repair of chin deformities (microgenia, macrogenia, asymmetric chin are a few of the defects)

 2. Description: repair done by open bone reduction, augmentation with synthetic or natural materials, or osteotomy with plate and screw fixation

H. Gingivectomy

 1. Purpose: to eradicate periodontal infection and reduce the gingival sulcus depth

 2. Description: excision of all loose infected and diseased gingival tissue

I. Implants

 1. Purpose: used to stabilize or totally support tooth replacements; prostheses may be fixed or fixed and removable

 2. Description

  a. Osseointegration screw technique (Branemark)

   (1) Titanium screw inserted into jaw bone, grows into the bone (osseointegrates)

   (2) After 3 months (mandible) or 6 months (maxilla), attached to and loaded with a prosthesis

  b. Transmandibular implant (Bosker)

   (1) Consists of a base plate, screws to fix the plate to the mandible, and posts that attach to a bar (Dolder) in the mouth

   (2) Lower prosthesis is attached to the bar; prosthesis started 4 to 6 weeks after surgery

J. Intraoral biopsy

 1. Purpose: removal of abnormal tissue for histopathological examination

 2. Description

  a. Excisional: complete removal of a lesion with primary closure

  b. Incisional: small representative portion of a lesion is removed if the lesion is large and the defect left from its removal could not be closed primarily.

K. Multiple dental extractions

 1. Purpose: may follow trauma, significant or recurring infection, nonrestorable teeth, or in preparation for prosthetic replacement

 2. Description: surgical removal of teeth

L. Odontectomy: tooth extraction

M. Open reduction and internal fixation of zygomatic fracture
1. Purpose: to realign fractured bone fragments and restore facial contour
2. Description: using a transconjunctival or lower eyelid subciliary incision with skin muscle flap and orbital floor exploration, the fracture reduced and fixated with wires or microplate system for the infraorbital rim and wires or miniplating fixation of the zygomaticomaxillary buttress

N. Osteotomy
1. Purpose: to correct maxillofacial deformities
2. Description
   a. Le Fort osteotomy: an osteotomy performed along the classic lines of fracture as described by Le Fort to correct a maxillary skeletal deformity; classified as Le Fort osteotomy I, lower maxillary; II, pyramidal nasoorbitomaxillary; or III, high maxillary (depending upon the location of the deformity); the maxilla is sectioned transversely and repositioned (see Chapter 50)
   b. Sagittal split mandibular osteotomy: an intraoral surgical procedure for correction of retrognathism, prognathism or open bite; the mandibular rami and posterior body are sectioned in the sagittal plane
   c. Segmental alveolar osteotomy: an intraoral surgical procedure in which segments of alveolar bone containing teeth are sectioned between, and apically to, the teeth for the repositioning of the alveolus and teeth; it may be maxillary or mandibular, and may be combined with ostectomy
   d. Sliding oblique osteotomy: an oral surgical procedure in which the mandibular ramus is cut vertically from the sigmoid notch to the angle to facilitate posterior repositioning of the mandible in correction of mandibular prognathism; it may be performed extraorally or intraorally, and is similar to vertical osteotomy
   e. Vertical osteotomy: an oral surgical procedure similar to sliding oblique osteotomy
3. Postanesthesia priorities
   a. Airway
   b. Bleeding
   c. Nausea and vomiting
   d. Swelling
   e. Pain management
4. Psychosocial concerns
   a. Facial swelling distorting appearance
   b. Reason for procedure (trauma or cosmetic and functional appearance)

O. Splint
1. Purpose: used in orthognathic surgical procedures to stabilize the maxillomandibular position (secured to the maxilla and mandible, interlocked, retain the desired position of the osteotomized units); used to reduce and stabilize maxillofacial fractures; may be used in the interim before MMF or plate and screw (rigid) fixation
2. Description: made of acrylic resin or metal, used as space maintainer or fixator; to hold teeth in alignment; temporarily, permanent, or removable

P. Temporomandibular joint (TMJ) arthroscopy
1. Purpose: diagnosis of internal joint pathology, lavage of joint, lysis of adhesions, biopsy of synovial tissue
2. Description: direct visual inspection and examination of the interior TMJ structures using an endoscopic instrument
3. Postanesthesia priorities
   a. Trismus may be problem.
   b. TMJ physiotherapy initiated
   c. Provide information on jaw-opening exercises.
4. Psychosocial concerns
   a. Chronic pain may be an issue; ongoing assessment and pain management essential

BIBLIOGRAPHY

1. Dimitroulis G: *A synopsis of minor oral surgery.* Oxford, England: Reed Educational and Professional Publishing, 1997.
2. Donoff RB: *Massachusetts General Hospital manual of oral and maxillofacial surgery,* ed 3. St Louis: Mosby, 1997.
3. *Dorland's illustrated medical dictionary,* ed 29. Philadelphia: WB Saunders, 2000.
4. Ferraro JW: *Fundamentals of maxillofacial surgery.* New York: Springer-Verlag, 1997.
5. Kaban LB, Pogrel MA, Perrott DH: *Complications in oral and maxillofacial surgery.* Philadelphia: WB Saunders, 1997.
6. Kwon PH, Laskin DM: *Clinician's manual of oral and maxillofacial surgery,* ed 3. Chicago: Quintessence Publishing, 2001.
7. Miller-Keane, O'Toole, MT: *Encyclopedia and dictionary of medicine, nursing, and allied health,* ed 7. Philadelphia: WB Saunders, 2003.
8. Riden K: *Key topics in oral and maxillofacial surgery.* Oxford, UK: BIOS Scientific, 1998.
9. *Stedman's medical dictionary,* ed 27. Philadelphia: Lippincott Williams & Wilkins, 2000.
10. White P: *Ambulatory anesthesia and surgery.* Philadelphia: WB Saunders, 1997.
11. Yates C, editor: *A manual of oral and maxillofacial surgery for nurses.* Oxford, UK: Blackwell Science, 2000.

49 Orthopedic Surgery

LORI HOWARD

OBJECTIVES

At the conclusion of this chapter the reader will be able to:

1. Identify nursing diagnosis specific to the orthopedic surgical patient.

2. Discuss the parameters of an orthopedic neurovascular assessment.

3. Describe common orthopedic surgical procedures and their associated nursing interventions.

4. Discuss the assessment and management of complications associated with orthopedic procedures.

5. Describe the pathophysiology and management of arthritic disorders.

6. Detail nursing care priorities for patients with casts.

7. Discuss the various types of traction and the nursing care priorities for patients in traction.

8. Describe the treatment and nursing management of the patient with a fracture.

9. Discuss the educational needs of the orthopedic patient.

■
■■ This chapter on orthopedic surgery covers surgical interventions to correct congenital and joint deformities as well as traumatic injuries to the skeletal system. Assessment parameters, common surgical interventions, and potential complications are reviewed.

ANATOMY AND PHYSIOLOGY

I. Skeletal system
   A. System of living connective tissue, high in mineral content
      1. Haversian system
         a. Nourishes bone tissue
         b. Made up of blood vessels and lymphatics
      2. Types of bone
         a. Cortical (compact) bone
            (1) Dense, hard outer layer of bone
            (2) Found in shafts of long bones
            (3) Poor blood supply
         b. Trabecular (cancellous) bone
            (1) Spongy, porous bone
            (2) Found at the ends of long bones and in vertebrae
            (3) Rich blood supply
      3. Types of cells
         a. Osteoblasts: form new bone
         b. Osteocytes: mature bone cell
         c. Osteoclast: resorb bone
   B. Functions of the skeleton
      1. Provides framework for the body
      2. Provides attachment and leverage for muscles, facilitating movement
      3. Protects vital organs and soft tissue
      4. Manufactures red blood cells
      5. Provides storage for minerals, calcium, phosphate ions, lipids, and marrow elements

    C. Divisions of skeleton
      1. Axial: framework of head and trunk
      2. Appendicular: framework of arms and legs
    D. Classification of bones
      1. Long bones
        a. Diaphysis: shaft of bone
        b. Epiphysis: ends of bone, helps with bone development, made of cancellous bone
        c. Metaphysis: flared portion between diaphysis and epiphysis, growing part of bone, has richest blood supply
        d. Physis or epiphyseal plate: growth plate between epiphysis and metaphysic of immature bone
        e. Periosteum: connective tissue that covers bone
      2. Short bones
        a. Sesamoid or accessory bones: carpals, tarsals, patella
        b. Primarily found in hands and feet
      3. Flat bones
        a. Skull
        b. Ribs
        c. Pelvic girdle
      4. Irregular bones
        a. Ossicles of ear
        b. Vertebrae
II. Tissue of musculoskeletal system
    A. Connective tissue
      1. Development
        a. Develops from mesenchymal cells
        b. Later differentiates into specialized connective tissue cell types
      2. Types (three)
        a. Collagenous tissue
          (1) Derived from dense fibrous connective tissue
          (2) Constructed primarily of collagen fibers
          (3) Includes tendons, ligaments, and fascia
          (4) Tendons
            (a) Dense fibrous connective tissue strands at the ends of muscles that attach muscles to bone
            (b) Characteristics of: flexibility, strength, extensibility
          (5) Ligaments
            (a) Dense connective tissue bands that attach bone to bone and provide stability to joints
          (6) Tendons and ligaments can withstand pulling forces.
            (a) Activity
            (b) Joint motion largely affects ligaments.
            (c) Muscle contraction largely affects tendons.
          (7) Fascia
            (a) Made of connective tissue
            (b) Has many proprioceptive endings
            (c) Covers muscles; provides network of nerves, blood, and lymph vessels
        b. Cartilage: nonvascular tissue composed of collagenous and elastic fibers
          (1) Hyaline cartilage—very elastic; found in the trachea, in synovial joints, in the larynx, nasal septum, and ribs
            (a) Tends to get calcified in old age
          (2) White fibrocartilage—thick, shock absorbing; found in symphysis pubis, between vertebrae, wrist and knee joints, and ends of clavicle

          (a) Interarticular fibrocartilage—flattened fibrocartilaginous plates between articular surfaces of joints, such as the menisci of the knee, temporomandibular, sternoclavicular, acromioclavicular, wrist, and knee joints

          (b) Connecting fibrocartilage—found in joints with limited mobility, such as the intervertebral discs

          (c) Circumferential fibrocartilage—rims surrounding sockets of articular surfaces such as the glenoidal labrum of the hip and the shoulder

          (d) Stratiform fibrocartilage—forms a coating on osseous groove that tendons pass through

        (3) Yellow or elastic cartilage—dense, more flexible and pliant than hyaline cartilage; strong

          (a) Found in the outer ear, epiglottis, and eustachian tube

        (4) Synovial membrane—covers and lines joints; forms synovial fluid responsible for lubricating and nourishing articular cartilage

     c. Bone

        (1) Osseous connective tissue

        (2) Predominantly made up of a fibrous component called collagen and an amorphous component called calcium phosphate

        (3) Highly porous and vascular

B. Muscular system

    1. Made up of muscle cell bundles

    2. Possess rich vascular supply

    3. Covered by fascia

    4. Attached to bone by tendons

    5. Produces bodily movement by contraction

    6. Controlled by complex interaction with the central nervous system

C. Joints: articulations where bones or two bone surfaces come together

    1. Diarthroses—freely movable, synovial

      a. Uniaxial—move in one axis and only one plane

        (1) Hinge—knee, elbow, finger

        (2) Pivot—radial head

      b. Biaxial—moves around two perpendicular axes, in two perpendicular planes

        (1) Saddle—base of the thumb

        (2) Condyloid—distal radius and wrist bones

      c. Multiaxial—moves in three or more planes and around three or more axes

        (1) Ball and socket—hip, shoulder

        (2) Gliding—vertebral joints

    2. Amphiarthroses—limited movement

      a. Symphysis pubis, intervertebral

    3. Synarthroses—immovable

      a. Sutures—fibrous tissue between skull bones

      b. Syndesmoses—ligaments connecting bones' distal radius and ulna, distal tibia and fibula

      c. Gomphoses—fibrous membrane connects to bone, tooth and mandible or maxilla

      d. Range of motion—degree of movement of a joint (refer to Figure 49-1)

        (1) Angular—changes the size of angles between articulating bones

          (a) Flexion—shortens the angle by bending forward

          (b) Extension—lengthens the angle by bending backward

          (c) Abduction—movement away from the midline

          (d) Adduction—movement toward the midline

          (e) Plantar flexion—increases the angle between the foot and the front of the leg by bending the foot and toes down and back

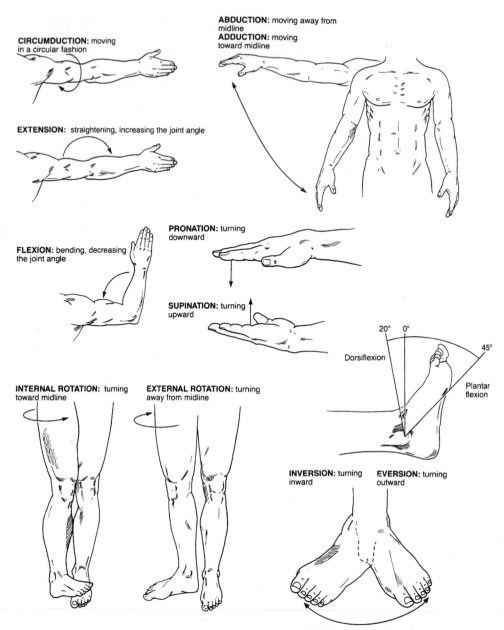

FIGURE 49-1 ■ Joint movements. (From Maher AB, Salmond SW, Pellino TA: *Orthopaedic nursing.* Philadelphia: WB Saunders, 2002, p 198.)

    (f) Dorsiflexion—decreases the angle between the foot and the back of the leg by bending the toes and foot upward

    (g) Hyperextension—stretching a part beyond its normal anatomic limits

  (2) Circular—movement around an axis

    (a) Rotation—moving or pivoting a bone around its axis (side to side of the head)

    (b) Circumduction—movement that resembles a cone shape; the distal part is a wider circle (winding up to throw)

    (c) Supination—palm turns upward while forearm rotates outward

    (d) Pronation—palm turns downward while forearm rotates inward

(3) Gliding—moving one joint surface over another with no circular or angular movement

(4) Miscellaneous movements

    (a) Elevation—moving upward, lifting

    (b) Depression—moving downward, lowering

    (c) Inversion—sole of the foot turns inward

    (d) Eversion—sole of the foot turns outward

    (e) Protraction—moving a part forward, such as the jaw or shoulder

    (f) Retraction—moving a part backward

    (g) Opposition—moving parts together (finger and thumb)

PATHOPHYSIOLOGY OF THE MUSCULOSKELETAL SYSTEM

I. Common congenital and developmental abnormalities

  A. Joint dysplasia

    1. Incomplete formation of diarthrodial joint

    2. May lead to chronic subluxation or dislocation of joint

    3. Developmental dysplastic hip (DDH), including congenital dislocated hip; may lead to early secondary osteoarthritis

  B. Torsional problems of the long bones

    1. Deformity related to abnormal development of bone

      a. Metatarsal adductus: metatarsal deviated medially

      b. Tibial torsion: tibia rotated externally or internally

      c. Femoral anteversion: leads to intoeing with internal or external rotation of leg

    2. In extreme cases, may require surgical intervention

  C. Clubfoot

    1. Anomaly characterized by inversion of foot and forefoot, adduction, and equinus

    2. Classified as fixed or rigid

  D. Osteogenesis imperfecta ("brittle bone disease")

    1. Genetic disease characterized by a defect in collagen synthesis, generalized osteopenia, and metabolic abnormalities

    2. Classified according to severity: types I to III

  E. Legg-Calve-Perthes disease

    1. Idiopathic avascular necrosis of femoral head

    2. Seen in school-aged children

    3. May lead to residual deformity of femoral head, fracture, or early secondary osteoarthritis

  F. Slipped capital femoral epiphysis

    1. Disruption of the growth plate leading to posterior displacement of the femoral head on the femoral neck

    2. Seen in preteen and teenage children

    3. May lead to avascular necrosis of the femoral head, limb shortening, or early secondary osteoarthritis

  G. Scoliosis

    1. Lateral curvature of spine with vertebral rotation

    2. Classified according to causative factors

      a. Idiopathic

        (1) Unknown origin: accounts for 90% of cases

        (2) Most frequent in children 10 to 12 years of age

        (3) Occurs 10 times more frequently in females

        (4) Familial pattern may be present.

      b. Congenital

        (1) Develops in early embryonic life (6 to 8 weeks)

        (2) Malformation of spine occurs, resulting in hemivertebrae or failure of segmentation of vertebrae

      c. Neuromuscular
        (1) Neuropathic (paralytic): associated with spina bifida, poliomyelitis, or cerebral palsy
        (2) Myopathic: associated with muscular dystrophy
      d. Additional types of scoliosis
        (1) Acquired: seen in rheumatoid arthritis, rickets, spinal cord tumors, and neurofibromatosis
        (2) Traumatic: resulting from vertebral fracture after radiation

II. Metabolic bone disease
  A. Osteoporosis
    1. Common disorder characterized by a generalized reduction in the mass and strength of bone leading to high risk for fracture
    2. Rate of bone resorption is greater than rate of bone formation.
    3. Risk factors are multiple and include Caucasian or Asian race, small skeletal frame, estrogen deficiency or postmenopausal condition, inactivity or immobility, high caffeine or alcohol consumption, low-calcium or high-protein diet.
      a. Fractures of wrists, femoral head, vertebrae, and pelvis common and may be induced by minor trauma
  B. Paget's disease (osteitis deformans)
    1. Slow, progressive disease caused by initial bone resorption, followed by period of reactive bone formation
    2. New bone has reduced strength and is highly vascular.
  C. Rickets
    1. An abnormal calcification of bone seen in childhood, leading to soft and deformed bones
    2. Related to deficiency in vitamin D caused by nutritional deficit or inability to absorb or use vitamin D
  D. Osteomalacia
    1. Demineralization of bone in the adult leading to soft, deformed bones ("adult rickets")
    2. Related to inadequate supply of calcium or phosphorus caused by nutritional deficit or absorptive problem

III. Neoplastic disorders
  A. Primary bone or soft tissue tumors
    1. Benign or malignant tumors of the bone, cartilage, connective tissue, or vascular tissue near bone
    2. May lead to local bone destruction and weakening of the tissue
    3. Relatively uncommon
  B. Bone metastasis
    1. Spread of malignancy from a primary site of origin to bone
    2. Lytic or blastic lesions may lead to bone destruction, weakening, and impending or actual fracture.
    3. Frequent sequelae of common malignancies of the breast, prostate, lung, kidney, thyroid, and bladder

IV. Infection
  A. Bone or joint tuberculosis
    1. Infection of the bone or joint by *Mycobacterium tuberculosis,* leading to cartilage or bone destruction
    2. Weight-bearing joints and vertebral bodies most common sites
    3. May require surgical drainage of abscesses in addition to aggressive pharmacologic treatment
  B. Osteomyelitis
    1. Microbial invasion of bone leading to acute or chronic infection
    2. Classified according to method of microbial invasion
      a. Hematologic: acute or chronic infection spread to the bone through circulatory system
        (1) More common in children

(2) More easily treated in children because of higher vascularity of their bones and supportive tissues
    b. Contiguous: infection of the bone by direct extension of bacteria from infected soft tissue or surgical site
        (1) More common in adults older than 50 years of age
        (2) Risk factors include orthopedic surgeries or soft tissue trauma.
    c. Traumatic: infection of the bone by direct contamination with environmental or bodily microbes
        (1) More common in young males and children
        (2) Risk factors include penetrating wounds, intramedullary rods, and open fractures.
  C. Septic arthritis
    1. Microbial invasion of the synovial membrane, commonly bacterial in origin, leading to joint infection
    2. Joint infection usually accompanied by signs and symptoms of systemic infection
    3. May lead to destruction of articular cartilage and early secondary osteoarthritis
V. Arthritic disorders
  A. Osteoarthritis (degenerative joint disease or osteoarthrosis)
    1. Progressive noninflammatory disorder of diarthrodial joints characterized by loss of articular cartilage, marginal osteophytes (spurs), subchondral cysts, and sclerotic changes
        a. Most common form of arthritis
        b. Primarily affect weight-bearing joints: hips, knees, spine, shoulders, interphalanges
    2. Classified by causative factor
        a. Primary osteoarthritis
            (1) Cause unknown
            (2) Increased with obesity, history of repetitive trauma to joint, and age
        b. Secondary osteoarthritis
            (1) Related to preexisting factors
            (2) Seen after trauma to joint, dysplasia, or other pediatric or congenital disorders of the joint, sepsis, or as a result of a primary disease involving the joint such as hemophilia
    3. Clinical findings
        a. Asymmetric distribution
        b. Pain or stiffness in joint, especially with weight-bearing activities
        c. Crepitation of joint
        d. Deformity of joint or decrease in range of motion
        e. Possible swelling and warmth of joint
        f. Gait disturbance (limp)
    4. Conservative treatment
        a. Reduction of risk factors
            (1) Weight loss if needed
            (2) Decrease in weight-bearing activities
        b. Gait rest devices (cane, crutch)
        c. Local application of heat or cold
        d. Pharmacologic therapy
            (1) NSAIDs (nonsteroidal antiinflammatory drugs)
                (a) Initial drug of choice for mild to moderate pain
                (b) NSAIDs inhibit prostaglandin formation through the cyclooxygenase enzyme.
                    (i) This enzyme exists in two isoforms.
                        [a] Cox-1
                        [b] Cox-2
                    (ii) NSAIDs primary therapeutic effect exhibited by blocking Cox-2

        (iii) Selectively blocking Cox-2 provides increased safety for the patient with fewer side effects.
- (c) Commonly prescribed NSAIDs—adult dosage guidelines
  - (i) Celecoxib, Celebrex—100 mg to 200 mg orally twice per day
  - (ii) Rofecoxib, Vioxx—12.5 mg to 25 mg orally daily. Cox-1 inhibitor
  - (iii) Ketorolac, Toradol—10 mg orally every 4-6 hours or 30 mg intravenous (IV) or intramuscular (IM) every 6 hours; if over 65 years of age, 15 mg IV or IM every 6 hours
  - (iv) Fenoprofen, Nalfon, Fenopron—300 mg to 600 mg orally three times per day or four times per day to a maximum of 3.2 g daily
  - (v) Nabumetone, Relafen, Relifex—1000 mg orally daily or twice per day with maximum of 2000 mg per day
  - (vi) Piroxicam, Feldene, Pirox—20 mg orally daily
  - (vii) Sulindac, Clinoril, Novo-Sundac—150 mg to 200 mg orally twice per day with maximum daily dose of 400 mg
  - (viii) Naproxen, Anaprox, Aleve—250 mg to 500 mg orally twice per day with a maximum daily dose of 1.5 g
  - (ix) Ketoprofen, Orudis, Actron—75 mg three times per day or 50 mg four times per day or 200 mg as extended-release form; maximum daily dose 300 mg or 200 mg as extended-release form
- (d) Possible side effects of
  - (i) Abdominal pain
  - (ii) Heartburn
  - (iii) Ulcers
  - (iv) Bleeding
  - (v) Renal failure
  - (vi) Decreased liver function
- (2) Opioids
  - (a) Added to NSAIDs or acetaminophen for mild to moderate pain; adult dosage guidelines:
    - (i) Codeine—15 mg to 60 mg orally every 4-6 hours as needed with maximum daily dose of 360 mg per day
    - (ii) Hydrocodone bitartrate, Lortab or Lorcet, combined in varying strengths with acetaminophen—500 to 650 mg
    - (iii) Oxycodone hydrochloride, Percodan, or Percocet combined in varying strengths with aspirin—325 mg or acetaminophen 500 mg to 600 mg
    - (iv) Propoxyphene hydrochloride, Darvon—65 mg orally every 4 hours, as needed with maximum daily dose of 390 mg
  - (b) For persistent pain, stronger opioid added along with antidepressants or antianxiety drugs to increase tolerance for pain
    - (i) Antidepressants helpful in reducing neuropathic pain
5. Nutritional supplements
  - **a.** Glucosamine and chondroitin reduces pain, improves health of cartilage.
6. Disease-modifying drugs
  - **a.** Current focus of pharmacologic research
    - (1) Pentosan
    - (2) Enzyme inhibitors
      - (a) Doxycycline
      - (b) Collagenase inhibitors
      - (c) Lipids
      - (d) Growth hormones
        - (i) Growth factor–1
7. Topical analgesics
  - **a.** Inexpensive, safe, effective

   b. Application of by massage releases endorphins

   c. NSAIDs

    (1) Salicylate

    (2) Benzydamine

    (3) Diclofenac

    (4) Ibuprofen

    (5) Indomethacin

    (6) Ketoprofen

    (7) Felbinac

    (8) Capsaicin

  8. Intraarticular injections

   a. Corticosteroids

   b. Local anesthetics

   c. Viscosupplements (hylagan products)

  9. Surgical options

   a. Arthroscopy: diagnostic or for removal of loose bodies

   b. Joint fusion (arthrodesis)

   c. Osteotomy: option in early arthritis accompanied by deformity

   d. Resection arthroplasty

   e. Hemiarthroplasty: common in hip (Austin-Moore type or bipolar prosthesis) and shoulder

   f. Total joint replacement

B. Rheumatoid arthritis

  1. Chronic systemic inflammatory disease potentially affecting multiple organs and joints, also considered an autoimmune disorder

   a. Extraarticular manifestations

    (1) Cardiovascular changes: fibrinous pericarditis, cardiac myopathy, vasculitis

    (2) Pulmonary changes: pulmonary nodules, pleuritis, pulmonary fibrosis, pleural effusion

    (3) Neurologic: peripheral neuropathy, carpal tunnel syndrome, nerve entrapment

    (4) Gastrointestinal: bowel and mesenteric vasculitis, malabsorption, enlarged spleen

    (5) Ocular: scleritis, episcleritis, Sjögren's syndrome

    (6) Integument: rheumatoid nodules, vasculitic skin lesions, purpura

    (7) Hematologic: anemia, thrombocytopenia, granulocytopenia, increased sedimentation rate

    (8) Constitutional: fatigue, malaise, fever

   b. Articular manifestations

    (1) Synovial proliferation

    (2) Pannus formation

    (3) Destruction of articular cartilage, with cartilage erosion, bone cysts, and osteophytes

    (4) Tendon and ligament scarring and shortening with ligamentous laxity, subluxation, and contracture

  2. Causative factors

   a. Etiology unknown; multiple theories exist

    (1) Infectious

    (2) Traumatic

    (3) Stress related

   b. Genetic predisposition exists.

   c. Seen in all ages, affecting females to males 3:1

  3. Clinical manifestations (musculoskeletal)

   a. Polyarticular symmetric joint distribution

    (1) Can affect any synovial joint

    (2) Most severe changes in weight-bearing joints

   b. Joint swollen, erythematous, and warm to touch

    c. Joint pain, stiffness, and possible contracture

    d. Joint deformity, laxity, or subluxation

       (1) Deformities of knees, feet, phalanges possible

       (2) Subluxation of cervical vertebrae

    e. Muscle atrophy

4. Conservative treatment

    a. Joint protection techniques

       (1) Weight loss if needed

       (2) Decrease in weight-bearing activities

       (3) Use of large, more proximal joints in more activities

    b. Gait rest devices (cane, crutch)

    c. Program of rest and exercise

    d. Application of heat or cold

    e. Splinting or bracing of joint

    f. Pharmacologic therapy

       (1) Oral nonsteroidal antiinflammatory drugs (NSAIDs) (see osteoarthritis)

       (2) Oral analgesics

       (3) Oral corticosteroids

       (4) Oral or parenteral gold therapy

       (5) Oral remittive agents: chloroquine phosphate

       (6) Oral immunosuppressives: methotrexate, cyclophosphamide, azathioprine

       (7) Intraarticular injection of steroid or local anesthetic

5. Surgical options

    a. Fusion of cervical spine or small joints (e.g., wrist)

    b. Synovectomy

    c. Osteotomy

    d. Tendon repair or transfer

    e. Hemiarthroplasty

    f. Total joint replacement

VI. Traumatic disorders

  A. Strain

    1. Musculotendinous injury caused by overstretching, repetitive stress, or misuse

    2. Classified according to degree of injury to musculotendinous unit

      a. First degree: mild stretching or injury

      b. Second degree: moderate stretching or tearing

      c. Third degree: severe stretching, leading to rupture of the body or insertion site of the musculotendinous unit

  B. Sprain

    1. Ligamentous injury caused by overstretching or overuse

    2. Classified according to degree of injury to ligament

      a. First degree: mild injury involving tear of few ligamentous fibers

      b. Second degree: moderate injury with tearing of up to one half of ligamentous fibers

      c. Third degree: severe injury leading to rupture of the body of the ligament or from its bony attachment

  C. Dislocation or subluxation

    1. Disruption of the contact of articulating surfaces of a joint caused by force to joint or development abnormality

      a. Dislocation: complete disruption of joint

      b. Subluxation: partial disruption of joint

    2. Most common in shoulder joint

    3. May be accompanied by soft tissue injury, including nerve palsy

    4. Recurrent dislocation may necessitate surgical repair of soft tissue or reconstruction of joint.

D. Fracture

　1. Disruption of the normal continuity of a bone, often accompanied by soft tissue trauma

　2. Classification of fractures

　　a. Severity of the fracture

　　　(1) Compound (open): bone is broken with communication of the fracture site with an external wound.

　　　(2) Simple (closed): bone is broken with skin intact.

　　　(3) Complete: continuous fracture line through entire section of bone

　　　(4) Incomplete: break in continuity of one side of cortex only, as in the "greenstick" fracture

　　　(5) Displaced: edges of fractured bone are not aligned, with higher risk for neurovascular damage.

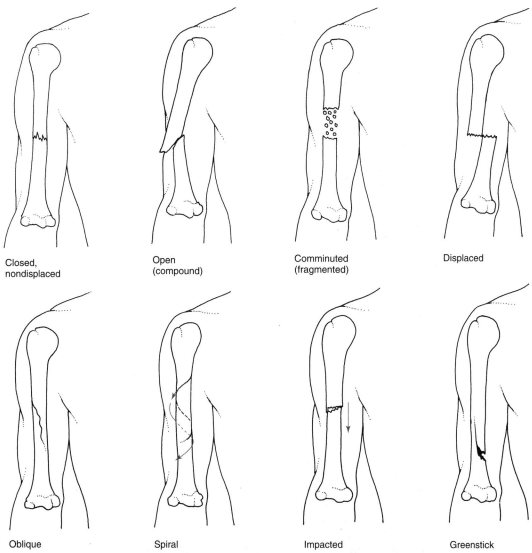

Closed,
nondisplaced
　　　　Open
(compound)
　　　　Comminuted
(fragmented)
　　　　Displaced

Oblique
　　　　Spiral
　　　　Impacted
　　　　Greenstick

FIGURE 49-2 ■ Types of fractures. (From Ignatavicius DD, Workman ML: *Medical surgical nursing,* ed 4. Philadelphia: WB Saunders, 2002, p 1126.)

   (6) Nondisplaced: edges of fractured bone remain aligned.
   (7) Impacted: fractured bone fragment forcibly driven into an adjacent bone ("telescoped").
   (8) Avulsion: separation of small fragment of bone at the site of a ligament or tendon attachment
  b. Direction of the line of fracture
   (1) Longitudinal (linear): fracture line runs parallel to the axis of the bone.
   (2) Oblique: fracture line runs at a 45° angle to the axis of the bone.
   (3) Spiral: fracture line encircles bone shaft.
   (4) Transverse: fracture line runs at a 90° angle to the longitudinal axis of the bone.
   (5) Comminuted: multiple fracture lines divide the bone into multiple fragments.
  c. Etiology of the fracture
   (1) Stress (fatigue): fracture occurs as result of repetitive microtrauma or an excessive musculotendinous pull that exceeds the strength of the bone.
   (2) Pathologic (spontaneous): fracture through an area of disease-weakened bone, usually related to minor trauma
   (3) Compression: fracture resulting from compressive force
  d. Fractures by name
   (1) Pott's fracture: a fracture at distal fibula associated with severe tibiofibular disruption
   (2) Colles' fracture: a fracture of the distal radius within 1 inch of joint in a characteristic manner
 3. Etiology of fractures: fractures occur when the bone is subjected to more stress than it can absorb.
 4. Predisposing factors for fractures: factors that reduce bone strength or forces that exceed bone strength
  a. Age: extremes in age
  b. Nutritional deficiency: diet low in calcium, low in vitamin D, or high in protein
  c. Metabolic diseases
  d. Inactivity or immobility: bone remains strongest under stress ("Wolff's Law").
  e. Physical abuse or trauma
 5. Fracture healing: healing maximized when bone edges are approximated
  a. Hematoma forms at site of fracture (first 24 hours).
  b. Leukocytes infiltrate site, followed by macrophages.
  c. Fibrous matrix of collagen proliferates at site.
  d. Highly vascular "callus" forms.
  e. Callus converts to loosely woven bone.
  f. Callus calcifies and remodels (full fracture "union").
 6. Goals of fracture management
  a. Reduce fracture to normal anatomic alignment.
  b. Promote bone healing.
  c. Maintain extremity function.
 7. Methods of fracture reduction
  a. Closed reduction: reduction achieved without surgical intervention
   (1) Continuous traction: skin or skeletal
   (2) Manual traction
   (3) Splints or casts
   (4) External fixation
  b. Open reduction and internal fixation—allows visualization of fracture site and uses pins, rods, nails, wire, screws, or plate and screw combinations to reduce the fracture

COMMON THERAPEUTIC DEVICES

I. Casts
- **A.** Purpose
  - **1.** Provide temporary immobilization
  - **2.** Prevent or correct deformities
  - **3.** Support bone and soft tissue during healing process
  - **4.** Promote early weight bearing
- **B.** Types of casts
  - **1.** Short extremity cast
    - **a.** Applied for stable fractures or tertiary sprains
    - **b.** May be weight bearing versus non–weight bearing
  - **2.** Long extremity cast
    - **a.** Applied for stable or unstable fractures
    - **b.** Immobilizes joint to protect soft tissue injuries: Achilles tendon rupture
  - **3.** Cylinder cast
    - **a.** Applied to treat stable fractures of long bones
  - **4.** Body cast
    - **a.** Immobilizes spine (e.g., postoperative spinal fusion)
    - **b.** Corrects deformities (e.g., scoliosis)
  - **5.** Spica cast
    - **a.** Immobilizes complex joint: shoulder, hip, thumb
    - **b.** Prevents dislocation of complex joint while promoting soft tissue healing
- **C.** Materials
  - **1.** Plaster of Paris
    - **a.** Applied by wrapping wet plaster strips
    - **b.** Easily molded
    - **c.** Heavier weight
  - **2.** Fiberglass—most common
    - **a.** Applied by wrapping wet plastic roll
    - **b.** More difficult to mold
    - **c.** Lightweight
  - **3.** Fiberglass-free, latex-free polymer
    - **a.** Use in latex allergy or latex sensitive patients.
  - **4.** Hybrid
    - **a.** Combination of Plaster of Paris and fiberglass
  - **5.** Polyester and cotton knit
  - **6.** Thermoplastic
    - **a.** Fabric tape composed of polyester polymer
- **D.** Early postcasting care
  - **1.** Promote cast drying.
    - **a.** Plaster of Paris: may take 24 hours or greater to dry
      - (1) Leave cast uncovered and open to air.
      - (2) Use fans to aid drying of large casts.
      - (3) Position casted part on pillow or smooth surface.
      - (4) Move cast on pillow or with palms to avoid plaster indentation.
      - (5) Advise patient to expect feeling of warmth as cast dries.
    - **b.** Fiberglass: dry within 30 minutes
      - (1) Blot moisture from surface with paper towel.
      - (2) Use blow dryer on cool or warm setting to aid drying of cast and skin.
  - **2.** Potential complications
    - **a.** Skin breakdown
    - **b.** Neurovascular compromise
    - **c.** Compartment syndrome
    - **d.** Fracture misaligned
    - **e.** Superior mesenteric artery syndrome (SMAS)

      (1) Only seen in body spica casts

      (2) A decreased blood supply to bowel resulting from compression of mesenteric artery; causes necrosis to gastrointestinal (GI) tract and hemorrhage

      (3) Symptoms of

        (a) Pain, distention, pressure in abdomen

        (b) Bowel obstruction

        (c) Nausea and vomiting

        (d) Presenting symptoms may appear days or weeks after cast applied because of retroperitoneal fat loss after patient immobilized.

      (4) Postcasting care

        (a) Prevent complications related to ineffective breathing pattern with body or spica cast.

          (i) Note rate and quality of respirations.

          (ii) Reposition patient in more upright position if possible.

          (iii) Teach relaxation techniques, deep controlled breathing.

          (iv) Remove cast, window or bivalve.

          (v) Place nasogastric tube to decompress stomach.

          (vi) Patient receives nothing by mouth (NPO), receiving intravenous fluids.

          (vii) Prone position optimal

          (viii) Ligament of Treitz released surgically

  3. Protect skin.

    a. Remove loose particles of plaster or plastic from cast edges and skin.

    b. Cover edges of cast to prevent skin irritation, especially important in personal area.

      (1) Turn edge of skin liner (stockinette) over cast edge and secure with tape.

      (2) If stockinette not used, "petal" edge with Transpore tape or moleskin.

      (3) Insert diaper at buttocks to prevent soiling in children with body or spica cast.

    c. Instruct patient to avoid putting any object between cast and skin.

  4. Reduce postoperative or postinjury swelling.

    a. Elevate extremity on pillow above level of heart.

    b. When cast dry, apply ice to area of injury or fracture.

  5. Assess neurovascular status of extremity.

    a. Perform "Integrated Bedside Assessment of Extremity."

      (1) Assessment of neurovascular status

        (a) Pain

        (b) Edema

        (c) Color

        (d) Capillary refill

        (e) Pulses

        (f) Temperature

        (g) Sensation

        (h) Motion

    b. Note amount and change in bloody drainage on cast and in dependent areas.

II. Traction

  A. Definition: Application of pulling force in the presence of a counterforce

  B. Purpose

    1. Aligns fragments of displaced bones, preventing further soft tissue injury

    2. Reduces muscle spasm

    3. Maintains limb length

    4. Maintains alignment of limb, while resting soft tissue

    5. Reduces contracture and deformity

C. Types of traction
   1. Skin traction
      a. Traction force applied wraps, straps, or prefabricated boots secured to body (e.g., Russell's or Buck's traction)
      b. Uses
         (1) Short-term immobilization of stable fractures (e.g., Buck's traction for proximal femoral fractures)
         (2) Intermittent traction (e.g., cervical neck traction)
      c. Techniques of application
         (1) Traction applied at bedside by trained individual
         (2) "Customized" devices applied using webril and moleskin
         (3) Prefabricated devices (e.g., boots)
         (4) Traction weight generally no more than 10 pounds (4.5 kg)
   2. Skeletal traction
      a. Traction applied directly to bone through transcortical or pericortical wires or screws (e.g., halo traction)
      b. Uses
         (1) Long-term immobilization of fractures (commonly greater than 1 week)
         (2) Short-term to long-term immobilization of unstable fractures of long bones or pelvis
      c. Techniques of application
         (1) Traction applied at bedside or in operative suite
         (2) Local anesthetic applied to skin and injected into periosteum
         (3) Conscious sedation also commonly used with pediatric patients
         (4) Amount of weight to traction according to patient's body weight and complexity of fracture, usually 15 to 40 pounds
         (5) Use of portable x-ray to confirm fracture reduction
   3. Manual traction
      a. Temporary traction applied by manual pull on extremity
      b. Uses
         (1) Maintenance of alignment and position of extremity when skin or skeletal traction is being readjusted
         (2) Short transport of patient
         (3) Dislocation or relocation of joint, casting of extremity, and reduction of fracture
      c. Techniques of application: firm manual pull placed on extremity while taking care to avoid pressure on bony prominences
D. Nursing care of the patient in traction
   1. Maintain traction apparatus to ensure proper alignment of body.
      a. Reposition patient in neutral alignment, usually supine.
      b. Obtain specific orders for amount of traction pull, position of extremity in bed, and head of bed (elevating head of bed decreases counterforce of body).
      c. Readjust skin traction if device dislodged.
      d. Apply manual traction to extremity whenever skeletal traction interrupted.
      e. Avoid heavy coverings (blankets) over extremities, which may disrupt traction.
      f. Inspect traction apparatus carefully every shift to ensure that bolts are tight on frame, knots are tight, and weights are free hanging.
   2. Assess skin integrity.
      a. Inspect pressure points between skin and apparatus.
      b. Inspect bony prominences of body in bed.
      c. Note redness, swelling, abrasion, pain caused by pressure.
   3. Assess for neurovascular compromise.
      a. Perform "Integrated Bedside Assessment of Extremity" as previously described.

       b. Compare affected to nonaffected side.

       c. Note potential problems caused by disrupted traction or inappropriately sized devices (e.g., boots).

    4. Assess for complications related to skeletal pin.

       a. Note redness, purulent drainage, "tenting" of skin surrounding pin, or pain at insertion of skeletal pin.

       b. Note signs and symptoms of infection in patient with long-standing traction.

III. External fixator

  A. Definition: method of rigid fixation applied using percutaneous pins and wire in bone that attach to a portable external frame

  B. Purpose

    1. Reduces fractures, especially complex or open fractures

    2. Permits care of soft tissue wounds associated with fractures

    3. Corrects bony deformity

    4. Stabilizes fractures with delayed union or nonunion

    5. Stabilizes arthrodesis (fusion) of a joint

  C. Types of external fixators

    1. Simple

       a. One or two bars on side(s) of limb (e.g., unilateral or bilateral frame)

       b. Used to treat less complex fractures

    2. Complex

       a. Multiple bars or semicircular rings placed in three-dimensional configuration around limb (e.g., triangular, quadrilateral, semicircular, or circular frame)

       b. Used to treat more complex fractures, often accompanied by soft tissue trauma

  D. Nursing care of the patient with an external fixator

    1. Maintain external fixator.

       a. Inspect device carefully every shift to ensure that bolts are tight on frame, with no movement of fixator pieces.

       b. Move device and limb using pillow beneath extremity or by grasping longitudinal bars on each side of limb.

    2. Assess for neurovascular compromise.

       a. Perform "Integrated Bedside Assessment of Extremity" as previously described.

       b. Compare affected to nonaffected side.

    3. Assess for complications related to skeletal pin.

       a. Note redness, purulent drainage, or pain at pin site.

       b. Note signs and symptoms of infection in patient with long-standing device.

       c. Note changes in sensory-motor status.

IV. Assistive devices

  A. Definition: devices prescribed to assist in mobility by providing support to an injured or weakened lower extremity by redistributing weight to the upper extremities

  B. Purpose

    1. Promote healing of traumatically fractured bones

    2. Promote healing of surgically osteotomized bones

    3. Support weakened or injured soft tissue

  C. Weight-bearing prescription

    1. Non–weight bearing (NWB): affected extremity should not touch floor.

    2. Touch-down weight bearing (TDWB): foot rests on floor with no weight.

    3. Partial weight bearing (PWB): 30% to 50% of body weight placed on affected extremity

    4. Weight bearing as tolerated (WBAT): as much weight as patient can tolerate without extreme pain

    5. Full weight bearing (FWB): full weight should be placed on affected extremity.

D. General instructions for patients
   1. Take small, controlled steps at all times.
   2. Wear sturdy, walking shoes with nonskid soles.
   3. Avoid wet or snowy areas.
   4. Remove throw rugs, electrical cords, excess furniture, and other obstructions from path of walking.
   5. Stand erect, looking forward when walking.
   6. Lead with strong, unaffected leg.
E. Types of assistive devices
   1. Crutches
      a. Selection criteria: prescribed for persons with good coordination, balance, and upper body strength
      b. Types of crutches
         (1) Axillary: most commonly crutch where weight is born on wrist and by triceps contraction; consists of a central post, handgrip, and axillary pad
         (2) Platform: crutch used to distribute weight to forearm; consists of a central post and forearm platform; reduces stress on arthritic wrist or fingers
         (3) Canadian or Lofstrand: crutch used to distribute weight to wrist and hand; consists of a central post with a band that fits around the forearm
      c. Proper fit of axillary crutches
         (1) Instruct patient to stand erect while wearing comfortable walking shoes.
         (2) Raise or lower central post so that two or three fingers can be inserted between the axilla and axillary pad.
         (3) Raise or lower handgrips so that elbows are bent 20° to 30°.
      d. Crutch gaits
         (1) Two-point gait: patient advances one crutch at the same time as the contralateral leg in alternating fashion (common with PWB).
         (2) Three-point gait: patient advances both crutches along with affected leg (common in PWB, TDWB, and NWB).
         (3) Four-point gait: patient advances right crutch, left foot, left crutch, right foot, with three "points" on ground at all times (used only in patient with high disability).
      e. Stair climbing
         (1) Climbing up stairs: patient holds banister on affected side and both crutches in contralateral hand; patient steps up with unaffected leg and follows with crutches and affected leg to same stair.
         (2) Climbing down stairs: patient holds banister on affected side and both crutches in contralateral hand; with weight on "good leg," patient steps down with affected leg and crutches; patient brings unaffected leg down to same stair.
   2. Walkers
      a. Selection criteria: prescribed for persons who require more stability than crutches, such as those with impaired balance or coordination
      b. Types of walkers
         (1) Simple walker: most common type of walker; consists of sturdy frame with handgrips
         (2) Platform walker: walker used to distribute weight to forearm; consists of a sturdy frame with forearm platform; reduces stress on arthritic wrist and fingers
      c. Proper fit of simple walker
         (1) Instruct patient to stand erect while wearing comfortable walking shoes, heels even with back of walker.
         (2) Raise or lower all four legs of walker equally so that elbows are bent 20° to 30°.

    d. Walker gait
      (1) Patient advances walker a short arm length forward, planting walker firmly on all four legs.
      (2) Patient advances affected foot, then advances body forward while supporting weight on arms.
    e. Stairs: performed with folded walker in manner similar to stair climbing with crutches

  3. Canes
    a. Selection criteria: prescribed for patients with minor disability and good balance, often after use of crutches or walker
    b. Types of canes
      (1) Simple cane: central post with curved handle
      (2) Quad cane: central post with four distal legs and curved handle
    c. Proper fit of cane
      (1) Instruct patient to stand erect while wearing comfortable walking shoes, cane 2 inches (5 cm) in front and 6 inches (15 cm) to the side of unaffected leg.
      (2) Raise or lower central post so that elbow is bent 20 to 30 degrees.
    d. Cane gait
      (1) Instruct patient to hold cane in hand opposite affected side.
      (2) Patient puts weight on "good leg," advancing affected leg and cane a comfortable distance.
      (3) Patient supports weight on both cane and affected leg, stepping through with "good leg."
    e. Stairs: performed with cane hand opposite affected leg in manner similar to stair climbing with crutches

ASSESSMENT PARAMETERS

I. Vascular assessment
  A. Pulses
    1. Assess operative extremity first; compare findings with the opposite extremity.
      a. Note rate, rhythm, quality.
      b. Compare distal to proximal pulses and side to side.
    2. Diminished neurovascular function requires prompt intervention to prevent complications and/or permanent damage.
  B. Skin color
    1. Note pallor or blanching, suggestive of insufficient arterial blood flow.
    2. Note duskiness or cyanosis, suggestive of insufficient venous return.
    3. Compare side to side.
  C. Skin temperature
    1. Note increase or decrease in temperature.
      (a) A cold hand or foot may indicate a diminished arterial blood supply to the area.
      (b) An extremity that is hot may indicate decreased venous return.
  D. Capillary refill
    1. Compress nail bed and quickly release; expect return of color within 2 to 3 seconds.
      a. Rapid refill suggests venous congestion.
      b. Slow refill suggests arterial insufficiency.
    2. Compare side to side.
  E. Edema
    1. Note location and severity of edema.
    2. Note effect of elevating extremity above heart level on extent of edema.
    3. Compare side to side.
  F. Pain
    1. Assess level of pain.

   a. Severe pain, particularly on passive motion, reliable sign of probable neurovascular compromise.
   b. If vascular status compromised, pain intensifies even with use of opioids and therapeutic measures.
II. Peripheral nervous system assessment
   A. Sensory component
      1. Note patient's ability to detect sensory stimulation (pain, light touch, deep touch, heat or cold, vibratory sense, proprioception, two-point discrimination).
      2. Note location and severity of any change.
      3. Compare side to side.
   B. Motor component
      1. Note patient's ability to move extremity actively through range of motion (ROM).
      2. Grade strength of major muscle groups.
         a. Grade 5: Active ROM against strong resistance (considered "normal" in well functioning adult)
         b. Grade 4: Active ROM against moderate resistance
         c. Grade 3: Active ROM against gravity only
         d. Grade 2: Weak, incomplete ROM against gravity
         e. Grade 1: No notable motion, but visible contractility of muscle group
         f. Grade 0: No motion or visible contractility
      3. Compare side to side.
III. Integrated peripheral nervous system assessment of extremities
   A. Upper extremity
      1. Radial nerve
         a. Sensory: touch web space between thumb and index finger
         b. Motor: extend wrist, hyperextend thumb
      2. Median nerve
         a. Sensory: touch tip of index finger
         b. Motor: oppose thumb to small finger
      3. Ulnar nerve
         a. Sensory: touch tip of small finger
         b. Motor: abduct fingers
   B. Lower extremity
      1. Peroneal nerve
         a. Sensory: touch lateral side of great toe, medial side of second digit
         b. Motor: dorsiflex ankle, hyperextend great toe
      2. Tibial nerve
         a. Sensory: touch each lateral and medial aspect on sole of foot
         b. Motor: plantar flex ankle, flex great toe

COMPLICATIONS COMMON TO ORTHOPEDICS

   I. Deep vein thrombosis (DVT)
   A. Definition: obstruction of deep venous circulation by a blood clot, usually distal to the cusp of a venous valve
   B. Etiology: Virchow's triad
      1. Venous stasis: immobilization, peripheral edema
      2. Vascular wall damage: trauma, traction of vessel during limb manipulation (dislocation), surgery
      3. Hypercoagulable state: clotting disorder, dehydration
   C. Incidence and risk factors
      1. Seen in 40% to 60% of patients with lower extremity surgery or injury
      2. Factors increasing risk for DVT: increased age, surgery (especially orthopedic, abdominal, gynecologic), immobility, lower extremity trauma, previous DVT, obesity, use of oral contraceptives, and coexistence of peripheral vascular disease, malignancy, stroke, pregnancy, cardiac disease, smoking, IV drug abuse, inflammatory bowel disease, dehydration, sickle cell disease

   3. Factors decreasing risk for DVT: high mobility, good hydration, use of epidural anesthesia, use of anticoagulants
   D. Postanesthesia care
      1. Assess for signs and symptoms of DVT: most common at least 48 to 72 hours after immobilization or surgery.
         a. Unilateral edema of the lower extremity, unrelieved with elevation
         b. Warmth, redness, tenderness, "fullness" of lower extremity
      2. Monitor results of diagnostic tests.
         a. Noninvasive: Doppler ultrasonography
         b. Invasive: ascending contrast venography (most diagnostic)
      3. Initiate interventions to prevent DVT.
         a. Provide adequate hydration.
         b. Encourage maximal mobility and early ambulation.
         c. Apply mechanical devices per order: antiembolic hose, sequential compression devices to lower leg or calf, plantar "foot pumps."
            (1) Apply device to both extremities in operating room or PACU if possible to combat early DVT formation.
            (2) Inconclusive data exist comparing device effectiveness with or without anticoagulation.
         d. Administer anticoagulants per order.
            (1) Oral warfarin: may be ordered day before, day of surgery, or in first 24 hours postoperatively
            (2) Low–molecular weight heparin: generally begun at least 12 hours postoperatively
            (3) Aspirin
            (4) Additional pharmacologic agents for high-risk patients
               (a) Danaparoid
               (b) Dextran
               (c) Thrombin inhibitors
               (d) Dermatan sulfate
      4. Initiate early interventions to treat patient with known DVT.
         a. Administer anticoagulation per order: bolus heparin, then adjust to achieve recommended international normalized ratio (INR).
         b. Decrease risk for clot embolization.
            (1) Maintain patient on bed rest per order: common with large proximal DVT.
            (2) Avoid aggressive massage of involved extremity.
            (3) Administer thrombolytic agent: uncommon therapy.
            (4) Prepare patient for surgical intervention: inferior vena cava filter inserted if multiple DVT.
            (5) Use noncemented prostheses if possible.
II. Pulmonary embolism (PE)
   A. Definition: complete or partial obstruction of the pulmonary artery or one of its branches by a systemically mobile thrombus or foreign body
   B. Causes: as listed for DVT
   C. Incidence and risk factors
      1. Seen clinically in 10% to 20% of patients undergoing major lower extremity surgery, fatal up to 10% of the time
      2. Factors increasing the risk for PE: unrecognized DVT and all other risk factors for DVT
   D. Postanesthesia care
      1. Assess for signs and symptoms of PE: most common 48 to 72 hours after injury or surgery; vary with degree of vessel occlusion.
         a. Dyspnea, tachypnea, restlessness
         b. Pleuritic chest pain, cough or hemoptysis, rales, pulmonary friction rub, hypoxemia
         c. Tachycardia
      2. Monitor results of diagnostic tests.
         a. Noninvasive

(1) ECG: may show T-wave inversion and ST depression.
(2) Chest x-ray film: may show wedge-shaped defect and accompanying diaphragmatic elevation
   b. Invasive
(1) Arterial blood gases: may be normal or show hypoxemia
(2) Lung scan (ventilation/perfusion studies): not reliable in absence of signs and symptoms
(3) Pulmonary angiography: highly diagnostic; usually performed only if lung scan nondiagnostic because of risk of examination
   3. Initiate interventions to prevent PE: see DVT.
   4. Initiate interventions to treat patient with known PE.
   a. Promote adequate gas exchange.
(1) Position patient in high Fowler's.
(2) Instruct on slow deep breathing.
(3) Provide oxygen: nonrebreathing mask common.
(4) Prepare for intubation if necessary.
   b. Administer anticoagulation per order: bolus heparin, then adjust to achieve recommended INR.
   c. Decrease risk for clot embolization: see DVT.
III. Fat embolism syndrome (FES)
   A. Definition: the mobilization of fat and free fatty acids that leads to acute pulmonary insufficiency
   B. Causes
   1. Mechanical theory: fat from the marrow of broken bones embolized to lung and occludes small pulmonary vessels
   2. Biochemical theory: stress response leads to release of catecholamines; free fatty acids mobilize; chylomicrons coalesce in lung and increase capillary permeability within the alveoli.
   C. Incidence and risk factors
   1. Seen clinically in 1% to 10% of patients with fractures; 5% to 10% of patients with multiple fractures or pelvic fractures; up to 50% of patients with fractures may have subclinical FES; seen rarely with insertion of intramedullary rods or stemmed prostheses
   2. Possible at any age, most prevalent in men age 20 to 40 and elderly between ages 70 to 80
   3. Factors that increase the risk for FES: invasion of the intramedullary canal, sepsis, shock
   D. Postanesthesia care
   1. Assess for signs and symptoms of FES: often present 12 to 48 hours after causative event, often rapidly progressing.
   a. Confusion, agitation, anxiety
   b. Tachypnea, dyspnea, pulmonary edema
   c. Hypoxemia, hypocarbia
   d. Tachycardia, dysrhythmias, substernal chest pain
   e. Hypotension
   f. Petechiae of trunk or conjunctiva: occur 50% of time
   g. Pyrexia
   2. Monitor results of diagnostic tests.
   a. Noninvasive
(1) ECG: may show atrial fibrillation
(2) Chest x-ray film: may show diffuse pulmonary infiltrate
   b. Invasive
(1) Arterial blood gases: may be normal or show hypoxemia
(2) Central venous pressure: elevated
(3) Pulmonary wedge pressure: initially reduced because of decreased perfusion of left atrium; later may rise
(4) Lung scan: may be performed in stable patient to rule out pulmonary embolism

(5) Pulmonary angiography: may be performed in stable patient to rule out pulmonary embolism

(6) Laboratory findings: elevated serum lipase, sedimentation rate, triglycerides, and glomerular filtration rate; decreased hematocrit, increased fat in urine

3. Initiate interventions to prevent FES.
   a. Maintain stability of fractured limbs.
   b. Treat sepsis and shock aggressively.
   c. Provide adequate hydration.
   d. Administer methylprednisolone to maintain the integrity of the pulmonary vascular system: controversial.

4. Initiate interventions to treat patient with known FES: early diagnosis and aggressive treatment critical.
   a. Promote adequate gas exchange.
      (1) Position patient in high Fowler's.
      (2) Instruct on slow deep breathing.
      (3) Provide oxygen: nonrebreathing mask common.
      (4) Prepare for intubation: common.
   b. Administer corticosteroids: creates antiadhesive effect on platelets, decreases inflammation of vascular membranes.
   c. Administer diuretics: reverses pulmonary edema.
   d. Support cardiovascular system.
      (1) Provide adequate fluid replacement.
      (2) Administer blood products.
      (3) Enhance blood pressure: dopamine.
      (4) Enhance pulmonary arterial pressure and right ventricle afterload: nitroglycerin drip.

IV. Compartment syndrome
   A. Definition: condition in which increased pressure within a muscle compartment may lead to severe neurovascular compromise; in cases of massive muscle destruction, may also see myoglobinuric renal function.
   B. Cause: any event that leads to increased extracompartmental or intracompartmental pressure, leading to edema and ischemia
   C. Pathophysiology: Edema-ischemia cycle
      1. Compromise of muscle compartment from overuse; extended compression of limb, fracture, or bleeding produces profound, quick response by surrounding tissue
      2. As edema of muscles increases, capillary bed perfusion compromised and venous congestion ensues.
         a. Edema compresses nerves and vessels.
         b. Progressive edema causes muscle ischemia.
         c. Histamine release by ischemic muscles causes capillary dilation and enhanced capillary permeability.
         d. Edema increases, resulting in greater compromised tissue perfusion and tissue oxygenation.
         e. Lactic acid formation increases, causing anaerobic metabolism to accelerate.
         f. Blood flow increases, causing increase in tissue pressure leading to greater compartmental pressures.
      3. If edema-ischemia cycle not arrested, irreversible muscle damage occurs in 4-8 hours, permanent nerve damage in 8 hours.
      4. Three types
         a. Acute compartment syndrome
            (1) Trauma related, limb threatening
         b. Chronic compartment syndrome
            (1) Overuse of muscles (i.e., weekend exercise enthusiast)
         c. Crush syndrome
            (1) Prolonged compression of limb

D. Incidence and risk factors

   1. Uncommon in general population; most commonly associated with fractures or injuries of the lower extremities

   2. Development within

      a. Thirty minutes to one half hour postinjury

      b. Postoperatively during first 7 days

   3. Factors that increase the risk for compartment syndrome

      a. Fracture

      b. Severe soft tissue injury (e.g., crush injury)

      c. Prolonged limb compression

         (1) Restrictive wraps, cast, brace, or apparatus

         (2) Prolonged compression of limb: unconscious victim lying on own limb, prolonged pressure from positioning device during lengthy surgery

         (3) Prolonged use of antishock trousers

         (4) Tight fascial closure

      d. Internal bleeding

      e. Increased capillary permeability: related to histamine release

         (1) Infiltrated intravenous fluids or medications

         (2) Some poisonous snake bites

         (3) Severe frostbite

   4. Postanesthesia care

      a. Assess for signs and symptoms of compartment syndrome: perform comprehensive neurovascular assessment, noting deterioration as follows.

         (1) Pain: most universal symptom related to muscle ischemia; pain extreme, unrelieved, aggravated by passive flexion or extension of digit or limb, not well localized, involves entire compartment

         (2) Pallor: seen in early stage related to compression of artery; later may be seen as cyanosis

         (3) Paresthesias: commonly seen change related to compression of sensory nerve; burning, searing, electric sensations

         (4) Pulselessness: in early stage pulse with decreased strength; later, pulse nonpalpable but audible on Doppler ultrasonography; in later stages no pulse found on Doppler ultrasonography (note: muscle and nerve ischemia can be occurring without occluding an artery; pulses may be palpable in the patient with acute compartment syndrome)

         (5) Paralysis: in early stage may be motor weakness related to compression of motor nerve; in later stage may be complete paralysis

         (6) Rigid or "tight" limb representing compartment engorgement

         (7) Decreased urine output, with dark urine

      b. Monitor results of diagnostic tests.

         (1) Direct measurement of compartment pressures: variety of methods in which catheter is inserted into the compartment; catheter is purged with normal saline; monitor intracompartmental pressure; pressures greater than 30 to 35 mm Hg considered diagnostic and warrant surgical intervention

         (2) Laboratory findings of muscle destruction and renal insufficiency: elevated serum creatine kinase MM-isoenzyme (CPK-MM), elevated white blood cells (WBC), potassium, phosphate, blood urea nitrogen (BUN), and creatinine; reduced serum calcium and pH; elevated urine myoglobin.

      c. Initiate interventions to prevent compartment syndrome.

         (1) Perform comprehensive neurovascular assessment on all patients at risk.

         (2) Provide early measures to decrease lower extremity edema: elevate limb above heart level, ice limb at site of injury or surgery.

       (3) Decrease potential for further injury: carefully handle injured part; maintain traction, brace, cast, for example.

    d. Initiate interventions to treat patient with suspected or diagnosed compartment syndrome.

       (1) Perform comprehensive neurovascular assessment every 15 minutes with special attention to compartment at risk.

       (2) Maintain limb in neutral at level of heart: enhances arterial blood flow, reduces possible neurovascular impingement.

       (3) Remove ice: reduce vasoconstriction.

       (4) Release or remove restrictive wraps, splints, or casts.

       (5) Assess pain and administer analgesics.

       (6) Maintain accurate input and output (I & O) records.

       (7) Provide emotional support.

       (8) Assist with compartment pressure checks.

       (9) Prepare patient for fasciotomy per order: extensive surgical decompression of compartment; high risk for infection as a result of ischemic conditions.

THE PERIANESTHESIA EXPERIENCE

  I. Preoperative phase—begins with patient's decision to have surgery and ends when he or she enters the operating room

    A. Goals of

      1. Thorough assessment of patient's physical and psychosocial condition

      2. Educating and preparing patient for surgery

    B. To include the following

      1. Complete history including preexisting conditions

      2. Medications

      3. Allergies to foods, medications, or latex

      4. Any family history of anesthetic complications such as pseudocholinesterase deficiency and malignant hyperthermia

      5. Social history—does the patient have assistance after surgery?

      6. Lab work dependent on procedure and age of patient

      7. Blood donation if replacement a possibility

      8. Informed consent

      9. NPO status

     10. Preoperative education

       a. Begin discharge teaching.

        (1) Use of assistive devices

        (2) Pain management

        (3) Signs of infection

        (4) Dressing and incisional management

  II. Intraoperative phase—time patient is in the operating room to admission to phase I postanesthesia care unit

    A. Goals of

      1. Appropriate surgical positioning

      2. Prevent infection

      3. Prevent injury

      4. Maintain sterile field

      5. Surgical counts

      6. Procure type of implant, traction, fixator, or cast as needed

      7. Assess fluids and vital signs

 III. Postoperative care, phase I—acute phase of recovery from anesthesia and surgical procedure

    A. Assessment of

      1. Airway

      2. Level of consciousness

3. Vital signs
   a. Hypothermia correction
4. Surgical site
   a. Position of operative site
   b. Neurovascular status
      (1) Temperature
      (2) Color
      (3) Capillary refill
      (4) Pulses
      (5) Movement
      (6) Sensation
      (7) Pain management (Box 49-1)
      (8) Control of nausea and vomiting
      (9) Initiate physician orders.
B. Discharge to phase II when
   1. Recovered from anesthesia
   2. Hemodynamically stable
   3. Pain managed
   4. Nausea and vomiting subsided
   5. Aldrete score of 10

IV. Postoperative care, phase II—observation period that includes preparing patient and support persons for home care
A. Teaching postoperative care critical to successful recovery
   1. Medications (pain control, antibiotics, resuming daily medications)
   2. Bowel management (stool softener with stimulant)
   3. Assessing neurovascular status
   4. Care of dressings, incision site, wounds, drains, casts, cryotherapy, continuous passive motion (CPM), pin sites
   5. Signs of infection
   6. When to call the physician (increasing pain, fever, edema, infection, bleeding, change in neurovascular status)
   7. Diet
   8. Mobility guidelines
   9. Reinforce instructions on assistive devices.
   10. Postoperative appointment with surgeon
   11. Driving considerations
   12. Self-care (showering, bathing)

V. Postoperative care, phase III
A. Extended stays
B. See Box 49-2: Patient Discharge Goals.

■ BOX 49-1
■ **THE HIERARCHY OF IMPORTANCE OF THE BASIC MEASURES OF PAIN INTENSITY**

1. The patient's pain rating using a self-reported pain rating scale (e.g., 0-10 numerical rating scale)
2. The patient has experienced a procedure or condition that is thought to be painful (e.g., surgery).
3. Behavioral signs (e.g., facial expression, crying, restlessness, fidgeting)
4. Proxy pain rating provided by a family member or other person who knows the patient well
5. Physiologic indicators (e.g., elevated vital signs)

From McCaffery M, Pasero C: Assessment: Underlying complexities, misconceptions, and practical tools. In Bowlus B, editor: *Pain clinical manual*, ed 2. St Louis: Mosby, 1999, p 95.

■ BOX 49-2
■ **PATIENT DISCHARGE GOALS FOLLOWING AMBULATORY SURGERY AND ANESTHESIA**

1. To promote patient satisfaction by minimizing disruptive influences associated with the patient's perioperative care
2. To optimize quality patient care such that patients can be safely discharged from the facility
3. To educate patients regarding the anticipated recovery process, thus facilitating patient participation and compliance with postoperative care plus early recognition of problems
4. To proficiently manage patients to minimize cost to the patient, medical facility, and third party payers

From Marley RA, Moline BM: Patient discharge issues. In Burden N, DeFazio Quinn DM, O'Brien D, Gregory Dawes BS, editors: *Ambulatory surgical nursing,* ed 2. Philadelphia: WB Saunders, 2000, p 505.

VI. Nursing diagnosis for the orthopedic patient
   A. Anxiety and fear related to surgical procedure, loss of control
   B. Knowledge deficit relating to surgical procedure and perianesthesia experience
   C. High risk for ineffective coping
   D. Risk for neurovascular compromise from perioperative positioning
   E. Pain management deficit
   F. Impaired physical mobility secondary to surgical procedure and postoperative pain management
   G. Knowledge deficits regarding mobility skills
   H. Self-care deficits
   I. Activity intolerance
   J. Potential for constipation from immobility and use of opioids
   K. High risk for skin breakdown
   L. Potential for infection
   M. Potential for neurovascular compromise related to cast or traction devices
   N. Knowledge deficit relating to use of CPM, cryotherapy, and/or assistive devices

COMMON OPERATIVE PROCEDURES

I. Definitions
   A. Upper extremity
      1. Carpal tunnel release—decompression of the median nerve by dividing the transverse carpal ligament
      2. Finger amputation and revision—generally for traumatic injuries, infection, or vascular compromise
      3. Joint replacement—small joints of the finger, hand, or wrist; performed to improve function in patients with rheumatoid arthritis or other degenerative diseases
      4. Olecranon bursectomy—excision of bursal wall and calcifications
      5. Open reduction, internal fixation—surgical placement of hardware such as pins, screws, or plates to maintain position of bones for healing
      6. Release of de Quervain's hand—decompression of the dorsal compartment of the hand to treat stenosing tenosynovitis of the wrist at the base of the thumb
      7. Release of Dupuytren's contracture—fasciotomy or fasciectomy to treat contracture in the palmar surface of the hand
      8. Rotator cuff repair—repair of muscles and tendons of the rotator cuff
      9. Synovectomy—removal of part or all of the synovial lining of a joint to retard progression of rheumatic destruction of the joint

B. Lower extremity
1. Anterior cruciate ligament reconstruction—replacement of damaged ligament with autograft, allograft, or synthetic ligament to return stability to the knee following ligament tear
2. Arthroscopic meniscectomy—removal of a part of the meniscus (cartilage) of the knee using arthroscopic technique
3. Osteotomy—cutting a bone to change its position for weight bearing or to correct an abnormal curvature
4. Prepatellar bursectomy—excision of bursal wall and calcifications
C. Miscellaneous
1. Arthroscopy: shoulder, wrist, knee, ankle
   a. Diagnostic arthroscopy can be performed in a variety of joints.
   b. It involves insertion of a fiber optic instrument into a joint to visualize the interior.
   c. Multiple procedures can be performed through a scope, including but not limited to debridement, biopsy, meniscectomy, ligament repair, and removal of loose bodies.
2. Bone biopsy—arthroscopic or open
3. Cast change
4. Closed reduction of fractures
5. Cyst removal
6. Debridement—arthroscopic or open
7. Excision of bone spurs—commonly formed as a result of osteoarthritic changes
8. Excision of ganglion—removal of a cystic mass found over a joint or tendon sheath
9. Excision of lesion
10. Hardware removal
11. Joint manipulation (e.g., following knee arthroplasty)
12. Muscle biopsy
13. Removal of foreign body
14. Simple tendon repair
15. Fasciotomy—surgical incision of fascia to relieve constriction and swelling in a muscle compartment
16. Bone graft—transfer of autologous or homologous bone from one site to another to replace bone, stabilize an internal fixation, or promote a bony fusion
17. Arthroplasty—surgical resection of a joint with placement of prosthesis; may be done as open repair or arthroscopically assisted repair
18. Tendon transfer—transference of tendon insertion point to different position to improve muscle function
19. Amputation—surgical removal of a body part
20. Replantation—microvascular surgery to restore a body part to its original site

TYPES OF ORTHOPEDIC SURGERY

I. Rotator cuff repair
A. Composed of four joints
1. Glenohumeral joint
   a. Ball-and-socket joint at end of humerus
   b. Most mobile joint in body
   c. Muscles and ligaments of rotator cuff strengthen this joint.
B. Areas of shoulder most easily seen arthroscopically
1. Glenohumeral joint
2. Subacromial space
3. Acromioclavicular joint
C. Procedure: arthroscopically assisted repair; also done as open repair if large enough tear involving more than one tendon

    D. Purpose
      1. Pain relief
      2. Improvement of functional abilities of joint
    E. Types of tears
      1. Four muscles and their tendons comprise the rotator cuff.
        a. Supraspinatus, infraspinatus, teres minor, subscapularis
        b. The subscapularis most frequently torn muscle, responsible for internal rotation of humerus
      2. Tears occur more in women and are seen most frequently after age 40.
      3. Etiology
        a. Degenerative weakened areas in cuff as a result of aging process
        b. Severe tears may result from
          (1) Heavy lifting
          (2) Throwing object
          (3) Fall on shoulder
          (4) Sudden adduction force applied to rotator cuff while arm is held in abduction
    F. Postanesthesia care
      1. Neurovascular assessment of affected arm
      2. Support surgical arm in sling or sling and swathe with abductor pillow to maintain joint alignment and diminish tension from operative shoulder.
      3. Ice packs or cryotherapy to decrease edema and pain
      4. Monitor dressing; reinforcing or changing of may be required as result of multiple puncture sites and leaking of irrigation fluids used intraoperatively to visualize joint.
      5. Pain management
        a. Intraoperative intraarticular injection of local anesthetic
        b. Interscalene block
        c. Opioids and NSAIDs
      6. Physical therapy and home mobility instructions reinforced
        a. Emphasize importance of following instructions to avoid exacerbation of condition.
        b. Rehabilitation usually takes 6 months to 1 year.
      7. Complications
        a. Contractures of elbow and shoulder if patient noncompliant with rehabilitation program
        b. Potential damage to deltoid muscle
        c. Repair work to cuff not holding because of misuse or overuse by patient
II. Spinal fusion and stabilization (thoracolumbar spine)
    A. Procedure: surgical stabilization of the spine using mechanical instrumentation with or without bone graft augmentation
    B. Purpose
      1. Prevent progression of spinal deformity
      2. Correct spinal deformity: lateral curves greater than 40°
      3. Reduce actual or potential neurologic or cardiopulmonary deficits
    C. Methods of spinal fusion
      1. Posterior spinal fusion with instrumentation
        a. Cotrel-Dubousset instrumentation: most common
        b. Harrington distraction rods or spinous process wiring
        c. Luque rods: most common for paralytic scoliosis
      2. Anterior spinal fusion
        a. Zielke instrumentation
        b. Harms instrumentation
      3. Combined anterior and posterior surgery
        a. Recommended for adults or children with severe deformities
        b. Anterior approach performed first, posterior approach commonly staged 5 days or more later

    4. Bone graft
        a. Autograft harvested from iliac crest
        b. Graft placed on decorticated spine to encourage osteoinduction
  D. Postanesthesia care
    1. Assess neurovascular status: perform comprehensive neurovascular assessment every 15 minutes for the first 2 hours, then hourly.
        a. Note bowel and bladder dysfunction.
        b. Assist with somatosensory evoked potential (SEP) monitoring as ordered.
    2. Assess for headache, possibly related to spinal fluid leak.
    3. Assess for wound drainage.
        a. Note dependent drainage on dressing and bed.
        b. Note formation and extent of hematoma.
        c. Maintain occlusive compression dressing to operative site.
        d. Maintain drainage device if present.
    4. Position patient for safety.
        a. Patient commonly positioned supine in regular hard bed: Stryker frame and CircOlectric bed not common
        b. Maintain patient in neutral body alignment.
        c. Log roll patient side to side with physician order.
        d. Assist patient's movement with draw sheet.
        e. Discourage patient use of trapeze or pulling under patient's axilla (to avoid rod displacement).
    5. Monitor for complications after spinal fusion (see previous section on complications common to orthopedics).
        a. Reduced gas exchange and ineffective breathing patterns
            (1) Encourage coughing and deep breathing hourly.
            (2) Assess equality and clarity of breath sounds.
            (3) Obtain chest x-ray film after anterior fusion to determine lung expansion.
            (4) Monitor arterial blood gases.
            (5) Turn patient side to side every hour.
        b. Gastric distension and decreased peristalsis
            (1) Auscultate for bowel sounds hourly.
            (2) Insert nasogastric tube if necessary.
            (3) Administer stool softener as needed.
III. Arthroplasty (joint reconstruction)
  A. Procedure: reconstruction of articulating surfaces of joint
  B. Purpose
    1. Relief of chronic disabling pain
    2. Improvement in joint function and activities of daily living
    3. Correction of deformity
    4. Prevention of further bone destruction
    5. Stabilization of joint
  C. Joints replaced
    1. Most common arthroplasties
        a. Hip
        b. Knee
        c. Shoulder
    2. Other joints replaced
        a. Elbows
        b. Fingers (proximal interphalangeal joint [PIP], metacarpophalangeal joint [MCP])
        c. Wrist and thumb
        d. Ankle
        e. Temporomandibular joint
  D. Common diagnosis prearthroplasty
    1. Degenerative arthritis (osteoarthritis or osteoarthrosis)
    2. Rheumatoid arthritis

      3. Avascular necrosis (osteonecrosis or ischemic necrosis)

      4. Posttraumatic arthritis

  E. Types of arthroplasties

    1. Hemiarthroplasty (one joint surface reconstructed with artificial part)

      a. Cup arthroplasty: placement of metal cup over femoral head (uncommon in modern arthroplasties)

      b. Endoprosthesis: replacement of femoral head with stemmed prosthesis stabilized in proximal medullary canal

        (1) Austin Moore prosthesis: prosthetic femoral head articulates with natural acetabulum.

        (2) Bipolar prosthesis: prosthetic femoral head articulates with plastic liner of large metal "shell" placed against acetabulum (greatest motion is within prosthetic device).

    2. Total joint arthroplasty: both joint surfaces reconstructed with artificial parts

  F. Materials commonly used

    1. Metals

      a. Cobalt chromium

      b. Titanium or titanium alloys

    2. Ceramics

    3. Plastics (high–molecular weight polymers)

    4. Polymethyl methacrylate ("bone cement")

  G. Methods of component fixation in bone

    1. Cement

      a. "Gold standard" of fixation

      b. Cement injected under pressure

      c. Cement hardens in minutes, emits heat in process.

      d. Allows for immediate full weight bearing on extremity

    2. Biologic ingrowth

      a. Microtextured surface of prosthesis allows bone to "grow into" and stabilize component.

      b. Bone ingrowth optimized with tight fit of prosthesis into bone, healthy dense bone, and reduction of prosthetic motion in early stages of bone incorporation

      c. Attempts at "tight fit" can cause intraoperative fracture.

      d. Postoperative weight-bearing restrictions generally continue for average of 2 months.

    3. Press fit

      a. Used for stemmed components only

      b. Stem impacted snugly into canal of bone with cement; stem mechanically supported by cortical bone

  H. Potential complications common to arthroplasties

    1. Deep vein thrombosis

      a. Single most common complication with lower extremity joint arthroplasty

      b. Prophylaxis generally given to all patients

    2. Pulmonary embolism

    3. Fat embolism: rare, possible during insertion of stemmed devices or in situations of acute traumatic injury

    4. Compartment syndrome: rare, may occur as a result of compression of contralateral limb during surgery or with large wound hematoma

    5. Peripheral neurovascular impairment

    6. Infection—number one causative organism, *Staphylococcus aureus*

      a. Superficial wound infection

        (1) Generally limited

        (2) May be related to stitch abscess

        (3) Treated with topical or oral antibiotics or both

    b. Deep wound infection
        (1) Acute: attributed to perioperative event
        (2) Late: attributed to hematologic spread of infection in body from remote site (e.g., urinary tract infection or abscessed tooth)
        (3) Acute deep infection requires open irrigation of joint and possible exchange of liner and long-term antibiotics
        (4) Late deep infection often requires removal of prosthesis, debridement of bone or tissue, and long-term antibiotics

I. Postanesthesia care of the hip arthroplasty patient

  1. Assess neurovascular status.
    a. Perform comprehensive neurovascular assessment at least every hour for first 4 hours.
    b. Note signs of peroneal nerve palsy, possibly resulting from stretch injury caused by intraoperative hip dislocation, limb lengthening, or hematoma.
        (1) Weak or absent dorsiflexion of foot and ankle against examiner resistance
        (2) Decreased or loss of sensation in lateral aspect of great toe, medial aspect of second toe

  2. Assess for signs of wound drainage: blood loss should not exceed 500 ml in first 8 hours.
    a. Note dependent drainage on dressing and bed.
    b. Note formation and extent of hematoma.
        (1) May suggest active hemorrhage
        (2) May require surgical evacuation
    c. Maintain occlusive compression dressing on operative site, reinforcing if necessary.
    d. Maintain drainage device if present.
        (1) Closed suction device such as a Hemovac: most common suction device used
        (2) Gravity device: uncommon
        (3) Autotransfusion device: used to collect and reinfuse blood according to hospital guidelines

  3. Position lower extremity to reduce risk of dislocation.
    a. Maintain operative extremity in neutral alignment.
    b. Avoid hip adduction.
        (1) Place pillow or abduction device between legs at all times.
        (2) Turn patient carefully to unaffected side, maintaining abduction, if allowed.
    c. Avoid hip flexion greater than 90°.
        (1) Avoid raising head of bed and foot of bed at same time.
        (2) Encourage use of overhead trapeze for support during position changes.
    d. Avoid extremes in hip rotation using trochanteric roll to side(s) of affected leg, considering surgical approach.
        (1) Avoid internal rotation if posterior approach.
        (2) Avoid external rotation if anterolateral approach.

  4. Provide aids to enhance patient compliance to position restrictions (e.g., long-handled reacher, long shoe horn, sock aid, elevated toilet seat, chair cushions).

  5. Provide for pain control.
    a. Instruct patient regarding use of parenteral patient-controlled analgesia.
    b. Expect intravenous or epidural opioids postoperatively.

  6. Prevent infection.
    a. Use strict aseptic technique for all invasive procedures.
    b. Insert Foley catheter if signs of bladder distension.
    c. Instruct patient in aggressive pulmonary hygiene.

J. Postanesthesia care of the knee arthroplasty patient
1. Assess neurovascular status.
   a. Perform comprehensive neurovascular assessment at least every hour for first 4 hours.
   b. Note signs of tibial nerve palsy: possibly caused by stretch injury from intraoperative knee dislocation, extensive swelling or hematoma.
2. Assess for signs of wound drainage: blood loss should not exceed 500 ml in first 8 hours (see interventions for hip arthroplasty, section I.2).
3. Position extremity to reduce edema and prevent contracture.
   a. Maintain operated extremity in neutral alignment.
   b. Elevate extremity on pillow above level of heart.
   c. Avoid placement of pillow beneath popliteal fossa.
   d. Avoid prolonged side lying with knee flexed.
4. Provide assistive devices to enhance patient's independence (e.g., long-handled reacher, long shoe horn, sock aid).
5. Encourage aggressive range of motion of knee.
   a. Activate CPM machine as ordered.
      (1) Supplied and adjusted by trained personnel
      (2) Degrees of flexion and extension ordered by physician
      (3) Gradually increase knee flexion and extension per order according to patient tolerance.
6. Provide for pain control (see interventions for hip arthroplasty, section I.5).
7. Prevent infection (see intervention for hip arthroplasty, section I.6)
K. Postanesthesia care of the shoulder arthroplasty patient
1. Assess neurovascular status.
   a. Perform comprehensive assessment at least every hour for first 4 hours.
   b. Note deficit in medial, radial, or ulnar nerve.
2. Assess for wound drainage: blood loss should not exceed 150 ml in first 24 hours.
   a. Note dependent drainage on dressing and bed.
   b. Note formation and extent of hematoma.
   c. Maintain occlusive compression dressing to operative site.
   d. Maintain drainage device if present.
      (1) Suction device: most common
      (2) Gravity device: uncommon
3. Positioning to reduce risk of dislocation
   a. Maintain postoperative extremity positioning.
      (1) Shoulder adduction and internal rotation using sling and swathe dressing with affected arm at side: most common
      (2) Shoulder abduction with abduction frame or airplane splint: less common
4. Assist with measures to reduce edema.
   a. Encourage range of motion of upper extremity joints distal to shoulder.
      (1) Range of motion of fingers and wrist commonly encouraged at least every hour
      (2) Range of motion of elbow often allowed: patient lightly stabilizes upper arm with unaffected hand during elbow range of motion.
5. Provide overhead trapeze and assistive devices to enhance patient ability to perform activities of daily living.
6. Encourage range of motion of shoulder as soon as possible.
   a. Activate CPM machine as ordered.
      (1) Supplied and adjusted by trained personnel
      (2) Used in supine position or in chair-sitting position
      (3) Degrees and direction of movement ordered by physician
      (4) Increase shoulder motion per order and according to patient tolerance.
7. Provide for pain control (see interventions for hip arthroplasty, section I.5).
8. Prevent infection (see intervention for hip arthroplasty, section I.6).

IV. Open reduction internal fixation (ORIF) of femoral fracture
  A. Procedure: operative reduction of a fracture of the femur and stabilization with hardware
  B. Purpose
    1. Attains and maintains reduction of fracture
    2. Enhances fracture healing through stability
    3. Allows for early mobilization of patient
  C. Types of femoral fractures
    1. Femoral neck fracture
      a. Basilar: fracture at the distal neck of the femur
      b. Subcapital: fracture directly under the femoral head
    2. Intertrochanteric fracture: fracture on a line through the greater and lesser trochanter
    3. Subtrochanteric fracture: transverse fracture between the lesser trochanter and a site an inch or more below the greater trochanter
    4. Femoral shaft fracture: fracture between the greater trochanter and the knee
  D. Commonly used fixation devices
    1. Wires and pins
    2. Bone screws
    3. Plates with screws
    4. Compression (sliding) hip screw
    5. Intramedullary rods and nails
  E. Postanesthesia care
    1. Assess neurovascular status: perform comprehensive neurovascular assessment.
    2. Maintain proper positioning.
      a. Place extremities in neutral position.
      b. Use trochanter roll (rolled sheet or blanket) or sandbag to prevent rotation of lower extremities.
      c. Turn patient on physician order only.
        (1) Usually approved to turn to unaffected side only
        (2) Maintain anatomic positioning by using pillows between legs and back for support.
      d. Prevent dislocation after ORIF for femoral neck fracture (less stable because capsule of hip is interrupted).
        (1) Avoid hip flexion greater than 90°.
        (2) Avoid hip adduction by placing abduction devices between legs.
        (3) Avoid extremes in rotation with trochanter roll.
        (4) Provide overhead trapeze to aid patient movement.
    3. Prevent extremity edema.
      a. Elevate extremity above level of heart using pillows.
      b. Avoid direct pressure in popliteal fossa.
    4. Monitor wound drainage.
      a. Maintain patency of drainage device if present.
      b. Expect pattern of decreasing drainage after first 2 to 4 hours postoperatively.
      c. Assess for dependent drainage underneath operative site and for drainage on dressing or cast.
      d. Maintain occlusive compression dressing, reinforcing if needed.
    5. Monitor for complications after femoral fracture (see previous section on complications common to orthopedics)
      a. Infection
        (1) Most common with open fracture
        (2) Assess for systemic signs or symptoms of infection.
        (3) Assess for local signs of infection (visibly reddened incision line).
        (4) Identify high-risk patient: malnourished or infirm patient, incontinent patient, patient with urinary tract infection or tooth abscess.

       b. Deep vein thrombosis (DVT): High risk in patients who are elderly, dehydrated, immobile, or have history of DVT.

       c. Pulmonary embolism (PE): High risk as for DVT

       d. Compartment syndrome: High risk in patients with prolonged limb compression, extensive soft tissue, vascular trauma, and sepsis

       e. Fat emboli syndrome (FES): High risk in patients with fracture of midshaft femur, fractures associated with sepsis or shock

V. Arthroscopy

  A. Procedure: examination of the interior of a joint with a small fiber optic tube in effort to visualize accurately or treat the joint cavity

  B. Purpose

    1. Diagnosis of pathologic condition

      a. Direct visualization of the articular surfaces, the synovium, supportive tissue, and foreign tissue

      b. Biopsy of synovium

    2. Treatment of pathologic condition

      a. Repair or resection of torn menisci

      b. Debridement of cartilage

      c. Removal of foreign body

      d. Arthroscopic-assisted ligament repair

      e. Fixation of minor damage to cartilage

  C. Joints amenable to arthroscopy

    1. Knee: Most common

    2. Hip

    3. Ankle

    4. Shoulder

    5. Elbow

    6. Temporomandibular joint

  D. Postanesthesia care

    1. Assess neurovascular status: perform comprehensive neurovascular assessment.

    2. Assess multiple portal sites.

      a. Monitor dressing for drainage.

      b. Maintain original dressing, reinforce with additional bulky dressing, and ACE wrap if needed.

    3. Prevent extremity edema.

      a. Elevate extremity above level of heart with pillows.

      b. Avoid direct pressure in popliteal fossa.

    4. Monitor for postarthroscopy complications (see previous section on complications common to orthopedics).

      a. Infection

        (1) Monitor portal sites for redness, swelling, pain, erythema: most common complication is superficial infection.

        (2) Instruct patient in manifestation of signs and symptoms of systemic and deep infection: uncommon, occurring more than 24 hours postoperatively.

      b. Major complications: rare but may include DVT, PE, and compartment syndrome

    5. Instruct patient regarding use of crutches.

    6. Provide for pain control.

      a. Oral opioids commonly used postoperatively

      b. Parenteral patient-controlled analgesia (PCA) may be used for 24 hours when more extensive joint repair is performed (e.g., anterior cruciate ligament repair).

    7. Position joint and allow for movement per order.

      a. Avoid direct pressure under joint and on bony prominences.

      b. Encourage active range of motion to all unaffected joints.

      c. Provide CPM machine per order.

        d. Provide for joint support with hinged brace or other device per order.

VI. Anterior cruciate ligament (ACL) repair

    A. Most frequently injured or torn ligament in knee joint

        1. Research supports increased ACL injury in female athletes.

            a. ACL contains hormone receptor sites for estrogen, progesterone, and relaxin. Injuries are seen more during menses, when estrogen causes the ligament to relax.

    B. Procedure: Reconstruction may be arthroscopically assisted or as open arthrotomy. Grafts choices for reconstruction include:

        1. Autogenous

            a. Patellar tendon—graft of choice, most reliable

            b. Semitendinous tendon

            c. Iliotibial band

            d. Gracilis muscle

            e. Fascia lata

        2. Allograft

        3. Ligament substitutes

            a. Stints—protect joint while ligament repair heals

            b. Scaffolds—protect soft tissue

            c. Synthetic ligaments—prone to mechanical failure, usually used as last resource

                (1) Gore-Tex

                (2) Dacron

                (3) Polyester

    C. Purpose

        1. Improve joint stability by strengthening anterior-posterior control of the knee.

    D. Complications of ACL repair

        1. Compartment syndrome

        2. Neurovascular impairment from inadvertent suturing of peroneal nerve, with a result of possible footdrop, decreased sensation to foot

        3. Prolonged tourniquet time could cause sciatic or femoral nerve palsy.

        4. Rare—fracture to femur or sprain to ligaments from leg brace used intraoperatively

        5. Pain from use of tourniquet and leg brace intraoperatively

        6. Rare—hemarthrosis and thromboembolism

    E. Postanesthesia care of the ACL repair patient

        1. Assess neurovascular status.

        2. Assess wound drainage; check dressing and drain.

        3. Position leg to decrease edema, pain.

        4. Begin cryotherapy, CPM as directed.

            a. The cold from cryotherapy decreases inflammation, pain, swelling, and the potential for postoperative bleeding with hematoma formation and muscle spasm.

        5. Keep knee immobilizer on to stabilize joint.

        6. Aggressively manage pain.

            a. Multimodal, preemptive pharmacologic approach most effective

                (1) Intraarticular injection of local anesthetics, opioids, NSAIDs, clonidine, and/or corticosteroids before incision is made

                (2) Opioid receptors, (mu, delta, kappa) found in peripheral nerves and play role in preventing and/or diminishing postoperative pain

                (3) Local anesthetics (bupivacaine) manage pain approximately 2-4 hours; opioids such as morphine 2-5 mg injected into the joint may last up to 8-12 hours without systemic side effects. Using a combination approach provides early onset and longer duration of analgesia (note: intraarticular meperidine has been shown to cause systemic side effects, but does appear to have a earlier onset than morphine).

(4) Corticosteroids (methylprednisone) and NSAIDs (ketorolac) provide analgesia by diminishing the inflammatory response after arthroscopic knee surgery.

(5) Clonidine increases the duration time of intraarticular morphine and local anesthetics.

(6) Effective pain management promotes quicker healing and increased compliance with rehabilitation programs and provides a more palatable experience overall for the patient.

(7) The use of preemptive analgesia reduces opioid use postoperatively.

   b. Femoral block, no weight bearing until worn off

     (1) Average length of analgesia: 29 hours

   c. Postoperative NSAIDs and opioids as directed

     (1) Controlled-release oxycodone (OxyContin) provides extended pain relief and promotes increased patient compliance with a twice per day dosing schedule.

   d. Epidural analgesia—allows for earlier ambulation, more comfort during rehabilitation, and improved pulmonary function postoperatively

VII. Amputation

  A. Procedure: surgical (or traumatic) removal of a body part

  B. Purpose

    1. Reduce risk of systemic sepsis

    2. Control pain of ischemia

    3. Maximize mobility

  C. Types of amputation

    1. Traumatic: results in extreme destruction of soft tissue and bone in the presence of infectious microorganisms

    2. Elective

      a. Closed (flap): performed in the absence of infection

      b. Open (guillotine): performed in presence of infection, allowing drainage of infectious material

  D. Indications for elective amputation

    1. Peripheral vascular disease: most frequent indication for lower extremity amputation, often associated with diabetes mellitus

    2. Severe trauma: most frequent indication for upper extremity amputation

    3. Other indications (in order of frequency)

      a. Acute or chronic infection: osteomyelitis or gas gangrene

      b. Trophic ulcers

      c. Severe crushing injuries

      d. Malignancies

      e. Frostbite

      f. Congenital deformities

  E. Postanesthesia care of the patient after amputation

    1. Assess neurovascular status: perform comprehensive neurovascular assessment.

    2. Assess for signs of wound drainage.

      a. Note dependent drainage on dressing and bed.

      b. Note unusual odors or color of drainage (important in presence of infection).

    3. Maintain stump dressing.

      a. Plaster cast: rigid dressing

        (1) Prevents swelling of stump

        (2) Protects stump from trauma

        (3) Used when patient will be fitted for immediate prosthesis (usually Pylon type)

      b. Soft dressing: gauze with elastic wrap

        (1) Prevents swelling of stump

        (2) Used when use of prosthesis unlikely

      4. Position extremity to minimize complications.

        a. Elevate stump to facilitate venous return first 24 to 48 hours.

        b. After 48 hours, position to prevent hip flexion contractures.

          (1) Avoid stump elevation.

          (2) Instruct patient to lie intermittently prone (encourages hip extension).

      5. Provide for pain control

        a. Administer parenteral opioids as ordered for postoperative surgical pain.

        b. Assess for phantom limb pain.

          (1) Pain sensation in area of absent, amputated limb

          (2) Common in first 24 to 48 hours postoperatively in traumatic amputation

          (3) Treated with opioids and phenytoin

          (4) Adequate treatment important to reduce risk of chronic phantom pain syndrome

      6. Instruct patient regarding phantom limb sensation: sensation that amputated limb is present.

        a. Inform patient that phenomenon is common in early postoperative period.

        b. Instruct patient that sensation is normal phenomenon.

        c. Treat with nonpharmacologic methods.

      7. Provide emotional support.

VIII. Replantation of amputated digits or limbs

    A. Procedure: reattachment of totally or partially amputated part involving restoration of vascular, nervous, bony, and soft tissue structures

    B. Possible sites for replantation

      1. Upper extremity

        a. Digits

          (1) Most common traumatic amputation

          (2) Replantation attempted in proximal digit amputations, amputation of multiple digits, amputation of index finger or thumb

          (3) Viability after replantation: 80% to 90%

          (4) Functional return after replantation: 65%

        b. Arms: less successful result

      2. Lower extremity

        a. Digits: great toe

        b. Leg

          (1) Amputation through tibia or fibula shows unfavorable results with high infection rate.

          (2) Leg length discrepancies common

    C. Factors influencing prognosis

      1. Positive factors

        a. Clean-cut (guillotine) amputation

        b. Young patient

        c. Hemodynamically stable patient

        d. Absence of systemic disease

        e. No history of smoking, alcohol, or drug abuse

        f. Absence of gross contamination of wound

        g. Amputated part wrapped in gauze and placed in cool environment

        h. Replantation attempted within 24 hours

      2. Negative factors

        a. Crushing injury

        b. Extremes of age

        c. History of peripheral vascular disease, hypertension, or other chronic illness

        d. History of smoking, alcohol, or drug abuse

      e. Grossly contaminated wound

      f. Delay in retrieval and care of amputated part

      g. Delay in replantation

D. Postanesthesia care of the patient postreplantation

    1. Assess neurovascular status at least every 15 minutes.

      a. Perform comprehensive bedside assessment.

      b. Perform technical monitoring as ordered.

        (1) Doppler ultrasonography

        (2) Temperature probes

        (3) Muscle contraction monitoring (evoked M wave)

        (4) Fluorometry readings (determines venous return)

      c. Promptly notify physician if negative change occurs.

    2. Promote circulation and prevent vasoconstriction.

      a. Elevate extremity above heart level.

      b. Administer thrombolytic agents to decrease clotting in peripheral vessels.

      c. Maintain room temperature at 78° to 90° F (26° to 30° C).

      d. Prevent patient exposure to nicotine and caffeine.

      e. Maintain patient hydration.

    3. Prevent infection.

      a. Administer antibiotics as ordered.

      b. Assess for signs and symptoms of infection.

      c. Provide for nutritional needs necessary for wound healing (high-protein diet).

    4. Provide for pain control.

      a. Provide oral opioids as needed.

      b. Assess pain caully, noting changes in pain pattern suggestive of ischemia.

    5. Provide emotional support.

    6. Complications

      a. Venous congestion

        (1) Massage digit.

        (2) Leech therapy

        (3) Revision of replantation

      b. Thrombosis

        (1) Anticoagulants

        (2) Revise surgically.

      c. Sepsis

      d. Renal failure

      e. Contractures

      f. Diminished or lost proprioception

IX. Nursing interventions

  A. Upper extremity

    1. Upper extremity procedures

      a. Position the hand above the heart.

      b. Provide a sling if ordered.

      c. Assess and protect cast and splint.

        (1) Cast should be kept dry.

        (2) Observe for cast defects that could lead to tissue compression damage.

      d. Apply ice packs as ordered.

      e. Check neurovascular status.

        (1) Nerve function

          (a) Radial—check sensation at the thumb–index finger web; have the patient hyperextend thumb or wrist.

          (b) Median—check sensation on the distal surface of the index finger; have patient oppose thumb and finger.

          (c) Ulnar—check sensation at distal end of small finger; have patient abduct all fingers.

(2) Vascular status—assess capillary refill.
  (a) Normal capillary refill: 3 seconds or less
  (b) Perform blanch test.
    (i) Compress and release nail bed quickly.
  (c) Compare capillary refill to unaffected extremity.
  (d) Rapid filling may indicate venous congestion.
  (e) Sluggish filling is a sign of arterial insufficiency.
  (f) Note color, comparing with unaffected extremity.
    (i) Blanching or pallor indicates arterial insufficiency.
  (g) Cyanosis indicates insufficient venous return.
(3) Mobility
  (a) Within limitations of casts, splints, and so forth, have patient wiggle fingers; this should be easy and not painful.

2. Lower extremities
  a. Position the extremity above the heart.
  b. Assess and protect cast and splint.
    (1) Cast should be kept dry.
    (2) Observe for cast defects that could lead to tissue compression damage.
  c. Apply ice packs or cooling device as ordered.
  d. Check neurovascular status frequently.
    (1) Nerve function—peroneal
      (a) Check sensation at lateral surface of great toe and medial surface of second toe.
      (b) Have patient dorsiflex ankle and extend toes.
      (c) Peroneal nerve damage results in foot drop.
    (2) Nerve function—tibial
      (a) Check sensation at the medial and lateral surfaces of the sole of the foot.
      (b) Have patient plantar flex the ankle and flex the toes.
      (c) Signs and symptoms of nerve damage include pain that is increasing, persistent, and localized; paresthesia; hyperesthesia; numbness; motor weakness; or paralysis.
    (3) Vascular status
      (a) Perform blanch test.
        (i) Compress and release nail bed quickly.
        (ii) Compare capillary refill with unaffected extremity.
        (iii) Rapid filling may indicate venous congestion.
        (iv) Sluggish filling is a sign of arterial insufficiency.
      (b) Note color, comparing with unaffected extremity.
        (i) Blanching or pallor indicates arterial insufficiency.
        (ii) Cyanosis indicates insufficient venous return.
      (c) Signs and symptoms of nerve damage include loss of pulse, sluggish or absent capillary refill, pallor, cyanosis, blanching, temperature decrease, paresthesia, or hyperesthesia.
    (4) Mobility
      (a) Within limitations of casts, splints, and so forth, have patient wiggle toes; this should be easy and not painful.
      (b) Severe pain on dorsiflexion of the toes can indicate compartment syndrome.

BIBLIOGRAPHY

1. Altizier L: Neurovascular assessment. *Orthop Nurs* 21(4):48-50, 2002.
2. American Society of periAnesthesia Nurses, Quinn D, editor: *Ambulatory surgical nursing core curriculum.* Philadelphia: WB Saunders, 1999.
3. Baird C: First line treatment for osteoarthritis, part 1: Pathophysiology, assessment, and pharmacologic interventions. *Orthop Nurs* 20(5):17-24, 2001.
4. Burden N: *Ambulatory surgical nursing,* ed 2. Philadelphia: WB Saunders, 2000.

5. Chapman MW: *Chapman's orthopaedic surgery,* ed 3, vol 1. Philadelphia: Lippincott Williams & Wilkins, 2001.

6. Childs S: Pathogenesis of anterior cruciate ligament injury. *Orthop Nurs* 21(4):35-40, 2002.

7. de Wit S: *Essentials of medical-surgical nursing,* ed 4. Philadelphia: WB Saunders, 1998.

8. Dunn D: Preoperative assessment criteria and patient teaching for ambulatory surgery patients. *J Post Anesth Nurs* 13(5):274-291, 1998.

9. Harvey C: Compartment syndrome: When it is least expected. *Orthop Nurs* 20(3):15-26, 2001.

10. Litwack K: *Core curriculum for perianesthesia nursing practice,* ed 4. Philadelphia: WB Saunders, 1999.

11. Mauer KA, Abrahams EB, Arslanian C, et al: National practice patterns for the care of the patient with total joint replacement, *Orthop Nurs* 21(3):37-47, 2002.

12. McCaffery M, Pasero C: *Pain clinical manual,* ed 2. St Louis, Mosby, 1999.

13. Nettina SM: *The Lippincott manual of nursing practice,* ed 7. Philadelphia: Lippincott Williams & Wilkins, 2001.

14. *Nursing 2000 drug handbook,* ed 22. Springhouse, PA: Springhouse, 2002.

15. Pellicci PM, Tria AJ Jr, Garvin KL: *Orthopaedic knowledge update: Hip and knee Reconstruction 2.* Rosemont, IL: American Academy of Orthopaedic Surgeons, 2000.

16. Reuben SS, Sklar J: Pain management in patients who undergo outpatient arthroscopic surgery of the knee. *J Bone Joint Surg* 82-A(12):1754-1766, 2000.

17. Rothrock JC: *Alexander's care of the patient in surgery,* ed 12. St Louis, Mosby, 2003.

18. Schoen DC: *NAON core curriculum for orthopaedic nursing,* ed 4. Pitman, NJ: Anthony J Jannetti, 2001.

19. Slowikowski RD, Flaherty SA: Epidural analgesia for postoperative orthopaedic pain. *Orthop Nurs* 19(1):23-33, 2000.

20. Sparks SM, Taylor CM: *Nursing diagnosis reference manual,* ed 5. Springhouse, PA, Springhouse, 2001.

21. Swearingen PL, Ross DG: *Manual of medical-surgical nursing care,* ed 4. St Louis: Mosby, 1999.

50 Otorhinolaryngologic Surgery

DONNA R. MCEWEN

OBJECTIVES
At the conclusion of this chapter the reader will be able to:

1. Identify the pathophysiologic ear, nose, throat, and head and neck conditions requiring surgical interventions.

2. Become familiar with the various surgical procedures performed in this specialty.

3. Become familiar with the postanesthesia problems encountered in the ear, nose, throat, and head and neck patient and the nursing interventions required in the management of these problems.

4. Be aware of the possible complications that can arise after ear, nose, throat, and head and neck procedures.

■■ Patients undergoing otorhinolaryngologic procedures present unique challenges to postanesthesia care unit (PACU) nurses. The severity and complexity of the procedures performed in this specialty range from relatively minor to extensive and major. Basic assessment skills common to all postanesthesia patients apply to this population; however, additional consideration must be given to communication needs because the outcome of the procedures frequently compromise one or more senses. This sensory compromise may be temporary or permanent. The patient may be unable to hear, smell, or speak. Procedures performed on the upper airway may create feelings of discomfort, pressure, and suffocation with each breath. Patients undergoing major procedures may arrive intubated or with tracheostomy or laryngostomy stomas. Frequent reassurance and explanations of nursing interventions are required.

ANATOMY AND PHYSIOLOGY

Ear

I. Structure and function
  A. Anatomy of ear (organ of hearing and equilibrium; Figure 50-1)
    1. Outer ear
      a. Visible portion consists of skin-covered flap of cartilage known as auricle or pinna.
        (1) Collects sound waves
        (2) Directs sound waves to external acoustic meatus
      b. Auditory canal—external acoustic meatus
        (1) Extends to tympanic membrane (eardrum)
      c. Tympanic membrane (eardrum)
        (1) Thin, transparent, pearly gray, cone-shaped membrane
        (2) Stretches across the ear canal
        (3) Separates the middle ear (tympanic cavity) from the outer ear
      d. Nerve supply
        (1) Auriculotemporal branch of the trigeminal nerve
          (a) General sensory
          (b) Innervates tympanic membrane, external acoustic meatus, anterior auricle

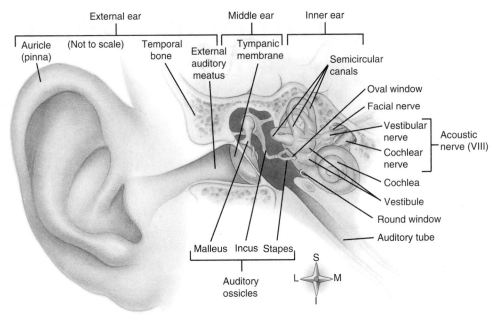

FIGURE 50-1 ■ The ear. (From Thibodeau G, Patton K: *Anthony's textbook of anatomy and physiology,* ed 16. St Louis: Mosby, 1999, p 455, Figure 15-5.)

2. Middle ear
   a. Structure
      (1) Ossicles
         (a) Malleus (hammer)
            (i) Largest of the three ossicles
         (b) Incus (anvil)
            (i) Middle ossicle
         (c) Stapes (stirrup)
            (i) Innermost ossicle
      (2) Eustachian tube
         (a) Channel connecting the tympanic cavity and the nasal part of the pharynx through which air reaches the middle ear
   b. Function
      (1) Ossicles form a chain from tympanic membrane to the oval window.
      (2) Transmits vibrations to inner ear, conducting sound to the inner ear
3. Inner ear
   a. Cochlea—spiral-shaped, forms the anterior part of the labyrinth of the inner ear; contains three compartments
      (1) Scala vestibuli
         (a) Part of the cochlea above the spiral lamina, which divides the canal
      (2) Scala tympani
         (a) Part of the cochlea below the spiral lamina
      (3) Cochlear duct (scala media)
         (a) Canal between the scala tympani and scala vestibuli
   b. Organ of Corti
      (1) Organ lying against the basilar membrane in the cochlear duct
      (2) Contains special sensory receptors for hearing
      (3) Consists of neuroepithelial hair cells that respond to vibration from the ossicles, converting mechanical energy to electrochemical impulses

      c. Vestibular labyrinth—controls equilibrium
        (1) Utricle
          (a) Larger of the two divisions of the membranous labyrinth of the inner ear
        (2) Saccule
          (a) Smaller of the two divisions of the membranous labyrinth of the vestibule
          (b) Communicates with the cochlear duct by way of the ductus reuniens
        (3) Semicircular canals
          (a) Description: Three canals—anterior, lateral, and posterior
          (b) Passages in the inner ear
          (c) Located in the bony labyrinth
          (d) Functions: Control sense of balance
          (e) Respond to movement of head
          (f) Can cause feeling of dizziness or vertigo after spinning
          (g) Motion sickness results from unusual movements of the head that result in stimulation of the semicircular canals.

Nose

I. Structure and function
   A. Anatomy of nose (organ of respiration and olfaction; Figure 50-2)
      1. External
        a. Upper—formed by nasal bones and maxilla
        b. Lower—formed by connective tissue
        c. Nares—separated by columella, formed from nasal cartilage
        d. Nasal septum
          (1) Nasal cartilage
          (2) Vomer bone
          (3) Perpendicular plate of ethmoid bone

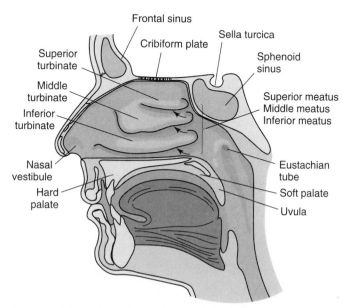

FIGURE 50-2 ■ Lateral wall of nose, showing superior, middle, and inferior turbinates. (From Phipps WJ: *Medical surgical nursing*, ed 7, St Louis: Mosby, 2003, p 456.)

    2. Internal—nasal cavity
        a. Nares (nostrils)
            (1) External opening of the nasal cavity
        b. Choanae
            (1) Paired openings between nasal cavity and oropharynx
        c. Nasopharynx
            (1) Part of the pharynx above the soft palate
        d. Eustachian tube
            (1) Narrow channel that connects tympanum with nasopharynx
        e. Paranasal sinuses
            (1) Arranged in four pairs
                (a) Maxillary
                (b) Frontal
                (c) Sphenoid
                (d) Ethmoid
        f. Nasal duct
            (1) Extends from the lower part of the lacrimal sac to the inferior meatus of the nose
            (2) Channel through which tear fluid is conveyed into the cavity of the nose
        g. Turbinate bones
            (1) Extend horizontally along the lateral wall of the nasal cavity
            (2) Separate the middle meatus of the nasal cavity from the inferior meatus
        h. Nasal septum
            (1) Separates the nasal cavity into two fossae
        i. Nerve supply
            (1) Trigeminal nerve
                (a) Cranial nerve V
                (b) General sensory, motor
                (c) Face, teeth, mouth, nasal cavity
            (2) Cranial nerve I (olfactory)
                (a) Special sensory
                (b) Nerve of smell
        j. Other nerves to consider
            (1) Cranial nerve II (optic)
                (a) Special sensory
                (b) Nerve of sight
                (c) Can be damaged in endoscopic sinus surgery
        k. Blood supply
            (1) Internal maxillary
            (2) Anterior ethmoid
            (3) Sphenopalatine
            (4) Nasopalatine
            (5) Pharyngeal
            (6) Posterior ethmoid

Throat

I. Structure and function
   A. Anatomy of oral cavity
      1. Mouth
         a. Lips
         b. Buccal cavity
         c. Lingual cavity
            (1) Tongue
            (2) Hard palate
            (3) Soft palate

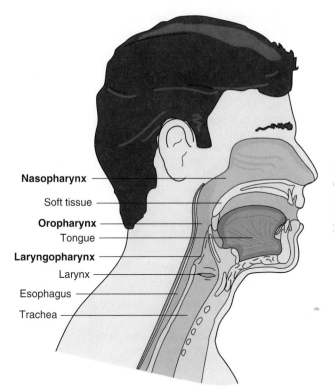

FIGURE 50-3 ■ Sagittal section of head showing pharynx and larynx. (From Phipps WJ: *Medical surgical nursing,* ed 7. St Louis: Mosby, 2003, p 456.)

Nasopharynx
Soft tissue
Oropharynx
Tongue
Laryngopharynx
Larynx
Esophagus
Trachea

2. Pharynx (see Figure 50-3)
   a. Throat
      (1) Nasopharynx (see Figure 50-3)
         (a) Lies posterior to the nose and above the level of the soft palate
         (b) Provides passageway for air
         (c) Contains opening of the eustachian tubes
      (2) Oropharynx (see Figure 50-3)
         (a) Extends from soft palate to the hyoid bone
         (b) Provides passageway for both air and food
      (3) Laryngopharynx (see Figure 50-3)
         (a) Extends from the hyoid bone to the lower border of the cricoid cartilage
         (b) Continues with the esophagus
         (c) Anterior entrance of the larynx is the epiglottis.
3. Tonsils
   a. Types
      (1) Palatine tonsils
         (a) Pair of oval-shaped structures
         (b) Size of almonds
         (c) Partially imbedded in mucous membrane
         (d) One on each side of the throat
      (2) Lingual tonsils
         (a) Below palatine tonsils
         (b) At base of tongue
      (3) Pharyngeal tonsils (adenoids)
         (a) Located in upper rear wall of oral cavity
         (b) Fair size in childhood, shrink after puberty
   b. Functions
      (1) Part of the lymphatic system

(2) Assist in filtering the circulating lymph of bacteria and other foreign material that may enter body through mouth or nose
  c. Nerve supply
    (1) Middle and posterior branches of the maxillary and glossopharyngeal nerves
    (2) Cranial nerve X (vagus)
      (a) Parasympathetic, visceral, afferent, motor, general sensory
      (b) Supplies sensory fibers to ear, tongue, pharynx, and larynx
      (c) Supplies motor fibers to pharynx, larynx, and esophagus
  d. Blood supply
    (1) External carotid branch (ascending palatine branch of facial artery)
4. Larynx
  a. Thyroid cartilage
    (1) Shield-shaped cartilage
    (2) Produces prominence on neck ("Adam's apple")
  b. Hyoid bone
    (1) Horse-shaped bone
    (2) Situated at the base of the tongue, just below the thyroid cartilage
  c. Cricoid cartilage
    (1) Ringlike cartilage
    (2) Forms lower and back part of larynx
  d. Epiglottis
    (1) Lidlike cartilage structure
    (2) Hangs over the entrance to the larynx
  e. Arytenoid cartilages
    (1) Jug-shaped cartilage of the larynx
  f. Corniculate cartilages
    (1) Two small conical nodules of yellow elastic cartilage
    (2) Articulate with the arytenoid cartilages
  g. Cuneiform cartilage
    (1) Elongated yellow elastic cartilage in the aryepiglottic fold
  h. Glottis
    (1) Vocal apparatus of the larynx
    (2) Consists of true vocal cords (vocal folds) and opening between them
  i. Nerve supply
    (1) Superior laryngeal nerve
      (a) Motor, general sensory, visceral afferent, parasympathetic
      (b) Cricothyroid muscle and inferior constrictor muscles of the pharynx, mucous membrane of back of tongue and larynx
    (2) Recurrent laryngeal nerve
      (a) Parasympathetic, visceral afferent, motor
      (b) Tracheal mucosa, esophagus, cardiac plexus
5. Thyroid gland
  a. Located in anterior portion of the neck
  b. Consists of right and left lobes united by isthmus
  c. Vascular supply: superior and inferior thyroid arteries
  d. Nerves in proximity
    1. Recurrent laryngeal nerve
    2. Superior laryngeal nerve

GENERAL NURSING CONCERNS FOR THE OTOLARYNGOLOGY PATIENT

I. Preoperative concerns
  A. Medical history assessment
  B. Nursing assessment
    1. Chief complaint

   2. Medications
       a. Allergies
       b. Current medications patient is taking
       c. Use of aspirin, ibuprofen, or drugs containing aspirin (increased risk of bleeding)
       d. Hormone therapy
       e. Preoperative medications
   3. Patient's understanding of surgical procedure and expected outcomes
   4. Patient's psychosocial status
   C. Laboratory and radiologic evaluations
       1. Complete blood count (CBC)
       2. Electrolytes based on patient history
       3. Urinalysis
       4. Coagulation studies
       5. Availability of designated units, type, and crossmatch
       6. Electrocardiogram (ECG)
       7. Chest radiograph
       8. Radiograph of sinuses, neck, mastoid
       9. Computed tomography (CT)
      10. Magnetic resonance imaging (MRI)
   D. Preoperative instructions
       1. Surgical procedure
       2. Expected outcomes
       3. Environment
       4. Alterations in lifestyle
       5. Self-care
       6. Suctioning
       7. Deep breathing
       8. Pain management
 II. Intraoperative concerns
   A. Nursing assessment
       1. Assess respiratory status.
       2. Determine patient's comfort.
       3. Identify positioning needs.
       4. Establish priorities.
       5. Reinforce preoperative teaching, orient to operating room (OR) environment, instruct patient in postoperative dressings.
       6. Determine patient's anxiety or apprehension.
   B. Aseptic technique
   C. Skin and tissue integrity
   D. Correct counts
   E. Medications given
   F. Intake and output
   G. Blood loss
   H. Patient's condition at time of transfer to PACU
III. Postanesthesia concerns: Phase I
   A. Nursing assessment
       1. Respiratory status
       2. Cardiovascular status
       3. Neurologic status
       4. Psychosocial status
   B. Report from anesthesiologist or certified registered nurse anesthetist (CRNA) or OR nurse
       1. Procedure, extent of surgery; complications
       2. Anesthetic agents and medications administered
       3. Blood loss and fluid replacement
       4. Placement of drains, packing
       5. Pertinent history, allergies

    C. Pain status

    D. Intake and output

    E. Patient's position

    F. Presence or absence of nausea

    G. Patient's ability to communicate

    H. Integrity of dressings and incision

    I. Patient's temperature

    J. Drainage from surgical site

IV. Postanesthesia concerns, discharge from phase I

    A. Patient

        1. Is conscious and able to maintain airway

        2. Is able to maintain oxygen saturation greater than 92% after 15 minutes on room air without being stimulated

        3. Remains in this condition for 30-45 minutes after extubation or administration of narcotic or narcotic antagonist

    B. No active bleeding from operative site or drains

V. Postanesthesia concerns: Phase II

    A. Prepare for discharge (criteria and polices vary among facilities).

        1. Ensure adequate pain control.

        2. Validate ability to retain fluids and maintain hydration status.

        3. Validate patient's ability to urinate.

        4. Assist patient with changing from hospital gown to personal clothing.

        5. Provide discharge instructions to patient and caregiver.

        6. Ensure that the patient is accompanied by responsible adult at discharge.

VI. Pediatric otolaryngology patients

    A. Special considerations

        1. Preoperative concerns

            a. Fear of separation, pain, injury, death: establish trust, reassure patient.

            b. Child's feelings of "loss of control": allow child to choose flavoring for anesthetic induction mask.

            c. Anxiety and fear of child and parents: prepare child and parents.

        2. Intraoperative concerns

            a. Airway management: increased risk of laryngospasm and vomiting if child is induced while crying

            b. Maintenance of body temperature (pediatric patient loses temperature faster than adult): warm OR, keep patient covered, use of warm blankets, insulated drapes, convection warming blanket to prevent loss of body heat

        3. Postoperative concerns

            a. Maintenance of body temperature: use of warm blankets, insulated drapes, keep patient covered, warm PACU, and so forth to prevent further heat loss and restore body temperature

            b. Increased risk for bleeding because of postoperative crying: administer pain medication as needed, provide reassurance to child and parents, involve parents as early postoperatively as possible.

            c. Fluid balance (pediatric patient dehydrates easier than adult): encourage fluid intake postoperatively, monitor intravenous (IV) fluids and output.

SURGICAL PROCEDURES

I. Ear

    A. Myringotomy with or without tympanostomy tubes

        1. Purpose

            a. Relieves pressure and allows for drainage of purulent or serous secretions from middle ear

            b. Aerates middle ear

            c. Relieves eustachian tube obstruction (thick, mucoid fluid)

      d. May be short-term or long-term
    2. Description
      a. Small incision made into posteroinferior aspect of tympanic membrane
      b. Polyethylene tube can be inserted into eardrum.
    3. Indications
      a. Acute otitis media unresponsive to antibiotics
      b. Bulging tympanic membrane
      c. Multiple episodes of acute otitis media along with chronic otitis media
    4. Preoperative concerns
      a. Frequently performed on children
        (1) Preoperative medication provided in oral form
        (2) Usually performed under mask anesthesia; no IV access established
    5. Intraoperative concerns
      a. General anesthetic essential for children to ensure accurate incision of tympanic membrane and placement of tube
      b. Parents may be present in OR for induction of pediatric patients, depending on institutional policy and practice.
    6. Postanesthesia priorities
      a. Phase I
        (1) Standard phase I activities as previously described
          (a) Nurse patient ratio 1:1 until consciousness and reflexes return for pediatric patients
          (b) Children may struggle against face tent; provide humidified oxygen by placing tubing near mouth and nose.
        (2) Depending on setting and institutional policy, patient may bypass phase I.
      b. Phase II
        (1) Standard phase II activities as previously described
        (2) Reunite parents with child as soon as possible to alleviate separation anxiety.
        (3) Discharge instructions
          (a) Avoid getting ears wet.
          (b) Change cotton balls as directed by physician.
          (c) Discuss pain management techniques.
          (d) Advise parents that tubes may fall out naturally.
    7. Psychosocial concerns
      a. Children may experience separation anxiety.
        (1) Allow for parent presence at induction if allowed by institutional policy.
      b. Allow child to assert control over situation when appropriate.
        (1) Remain in pajamas or street clothes.
        (2) Select flavor and scent of mask used for induction.
    8. Complications
      a. Hearing loss
      b. Persistent otorrhea
      c. Chronic perforation
      d. Bleeding
      e. Premature tube extrusion
B. Tympanoplasty
    1. Purpose
      a. Improve hearing
      b. Prevent recurrent infection
    2. Description
      a. Refers to a variety of reconstructive surgical procedures performed on deformed or diseased middle ear components
      b. Some tympanoplasties carried out in two stages
        (1) First procedure removes diseased tissue; second procedure involves reconstruction of hearing and middle ear function.

    d. Involves tissue grafts of cartilage, bone, fascia, skin, silicone, Teflon or hydroxyapatite

    e. Types

        (1) Tympanoplasty, type I (myringoplasty): repair of tympanic membrane

        (2) Tympanoplasty, type II: graft rests on incus.

        (3) Tympanoplasty, type III: graft attaches to head of stapes.

        (4) Tympanoplasty, type IV: graft attaches to footplate of stapes.

3. Indications

    a. Defects in tympanic membrane

    b. Necrotic destruction of ossicles

    c. Cholesteatoma (epidermal pocket or cystlike sac filled with keratin debris)

    d. Chronic drainage from ear canal

    e. Conductive hearing loss

    f. Trauma

4. Preoperative concerns

    a. Hearing deficits may be present; adjust communication methods as appropriate.

    b. Shampoo hair morning of surgery or night before surgery.

    c. Advise patient that postoperative hearing may be diminished initially because of packing and dressing.

5. Intraoperative concerns

    a. Allow patient to wear hearing aids (if present) to the OR to enhance communication.

    b. Involves use of microscope for work on minute, delicate structures

    c. Postauricular (behind ear) and/or endaural (through ear canal) approach used to expose structures of middle ear

    d. Facial nerve monitoring may be used.

    e. Positioning involves tilting OR bed at an angle to provide optimum exposure to operative ear; may cause pressure injury to dependent structures

6. Postanesthesia concerns

    a. Phase I

        (1) Standard phase I activities as previously described

        (2) Elevate head of bed at least 30° to minimize eustachian tube edema; clarify positioning with surgeon for specific instructions.

        (3) Position with operative ear upward to prevent pressure and graft displacement.

        (4) Assess facial nerve function—assess facial symmetry by asking patient to

            (a) Smile enough to show teeth.

            (b) Wrinkle forehead.

            (c) Pucker lips.

            (d) Wrinkle nose.

            (e) Squeeze eyelids shut.

            (f) Stick out tongue.

        (5) Prepare to treat nausea, vomiting, vertigo.

        (6) Avoid excess motion; transfer patient slowly and smoothly to minimize vertigo.

    b. Phase II

        (1) Standard phase II activities as previously described if patient discharged to home

        (2) Discharge instructions

            (a) Avoid getting ears wet.

            (b) Avoid sudden turning; encourage slow, smooth motion.

            (c) Sneeze with mouth open to avoid pressure on eustachian tubes.

            (d) Gentle nose blowing only

            (e) Noises such as popping and/or cracking may be heard in the ear by the patient and are considered normal.

7. Psychosocial concerns
   a. Anxiety related to hearing loss
8. Complications
   a. Facial nerve injury
   b. Hearing loss caused by drill trauma to ossicles

C. Stapedectomy
   1. Purpose
      a. Restoration of stapes bone function
   2. Description
      a. Removal of diseased stapes and replacement with prosthetic graft
   3. Indications
      a. Procedure of choice for treatment of otosclerosis, a condition of unknown etiology characterized by the formation of spongy bone around the round window, which causes stiffening and hardness of the stapes
   4. Preoperative concerns
      a. Hearing deficits may be present; adjust communication methods as appropriate.
      b. Advise patient that postoperative hearing may be diminished initially because of packing and dressing.
   5. Intraoperative concerns
      a. May be performed under local anesthesia with moderate sedation in adult patients
      b. Involves use of microscope
      c. May involve the use of the laser
      d. Profound intraoperative vertigo may be noted in patients under local anesthesia.
      e. Prosthesis fabricated from Teflon, stainless steel, or other synthetic material
   6. Postanesthesia priorities
      a. Phase I
         (1) Standard phase I activities as previously described
         (2) Elevate head of bed at least 30° to minimize eustachian tube edema; clarify positioning with surgeon for specific instructions.
         (3) Position with operative ear upward to prevent pressure and graft displacement.
         (4) Nausea, vomiting, and vertigo should be anticipated.
      b. Phase II
         (1) Standard phase II activities as previously described
         (2) Discharge instructions
            (a) Avoid getting ears wet.
            (b) Avoid sudden turning; encourage slow, smooth motion.
            (c) Sneeze with mouth open to avoid pressure on eustachian tubes.
            (d) Gentle nose blowing only
   7. Psychosocial concerns
      a. Patient may report immediate improvement in hearing, but hearing may decrease postoperatively because of accumulation of drainage.
   8. Complications
      a. If chorda tympani is cut to expose stapes and footplate, loss of taste to anterior two thirds of tongue will occur on the affected side.
      b. Facial nerve dehiscence
      c. Ossicular chain dislocation
      d. Perilymph leak
      e. Dizziness

D. Mastoidectomy
   1. Purpose
      a. To eradicate infected or diseased mastoid air cells

2. Description
   a. Simple mastoidectomy
      (1) Removal of mastoid air cells only
   b. Modified radical mastoidectomy
      (1) Removal of mastoid cells, posterior and superior external bony canal walls
      (2) Conversion of mastoid and epitympanic space into one common cavity
   c. Radical mastoidectomy
      (1) Removal of mastoid cells, posterior wall of external auditory canal, remnants of tympanic membrane, ossicles (except stapes), and middle ear mucosa
      (2) Removal of infected or diseased mucosa from middle ear orifice of the eustachian tube
      (3) Conversion of middle ear and mastoid space into one cavity
3. Indications
   a. Acute or chronic infection
   b. Extension of cholesteatoma into mastoid cells
4. Preoperative concerns
   a. Hearing deficits may be present; adjust communication methods as appropriate.
   b. Advise patient that postoperative hearing may be diminished initially because of packing and dressing.
5. Intraoperative concerns
   a. Involves use of microscope
   b. Positioning involves tilting OR bed at an angle to provide optimum exposure to operative ear; may cause pressure injury to dependent structures
6. Postanesthesia concerns
   a. Phase I
      (1) Standard phase I activities as previously described
      (2) Elevate head of bed at least 30°; clarify positioning with surgeon for specific instructions.
      (3) Position with operative ear upward to prevent pressure.
      (4) Assess facial nerve function—assess facial symmetry by asking patient to
         (a) Smile enough to show teeth.
         (b) Wrinkle forehead.
         (c) Pucker lips.
         (d) Wrinkle nose.
         (e) Squeeze eyelids shut.
         (f) Stick out tongue.
      (5) Prepare to treat nausea, vomiting, vertigo.
      (6) Avoid excess motion; transfer patient slowly and smoothly to minimize vertigo.
   b. Phase II
      (1) Standard phase II activities as previously described if patient discharged to home
      (2) Discharge instructions
         (a) Avoid getting ears wet.
         (b) Avoid sudden turning; encourage slow, smooth motion.
         (c) Sneeze with mouth open to avoid pressure on eustachian tubes.
         (d) Gentle nose blowing only
         (e) Noises such as popping and/or cracking may be heard in the ear by the patient and are considered normal.
7. Psychosocial concerns
   a. Patient may report immediate improvement in hearing, but hearing may decrease postoperatively from accumulation of drainage.

8. Complications
   a. Facial nerve dehiscence and damage
   b. Dizziness
E. Endolymphatic shunt
   1. Purpose
      a. To relieve pressure in endolymphatic sac
   2. Description
      a. Placement of shunt (commercially prepared or fashioned by surgeon) into endolymphatic sac via a mastoidectomy to allow for drainage of excess endolymph
   3. Indications
      a. Treatment of Meniere's disease
   4. Preoperative concerns
      a. Vertigo may be present preoperatively; a quiet, dark environment is advised to minimize stimuli.
   5. Intraoperative concerns
      a. Transfer patient slowly to avoid exacerbation of vertigo.
      b. See information on mastoidectomy (preceding section D.5).
   6. Postanesthesia concerns
      a. Phase I
         (1) Standard phase I activities as previously described
         (2) Elevate head of bed at least 30°; clarify positioning with surgeon for specific instructions.
         (3) Position with operative ear upward to prevent pressure.
         (4) Prepare to treat nausea, vomiting, vertigo.
         (5) Avoid excess motion; transfer patient slowly and smoothly to minimize vertigo.
      b. Phase II
         (1) Standard phase II activities as previously described if patient discharged to home; generally patients will require 24-hour admission because of vertigo
         (2) Discharge instructions
            (a) Avoid getting ears wet.
            (b) Avoid sudden turning; encourage slow, smooth motion.
            (c) Sneeze with mouth open to avoid pressure on eustachian tubes.
            (d) Gentle nose blowing only
            (e) Noises such as pulsations, popping, and/or cracking may be heard in the ear by the patient and are considered normal.
   7. Psychosocial concerns
      a. Meniere's sufferers may experience feelings of loss of control, depression, and powerlessness related to the unpredictability of the condition.
      b. Life style modifications may be necessary to cope with vertigo and hearing deficits.
   8. Complications
      a. Deafness or profound hearing loss
      b. Labyrinthitis
F. Vestibular neurectomy
   1. Purpose
      a. To interrupt transmission of the vestibular branch of the acoustic nerve, reducing stimuli to the vestibule and alleviating vertigo
   2. Description
      a. Resection of the vestibular portion of the acoustic nerve with preservation of the cochlear portion via transcochlear, translabyrinthine, middle fossa, retrolabyrinthine, or retrosigmoid approaches
   3. Indications
      a. Meniere's disease
      b. Traumatic labyrinthitis
      c. Vestibular neuronitis

4. Preoperative concerns
   a. Vertigo may be present preoperatively; a quiet, dark environment is advised to minimize stimuli.
5. Intraoperative concerns
   a. A fat graft is obtained from either the abdomen or lateral thigh to obliterate the mastoid cavity at the end of the procedure.
6. Postanesthesia concerns
   a. Phase I
      (1) Standard phase I activities as previously described
      (2) Elevate head of bed at least 30°; clarify positioning with surgeon for specific instructions.
      (3) Position with operative ear upward to prevent pressure.
      (4) Prepare to treat nausea, vomiting, vertigo.
      (5) Avoid excess motion; transfer patient slowly and smoothly to minimize vertigo.
      (6) Assess facial nerve function—assess facial symmetry by asking patient to
          (a) Smile enough to show teeth.
          (b) Wrinkle forehead.
          (c) Pucker lips.
          (d) Wrinkle nose.
          (e) Squeeze eyelids shut.
          (f) Stick out tongue.
   b. Phase II
      (1) Patient may be transferred to intensive care unit (ICU) if middle fossa approach utilized.
      (2) Standard phase II activities as previously described if discharged to home after transcochlear or translabyrinthine approaches; may require 24-hour admission
      (3) Discharge instructions
          (a) Avoid getting ears wet.
          (b) Avoid sudden turning; encourage slow, smooth motion.
          (c) Sneeze with mouth open to avoid pressure on eustachian tubes.
          (d) Gentle nose blowing only
          (e) Noises such as pulsations, popping, and/or cracking may be heard in the ear by the patient and are considered normal.
7. Psychosocial concerns
   a. Vertigo sufferers may experience feelings of loss of control, depression and powerlessness related to the unpredictability of the condition.
   b. Life style modifications may be necessary to cope with vertigo and hearing deficits.
8. Complications
   a. CSF leak
   b. Dural herniation

G. Labyrinthectomy
   1. Purpose
      a. Alleviation of severe vertigo
   2. Description
      a. Destruction of the membranous labyrinth of the horizontal semicircular canal via transcanal or transmastoid approach
   3. Indications
      a. Refractive unilateral Meniere's disease in a deaf or near deaf ear.
   4. Preoperative concerns
      a. Causes total deafness in operative ear
      b. Vertigo may be present preoperatively; a quiet, dark environment is advised to minimize stimuli.
   5. Intraoperative concerns
      a. Transfer patient slowly to avoid exacerbation of vertigo.
      b. See information on tympanoplasty (preceding section I.B.5).

6. Postanesthesia priorities
   a. Phase I
      (1) Standard phase I activities as previously described
      (2) Elevate head of bed at least 30°; clarify positioning with surgeon for specific instructions.
      (3) Position with operative ear upward to prevent pressure.
      (4) Prepare to treat nausea, vomiting, vertigo.
      (5) Avoid excess motion; transfer patient slowly and smoothly to minimize vertigo.
      (6) Assess facial nerve function—assess facial symmetry by asking patient to
         (a) Smile enough to show teeth.
         (b) Wrinkle forehead.
         (c) Pucker lips.
         (d) Wrinkle nose.
         (e) Squeeze eyelids shut.
         (f) Stick out tongue.
   b. Phase II
      (1) Standard phase II activities as previously described if discharged to home; may require 24-hour admission
      (2) Discharge instructions
         (a) Avoid getting ears wet.
         (b) Avoid sudden turning; encourage slow, smooth motion.
         (c) Sneeze with mouth open to avoid pressure on eustachian tubes.
         (d) Gentle nose blowing only
         (e) Noises such as pulsations, popping, and/or cracking may be heard in the ear by the patient and are considered normal.
         (f) Severe dizziness may be expected for several days as the brainstem must accommodate to labyrinth destruction and compensate.
         (g) Temporary taste disturbances can occur, but normal functioning will generally return.
7. Psychosocial concerns
   a. Vertigo sufferers may experience feelings of loss of control, depression, and powerlessness related to the unpredictability of the condition.
   b. Life style modifications may be necessary to cope with vertigo and hearing deficits.
8. Complications
   a. Meningitis
   b. Cerebrospinal fluid (CSF) leak
   c. Tinnitus
   d. Facial nerve paralysis
   e. Taste disturbances
H. Facial nerve decompression and exploration
   1. Purpose
      a. To relieve facial nerve pressure caused by edema or other compromise
      b. Repair of facial nerve transection
   2. Description
      a. Incision of facial nerve sheath at area of compromise via transmastoid, translabyrinthine, or middle cranial fossa approach
      b. Repair of transected nerve with nerve graft
   3. Indications
      a. Bell's palsy; an idiopathic edema and inflammation of the facial nerve, possibly viral in origin
      b. Trauma; skull or mandibular fractures, gunshot wounds
   4. Preoperative concerns
      a. Eye on affected side must be protected to guard against corneal dryness

    5. Intraoperative concerns

        a. Eye on affected side protected with ointment or tarsorrhaphy

        b. Nerve monitoring via electromyography (EMG)

        c. Auditory brainstem evoked potentials may also be used.

    6. Postanesthesia priorities

        a. Phase I

            (1) Standard phase I activities as previously described

            (2) Elevate head of bed at least 30°; clarify positioning with surgeon for specific instructions.

            (3) Place patient on side to prevent aspiration.

            (4) Assess facial nerve function—assess facial symmetry by asking patient to

                (a) Smile enough to show teeth.

                (b) Wrinkle forehead.

                (c) Pucker lips.

                (d) Wrinkle nose.

                (e) Squeeze eyelids shut.

                (f) Stick out tongue.

        b. Phase II

            (1) Patient may be transferred to ICU if middle fossa cranial approach is utilized.

            (2) Discharge instructions

                (a) Discuss aspiration risks and preventative measures.

                (b) Review oral care procedures.

                (c) Discuss importance of eye care and eye protection.

    7. Psychosocial concerns

        a. Body image disturbances related to appearance

        b. Regeneration time of repaired nerves may be lengthy, resulting in slow changes to appearance and function.

    8. Complications

        a. Scarring of nerve after repair

        b. CSF leak (cranial approach)

        c. Infection

        d. Dizziness

I. Removal of acoustic neuroma (vestibular schwannoma)

    1. Purpose

        a. To remove tumor mass while preserving nerve function

    2. Description

        a. Vestibular schwannomas are benign tumors arising from the Schwann cells of the vestibular portion of the acoustic nerve that may cause a myriad of symptoms including hearing loss, headache, vertigo, tinnitus, gait disturbance, and ocular disorders.

        b. Procedure involves resection of tumors usually via a translabyrinthine or middle cranial approach.

    3. Indications

        a. Diagnosed vestibular schwannoma

        b. Neurofibromatosis

    4. Preoperative concerns

        a. Hair removal may range from partial to complete head shave.

    5. Intraoperative concerns

        a. Middle cranial approach may be performed in sitting or prone position.

        b. Risk for air embolism related to surgical positioning.

    6. Postanesthesia priorities

        a. Phase I

            (1) Standard phase I activities as previously described

            (2) Elevate head of bed at least 30°; clarify positioning with surgeon for specific instructions.

(3) IV fluid infusion strictly monitored to prevent overload and possible cerebral edema.
  b. Phase II
   (1) Patient will be transferred to ICU after phase I care.
 7. Psychosocial concerns
  a. Partial or total hearing loss may necessitate life style adjustments.
  b. Body image disturbances related to hair removal
 8. Complications
  a. CSF leak
  b. Dural herniation
  c. Air embolism
  d. Tinnitus
  e. Facial nerve paralysis
  f. Vertigo
  g. Hearing loss or dead ear
  h. Meningitis

II. Nose
 A. Septoplasty, submucous resection
  1. Purpose
   a. To repair acquired or congenital intranasal and septal defects that interfere with normal respiratory function
  2. Description
   a. Excision of deviated septal cartilage and bone via intranasal incision
   b. Removal of polypoid tissue if present
   c. May include turbinectomy (reduction of turbinate size)
   d. Restoration of functional septal architecture
  3. Indications
   a. Deviated nasal septum
   b. Nasal polyps
   c. Hypertrophied nasal turbinates
  4. Preoperative concerns
   a. Discuss expected postoperative events.
    (1) Nasal packing may be in place and cause feeling of suffocation; patient will have to breathe through his or her mouth.
  5. Intraoperative concerns
   a. May be performed under local anesthesia for adults
   b. Nasal packing and/or nasal splints inserted
    (1) Nasal packing prevents hematoma.
    (2) Nasal splints help prevent synechiae.
  6. Postanesthesia priorities
   a. Phase I
    (1) Standard phase I activities as previously described
    (2) Progress from side lying to semi-Fowlers with head of bed elevated 30°.
    (3) Monitor patient closely for hypoventilation and hypoxia related to nasal packing and mouth breathing.
    (4) Apply ice packs as ordered to promote vasoconstriction and minimize edema.
    (5) Change moustache dressing as needed.
    (6) Observe for hemorrhage and/or septal hematoma.
     (a) Frequent swallowing may indicate bleeding.
     (b) Blood from septal hematoma dissects into cheeks, upper lip, and nose.
    (7) Excessive gagging may be indication that packing has dislodged and migrated to pharynx.
     (a) Provide equipment for reinsertion.
      (i) Bayonet forceps
      (ii) Nasal speculum

          (iii) Scissors

          (iv) Nasal packing

          (v) Headlight

          (vi) Tongue depressor

  b. Phase II

    (1) Standard phase II activities as previously described

    (2) Offer frequent mouth rinses to combat mouth dryness.

    (3) Discharge instructions

      (a) Change moustache dressing when soiled.

      (b) Use a humidifier to moisten the air.

      (c) No nose blowing; sniff secretions to the back of the nose; swallow or expectorate

      (d) No bending, straining, or lifting

      (e) Sneeze with the mouth open.

      (f) Bloody or tarry stools may be expected because of swallowed blood.

7. Psychosocial concerns

  a. Nasal packing may cause feelings of claustrophobia and anxiety.

8. Complications

  a. Bleeding

  b. Infection

  c. Edema

  d. Septal perforation

  e. Intranasal synechiae

  f. Septal hematoma

B. Rhinoplasty

  1. Purpose

    a. Restoration and improvement of respiratory function

    b. Alteration of appearance of the nose

  2. Description

    a. Nasal cartilage and bony structure reduced, realigned, or augmented via intranasal or small external skin incisions

    b. Surgical fracture of nasal bones

    c. May change appearance of sides, tip, or hump of nose

  3. Indications

    a. Traumatic or congenital deformity

    b. Cosmetic appearance

  4. Preoperative concerns

    a. Discuss expected postoperative events.

      (1) Nasal packing may be in place and cause feeling of suffocation; patient will have to breathe through his or her mouth.

    b. Careful screening of cosmetic patients to ensure that expectations of surgery are realistic

  5. Intraoperative concerns

    a. May be combined with septoplasty to correct defects

    b. May be performed under local anesthesia in adult patients

    c. External nasal splint and dressing will be applied to maintain correction.

  6. Postanesthesia priorities

    a. Phase I

      (1) Standard phase I activities as previously described

      (2) Progress from side lying to semi-Fowlers with head of bed elevated 30°.

      (3) Monitor patient closely for hypoventilation and hypoxia related to nasal packing and mouth breathing.

      (4) Apply ice packs as ordered to nose and eyes to promote vasoconstriction and minimize edema.

      (5) Change moustache dressing as needed.

      (6) Observe for hemorrhage.

        (a) Frequent swallowing may indicate bleeding.

(7) Excessive gagging may be indication that packing has migrated to pharynx.

　　(a) See information on septoplasty (preceding section II.A.6).

　b. Phase II

　　(1) Standard phase II activities as previously described

　　(2) Offer frequent mouth rinses to combat mouth dryness.

　　(3) Discharge instructions

　　　(a) Change moustache dressing when soiled.

　　　(b) Use a humidifier to moisten the air.

　　　(c) No nose blowing; sniff secretions to the back of the nose; swallow or expectorate

　　　(d) No bending, straining, or lifting

　　　(e) Sneeze with the mouth open.

　　　(f) Bloody or tarry stools may be expected because of swallowed blood.

　　　(g) External splint should not be disturbed or removed by patient.

7. Psychosocial concerns

　a. Cosmetic results may not meet patient expectations.

　b. Mild edema may persist for several months, obscuring final results of surgery.

8. Complications

　a. CSF leak

　b. Bleeding

　c. Edema

　d. Undesirable cosmetic appearance

C. Reduction of nasal fracture

　1. Purpose

　　a. Restoration of nasal architecture

　　b. Prevent nasal deformity

　2. Description

　　a. Tactile manipulation of external nose to realign cartilaginous structures

　　b. Intranasal reduction of fracture with instrumentation

　3. Indications

　　a. Nasal trauma

　4. Preoperative concerns

　　a. Procedure may be delayed to allow swelling from injury to subside.

　5. Intraoperative concerns

　　a. May be performed under local anesthesia in adult patients

　　b. Generally does not require postoperative nasal packing

　6. Postanesthesia priorities

　　a. Phase I

　　　(1) Standard phase I activities as previously described

　　　(2) Progress from side lying to semi-Fowlers with head of bed elevated 30°.

　　　(3) Apply ice packs as ordered to nose and eyes to promote vasoconstriction and minimize edema.

　　b. Phase II

　　　(1) Standard phase II activities as previously described

　　　(2) Discharge instructions

　　　　(a) No nose blowing; sniff secretions to the back of the nose; swallow or expectorate

　　　　(b) No bending, straining, or lifting

　　　　(c) Sneeze with the mouth open.

　　　　(d) Bloody or tarry stools may be expected because of swallowed blood.

　7. Psychosocial concerns

　　a. Additional procedures may be necessary if acceptable cosmetic results are not achieved.

8. Complications
   a. Incomplete reduction of fracture
      (1) Undesirable cosmetic appearance

III. Paranasal sinuses
   A. Functional endoscopic sinus surgery (FESS)
      1. Purpose
         a. Removal of diseased sinus mucosa
         b. Establishment or reestablishment of airflow, mucociliary clearance, and drainage from osteomeatal complex
      2. Description
         a. Nasal cavity examined via a rigid telescope inserted through the nares
         b. Sinuses entered via fenestrations
         c. Under direct vision, mucosa and/or polyps stripped and removed
         d. Sinus osteomeatal complex enlarged as needed and bony structure altered to achieve functional drainage
         e. Mucopurulent fluid drained
      3. Indications
         a. Nasal polyps
         b. Chronic sinusitis
         c. Mucocele
         d. Tumor masses
      4. Preoperative concerns
         a. Discuss expected postoperative events.
            (1) Nasal packing may be in place and cause feeling of suffocation; patient will have to breathe through his or her mouth.
      5. Intraoperative concerns
         a. May be performed under local anesthesia with sedation in adult patients
         b. Uses telescopes and video equipment to visualize intranasal structures
         c. Powered instrumentation may be used to remove diseased mucosa.
         d. Care is taken to maintain integrity of orbit to avoid ophthalmic injury.
         e. Packing may extend into sinus cavity.
      6. Postanesthesia priorities
         a. Phase I
            (1) Standard phase I activities as previously described
            (2) Progress from side lying to semi-Fowlers with head of bed elevated 30°.
            (3) Monitor patient closely for hypoventilation and hypoxia related to nasal packing and mouth breathing.
            (4) Apply ice packs as ordered to nose and eyes to promote vasoconstriction and minimize edema.
            (5) Change moustache dressing as needed.
            (6) Observe for hemorrhage.
               (a) Frequent swallowing may indicate bleeding.
            (7) Excessive gagging may be indication that packing has migrated to pharynx.
               (a) See information on septoplasty (preceding section II.A.6).
            (8) Observe for excessive orbital swelling, bruising, changes to visual acuity, impairment of extraocular movements.
         b. Phase II
            (1) Standard phase II activities as previously described
            (2) Discharge instructions
               (a) No nose blowing; sniff secretions to the back of the nose; swallow or expectorate
               (b) No bending, straining, or lifting
               (c) Sneeze with the mouth open.
               (d) Bloody or tarry stools may be expected because of swallowed blood.
      7. Psychosocial concerns
         a. Patient may have altered postoperative appearance (orbital bruising "raccoon eyes") if extensive surgery performed in ethmoid cavity.

8. Complications
   a. Orbital hematoma
   b. Optic nerve damage
   c. CSF leak
   d. Hemorrhage
   e. Infection
   f. Recurrence of nasal polyps
B. Caldwell Luc antrostomy
   1. Purpose
      a. To access the maxillary sinus for removal of diseased sinus mucosa or polyps and/or to ligate the maxillary artery
      b. Establishment or reestablishment of drainage from osteomeatal complex
   2. Description
      a. Sublabial and nasal mucosal incisions created
      b. Bone removed from antral wall to create opening for drainage
      c. Mucosal material stripped from walls of maxillary sinus
      d. Division and ligation of maxillary artery where indicated
      e. Packing placed in maxillary sinus cavity and nasal cavity
   3. Indications
      a. Chronic sinusitis unresponsive to medical therapy
      b. Maxillary polyps
      c. Maxillary tumors
      d. Acute or chronic epistaxis
   4. Preoperative concerns
      a. Discuss expected postoperative events.
         (1) Nasal packing may be in place and cause feeling of suffocation; patient will have to breathe through his or her mouth.
   5. Intraoperative concerns
      a. May be performed under general or local anesthesia
   6. Postanesthesia priorities
      a. Phase I
         (1) Standard phase I activities as previously described
         (2) Progress from side lying to semi-Fowlers with head of bed elevated 30°.
         (3) Monitor patient closely for hypoventilation and hypoxia related to nasal packing and mouth breathing.
         (4) Apply ice packs as ordered to face to promote vasoconstriction and minimize edema.
         (5) Change moustache dressing as needed.
         (6) Offer frequent mouth rinses to combat mouth dryness and eliminate bloody secretions from intraoral incisions.
         (7) Observe for hemorrhage.
            (a) Frequent swallowing may indicate bleeding.
         (8) Excessive gagging may be indication that packing has migrated to pharynx.
            (a) See information on septoplasty (preceding section II.A.6).
      b. Phase II
         (1) Standard phase II activities as previously described
         (2) Discharge instructions
            (a) No nose blowing; sniff secretions to the back of the nose; swallow or expectorate
            (b) No bending, straining, or lifting
            (c) Sneeze with the mouth open.
            (d) Continue to brush teeth, but avoid intraoral incisions; avoid excessive brushing pressure to teeth and gums.
            (e) Bloody or tarry stools may be expected because of swallowed blood.
   7. Psychosocial concerns
      a. Numbness to lip may result in uneven smile or altered appearance to lip and mouth.

8. Complications
   a. Persistent numbness to cheek, upper lip, gums, and teeth
   b. Damage to maxillary division of the trigeminal nerve (cranial nerve V) will cause permanent loss of sensation to upper lip.
   c. Oral antral fistula
C. Ethmoidectomy
   1. Purpose
      a. Promotion of drainage of the ethmoid sinus
      b. Used in conjunction with orbital decompression for exophthalmos
   2. Description
      a. Intranasal or external medical canthal incision
      b. Removal of bony walls between ethmoid air cells
      c. Creation of common ethmoid cavity to promote drainage
   3. Indications
      a. Chronic ethmoid sinusitis
      b. Mucoceles
      c. Polyps
   4. Preoperative concerns
      a. Discuss expected postoperative events.
         (1) Nasal packing may be in place and cause feeling of suffocation; patient will have to breathe through his or her mouth.
   5. Intraoperative concerns
      a. May use operating microscope
      b. May use endoscopes
   6. Postanesthesia priorities
      a. Phase I
         (1) Standard phase I activities as previously described
         (2) Progress from side lying to semi-Fowlers with head of bed elevated 30°.
         (3) Monitor patient closely for hypoventilation and hypoxia related to nasal packing and mouth breathing.
         (4) Apply ice packs as ordered to nose and eyes to promote vasoconstriction and minimize edema.
         (5) Change moustache dressing as needed.
         (6) Observe for hemorrhage.
            (a) Frequent swallowing may indicate bleeding.
         (7) Excessive gagging may be indication that packing has migrated to pharynx.
            (a) See information on septoplasty (preceding section II.A.6).
         (8) Observe for excessive orbital swelling, bruising, changes to visual acuity, impairment of extraocular movements.
      b. Phase II
         (1) Standard phase II activities as previously described
         (2) Discharge instructions
            (a) No nose blowing; sniff secretions to the back of the nose; swallow or expectorate
            (b) No bending, straining, or lifting
            (c) Sneeze with the mouth open.
            (d) Sleep with head elevated to minimize edema.
            (e) Apply ice packs to face to minimize bruising.
            (f) Bloody or tarry stools may be expected because of swallowed blood.
   7. Psychosocial concerns
      a. If eye pads and eye dressings are applied in the OR, patient may experience panic because of inability to see.
      b. Patient will have altered postoperative appearance from edema and orbital bruising ("raccoon eyes").
   8. Complications
      a. CSF leak
      b. Orbital injury

        c. Optic nerve injury and loss of vision

        d. Diplopia

        e. Hemorrhage

D. Frontal sinusotomy and obliteration

  1. Purpose

        a. To eradicate diseased mucosa from the frontal sinus and obliterate the space to prevent communication with the nasal cavity

  2. Description

        a. Approached through brow or scalp (bicoronal) incision

        b. Periosteum elevated; bone cut superiorly and laterally

        c. Fat graft removed from abdomen to pack sinus cavity

        d. Pressure dressing applied

  3. Indications

        a. Chronic frontal sinusitis

  4. Preoperative concerns

        a. May require hair removal to accomplish bicoronal incision

  5. Intraoperative concerns

        a. May require team approach from otorhinolaryngology and neurosurgery

  6. Postanesthesia priorities

        a. Phase I

           (1) Standard phase I activities as previously described

           (2) Elevate head of bed at least 30°; clarify positioning with surgeon for specific instructions.

           (3) Place patient on side to prevent aspiration.

           (4) Monitor patient closely for hypoventilation and hypoxia related to nasal packing and mouth breathing.

           (5) Apply ice packs as ordered to face to promote vasoconstriction and minimize edema.

           (6) Observe for hemorrhage.

              (a) Frequent swallowing may indicate bleeding.

           (7) Excessive gagging may be indication that packing has migrated to pharynx.

              (a) See information on septoplasty (preceding section II.A.6).

        b. Phase II

           (1) Standard phase II activities as previously described if patient discharged to home; may require 24-hour admission

           (2) Discharge instructions

              (a) No nose blowing; sniff secretions to the back of the nose; swallow or expectorate

              (b) No bending, straining, or lifting

              (c) Sneeze with the mouth open.

              (d) Sleep with head elevated to minimize edema.

              (e) Report signs and symptoms of infection to surgeon.

  7. Psychosocial concerns

        a. Unacceptable cosmetic appearance from hair removal, scarring, and/or prolonged edema

  8. Complications

        a. CSF leak

        b. Meningitis

        c. Brain abscess

        d. Scalp hematoma

        e. Fat necrosis

        f. Infection to donor site

IV. Oropharyngeal

  A. Adenoidectomy

    1. Purpose

        a. To remove infected or hypertrophied adenoidal tissue

    2. Description

3. Indications
   a. Chronic infection (adenoiditis or otitis media)
   b. Lymphoid hypertrophy
4. Preoperative concerns
   a. Discuss expected postoperative events.
   b. Frequently performed in pediatric population; use age appropriate teaching techniques and interventions.
5. Intraoperative concerns
   a. Performed under general anesthesia
   b. Often performed in conjunction with tonsillectomy
   c. Parents may be present in OR for induction of pediatric patients, depending on institutional policy and practice.
6. Postanesthesia priorities
   a. Phase I
      (1) Standard phase I activities as previously described
      (2) Place patient on side to prevent aspiration; advance to semi-Fowlers with head of bed elevated 30° when patient awake.
      (3) Monitor closely for hemorrhage.
         (a) Bright red emesis
         (b) Frequent and repeated swallowing
         (c) Agitation and restlessness
      (4) Pediatric considerations
         (a) Nurse patient ratio 1:1 until consciousness and reflexes return for pediatric patients
         (b) Children may struggle against face tent; provide humidified oxygen by placing tubing near mouth and nose.
   b. Phase II
      (1) Standard phase II activities as previously described
      (2) Discharge instructions
         (a) Avoid throat clearing, coughing, vigorous nose blowing.
         (b) No bending, straining, or lifting
         (c) Bland and soft diet
         (d) Bloody or tarry stools may be expected because of swallowed blood.
         (e) Throat discomfort increases between postoperative days 4 and 8 because of separation of eschar from pharyngeal bed.
7. Psychosocial concerns
   a. Children may experience separation anxiety.
      (1) Allow for parent presence at induction if allowed by institutional policy.
   b. Allow child to assert control over situation when appropriate.
      (1) Remain in pajamas or street clothes
      (2) Select flavor and scent of mask used for induction
8. Complications
   a. Otalgia
   b. Velopharyngeal insufficiency
   c. Hemorrhage
   d. Hypernasality
   e. Nasopharyngeal stenosis
B. Tonsillectomy
   1. Purpose
      a. To remove tonsillar tissue
   2. Description
      a. Removal of tonsils with sharp and blunt dissection via intrapharyngeal incisions
   3. Indications
      a. Chronic tonsillitis
      b. Peritonsillar abscess

      c. Tonsillar hypertrophy

      d. Ulcerations, lesions, and masses

    4. Preoperative concerns

      a. Discuss expected postoperative events.

      b. Frequently performed in pediatric population; use age appropriate teaching techniques and interventions

    5. Intraoperative concerns

      a. May be performed under local in adults

    6. Postanesthesia priorities

      a. Phase I

        (1) See information on adenoidectomy (preceding section IV.A.6).

      b. Phase II

        (1) See information on adenoidectomy (preceding section IV.A.6).

    7. Psychosocial concerns

      a. See information on adenoidectomy (preceding section IV.A.6).

    8. Complications

      a. Hemorrhage

C. Uvulopalatopharyngoplasty

    1. Purpose

      a. To reduce the amount of redundant pharyngopalatal mucosa

    2. Description

      a. Removal of tissue, reduction of or removal of uvula via intrapharyngeal incisions; sharp and dull dissection

      b. Tonsillectomy may also be performed.

    3. Indications

      a. Obstructive sleep apnea

      b. Snoring

    4. Preoperative concerns

      a. Discuss expected postoperative events.

        (1) Prepare patient for possibility of tracheostomy if edema is excessive.

    5. Intraoperative concerns

      a. May be intubated awake if obstruction and amount of redundant tissue is severe

      b. May be performed under local anesthesia with moderate sedation

      c. Laser may be used.

      d. Tracheostomy may be placed as temporary measure if extensive dissection performed or excessive airway edema is anticipated.

    6. Postanesthesia priorities

      a. Phase I

        (1) Standard phase I activities as previously described

        (2) Progress from side lying to semi-Fowlers with head of bed elevated 30°.

        (3) Monitor patient closely for hypoventilation and hypoxia related to edema.

        (4) Perform intraoral suctioning with care to avoid trauma to mucosal incision lines.

      b. Phase II

        (1) Often transferred to ICU for observation because of risk of airway edema and compromise

        (2) Generally will be admitted for minimum of 24 hours because of risk of airway edema

        (3) Discharge instructions

          (a) Avoid throat clearing and coughing.

          (b) No bending, straining, or lifting

          (c) Bland or soft diet

          (d) Bloody or tarry stools may be expected because of swallowed blood.

          (e) Use humidifier to moisten the air.

7. Psychosocial concerns
   a. Tracheostomy will temporarily affect verbal communication.
   b. Patient and/or caregivers will require tracheostomy care instructions.
   c. Procedure may alleviate snoring, but sleep apnea may still be present.
8. Complications
   a. Airway edema
   b. Hemorrhage
   c. Infection

D. Salivary gland surgery
   1. Purpose
      a. To remove infected salivary glands, sialoliths, cysts, or neoplasms
      b. Correction of ductal stenosis
   2. Description
      a. Types
         (1) Submandibular gland excision
         (2) Parotidectomy
   3. Indications
      a. Malignant and benign neoplasms
      b. Sialoliths and sialolithiasis
      c. Trauma causing stenosis of the duct
      d. Cysts
   4. Preoperative concerns
      a. Discuss expected postoperative events.
   5. Intraoperative concerns
      a. Facial nerve monitoring may be used.
   6. Postanesthesia priorities
      a. Phase I
         (1) Standard phase I activities as previously described
         (2) Progress from side lying to semi-Fowlers with head of bed elevated 30°.
         (3) Monitor patient closely for hemorrhage.
         (4) Assess facial nerve function—assess facial symmetry by asking patient to
            (a) Smile enough to show teeth.
            (b) Wrinkle forehead.
            (c) Pucker lips.
            (d) Wrinkle nose.
            (e) Squeeze eyelids shut.
            (f) Stick out tongue.
      b. Phase II
         (1) Standard phase II activities as previously described if patient discharged to home; may require 24-hour admission
         (2) Discharge instructions
            (a) Avoid throat clearing and coughing.
            (b) No bending, straining, or lifting
            (c) Bland and soft diet
   7. Psychosocial concerns
      a. Frey's syndrome
   8. Complications
      a. Hemorrhage
      b. Facial nerve paralysis
      c. Gustatory sweating (Frey's syndrome)
      d. Salivary fistula

E. Esophagoscopy
   1. Purpose
      a. To assess the structure and function of the esophagus and cardia of the stomach
      b. Obtain tissue biopsy to facilitate diagnoses
   2. Description
      a. Direct visualization with a rigid or flexible scope

  3. Indications
      a. Suspected carcinoma
      b. Stricture and stenosis
      c. Reflux
      d. Bleeding
  4. Preoperative concerns
      a. Discuss expected postoperative events.
  5. Intraoperative concerns
      a. May occasionally be performed under topical anesthesia and moderate sedation
  6. Postanesthesia priorities
      a. Phase I
          (1) Standard phase I activities as previously described
          (2) Progress from side lying to semi-Fowlers with head of bed elevated 30°.
          (3) Assess return of swallowing and gag reflex.
          (4) Observe for perforation and hemorrhage.
              (a) Frank blood in emesis
              (b) Agitation and restlessness
              (c) Complaints of severe pain
      b. Phase II
          (1) Standard phase II activities as previously described
          (2) Discharge instructions
              (a) Avoid throat clearing and coughing.
              (b) Bland and soft diet when gag reflex returned
  7. Psychosocial concerns
      a. Anxiety related to diagnostic findings
  8. Complications
      a. Bleeding
      b. Edema
      c. Esophageal perforation
V. Laryngeal surgery
  A. Tracheotomy
    1. Purpose
        a. To create a surgical opening in the trachea for airway maintenance
    2. Description
        a. Incision over the trachea
        b. Insertion of a catheter or cannula through tracheal rings
    3. Indications
        a. Acute airway obstruction
        b. Prolonged ventilator dependency
        c. Prevention of aspiration
        d. Bypass of upper airway obstruction because of tumor
    4. Preoperative concerns
        a. May be emergent procedure
    5. Intraoperative concerns
        a. Send obturator and ventilator adaptors to PACU with patient.
    6. Postanesthesia priorities
        a. Phase I
            (1) Standard phase I activities as previously described
            (2) Elevate head of bed 30°.
            (3) Ensure that tracheostomy tube ties are secure.
            (4) Prepare to reinsert tracheostomy tube or obturator if tube is coughed out.
            (5) Observe for hemorrhage.
            (6) Assess for pneumothorax.
            (7) Provide alternate means of communication for patient (e.g., magic slate, pen and paper, communication board).

  b. Phase II

   (1) May be transferred to ICU for observation; otherwise will require 24 hour admission at minimum.

   (2) Discharge instructions

    (a) Discuss need for humidification.

    (b) Teach tracheostomy care to patient, family, and/or caregivers.

 7. Psychosocial concerns

  a. Reduces ability to communicate verbally; alternate methods of communication must be used unless speaking valve is in place

 8. Complications

  a. Hemorrhage

  b. Dislodgement of tracheotomy tube

  c. Tracheoesophageal fistula

  d. Subcutaneous emphysema

  e. Pneumothorax

  f. Tracheostenosis

B. Laryngoscopy

 1. Purpose

  a. To visualize the interior of the larynx

  b. Obtain tissue biopsy for diagnosis

  c. Removal of vocal cord lesions

 2. Description

  a. Types

   (1) Direct laryngoscopy

    (a) Rigid

    (b) Flexible

   (2) Microsuspension

 3. Indications

  a. Suspected carcinoma

  b. Vocal cord polyps and nodules

 4. Preoperative concerns

  a. Discuss expected postoperative events.

 5. Intraoperative concerns

  a. Prepare for laryngospasm on extubation.

 6. Postanesthesia priorities

  a. Phase I

   (1) Standard phase I activities as previously described

   (2) Progress from side lying to semi-Fowlers with head of bed elevated 30°.

   (3) Be alert to possibility of laryngospasm.

   (4) Assess for return of swallowing and gag reflexes.

   (5) Mild hemoptysis may be anticipated after vocal cord procedures or biopsies.

  b. Phase II

   (1) Standard phase II activities as previously described

   (2) Discharge instructions

    (a) Avoid throat clearing, and start bland and soft diet when gag reflex returned.

    (c) Voice rest as directed by physician

    (d) Avoid whispering.

 7. Psychosocial concerns

  a. Anxiety related to diagnostic findings

  b. Anxiety related to vocalization changes

 8. Complications

  a. Vocal cord trauma and paralysis

  b. Laryngospasm

C. Phonosurgery

 1. Purpose

  a. To improve voice quality and vocal cord mobility

2. Description
   a. Insertion of Silastic shim or prosthesis to maintain vocal cord position
      (1) Type I
          (a) Improves or changes voice quality
      (2) Types II and III
          (a) Improves or changes pitch
          (b) Alters vocal cord tension
3. Indications
   a. Vocal cord paralysis caused by
      (1) Trauma
      (2) Neoplasms
      (3) Thyroidectomy
      (4) Mechanical dysfunction
4. Preoperative concerns
   a. Discuss expected postoperative events.
   b. Assess quality of patient's voice.
5. Intraoperative concerns
   a. Performed under local anesthesia with light sedation to allow patient to speak as a test of voice quality
   b. Voice quality tested as shim or prosthesis manipulated to find best position to reapproximate vocal cords
6. Postanesthesia priorities
   a. Phase I
      (1) May bypass phase I
   b. Phase II
      (1) Standard phase II activities as previously described
      (2) Provide alternate means of communication for patient (e.g., magic slate, pen and paper, communication board) to allow patient to rest voice.
      (3) Observe for laryngeal edema.
      (4) Discharge instructions
          (a) Voice rest as directed by physician
          (b) Avoid whispering.
7. Psychosocial concerns
   a. Speech therapy may be needed to improve quality of voice.
8. Complications
   a. Airway edema
   b. Infection
   c. Need for revision surgery
D. Laryngectomy
   1. Purpose
      a. Removal of larynx
   2. Description
      a. Types
         (1) Hemilaryngectomy
             (a) Removal of false vocal cord, arytenoids, and one side of thyroid cartilage
             (b) Patient has hoarse voice postoperatively.
         (2) Supraglottic laryngectomy
             (a) Removal of laryngeal tissues and structures above the epiglottis, hyoid bone, and false vocal cords
             (b) Normal voice postoperatively
         (3) Total laryngectomy
             (a) Removal of larynx, hyoid bone, laryngeal muscles, and preepiglottic space
             (b) Permanent stoma
             (c) Loss of natural voice postoperatively
   3. Indications
      a. Malignant neoplasm

    4. Preoperative concerns

      a. Discuss expected postoperative events.

      b. Discuss method to be used for communication in postoperative period.

      c. Patients with the presenting disorder of laryngeal neoplasms may have other chronic health conditions (e.g., smoking, diabetes, pulmonary disease; adjust planned interventions accordingly).

    5. Intraoperative concerns

      a. May be lengthy procedures, provide attention to patient positioning to avoid pressure injury

      b. May involve multiple specimens and frozen sections

      c. May be combined with tracheoesophageal puncture to allow for postprocedure speech prosthesis

        (1) Creates small fistula from superior wall of trachea to proximal wall of esophagus

        (2) Red rubber catheter inserted; after healing, silicone voice prosthesis with one-way valve is inserted

    6. Postanesthesia priorities

      a. Phase I

        (1) Standard phase I activities as previously described

        (2) Elevate head of bed at least 30° to minimize edema; clarify positioning with surgeon for specific instructions.

        (3) Provide alternate means of communication for patient (e.g., magic slate, pen and paper, communication board).

        (4) Frequent oral care when patient awake and alert

        (5) Promote coughing and deep breathing.

      b. Phase II

        (1) May be transferred to ICU if patient has concomitant health problems; otherwise will be transferred to medical-surgical nursing unit

        (2) Discharge instructions

          (a) Discuss need for humidification.

          (b) Teach stoma care to patient, family, and/or caregivers

    7. Psychosocial concerns

      a. Depression related to alteration in body image and communication difficulties

      b. Esophageal or electronic speech (i.e., from mechanical larynx) may be difficult to understand.

      c. Patient will require speech rehabilitation.

      d. Provide referral to support groups (American Cancer Society, Lost Cord Club, etc.).

    8. Complications

      a. Hemorrhage

      b. Pharyngocutaneous fistula

      c. Pneumothorax

VI. Neck procedures

  A. Neck dissection

    1. Purpose

      a. To remove cancerous and metastatic tissue and lymph nodes from the neck

    2. Description

      a. Types

        (1) Radical

          (a) Removal of lymph nodes, soft tissue, sternocleidomastoid muscle, eleventh cranial nerve, and internal jugular vein

        (2) Modified radical

          (a) Removal of soft tissue of neck and lymph nodes with preservation of other structures

    3. Indications

      a. Malignant neoplasms

      b. Prophylaxis against metastasis

4. Preoperative concerns
   a. Discuss expected postoperative events.
   b. Patients often have other health concerns (see laryngectomy).
5. Intraoperative Concerns
   a. Usually combined with laryngectomy procedures
   b. May be lengthy procedures; provide attention to patient positioning to avoid pressure injury
   c. May involve multiple specimens and frozen sections
6. Postanesthesia priorities
   a. Phase I
      (1) See information on laryngectomy (section V.D.4).
      (2) Support affected arm on pillow to minimize pain.
   b. Phase II
      (1) May be transferred to ICU for observation; otherwise will be transferred to general medical-surgical nursing unit.
7. Psychosocial concerns
   a. Unacceptable cosmetic appearance (radical dissection)
   b. Depression related to appearance, concern about prognosis
   c. Physical therapy required to regain strength in remaining neck muscles
8. Complications
   a. Hemorrhage
   b. Impaired circulation to tissue flaps
   c. Pneumothorax
   d. Chyle leak
B. Thyroidectomy
   1. Purpose
      a. To remove a hypertrophied thyroid gland and/or parathyroid glands
      b. Removal of thyroid tumors and nodules
   2. Description
      a. Excision of the thyroid gland and parathyroid gland via a neck incision
   3. Indications
      a. Tumor and nodules
      b. Hyperthyroidism (Graves' disease)
      c. Hashimoto's thyroiditis
   4. Preoperative concerns
      a. Discuss expected postoperative events.
      b. Hypothyroidism may predispose patient to skin breakdown and edema.
   5. Intraoperative concerns
      a. May be performed as video-assisted procedure utilizing harmonic scalpel
      b. Positioning is critical to expose gland. Neck is hyperextended with head resting on headrest.
      c. Electrocautery not used in vicinity of recurrent laryngeal nerve to avoid thermal damage to nerve
   6. Postanesthesia priorities
      a. Phase I
         (1) Standard phase I activities as previously described
         (2) Elevate head of bed at least 30° to minimize edema; clarify positioning with surgeon for specific instructions.
         (3) Obtain tracheostomy tray at bedside if signs and symptoms indicate respiratory distress.
         (4) Encourage deep breathing.
         (5) Observe for low calcium levels (have calcium gluconate at bedside).
            (a) Cramping, tingling of extremities
            (b) Numbness around lips
         (6) Monitor for thyroid storm.
            (a) Rare if patient is euthyroid (normal) before surgery

      (b) Characterized by increased heart rate, increased blood pressure, heat intolerance, high oxygen consumption, sweating

      (c) Treated with beta-blockers, usually propranolol

  b. Phase II

    (1) Standard phase II activities as previously described; will generally be admitted for 24-hour observation

    (2) Discharge instructions

      (a) Discuss symptoms of hypocalcemia, and instruct patient to notify surgeon if these symptoms occur.

      (b) Keep all follow-up appointments; laboratory monitoring of thyroid levels and hypothyroidism imperative

      (c) Encourage range of motion exercises for neck.

      (d) Soft diet until dysphagia eases

      (e) Voice rest as directed by surgeon

7. Psychosocial concerns

  a. Alteration in body image because of neck scar

8. Complications

  a. Recurrent laryngeal nerve injury

  b. Hemorrhage

  c. Hypoparathyroidism

BIBLIOGRAPHY

1. Burden N: *Ambulatory surgical nursing.* Philadelphia: WB Saunders, 2000.
2. Lewis SM, Heitkemper MM, Dirksen SR: *Medical surgical nursing: Assessment and management of clinical problems.* St Louis: Mosby, 2000.
3. Phipps WJ, Sands JK, Marek JF: *Medical surgical nursing: Concepts and clinical practice.* St Louis: Mosby, 1999.
4. Rothrock JC: *Alexander's care of the patient in surgery.* St Louis, Mosby, 2003.

51 Peripheral Vascular Surgery

MAUREEN E. LISBERGER

OBJECTIVES

At the conclusion of this chapter the reader will be able to:

1. Explain three factors that affect peripheral circulation

2. Describe three causes of arteriosclerosis.

3. Compare the signs and symptoms of arterial and venous vascular disease.

4. Identify the risk factors that contribute to the development of peripheral vascular disease.

5. List three postarteriography assessment criteria.

6. Identify the most common sites of occurrence of peripheral vascular disease.

7. Describe the 19 operative procedures performed on patients with peripheral vascular disease as outlined in this chapter.

8. Describe the immediate postoperative nursing considerations for each operative procedure.

9. State at least six major postoperative complications of vascular surgery.

10. List at least two postanesthesia nursing interventions for each of the surgical procedures described.

11. By use of the nursing process, describe how you would synthesize the preoperative assessment and intraoperative concerns of the surgical team into a rationale for postanesthesia care of the vascular patient.

The most common causative factor in the development of peripheral vascular disease (PVD) is atherosclerosis. The most common form of arteriosclerosis is obliterans. Atherosclerotic occlusive disease affects not only the peripheral vascular system but also the coronary arterial circulation. The presence of vascular disease in the extremities may precipitate the development of acute or chronic disability with a diminished quality of life, whereas the coexisting cardiac problems may complicate the prognosis of the patient with PVD.

Cardiac monitoring is an integral part of the postoperative (postanesthesia) care of the patient with PVD. This chapter discusses atherosclerosis in addition to the other common causes of PVD, related surgical interventions, and appropriate nursing management criteria.

    I. Anatomy and physiology
        A. Peripheral vascular anatomy:
            1. Includes
                a. Peripheral arterial
                b. Venous systems
            2. Excludes
                a. Cardiac
                b. Pulmonary
                c. Cerebral systems

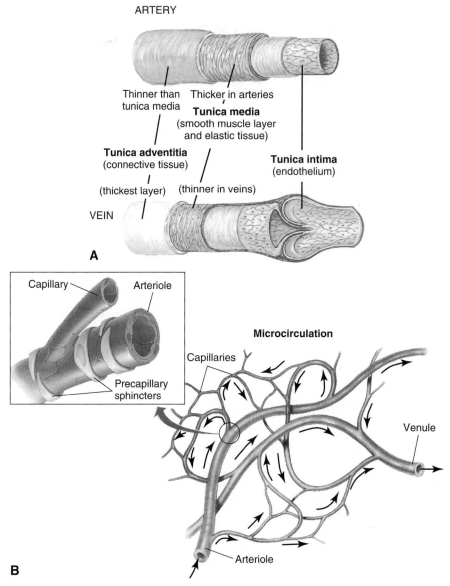

FIGURE 51-1 ■ **A,** Arterial and venous wall structure. **B,** Microcirculation (From Rothrock JC, Smith DA, McEwen DR: *Alexander's care of the patient in surgery,* ed 12. St Louis: Mosby, 2003, p 1083.)

    B. Arterial and venous wall structure contains three layers (Figure 51-1A)
        1. Adventitia: thin outer layer containing
            a. Collagen
            b. Lymphatics
        2. Media: thick middle layer containing smooth muscle cells arranged into strong, intertwining sheets of elastin that constrict or dilate. The medial layer is thinner in veins.
        3. Intima: thin, inner, single endothelial layer; easily traumatized
    C. Circulatory path (Figure 51-1B)
        1. Artery → Arteriole → Precapillary sphincter → Capillary
            a. Artery: high pressure, low volume
            b. Arteriole (diameter <0.5 mm)

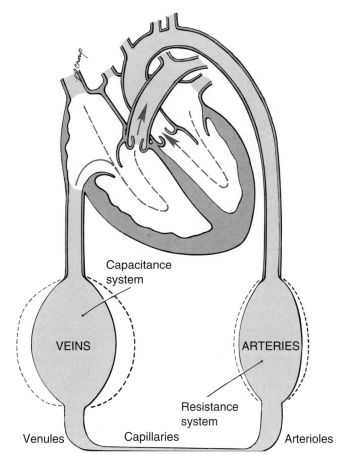

FIGURE 51-2 ■ Systemic circulation. (From Price SA, Wilson LM: *Pathophysiology: Clinical concepts of disease processes,* ed 6. St Louis: Mosby, 2003, p 2082.)

      (1) Offers resistance to blood flow
      (2) Regulates blood flow into capillary bed
   c. Precapillary sphincters
      (1) Rings of smooth muscle located at proximal end of a true capillary
      (2) Regulates flow of blood and oxygen (Figure 51-2)
   d. Capillary: site of gas and nutrient exchange
 2. Capillary → Venule → Vein
   a. Venule: as venules merge, the rate of blood flow increases.
   b. Vein
      (1) Low pressure
      (2) High volume
      (3) Veins are capacitance vessels because they accommodate large volumes of blood.
      (4) Unidirectional valves direct venous flow from feet toward heart and prevent reflux.
      (5) Approximately 70% of blood volume contained in venous circulation (Figure 51-3)
D. Arterial circulation (Figure 51-4)
 1. Aorta: largest peripheral vessel, which includes four sections (Figure 51-5)
   a. Ascending aorta: from aortic valve to arch
   b. Arch: where brachiocephalic and carotid vessels originate

      c. Descending thoracic aorta: from aortic arch to level of diaphragm

      d. Abdominal aorta: from thoracic to aortic bifurcation

  2. Aortic bifurcation: where aorta divides into common right and left iliac arteries

      a. Common iliac divides

        (1) Internal iliac (hypogastric)

        (2) External iliac: continuation of common iliac artery that becomes the common femoral artery in the thigh

      b. Common femoral (thigh) (Figure 51-6)

        (1) Lateral and medial femoral circumflex

        (2) Profunda (deep) femoral

      c. Popliteal: continuation of common femoral located posterior to knee surface divides

        (1) Anterior tibial

          (a) Dorsalis pedis

          (b) Posterior tibial

            (i) Medial and lateral plantar

            (ii) Peroneal

      d. Venous circulation (see Figure 51-7)

        (1) Superficial system: in subcutaneous tissue

          (a) Greater saphenous: longest vein in the body extending from malleolus of the ankle to the femoral vein (saphenous junction)

          (b) Lesser saphenous: extends from the ankle to the popliteal vein in the knee (saphenopopliteal junction)

        (2) Deep veins: in muscular layers

          (a) Anterior and posterior tibial

          (b) Peroneal

          (c) Popliteal

          (d) Femoral, profunda femoris

          (e) Iliac

        (3) Perforating (communicating): vascular channels (Figure 51-8)

          (a) Communicate between deep and superficial veins

          (b) Flow is shunted from superficial to deep system with the help of unidirectional valves and finally to the inferior vena cava.

          (c) Muscle contraction promotes forward flow; valves prevent backflow during muscular relaxation.

II. Factors affecting circulation

  A. Cardiac output (Cardiac output = Stroke volume × Heart rate): Venous capacity will determine venous return that will affect stroke volume of the heart.

  B. Arteriolar resistance: systemic vascular resistance (SVR) depends on

    1. The degree of arteriolar constriction

    2. Resistance

      a. Increases as vessels constrict

      b. Decreases as vessels dilate

    3. High SVR will

      a. Decrease blood flow

      b. Increase myocardial workload

  C. Vessel wall elasticity

    1. With low compliance, the pressure is greater.

    2. Increased pressure will increase myocardial oxygen consumption.

  D. Fluid volume status: low fluid volume will reduce peripheral resistance.

  E. Diameter of vessel (arteriole diameter <0.5 mm)

    1. Vasoconstriction: exposure to cold, vasoconstrictive agents

    2. Vasodilation: exposure to heat, vasodilator agents

  F. Sympathetic nervous system: regulates amount of vasoconstriction.

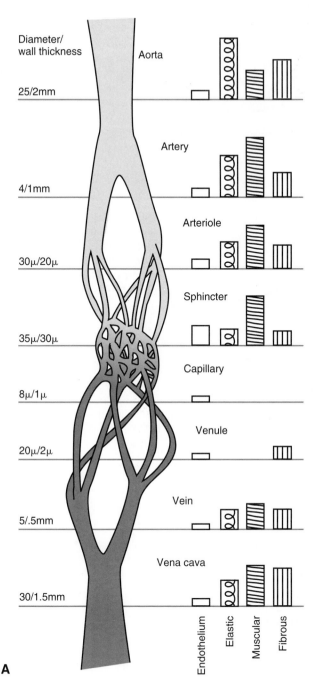

FIGURE 51-3 ■ **A,** Structural characteristics of blood vessels in the systemic circulation, including a comparison of the endothelial, elastic, muscle, and fibrous layers. (From Dolan JT: *Critical care nursing: Clinical management through the nursing process.* Philadelphia: Davis, 1991, p 742.)

A

III. Common sites of vascular disease (Figure 51-9)
  A. Internal carotid arteries
  B. Aorta
  C. Aortoiliac: bifurcation of aorta and iliac arteries
  D. Superficial femoral: middle to distal thigh
  E. Popliteal artery
  F. Tibial arteries: common in patients with diabetes
IV. Pathophysiology of peripheral vascular disease
  A. Arterial occlusive disease
    1. Obstruction or stenosis of vessel
      a. Decreased peripheral vessel blood flow

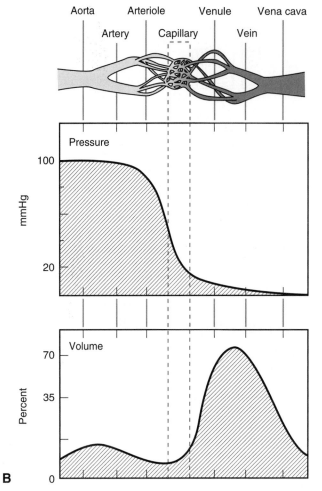

FIGURE 51-3 ▪ **B**, Resistance and capacitance. (From Dolan JT: *Critical care nursing: Clinical management through the nursing process.* Philadelphia: Davis, 1991, p 742.)

      b. Decreased vessel diameter
      c. Increased peripheral vascular resistance
      d. Decreased blood flow velocity
    2. Degenerative changes
      a. Reduced tissue oxygen and nutrient supply
        (i) Inadequate tissue integrity
        (ii) Ischemic tissue
        (iii) Destruction of muscle and elastic fibers
      b. Formation of calcium and/or cholesterol deposits
        (i) Thickening of arterioles
        (ii) Loss of elasticity
  B. Venous disease
    1. Deep vein thrombosis (DVT): disease of the deep veins of the lower extremity, often accompanied by intraluminal clot
    2. Superficial thrombophlebitis: inflammation and clot in the superficial veins
    3. Virchow's triad: three factors that increase incidence of venous thrombosis
      a. Hypercoagulability caused by alteration of platelet and clotting factors
      b. Venous stasis caused by incompetent venous valves
      c. Intimal damage caused by trauma, intravenous infusions, ischemia
    4. Pulmonary embolism: dislodged DVT with migration to pulmonary vasculature

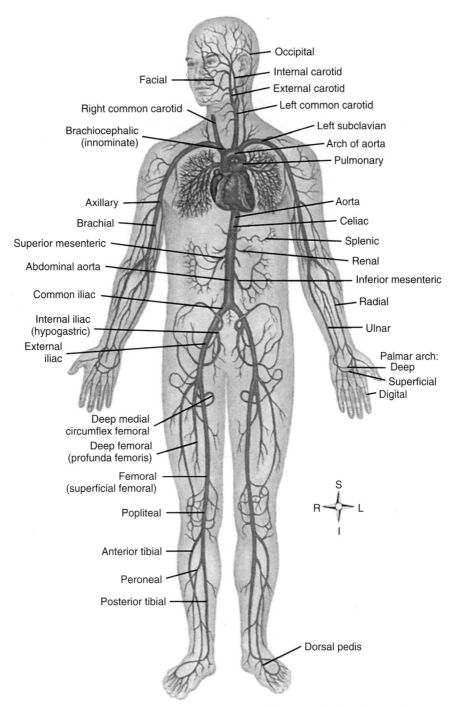

FIGURE 51-4 ■ Principle arteries of the body. (From Rothrock JC, Smith DA, McEwen DR: *Alexander's care of the patient in surgery*, ed 12. St Louis: Mosby, 2003, p 1081.)

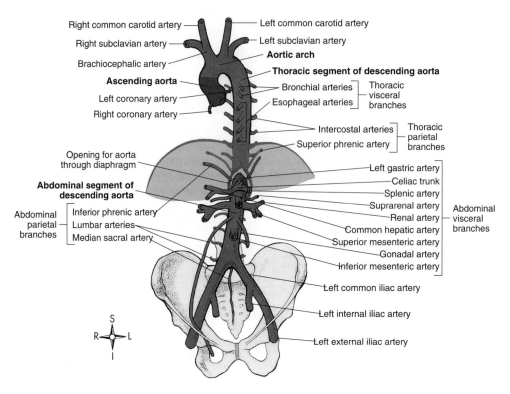

FIGURE 51-5 ■ ■ The aorta. (From Rothrock JC, Smith DA, McEwen DR: *Alexander's care of the patient in surgery*, ed 12. St Louis: Mosby, 2003, p 1084.)

5. Varicose veins
   a. Structural weakness
   b. Vessel tortuosity
   c. Dilation
      (1) Incompetent venous valves
      (2) Reflux of blood results in venous pooling
6. Venous hypertension: hereditary
   a. Incompetent valves results in reduced blood return to the heart.
   b. Venous stasis and pooling of the blood results in venous hypertension.
V. Arterial insufficiency: Arterial occlusive disease
   A. Arteriosclerosis obliterans
      1. Atherosclerosis: most common form of arteriosclerosis obliterans
         a. Accumulation of lipids and connective tissue
         b. Intraluminal plaque formation
         c. Platelet aggregation
         d. Thrombus formation
         e. Loss of elasticity
      2. Möönckeberg's arteriosclerosis: arteriosclerosis of peripheral arteries
         a. Characterized by calcium deposits within medial layer
      3. Arteriolosclerosis: sclerosis of arterioles
   B. Aneurysm: abnormal dilation of vessel wall with high incidence of rupture and mortality when greater than 6 cm in diameter (Figure 51-10) (Figure 51-11)
      1. Fusiform: diffuse circumferential dilation of artery
      2. Saccular: area of pouching; affects localized part of arterial wall
      3. Dissecting: intimal layer torn; blood accumulates between layers

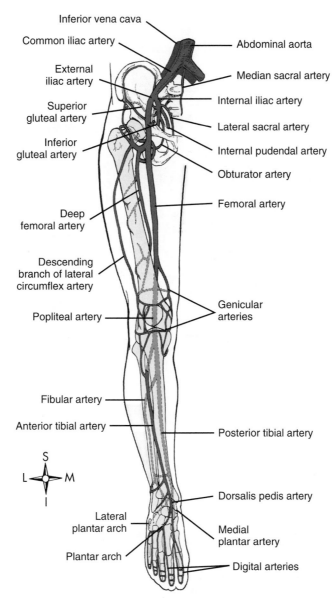

Inferior vena cava

Common iliac artery

Abdominal aorta

External iliac artery

Median sacral artery

Superior gluteal artery

Internal iliac artery

Lateral sacral artery

Inferior gluteal artery

Internal pudendal artery

Obturator artery

Femoral artery

Deep femoral artery

Descending branch of lateral circumflex artery

Genicular arteries

Popliteal artery

Fibular artery

Anterior tibial artery

Posterior tibial artery

S
L ← ⊕ → M
I

Dorsalis pedis artery

Lateral plantar arch

Medial plantar artery

Plantar arch

Digital arteries

FIGURE 51-6 ■ Major arteries of the lower extremity. (From Rothrock JC, Smith DA, McEwen DR: *Alexander's care of the patient in surgery*, ed 12. St Louis: Mosby, 2003, p 1101.)

    4. False aneurysm: when palpable hematoma often present, a complete tear of all three layers of arterial wall occurs caused by
      a. Trauma
      b. Needle puncture
      c. Suture failure at anastomosis site of prosthetic graft
    5. Pseudoaneurysm: dilated or tortuous segment of arterial wall without interruption of layers
  VI. Vascular diseases and conditions
    A. Acute
      1. Arterial embolism: sudden onset of symptoms of acute arterial insufficiency
        a. Originates in myocardium or arterial aneurysm

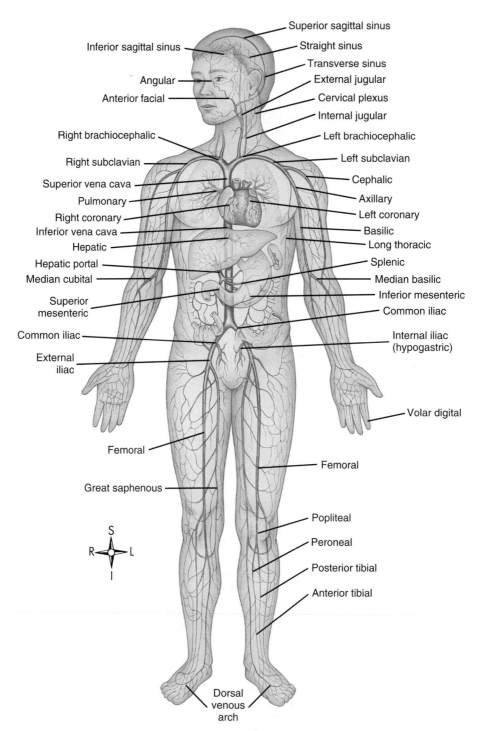

FIGURE 51-7 ■ Principle veins of the body. (From Rothrock JC, Smith DA, McEwen DR: *Alexander's care of the patient in surgery*, ed 12. St Louis: Mosby, 2003, p 1082.)

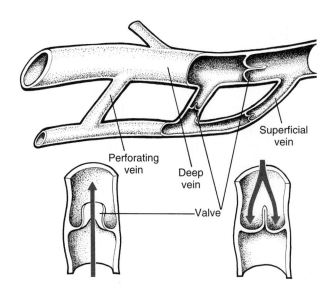

FIGURE 51-8 ■ Perforating (communicating): vascular channels. (From Price SA, Wilson LM: *Pathophysiology: Clinical concepts of disease processes,* ed 6. St Louis: Mosby, 2003, p 527.)

Superficial vein

Perforating vein

Deep vein

Valve

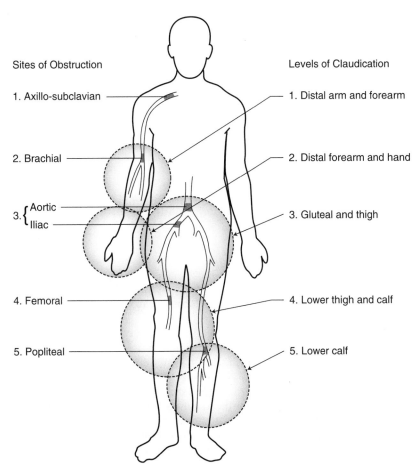

Sites of Obstruction

1. Axillo-subclavian

2. Brachial

3. { Aortic
      Iliac

4. Femoral

5. Popliteal

Levels of Claudication

1. Distal arm and forearm

2. Distal forearm and hand

3. Gluteal and thigh

4. Lower thigh and calf

5. Lower calf

FIGURE 51-9 ■ Sites of arterial obstruction and corresponding levels of claudication. (From Fahey VA: *Vascular nursing,* ed 3. Philadelphia: WB Saunders, 1999, p 61.)

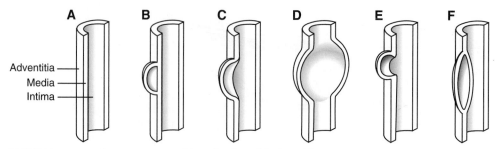

FIGURE 51-10 ■ Aneurysm types. (From Smeltzer SC, Bare BG: *Brunner and Suddarth's textbook of medical-surgical nursing,* ed 8. Philadelphia: Lippincott, 1996, p 739.)

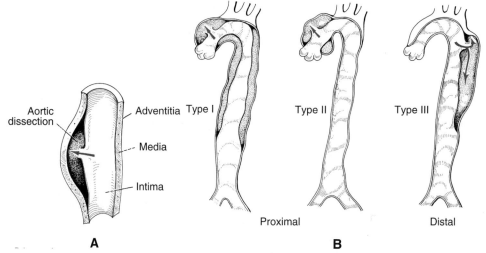

FIGURE 51-11 ■ Aortic dissection. (From Price SA, Wilson LM: *Pathophysiology: Clinical concepts of disease processes,* ed 6. St Louis: Mosby, 2003, p 526.)

    b. May be secondary to external or iatrogenic trauma (catheter placement)

  2. Trauma: arterial wall tear or dissection

B. Chronic

  1. Diabetes mellitus: medial layer calcification; arteries become noncompressible

  2. Hypertension: increases permeability of intimal endothelium

  3. Polycythemia: increased blood viscosity caused by increase in red blood cell count

  4. Inflammatory processes: may cause occlusive lesions

    a. Arteritis: inflammation of arterial wall

      (1) Polyarteritis nodosa (PAN): systemic disease causing arterial inflammation and aneurysm rupture in adults

      (2) Kawasaki: similar to PAN, occurs in children

      (3) Cogan's: (rare condition) similar to PAN, inflammatory infiltration of large veins and muscular arteries

      (4) Behcet's: similar to PAN; affects both arteries and veins

      (5) Drug abusers: similar to PAN, necrotizing arteritis (intraarterial injection of drugs)

    b. Fibromuscular dysplasia (FMD): multiple areas of arterial stenosis and dilation

        c. Buerger's disease: thromboangiitis obliterans
          (1) Inflammation of arterial walls
          (2) Thrombus formation caused by intimal thickening
          (3) Affects plantar and digital vessels
          (4) Extremity cold, cyanotic, and painful
     5. Raynaud's phenomenon: vasospastic disease
        a. Intense vasospasm of arteries and arterioles
        b. Precipitated by exposure to cold
        c. Ischemic changes: cyanosis, numbness, tingling
        d. Occurs in 40% of patients with systemic lupus erythematosus (SLE)

VII. Clinical signs and symptoms
    A. Arterial insufficiency
      1. Decreased blood flow may cause inadequate tissue oxygenation distal to lesion.
      2. A 70% to 90% occlusion of a large artery usually must occur before a decrease in blood flow or pressure causes symptoms at rest.
      3. A 60% obstruction may be sufficient to precipitate signs and symptoms during exercise.
      4. Acute
        a. Peripheral pulses diminished, weak, or absent
        b. Cold and pale extremity (sudden onset)
          (1) Pallor when elevated
          (2) Rubor when dependent
        c. Sudden severe pain may occur during exercise or at rest.
        d. Limited sensory and motor function
          (1) Possible paresthesia
          (2) Atrophied skeletal muscle: restricted limb movement
        e. Minimal edema: usually unilateral
        f. Bruit present with partial occlusion; no bruit with total occlusion
      5. Chronic
        a. Diminished or weak distal pulses
        b. Pain at rest related to severe ischemia
        c. Tissue necrosis: gangrene
        d. Intermittent claudication
        e. Skin
          (1) Skin ulceration
          (2) Delayed healing of skin lesions
          (3) Skin texture: thin, shiny, dry
          (4) Cool skin: poikilothermic
        f. Color: pale extremity
          (1) Increased pallor when elevated
          (2) Rubor or cyanosis or both when dependent
        g. Possible paresthesia of limb
        h. Edema: none or mild
          (1) Hair loss distal to occlusion
        j. Nails: thick, brittle
        k. Impotence: associated with aortoiliac disease
    B. Venous insufficiency
      1. Acute
        a. Moderate pain localized to area of inflammation
        b. Pulses present or diminished (absent in presence of concomitant disease)
        c. Skin warm, cyanotic, mottled, or pale
        d. Engorged veins when legs slightly dependent
        e. Moderate to severe peripheral edema
      2. Chronic
        a. Minimal to moderate pain
        b. Moderate to severe edema, unilateral or bilateral

        c. Sensation of heaviness at site of occlusion

        d. Muscle cramps, aching

        e. Ulceration of ankle area

        f. Superficial veins may be prominent.

        g. Skin

           (1) Warm

           (2) Brawny (reddish brown) color

           (3) Pronounced lower leg pigmentation

           (4) Texture: thickening, scaling, and/or scarring

VIII. Incidence and risk factors associated with peripheral vascular disease

    A. Highest incidence among elderly, male, diabetic, smokers

    B. Gender

      1. More common in males

      2. Earlier onset in males

      3. Postmenopausal women susceptible

    C. Age

      1. Occurs beyond 30 years of age

      2. Symptoms worsen after 65 years of age

IX. Risk factors of atherosclerosis

    A. Lifestyle habits

      1. Psychophysiologic stress triggers vasoconstriction.

      2. Sedentary; lack of exercise

      3. Smoking (major risk factor) for smokers and passive smoking (environmental tobacco smoke exposure)

        a. Vasoconstrictive effect of nicotine

        b. Inhalation of carbon monoxide in cigarette smoke

           (1) Increases carboxyhemoglobin levels (carbon monoxide binds with hemoglobin)

           (2) Impaired oxygen transport

           (3) Hypoxic injury to intimal lining of artery

           (4) Increased platelet aggregation caused by enhanced platelet adhesiveness

      4. Diet

        a. Hyperlipidemia (hyperlipoproteinemia): accumulation of lipids in arterial wall

           (1) Elevated cholesterol: total serum levels

           (2) Elevated triglycerides

              (a) Low-density lipoproteins (LDL): high serum levels related to premature development of atherosclerotic process

              (b) High-density lipoproteins (HDL): high serum levels demonstrate protective effect against atherosclerosis.

        b. Obesity

    B. Positive family history

    C. Disease processes

      1. Diabetes mellitus

      2. Hypertension (major risk factor)

X. Indications for surgical intervention

    A. Ischemic pain at rest

    B. Significant limb ischemia

    C. Limiting claudication

XI. Diagnostic assessment

    A. Arterial tests

    B. Noninvasive laboratory studies

      1. Segmental pressure measurement: measurement of systolic blood pressure along selected segments of each extremity

        a. A gradient >20 mm Hg is evidence of arterial stenosis in the lower extremity.

      b. A gradient >10 mm Hg is evidence of arterial stenosis in the upper extremity.
  2. Ankle/brachial index (ABI): ratio of ankle to brachial pressure. (normal ABI is 1.0 or greater)
      a. One limitation is calcified vessels as in renal failure or diabetes.
  3. Toe pressure measurements: assess distal arterial flow
      a. Useful in diabetics with calcification of larger vessels
  4. Pulse volume recording (PVR): quantifies arterial flow to determine the location of the lesion and the severity
  5. Doppler ultrasound: determines blood flow and velocity
  6. B-mode ultrasonography: projects a two-dimensional image in real time
  7. Duplex ultrasound imaging: assesses both anatomic characteristics and stenosis of peripheral arteries; combination of Doppler and B-mode ultrasonogram
  8. Air plethysmography (APG) and photoplethysmography (PPG) records volume changes in the limb.
  9. Treadmill exercise testing: objective evidence of walking capacity and evaluate peripheral stenosis
  10. Computed tomography (CT): A tomograph is an image of a cross-sectional slice of a body part
      a. CT image is three dimensional: a camera rotates around the selected body part taking two-dimensional images at multiple angles, which are converted to a composite three-dimensional image by a computer.
      b. Contrast material (usually iodine) is injected to heighten the contrast between the vessel wall and the blood.
      c. Used for diagnosis of aortic aneurysms and aortic dissection
      d. Able to detect hematomas or thrombi better with CT than with arteriography
  11. Magnetic resonance imaging (MRI): detailed and three-dimensional imaging of vessel lumen where contrast is not needed; contraindicated in patients with pacemakers and cerebral aneurysm clips
  12. Magnetic resonance angiography (MRA): technology is developing; has replaced angiography for severe carotid stenosis; uses intravenous gadolinium; no arterial puncture required
C. Invasive laboratory studies
  1. Arteriography: Invasive radiographic procedure in which radiopaque contrast is injected into artery
  2. Transcatheter therapy: percutaneous transluminal angioplasty (PTA), stenting, lyse clot, therapeutic embolization
      a. Purposes
         (1) Depict location of stenosis, occlusion, or view aneurysm
         (2) Visualize collateral, proximal, and distal arterial circulation to determine surgical treatment options
      b. Complications
         (1) Intimal disruption
            (a) Hematoma formation at puncture site
            (b) Plaque dislodgment
            (c) Arterial occlusion: thrombosis
            (d) Distal embolization
            (e) Arteriovenous fistula
            (f) Arterial dissection
            (g) Renal failure
         (2) Transient ischemic attack (TIA) or cerebrovascular accident (CVA)
         (3) Toxic reaction to contrast media: renal or cardiac
         (4) Allergic reaction
            (a) Skin rash
            (b) Bronchospasm

            (c) Altered consciousness

            (d) Convulsions

            (e) Anaphylaxis

            (f) Cardiac arrest

     c. Postarteriography assessment and intervention

        (1) Assessment

            (a) Vital signs

            (b) Hematoma and/or bleeding at puncture site

            (c) Signs and symptoms of acute arterial insufficiency

               (i) Skin: color, temperature

               (ii) Pulses distal to puncture site

               (iii) Pain

               (iv) Urinary output

               (v) Neurologic status

               (vi) Signs of heart failure or respiratory distress

        (2) Intervention

            (a) Observe for skin rash.

            (b) Maintain adequate hydration to flush contrast.

            (c) Head of bed at 30° or less

            (d) Keep affected extremity straight for 4 to 6 hours after the procedure.

            (e) Wait a minimum of 4 hours to resume heparin if previously on heparin.

XII. Venous tests

  A. Noninvasive laboratory studies

     1. Venous Doppler ultrasonography examinations: used to determine blood flow patterns and velocity

       a. During inspiration, intrathoracic pressure decreases and venous return to the heart increases.

       b. During expiration, venous flow to the lower extremities will increase.

     2. Air plethysmography (APG)

       a. Used to evaluate venous obstruction, reflux, and calf muscle pump function

       b. Able to differentiate deep and superficial venous insufficiency

     3. Duplex imaging of valvular closing times indicate severity of venous reflux.

     4. Arm/foot pressure gradient measures outflow obstruction: normal difference between arm and foot is <4 mm Hg.

  B. Invasive testing

     1. Ascending phlebography: used to assess venous patency

     2. Descending phlebography: used to assess valvular function

XIII. Operative procedures

  A. Endarterectomy

     1. Opening of occluded portion of artery

     2. Removal of atheromatous material or plaque

     3. Excision of artery's intimal lining

     4. Performed on carotid, subclavian, iliac, or femoral artery

  B. Carotid-subclavian bypass

     1. Anastomosis of carotid and subclavian arteries to improve circulation

     2. Common carotid used as donor for subclavian lesions

     3. Subclavian used to restore circulation for carotid lesions

  C. Aortocarotid-subclavian bypass

     1. Insertion of bypass graft from ascending aorta into carotid or subclavian artery

     2. For occlusive lesions of both common carotid or innominate and subclavian arteries

D. Carotid artery ligation
   1. Surgical occlusion of carotid artery
   2. Temporary control of hemorrhaging during intracranial vessel surgery
   3. Permanent control of intracranial or nasal hemorrhaging
   4. Treatment of carotid-cavernous fistula
E. Aorto-innominate-subclavian bypass: Thoracic aortic graft into innominate, subclavian arteries
F. Aneurysmectomy
   1. Excision of weakened dilated area of artery
   2. Insertion of synthetic prosthesis to reestablish circulatory continuity
   3. Usually occurring in abdominal aorta, thoracic aorta, or carotid, popliteal, or femoral artery
G. Thoracoabdominal aortic aneurysm repair
   1. Clots are removed before anastomosis of Dacron graft.
   2. A spinal catheter is placed at L1 to L2 to allow for cerebrospinal fluid (CSF) drainage.
   3. Spinal cord ischemia is evaluated by monitoring CSF pressure.
H. Bypass approaches for aortoiliac occlusions (Figure 51-12)
   1. Aortoiliac bypass: insertion of vascular graft from distal aorta into iliac artery or arteries
   2. Aortofemoral bypass
   3. Anastomosis of distal aorta to femoral arteries
   4. Lesion bypassed with vascular graft
I. Axillofemoral bypass (Figure 51-13)
   1. Superficial flank placement
   2. Anastomosis of prosthetic graft from one axillary artery to one or both femoral arteries
   3. Restores blood flow beyond occlusive lesion
J. Femorofemoral bypass: femoral crossover graft (Figure 51-14)
   1. Extraanatomic bypass procedure with subcutaneous placement across suprapubic area
   2. End-to-side anastomosis from patent femoral to stenotic femoral artery
   3. Diverts blood flow from one donor femoral artery to recipient stenotic artery
K. Aortorenal bypass: Anastomosis of abdominal aorta to renal artery with vascular graft
L. Femoropopliteal bypass
   1. Establishes adequate circulation to leg and foot through popliteal artery and branches
   2. Graft used for superficial femoral artery occlusion
M. Femorotibial bypass
   1. Autogenous saphenous vein graft from common femoral artery to proximal anterior tibial artery
   2. Procedure indicated for superficial femoral and popliteal artery occlusion
N. Angioplasty: Percutaneous insertion of balloon-tipped catheter to dilate areas of localized vessel stenosis
O. Vena cava ligation
   1. Partial or total surgical occlusion of vena cava to prevent emboli from entering pulmonary vasculature
   2. Common ligation sites
      a. Superficial femoral
      b. Inferior vena cava below renal veins
P. Vena caval umbrella filter
   1. Insertion of intravascular device through jugular or femoral vein to occlude inferior vena cava
   2. Prevents emboli from entering pulmonary vessels
Q. Vein ligation and stripping: Surgical ligation and removal of varicose vein(s) of leg(s)

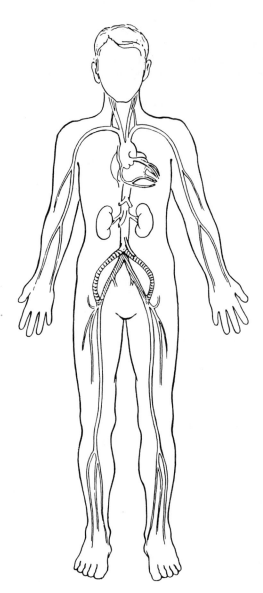

FIGURE 51-12 ■ Aortoiliac occlusion and revascularization. **A,** Aortobifemoral prosthetic bypass graft. **B,** Unilateral aortofemoral prosthetic bypass graft. (From Kinney MR, Dunbar SB, Brooks-Brunn JA, et al: *AACN's clinical reference for critical care nursing,* ed 4. St Louis: Mosby, 1998, p 422.)

R. Sympathectomy
  1. Interruption of some portion of sympathetic nervous system pathway
  2. Causes vasodilation, improvement in circulation to extremity
  3. Treatment for partial arterial obstruction with resultant distal trophic changes
S. Interventional radiology
  1. Catheter-directed thrombolysis
  2. Urokinase has been unavailable in the United States since 1999. Food and Drug Administration (FDA) pulled off the market because screening for viral vectors was inadequate.
  3. Streptokinase has a high rate of allergic reactions.
  4. Recombinant tissue plasminogen activator (rtPA)
  5. Alteplase weak plasminogen
  6. Reteplase plasminogen activator penetrates and destroys fiber in matrix.
T. Percutaneous mechanical thrombectomy used in combination with thrombolytics

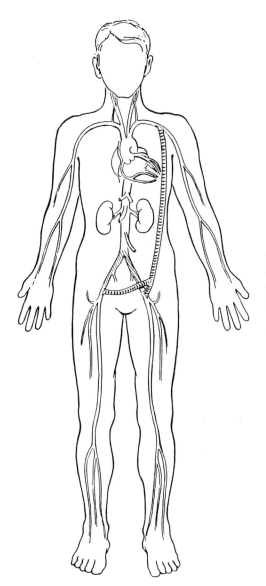

FIGURE 51-13 ■ Aortoiliac occlusion and revascularization. Left axillofemorofemoral prosthetic bypass graft. (From Kinney MR, Dunbar SB, Brooks-Brunn JA, et al: *AACN's clinical reference for critical care nursing,* ed 4. St Louis: Mosby, 1998, p 423.)

XIV. General systems assessment of vascular patients
  A. Cardiovascular:
    1. Myocardial infarction remains leading cause of death after peripheral vascular procedures because of coexisting cardiovascular disease.
  B. Evaluation of cardiac status
    1. Hemodynamic profile: cardiac output (CO), SVR
    2. Electrocardiogram (ECG); dysrhythmias
      a. Increased myocardial oxygen demands
      b. Increased cardiac ischemia: angina
    3. Signs and symptoms of myocardial infarction
      a. Chest pain
      b. Dysrhythmias
      c. Diaphoresis
      d. Nausea and vomiting
      e. Dyspnea
      f. Hypotension
    4. Chest x-ray film to assess heart size and fluid status

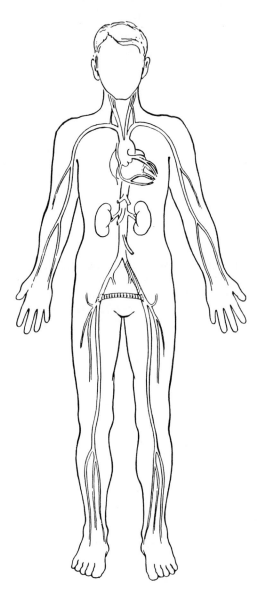

FIGURE 51-14 ■ Left iliac occlusion and revascularization. Right-to-left femorofemoral prosthetic bypass graft. (From Kinney MR, Dunbar SB, Brooks-Brunn JA, et al: *AACN's clinical reference for critical care nursing,* ed 4. St Louis: Mosby, 1998, p 423.)

C. Cardiac enzymes
   1. Creatine kinase (CK)
   2. CK-MB isoenzyme
   3. Troponin T (cTnT) and troponin I (cTnI)
   4. Myoglobin never used alone but in conjunction with cardiac specific markers
D. Serum electrolytes
   1. Hyperkalemia
      a. Oliguric renal failure
      b. Volume depletion
      c. Decreased effect of aldosterone: Addison's disease, chronic heparin administration
   2. Hypokalemia
      a. Diuretic or digitalis therapy
      b. Stress
      c. Gastrointestinal disorders

(1) Long-term steroid therapy: arthritis, chronic obstructive pulmonary disease (COPD)

(2) Hypoaldosteronism

3. Hypernatremia
   a. Mechanical ventilation without humidification
   b. Fever

4. Hyponatremia
   a. Diuretics
   b. Gastrointestinal disorders
   c. Hypotonic irrigating solutions
   d. Hyperlipidemia
   e. Hyperglycemia

5. Hypermagnesemia
   a. Renal failure
   b. Adrenal insufficiency
   c. Shock
   d. Hypothermia

6. Hypomagnesemia
   a. Excessive loss of body fluids
   b. Diuretics
   c. Cardiac glycosides, aminoglycosides
   d. Decreased intestinal absorption
   e. Primary hyperaldosteronism
   f. Hypercalcemia associated with hyperparathyroidism and hyperthyroidism
   g. ECG reflects prolonged QT interval, decreased T-wave amplitude, shortened ST segment.

XV. Accompanying cardiovascular disorders
   A. Hypertension
      1. High incidence (40% to 60%) associated with PVD
      2. Adds stress to anastomotic sites
      3. Precipitates postoperative incisional bleeding
   B. Hypotension
      1. Decreases cerebral, coronary, and renal artery perfusion
      2. Decreases stroke volume: decreased cardiac output
   C. Valvular disease: associated with decreased cardiac output and left ventricular failure
      1. Mitral valve stenosis: associated with pulmonary fibrosis and hypertension
      2. Aortic insufficiency: associated with circulatory collapse with sudden hypotension

XVI. Pulmonary status
   A. Baseline parameters
      1. Respirations
         a. Rate, quality
         b. Pattern, excursion
      2. Auscultation of lungs
         a. Wheezes
         b. Rales
         c. Rhonchi
         d. Crackles
      3. Arterial blood gases (ABGs), SvO_2 monitoring
      4. Pulmonary function studies
         a. Forced vital capacity (FVC)
            (1) Measurement of volume of air expelled by fully inflated lung
            (2) Compromised FVC indicative of lung parenchymal restriction
         b. Forced expiratory volume (FEV)
            (1) Decreased FEV indicative of impaired elastic recoil (emphysema)

(2) Increased FEV indicative of airway resistance (chronic bronchitis or asthma)

    c. Ventilation to perfusion ratio

  5. Chest x-ray film

    a. Pulmonary infiltrate or lesion

    b. Heart size

    c. Congestive heart failure (CHF)

    d. Fibrosis or effusion

B. Pulmonary history

  1. Obstructive disorders (COPD, emphysema, asthma)

  2. Infections (bronchitis, tuberculosis)

  3. Presence of cough (lesions, smoking, bronchitis)

  4. Complaints of shortness of breath

  5. Orthopnea

XVII. Neurologic status

A. Postoperative assessment: compare with preoperative baseline.

  1. Level of consciousness

  2. Pupillary reactions

  3. Sensory and motor ability

  4. Evaluation of following cranial nerves

    a. Facial (VIII): controls facial muscles; affects ability to smile, show teeth, wrinkle forehead, raise eyebrows

    b. Hypoglossal (XII): most frequently traumatized; controls tongue; affects side-to-side motion of tongue

    c. Glossopharyngeal (IX): controls posterior third of tongue, uvula; affects gag reflex

    d. Vagus (X): controls pharynx, larynx, soft palate; affects gag reflex

    e. Spinal accessory (XI): controls trapezius and sternocleidomastoid muscles; affects strength and tone of shoulder muscles

    f. Phrenic nerve: controls diaphragm; affects diaphragmatic function in respiratory excursion

B. Neurologic history

  1. Vertigo

  2. Syncope

  3. Transient ischemic attacks (TIA)

  4. CVA

  5. Spinal cord ischemia with descending thoracic aorta repair

XVIII. Renal status

A. Preoperative baseline studies

  1. Blood urea nitrogen (BUN)

  2. Creatinine

  3. Electrolytes

  4. Calcium

  5. Phosphorus

  6. Urinalysis

B. Specific renal function studies, if indicated

  1. Osmolar, free water, and sodium clearances

  2. Creatinine or insulin clearance to evaluate glomerular filtration

  3. Para-aminohippurate clearance to evaluate renal blood flow

  4. Postangiographic renal function to evaluate possibility of renal failure caused by radioactive dye

C. Compromised renal system during vascular surgery caused by

  1. Hemorrhage

  2. Trauma

  3. Renal vessel damage, tubular damage

  4. Anoxia

  5. Prolonged hypotension

XIX. Diabetes
- **A.** Relationship to PVD
  1. High incidence of occurrence in patients with PVD
  2. Higher incidence of postoperative complications
  3. Altered fluid requirements
- **B.** Management of diabetes in a surgical patient (insulin regimen dependent on institutional policy)
  1. Preoperative dose: usually less than routine daily dose
  2. Stress of surgery with release of epinephrine and glucocorticoids increases need for insulin.
  3. Diet-controlled diabetics may require insulin in immediate postoperative period.
- **C.** Laboratory assessment
  1. Fasting glucose levels
  2. Electrolyte series
  3. Serum ketones and acetones
  4. Renal function studies
  5. ABGs

XX. Hematologic evaluation
- **A.** Laboratory studies
  1. Prothrombin time, partial thromboplastin time
  2. D-dimer assay
  3. Platelet count
  4. Bleeding time, clotting time
  5. Type and crossmatch
  6. Complete blood count
- **B.** Anticoagulant medications
  1. Heparin (sodium warfarin, Coumadin)
  2. Aspirin
  3. Dipyridamole (Persantine)
  4. Ticlopidine (Ticlid)
- **C.** Previous postoperative bleeding and clotting problems
  1. Disseminated intravascular coagulopathy (DIC)
  2. Blood transfusion reactions
  3. Thrombophlebitis
  4. Pulmonary emboli
  5. History of any postoperative bleeding

XXI. Intraoperative concerns
- **A.** Carotid and other neck vessel procedures
  1. Anesthesia choices
     - **a.** Local anesthesia
       - (1) Advantages
         - (a) Quick evaluation of level of consciousness and neurologic changes
         - (b) Minimizes risk of cerebral ischemia
       - (2) Disadvantages
         - (a) Difficult to manage systemic complications (convulsions, dysrhythmias, hypotension, hypertension)
         - (b) Positional discomfort
     - **b.** General anesthesia
       - (1) Advantages
         - (a) Facilitates control of
           - (i) Hypertension
           - (ii) Hypoxia
           - (iii) Dysrhythmias
           - (iv) Blood loss
         - (b) Temperature control
       - (2) Disadvantages

          (a) Inability to assess immediate neurologic status
          (b) May require postoperative ventilatory support
          (c) Anesthetic side effects

       c. Extubation as soon as possible allows for accurate neurologic evaluation.

       d. Maintenance of adequate cerebral blood flow: avoidance of hypotension

       e. Intraoperative complications of carotid surgery
          (1) Hemorrhage
          (2) Acute CVA: higher incidence when stenosis of opposite carotid and vertebral artery prevents adequate cerebral perfusion
          (3) Facial and hypoglossal nerve damage (refer to neurologic assessment section)

XXII. Intrathoracic vascular procedures
  A. Lung deflation during procedure
    1. To protect lung from injury
    2. For adequate exposure to operative site
  B. Use of extracorporeal circulation, depending on location of lesion
  C. Use of hypothermia and/or temporary shunts to minimize organ ischemia
  D. Intraoperative complications
    1. CVA
    2. Pneumothorax, hemothorax
    3. Myocardial injury
    4. Severe hypotension
    5. Renal failure
    6. Spinal cord ischemia

XXIII. Abdominal vessel procedures
  A. Bowel preparation
    1. Decreases incidence of ischemic bowel injury
    2. Minimizes postoperative ileus
  B. Anesthesia choices
    1. Spinal and epidural for elective lower abdominal procedures
      a. Advantages
        (1) Elimination of vasospasm
        (2) Reduction of respiratory complications
      b. Disadvantages
        (1) Positional discomfort if procedure prolonged
        (2) Anxiety increases tachycardia, dysrhythmias.
        (3) Prolonged decreased sensory and motor function
      c. General anesthesia (as previously outlined)
  C. Aortic crossclamping
    1. Extreme hypertension can occur as aorta is clamped.
    2. Hypotension occurs after clamping released because of
      a. Vasodilation of lower extremities
      b. Third space fluid shifting
      c. Metabolic acidosis: products of catabolism and ischemia released systemically
  D. Renal status changes
    1. Approximately 20% of postoperative abdominal vessel patients have acute renal failure develop.
    2. Transient oliguria if hypovolemia occurs
      a. Fluid challenge
      b. Mannitol: osmotic diuretic
      c. Furosemide (Lasix): loop diuretic
    3. Hematuria
      a. Possible reaction to transfusion
      b. Ureteral damage
      c. Dislodged microemboli in renal arteries (renal failure)

    E. Decreased core temperature related to
        1. Massive fluid replacement
        2. Length of procedure
        3. Extensive viscera exposure
        4. Cold irrigation fluid
        5. Rapid heat loss in elderly patients
        6. General anesthesia
    F. Intraoperative complications
        1. Hemorrhage: abdominal aorta, iliac vessels, inferior vena cava
        2. Injury to ureters
        3. Injury to duodenum, renal arteries and veins, kidney, or spleen
        4. Hemiplegia
        5. Ischemic bowel
    G. Anticoagulation and reversal
        1. Heparin administered during vessel clamping and anastomosis
        2. Protamine sulfate administered to reverse effects of heparinization before completion of procedure
XXIV. Sympathectomy: A palliative surgical option for patients with peripheral vascular disease
    A. Peripheral blood vessels: under continuous control of sympathetic nervous system
        1. With normal vasculature, sympathetic system regulates amount of vasoconstriction.
           a. To keep extremities warm, dry, and comfortable
           b. To supply adequate amount of blood to periphery
        2. With compromised peripheral circulation
           a. Surgical division of sympathetic chain (variable response in patients with PVD)
              (1) Permits permanent, maximal vasodilation
              (2) Allows for maximal blood supply to affected extremity
              (3) Not primary treatment for vascular obstructive disease
           b. Benefits of sympathectomy
              (1) Increases warmth and comfort of extremity
              (2) Infection subsides; ulcers heal.
              (3) Small areas of gangrene or fibrosis improve.
              (4) Ischemic pain less severe
    B. Surgical approaches
        1. Lumbar sympathectomy: resection of ganglions L2, L3, L4
           a. Indications for surgery
              (1) Vasospastic disease
              (2) Ischemic ulcers with pain at rest
              (3) Certain forms of causalgia (severe sensation of burning skin)
           b. Specific surgical risks
              (1) Hemorrhage caused by lumbar arterial or venous damage
              (2) Impotence related to genitofemoral nerve damage
              (3) Ureteral damage: inadvertent ligation or clipping during excision of lumbar sympathetic chain
           c. Nursing considerations
              (1) Supine, lateral recumbent position
              (2) Increased sensitivity to position change; turning, elevating of head must be performed slowly
              (3) Flank dressing should remain dry.
              (4) Presence of urine on dressing: ureteral damage
              (5) Presence of blood on dressing: lumbar vessel damage
              (6) Nasogastric decompression to prevent paralytic ileus
              (7) Pain: usually moderate, relieved by analgesics; severe flank pain indicative of ureteral ligation, hydronephrosis; requires surgical reexploration

        (8) Urine output: bladder distension and acute retention associated with operative discomfort

    d. Neurovascular assessment: both lower extremities

        (1) Increase in warmth and vasodilation: desired result

        (2) Neuralgia may occur from damaged nerve.

  2. Cervical sympathectomy: resection of thoracic ganglia T2 to T6 and half of stellate ganglia C8 to T1

    a. Effectively denervates upper extremity of all extrinsic vasoconstrictor influences arising in sympathetic nervous system, permitting return of normal vasodilation

    b. Surgical approach: usually supraclavicular; may use thoracic, transaxillary, or transpleural approach

    c. Specific surgical risks

        (1) Hemothorax or pneumothorax

        (2) Phrenic nerve dysfunction: ipsilateral paralysis of diaphragm

        (3) Chylous leak caused by ligation of divided thoracic duct

    d. Nursing considerations: cervical sympathectomy

        (1) Elevation of head enhances respiratory exchange.

        (2) Position on side opposite chest tube; permits optimal lung inflation

        (3) Chest tube drainage should be less than 200 ml in first 8 hours.

        (4) Vital signs: changes may indicate intrathoracic or intercostals bleeding.

    e. Cardiopulmonary assessment: includes care of mechanically ventilated patients and monitoring of cardiac parameters

    f. Neurovascular assessment

        (1) Palpable radial pulse: confirm with Doppler apparatus if necessary.

        (2) Circulation to affected extremity: warm, dry, pink

        (3) Observe for Horner's syndrome: common after cervical sympathectomy

            (a) Ptosis of upper eyelid

            (b) Slight elevation of lower lid

            (c) Constriction of affected pupil

            (d) Increased salivation and drooping of mouth on affected side

    g. Pain management: per nursing diagnosis and intervention appropriate to unit policy

    h. Complications

        (1) Persistent pneumothorax: damage to underlying lung during thoracotomy

        (2) Intrathoracic bleeding: undetected intercostal vessel interruption

        (3) Radial nerve and artery damage

        (4) Pleural effusion

    i. Postanesthesia concerns: Examples of related nursing diagnostic categories include

        (1) Ineffective airway clearance

        (2) Pain

        (3) Ineffective breathing pattern

        (4) Altered peripheral tissue perfusion

        (5) Decreased cardiac output

        (6) Hypothermia

        (7) Paralysis

XXV. General PACU care of vascular patient

  A. Postoperative report includes

    1. Preoperative preparation

      a. Sedation: control of anxiety

      b. Anticholinergics for reduction of secretions

      c. Antibiotics

      d. Insulin: adjusted dose (according to regimen of institution)

      e. Heparin infusion rate

  2. Preoperative medications: often continued until time of surgery

      a. Nitroglycerin

        (1) Increases coronary perfusion

        (2) Decreases peripheral resistance

      b. Antihypertensives

        (1) Beta-blocker

        (2) Calcium channel blocker

        (3) Angiotensin-converting enzyme (ACE) inhibitors

      c. Antidysrhythmics

  3. Background information

      a. Patient identification

      b. Baseline vital signs

      c. Procedure performed

      d. Anesthesia administered

      e. Drugs received

      f. Length of procedure

      g. Estimated blood loss

  4. Intraoperative vital signs and monitoring data

  5. Intraoperative problems encountered

  6. Anticipated problems

B. Postoperative monitoring data: observe for compensatory mechanisms.

  1. ECG: rhythm, ST segment changes

  2. Arterial line and/or noninvasive blood pressure

  3. Central venous pressure (CVP)

  4. Pulmonary artery pressures (Swan-Ganz catheter)

  5. Core temperature

  6. Ventilation and oxygen support

      a. Mechanical ventilation; parameters:

        (1) Fio_2

        (2) Mode-continuous mechanical ventilation (CMV)

        (3) Synchronous intermittent mechanical ventilation (SIMV)

        (4) Continuous positive airway pressure (CPAP)

        (5) Tidal volume (TV)

        (6) Rate

        (7) Positive end-expiratory pressure (PEEP)

        (8) Pressure support

      b. Spontaneous ventilation: face mask

      c. Oxygen saturation (pulse oximetry)

      d. End-tidal CO_2

      e. Svo_2

C. Vascular assessment

  1. Skin

      a. Temperature: warm, cool, or cold

      b. Skin color: pink, ruddy, dusky, pale, or mottled

  2. Capillary refill

      a. Normal color return after nail bed blanching

      b. Color return should occur within 2 seconds.

  3. Peripheral pulses

      a. Head and neck arteries

      b. Carotid

      c. Temporal

      d. Upper extremity arterial pulses

        (1) Radial

    (2) Brachial
    (3) Axillary
   e. Lower extremity arterial pulses
    (1) Femoral artery
    (2) Popliteal artery
    (3) Posterior tibial artery
    (4) Dorsalis pedis artery
  4. Quality of pulse
   a. Reflection of cardiac output and peripheral vascular patency
   b. Use of objective pulse quality scale for charting purposes
    (1) 0: Absent pulse
    (2) 1+: Fleeting pulse
    (3) 2+: Weak thready pulse
    (4) 3+: Normal quality
    (5) 4+: Increased volume, strong and bounding
  5. Doppler ultrasound confirmation: device amplifies sound waves produced by pulsating blood flow in vessel and allows for detection of pulsatile flow in absence of palpable pulse.
  6. Marking of pulses: facilitates comparison of pulses and promotes continuity of care
  7. Extraanatomic graft pulses: placed subcutaneously to improve recipient vessel circulation
 D. Neurologic assessment (vital signs)
  1. Level of consciousness: orientation to person, place, time
  2. Motor and sensory function
   a. Motion and sensation of all extremities
   b. Bilateral and equal hand grasp
  3. Pupillary function: equal reaction and accommodation to light
  4. Abnormal findings
   a. Tics
   b. Tremors
   c. Gazing
   d. Seizures
 E. Neurovascular assessment: evaluate the 6 Ps.
  1. Pulses and pulselessness
  2. Pain
  3. Paresthesia
  4. Paralysis
  5. Pallor
  6. Poikilothermia (coldness)
 F. Fluid volume status
  1. CVP, pulmonary artery pressures
  2. Assessment of vital signs
  3. Laboratory data
   a. Hemoglobin, hematocrit
   b. Serum sodium, potassium
   c. Coagulation studies
  4. Replacement of blood and (third space) fluid loss
   a. Colloid
   b. Crystalloid
   c. Plasma expanders
 G. Operative site observation
  1. Dressing site and condition
  2. Drains and drainage
  3. Presence of abnormalities
   a. Hematoma formation
   b. Discolorations
  4. Changes in abdominal girth, diameter

H. Limb protection
   1. Bed cradle
   2. Heel and elbow padding
   3. Lanolin for dry skin
   4. Lamb's wool between toes
   5. No pressure under knee
   6. Avoidance of joint (graft) flexion at hip or knee

XXVI. PACU care for specific vascular procedures
   A. Carotid vessel procedures
      1. Neurologic assessment
         a. Presence of swallow and gag reflexes
         b. Cranial nerve function: affected by intraoperative retraction and stretching of nerves
      2. Respiratory concerns
         a. Instruct patient to inhale deeply and minimize deep cough response to avoid elevation of venous pressure.
         b. Incentive spirometry encourages deep inhalation.
         c. Assess for possible respiratory obstruction.
            (1) Vocal cord edema and injury, surgical trauma
            (2) Tracheal deviation: hematoma development at operative site; may present with stridor
      3. Blood pressure concerns: maintain adequate blood pressure to maximize cerebral perfusion and minimize possible sequelae of hypertension or hypotension
         a. Hypertension
            (1) Sequelae
               (a) Suture line disruption: tension at site of anastomosis may cause bleeding.
               (b) Hematoma formation: tracheal compression
               (c) Cerebral hemorrhage, edema
            (2) Nursing interventions
               (a) Elevate head of bed to decrease venous pressure.
               (b) Comfort measures to minimize pain and maintain desired blood pressure parameters
               (c) Ensure adequate ventilation.
         b. Hypotension
            (1) Sequelae resulting from hypersensitive carotid sinus
               (a) Sluggish blood flow through operative artery and graft
               (b) Difficult pulse assessment
               (c) Decreased cerebral or coronary artery perfusion
            (2) Nursing interventions
               (a) Increase fluids if indicated.
               (b) Reduce high Fowler's to more moderate position.
               (c) Titration of vasopressor
         c. Pharmacologic intervention
            (1) Sodium nitroprusside (Nipride): vasodilator
               (a) Direct effect on arterial and venous smooth muscle
               (b) Used to treat severe acute hypertension: rapid onset
               (c) Reduces peripheral resistance and increases cardiac output
            (2) Nitroglycerin: vasodilator
               (a) Relaxes smooth muscle in small blood vessels
               (b) Causes venous and arterial dilation; increases coronary artery perfusion
               (c) Used for treatment of myocardial ischemia and hypertension
            (3) Trimethaphan (Arfonad): antihypertensive
               (a) Ganglionic blocking agent
               (b) Causes peripheral vasodilation; used to treat hypertension

(4) Dopamine (Intropin): vasopressor
  (a) Directly stimulates beta-receptors and dopaminergic receptors
  (b) Low dose causes renal and mesenteric vasodilation and subsequently increases urine output.
  (c) Midrange dose produces a positive inotropic effect on myocardium.
  (d) High dose stimulates alpha-adrenergic receptors and causes renal vasoconstriction, increased peripheral resistance, and increased blood pressure.
(5) Milrinone (Primacor)
  (a) Positive inotropic agent with vasodilator properties
  (b) Causes thrombocytopenia and may be contraindicated for some patients
(6) Phenylephrine (Neo-Synephrine): vasopressor
  (a) Acts on alpha-adrenergic receptors
  (b) Produces vasoconstriction and increased peripheral resistance
  (c) Increases systolic and diastolic blood pressure
  (d) Reflex bradycardia occurs because of increased vagal activity.
(7) Labetalol hydrochloride (Normodyne, Trandate): alpha-receptor and nonspecific beta-receptor blocking agent
  (a) Used for treatment of hypertension
  (b) Administer supine to avoid orthostatic hypotensive effect.
(8) Esmolol (Brevibloc): beta-blocking agent used to treat supraventricular tachyarrhythmias
  (a) Rapid onset of action, short half-life
  (b) Hypotension is most common side effect.
(9) Nifedipine (Procardia): calcium channel blocker used for treatment of chronic hypertension, acute hypertensive emergencies, and angina
  (a) Decreases systemic vascular resistance
  (b) Augments cardiac output
3. Bradycardia
  a. Causes
    (1) Altered baroreceptor responses
    (2) Vagal manipulation
    (3) Vagal pressure from hematoma formation
    (4) Myocardial infarction
  b. Interventions
    (1) Pharmacologic
      (a) Atropine (anticholinergic, parasympatholytic): inhibits action of acetylcholine; stimulates or depresses central nervous system depending on dose; used to treat bradycardia
      (b) Glycopyrrolate (Robinul; anticholinergic): inhibits action of acetylcholine; used to treat bradycardia
    (2) Surgical
      (a) Excision of hematoma
      (b) Reexploration of wound
4. Positioning: elevation of head
  a. Decreases venous pressure
  b. Facilitates respiratory excursion
5. Dressings and drains
  a. Dressings: light, nonconstricting
  b. Drains: Penrose, Jackson-Pratt, Hemovac
B. Intrathoracic vessel procedures
  1. Respiratory support
    a. Principles of care of intubated and mechanically ventilated patient

      b. Head elevation permits respiratory excursion and allows proper chest tube function.

      c. Turn, cough, deep breathe every 2 hours and as needed.

  2. Assess for complications.

      a. Atelectasis

      b. Pneumothorax, hemothorax

      c. Adult respiratory distress syndrome (ARDS)

      d. CHF and pulmonary edema

  3. Ensure proper chest tube functioning.

      a. Secure connections

      b. Observe for air leaks.

      c. Measure drainage.

      d. Keep bottles below chest level.

      e. Auscultate lung sounds.

      f. Palpate for subcutaneous emphysema (crepitus).

  4. Neurovascular assessment (as previously outlined)

      a. Pulse assessment: upper and lower extremities

      b. Motor and sensory function

         (1) Spinal cord ischemia

            (a) Paraplegia can occur with prolonged thoracic and aortic occlusion.

            (b) Decreased perfusion pressure to spinal cord

         (2) Embolization to distal arteries, originating from aortic clot

  5. Monitor for cardiac, pulmonary, renal function (as previously outlined).

  6. Pain management (according to unit policy)

      a. Prevent splinting and permit lung expansion.

      b. Allay apprehension and fear.

      c. Decrease tachycardia and hypertension.

      d. Enhance mechanical ventilation compliance.

C. Abdominal vessel procedures

  1. Continuous cardiopulmonary assessment (as previously outlined)

  2. Observe for signs and symptoms of hypovolemic shock caused by hemorrhage.

  3. Gastrointestinal assessment

      a. Nasogastric tube: decompresses stomach, prevents paralytic ileus

      b. Complications

         (1) Ileus

         (2) Occlusion of inferior mesenteric artery, causing colon ischemia

         (3) Hemorrhage: measure and monitor abdominal girth.

  4. Renal assessment (as previously outlined)

      a. Hematuria: aortic crossclamping, kidney and/or bladder trauma

      b. Oliguria: renal failure, tubular necrosis

  5. Neurovascular status (as previously outlined)

      a. Pedal pulses may be absent for 6 to 12 hours postoperatively.

         (1) Vascular spasm

         (2) Peripheral vasoconstriction

         (3) Vessel patency, verified by surgeon

         (4) Confirm absence with Doppler ultrasonography.

      b. Absence of previously palpable pulse

         (1) Signifies occlusion of vessel or graft

         (2) Requires immediate surgical reexploration

  6. Positioning

      a. Abdominal procedures: head elevation

         (1) Facilitates respiratory excursion

         (2) Decreases suture line stress

      b. Vena cava plication: supine to slight Trendelenburg

         (1) Prevents further reduction of venous return

         (2) Decreased venous return results in decreased cardiac output.

7. Pain or vascular spasm
   a. Severe pain indicative of retroperitoneal bleeding
   b. Spasms
      (1) Usually follow aortic surgery
      (2) Aggravated by
         (a) Hypotension
         (b) Hypothermia
         (c) Pain
         (d) CO_2 retention
8. Hypothermia or shivering
   a. Sequelae
      (1) Increases oxygen requirement
      (2) ST segment depression can occur with increased myocardial oxygen requirement.
      (3) Prolonged somnolence occurs with decreased cerebral perfusion.
      (4) Increases vasoconstriction and vasospasm
         (a) Increases difficulty in palpating pulses
         (b) Aggravates hypertension
      (5) Increases patient anxiety and discomfort
   b. Corrective nursing interventions
      (1) Heated blankets, automatic hyperthermia blanket
      (2) Warming lights
      (3) Heated aerosol nebulizers with oxygen delivery
9. Complications
   a. Acute arterial occlusion
   b. Debris embolization: pulmonary, cerebral, peripheral
   c. Graft suture line hemorrhage
   d. Cardiopulmonary complications
      (1) Dysrhythmias
      (2) Myocardial infarction (MI)
      (3) CHF
   e. Third space fluid accumulation
   f. Renal complications: failure, trauma
D. Extraanatomic vessel bypasses (femoral crossover, axillofemoral bypass)
   1. Positioning: turn only to unoperated side.
      a. Avoid external pressure on graft.
      b. Avoid flexion of graft; careful pillow positioning
   2. Pulse checks with femoral crossover
      a. Across symphysis pubis (femoral to femoral)
      b. Both lower extremities
   3. Pulse checks with axillofemoral bypass: monitor donor arm and revascularized limb.
      a. Avoid damage to donor artery; obtain blood pressure, draw blood from opposite arm.
      b. Specific complications of axillofemoral bypass
         (1) Brachial plexus injury
         (2) Subclavian or axillary artery injury
         (3) Upper extremity embolization
E. Extremity vessel procedures (arterial bypass grafts, embolectomies; vein stripping and ligation)
   1. Nursing concerns: arterial procedures
      a. Positioning: avoid severe joint flexion, crossing of legs, pillows under popliteal area.
      b. Nonrestrictive dressings
      c. Neurovascular assessment
         (1) Comparison of both extremities

      (2) Doppler confirmation

      (3) If no pulses expected by surgeon, successful revascularization assessed by dry, pink, warm legs and feet

   d. Limb protection (as previously outlined)

   e. Laboratory data

      (1) Monitor glucose in diabetic patient: control of blood sugar can prevent infection.

      (2) Monitor potassium: extracellular potassium increases with limb ischemia and infection.

      (3) Monitor for metabolic acidosis: causes increased serum potassium

   f. Administer low–molecular weight dextran (500 ml over 10 to 24 hours)

      (1) Anticoagulation effect: interrupts action of fibrinogen and clotting factors

      (2) Reduces platelet accumulation and adhesiveness

      (3) Increases tissue perfusion

      (4) Reduces blood viscosity

      (5) Increases colloid osmotic pressure

   g. Control of pain to prevent spasms

2. Complications of extremity vessel procedures

   a. Graft occlusion

   b. Vein, nerve injury

   c. Pulmonary or cerebral emboli

3. Nursing concerns: vein procedures

   a. Positioning

      (1) Supine to slight head elevation with leg elevation

      (2) Avoidance of knee bending or leg crossing

   b. Dressing: multiple wounds covered by ACE bandages

   c. Neurovascular assessment: bilateral comparison as previously outlined

   d. Pain assessment: incisional discomfort versus deep calf pain of thrombophlebitis

4. Complications of vein ligation, stripping procedures

   a. Hematoma and wound bleeding

   b. Femoral vein or femoral saphenous nerve damage

   c. Thrombophlebitis

   d. Edema

BIBLIOGRAPHY

1. Ahijevych K, Wewers ME: Passive smoking and vascular disease. *J Cardiovasc Nurs* 4(1):69-74, 2003.

2. Allen A, editor: *Core curriculum for post anesthesia nursing practice,* ed 2. Philadelphia: WB Saunders, 1991.

3. Alspach JG, editor: *Core curriculum for critical care nursing,* ed 5. Philadelphia: WB Saunders, 1998.

4. Barash PG, Cullen BF, Stoelting RK: *Handbook of clinical anesthesia,* ed 4. Philadelphia: Lippincott Williams & Wilkins, 2001.

5. Bates B, Bickley LS, Hoekelman RA, et al: *A guide to physical examination and history taking,* ed 6. Philadelphia: Lippincott, 1995.

6. Beckman JA: Diseases of the veins. *Circulation* 106(17):2170-2172, 2002.

7. Black JM, Nawks JH, Keene AM: *Medical-surgical nursing clinical management for positive outcomes,* ed 6. WB Saunders, 2001.

8. Bojar RM: *Manual of perioperative care in cardiac and thoracic surgery,* ed 3. Cambridge: Blackwell Science, 1999.

9. Boyer MJ: *Study guide to Brunner and Suddarth's textbook of medical-surgical nursing,* ed 9. New York: Lippincott, Williams, Wilkins, 2000.

10. Braunwald E, Zipes DP, Libby P: *Heart disease textbook of cardiovascular medicine,* vol 2. Philadelphia: WB Saunders, 2001.

11. Bright LD, Georgi S: Peripheral vascular disease: Is it arterial or venous? *Am J Nurs* 92(9):34-43, 1992.

12. Bussard ME: Reteplase: Nursing implications for catheter-directed thrombolytic therapy for peripheral vascular occlusion. *Crit Care Nurse* 22(3):57-63, 2003.

13. Chulay M, Guzzetta C, Dosey B: *AACN Handbook of critical care nursing.* Stamford, CT: Appleton & Lange, 1997.

14. Church V: Staying on guard for DVT and PE. *Nursing* 30(2):34, 2002.

15. Civetta JM, Taylor RW, Kirby RR: *Critical care,* ed 2. Philadelphia: Lippincott, 1992.

16. Clochesy JM, Breu C, Cardin S, et al: *Critical care nursing,* ed 2. Philadelphia: WB Saunders, 1996.

17. Creager MA, Libby P: Peripheral arterial diseases. In Braunwald E, Zipes DP, Libby P, editors: *Heart disease: A textbook of cardiovascular medicine,* ed 6, vol 2. Philadelphia: WB Saunders, 2001, pp 1457-1478.

18. DeSanctis JT: Percutaneous interventions for lower extremity peripheral vascular disease. *Am Fam Physicians* 64 (12): 1965-1972, 2001.

19. Eckman M, Priff N, editors: *Diseases,* ed 2. Springhouse, PA: Springhouse, 1997.

20. Emma LA: Chronic arterial occlusive disease. *J Cardiovasc Nurs* 7(1):14-24, 1992.

21. Estes MEZ: *Health assessment and physical examination,* Albany, NY: Delmar, 2002.

22. Fahey VA: *Vascular nursing,* ed 3. Philadelphia: WB Saunders, 1999.

23. Fauci AS, Braunwald E, Isselbacher KJ, et al, editors: *Harrison's principles of internal medicine,* ed 14. New York: McGraw-Hill, 1998.

24. Guilmet D, Bachet J, Goudot G, et al: Aortic dissection: Anatomic types and surgical approaches. *J Cardiovasc Surg* 34(1):23-32, 1993.

25. Hoekstra JW, editor: *Handbook of cardiovascular emergencies,* ed 1. Boston: Little, Brown, 1997.

26. Hollier LH, Procter CD, Naslund TC: Spinal cord ischemia. In Bernhard VM, Towne FB, editors: *Complications in vascular surgery.* St Louis: Quality Medical, 1991.

27. Hudak CM, Gallo BM, Morton PG: *Critical care nursing: A holistic approach,* ed 7. Philadelphia: Lippincott, 1998.

28. Joffe HV, Goldhaber SZ: Upper extremity deep vein thrombosis. *Circulation* 106: 1874-1880, 2002.

29. Keller KB, Lemberg L: The importance of magnesium in cardiovascular disease. *Am J Crit Care* 4(2):348–350, 1993.

30. Kinney MR, Packa DR, Dunbar SB: *AACN's clinical reference for critical-care nursing.* St Louis: Mosby, 1998.

31. Kristt AM: *Post anesthesia care nursing: The peripheral vascular surgical patient,* ed 2. St Louis: Mosby–Year Book, 1995.

32. Kuhn JK, McGovern M: Peripheral vascular assessment of the elderly client. *J Gerontol Nurs* 18(12):35-38, 1992.

33. Litwack K: *Post anesthesia care nursing,* ed 2. St Louis: Mosby–Year Book, 1995.

34. Luckmann J: *Saunders manual of nursing care.* Philadelphia: WB Saunders, 1997.

35. Marston WA: PPG, APG, duplex. Which noninvasive tests are most appropriate for the management of patients with chronic venous insufficiency? *Semin Vasc Surg* 15(1):13-20, 2002.

36. Merli GJ, Weitz HH: *Medical management of the surgical patient.* Philadelphia: WB Saunders, 1998.

37. Moneta LG, Foley MI, Giswold ME, et al: Vascular surgery for peripheral arterial disease. *Clin Cornerstone* 4(5):41-55, 2002.

38. Morris B, Colwell CW, Hardwick ME: The use of flow molecular weight heparins in the prevention of venous thromboembolic disease. *Orthop Nurs* 17(6):23-29, 1998.

39. Owens MW, Daniel J: IV magnesium sulfate in the treatment of ventricular tachycardia and acute myocardial infarction. *Crit Care Nurse* 13(6):83-85, 1993.

40. Pagana KD, Pagana TJ: *Diagnostic testing and nursing implications: A case study approach,* ed 5. St Louis: Mosby, 1999.

41. Price SA, Wilson LM: *Pathophysiology: Clinical concepts of disease processes,* ed 6. St Louis: Mosby, 2003.

42. Procter CD, Kazmier FJ, Hollier LH, et al: Selection of patients for peripheral revascularization surgery. *Med Clin North Am* 76(5):1159-1168, 1992.

43. Quaal SJ: Interactive hemodynamics of IABC. In *Comprehensive intraaortic balloon counterpulsation,* ed 2. St Louis: Mosby–Year Book, 1993, pp 101-117.

44. Rothrock JC, Smith DA, McEwen DR: *Alexander's care of the patient in surgery,* ed 12. St Louis: Mosby, 2003.

45. Ruppert SD, Kernicki J, Dolan JT: *Dolan's critical care nursing: Clinical management through the nursing process,* ed 2. Philadelphia: Davis, 1996.

46. Shettigar UR, Toole JG, Appunn DO: Combined use of esmolol and digoxin in the acute treatment of atrial fibrillation or flutter. *Am Heart J* 126(2):368-374, 1993.

47. Siedlecki B: Peripheral vascular disease. *Can Nurse* 88(11):26-28, 1992.

48. Stone DJ, Bogdonoff D, Leisure G, et al: *Perioperative care anesthesia, medicine, and surgery,* St Louis: Mosby, 1998.

49. Stoney RJ, Effeney DJ: *Wylie's atlas of vascular surgery: Thoracoabdominal aorta and its branches.* Philadelphia: Lippincott, 1992.

50. Tran NT, Meissner MH: The epidemiology, pathophysiology, and natural history of chronic venous disease. *Semin Vasc Surg* 15(1):5-12, 2002.

51. Urden LD, Stacy KM, Lough ME: *Thelan's critical care nursing: Diagnosis and management,* ed 4. St Louis: Mosby, 2002.

52. Veith FJ, Hobson RW, Williams RA, et al: *Vascular surgery: Principles and practice,* ed 2. New York: McGraw-Hill, 1994.

53. Venes D, Thomas CL, editors: *Taber's cyclopedic medical dictionary,* ed 19. Philadelphia: Davis, 2001.

54. Waugaman WR, Foster SD, Rigor BM, editors: *Principles and practice of nurse anesthesia,* ed 3. Norwalk, CT: Appleton & Lange, 1999.

52 Plastic and Reconstructive Surgery

THERESA L. CLIFFORD

OBJECTIVES

At the conclusion of this chapter the reader will be able to:

1. Describe the anatomy of skin.

2. Describe the physiology of wound healing.

3. Describe common medical conditions affecting surgical outcomes.

4. Discuss the psychological factors that affect the plastic surgery patient.

5. Describe common plastic and reconstructive surgeries.

6. Describe preoperative preparation of the plastic and hand surgical patient.

7. Identify anesthesia administration concerns for the plastic surgery patient.

8. Discuss postoperative management concerns for the plastic surgery patient.

9. Discuss the nursing care for the individual surgical procedures outlined.

10. Discuss patient education related to various surgical procedures.

11. Discuss the clinical management of burn injury.

■
■■ Plastic and reconstructive surgery may be performed for a variety of reasons. These procedures impact physical appearance as well as emotional well-being and body image. Plastic surgery may be elective and cosmetic, or it may be reconstructive, correcting congenital or acquired abnormalities to restore normal function and appearance. Anesthetic needs vary on the basis of the complexity of the procedure, from local anesthesia for simple lesion removal to prolonged general anesthesia for complex reconstruction.

This chapter discusses the perioperative needs of the plastic surgery and burn patient. The purpose, procedure, perianesthesia nursing care management, and patient education for specific surgical interventions will be outlined.

I. Physiology
 A. Physiology of wound healing
  1. Wound
   a. An alteration in the integrity and function of tissues in the body
   b. Intentional wounds are surgically caused.
   c. Unintentional wounds include pressure ulcers and failed wound closure, for example.
  2. Process of wound healing
   a. Hemostasis
    (1) Injury causes blood cells to enter wound and release coagulation factors to promote platelet aggregation.
   b. Inflammation
    (1) Histamines are released from mast cells to cause vasodilation and increased capillary permeability.

      (2) Epithelialization occurs; white blood cells (WBCs) cleanse wound (phagocytosis).

      (3) Stage of exudate and wound drainage

      (4) Stage lasts up to four days.

   c. Proliferation

      (1) Collagen synthesis occurs giving strength to the wound; granulation tissue forms.

      (2) Stage lasts up to three weeks.

   d. Remodeling and maturation

      (1) Collagen fibers are remodeled, and scar matures.

        (a) Becomes flat, thin, silver in color

        (b) Stage lasts 1 to 2 years.

        (c) Comorbidities affecting wound healing

          (i) Local factors

           [a] Presence of necrotic tissue or foreign bodies

           [b] Desiccation or dehydration of wound

           [c] Incontinence or other chronic skin irritants

           [d] Mechanical trauma such as prolonged or excessive pressure or friction to surface of wound

           [e] Use of cytotoxic products near wound

          (ii) Age

           [a] Children heal rapidly.

           [b] Geriatrics heal slower because of decreased circulation and higher incidence of chronic illnesses.

         (iii) Nutrition—malnutrition, dehydration, and vitamin deficiency slow healing process.

         (iv) Nicotine—causes poor healing because of oxygen deprivation and vasoconstriction

         (v) Psychological stress—corticosteroids decrease inflammatory response, and catecholamines suppress microcirculation.

         (vi) Infection—slows healing because of prolonged inflammatory response

        (vii) Dead space—accumulation of air or fluid slows healing, promotes infection.

        (viii) Chronic use of aspirin-containing products or steroids

         (ix) Immunosuppression—patient with cancer, diabetes, HIV, for example.

         (x) Peripheral vascular disease—venous stasis common

        (xi) Psychological stress—higher level

II. Other medical conditions affecting surgical outcomes

  A. Pulmonary disease

    1. Prone positioning intraoperatively may affect ventilation.

    2. Prolonged anesthesia increases pulmonary hygiene needs postoperatively.

    3. Hypoxemia causes tissue hypoxia, which will divert necessary oxygen and nutrients from tissues.

  B. Cardiac disease

    1. Coronary insufficiency may affect tolerance of hypotensive anesthesia.

    2. Cardiac function affects tolerance of prolonged reconstructive procedures.

  C. Diabetes mellitus

    1. Affects wound healing by decreasing phagocytosis in the presence of hyperglycemia

    2. Optimal glucose control required

  D. Medication history

    1. Use of steroids

    2. Use of aspirin products

    3. Chemotherapeutic agents

  E. History of bleeding disorders

    F. Presence of infection
       1. Infection prolongs inflammatory stage of wound healing.
       2. Children with concurrent or recent upper respiratory infection are more likely to have laryngospasm or to cough during induction or emergence.
    G. Nutritional status
       1. Wound healing depends on adequate nutritional status particularly vitamin C, zinc, iron, and protein.
       2. Poor nutritional status decreases ability to prevent infection.

III. Preoperative assessments
    A. Local procedures
       1. Complete blood cell count
       2. Chemistry profile
    B. General anesthesia
       1. Complete blood cell count
       2. Chemistry profile
       3. Electrocardiogram (ECG) in adults
       4. Pulmonary function testing if necessary
       5. Chest x-ray film (in adults or in children with pulmonary pathologic findings)
       6. Bleeding profile: prothrombin time and partial thromboplastin time (international normalized ratio [INR])
       7. Pregnancy testing if indicated or desired

IV. Psychological considerations
    A. Body image—the mental picture we possess of our own body
       1. Body image is a changing dynamic entity influenced by internal and external factors.
       2. Body image is a component of how we feel about ourselves.
    B. Motivation for plastic surgery
       1. Internal motivation—surgery to change physical appearance of oneself
       2. External motivation—surgery to change physical appearance at recommendation of others
       3. Patients who are internally motivated are most pleased with surgical outcomes.
    C. Preoperative assessment related to body image
       1. Understand patient's perception of body deformity
       2. Understand patient's expectation of surgical outcome
       3. Explore significant other's feelings regarding procedure.
       4. Assess postoperative support and coping mechanisms.
    D. Integration of surgical changes into body image
       1. Patients may progress through the stages of grieving.
       2. Changed physical appearance slowly integrates into body image and then self-concept.
       3. Some patients never integrate changes into body image; may request more surgery or require counseling
    E. Nursing care related to body image
       1. Encourage patient to verbalize feelings.
       2. Reassure patient that it is normal to desire physical attractiveness.
       3. Support the stages of grieving.
       4. Be nonjudgmental with verbal and nonverbal communication.
    F. Determine patient's expectations of surgery.
       1. Expectations realistic?
       2. Motivation for surgery?
       3. Reinforce that immediate results may not meet patient's expectations because of swelling, color changes, and suture lines.
       4. Family expectations
       5. Reinforce that long-term results may not meet expectations.
    G. Impact of deformity on patient's self-perception
       1. How does patient view it as changing his or her life?

      2. How important is it to be attractive?

      3. Effect of others' reactions on patient

  H. Psychological evaluation may be appropriate before procedure.

V. Perioperative concerns for the plastic surgery patient

  A. Preprocedural teaching

      1. Preemptive medications should be reviewed with patient.

      2. NPO instructions

      3. Review any over-the-counter medications and herbal remedies patient uses to determine if any need to be stopped.

      4. Encourage patient to stop smoking prior to surgery.

      5. Encourage to wear loose, button up clothing with preferably slip-on shoes for comfort.

      6. Have patient arrange for a ride and home care support.

  B. Procedural concerns

      1. Primary goal for plastic surgery procedures

         a. Provide cosmetically acceptable results.

         b. Restore function.

         c. Promote healing with minimal scarring.

         d. Prevent infection.

      2. Procedures are carefully planned before surgery using photography, computerized imaging, and so forth.

      3. Patient positioning requirements

         a. Provide comfortable access to surgical field.

            (1) Optimal position on table to allow for repositioning during procedure to evaluate results (e.g., mammoplasty)

         b. Prevent nerve decompression from improper positioning.

            (1) Careful positioning

            (2) Padding of pressure points

      4. Promote venous drainage.

         a. Use of sequential compression devices, TEDS, for example.

      5. Provide for greatest hypotensive advantages (reduction of bleeding) if deliberate hypotensive technique is used.

      6. Incision placement

         a. Incisions placed so that scar lines lie parallel to existing skin lines or behind hairline

         b. Skin lines represent areas with minimal tension.

         c. Cosmetic effect better if tension is minimized

         d. Frequently found under long axis of muscle

      7. Hemostasis

         a. Must be obtained and maintained to promote good cosmetic effect

         b. Bleeding under skin potentiates inflammation, infection, pressure, and dehiscence.

         c. Achieved with ligation, electrocautery, pressure

      8. Instrumentation

         a. Microinstrumentation for nontraumatic repair

         b. Use of operating microscope

            (1) Provides three-dimensional view (stereoscopic) that must be clearly seen by surgeon and assistants

            (2) Careful movements in vicinity of operating table

            (3) May require separate instrument tables for donor and recipient sites

         c. Lasers

            (1) LASER acronym for Light Amplification by the Stimulated Emission of Radiation

            (2) CO_2 laser, argon laser, Nd:YAG lasers may be used in aesthetic (cosmetic) surgery.

            (3) Uses

               (a) Removal of professional tattoos and traumatic tattoos caused by friction, scraping, or explosives

    (b) Alternative for skin resurfacing (CO_2 laser)

     (i) Laser blepharoplasty

  d. Endoscopy

   (1) Endoscope requires body cavity for insertion of scope and visualization.

    (a) No natural cavities in plastic surgery operative areas

     (i) Cavity created by use of umbrella or balloonlike retractor on soft tissues

   (2) Uses

    (a) Endoscopic forehead lift

    (b) Facelift

    (c) Augmentation or reduction mammoplasty

    (d) Abdominoplasty

C. Anesthesia concerns

 1. Selection of anesthetic routes and agent

  a. Local anesthesia

   (1) Suitable for minor plastic surgical procedures (e.g., skin lesions, rhinoplasty)

   (2) Often used for outpatients or office patients

   (3) Indicated for procedures that require patient participation (e.g., patients may need to open and close eyes during blepharoplasty)

   (4) Selection of agent that lasts 50 to 100 minutes longer than anticipated length of surgery

  b. Regional anesthesia

   (1) Suitable for procedures localized to extremity

    (a) Axillary, plexus blocks for upper extremities

    (b) Sciatic block for feet

    (c) Lumbar epidural or spinal for leg procedures

  c. General anesthesia

   (1) Suitable for long procedures, pediatrics, and anxious patients

   (2) Long plastic procedures generally require lighter general anesthesia.

   (3) Selection of inhalation agents

    (a) Agents that do not sensitize the heart to catecholamines because of large doses of epinephrine used in plastic procedures (e.g., isoflurane)

    (b) Agents that are less likely to precipitate coughing and laryngospasm, particularly in procedures of face and neck

    (c) Length of time required for elimination for short procedures (e.g., enflurane is rapidly eliminated if used in procedures that last less than 40 minutes)

    (d) Inducing deliberate hypotension

     (i) Selection of agents that induce hypotension

      [a] Reduces blood loss

      [b] Improves visibility at surgical field

     (ii) May be accomplished with volatile agents alone or in combination with ganglionic blocking agents, vasodilators, alpha-blockers, or beta-blockers

     (iii) Used for reconstruction of head and neck

     (iv) Hypotension onset and reversal performed slowly to prevent rapid blood pressure fluctuations (e.g., perfusion to organ is maintained)

 2. Intraoperative management

  a. Airway management

   (1) Method of intubation (oral or nasal) depends on access to surgical field.

    (a) Nasal intubation for oral procedures

    (b) Use of oral or nasal RAE tube for cleft lip and palate repair (endotracheal tubes with sharp curves that promote access to field by surgeon)

(c) Intubation may be difficult and require fiber optic bronchoscope in patients, particularly children, with maxillofacial deformities.

(2) Ensure vigorous spontaneous breathing before extubation in patients with maxillofacial surgery.

(3) Esophageal or precordial stethoscope to assess ventilation

(4) Monitor oxygenation.

    (a) Transcutaneous oxygen measurement

    (b) Direct arterial blood gas measurement

    (c) Pulse oximetry

(5) Carbon dioxide monitoring; end-tidal carbon dioxide

    (a) Elevated carbon dioxide levels result in vasodilation, which increases bleeding and intracranial pressure.

  b. Cardiovascular management

(1) ECG monitoring (including ST segment analysis) for patients at risk for coronary ischemia

    (a) From use of epinephrine

    (b) As result of deliberate hypotensive technique

(2) Direct or indirect blood pressure monitoring

    (a) Large blood loss common in plastic procedures

        (i) Crystalloids

        (ii) Colloids

        (iii) Blood products

    (b) Significant hypotension may result in graft or flap failure.

(3) Positioning and position change

    (a) Anesthetic agents affect vascular homeostasis and reflect pressure control mechanisms.

    (b) Position changes during procedure may be necessary.

        (i) To access donor and recipient sites

        (ii) To evaluate cosmetic result of procedure (e.g., mammoplasty)

    (c) Minimizing excessive hypotension

        (i) Slow, careful movement of patient

        (ii) Maintain light anesthesia.

(4) Emergence from anesthesia

    (a) Smooth emergence desired to prevent thrashing that may disrupt delicate suture lines

    (b) Prevent excessive coughing, particularly in head and neck procedures.

    (c) Minimize nausea and vomiting.

COMMON PROCEDURES

  I. Aesthetic: Body

    A. Abdominoplasty

      1. Purpose

        a. Surgical correction of deformities of anterior abdominal wall

        b. Removal of apron deformities (panniculus)

        c. Repair of muscle wall from previous abdominal surgeries

        d. Improve body shape

      2. Procedure

        a. Surgical removal of redundant tissue of the abdomen

        b. Involves skin, fascia, and adipose tissue

        c. May include closure of abdominal wall muscles

      3. Perianesthesia care

        a. Anesthesia-general

        b. Patient selection important for ambulatory abdominoplasty

        (1) Must stay within close proximity to surgery center

        (2) Patient must be motivated.

        (3) Home support must be adequate.

      c. Maintain good pain control so patient can ambulate, cough, and deep breathe.

      d. Control nausea so pain medications will be tolerated.

      e. Maintain correct positioning.

        (1) Head of bed elevated

        (2) Pillow under knees

        (3) Use pillow splint for coughing and moving.

        (4) Walk in stooped position for 1 week.

      f. Empty drains as needed.

        (1) Two Jackson-Pratt drains not unusual

        (2) Empty and record drainage.

        (3) Maintain patency of drains.

          (a) Clots can be signs of hematoma formations.

      g. Patient will wear a compression girdle for 2 to 3 weeks.

   4. Patient education

      a. Review instructions with patient and caregiver.

        (1) Demonstration for positioning and moving

        (2) Activity restrictions: no straining, lifting, exercising for 4-6 weeks

        (3) Drain-emptying demonstration

        (4) Hematoma assessment

        (5) Pain-management techniques

        (6) Keep compression garment on as directed.

        (7) Report signs and symptoms of infection.

B. Buttock, thigh, upper arm lifts

   1. Purpose

      a. Eliminate loose and sagging skin.

      b. Improve appearance and boost self-confidence.

   2. Procedure

      a. Excision of redundant skin and tissue

      b. Excisional surgery can be performed in conjunction with liposuction.

   3. Perianesthesia care

      a. Anesthesia—local or general

      b. Maintain good pain control so patient can ambulate, cough, and deep breathe.

      c. Monitor drains if used.

        (1) Maintain patency of drains.

        (2) Clots can be a sign of hematoma formation.

      d. Patient will wear a compression girdle for 2 to 3 weeks.

   4. Patient education

      a. Review instructions with patient and caregiver.

        (1) Demonstration for positioning and moving

        (2) Activity restrictions: no straining, lifting, exercising for 4-6 weeks

        (3) Drain-emptying demonstration

        (4) Hematoma assessment

        (5) Pain-management techniques, including cold compress applications (avoid aspirin)

        (6) Keep compression garment on as directed.

        (7) Report signs and symptoms of infection.

C. Liposuction

   1. Purpose

      a. To remove pockets of adipose tissue for body contouring

   2. Procedure

      a. Removal of adipose tissue with suction-assisted device from face, neck, abdomen, thighs, buttocks, flanks, and extremities

      b. Small (1 to 2 cm) incisions are used to minimize scarring.

      c. Adipose tissue is aspirated using crisscross technique.

      d. Compression dressing applied to collapse tunnels created

        e. Accurate volume loss recorded to monitor for hypovolemia and third spacing

   3. Perianesthesia care

        a. Anesthesia—general or local

        b. Preprocedure patient is marked in standing position.

        c. Often performed on outpatient basis unless more than 2500 ml of fat is removed

           (1) Admit for fluid replacement.

        d. Medicate for pain

           (1) Usually described as mild to moderate

        e. Maintain fluid balance.

        f. Observe for hypovolemia.

           (1) Replace fluids as indicated by clinical signs and symptoms.

           (2) Autologous blood should be available when high blood loss is expected.

           (3) EBL will be decreased with the tumescent technique versus the nontumescent technique.

              (a) Tumescent technique I

                 (i) Involves infusion of saline, lidocaine, and epinephrine into area to be suctioned

                 (ii) Lipolysis is improved and blood loss is decreased.

                 (iii) Third spacing can occur with removal of large volumes of adipose tissue.

        g. Assess for hematoma and seroma formation.

        h. Compression applied with compression garment or ACE wraps

           (1) Keep dressings flat and smooth for even contouring.

   4. Patient education

        a. Instruct patient to push fluids to cover third space fluid shifts.

        b. Patient should avoid aspirin-containing products.

        c. Compression garment will be worn for 24 hours to several weeks (physician preference).

        d. Activity

           (1) Rest; minimal activity for first week

           (2) Avoid strenuous activity for 1 month.

        e. Observe for hematoma and seroma formation.

        f. Bruising and swelling are expected.

        g. Female urinal can aid in elimination while compression garment is worn.

        h. Instruct patient to protect bedding the first 24 hours because copious serous-sanguinous drainage is not unusual.

        i. Sponge bathing may be required while patient is restricted to compression garment.

D. Spider vein therapy

   1. Purpose

        a. To treat spider veins (telangiectasia) and varicose veins

   2. Procedure

        a. Sclerotherapy

           (1) Injection of chemical agents to eliminate unsightly veins

           (2) Three categories of agents

               (a) Detergents

               (b) Osmotic agents

               (c) Chemical irritants

        b. Other treatment options include laser surgery, electrodesiccation.

   3. Perianesthesia care

        a. Anesthesia—local

        b. Observe for itching and burning at injection site.

   4. Patient education

        a. Keep compression bandages on as directed.

        b. Early return to walking regimens encouraged to promote aerobic circulation

        c. Mild analgesics may be required initially for cramplike discomfort.

        d. Reinforce with patient that area will "look and feel worse before it gets better."

II. Aesthetic: Breast

  A. Augmentation mammoplasty

    1. Purpose

      a. To improve body image and self confidence

      b. Increase size and modify shape of breast to increase breast size or correct surgical defects with the use of a prosthesis

    2. Procedure

      a. Insertion of prosthetic devices (e.g., tissue expanders that are inflated with normal saline)

      b. Prosthesis placed under the pectoral muscle or mammary tissue through an inframammary, axillary, areolar incision, or endoscope

        (1) Submammary: beneath breast tissue on anterior surface of pectoralis muscle

        (2) Submuscular: beneath pectoralis major and serratus anterior muscles

    3. Perianesthesia care

      a. Anesthesia—general or local with monitored anesthesia care (MAC)

      b. Assess for hematoma.

        (1) Palpate superior aspect of pectoralis muscle over the third rib to the clavicle.

        (2) Breast size should remain equal.

      c. Assess for signs of pneumothorax.

        (1) More common with axillary incision

        (2) Have chest tube and drainage setup available.

        (3) Auscultate lung sounds.

      d. Provide pain relief.

        (1) Pain is moderate to severe.

        (2) Prosthesis beneath chest muscle is more painful.

        (3) Multimodal drug therapy effective

          (a) Preemptive oral narcotics

          (b) Toradol and narcotics intravenous (IV) or oral

          (c) Local anesthesia in wounds

          (d) Muscle relaxants for spasm

          (e) Ice may be helpful for pain control.

      e. Prevent and treat nausea so oral pain medications can be tolerated.

    4. Patient education

      a. Observe for hematoma.

      b. ACE wrap or soft-support bra may be worn for 1 week.

      c. Observe for capsule formation.

        (1) May occur months after surgery

      d. Massage instructions per physician preference

        (1) Massage usually begins within first 2 weeks.

        (2) Massage keeps prosthesis mobile in pocket.

        (3) Postmassage ice packs helpful

      e. Activity

        (1) Restrict arm activity for 3 to 4 weeks.

  B. Pectoral implantation

    1. Purpose

      a. To provide an athletic chest contour for male patients

      b. To treat underdevelopment of the muscles of one side of the chest as a result of congenital defects or injury

    2. Procedure

      a. Small transaxillary incisions are made.

      b. Implants are inserted under pectoralis muscles.

      c. Can be done endoscopically to minimize risk of bleeding and infection

3. Perianesthesia care
   a. Similar to breast augmentation surgery
   b. Usually no drains are required.
   c. Assess for hematoma formation.
4. Education
   a. Pain is usually mild to moderate soreness.
   b. Normal activity can be resumed within a week, but strenuous exercise should be restricted for at least 6 weeks.
C. Gynecomastectomy
   1. Purpose
      a. To improve self confidence and body image
   2. Procedure
      a. Removal of excessive breast tissue in male patient
      b. May combine excision of excess skin and tissue with liposuction
   3. Perianesthesia care
      a. Anesthesia-general or local (for small excision)
      b. Assess for hematoma formation.
      c. Maintain patency of drains (Jackson-Pratt not unusual).
      d. Pain usually described as moderate
   4. Education
      a. Observe for hematoma.
      b. Provide instruction and demonstration of drain care.
      c. Usually removed after 48 hours
      d. Arm activity limited for one month
      e. ACE wrap or compression vest usually worn for compression
D. Mastopexy
   1. Purpose
      a. Reshaping (uplifting) of redundant, sagging breast skin
      b. Generally less than 300 g of tissue removed
   2. Procedure
      a. Incisions usually placed in the inferior pedicle, maintaining nerve innervation to the nipple
   3. Perianesthesia care
      a. General anesthesia most common
      b. Usually same-day procedure
      c. Position supine or semi-Fowler's for comfort.
      d. Assess for hematoma formation.
      e. Maintain patency of drains if used (rarely).
      f. Pain usually described as mild
   4. Education
      a. Observe for hematoma.
      b. Surgical support bra may be worn.
      c. Inform patient about potential for scarring.
III. Aesthetic: Head and neck
   A. Blepharoplasty
      1. Purpose
         a. Repair or reconstruction of upper or lower eyelid to correct "baggy" appearance
         b. To provide patient with a more youthful and less fatigued look
         c. To improve vision fields
      2. Procedure
         a. Surgical removal of redundant skin and adipose tissue with shortening of muscles of the upper and lower eyelids
         b. Incisions placed in the crease of the upper lid and in the lower lid below lash margin
         c. Surgical incisions may be done with laser or scalpel.
      3. Perianesthesia care
         a. Anesthesia—local

        b. Assess for signs of retrobulbar hematoma formation.

           (1) Medical emergency

               (a) Signs

                  (i) Pressure behind eye

                  (ii) Loss of vision

           (2) Observe for

               (a) Pallor, ecchymosis, firmness, or complaints of pain or tightness around eyes

               (b) Proptosis: forward displacement or bulging eye

        c. Maintain normal blood pressure.

           (1) Retards hematoma formation

           (2) Avoid straining, lifting, bending at least 1 week.

           (3) Elevate head of bed.

        d. Pain usually described as mild to moderate

           (1) Control with moderate strength narcotics (codeine or hydrocodone usually effective).

           (2) Ice packs provide pain control and decrease swelling.

    4. Education

      a. Activity

        (1) Avoid activities that will increase blood pressure.

        (2) Keep head elevated.

        (3) Limit reading and television for 48 hours.

      b. Observe for hematoma formation.

      c. Use ice or cool, moist compresses as ordered.

        (1) Keep cloth between ice bag and skin.

        (2) Frozen peas in the bag work well.

      d. Eyes may be dry and lashes crusty with bloody drainage.

      e. Expect periorbital ecchymosis and swelling.

        (1) Mild blurring is expected.

        (2) Call immediately for loss of vision or pressure behind eye.

        (3) Use sterile saline drops to moisten eyes and separate lashes.

      f. Sutures usually removed in 5 days or surgeon preference

B. Genioplasty and mentoplasty

    1. Purpose

      a. Surgical reshaping of chin

      b. Modifications in mandible or insertion of prosthesis

      c. May be performed in conjunction with rhinoplasty to provide a balanced facial profile

    2. Procedure.

      a. Incisions placed inside mouth or beneath chin

    3. Perianesthesia care

      a. Maintain dressing.

      b. Liquid or soft diet

      c. Meticulous oral hygiene if oral incisions placed

    4. Education

      a. Minimize facial movements.

      b. Offer suggestions for nutritional alternatives.

      c. Meticulous oral hygiene if oral incisions placed

C. Otoplasty

    1. Purpose

      a. Surgical reshaping or repositioning of ears

      b. To correct prominent or malformed ears (i.e., microtia)

      c. To improve body image and self confidence

      d. May be performed on children after 6 years of age, when ears have reached most of their adult size

    2. Procedure

      a. Reshaping of the cartilage and skin of the outer ear

      b. May require harvesting cartilage from the ribs

  3. Perianesthesia care
   a. Anesthesia—local or general, depending on age of patient
   b. Frequently a procedure for school-age children
   c. Assess for hematoma formation.
    (1) Use severe pain as an indicator because of bulky head dressing.
   d. Maintain patency of any drains.
   e. Medicate for pain with oral narcotics.
    (1) Usually described as moderate pain
   f. Children have usually suffered teasing because of ears.
    (1) Assure them that surgical outcome is good.
  4. Education
   a. Activity
    (1) Elevate head with two pillows.
    (2) No strenuous activity for 2 to 4 weeks
   b. Ears will be sensitive to cold and swell in heat for 3 to 6 months.
   c. Observe for hematoma.
   d. Teach drain care.
   e. Bulky head dressing usually worn for 1 week
 D. Rhytidoplasty, rhytidectomy, browlift
  1. Purpose
   a. To remove wrinkle and facial laxity giving a more rested, youthful appearance
   b. To tighten loose tissue in face
    (1) May involve skin, fat, subcutaneous tissue, and muscle
  2. Procedure
   a. Standard incisions placed in the temporal area behind hairline
   b. Additional procedures may be performed in conjunction with rhytidectomy.
    (1) Tightening of underlying fascia in the superficial musculoaponeurotic system (SMAS)
    (2) Blepharoplasty, brow lifting, chemical peel, suction-assisted lipectomy or lipolysis (SAL)
   c. Rhytidectomy—facelift
    (1) Tightening of all tissue of the face and neck with excision of redundant tissue
   d. Coronal browlift
    (1) Tightening the tissue of the forehead and brow with excision of redundant tissue
   e. Endoscopic surgery of the head and neck
    (1) Face, neck, and brow lift may be performed with the endoscopic technique when redundant tissue excision is not required.
    (2) Endoscopic techniques generally involve minimal bleeding.
  3. Perianesthesia care
   a. Anesthesia—MAC or general
   b. Assess for hematoma formation.
    (1) Palpate neck, forehead, and check frequently.
    (2) Bulky dressings common
     (a) Assess for absence of increasing tightness, difficulty breathing, or swallowing.
     (b) If any question of hematoma, notify surgeon so dressing can be taken down.
   c. Maintain patency of drains.
    (1) May have Jackson-Pratt or Penrose
   d. Maintain normal blood pressure.
    (1) To prevent hematoma formation
    (2) Manage pain before it increases blood pressure.
    (3) Treat uncontrolled hypertension with antihypertensives if pain management not the cause.

      e. Prevent nausea and vomiting.

      f. Provide calm, reassuring environment to decrease anxiety.

      g. Maintain comfort.

         (1) Pain can be considered moderate to severe for facelift.

         (2) Browlift pain usually described as severe headache

         (3) Begin medications before all local anesthesia has resolved.

         (4) Combination of oral and IV narcotics may be required.

         (5) Toradol very effective but contraindicated by some physicians because of bleeding potential

         (6) Cold compresses or ice can be effective.

      h. Positioning

         (1) Elevate head of bed to decrease swelling.

         (2) Avoid activities that increase blood pressure.

         (3) Avoid turning head side to side or nodding.

      i. Assess cranial nerve VII.

         (1) Temporary numbness of ears and cheeks are normal sequelae.

         (2) Ask patient to smile, frown, wrinkle forehead and nose.

         (3) Assess facial symmetry.

         (4) Assess sensation of earlobes.

            (a) If facial nerve is damaged, it will regenerate with time.

4. Education

    a. Activity

      (1) Avoid strenuous activity for 1 month.

    b. Elevate head and torso with two pillows at bedtime.

    c. Observe for hematoma formation.

      (1) Drain care demonstration

      (2) If drains are present, they are usually removed in 24 hours.

    d. Hair washing per physician

      (1) Usually after sutures are removed in 1 week

    e. Soft diet with little chewing

    f. Appropriate use of pain medications and ice for pain control

    g. Signs to report

      (1) Increased facial pain or unilateral numbness

      (2) Signs and symptoms of infection

E. Rhinoplasty

  1. Purpose

    a. Surgical reshaping of nose

    b. To improve body image and self confidence

  2. Procedure

    a. Excision of fat, cartilage, and skin with fracturing of nasal bones to reshape the nose

  3. Perianesthesia care

    a. Anesthesia-general or MAC with local anesthesia

    b. Provide comfort measures

      (1) Pain usually described as moderate but may be severe

      (2) Medicate with oral or IV narcotics as needed.

         (a) Nonsteroidal antiinflammatory drugs (NSAIDs) can be helpful.

         (b) Begin medications before local anesthesia resolves.

         (c) Ice mask to reduce swelling and pain

    c. Provide calm, reassuring environment.

    d. Patient may have packing in both nares.

      (1) Maintain nasal packing, and avoid removal of clots from nose.

      (2) Change "drip pad" as needed.

      (3) Avoid pressure to nose, including glasses.

      (4) Sneeze through mouth.

      (5) Inability to breathe through nose can be anxiety producing.

         (a) Provide reassurance.

(6) Mouth will be very dry.
    (a) Give frequent mouth care.
  e. Position patient with head of bed elevated.
  f. Prevent postoperative nausea and vomiting.
    (1) Encourage patient to expectorate any postnasal bloody secretions.
    (2) Medicate with antiemetics as needed.
4. Education
  a. Activity
    (1) No strenuous activity for 1 month
    (2) No flexing from waist
    (3) No flexing head
  b. Nasal packing usually removed in 24 to 72 hours
  c. Continue ice mask at home.
    (1) Swelling and bruising may be worse on second or third postoperative day.
  d. Use humidifier at home to prevent drying of mucous membranes.
  e. Force fluids.
F. Skin enhancement and chemosurgery
  1. Purpose
    a. To remove signs of aging and give a youthful appearance
    b. Use of chemical agents to remove or destroy tissue to improve tone and texture of skin
    c. Removal of facial epidermis and part of superficial dermis to correct skin defects
      (1) Acne or depressed scarring
      (2) Wrinkles
      (3) Irregular skin pigmentation
  2. Procedures
    a. Chemical peels
      (1) Phenol: creates a controllable superficial thickness burn
      (2) Trichloroacetic acid: medium depth peel causing temporary blanching of skin
      (3) Alphahydroxy acid ("fruit peel"): Better choice for "sensitive" skin because it causes less irritation and photosensitivity postapplication
      (4) Retin A: Common topical treatment for acne
    b. Dermabrasion
      (1) Helpful for skin resurfacing: to make the skin smoother, improve mild pigmentation problems, reduce pore size and treat acne, and give skin a smoother contour
      (2) Uses sanding with microparticles or rotating wire brushes on skin
    c. Collagen injections: injections of autologous or bovine collagen to enhance or remodel skin and tissue appearance
      (1) Scar revisions
      (2) Lip enhancement
      (3) Minor facial corrections
  3. Perianesthesia care
    a. Anesthesia—usually local, general if combined with total facial resurfacing
    b. Provide comfort measures.
      (1) NSAIDs helpful
      (2) Pain can be mild to moderate.
        (a) Ice to affected area or cold gel mask decreases discomfort and swelling.
    c. Elevate head of bed.
    d. Continue prophylactic antibiotics and antiviral agents as ordered.
    e. Skin care will vary according to physician preference.

4. Education
   a. Activity
      (1) Elevate head of bed.
      (2) Minimize facial movement to decrease cracking of dead tissue.
   b. Skin and dressing care per physician's preference.
      (1) Avoid picking or scratching of skin.
      (2) Expect erythema.
      (3) Expect mild weeping serous fluid.
   c. Continue antiviral and antibiotic agents if ordered.
      (1) Application of antibiotic or hydrocortisone ointments or powders if indicated
   d. Observe and report any signs of infection.
   e. Encourage patient to call office with any questions on skin care.
   f. Instruct patient to avoid sun while skin is healing.
      (1) When healed, use at least a sun protection factor (SPF) 15 sunscreen.
   g. Instruct patient to notify physician if any hyperpigmentation changes are noted.
      (1) Face will remain pink for 4 to 6 weeks.
      (2) Camouflage makeup is helpful.
G. Laser resurfacing
   1. Purpose
      a. To remove signs of aging and give a youthful appearance
      b. Removal of facial epidermis and part of superficial dermis to correct skin defects
         (1) Acne or depressed scarring
         (2) Wrinkles and sun damaged skin
         (3) Irregular skin pigmentation: Freckles, liver spots, keratoses
   2. Procedure
      a. Short blasts of invisible light vaporizes a thin layer of epidermis.
         (1) CO_2 and Er:YAG lasers remove the epidermis.
         (2) Nd:YAG penetrates more deeply to dermis.
         (3) Pulsed-dye laser and intense pulse light both stimulate collagen growth and improve skin's appearance with less blanching.
      b. The deeper the laser penetrates, the more lines and wrinkles will be removed.
      c. Penetration that is too deep will cause scarring.
      d. Contraindicated in dark-skinned people
   3. Perianesthesia care
      a. Anesthesia—local or general
      b. Provide comfort measures.
         (1) Medicate with narcotics as needed.
            (a) NSAIDs helpful
         (2) Pain can be mild to severe.
            (a) Ice to affected area or cold gel mask decreases discomfort and swelling.
      c. Elevate head of bed.
      d. Continue prophylactic antibiotics and antiviral agents as ordered.
      e. Provide nourishment through a straw.
      f. Full face resurfacing will cause swelling around the mouth.
      g. A child's toothbrush can assist with mouth care.
      h. Skin care will vary according to physician preference.
         (1) Open technique (no dressing)
            (a) Cool saline compresses on the face for the first night
            (b) On day one, four times per day, vinegar and water soaks with gentle removal of crusts
            (c) Frequent application of petroleum jelly, antibiotic ointment, Aquaphor, or Preparation H
            (d) Goal is to keep skin soft, pink, and free of crusts.

> > > (e) Soaks are continued until the crusting ceases (7 to 10 days), then a moisturizer is used.
> > (2) Closed technique
> > > (a) Flexan (biomembrane dressing) is applied to the affected area.
> > > > (i) Any exposed areas are treated with the open technique.
> > > > (ii) Flexan dressing is changed according to the physician's preference.
> > > (b) N-terface dressing can be applied to affected areas.
> > > > (i) It is held in place with tube gauze and 4×4 inch bandages to absorb drainage.
> > > > (ii) Soaks may be done through the dressing, and application of petroleum jelly or other lubricant is put on over the dressing.
> > > > (iii) N-terface is changed according to physician's preference.

4. Education
   a. Activity
      (1) Elevate head of bed.
   b. Skin and dressing care per physician's preference
      (1) Laser resurfacing patients require reassurance and reinforcement of skin care instructions.
      (2) Avoid picking or scratching of skin.
      (3) Expect erythema.
      (4) Expect weeping serous fluid.
   c. Continue antiviral and antibiotic agents as ordered.
      (1) Application of antibiotic or hydrocortisone ointments or powders if indicated
   d. Observe and report any signs of infection.
   e. Encourage patient to call office with any questions on skin care.
   f. Instruct patient to avoid sun while skin is healing.
      (1) When healed, use at least an SPF 15 sunscreen.
   g. Instruct patient to notify physician if any hyperpigmentation changes are noted.
      (1) Face will remain pink for 4 to 6 weeks.
      (2) Camouflage makeup is helpful.
   h. Pain management

IV. Reconstructive: General
   A. Cleft lip and palate
      1. Purpose
         a. Repair of congenital cleft lip or palate defects
         b. Repair of congenital defects from early closure of sutures (craniosynostosis)
         c. Repair of congenital maxillofacial deformities
         d. Obtain nostril symmetry and Cupid's bow of upper lip, and repair lip muscle.
            (1) Commonly performed when child (rule of 10s):
               (a) Is at least 10 weeks old
               (b) Weighs at least 10 pounds (4500 g)
               (c) Has a hemoglobin of 10 g/dl
      2. Procedure
         a. May require extensive skeletal reconstruction
         b. May be performed in staged procedures
      3. Perianesthesia care
         a. Anesthesia—general
         b. Position side to side, never prone.
         c. Avoid crying and restlessness that strain suture lines.
            (1) Allow parents to hold the child.
            (2) Offer cool compresses to suture areas to reduce swelling and promote comfort.

      d. Monitor for bleeding.
        (1) Swelling or hematoma at lip
        (2) Excessive swallowing
      e. Maintain in elbow extension splints to protect incisions.
      f. Gentle oral suctioning with soft-tip catheter
      g. Provide mist humidifiers if possible to keep airway moist.
      h. Maintain elevation of head of bed to decrease intracranial pressure.
      i. Place on seizure precautions.
      j. Minimize activities that increase intracranial pressure.
        (1) Crying in children
        (2) Straining
      k. Medicate to provide comfort but not enough to mask neurologic symptoms.
    4. Education
      a. Feeding routines by physician preference
      b. Pain management
  B. Genitourinary
    1. Purpose
      a. Surgical interventions for "intersex" children
        (1) The most frequent disorder is genital ambiguity (congenital adrenal hyperplasia).
        (2) Highly controversial circumstance concerning the appropriate developmental stage to pursue intervention
      b. Sex reassignment surgery for transsexual individuals
    2. Procedure
      a. Surgical restructuring of genitalia
        (1) Feminizing genitalia involves clitoral reduction and/or vaginoplasty.
        (2) Penile reconstruction
    3. Perianesthesia care
      a. Same as any major genitourinary procedure
    4. Education
      a. Patients and family require extensive counseling and education regarding treatment options and to address any underlying issues of self-esteem and psychological stress.
  C. Hand surgery
    1. Purpose
      a. To correct deformities of the hand
      b. To restore function
    2. Procedures
      a. Ganglionectomy: Excision of painful fluid-filled cyst attached to a joint capsule or tendon
      b. Palmar fasciectomy: Release of flexion contractures of the metacarpophalangeal joints
      c. Carpal tunnel release: Decompression of the carpal tunnel releasing pressure on the median nerve
        (1) May be done open or endoscopically
      d. Trauma repair: May involve open reduction, internal fixation (ORIF) of fractures or microvascular surgery
    3. Perianesthesia care
      a. Anesthesia: Local, axillary or bier block, general
      b. Assess extremity for circulation and neurologic status.
        (1) Include sensory, motor, color, and capillary refill.
      c. Apply temporary sling after axillary block.
      d. Elevate extremity above level of heart using pillows.
      e. Provide adequate analgesia.
        (1) Consider multimodal therapies.
      f. Maintain patency of drains.

    4. Education

      a. Activity restrictions as directed

      b. Maintain elevation of affected limb.

      c. Observe for changes in circulation and neurologic status.

      d. Teach signs and symptoms of infection.

D. Microvascular surgery

    1. Purpose

      a. Generally employed to replant severed body parts

    2. Procedure

      a. Tedious anastomosis of severed blood vessels, nerves, and other injured structures

      b. Reconstruction of absent digits using transplanted body parts

        (1) Example: reconstruction of absent finger using patient's toe

    3. Perianesthesia care

      a. Procedure-specific care

        (1) Special attention given to observation of skin color at operative site

          (a) White indicates no blood is perfusing to area because of arterial obstruction.

          (b) Pink is normal.

          (c) Blue indicates hypoxemia in the tissues.

          (d) Dark blue to black indicates impending tissue infarct from venous obstruction.

      b. Often require posttraumatic counseling

    4. Education

      a. Procedure-specific and site-specific patient education to include but not be limited to activity, pain management, and wound care.

E. Scar revisions (Z-plasty, V-plasty)

    1. Purpose

      a. Remove or reduce scar tissue.

    2. Procedure

      a. Z-plasty

        (1) Use of Z-shaped incision to remove scar tissue

        (2) Requires tissue with elasticity

      b. V-plasty

        (1) Used to repair skin defects

        (2) Two triangular flaps of adjacent skin transposed

      c. Laser therapy can be used.

      d. All procedures can be offered in combination.

    3. Perianesthesia care

      a. Anesthesia—local or general

      b. Wound and dressing assessments to observe for hematoma formation

      c. Analgesia as required

      d. Minimal activity involving operative site to reduce tension on operative sutures

    4. Education

      a. Signs and symptoms of infection

      b. Activity restrictions

      c. Pain management

F. Skin lesions

    1. Purpose

      a. Removal of skin lesions whether benign or malignant

        (1) Benign skin lesions

          (a) Nevus

            (i) Most common skin lesion

              [a] Round

              [b] Brown or black in color

              [c] Flat or raised

              [d] With or without hair

(ii) Three types
    [a] Intradermal
    [b] Junctional
    [c] Compound
        [1] Most need no treatment unless a change is noted or if there is constant irritation.
        [2] Junctional may convert to malignant melanoma.
(2) Malignant skin lesions
  (a) Basal cell carcinoma
    (i) Most common skin cancer
    (ii) May be nodular with an ulcerated center or crusted, dermatitis-like
  (b) Squamous cell carcinoma
    (i) Begins as a red papule
    (ii) Progresses to an area that ulcerates, then crusts
    (iii) Invades underlying tissue
  (c) Malignant melanoma
    (i) Suspicious lesions with
      [a] Change in size
      [b] Change in color (brown to black)
      [c] Change from smooth to rough
      [d] Irregular borders
      [e] Change in sensation
      [f] Satellite lesions

2. Procedure
  a. Simple excision
  b. Laser therapy
  c. Wide excision, possible flap graft, node dissection, radiation, topical chemotherapy, or cryosurgery

3. Perianesthesia care
  a. Anesthesia—local or general
  b. Provide reassurance, and allow patient to verbalize any fears or concerns regarding body image, diagnosis, and so forth.
  c. Elevated extremities
  d. Monitor dressings and assess for hematoma.
  e. Position for comfort.

4. Education
  a. Teach patient proper dressing and wound care per physician preference.
  b. Protect healing incisions from sun.
  c. Minimize activity of affected areas for 1-2 weeks.
  d. Encourage proper follow-up care to monitor for new lesions.

V. Reconstructive: Breast
  A. Breast reconstruction
    1. Purpose
      a. Breast reconstruction following wide local excision and mastectomy for breast cancer to achieve breast symmetry
      b. Repair of traumatic injury
      c. Repair of defects from cancer treatment
    2. Procedure
      a. Insertion of breast implants
        (1) Creation of a pocket space under remaining breast tissues into which a soft prosthetic breast implant can be placed
        (2) Pocket can be created by means of inflatable tissue expander used to gradually increase the volume of pocket space to receive prosthesis.
      b. Transplantation of skin, muscle, and blood supply from autologous donor site to repair congenital or acquired tissue defects

(1) Flaps or tissue transfer
    (a) At time of procedure, absence of infection is required at recipient site.
    (b) Donor muscle or skin for flap is selected to appropriately fit defect and minimally impact patient's activity and function after removal.
        (i) Muscle size will decrease at recipient site after denervation.
    (c) Pedicle flap (delayed) flap is selected to reach defect comfortably.
    (d) Preparation of recipient vessels
        (i) Devitalized tissue carefully removed
        (ii) Selection of recipient blood vessels that have been minimally impacted by trauma of defect
    (e) Anastomosis of vessels
        (i) Avoid twisting of vessels.
        (ii) Vessels must be delicately handled.
        (iii) Use of heparin-containing irrigating solutions

(2) Types of flaps
    (a) Delayed flap
        (i) Donor tissue attached to recipient site without being separated from its blood supply
        (ii) Remains attached to donor site (by pedicle) until recipient circulation is established
    (b) Local flaps
        (i) Moved from location immediately adjacent to defect
        (ii) Maintains blood supply from original source
    (c) Free flap
        (i) Entire tissue and blood supply detached from donor site
        (ii) Requires prolonged microsurgery (6 to 12 hours)

(3) Common sources of flaps
    (a) Skin flaps
        (i) Consists of skin and subcutaneous tissue
        (ii) May be placed to a remote area by means of pedicle
        (iii) May be advanced into a defect close to the donor site or moved at a pivotal point and rotated into the tissue defect
        (iv) Sources
            [a] Temporalis fascia: may be used to cover dorsum of hand or foot
            [b] Lateral forearm: skin and fascia used to cover areas requiring a thicker coverage
            [c] Omentum: for areas that require pliable tissue (e.g., frontal sinuses)
    (b) Muscle and myocutaneous flaps
        (i) Movement of muscle with or without skin to cover defect
            [a] Local transfer
            [b] Free transfer
        (ii) May require additional skin grafting at recipient site
        (iii) Sources
            [a] Latissimus dorsi
            [b] Pectoralis major
            [c] Tensor fascia lata
            [d] Rectus abdominus
            [e] Gluteus maximus
            [f] Gracilis

3. Perianesthesia care
  a. Anesthesia—general
  b. Monitor for and prevent factors that promote vasospasm and thrombosis.
    (1) Hypothermia
        (a) Results in vasoconstriction

       (b) Arterial flow compromised

       (c) Use warming blankets, lights, warmed fluids, increased room temperature.

    (2) Hypotension

    (3) Hypovolemia

       (a) Large blood loss may have occurred.

       (b) Replacement with crystalloids and colloids

       (c) Excessive red cell replacement may raise hematocrit, causing sluggish capillary flow.

    (4) Agents that increase vasoconstriction and vasospasm (e.g., nicotine, caffeine)

  c. Maintenance of normal body temperature

    (1) Warmed intravenous and irrigating fluids

    (2) Room temperature regulation

    (3) Warming blankets

  d. Assess condition of flap.

    (1) Skin temperature

       (a) Should be warm to touch

       (b) Coolness reflects reduced blood flow.

    (2) Capillary refill

       (a) Blanching within 2 seconds

       (b) Rapid blanching may indicate venous engorgement.

       (c) Delayed blanching may indicate arterial insufficiency.

       (d) Arterial and venous flow may be obtained by Doppler ultrasonography and are marked by surgeon with a marker or suture.

       (e) Venous congestion frequently results in failure before arterial insufficiency.

    (3) Color

       (a) Normally white or gray immediately postoperatively

       (b) Increasingly pale flaps suggest arterial insufficiency.

       (c) Bluish color suggests venous congestion.

       (d) Color of flap may be different from other skin in recipient area if obtained from tissue far removed.

    (4) Edema

       (a) Slight swelling is expected.

       (b) Significant swelling may indicate hematoma or venous congestion.

    (5) Monitor drainage from drains every 30 to 60 minutes.

       (a) Gentle continuous suction

       (b) Greater than 50 ml/hour is problematic.

    (6) Monitor muscle donor site for bleeding

    (7) Antiplatelets or anticoagulants may be used to decrease platelet aggregation and thrombosis.

       (a) Low–molecular weight dextran

       (b) Heparin drip

       (c) Aspirin

    (8) Flap failure is usually caused by inadequate circulation or infection.

       (a) Prevent patient from lying on operative site.

       (b) Prevent compression of operative site by blankets.

    (9) Patient care for patient with tissue expander or prosthetic implant same as augmentation mammoplasty

       (a) When expansion complete

         (i) Prosthesis inserted

         (ii) Nipple reconstruction done

         (iii) Nipple tattoo or graft reconstruction

       (b) Pain can be severe with initial insertion of expander.

        e. Anesthesia—general

        f. Psychological support crucial as patients have had multiple procedures and cancer diagnosis

    4. Education

        a. Observe for hematoma formation.

        b. Report deflation of tissue expander.

          (1) Could mean rupture

        c. Limit arm activity for 1 month.

        d. Frequent appointments required for inflation of expander with saline

B. Reduction mammoplasty

    1. Purpose

        a. Removal of excess breast mass to decrease neck, back, and shoulder pain

        b. To improve body image and self confidence

        c. May be performed to correct severe asymmetry as in Poland's syndrome

    2. Procedure

        a. Surgical excision of redundant breast tissue and skin with recontouring of breast shape

        b. Areolar transplantation can be done through free tissue transfer to pedicle.

        c. On occasion, areola may be replaced as free graft resulting in loss of breast-feeding abilities and sensation.

    3. Perianesthesia care

        a. Anesthesia—general

        b. Assess for hematoma.

          (1) Palpate superior aspect of pectoralis muscle over the third rib to the clavicle.

        c. Drains may be used postoperatively.

          (1) Monitor drainage.

          (2) Reinforce to keep clothing and bedding dry.

        d. Treat pain.

          (1) Usually described as moderate

          (2) May need IV narcotic on emergence

            (a) Control with strong narcotics at home (e.g., oxycodone for first day or two).

        e. Surgical bra or compression dressing applied postoperatively to maintain new breast contour and decrease fluid accumulation; compression bra

          (1) Tube gauze over the bra assists in holding reinforcement ABD pads in place.

        f. Prevent and treat nausea and vomiting.

          (1) Vomiting can cause hematoma formation.

        g. Provide aggressive fluid replacement for blood loss.

          (1) Usual blood loss, 400 ml

          (2) Replace with crystalloid or colloid as needed.

          (3) Some patients may require hospitalization if symptomatic after blood loss and fluid replacement.

    4. Education

        a. Observe for hematoma formation.

        b. Activity

          (1) No heavy lifting or strenuous activity for 1 month

          (2) No pushing self up with arms

          (3) Instruct patient and caregiver on how to make position changes.

        c. Usually a return appointment in 24 hours for drain removal

        d. Steristrips or sutures may be removed in 1 week.

        e. Compression bra for 2 to 3 weeks

          (1) Demonstrate how to reinforce dressing.

OVERVIEW OF BURNS

I. Anatomy and physiology
- A. Overview of burn injury
  - 1. Function of skin
    - a. Largest organ of the body
    - b. First line of defense against trauma and infection
    - c. Retention of body fluids
    - d. Regulation of body temperature
      - (1) Vasoconstriction and vasodilation
      - (2) Evaporation of water
    - e. Secretion and excretion
      - (1) Secretion of oil from sebaceous glands to lubricate skin, preventing cracks and organism invasion
      - (2) Excretion of water, sodium chloride, cholesterol, and urea from sweat glands
    - f. Metabolizes and produces vitamin D
    - g. Sensation and communication
      - (1) Pressure, pain, touch, temperature
      - (2) Reaction to environmental stimuli
    - h. Generates new skin
      - (1) Contributes to self-image
  - 2. Anatomy of the skin
    - a. The largest organ of the body
    - b. Structure of the skin
      - (1) Epidermis
        - (a) Outermost layer
          - (i) Made up of five layers
            - [a] Stratum corneum
            - [b] Stratum lucidum
            - [c] Stratum granulosum
            - [d] Stratum spinosum
            - [e] Stratum germinativum
        - (b) Surface and deepest layers of most importance in burn care
        - (c) Stratum corneum
          - (i) Dead keratinized cells
          - (ii) Provides vapor barrier and protects body from microorganisms and chemical irritants
        - (d) Stratum germinativum
          - (i) Regenerates epithelial covering
          - (ii) Necessary for spontaneous healing
        - (e) Blood supplied by dermis
        - (f) Lines skin appendages (e.g., sebaceous glands, sweat glands, and hair follicles)
        - (g) New skin can be generated from lining of skin appendages even if epidermis is destroyed.
        - (h) Varies in thickness
          - (i) Thickest at soles of feet, palms, scapula
          - (ii) Thinnest at eyelids
      - (2) Dermis—true skin
        - (a) Outer layer
          - (i) Varies in thickness—thickest over soles of feet and thinnest over eyelids
          - (ii) Contains nerve endings, capillaries, and the lymph system
          - (iii) Composed of connective tissue and collagen
        - (b) Subcutaneous tissue
          - (i) Contains adipose tissue and connective tissue

(ii) Attached to dermis by collagen

(iii) Holds burn tissue (eschar) tightly, making eschar removal difficult

(c) Deep fascia—surrounds muscle and bone

(i) Connects periosteum to bone

(ii) Skin also includes hair, nails, and sweat and sebaceous glands.

B. Determining severity of burn injury

    1. Size of percent of body surface involved (TBSA, or total body surface area)

      a. Rule of 9s (Figure 52-1)

        (1) Body areas divided into equal multiples of 9

        (2) Head and each arm equal 9%.

        (3) Chest, back, and leg equal 18% each.

        (4) Perineum equals 1%.

      b. Berkow's method, or Lund and Browder chart

        (1) Used for children

        (2) Adjusts for differences in body part sizes between adults and children

          (a) Head in child <2 years equals 18%.

          (b) Each leg in child <2 years equals 13%.

      c. One percent method

        (1) Used for quick assessment

        (2) Palmar surface of patient's hand equals approximately 1% TBSA.

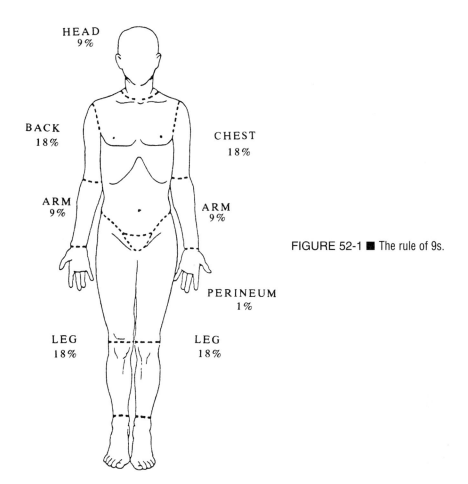

FIGURE 52-1 ■ The rule of 9s.

    d. Major burn injury
        (1) Adults
            (a) Greater than 25% TBSA: partial-thickness burn, age <40 years
            (b) Greater than 20% TBSA: partial-thickness burn, age >40 years
            (c) Greater than 10% TBSA: full-thickness burn
        (2) Children
            (a) Greater than 20% TBSA: partial-thickness burn
            (b) Greater than 10% TBSA: full-thickness burn
        (3) Other factors
            (a) Burns of face, eyes, ears, hands, feet, and perineum
            (b) Electrical burns
            (c) Burns complicated by inhalation injury or major trauma
            (d) Patients' preexisting diseases may impact recovery (e.g., diabetes, congestive heart failure).

C. Depth of injury
   1. Superficial injury (first degree)
     a. Affects epidermis only
     b. Appearance: skin intact, red, blanches
     c. Painful
     d. Healing time: 2 to 10 days
     e. Causes: flash burns, sunburn
   2. Partial-thickness injury (second degree)
     a. Affects epidermis and part of dermis, leaving skin appendages intact
     b. Levels
        (1) Superficial partial-thickness: affects upper layers of dermis
        (2) Deep partial-thickness:
            (a) Affects lower layers of dermis
            (b) May convert to full-thickness injury
     c. Appearance
        (1) Superficial partial-thickness: red, moist, blistered, blanches
        (2) Deep partial-thickness: deep red, moist, areas of white or yellow tissue, delayed capillary refill
     d. Very painful
     e. Healing time
        (1) If affecting outer layers of dermis, 5 to 21 days
        (2) If affecting deeper layers of dermis, 21 to 35 days
            (a) May convert to full-thickness burn in first few days after burn
            (b) May require skin grafting
     f. Causes: scald, flame, chemicals
   3. Full-thickness injury (third degree)
     a. Affects epidermis and entire dermis and may extend to subcutaneous tissue, muscle, or bone
     b. Appearance: hard, dry, leathery; color may be black, tan, white; nonblanching
     c. Minimal to no pain
     d. Healing time: requires excision and skin grafting
     e. Causes: flame, scald, chemicals, electrical, contact with hot surfaces

D. Part of body involved
   1. Specific areas of body have significant impact on healing, cosmetic appearance, and function.
   2. Head, face, and chest burns significantly related to respiratory function
   3. Hand, face, and feet burns significantly related to cosmetics and function
   4. Perineal burns significantly related to infection
   5. Circumferential burns significant because of compromised circulation

E. Burning agent
   1. Scald
     a. Most common type of burn, especially in children
     b. Caused by immersion, splash, or steam

    2. Flame and flash burns
        a. Second most common type of burn
        b. Commonly associated with smoke inhalation
        c. Frequently full thickness in nature
        d. From house fires, kerosene or gasoline ignition
    3. Contact burns
        a. Area burned is well defined in appearance in shape of item contacted.
        b. May occur from hot metal, asphalt, or sand
    4. Chemical burns
        a. Less than 10% of all injuries
        b. Acid or alkali
        c. May be topical or ingested
        d. More commonly from industrial accidents
    5. Electrical
        a. Least common
        b. May cause significant internal or external damage
        c. Direct current or alternating current
        d. Alternating current more dangerous than direct current because of increased risk for cardiopulmonary arrest
        e. Cataracts may occur 1 to 2 days to 3 years after burn.
        f. May require extensive reconstructive surgery (e.g., myocutaneous flaps)
 F. Age of victim
    1. Higher mortality in patients less than 2 years or older than 60 years
    2. Thinness of skin in very young and very old makes injury more likely.
    3. Changes in immune status alter ability to heal.
 G. Preexisting medical conditions that impair healing process
    1. Cardiovascular disease
    2. Diabetes
    3. Pulmonary disease: asthma, chronic obstructive pulmonary diseases (COPD)
 H. Other associated injuries at time of burn that might affect healing
    1. Smoke inhalation
    2. Traumatic injury (e.g., fractures, closed head injury)
    3. Need for tracheostomy significantly increases mortality risk.
II. Physiologic changes after burn injury
 A. Burn shock
    1. Massive fluid and protein shifts from intravascular space to interstitium
        a. Vasodilation, increased capillary permeability, and altered cell membrane at injury site
        b. Hypovolemic shock occurs because of volume loss.
        c. Edema of tissues occurs from increased capillary permeability.
    2. Hypovolemia stage lasts for first 48 hours after injury.
    3. Sodium and protein lost from intravascular space into interstitium
 B. Hypothermia
    1. Loss of water and heat by evaporation
    2. Loss of skin's ability to vasoconstrict or vasodilate in response to environmental temperature
 C. Cardiovascular
    1. Decreased cardiac output related to hypothermia, uncompensated hypovolemia, and release of myocardial depressant factor
    2. Catecholamine release from stress response causes vasoconstriction and increases systemic vascular resistance.
    3. Potential for decreased organ perfusion exists.
 D. Pulmonary
    1. Potential airway obstruction from edema of face and neck
    2. Decreased chest wall compliance if chest expansion is impaired by chest burns
    3. Bronchopulmonary mucosal damage from smoke inhalation

    E. Metabolic
       1. Hypermetabolic state occurs as result of stress response.
       2. Patient develops catabolic state.
    F. Immunologic
       1. Postburn immunosuppression occurs from changes in humoral and cell-mediated immunity.
       2. Loss of skin as first line of defense
    G. Hematologic
       1. Potential red cell hemolysis from thermal injury
       2. Decreased coagulation ability from loss of clotting factors into interstitium
    H. Gastrointestinal
       1. Development of paralytic ileus
       2. Prone to stress ulcer development
    I. Renal failure
       1. Related to inadequate fluid resuscitation
       2. Related to myoglobinuria from muscle damage in electrical and severe flame burns

COMMON SURGICAL BURN PROCEDURES

  I. Escharotomy
    A. Indicated for circumferential full-thickness burns
       1. Burn eschar acts as tourniquet.
          a. Decreases arterial flow
          b. Causes venous congestion
       2. Common sites are extremities or trunk.
    B. Linear incisions placed extending through burn eschar down to superficial fascia releasing constriction
    C. May be performed with or without anesthesia
       1. Nerve endings in eschar are dead.
       2. Premedication to relieve anxiety and discomfort
  II. Excision and skin grafting
    A. Goal is to restore function and maximize cosmetic appearance.
       1. Performed in burns with limited or inability to heal
       2. May require grafting months to years after injury to revise scar tissue
       3. Principles of grafting similar for burns and nonburn wounds requiring skin coverage
    B. Nonviable tissue removed
    C. Graft sources
       1. Autograft
          a. Patient's own skin used
          b. Permanent
       2. Cultured autologous human epithelium
          a. Biopsy of patient's skin obtained
          b. Skin grown in petri dish and then grafted to patient
       3. Homograft (allograft)
          a. Skin obtained from another human
          b. Fresh cadaver
             (1) Provides a temporary covering to excised tissue awaiting permanent grafting
             (2) May be placed over a widely meshed autograft to promote graft take
             (3) Patient will eventually reject.
          c. Processed human dermis (AlloDerm)
             (1) Donated skin processed to remove components that cause rejection
                (a) Epidermis removed
                (b) Cells that contain antigen targets for rejection removed
                (c) Tissue (dermal matrix) freeze dried for storage

          (2) Procedure
             (a) Wound excised
             (b) AlloDerm applied to wound bed
             (c) Thin autograft applied over AlloDerm
    4. Skin substitutes
        a. Integra
          (1) Bilaminate skin substitute
             (a) Dermal analog of collagen fibers
             (b) Epidermal analog is Silastic membrane.
          (2) Applied to excised wound
             (a) Dermal analog develops vasculature.
             (b) Silastic membrane removed after dermal vascularity established (approximately 2 weeks)
             (c) Thin autograft applied after Silastic membrane is removed
          (3) Requires a two-step process
             (a) Excision and application of Integra
             (b) Removal of Silastic membrane and autograft
        b. Biobrane
          (1) Synthetic polymer dressing
          (2) Porcine collagen base with nylon covering
          (3) Placed over excised tissue
          (4) Patient's dermis binds with collagen base.
          (5) Biobrane removed after dermal healing
          (6) Patient must have capacity for dermal regeneration.
          (7) May be placed over donor sites
    5. Heterograft (xenograft)
        a. Tissue from another species, usually pigskin
        b. Temporary covering over excised wounds
III. Primary closure
    A. May be used for small burns
    B. Burn tissue is excised and closed primarily.

INTRAOPERATIVE CONSIDERATIONS FOR THE BURN PATIENT

  I. Surgical concerns
    A. Minimize physiologic stress experienced by patient.
        1. Limit operative time to 2-hour to 3-hour sessions.
        2. Limit excision to 20% of total body surface at any one operative session.
    B. Selection of donor sites
        1. Preferred sites: thighs, buttock, abdomen, back, scalp
        2. Best color match if skin is obtained from area near burn
    C. Types of grafts
        1. Split-thickness skin graft
          a. Donor skin contains epidermis and part of dermis.
          b. Thickness: 0.012-inch
          c. Graft "takes" as capillaries grow in from granulation bed into graft (begins to occur after 48 hours).
          d. Donor site reepithelializes in 10 to 14 days and may be ready as donor site again in 21 days (scalp donor sites may heal in 7 days).
        2. Full-thickness graft
          a. Entire epidermis and dermis used as donor
          b. Used to cover deep defects, tendons, bone
          c. Requires split-thickness skin graft on donor area from which full-thickness skin was removed
          d. Less hyperpigmentation and contractures than with split-thickness skin graft

    3. Mesh graft
      a. Split-thickness skin graft in which donor skin is passed through mesher to produce slits in skin
      b. Allows for donor skin to be stretched covering large area
        (1) May be meshed 1.5 to 3 times original size
        (2) Useful in large burns
      c. Meshing helps prevent fluid or blood from accumulating under graft, which prevents "take."
      d. Less cosmetically perfect than sheet graft
    4. Sheet graft
      a. Split-thickness skin graft placed on wound without meshing
      b. Provides better cosmetic result, especially for hands, face, and neck
      c. Fluid and blood can accumulate under graft, affecting "take."
  D. Burn wound excision
    1. Tangential (sequential) excision
      a. Sequential removal of tissue until viable dermis is reached
      b. Provides optimal functional and cosmetic result
      c. Large blood loss may occur.
      d. May be difficult to determine end point of excision—too much or too little may be excised
    2. Fascial excision
      a. Used in deep full-thickness burns that may extend into fat or underlying tissues
      b. Tissue is sharply dissected to fascia.
      c. Blood loss is less than if tangentially excised.
      d. Easier to determine end point of excision
      e. Risk of injury to nerves, joints, tendons
      f. Results in cosmetic defects
  E. Control of bleeding
    1. Patient may have considerable blood loss.
    2. Controlled with thrombin, epinephrine soaks, electrocautery
    3. Hemostasis must be obtained before graft is placed.
  F. Factors promoting graft "take."
    1. Hemostasis
    2. Graft secured and immobilized
    3. Prevention of infection
    4. Good nutrition
II. Anesthesia concerns
  A. Anesthetic agents
    1. Pharmacokinetics may be altered because of physiologic changes that occur after major burn injury.
    2. Serum protein levels decrease, making agents that bind to albumin more pharmacologically active.
    3. Narcotic anesthesia amounts may be high because of developed tolerance.
    4. Amount of cardiac depression must be weighed if inhalation agents are used.
    5. Increased sensitivity to depolarizing neuromuscular blocking agents occurs and may result in hyperkalemic response.
      a. Succinylcholine use contraindicated because of hyperkalemic response
    6. Hyposensitivity to nondepolarizing neuromuscular blocking agents
  B. Ventilatory needs
    1. Intubation may be difficult because of burns of face and neck or limited oral mobility requiring use of fiber optic bronchoscope.
    2. Hypermetabolic response results in increased oxygen consumption and carbon dioxide production.
    3. Chest wall compliance may be decreased if chest burns are present.
    4. Ventilation/perfusion mismatches may occur with pulmonary injuries.

      5. Patient may need increased minute ventilation because of hypermetabolic state and positive end-expiratory pressure (PEEP).

      6. Monitor oxygen saturation and end-tidal carbon dioxide.

  C. Prevention of hypothermia

      1. Room temperature maintained at 85° F

      2. Use of warming blankets and warmed fluids

      3. Temperature monitoring

      4. Warmed inspired gases

  D. Maintaining hemodynamic stability

      1. May be prone to hypotension because of position changes as donor skin is obtained and burn wound is prepared

      2. Fluid loss through evaporation and bleeding

        a. Replacement with red blood cells and fresh frozen plasma

        b. Crystalloids to maintain adequate urine output without giving excess salt

  E. Fluid resuscitation criteria

      1. Calculated fluid requirements for first 24 to 48 hours after injury

      2. Thermal injuries uncommonly taken to operating room during burn shock period (first 24 to 48 hours)

        a. Early excision after 24 hours to begin wound coverage to decrease metabolic rate and decrease wound infection

      3. Calculated requirements (Parkland formula)

        a. 4 ml/kg per TBSA percent of injury

        b. One half of calculated requirements given over first 8 hours from time of injury

        c. One half of calculated requirements given over next 16 hours

        d. Fluids adjusted to maintain urinary output

          (1) Adult: 0.5 to 1 ml/kg per hour

          (2) Children: 1 to 2 ml/kg per hour

      4. Fluids used

        a. Isotonic crystalloid

          (1) Normal saline

          (2) Lactated Ringer's

        b. Hypertonic saline may be used.

          (1) Increases osmotic pull back to intravascular space

          (2) Decreases total fluid requirements and assists to minimize edema formation

        c. Colloids rarely used in first 12 hours after burn injury because of increased capillary permeability

      5. Electrical injury fluid requirements

        a. More difficult to estimate fluid needs

        b. Injury greater internally than what is seen externally

        c. Calculate on the basis of Parkland formula.

        d. Adjust fluids to maintain urinary output of 75 to 100 ml/hour in adults or 2 to 3 ml/kg per hour in children.

        e. Add sodium bicarbonate to alkalinize urine, promoting myoglobin excretion.

        f. Administer mannitol to increase urinary flow, promoting myoglobin excretion.

      6. Inadequate fluid resuscitation is primary cause of death in first 24 to 48 hours after injury.

POSTOPERATIVE CONCERNS FOR THE BURN PATIENT

  I. Airway and ventilatory needs

    A. Upper airway injuries

      1. Caused from heat injury to oronasopharynx and vocal cords

      2. Swelling usually peaks 48 hours after injury.

  3. Edema may lead to obstruction.
  4. Intubation performed early, often prophylactically
  5. If patient is extubated postoperatively, observe for signs of obstruction (e.g., stridor, tachypnea, increased work of breathing, low Sao_2, low Svo_2).
  6. Secure endotracheal tube.
   a. Use ties in patients with face burns.
   b. Tape will not adhere.
   c. Avoid pressure on burned nose or ears.
   d. Monitor ties for constriction as facial swelling increases.
 B. Lower airway injuries
  1. Injuries below glottis are caused by chemical irritants released from smoke.
  2. Lower airway damage results in
   a. Increased airway irritability, laryngospasm, bronchospasm
   b. Bronchiolar edema and impaired airway flow
   c. Increased mucus production caused by chemical irritants
   d. Damage to epithelial lining of bronchial tree and alveolar cells
  3. Management considerations
   a. Frequent assessment of respiratory function and airway patency
    (1) Respiratory effort
    (2) Chest wall expansion and symmetry
    (3) Monitor oxygenation with pulse oximeter and arterial blood gases.
    (4) Monitor end-tidal CO_2
   b. Assess need for bronchodilator therapy.
   c. Assess chest expansion.
    (1) Constriction of nonexcised chest burns
    (2) Constriction of chest dressings
   d. Deep breathing and coughing to facilitate mucus mobilization
   e. Provide for oxygen and ventilatory needs.
    (1) May need increased minute ventilation (rate or tidal volume or both) because of hypermetabolic state
    (2) Humidified oxygen
    (3) Prevent oxygen administration device from applying pressure if grafts have been placed on face or neck.
II. Circulatory function
 A. Blood and fluid loss may be significant.
 B. Monitor for signs of hypovolemia.
  1. Tachycardia
  2. Decreased blood pressure and presence of pulsus paradoxus
  3. Delayed capillary refill
  4. Monitor urinary output.
   a. Maintain 30 to 50 ml/hour in adult
   b. Maintain 1 to 2 ml/kg per hour in children.
 C. Provide fluid replacement.
  1. Isotonic or hypertonic crystalloids
  2. Colloids: red blood cells, fresh frozen plasma, albumin
 D. Monitor circulatory function distal to burn.
  1. Distal to escharotomy sites every 15 to 30 minutes
  2. Assess circulatory compromise caused by constricting dressings or splints.
  3. Assessment
   a. Pulses
   b. Capillary refill
   c. Movement and sensation
   d. Color
III. Infection
 A. Thorough hand washing and gloves are essential.
 B. Prevent cross-contamination with other patients.
 C. Isolation precautions, including gowns, mask, and gloves, may be necessary in large burns.

D. Aseptic wound technique

E. Frequent change of invasive catheters

IV. Temperature control

    A. Assess body temperature every 30 minutes.

    B. Warm fluids and blood products before infusion.

    C. Use heat shields or warming blankets.

    D. Adjust room temperature to 75° to 85° F.

    E. Monitor for ST segment changes caused by myocardial ischemia.

V. Wound care

    A. Monitor graft and donor sites for bleeding.

        1. Grafts will fail if blood collects beneath them.

        2. Dressings usually not changed for first few days.

    B. Monitor status of sheet grafts that do not have dressing.

        1. Assess for fluid and blood collection under graft.

            a. Aspiration of fluid using syringe and small-gauge needle

            b. Remove fluid by "rolling" fluid to edges of graft with cotton tip applicator.

        2. Avoid pressure or shearing.

        3. Antimicrobial ointment may be applied to the edges and seams of graft.

    C. Maintain joint immobility if graft is over joint.

    D. Elevate grafted extremities to minimize edema and promote venous return.

VI. Pain control

    A. Pain is usually more severe at donor site than at grafted areas.

    B. May have high analgesic needs because of previous narcotic needs during wound care

    C. Intravenous administration preferred over intramuscular in large burns because of poor absorption

    D. Avoid aspirin-containing products.

VII. Emotional support for patients and families

    A. Patients and families must deal with change in physical appearance from first day after injury.

    B. Ongoing emotional support required

        1. Change in physical appearance

            a. Long-term results may be uncertain.

            b. Must begin to adjust to fact that even with the best cosmetic results patients will never look the same again

        2. Possible changes in function if severe burns of extremities, hands, feet, face

    C. Surgical procedure may be the first or one of many.

        1. Expectations of each may differ.

        2. May view regrafting as a setback because of graft failure or poor cosmetic result

    D. Provide support appropriate to stage of adjustment that patient or family is experiencing.

    E. Use additional health care workers to assist in support (e.g., child life specialists, clergy, mental health practitioners, social worker).

    F. Priorities of care: life, limbs, looks (in that order)

VIII. Discharge instructions for the ambulatory skin graft patient

    A. Maintain dressing dry and intact.

        1. Donor site dressing may exhibit some bloody drainage.

        2. Avoid getting dressings wet.

    B. Keep grafted area immobile.

        1. Avoid activities that would cause sheer.

        2. Grafts over joint must remain immobile—may have splints in place.

        3. Reinforce weight-bearing status or crutch walking for lower extremity grafts.

        4. Elevate grafted extremity to limit edema.

    C. Pain management

        1. Reinforce that donor site may be more painful.

        2. Instruct on use of prescribed analgesia.

    D. Notify physician of
        1. Temperature >38.5° C (101.3° F)
        2. Numbness, paresthesia of grafted extremity
        3. Pain that is not controlled by analgesia
        4. Bleeding of graft or donor site
    E. Reinforce follow-up instructions.
        1. Dressing usually changed and graft evaluated 3 to 5 days after grafting

BIBLIOGRAPHY

1. Amadio PC: What's new in hand surgery. *J Bone Joint Surg* 83-A(3):473-477, 2001.
2. Ancira M: Chemical peels: An overview. *Plast Surg Nurs* 19(4):179-184, 1999.
3. Anthony ML: Surgical treatment of non-melanoma skin cancer. *AORN J* 71(3): 552-570, 2000.
4. Clark JJ: Wound repair and factors influencing healing. *Crit Care Nurs Q* 25(1):1-12, 2002.
5. Goodman T, editor: *Core curriculum for plastic and reconstructive surgical nurses.* Pitman, NJ: Anthony J Janetti, 1996.
6. Guttman C: Endoscopic approach alternative to facelift. *Dermatol Times* 20(9):30, 1999.
7. Harcourt D, Rumsey N: Psychological aspects of breast reconstruction: A review of the literature. *J Adv Nurs* 35(4):477-487, 2001.
8. Hilton L: What to look for, how to deal with chemical peel complications. *Dermatol Times* 22(9):70, 2001.
9. Johnson D, Whitworth IH: Recent developments in plastic surgery. *BMJ* 325(7359): 319, 2002.
10. Judkins K: Current consensus and controversies in major burns management. *Trauma* 2:239-251, 2000.
11. Kagan RJ: Evaluation and treatment of thermal injuries. *Dermatol Nurs* 12(5): 334-335, 338-344, 347-350, 2000.
12. Li V: Sclerotherapy: Disappearing act for spider veins. *Harv Womens Health Watch* 7(11): 2000.
13. Markey AC: Liposuction in cosmetic dermatology. *Clin Experiment Dermatol* 26:3-5, 2001.
14. Melton L: New perspectives on the management of intersex. *Lancet* 357(927): 2110, 2001.
15. Moran SL, Herceg S, Kurtelawicz K, et al: TRAM flap breast reconstruction with expanders and implants. *AORN J* 71(2): 354-368, 2001.
16. Nelson DB, Dilloway MA: Principles, products, and practical aspects of wound care. *Crit Care Nurs Q* 25(1):33-54, 2002.
17. Putting on a new face: Laser resurfacing. *Harv Womens Health Watch* 9(5):4, 2002.
18. Quinn DM: *Ambulatory surgical nursing core curriculum.* Philadelphia: WB Saunders, 1999.

53 Podiatric Surgery

LINDA BOYUM

OBJECTIVES

At the conclusion of this chapter the reader will be able to:

1. Identify the skeletal structure of the foot.

2. Incorporate specific physical and psychosocial changes into the assessment of persons with foot disease.

3. Understand operative procedures of the foot.

4. Prioritize postanesthesia care to be provided following surgical procedures on the foot.

The foot is the terminal portion of the lower extremity. It is a complex combination of bones, joints, ligaments, and tendons working as one.

I. Anatomy and physiology of the skeletal structure of the foot (see Figure 53-1)
   A. Bony structure—7 tarsal, 5 metatarsal, 14 phalanges
      1. Tarsals—seven bones of the ankle, hind foot and midfoot
         a. Talus—irregularly shaped bone
            (1) Located between bimalleolar fork and tarsus
            (2) Ligament attachments, no tendons
         b. Calcaneus
            (1) Largest bone in foot
         c. Cuboid
            (1) Wedge shaped
         d. Scaphoid (navicular)
            (1) Bound with ligaments
         e. Three cuneiforms
            (1) Interposed between scaphoid, first three metatarsals, and cuboid
            (2) Wedge shaped
      2. Metatarsals—five
         a. First toe (great toe)
         b. Four lesser toes
         c. Articulates with three cuneiforms
         d. Form tarsometatarsal or Lisfranc's joint
      3. Phalanges
         a. Great toe, proximal, and distal
         b. Lesser toes (2, 3, 4, 5), proximal, middle, distal
      4. Sesamoids
         a. Small, round bones
         b. Embedded (partially or totally) in substance of corresponding tendon
         c. Pressure-absorbing mechanism
   B. Arches
      1. Formed by bony structure
      2. Longitudinal (lengthwise) arches
         a. Medial longitudinal arch
            (1) Formed by calcaneus, talus, navicular, three cuneiforms, and first three metatarsals
         b. Lateral longitudinal arch
            (1) Formed by calcaneus, cuboid, and fourth and fifth metatarsals
      3. Transverse—across the ball (top) of the foot
   C. Muscles, ligaments, and tendons; nerves (multiple structures)

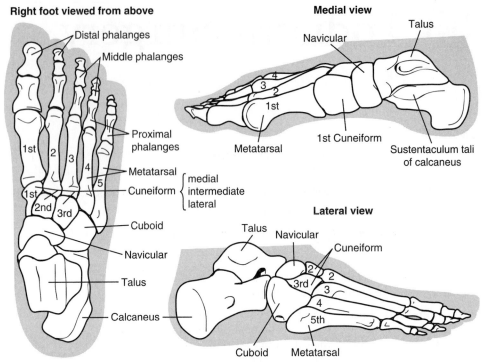

FIGURE 53-1 ■ Bones of the right foot. (Redrawn from Jacob S, Francone C: *Elements of anatomy and physiology,* ed 2. Philadelphia: WB Saunders, 1989, p 64.)

II. Assessment parameters (procedure specific)
  A. Structural disorders
    1. Causes
      a. Weakness of muscles, ligaments, and tendons
      b. Imbalance between bone support and supporting structure
      c. Constant wear, rub
  B. Identified disorders (see Table 53-1 for podiatric definitions)
    1. Hallux valgus (also called bunion): deformity of the foot involving the first metatarsal and great toe
      a. Lateral angulation of great toe
      b. Progresses, resulting in medial deviation of first metatarsal
      c. Often accompanied by multiple disorders and symptoms; commonly affects lesser toes
      d. Adults—chief complaint is dull ache over medial eminence; occurs in females more frequently than males
      e. Adolescent—chief complaint is unrelated to pain; cosmesis desired, family history prevalent
    2. Hallux varus
      a. First metatarsal deviates medially, and the great toe deviates laterally.
      b. Condition may start in late childhood or early adult life.
      c. More common in females
      d. Not evidenced the cause is tight footwear; however, it could be agitated by improperly fitting footwear.
    3. Hallux rigidus—"stiff big toe"
      a. Painful stiffness of first metatarsophalangeal joint of the toes when walking; toe becomes rigid
      b. Caused by arthritis

    4. Corns

      a. Conical thickening of skin in areas of constant irritation

    5. Bursal hypertrophy

      a. Inflammation of the joint

    6. Digital deformity

      a. Mallet toe—congenital abnormality of the distal interphalangeal joint, usually genetic

        (1) Flexion posture of the distal interphalangeal joint

        (2) Most commonly affects second toe

        (3) Associated with a long digit

        (4) Caused by pressure at tip of toes

        (5) Occurs in persons with peripheral neuropathy, no known reason

      b. Varus toes

        (1) Curly or overlapping toes

        (2) Flexion and varus rotation

        (3) Commonly affects 3, 4, 5

      c. Hammer toe deformity

        (1) Affects one of the lesser four toes (commonly second toe)

        (2) Hyperextension at metatarsophalangeal joint, flexion at proximal interphalangeal joint

        (3) Etiology unknown

      d. Clawtoe

        (1) Hyperextension of metatarsophalangeal joint with flexion of the proximal interphalangeal joint

        (2) Associated with cavus foot deformity and neuromuscular conditions

    7. Interdigital deformity (Morton's neuroma)

      a. Benign enlargement of third common digital branch at site of bifurcation of interdigital nerves (medial plantar nerve)

      b. Frequently between and distal to third and fourth metatarsal heads

      c. Symptoms and common findings

        (1) Pain in plantar forefoot area (sharp, dull, throbbing, or burning sensation)

        (2) Swelling of plantar metatarsal

        (3) Affects females more than males

        (4) Overweight person

    8. Pes planus (flatfoot)

      a. Loss of normal medial longitudinal arch

      b. Initial treatment is conservative therapy with shoes, arch supports.

      c. Surgical treatment with onset of disabling pain

      d. Correction procedures include Miller, Durham flatfoot plasty, triple arthrodesis, calcaneal displacement osteotomy.

    9. Pes cavus (hollow foot, clawfoot)

      a. Occurs with neuromuscular conditions as spina bifida, cerebral palsy, muscular dystrophy, congenital clubfoot

      b. Muscular weakness in foot

      c. Several procedures required for repair

        (1) Soft tissue release, decrease contracture

        (2) Tendon transfer to correct muscle imbalance

        (3) Osteotomy—incision into a bone

        (4) Arthrodesis—surgical immobilization or fusion of a joint

III. Elective operative procedures

  A. Treatment of disorders

    1. Determined by the degree of involvement

    2. Goals toward alignment, shortening, stabilization

    3. Multiple procedures may be indicated.

  B. General intraoperative care

    1. Tourniquet application

    2. Operative site cleansing (including hair removal and cleaning toenails)

3. Provision of sterile instruments, supplies
4. Availability of implants including joint replacement, K-wire (pins), screws
   C. Procedures
   1. Arthrodesis
      a. Excision of bone wedges with fusion
      b. Indicated for severe compromise of muscle function; digital and metatarsophalangeal joint stability inadequate
      c. Treatment for hallux valgus
         (1) Method: divide tendon, resect cartilage, provide stability to joint with K-wire or other means
      d. Triple arthrodesis—subtalar joint, talonavicular joint, tarsometatarsal joint
         (1) Treatment for equinus deformity, cavus deformity, flatfoot, or forefoot cavus
   2. Arthroplasty
      a. Resection or replacement of bony structure of joint
      b. Indicated for alleviation of pain and correction of digits with flexor to rigid deformity as
         (1) Inflammatory arthritis
         (2) Degenerative arthrosis
         (3) Congenital deformity
         (4) Flail toes
         (5) Revision of previous surgery
      c. Keller resection arthroplasty: tissues released around the joint, expose articular surface, resect medial eminence, implant (K-wire) seated, capsulorrhaphy completed
   3. Bunion procedures
      a. Revision of soft tissue structures and/or bone to correct deformity
      b. Soft tissue procedures correct muscle imbalance: McBride, DuVries, Mann, Silver.

■ **TABLE 53-1**
■ ■ **Podiatric Definitions**

Arthrodesis	Surgical immobilization or fusion of a joint
Arthrolysis	Surgical procedure in which mobility is restored to an ankylosed (fused/immobile) joint
Arthroplasty	Surgical repair or reformation of a joint
Arthrotomy	Incision into a joint
Bunion	Enlargement and inflammation of the joint bursa at the base of the great toe, usually causing the toe to displace laterally; usual etiology is long-term wearing of tight-fitting shoes
Capsulotomy	Incision into the joint capsule
Exostosis	A bony growth on the surface of a bone, also called "osteoma" or "hyperostosis"
Hallux	The great toe
Hallux valgus	Displacement of the great toe laterally toward the other toes; often coexists with a bunion, but often the two terms are inaccurately used synonymously.
Hammer toe	A deformity in which there is dorsiflexion of the metatarsophalangeal joint (joint between the foot and the toe) or plantar flexion of interphalangeal (IP) joints; when the most distal IP joint is the only one involved, it is called mallet toe.
Morton's neuroma	Interdigital nerve entrapment within a metatarsal interspace that causes pain, particularly with weight-bearing
Osteotomy	Incision into a bone
Plantar	Regarding the sole of the foot
Tenotomy	Incision of a tendon, often used to correct hammer toe

From Burden N, Quinn DMD, O'Brien D, et al: *Ambulatory surgical nursing*, ed 2. Philadelphia: WB Saunders, 2002, p 794.

        c. Soft tissue and bone procedure: Keller resection arthroplasty, Chevron osteotomy, Akin procedure

        d. Purpose: simple treatment of hallux valgus causing impaired function and/or pain; cosmetic improvement

        e. Satisfactory for older adult, less mobile

    4. Capsulotomy

        a. Incision of capsule

        b. Treatment of equinovarus foot

        c. Performed in conjunction with other procedures

        d. Method: incision through superficial fascia, expose joint, incise capsule

    5. Endoscopic plantar fasciotomy

        a. Operative tissue repair using a less invasive procedure

        b. Completed using fluoroscopy

        c. Procedure: stab incision, blunt dissection to create a channel, pass a trocar, release the plantar fascia

        d. Open procedure more invasive; appropriate procedure for fascia release

    6. Exostectomy

        a. Resection of lateral prominences (callus) of toes

        b. Commonly fifth toe

    7. Hammer toe repair

        a. Abnormal flexion posture of the proximal interphalangeal joint of one of the lesser four toes

        b. Second toe most frequently affected

        c. Metatarsophalangeal joint

        d. Stage of deformity depends on joint involvement and degree of contracture.

        e. Treatment

           (1) Soft tissue procedures: Girdlestone, Taylor, Parrish, Mann, Coughlin

           (2) Soft tissue and bone procedures

    8. Mallet toe repair

        a. Flexion posture of the distal interphalangeal joint

        b. Second toe most frequently affected

        c. Etiology

           (1) Pressure at tip of toes, possibly caused by shoes

           (2) Persons with peripheral neuropathy, no known reason

        d. Treatment

           (1) Flexor tenotomy at distal interphalangeal flexion crease

           (2) Subtotal or total resection of middle phalanx

    9. Osteotomy

        a. Removal or addition of a bone wedge

        b. Extraarticular or intraarticular

        c. Extraarticular most commonly in the calcaneus for cavovarus heel

        d. Metatarsal osteotomy for plantar calluses, hallux valgus: many types including wedge resection, Chevron, "Z," Reverdin, Mitchell

        e. Mitchell osteotomy: capsular incision, medial eminence removed, drill holes offset and suture passed; double osteotomy completed with excision of bone between, capital fragment displaced and suture tied; medial capsulorrhaphy completed

    10. Tenotomy

        a. Incision of tendon; eliminates tendon function; relieves contracture

        b. Completed in conjunction with other procedures

IV. Postanesthesia priorities (see Box 53-1)

  A. Phase I

    1. Predisposing factors

        a. Congenital, acquired, or traumatic

        b. Older adults and children included in the spectrum

        c. Existing conditions—neuromuscular disease, effect on other systems, neuropathy, diabetes, arthritis

   d. Previous procedures or anticipated future procedures (bilateral treatment needs)
2. Condition of foot
   a. Appearance and sensation
      (1) Soreness, tenderness, edema
      (2) Temperature equal on each foot
3. Color
   a. Blanching of nail beds
4. Vascular status
   a. Presence of dorsalis pedis pulse on dorsal center of metatarsal area of each foot
   b. Poor vascularity may impede healing.
5. Goals of procedure
   a. Pain relief
   b. Return or improvement of mobility
   c. Cosmetic improvement
   d. Extent of procedure influences outcome.
6. Support system
   a. Available assistance
   b. Impaired mobility related to other disease processes
7. Awareness of procedure and expected outcomes
   a. Procedure to be performed
   b. Anesthetic type
      (1) General anesthetic
      (2) Ankle block with IV conscious sedation
         (a) Procedure for block
         (b) Sensory deficit—length and precautions
   c. Complications
      (1) Loss of function, muscular imbalance
      (2) Neurovascular compromise, swelling
B. Phase II
   1. Neurovascular status
      a. Sensation in affected and opposite extremity
      b. Pulses
      c. Coloration, blanching of nail beds
   2. Preventive measures
      a. Elevation of extremity
      b. Ice pack
C. Phase III
   1. Ambulation and mobility
      a. Home care availability
      b. Sensory deficit with use of ankle block up to 8 hours

■ BOX 53-1
■ **KEY PATIENT EDUCATIONAL OUTCOMES**

Patient will demonstrate proper use of supportive devices (crutches, walker, walking shoe).
Patient will describe proper dosing procedure for prescribed analgesic medication(s) and report uncontrolled pain.
Patient will report excessive drainage on dressings.
Patient will describe signs and symptoms of infection and report findings to physician immediately.
Patient will report any neurological or circulatory impairment.
Patient will describe understanding of need for limited mobility for 6 to 8 weeks.

    c. Support devices—crutches, walker, walking shoe
      (1) Proper fit
        (a) Walking shoe long enough to protect toe, short enough to prevent tripping
      (2) Return demonstration of use
    d. Non–weight-bearing ambulation 3 to 5 days
    e. Limited mobility 6 to 8 weeks (longer depending upon procedure)
2. Wound care
    a. Incision site clean, dry
      (1) Report bleeding, discharge.
      (2) Protect K-wire(s) if used.
        (a) Clean around site with alcohol daily.
        (b) Removal time depends on procedure; possibly 6 to 8 weeks
    b. Dressings remain intact, clean, dry (no showering).
    c. Soft tissue procedures
      (1) Bulky, soft dressing for support
      (2) Three to 6 weeks with bandages in place (more involved procedures, longer bandage remains)
      (3) Compression dressing after 2 to 4 weeks
    d. Soft tissue and bone procedures
      (1) Six to 8 weeks with bandages in place, guarded ambulation
      (2) External support several additional weeks
      (3) If bone graft used, may immobilize 3 to 6 months
    e. Skin care beneath cast, dressing
3. Return of function
    a. Pain relief
      (1) Nonsteroidal antiinflammatory medications (NSAIDs)
        (a) Pain following foot surgery intense
        (b) Evaluate medication interactions.
      (2) Elevation of extremity
      (3) Ice packs
    b. Ambulation to tolerance
    c. Preventive measures
      (1) Eliminate pressure, rub on toes from footwear.

BIBLIOGRAPHY

1. Burden N, Dawes B, O'Brien D, Quinn D: *Ambulatory surgical nursing*, ed 2. Philadelphia: WB Saunders, 2000.
2. Fulkerson JP: Arthroscopy of the foot and ankle. In Cooper PS, Murray TF, editors: *Clinics in sports medicine.* Philadelphia: WB Saunders, 1996.
3. Laurin CA, Riley LH, Roy-Camille R: *Atlas of orthopaedic surgery,* vol 3. Paris, France: Masson, 1991.
4. McGlamery ED, Banks AS, Downey MS: *Comprehensive textbook of foot surgery,* ed 2. Baltimore: Williams & Wilkins, 1992.
5. Meeker MH, Rothrock JC: *Alexander's care of the patient in surgery,* ed 11. St Louis: Mosby, 1999.
6. Neyyoms, SM: *The Lippincott manual of nursing practice,* ed 7. Philadelphia: Lippincott, 2001.
7. Phippen ML, Wells MP: *Patient care during operative and invasive procedures.* Philadelphia: WB Saunders, 2000.
8. Pudner R: *Nursing the surgical patient.* Edinburgh, UK: Bailliere Tindall, 2000.

54 Trauma Surgery

JUDY STEVENSON

OBJECTIVES

At the conclusion of this chapter the reader will be able to:

1. Identify impact mechanism of injury has on actual injury.

2. Discuss continuum of trauma care from prehospital to postanesthesia care unit (PACU).

3. Prioritize elements of primary and secondary assessments in PACU as they relate to trauma care.

4. Incorporate care of total body systems into management of the trauma patient.

5. Discuss potential complications as they relate to trauma care and appropriate interventions to treat and/or prevent.

6. Describe the value of collaborative approach to care and communication.

7. Identify types of shock and how they impact the trauma patient.

In the United States, trauma continues to impact the lives of millions each year, and unfortunately many do not survive each day. In addition, of the patients who do survive, many have life-altering injuries. Swiftly and without warning, traumatic injuries span all ages, cultures, and races, reaching epidemic proportions.

Trauma accounts for more deaths in the United States during the first four decades of life than any other disease. Documented mortality from trauma may only be the tip of the iceberg because many patients initially survive but succumb to other disease processes resulting in death.

Many deaths from traumatic injury occur within minutes to hours after the event, with many dying within 48 hours from neurological complications. Additional traumatized patients will die from complications. Complications can include but are not limited to neurological, respiratory, circulatory, renal failure, and sepsis.

Those patients who survive and arrive at the hospital often will require surgical intervention. This intervention can range from the simple to the complex and from the single procedure to multiple procedures. All complications that can occur following anesthesia can occur in the trauma patient following anesthesia.

Nursing care of postanesthesia trauma patients requires a general knowledge of trauma care and intervention. Depending upon time from injury to the arrival in the operating room, new or previously unidentified injuries can make themselves known. The PACU nurse is an integral part of the trauma team in his or her approach to postoperative assessment. Swelling, bruising, and pain do not always occur upon impact and can be delayed during the surgical procedure, making an appearance while in the PACU. It is the PACU nurse's responsibility to identify abnormalities and report to the trauma physician prior to transporting the patient to the floor or discharge.

PREHOSPITAL

I. Goal of emergency medical services
   A. Improve field stabilization
   B. Resuscitation
   C. Transportation to the appropriate level trauma center
II. The Golden Hour
   A. Introduced by R. Adams Crowley, MD

   B. Emphasizes the importance of time in resuscitation
   C. Goal is to achieve maximal survival
   D. Represents the window of opportunity to institute life-saving and limb-saving measures
III. Prehospital phase
   A. Vital information
     1. Condition at the scene
       a. Age of victim
       b. Sex of victim
       c. Mechanism of injury
       d. Obvious injuries
       e. Questionable injuries
       f. Vital signs
       g. Intervention at the scene
       h. Intravenous (IV) fluids
       i. Response to interventions
       j. Stabilization
       k. Presence of drugs or alcohol
       l. Pertinent past medical history
       m. Transport time
       n. Any other pertinent information
     2. Mechanism of injury (factors that can influence outcome)
       a. Motor vehicle
         (1) Restraint devices
         (2) Air bag deployment
         (3) Patient ejection
         (4) Car rolling
         (5) Windshield star or shatter
         (6) Speed of vehicle
         (7) Where impact occurred on vehicle
         (8) Other fatalities at the scene
       b. Motorcycle
         (1) Speed of cycle
         (2) Object with impact
         (3) Front, rear, or side impact
         (4) Ejection from cycle (front, rear, or side)
         (5) Helmet usage
         (6) Protective covering (e.g., leather jacket, gloves)
         (7) Other fatalities at the scene
       c. Strike with blunt object (e.g., fist, ball bat, ball)
         (1) Object that struck
         (2) Place struck
         (3) Speed at which struck
         (4) Presence of protective covering
         (5) One strike or multiple strikes
         (6) Injury after initial injury (e.g., fall to the ground)
       d. Strike with penetrating object (e.g., gunshot, knife, screwdriver)
         (1) Object penetrated
         (2) Depth of object
         (3) Diameter of object
         (4) Twisting or stationary
         (5) Direction of penetration
         (6) Location of penetration
         (7) One wound or multiple wounds
         (8) Injury after initial injury (e.g., fall to the ground)
       e. Fall
         (1) Height from fall
         (2) Body position upon landing (e.g., feet, buttock)

        (3) Incident prior to landing (e.g., hit head, slipped)
        (4) Protective equipment (e.g., hard hat)
    f. Crush injury
        (1) Weight of object
        (2) Area compressed
        (3) Other injuries
        (4) Protective equipment
  3. Victim assistance
    a. Bystanders prior to emergency medical services (EMS)
        (1) Movement of victim prior to treatment
    b. EMS providers
        (1) Dressings
        (2) Stabilization of possible fractures
        (3) Cervical collar
        (4) Spine board
        (5) Safety straps

MECHANISM OF INJURY

  I. Basic understanding
    A. Related to the type of injuring forces and subsequent tissue response
    B. Helps to determine the extent of potential injuries
 II. Factors that influence injury
    A. Amount of force
      1. Energy is unloaded onto the body.
    B. Mass of the object
    C. Mass of the body
    D. Velocity at which the object is moving
    E. Deceleration forces
      1. Stop or decrease velocity of moving object
      2. Examples: falls, person striking dashboard
    F. Acceleration forces
      1. Stationary person struck by object
      2. Examples: pedestrian struck by car
    G. Multiple forces
      1. Both deceleration and acceleration forces together
      2. Example: pedestrian struck by car pushing into another vehicle
      3. Three impacts involved in auto crash
        a. Automobile to object
        b. Body into automobile
        c. Organs within body
    H. Blunt injury
      1. Direct impact
      2. Acceleration or deceleration
      3. Continuous pressure, shearing, or rotary forces
      4. May be less obvious and therefore more serious
      5. Can leave little outward evidence of internal damage
      6. Underlying tearing by rotary and shearing forces
      7. Disrupts blood vessels and nerves
      8. Can cause widespread epithelial and endothelial damage
      9. Stimulates cells to release their constituents activating the complement
     10. Coagulation cascade can begin.
     11. Masks more serious complications
    I. Penetrating injury
      1. Definition: that which cuts or pierces
      2. Multiple objects can be impaled (e.g., knife, firearms, handlebars).
      3. Causes penetrating and crushing of underlying tissue
      4. Produces capillary injury and destruction of tissue

5. Bullets (important factors affecting injury)
   a. Size and type of gun
   b. Velocity
   c. Range
   d. Mass
   e. Trajectory
   f. Entrance and exit wound
6. Stab wounds
   a. Length of object
   b. Force applied
   c. Angle of entry
   d. Twisting or stationary
   e. Penetrating object left in place or removed
7. Firearms
   a. More than bullets
   b. Include explosives such as bottle rockets, missiles, bombs
   c. Occurs many times more than penetrating injury occurs
8. Wounds cause disruption of tissue and cellular function.
9. Introduces debris and foreign bodies into wounds
10. May occur as local ischemia or may extend to fulminate hemorrhage

J. Compression injury
   1. Blunt trauma significant to produce capillary injury and destruction
   2. Contusion of tissue occurs
   3. Extravasation of blood causes discoloration, pain, and swelling.
   4. Massive hematoma increases myofascial pressure.
   5. Significant myofascial pressure can result in compartment syndrome.
      a. Increased pressure inside an osteofascial compartment
      b. Impedes circulation and causes cellular ischemia
      c. Results in alteration in neurovascular function
      d. Damaged muscular vessels dilate in response to histamine.
      e. Dilated vessels leak fluid into tissue, loss of capillary integrity
      f. Microvascular perfusion is impeded, and edema increases.
      g. Tissue pressure occurs.
      h. Most commonly occurs in lower leg or forearm
      i. Compartment pressure can be measured.
         (1) Normal is >10.
         (2) Greater than 35 is significant.
      j. Fasciotomy is treatment to prevent muscle or neurovascular damage.

K. Chemical
   1. Can be topical, ingested, or inhaled
   2. Caustic agent
      a. Alkaline
      b. Acids
      c. Petroleum-based products
   3. Damage often limited to localized area
   4. Factors to include
      a. Route
      b. Amount
      c. Concentration of substance
      d. Type of substance
      e. Time lapse after exposure
      f. Prehospital treatment

L. Electrical
   1. Always think of safety of rescuer.
   2. Internal burn not obviously seen
   3. Presents in unusual ways
      a. Burned hair on affected extremity

  b. Chest pain

  c. Thermal burn

  d. Enter and exit wounds (often hands or feet)

 4. Factors that influence

  a. Voltage

  b. Time of exposure

  c. Area affected

  d. Systemic symptoms

M. Radiant

 1. Events generating heat and or flames

 2. Topical or inhalation

 3. Can occur in combination with other injuries

 4. Burn can occur to skin and underlying structures.

 5. Vasoactive chemicals are released from mast cells.

 6. Intravascular volume is lost because of tissue disruption and protein leakage.

 7. Hyperemia increases blood flow and increases fluid loss.

 8. Seriousness of injury is dependent upon

  a. Surface area

  b. Degree of burn

  c. Presence of systemic problems

  d. Prehospital treatment

 9. Inhalation reaction from radiant event

  a. Damage to respiratory vasculature can occur.

  b. Low inhaled O_2 and increased inhaled CO_2 can cause hypoxia.

  c. Smoke inhalation causes

   (1) Edema of small airways

   (2) Atelectasis

N. Predicable injuries

 1. Can be based on specific mechanism of injury

 2. All injuries cannot be predicted based upon mechanism of injury.

III. Scoring systems

 A. Numerous scoring mechanisms can be used.

 B. Assists in determining severity of injuries

 C. Assists in determining likelihood of outcome

 D. Accuracy limitations can occur despite score used.

STABILIZATION PHASE

 I. Initial assessment, resuscitation, and stabilization

  A. Initiated in the emergency room (ER) or trauma center

  B. Extend into the operating room (OR)

  C. Continue on into the PACU

  D. Will further continue in the critical area or the surgical floor

  E. Can extend even beyond discharge

   1. Significance of discharge instructions cannot be overstressed..

 II. Hypovolemia in the trauma patient

  A. Most common cause of shock

   1. Result of acute blood loss

   2. Result of fluid redistribution

  B. Fluid resuscitation necessary

   1. Prompt fluid replacement

    a. Assists in tissue perfusion

    b. Assists in delivery of oxygen to the tissues

    c. Often requires use of rapid-volume fluid infuser

     (1) Can deliver IV fluids at rate of 500-700 ml/minute

    d. Beneficial to give warm IV fluids

     (1) Prevents hypothermia

2. Fluid selection
   a. Crystalloids
      (1) Electrolyte solution
      (2) Diffuses through capillary endothelium
      (3) Distributed throughout extracellular compartment
      (4) Common selections are lactated Ringer's (LR) and normal saline.
      (5) Recommended first line for replacement
      (6) Administration should be three to four times blood loss.
      (7) Use LR in caution with suspected liver injury.
      (8) Cheaper than colloids
   b. Colloids
      (1) Contain protein or starch molecules
      (2) Molecules remain in intravascular space.
      (3) Increase osmotic pressure gradient within vascular compartment
      (4) Administration is volume per volume.
      (5) Half-life is longer than crystalloids.
      (6) Common selections are
          (a) Plasma protein fraction
          (b) Dextran
          (c) Albumin
          (d) Hetastarch
   c. Hypertonic solutions
      (1) Controversial in treatment
      (2) Resuscitative in shock
      (3) Common selections are hypertonic or isotonic saline.
      (4) Pulls fluids from extracellular space to support blood pressure (BP)
      (5) Can be helpful in head injury patients
   d. Blood products
      (1) Only blood can replace blood.
      (2) Restores capacity to carry oxygen
      (3) Given following fluid administration
      (4) Packed red blood cells most common
      (5) Universal donor is O negative.
      (6) O positive can be given to nonchildbearing females and males.
      (7) Type specific blood is preferred when waiting is an option.
      (8) Platelets may be indicated if coagulopathy suspected.
3. Delayed fluid administration
   a. Can be useful in hemorrhagic patients
   b. Fluids are delayed until the start of surgery.
   c. Early fluid administration may delay transport.
   d. Restoration of volume can have adverse complication.
   e. Exacerbation of blood loss can occur from increased BP.
   f. Controversial among trauma surgeons
C. Other causes of shock in trauma patient
1. Cardiogenic
   a. Can result from cardiac tamponade
   b. Can result from tension pneumothorax
2. Neurogenic shock
   a. Related to spinal cord injury
3. Septic shock
   a. Usually late
   b. Caused by infectious process

DIAGNOSTIC STUDIES AND PROTOCOLS

I. Diagnostic tests
   A. Vital role in establishing injury
   B. Necessary for accurate diagnosis

  C. Assists in planning effective treatment
  D. X-rays
   1. Lateral cervical spine
   2. Upright chest anteroposterior
   3. Anteroposterior pelvis
   4. Any extremity with questionable injury
   5. Thoracic and lumbar spine
   6. Any other identified injured area
   7. Soft tissue films can be helpful if impaled object suspected.
  E. Computed tomography (CT) scan
   1. Head (without contrast)
   2. Chest
   3. Abdomen
   4. Pelvis
  F. Ultrasound
   1. Abdominal
  G. Twelve lead electrocardiogram (ECG)
   1. Useful with chest injury
   2. May be needed if chest pain resulted in additional trauma
  H. Diagnostic peritoneal lavage (DPL)
   1. Controversial
   2. Used only with suspected abdominal injury and severe hypotension
   3. Abdominal CT scan more useful with specific injury information
  I. Arteriogram
   1. Suspected vascular injury
II. Laboratory studies
  A. Vital role in establishing current status
  B. Common laboratory studies
   1. Arterial blood gases
   2. Electrolytes
   3. Glucose
   4. Lactate level
   5. Renal function studies
   6. Liver function studies
   7. Coagulation studies
   8. Complete blood count
   9. Type and cross match
   10. Urinalysis
   11. Pregnancy test (females ages 11-55)
   12. Alcohol and drug testing are controversial.
  C. Assist in planning effective treatment

COLLABORATIVE APPROACH

 I. Essential in care of trauma patient
  A. Begins with prehospital personnel
   1. Witnesses at scene
   2. First responder
   3. Paramedic
   4. Police
   5. Fire department
   6. Air ambulance personnel if activated
  B. Emergency room or trauma center
   1. Emergency physician
   2. Registered trained trauma nurse
   3. Emergency technician and paramedic
   4. Respiratory therapist

        5. X-ray personnel
        6. Trauma surgeon
        7. Anesthesiologist
        8. OR personnel
        9. Chaplain
    C. OR
        1. OR nurse
        2. Scrub technicians
        3. Anesthesia provider
        4. Postanesthesia care nurse
    D. Following the OR
        1. Critical care
        2. Surgical floor
        3. Discharge nurse
II. Communication is the key.
    A. Vital communication initiated prehospital
    B. Continues throughout hospital stay
    C. Comprehensive in approach
        1. Doctor to doctor
        2. ER nurse to OR nurse
        3. OR nurse to PACU nurse
        4. PACU nurse to floor nurse
        5. Physician to family
        6. Nurse to family
    D. Systematic reports
        1. Mechanism of injury
        2. Past medical history
        3. Airway, breathing, circulation
        4. Vital signs
        5. Include diagnostic findings
        6. Treatments
        7. Suspected injuries
        8. Abnormal assessment
        9. Vital nursing information
       10. Fluids and/or blood products

POSTANESTHESIA CARE

I. Anesthesia report
    A. Valuable information
        1. Presenting status
           a. Name
           b. Age
           c. Surgeon
           d. Anesthesiologist
           e. Level of consciousness preoperatively
        2. Significant facts pertaining to mechanism of injury
        3. Prehospital phase
        4. ER course
           a. Cervical spine (C spine) clearance documentation
        5. Operative procedure
           a. Single procedure
           b. More than one procedure
         6. Intubation
           a. Routine intubation
           b. Difficult intubation
           c. Rapid sequence intubation

      d. Full stomach

      e. Airway stability

      f. Intubation time and tolerance

    7. Anesthetic agents

      a. Rapid sequence intubation

      b. Inhalation agents

      c. IV agents

      d. Balanced anesthesia

      e. Narcotic usage (with time of last dose)

      f. Muscle relaxants (with time of last dose)

      g. Reversal agents (with time of last dose)

    8. Estimated blood loss

      a. Prehospital

      b. Emergency department

      c. OR

    9. Fluid resuscitation

      a. Prehospital

      b. Emergency department

      c. OR

      d. Crystalloids

      e. Blood products

      f. Chest drains

      g. Cell saver usage

      h. Ortho refuser (orthopedic refuser system)

      i. Other drains

   10. Cardiopulmonary status

      a. Vital signs

      b. Pulse oximetry

      c. Vasopressors

      d. Antiarrhythmics

      e. Arterial line

      f. Swan-Ganz catheter

      g. Urine output (to ensure end-organ perfusion)

   11. Other identified injuries

      a. Surgical interventions

      b. Nonsurgical interventions

   12. Treatment abnormalities

      a. Hypothermia

      b. Abnormal laboratory values

      c. Abnormal x-ray results

   13. Treatment plans

II. Nursing assessment, primary survey

  A. Airway

    1. Patency

    2. Proper head position

    3. Ensure cervical spine protection until cleared.

      a. *Do not remove cervical collar if not cleared.*

    4. Suctioning as needed for removal of secretions

    5. Airway management as indicated

      a. Nasopharyngeal

      b. Oropharyngeal

      c. Oral or nasal endotracheal tube

  B. Breathing

    1. Consider mechanism of injury.

      a. Blunt

      b. Penetrating

    2. Location of injury

        a. Chest injury may indicate pulmonary injury.

        b. Rib fractures

        c. Pulmonary contusion

        d. Pneumothorax

        e. Tension pneumothorax

        f. Neurological event affecting respiratory status

    3. Spontaneous respirations

    4. Chest wall movement

    5. Respiratory accessory muscle use

    6. Work of breathing

    7. Palpation

        a. Subcutaneous emphysema

        b. Trachea position

    8. Auscultation

        a. Bilateral breath sounds

        b. Adventitious breath sounds

    9. Pulse oximetry continuous

    10. End tidal CO_2

C. Circulation

    1. Pulses

        a. Carotid beats per minute (BPM)

           (1) BPM at least 60

        b. Radial

           (1) BPM at least 80

        c. Femoral

           (1) BPM at least 70

        d. Popliteal and dorsalis pedis (PT/DP) pulses

        e. Bilateral

        f. Quality

        g. Rate

        h. Upper extremities to lower extremities

        i. Pulseless electrical activity (PEA) can occur in trauma patient.

           (1) Tension pneumothorax

           (2) Cardiac tamponade

           (3) Hypovolemia

           (4) Hypothermia

           (5) Hypoxia

    2. Cardiac monitor

        a. Rate

        b. Rhythm

        c. Arrhythmia presence

        d. Continual cardiac monitor observance

    3. BP

        a. Hypertension

        b. Hypotension

        c. Normal BP range for patient

        d. Vasopressors

        e. Monitor every 10 minutes if stable.

        f. Monitor every minute if unstable.

        g. Noninvasive cuff

        h. Arterial line

        i. Capillary refill may be more beneficial in pediatric patient.

    4. Vascular access

        a. Number of sites

        b. Location of sites

        c. Type of fluids presently hanging

        d. Intake

   5. Dressings
      a. Surgical dressings for drainage
      b. Drainage from nonsurgical wounds
      c. Surgical drain placement and volume of drainage
      d. Bloody drainage versus nonbloody drainage
      e. Total output
   6. Urine output
      a. Ensures end-organ perfusion
      b. Essential for input and output (I and O) balance
III. Nursing assessment, secondary survey
   A. General information
      1. Done only after primary assessment
      2. High degree of suspicion concerning mechanism of injury
      3. Note any injuries not previously addressed.
         a. Swelling and bruising can take time to develop.
      4. Life-threatening injuries may limit time for secondary survey in ER.
         a. Initial surgery may be needed for life-threatening injuries.
   B. Head to toe assessment
      1. Neurological evaluation
         a. Level of consciousness
         b. Appropriate verbal response
         c. Pupil reactivity and symmetry
         d. Following commands
         e. Movement of all four extremities
      2. Examination of head and face
         a. Abrasions
         b. Lacerations
         c. Puncture wounds
         d. Ecchymosis
            (1) Raccoon eyes (periorbital bruising)
         e. Edema
            (1) Facial edema can result in potential airway compromise.
         f. Gross vision exam
         g. Check for presence of contact lens.
      3. Ears
         a. Ecchymosis
            (1) Battle sign (bruising behind ear)
         b. Drainage from nose
            (1) Bloody
            (2) Clear fluid (potential for cerebrospinal fluid [CSF] leak)
               (a) Check for presence of glucose.
         c. Never pack or suction nose if CSF leak suspected.
         d. If CSF leak suspected and/or Battle's sign, *never* insert nasogastric (NG) tube; consider oral gastric tube if needed.
      4. Evaluate neck.
         a. Edema
         b. Ecchymosis
         c. Tracheal deviation
         d. Pulsating or distended neck veins
         e. Subcutaneous emphysema
      5. Chest assessment
         a. Anterior, lateral, and axilla examination
         b. Lacerations
         c. Abrasions
         d. Contusions
            (1) Seat belt bruising can be seen on the chest.
         e. Puncture wounds
         f. Edema

g. Subcutaneous emphysema
h. Chest wall symmetry
i. Depth of respirations
j. Reevaluation of breathing
k. Auscultation of breath and heart sounds
  (1) Adventitious sounds
  (2) Murmurs
  (3) Bruits
  (4) Muffled heart sounds
l. Chest pain that may indicate
  (1) Pulmonary contusion
  (2) Rib fractures
  (3) Cardiac contusion
6. Abdomen, pelvis, and genitalia evaluation
  a. Abrasions
  b. Contusions
  c. Edema
  d. Ecchymosis
    (1) Seat belt bruising is often seen across abdomen.
  e. Tenderness
  f. Presence of bowel sounds
  g. Abdominal girth
  h. Pelvis examined for stability over crests and pubis
  i. Presence of priapism could indicate spinal cord injury.
  j. Urinary catheter
    (1) Should be in place on all multiple trauma patients
    (2) Examine urine
    (3) I and O documented
    (4) Ensure adequate output to prevent rhabdomyolysis.
  k. Rectal exam
    (1) Presence of blood
    (2) Rectal tone
    (3) Trauma surgeon or emergency department (ER) physician
7. Extremity assessment
  a. Circulatory
  b. Sensory
  c. Motor function
  d. Range of motion
  e. Edema
  f. Ecchymosis
  g. Lacerations
  h. Abrasions
  i. Reexamine if intervention activated.
8. Back evaluation
  a. Log roll with cervical spine support.
  b. Inspect and palpate back, flanks, and buttock.
  c. Lacerations
  d. Abrasions
  e. Ecchymosis
  f. Edema
  g. Pain
9. ER intervention assessment
  a. Open wounds need tetanus booster.
  b. Antibiotics often started preoperatively
  c. Pain medication
  d. Antianxiety medication
  e. Nausea medication
  f. Wound cleansing and dressings

IV. Nursing interventions
    A. Pain control (trauma considerations)
        1. Note preoperative medications given in ER.
            a. Intramuscular medications can have long half-life.
        2. Pain may be inclusive of more than the surgical site.
            a. Musculoskeletal injuries
            b. Sutured lacerations
            c. Extremity fractures
            d. Rib fractures
            e. Contusions and bruising
        3. Pain evaluation
            a. Subjective
            b. Verbal
            c. Nonverbal
            d. Hemodynamic changes (increased heart rate [HR] and BP)
            e. Splinting
            f. Nausea
            g. Crying
            h. Guarding
            i. Utilize standard pain scale to assess.
        4. Pain management
            a. IV injection
            b. Patient-controlled analgesia
            c. Epidural catheter
            d. Major plexus block
            e. Music therapy
            f. Guided imagery
            g. Relaxation techniques
            h. Visitors
        5. Pain goals
            a. Minimize cardiovascular depression.
            b. Minimize intracranial hypertension.
            c. Substance abusers may require higher pain doses.
            d. Pain management is vital to optimal care.
    B. Nausea management (trauma considerations)
        1. Can be of great concern for the trauma patient
        2. Seldom are trauma patients prepared with nothing by mouth (NPO).
        3. Enter anesthesia with potentially full stomach
        4. Vomiting can lead to aspiration.
        5. Extubation may be delayed until gag reflux returns.
        6. NG tube does not always function if food particles are large.
        7. Nausea has higher incidence in trauma patient.
        8. Nausea can be indication of increased intracranial pressure.
    C. Psychological management
        1. Emotional consideration increases postoperatively.
        2. Life-threatening interventions have been implemented.
        3. May be challenging postoperatively
            a. Initial shock may have worn off.
            b. Questions concerning others involved
            c. Fear of consequences
            d. Life-changing injuries
            e. Preevent drug or alcohol use can complicate.
        4. Emergence from anesthesia
            a. Orientate to place and time.
            b. Brief explanation of the event
            c. Acknowledges fears
                (1) Death
                (2) Mutilation

(3) Change in body image
(4) Loss of control
(5) Loss of family members and friends
d. Same information may need to be repeated several times.
e. Be honest with information.
f. Encourage appropriate coping skills.
g. Psychological concepts of trauma
(1) Need for information
(2) Need for compassion
(3) Need for hope
D. Infection risks (related to trauma care)
1. May have limited past medical history
2. Large amount of unknown information may exist.
3. High risk for
a. Communicable diseases
b. Human immunodeficiency virus (HIV)
c. Hepatitis
d. Sexually transmitted diseases
e. Chicken pox
4. Universal precautions should be observed.
5. Handwashing is the best defense.
E. Nursing diagnosis
1. Potential for ineffective airway clearance
2. Potential for ineffective gas exchange
3. Potential for alterations in cardiac output
4. Potential for alteration in tissue perfusion
5. Potential for fluid volume deficit
6. Potential for hypothermia
7. Potential for risk of injury
8. Potential for altered comfort
9. Potential for altered thought process
10. Potential for altered communication
11. Potential for anxiety
12. Potential for ineffective coping
13. Potential for disturbance in self-concept
14. Potential for posttraumatic stress
15. Additional potentials dependent upon surgical interventions and injuries
F. Nursing care
1. Vigilant continuous reassessment
2. Treatment priorities
3. Recognition of complex pathophysiologic responses
4. Anticipation of subtle or overt signs of shock
5. Prevention of complications
a. Acute respiratory distress syndrome
b. Sepsis
c. Acute renal failure
d. Hypoxic liver
e. Multisystem organ failure

SHOCK AS A COMPLICATION IN THE MULTITRAUMA PATIENT

I. Shock as a complication
A. Most common complication associated with traumatic injury
B. Different types of shock all exhibit a problems with
1. Delivery of oxygen to the cell
2. Delivery of nutrients to the cell

       3. Inadequate tissue perfusion (cellular hypoxia)
       4. Increased lactic acid level (caused by oxygen debt)
         a. Degree of rise correlates with severity and prognosis.
       5. Functional impairment of cells
       6. Functional impairment of organs
       7. Functional impairment of body systems
       8. Heat, brain, liver, kidneys, and lungs require increased oxygen.
       9. Ischemia initiates complex events.
         a. Energy-dependent functions cease.
         b. Protein synthesis is depleted.
         c. Loss of intracellular potassium
         d. Production of lactic acid
         e. Death of vital tissue
    C. Clinical manifestations of shock
       1. Cool, clammy skin
       2. Cyanosis
       3. Restlessness
       4. Altered level of consciousness
       5. Altered skin temperature
       6. Tachycardia
       7. Dysrhythmias
       8. Tachypnea
       9. Pulmonary edema
      10. Decreased urine output
      11. Decreased end-organ perfusion
      12. Increased platelet, leukocyte, and erythrocyte counts
      13. Sludging of the blood
      14. Metabolic acidosis
  II. Types of shock
    A. Hypovolemic
       1. Most common type
       2. Results from acute hemorrhagic loss
    B. Cardiogenic
       1. Rare in trauma patients
       2. Inadequate contractility of cardiac muscle
       3. May be secondary to blunt cardiac injury or myocardial infarction (MI)
    C. Distributive
       1. Includes neurogenic, anaphylactic, and septic
       2. Abnormality in vascular system and maldistribution of blood volume
       3. Neurogenic most common in trauma patient from spinal cord injury
    D. Obstructive
       1. Compression of great vessels or heart
         a. Results from tension pneumothorax or cardiac tamponade
 III. Hypovolemic shock
    A. Defined
       1. Decrease in intravascular volume
       2. Decrease in filling the intravascular compartment
    B. Causes
       1. Internal hemorrhage
       2. External hemorrhage
       3. Plasma volume loss
       4. Third spacing of fluids
       5. Decreased venous return
    C. Classification of hemorrhage
       1. Characteristic clinical manifestations according to approximate loss
       2. American College of Surgeons' Advanced Trauma Life Support Course
       3. Class I

   a. Early phase
   b. Loss of as much as 750 ml
   c. Approximately 1% to 15% total blood volume loss
   d. Minimal physiologic changes in
      (1) HR
      (2) BP
      (3) Capillary refill
      (4) Respiratory rate
      (5) Urine output
   e. Mild anxiety in response to sympathetic nervous system
   f. Treatment
      (1) Rapid infusion of 1 or 2 L of balanced salt solution
      (2) Maintaining renal output of more than 0.5 ml/kg per hour
4. Class II
   a. Moderate phase
   b. Loss of 750-1500 ml blood
   c. Approximately 15% to 30% total blood volume loss
   d. Multiple incremental physiologic changes
      (1) Increased anxiety
      (2) Restlessness
      (3) Catecholamine release
      (4) HR >100
      (5) Minimal BP changes
         (a) Rise in diastolic BP
         (b) Decreasing pulse pressure
      (6) Slight capillary refill delay
      (7) Cool, pale skin
      (8) Slight depression in urine output
   e. Treatment
      (1) Rapid infusion of 1 or 2 L of balanced salt solution
      (2) Maintaining renal output of more than 0.5 ml/kg per hour
5. Class III
   a. Progressive phase
   b. Loss of 1500-2000 ml blood
   c. Approximately 30% to 40% total blood volume loss
   d. Obvious physiologic changes
      (1) Cerebral hypoperfusion—decreased level of consciousness
      (2) Confusion
      (3) Agitation
      (4) Anxious
      (5) HR greater than 120
      (6) Hypotension
      (7) Capillary refill greater than 4 seconds
      (8) Deep, rapid respirations
      (9) Metabolic acidosis
      (10) Decreased urine output (approximately 5-15 ml/hour)
   e. Treatment
      (1) Fluid administration, but consider blood transfusion
6. Class IV
   a. Hemorrhage
   b. More than 2000 ml blood loss
   c. Approximately 40% total blood volume loss
   d. Profound impact
      (1) Lethargic
      (2) Stuporous
      (3) Unresponsive
      (4) HR 140 or higher

        (5) Peripheral pulses weak and difficult to palpate

        (6) Capillary refill more than 10 seconds

        (7) Severe hypotension, BP difficult to obtain

        (8) Cold, clammy, diaphoretic, or cyanotic skin

        (9) Shallow, irregular respirations greater than 35 per minute

        (10) No renal end-organ perfusion, resulting in anuria

     e. Treatment

        (1) Fluid administration and blood administration

  7. The Golden Hour

     a. Treatment within the first hour is associated with lower mortality.

     b. Filling the vascular tank allows

        (1) Adequate cardiac output

        (2) Perfusion of tissues

IV. Cardiogenic shock

  A. Defined

    1. Inadequate cardiac output

    2. Circulatory failure

    3. Impaired contractility

    4. Shock secondary to acute myocardial dysfunction

      a. Systolic BP less than 80 mm Hg (less than 30% baseline)

      b. Cardiac index less than 2.1 L/minute

    5. Mortality ranges 80% to 100%

  B. Causes

    1. In trauma secondary to blunt injury to heart muscle

    2. Occasionally myocardial infarction occurs preceding trauma event.

    3. History of heart disease in association with trauma and/or anesthesia can increase likelihood of myocardial infarction.

    4. Rapid fluid administration and ensuing cardiac failure

    5. Disruption in normal conduction sequence (heart block, dysrhythmias)

  C. Classifications of cardiogenic shock

    1. Coronary

      a. Obstructive coronary artery disease interrupting blood flow

      b. Interruption of blood flow causing ischemic heart muscle

      c. Ischemic heart muscle results in decreased contraction.

      d. Decreased contraction results in inadequate cardiac output.

      e. Incidence rises with compromise of 40% left ventricular function.

      f. Increased left atrial pressure

      g. Increased pulmonary venous pressure

      h. Increased pulmonary capillary pressure

      i. Pulmonary edema

    2. Noncoronary

      a. Absence of coronary artery disease

      b. Cardiac muscle damage

        (1) Cardiomyopathy

        (2) Valvular heart abnormalities

        (3) Cardiac dysrhythmias

  D. Clinical indicators

    1. Systolic BP less than 80 mm Hg (less than 30% baseline)

    2. Cardiac index less than 2.1 L/minute

    3. Urine output less than 20 ml/hour

    4. Diminished cerebral perfusion evidenced by confusion

    5. Cold, clammy, cyanotic skin

    6. Classic signs and symptoms

      a. May not be seen in the hypovolemic trauma patient

      b. Pulmonary edema

      c. Jugular vein distention

      d. Hepatic congestion

      7. Decreased cardiac, stroke, and left-ventricular stroke work index
      8. Increased pulmonary capillary wedge pressure
      9. Increased pulmonary artery pressure
    10. Increased systemic vascular resistance
    11. Decreased systemic venous oxygen saturation
    12. Decreased cardiac output
    13. Respiratory and metabolic acidosis

  E. Treatment
      1. Early recognition
      2. Improvement of myocardial oxygen supply
      3. Improvement of tissue perfusion
      4. Airway management, ventilation, and oxygenation
      5. Correct acidosis.
      6. Pain relief
      7. Pharmacological support to improve or correct rhythm
      8. Increasing cardiac output by increasing intravascular volume
      9. Vasoactive medications
        a. Epinephrine
        b. Dopamine
        c. Dobutamine
    10. Decrease afterload.
    11. When pharmacologic support fails
      a. Intraaortic balloon pump
      b. Right-ventricular assist device

V. Distributive shock
  A. Defined
      1. Also called vasogenic shock
      2. Abnormal placement of the vascular volume
      3. Heart pump and blood volume are normal.
      4. Alteration exists within the vascular circulatory network.
      5. Three types
        a. Neurogenic
        b. Anaphylactic
        c. Septic

  B. Neurogenic shock
      1. Defined
        a. Tremendous increase in vascular capacity
        b. Normal amount of blood incapable of adequately filling vasculature
        c. Loss of sympathetic vasomotor tone causes massive vasodilation.
        d. Venous pooling and decreased return to right heart
        e. Frequently transitory
        f. Not common in occurrence
      2. Causes
        a. Deep general or spinal anesthesia
        b. Loss of sympathetic vasomotor tone in the trauma patient
          (1) Brain concussion or contusion of basal regions
          (2) Spinal cord injury above level of T6
      3. Clinical symptoms
        a. Decreased peripheral vascular resistance
        b. Decreased stroke volume
        c. Decreased cardiac output
        d. Hypotension
        e. Decreased tissue perfusion
        f. Differs from hypovolemic shock
          (1) Bradycardia
          (2) Warm, dry, flushed skin

    4. Treatment

        a. Extensive volume expansion

        b. Vasopressors

            (1) Ephedrine

        c. Spinal anesthesia as causative event

            (1) Head of bed flat

            (2) Supine position

            (3) Elevate legs if possible.

C. Anaphylactic shock

    1. Defined

        a. Severe antigen-antibody reaction

        b. Relates to inflammatory process

        c. Activation of complement and arachidonic cascade

            (1) Immunoglobulin E produced and binds to mast cells and basophiles

            (2) Mast cells trigger vasoactive contents.

            (3) Histamine and vasoactive mediators released by mast cells

            (4) Vasoactive mediators cause massive vasodilation.

            (5) Vasoactive mediators cause increased capillary permeability.

        d. Rarely occurs in the trauma patient but should be of concern if no past medical history

    2. Causes

        a. Antigen-antibody reaction

        b. Can occur with exposure to any allergen, in the trauma patient consider

            (1) Antibiotics

            (2) Contrast medium

            (3) Blood transfusions

    3. Clinical symptoms

        a. Vary with severity

        b. Conjunctivitis

        c. Angioedema

        d. Hypotension

        e. Laryngeal edema

        f. Urticaria

        g. Bronchoconstriction

        h. Dysrhythmias

        i. Cardiac arrest

        j. One or any combinations of the preceding signs can occur.

        k. Repeat exposures can increase symptoms.

    4. Treatment

        a. Removal of causing agent

        b. Discontinue blood transfusion.

        c. Oxygen

        d. Epinephrine

            (1) Bronchodilator

            (2) Helps restore vascular tone

            (3) Increases arterial BP

        e. Aminophylline

            (1) If wheezing

        f. Benadryl

            (1) Antihistamine

        g. Steroids

            (1) Decrease inflammatory process

        h. Gastric acid blocker

D. Septic shock

    1. Defined

        a. Acute systemic response to invading blood-borne microorganisms

        b. Clinical syndrome on a continuum

    c. Begins with sepsis and ends with multisystem organ failure

    d. Complex cellular disease

    e. Loss of autoregulation and tissue dysfunction despite increased cardiac output

    f. Activation of kinins, complement, arachidonic, and coagulation cascades

    g. Hemodynamic instability
- (1) Initial phase
  - (a) High cardiac output
  - (b) Low systemic vascular resistance
- (2) Later phase
  - (a) Low cardiac output
  - (b) Extremely high systemic vascular resistance

    h. Myocardial depression related to severity of sepsis

    i. Release of vasoactive chemical mediators and endotoxins

    j. Decreased ventricular preload

    k. Increased capillary permeability augments myocardial depression.

    l. Increased capillary permeability produces decreased vascular volume.

    m. Endotoxin stimulates complement split products.

    n. Neutrophil and platelet aggregation to the lungs

    o. Fluid collects within the pulmonary interstitium.

    p. Pulmonary compliance is decreased.

    q. Acute respiratory distress syndrome ensues.

    r. Profound alteration in metabolism

    s. Increased oxygen debt

    t. Rising blood lactate levels

    u. Trauma patient is predisposed because of
- (1) Contaminated wounds
- (2) Poor nutritional status
- (3) Preexisting disease states
- (4) Altered integrity of body's defense mechanism

    v. Principal cause of death in trauma patient surviving first 3 days

2. Causes

    a. Gram-positive microorganisms less common

    b. Gram-negative microorganisms most common

    c. Viruses

    d. Fungi

    e. Parasites

3. Clinical symptoms

    a. Warm, flushed, and dry skin

    b. Rapid respiratory rate

    c. Confusion

    d. Increased HR

    e. Hypotension

    f. High cardiac output

    g. Low systemic vascular resistance

    h. Late clinical signs: skin changes to cold and clammy.

4. Treatment

    a. Identification and elimination of infection

    b. Cultures

    c. Proper definitive antimicrobial therapy

    d. Hemodynamic monitoring

    e. Oxygenation and ventilation support

    f. Fluid administration

    g. Pharmacological support
- (1) Positive inotropes
- (2) Vasopressors

    E. Obstructive shock
       1. Defined
          a. Myocardium is normal.
          b. Compression to the atria
          c. Obstruction in venous return
          d. Prevents atrial filling
          e. Decrease in stroke volume
       2. Causes
          a. Obstructive source
          b. Pulmonary embolism
          c. Dissecting aortic aneurysm
          d. Vena cava obstruction
          e. Cardiac tamponade
          f. Tension pneumothorax
       3. Clinical symptoms will be dependent on causative mechanism and can include
          a. Muffled heart sounds
          b. Jugular vein distension
          c. Tracheal deviation
          d. Diminished or absent lung sounds
          e. Hypotension
          f. PEA
       4. Treatment
          a. Correct the cause
          b. Dissecting aneurysm: surgical intervention
          c. Vena cava obstruction: surgical intervention
          d. Cardiac tamponade: cardiocentesis until surgical intervention
          e. Tension pneumothorax: needle decompression, chest tube
VI. Summary
    A. Trauma care is complex.
       1. Many pathophysiologic responses
       2. May be single surgical intervention
       3. May need repetitive surgical interventions
       4. Consider multiple disciplines.
    B. PACU nurse
       1. Focus on vigilant continuous assessment.
       2. Anticipate problems.
       3. Identify subtle changes.
          a. Remember medications can alter suspected responses.
       4. Intervene appropriately and promptly.
       5. Prevent complications.
       6. Offers challenge in caring
       7. Requires knowledge of current research and treatment
       8. Expect the unexpected.
          a. Trauma happens to children.
          b. Trauma happens to pregnant women.
          c. Trauma happens to the elderly.
          d. Trauma happens to the sick.
          e. Trauma happens to the wealthy.
          f. Trauma happens to the impoverished.
          g. Trauma happens to families.
          h. Trauma changes lives.
          i. Trauma happens.

BIBLIOGRAPHY

1. *Advanced cardiac life support provider manual,* ed 4. Dallas: American Heart Association, 2001.

2. *Advanced trauma life support course,* ed 7. Chicago: Committee on Trauma of the American College of Surgeons, 2003.

3. Alspach J, Epgang T, editors: *Core curriculum for critical care nursing,* ed 5. Philadelphia: WB Saunders, 1998.

4. Atlee J: *Complications in anesthesia.* Philadelphia: WB Saunders, 1999.

5. *Course in advanced trauma nursing: A conceptual approach.* Park Ridge, IL: Emergency Nurses Association, 1995.

6. Drain CB: *Post anesthesia care unit: A critical care approach to post anesthesia nursing.* Philadelphia: WB Saunders, 2002.

7. *Emergency nurse pediatric course,* ed 2. Park Ridge, IL: Emergency Nurses Association, 1998.

8. Feliciano D, Moore E, Mattox K: *Trauma.* Stanford, CN: Appleton and Lange, 1996.

9. Kwan I, Bunn F, Roberts I, on behalf of the WHO Pre-Hospital Trauma Steering Committee: Timing and volume of fluid administration for patients with bleeding following trauma. In *The Cochran library,* issue 2. Oxford, UK: Wiley, 2002.

10. Litwack K: *Core curriculum for perianesthesia nursing practice,* ed 4. Philadelphia: WB Saunders: Philadelphia, 1999.

11. Miller RD, editor: *Anesthesia,* ed 5. Philadelphia: Churchill Livingstone, 2000.

12. Swearingen, PL, Keen JH, editors: *Manual of critical care nursing,* ed 4. St Louis: Mosby, 2001.

13. *Trauma nursing core course,* ed 5. Park Ridge, IL: Emergency Nurses Association, 2000.

14. Urden LD, Stacy KM: *Priorities in critical care nursing,* ed 3. St Louis: Mosby, 2001.

55 Special Procedures

LINDA BOYUM

∎ ∎ ∎

OBJECTIVES

At the conclusion of this chapter the reader will be able to:

1. List the common ambulatory nonsurgical procedures.

2. Describe assessment parameters pertinent to the patient undergoing special procedures.

3. Identify nursing interventions appropriate to the care of the patient undergoing a gastrointestinal (GI) procedure.

4. Describe six types of reactions that can occur as a result of a blood transfusion.

5. Identify three potential complications for the patient undergoing electroconvulsive therapy (ECT) and discuss appropriate nursing interventions for each.

∎
∎ ∎ Because of the extensive number of procedures that can be classified as "special procedures," the emphasis of this chapter will include only those procedures commonly encountered in the ambulatory surgery center (ASC) or outpatient unit. These include endoscopic procedures, radiologic procedures, and ECT.

I. Overview
   A. Definition
      1. Variety of procedures performed throughout facility may be termed "special procedures."
      2. May include nonsurgical diagnostic procedures as well as invasive procedures
      3. May be performed in
         a. Endoscopy
         b. Radiology
         c. Nursing unit
         d. PACU
      4. Procedures include
         a. Endoscopy
         b. Radiologic exams
         c. ECT
   B. Involvement of postanesthesia care unit (PACU), ASC staff
      1. May or may not participate in
         a. Preprocedure preparation of patient
         b. Intraprocedure assessment and monitoring
         c. Postprocedure recovery and discharge
      2. Varies according to facility protocols
II. Anatomy and physiology
   A. GI procedures (see Chapter 42)
      1. Anatomy of GI tract
         a. Mouth (oral or buccal cavity)
            (1) Teeth, tongue, hard and soft palates, cheeks, lips, pharynx
            (2) Salivary glands
               (a) Parotid
               (b) Sublingual
               (c) Submandibular
         b. Esophagus
            (1) Hollow muscular tube

(2) Approximately 23-25 cm (10 inches) long

(3) Approximately 2-3cm (1 inch) in diameter

(4) Extends from pharynx to stomach
  (a) Passes through diaphragm into the abdomen opening called diaphragmatic hiatus

(5) Positioned posterior to trachea and anterior of vertebral column

(6) Wall made up of three layers
  (a) Mucosa
  (b) Submucosa
  (c) Muscularis

(7) Sphincters
  (a) Upper pharyngoesophageal
  (b) Lower esophagogastric (cardiac)

(8) Disorders
  (a) Gastroesophageal reflux disease (GERD)
  (b) Esophageal varices
  (c) Tumors
  (d) Diverticula
  (e) Motility disorders
  (f) Foreign bodies
  (g) Strictures, rings, and webs
  (h) Infectious disease

c. Stomach

(1) J-shaped distensible organ

(2) Located in left upper quadrant of abdomen (just below diaphragm, between esophagus and duodenum)

(3) Approximately 25-30 cm (l0-12 inches) long

(4) Approximately 10-15 cm (4-6 inches) wide at widest point

(5) Function
  (a) Digests food and prepares nutrients for absorption
  (b) Serves as reservoir for swallowed food, drink, and digested secretions
  (c) Mixes and delivers chyme to the small intestine for further digestion and absorption
  (d) Originates signals for hunger and satiety

(6) Consists of
  (a) Fundus
  (b) Body
  (c) Pylorus (antrum)
  (d) Cardiac region

(7) Sphincters
  (a) Esophagogastric (cardiac)
    (i) Prevents backward reflux of stomach contents
  (b) Pyloric
    (i) Works with duodenum to create pressure gradient, which allows emptying of stomach

(8) Disorders
  (a) Acid-peptic disorders
  (b) *Helicobacter pylori*
  (c) Polyps
  (d) Gastritis
  (e) Gastric cancer
  (f) Gastric varices
  (g) Hiatal hernia
  (h) Gastric outlet obstruction
  (i) Stress ulcers
  (j) Motor dysfunction
  (k) Bezoars (concretions of foreign material found in stomach)

    d. Small intestine
- (1) Tube-shaped structure
- (2) Approximately 18 feet long, 1 inch in diameter
- (3) Three sections
    - (a) Duodenum
        - (i) C shaped
        - (ii) First section
        - (iii) Begins at the pyloric sphincter
        - (iv) Ends at the ligament of Treitz
    - (b) Jejunum
        - (i) Middle section (proximal two fifths)
    - (c) Ileum
        - (i) Last section
        - (ii) Distal three fifths of small bowel
- (4) Properties
    - (a) Circular folds increase absorptive surfaces of small intestine.
- (5) Disorders
    - (a) Duodenal ulcer
    - (b) Bacterial and viral infections
    - (c) Parasitic disease
    - (d) Crohn's disease
    - (e) Meckel's diverticulum
    - (f) Malabsorption syndromes
    - (g) Celiac spruce (poor food absorption and gluten intolerance)
    - (h) Tropical sprue (chronic disorder acquired in endemic tropical areas)
    - (i) Whipple's disease
        - (i) Rare disorder characterized by chronic diarrhea and progressive wasting
        - (ii) Short bowel syndrome
        - (iii) Lactase deficiency
        - (iv) Small bowel tumors
        - (v) Motility disorders

    e. Large intestines
- (1) Tube-shaped structure
    - (a) Approximately 4-6 cm (2 inches) in diameter
    - (b) Approximately 90-150 cm (4-5 feet) long
    - (c) Extends from ileocecal value to the anus
- (2) Consists of
    - (a) Cecum
        - (i) Positioned at junction of ileum and colon
    - (b) Contains ileocecal valve and appendix
    - (c) Ascending colon
        - (i) Portion from cecum to hepatic flexure
    - (d) Transverse colon
        - (i) Segment from hepatic flexure to splenic flexure
    - (e) Transverses abdominal cavity
    - (f) Descending colon
        - (i) Segment from splenic flexure to iliac crest
    - (g) Located on left side of abdomen
    - (h) Sigmoid colon
        - (i) S-shaped segment
        - (ii) Ends at rectum
    - (i) Rectum
        - (i) Last portion of large intestine
        - (ii) Approximately 5 inches long
        - (iii) Segment after sigmoid colon
        - (iv) Connects to anal canal

    f. Disorders of the large intestine
      (1) Polyps
      (2) Angiodysplasia (vascular dilations in the submucosa)
      (3) Colitis
      (4) Necrotizing enterocolitis (NEC)
      (5) Ulcerative colitis
      (6) Pseudomembranous colitis
      (7) Crohn's colitis
      (8) Irritable bowel syndrome (IBS)
      (9) Diverticular disease
      (10) Diverticulosis
      (11) Colorectal cancer
      (12) Hemorrhoids
      (13) Anorectal disorders
      (14) Encopresis (chronic constipation that results in involuntary leaking of feces)
      (15) Anal fissure
      (16) Rectal prolapse
      (17) Anorectal abscess
      (18) Anoarectal fistula
      (19) Anorectal fissure

  2. Nerve supply—occurs two ways
    a. Neural transmission to smooth muscle
      (1) Stimulates movement of food through GI tract
      (2) Occurs as a result of distention of myenteric plexus or submucosal plexus
    b. Autonomic nervous system
      (1) Sympathetic
        (a) Thoracic and lumbar splenic nerves
        (b) Inhibit secretions and movement
        (c) Cause contraction of sphincters
      (2) Parasympathetic
        (a) Vagus nerve: Causes increase in motor activity
        (b) Causes increase in secretions
        (c) Causes sphincters to relax
        (d) Results in peristalsis

  3. Function of GI system
    a. Ingestion
    b. Transport
    c. Digestion
    d. Absorption
    e. Elimination

III. Common procedures
  A. Abdominal paracentesis
    1. Removal and drainage of ascitic fluid in the peritoneal cavity
    2. Diagnostic tool to examine ascitic fluid
    3. Palliative measure to relieve abdominal pressure that may be interfering with respiratory function
    4. Fluid withdrawn with a large-bore needle or a trocar and cannula inserted in the abdominal wall
    5. Before paracentesis, it is important to have patient void to reduce risk of accidental injury to the bladder.
  B. Endoscopy—overview
    1. Direct visual examination of the lumen of the GI tract
    2. Usually performed with lighted flexible fiber optic scope or video scope
    3. Provides undistorted image of body cavity
    4. Illumination provided by external light source

    5. Scope designed to allow for passage of instruments
      a. Allows for
        (1) Pictures to be taken
        (2) Biopsies to be obtained
        (3) Polyps to be removed
        (4) Foreign objects to be removed
        (5) Bleeding areas to be cauterized

C. Anoscopy
  1. Anoscope is a clear plastic or metal speculum designed to examine the anus and lower rectum

D. Anal manometry
  1. Used to assess
    a. Anal and rectal muscles
    b. Sphincter problems
      (1) Can be associated with several disorders, especially fecal incontinence
    c. Chronic constipation

E. Colonoscopy
  1. Direct visualization of the lower GI tract from the rectum to ileocecal valve using a long flexible endoscope (length 120-180 cm)
  2. Used to evaluate for
    a. Malignancy
    b. Polyps
    c. Inflammatory bowel disease
    d. Diverticulitis
    e. Strictures
    f. Bleeding

F. Endoscopic retrograde cholangiopancreatography (ERCP)
  1. Invasive exam using both endoscopic and radiologic techniques to visualize the pancreatic ducts, hepatic ducts, and common bile ducts
  2. Uses a flexible fiber optic duodenoscope
  3. Contrast material is injected.
  4. May include removal of stones, sphincterotomies, or dilation

G. Esophageal dilation
  1. Enlargement of the lumen of the esophagus
  2. Accomplished by forcing a series of increasingly larger dilators through a narrowed area (axial force)
  3. May use a balloon dilator to accomplish opening of a narrowed area (radial force)

H. Esophagogastroduodenoscopy (EGD)
  1. Direct visualization of esophagus, stomach, and proximal duodenum
  2. Flexible fiber optic endoscope (less than 10 mm in diameter) passed through mouth allows for direct vision with still and video photography.
  3. Used to diagnose
    a. Esophageal or gastric lesions
    b. Hiatus hernia
    c. Esophageal varices
    d. Esophagitis
    e. Ulcer disease
    f. Polyps
    g. Strictures (achalasia)
    h. Bleeding
      (1) Motility disorders

I. Percutaneous endoscopic gastrostomy (PEG)
  1. Placement of feeding tube via endoscopy for enteral nutrition
  2. Procedure
    a. Lighted endoscope inserted into stomach

      b. Light shines against abdominal wall.

        (1) Allows visualization of tube placement site

      c. Large-gauge needle and suture passed through abdominal wall and stomach wall

        (1) Snare or biopsy forceps used to bring inner end of suture up through patient's mouth (via endoscope)

      d. PEG tube is tied to suture.

        (1) Pulled through mouth into stomach

        (2) Pulled out abdominal wall

      e. Tube is anchored using internal and external rubber bumpers or internal retention balloon and outer disk.

    3. Advantages

      a. Less risk than surgical gastrostomy

      b. Procedure done under sedation rather than general anesthesia

      c. Faster recovery

      d. Feedings can begin within 24 hours.

      e. Can be performed in endoscopy suite or at bedside

      f. Less costly

J. Percutaneous endoscopic jejunostomy (PEJ)

    1. Tube is passed into jejunum through opening in abdominal wall.

    2. Approach can be surgical or percutaneous.

    3. Procedure

      a. Small tube passed through percutaneous endoscopic gastrostomy tube

      b. Guided via endoscope into duodenum

      c. Tube propelled by peristalsis into jejunum

      d. Placement confirmed by x-ray

        (1) Contrast medium injected

    4. Considerations

      a. Small diameter of tube predisposes it to clogging.

      b. Tube can migrate back to stomach as a result of vomiting.

      c. Feedings are continuous because of jejunum not being a normal reservoir for nutrients.

K. Polypectomy

    1. Removal of a protruding growth or mass of tissue that protrudes from a mucous membrane; usually performed via endoscope

      a. Pedunculated—attached to mucous membrane by a slender stalk or pedicle

      b. Sessile—broad-based polyp

L. Proctosigmoidoscopy (also called rectosigmoidoscopy)

    1. Endoscopic exam of distal sigmoid colon, rectum, and anal canal using a small hollow stainless steel tube approximately 1.5 cm in diameter

    2. Performed to evaluate

      a. Rectal bleeding

      b. Polyps

      c. Tumors

      d. Persistent diarrhea

      e. Fissures

      f. Fistulas

      g. Abscesses

      h. Inflammatory bowel disease

    3. Performed as an initial colorectal cancer screen

    4. Advantages

      a. Better tolerated than rigid proctosigmoidoscopy

      b. Allows for examining more of colon than possible with proctoscope

M. Other diagnostic or therapeutic procedures

    1. Blood transfusion

      a. Types

        (1) Whole blood

        (2) Packed red cells

        (3) Frozen red blood cells

        (4) Platelets

        (5) Granulocytes

        (6) Plasma

        (7) Albumin

        (8) Coagulation factor concentrates

        (9) Prothrombin complex

        (10) Cryoprecipitate

        (11) Immune serum globulins

    b. Collected from

        (1) Donor (homologous)

        (2) Recipient (autologous)

        (3) Donor designated by recipient (designated direct blood)

  2. Bronchoscopy

    a. Direct visualization of walls of trachea, the main-stem bronchus, and the major subdivisions of the bronchial tubes through a bronchoscope

        (1) Rigid bronchoscopy—performed under general anesthesia

        (2) Fiber optic (flexible) bronchoscopy

    b. Indications

        (1) Diagnosis

           (a) Lesions, bleeding sites

           (b) Obtain biopsies, bronchial brushing, bronchial washing.

        (2) Treatment

           (a) Destroy or remove lesions.

           (b) Clear airway of retained secretions.

           (c) Foreign body

        (3) Evaluation of disease progression

        (4) Evaluation of effectiveness of therapy

        (5) May be combined with laser (YAG) therapy for ablation of tracheal and bronchial obstructions

  3. ECT

    a. Application of brief electrical stimulus to induce a cerebral seizure

        (1) Used to treat major psychiatric disorders (e.g., severe depression)

  4. Thoracentesis

    a. Withdrawal of fluid or air from the pleural space

        (1) Amount of removal limited to 1 to 2 L at one time to avoid mediastinal shift and impaired venous return

    b. Indications

        (1) Diagnostic

           (a) Obtain specimen—fluid is evaluated for chemical, bacteriologic, and cellular composition.

        (2) Therapeutic

           (a) Relieve respiratory distress

           (b) Instill medication into pleural space

IV. Education content

  A. Preprocedure

    1. General

      a. Nothing by mouth (NPO) instructions as appropriate

      b. Hygiene

      c. Environment

      d. Facility protocols

      e. Aftercare arrangements

      f. Amnesic effects of conscious sedation

      g. Medication—discontinue or dose as usual.

    2. Procedure specific

      a. GI

        (1) Bowel preparation as appropriate

          (2) Course of procedure
          (3) Expectations
          (4) Recovery period
    b. ECT
          (1) Preprocedure emphasis includes screening for
             (a) Baseline mental status
             (b) Confusion
             (c) Disorientation
             (d) Cardiovascular disease
             (e) Cerebral pathology and/or suspected increased intracranial pressure
          (2) Instruct patient to wash hair night before procedure to remove hair products that may interfere with conduction.
    c. Blood transfusion
          (1) Patient's level of understanding regarding procedure
          (2) History of transfusion reactions
V. General assessment parameters
  A. GI procedures
    1. Preprocedure
      a. Preprocedure emphasis on screening for
          (1) Bleeding disorders in patient or family
          (2) Medications affecting clotting
          (3) Bowel activity
          (4) Swallowing ability
      b. Ensure understanding of preprocedure preparation.
          (1) NPO status
          (2) Diet
          (3) Enema
    2. Postprocedure
      a. General
          (1) Airway and respiratory status
          (2) Vital signs
          (3) Level of consciousness
    3. Procedure specific
      a. Upper GI tract
          (1) Swallowing ability
          (2) Pain
          (3) Bleeding
          (4) Reaction to local anesthetic
          (5) Temperature
      b. Lower GI tract
          (1) Pain
          (2) Flatus
          (3) Bleeding
  B. ECT
    1. Preprocedure assessment per routine protocol
    2. Postprocedure
      a. Assess for hypotension and bradycardia.
      b. Orientation to time, place, and person
  C. Blood transfusion
    1. Preprocedure
      a. Ensure informed consent and/or specific transfusion consent form is complete.
      b. Obtain baseline vital signs, including temperature.
      c. Assess patient history of transfusion reactions.
      d. Educate patient to signs and symptoms of potential reactions.
          (1) Inform patient to immediately report any unusual feelings.
    2. Administration

      a. Ensure blood has been typed and cross matched and that ABO group and Rh factor match patient's type.

      b. Check blood for abnormal color or cloudiness (indicates hemolysis).

      c. Check for presence of gas bubbles (indicates bacterial growth).

      d. Check expiration date on blood bag.

      e. Confirm information with another professional.

      f. Document confirmation.

      g. Administration of unrefrigerated blood should begin within one hour.

      h. Total administration time should generally not exceed four hours.

  3. Nursing interventions during procedure

      a. Assess vital signs per protocol.

      b. Be alert for signs of transfusion reaction.

      c. Types of reactions

         (1) Acute hemolytic

            (a) Caused by infusion of ABO-incompatible blood

            (b) May cause most severe symptoms

         (2) Febrile, nonhemolytic

            (a) Most common

            (b) Treat symptomatically.

         (3) Mild allergic

            (a) Rash, itching, low-grade fever

            (b) May administer antihistamines

         (4) Anaphylactic

            (a) Mild to severe symptoms

         (5) Circulatory overload

            (a) Rare

            (b) Caused by rapid infusion in patient unable to accommodate volume

            (c) Patient may have history of cardiac disease.

         (6) Septic reaction

            (a) Caused by contaminated blood

            (b) Symptoms are immediate.

            (c) Fever, chills, hypotension, shock

            (d) Treat with intravenous antibiotics.

         (7) Delayed

            (a) Can occur several days to two weeks following transfusion

D. Bronchoscopy

  1. Preprocedure

      a. NPO for 6 hours prior to procedure

         (1) Decrease risk of aspiration.

         (2) Remove dentures.

  2. Postprocedure

      a. Assess for return of swallow and gag reflex.

      b. Assess and prepare to treat potential complications.

         (1) Bronchospasm

         (2) Hypoxemia

         (3) Bleeding

         (4) Perforation

         (5) Aspiration

         (6) Cardiac dysrhythmias

         (7) Infection

         (8) Reaction to local anesthetic

      c. Blood-streaked sputum is expected for several hours postprocedure.

      d. Frank bleeding is indicative of hemorrhage.

VI. General perianesthesia priorities

  A. Phase I, preprocedure

    1. Objectives

      a. Assess and prepare patient for procedure.

  b. Obtain baseline data.
  c. Allow for development and implementation of nursing care.
  d. Initiate educational process.
  (1) Continues throughout the continuum of care
2. Nursing process
  a. Assessment parameters
  (1) Physical assessment as noted previously
  (2) Assess for educational needs.
  (3) Assess for psychosocial needs related to developmental age including
    (a) Availability of family member or responsible adult companion
    (b) Community resources needed
3. Plan of care
  a. Include patient, family, responsible adult companion in developing plan of care appropriate to the age of the patient.
  b. Nursing diagnosis might include
  (1) Anxiety and fear related to
    (a) Knowledge deficit
    (b) Unfamiliar environment
    (c) Separation from family
    (d) Lack of control
  (2) Pain related to procedural intervention
  (3) Potential for injury
  (4) Potential for infection
4. Interventions
  a. Nursing interventions might include
  (1) Ensure that all laboratory studies are completed as ordered and indicated.
  (2) Provide information on preprocedure preparation.
    (a) NPO status
    (b) Medications
    (c) Hygiene
    (d) Discharge arrangements
      (i) Ride
      (ii) Aftercare
  (3) Obtain baseline vital signs.
  (4) Ensure legal authorization is appropriate (informed consent).
  (5) Provide orientation to surroundings.
  (6) For ECT patients
    (a) Have patient void immediately prior to procedure.
    (b) Helps prevent incontinence and bladder distention
  (7) Apply monitoring devices as indicated.
    (a) ECG
    (b) Pulse oximetry
    (c) EEG according to facility policy
    (d) Nerve stimulator
5. Evaluation
  a. Evaluation of interventions and patient response might include
  (1) Laboratory results are reviewed, and follow-up completed as indicated.
  (2) Patient, family, responsible adult companion is questioned to determine understanding of preoperative instructions.
  (3) Determine that patient has arranged for aftercare as appropriate.
B. Phase II, PACU
1. Objectives
  a. Ensure that the patient safely recovers from the immediate effects of procedure and anesthesia.
  b. Patient may or may not receive care in PACU, depending on facility policy.

    c. Patient may be transported directly to PACU phase II, depending on facility policy.

2. Nursing process
    a. Assessment parameters
        (1) General
            (a) Routine PACU protocol
            (b) Airway status—patient is at high risk for airway compromise.
            (c) Vital signs are monitored frequently during and after procedure.
            (d) Effects of medications administered
            (e) IV conscious sedation protocol

3. Plan of care
    a. Include patient, family, responsible adult companion in developing a plan of care appropriate to the age of the patient.
    b. Nursing diagnoses might include those listed previously.
    c. Provide for patient safety.
    d. Be alert for potential complications.

4. Nursing interventions
    a. Monitor vital signs per protocol.
    b. Administer medications as ordered.
    c. Observe for potential complications.
    d. Ensure a safe environment.

5. Evaluation
    a. Response to interventions are evaluated continually throughout the patient's stay.
    b. Alterations to plan of care are made as indicated.

6. For ECT patients (patient may have procedure performed in PACU setting)
    a. Assessment parameters
        (1) Airway status
            (a) Patient is at high risk for airway compromise.
        (2) Vital signs are monitored frequently (per protocol) during and after ECT procedure.
        (3) Effects of medications
        (4) IV sedation and analgesia protocol
    b. Plan of care
        (1) Include patient, family, responsible adult companion in developing a plan of care appropriate to the age of the patient.
        (2) Nursing diagnoses might include those listed previously.
        (3) Provide for safety.
        (4) Be alert for potential complications.
    c. Nursing interventions
        (1) Monitor vital signs per protocol.
        (2) Administer medications as ordered.
        (3) Observe for complications.
            (a) Dysrhythmias
            (b) Aspiration
            (c) Hypotension
            (d) Prolonged seizure
        (4) Ensure a safe environment.
            (a) Bite block to prevent damage to teeth and oral cavity during seizure
    d. Evaluation
        (1) Response to interventions are evaluated continually throughout the patient's stay.
        (2) Alterations to plan of care are made as indicated.

7. Blood transfusion
    a. Vital signs per protocol
    b. Assess for latent reaction.

C. Phase III, preparation for discharge
   1. Objective
      a. Ready the patient to return to home.
      b. Patient and caregiver adequately prepared to successfully manage postprocedure care
      c. Education of patient and caregiver is critical to success of ambulatory procedure outcome.
   2. Nursing process
      a. Assessment parameters
         (1) General
            (a) Airway and respiratory status
            (b) Bleeding
            (c) Vital signs
            (d) Discomfort
            (e) Reactions to local anesthetics
            (f) Level of consciousness
   3. Plan of care
      a. Include patient, family, responsible adult companion in developing plan of care.
      b. Plan should be appropriate to the age of the patient.
      c. Nursing diagnoses might include
         (1) Anxiety and fear related to
            (a) Knowledge deficit
            (b) Unfamiliar environment
            (c) Separation from family
            (d) Lack of control
         (2) Alteration in comfort level
         (3) Ineffective breathing patterns related to sedation
         (4) Potential for infection
      d. Be alert for potential complications.
         (1) GI
            (a) Bleeding
            (b) Perforated viscus
               (i) Signs include
                  [a] Increased temperature
                  [b] Abdominal distention
                  [c] Pain
                  [d] Shortness of breath
                  [e] Subcutaneous emphysema
            (c) Respiratory depression
            (d) Vasovagal reaction
         (2) Blood transfusion
            (a) Transfusion reaction signs and symptoms
               (i) Delayed transfusion reaction
               (ii) Integumentary
                  [a] Itching
                  [b] Rashes
                  [c] Swelling
                  [d] Cyanosis
                  [e] Excessive perspiration
               (iii) Respiratory
                  [a] Tachypnea
                  [b] Dyspnea
                  [c] Apnea
                  [d] Wheezing
                  [e] Cyanosis
                  [f] Rales

           (iv) Urinary
              [a] Pain on or during urination
              [b] Oliguria
              [c] Changes in urine color
                  [1] Dark, concentrated
                  [2] Shades of red, brown, amber
          (v) Circulatory
              [a] Chest pain
              [b] Increased heart rate
              [c] Palpitations
              [d] Hypotension
              [e] Hypertension
              [f] Bleeding
         (vi) General
              [a] Muscle aches, pain
              [b] Back pain
              [c] Chest pain
              [d] Headache
              [e] Fever
              [f] Chills
        (vii) Nervous system
              [a] Tingling
              [b] Numbness
              [c] Apprehension, impending doom
    (3) Liver biopsy
      (a) Hemorrhage
      (b) Fluid leakage
      (c) Subcutaneous emphysema
      (d) Perforation of viscus
    (4) Bronchoscopy
      (a) Bronchospasm or laryngospasm
      (b) Hypoxia
      (c) Bleeding
      (d) Pneumothorax
    (5) Thoracentesis
      (a) Hemothorax
      (b) Pneumothorax
      (c) Air embolism
      (d) Subcutaneous emphysema
      (e) Bleeding
    (6) ECT
      (a) Bradycardia
      (b) Taachycardia
      (c) Hypotension
      (d) Hypertension
      (e) Airway management problems
4. Nursing interventions
  a. General
    (1) Monitor vital signs per protocol.
    (2) Administer medications for pain and nausea as ordered.
    (3) Observe for bleeding and other complications.
    (4) Ensure a safe environment.
  b. Procedure specific
    (1) GI
      (a) Withhold fluid until gag reflex intact.
      (b) Observe for complications.
    (2) Other

(a) Observe for complications.
(b) Activity restriction per physician orders
  c. Educational interventions
    (1) Discussion, demonstration, written materials
    (2) Copies of all materials given to patient should be maintained in medical record or on unit.
5. Evaluation
  a. Evaluation of clinical interventions is ongoing until patient is stable and ready for discharge
  b. Evaluation of learning
    (1) Patient and caregiver verbalize understanding.
    (2) Patient and caregiver able to demonstrate skill
      (a) Patient and responsible adult companion should sign that they have been instructed and had the opportunity to have questions answered.

VII. Education content
  A. Postprocedure
    1. General
      a. Activity
      b. Diet
      c. Medication
      d. Complications
      e. Follow-up care
      f. Emergency contact information
  B. Key patient educational outcomes
    1. Patient undergoing a blood transfusion will be able to accurately relate information regarding the transfusion and the signs and symptoms of a latent reaction.
    2. Patients undergoing a GI procedure will be able to identify the signs and symptoms of a perforation (abdominal/chest pain, dyspnea, fever, light-headedness, and distended abdomen).

BIBLIOGRAPHY

1. Brandt B, Ugarriza DN: (1996) Electroconvulsive therapy and the elderly client. *J Gerontol Nurs* 22(12):14-20, 1996.
2. Domkowski K, Schlossberg N: *Gastroenterology nursing, A core curriculum,* ed 2. St Louis: Mosby, 1998.
3. Enns MW, Reise JP: Electroconvulsive therapy. *Can J Psychiatry* 37:671-678, 1992.
4. Gregoratos G: Cardiac catheterization: Basic techniques and complications. In Peterson KL, Nicod P, editors: *Cardiac catheterization: Methods, diagnosis, and therapy.* Philadelphia: WB Saunders, 1997.
5. Meeker MH, Rothrock JC: *Alexander's care of the patient in surgery,* ed 11. St Louis: Mosby, 2000.
6. Mettoma SM: *The Lippincott manual of nursing practice,* ed 7. Philadelphia: Lippincott Williams & Wilkins, 2001.
7. Monahan FD, Neighbors M: *Medical surgical nursing: Foundations for clinical practice,* ed 2. Philadelphia: WB Saunders, 1998.
8. O'Brien D, Burden N: The ASC as a special procedures unit. In Burden N: *Ambulatory surgical nursing,* ed 2. Philadelphia: WB Saunders, 2000.
9. Phippwn M, Wells M: *Patient care during operative and invasive procedures,* Philadelphia: WB Saunders, 2000.
10. Pudner R: *Nursing the surgical patient.* London: Bailliere Tindall, 2000.

AMBULATORY SURGICAL NURSING COMPETENCIES

56 Postanesthesia Assessment Phase II

MARY C. REDMOND

OBJECTIVES

At the conclusion of this chapter the reader will be able to:

1. Explain staffing ratios for postanesthesia care unit (PACU) phase II.
2. Explain concepts of care: rapid postanesthesia care unit progression (RPP), fast-tracking.
3. Identify key points of report at patient admission to phase II.
4. Identify key points of ongoing patient assessment.
5. Explain content of discharge instructions.
6. Identify key points of discharge assessment.

I. General information
 A. Environment of care
  1. Perianesthesia nursing practice promotes and maintains a safe, comfortable, and therapeutic environment for patients, staff, and visitors.
  2. Criteria
   a. Unit specific written policies and policies for
    (1) Fire
    (2) Safety
    (3) Infection control
    (4) Internal and external disasters
    (5) Hazardous materials
   b. Preanesthesia, phase I, phase II, and phase III are distinct levels of care.
   c. Space allocation allows for separate and distinct needs of the perianesthesia patient.
    (1) Each area maintains privacy to ensure patient confidentiality.
    (2) Phase II has no restriction on proximity to phase I or where anesthesia is administered.
    (3) Preanesthesia patients are separated from patients undergoing procedures and/or recovery from anesthesia and sedation.
   d. Personnel and visitor dress codes determined by proximity and frequency of access to operating rooms (ORs)
   e. Supplies and equipment available to meet needs of patients and staff in each area
   f. Professional nurses maintain knowledge of current health care technology and information and participate in evaluation and selection for each area.
   g. Appropriate emergency drugs, equipment, supplies present, readily available, checked in each area
   h. Policy ensures safe transportation of patients.
   i. Professional nurse determines mode of transport and competency level of accompanying personnel based on patient needs.
   j. Professional nurse ensures availability of appropriate transportation from facility.

     k. Appropriate means of transportation from freestanding facility to full-service hospital will be used in emergency situations.

B. Staff

  1. Perianesthesia nurses strive to ensure

    a. Competency

      (1) Integrates knowledge, attitudes, skills, behaviors

    b. Responsibility to patients

      (1) Preserves human dignity, autonomy, confidentiality and worth, protects patient rights, supports patient well being

    c. Professional responsibility

      (1) Responsible and accountable for care provided and maintaining compliance with regulatory and professional agencies

    d. Collegiality

      (1) Member of multidisciplinary health care team

    e. Research

      (1) Participates in and conducts research to improve practice and education

  2. Staff characteristics and educational background

    a. Organized, energetic, versatile, independent thinkers

    b. Possess common sense and caring attitude

    c. Work efficiently, independently, and collaboratively

    d. Positive attitude, physically and emotionally supportive

    e. Previous medical-surgical nursing experience

    f. Strong teaching skills

    g. Basic understanding of anesthetic agents and side effects

    h. Strong clinical assessment skills

    i. Critical care background is advantageous.

    j. Certification in basic life support (BLS) in all areas

    k. Certification in advanced cardiac live support (ACLS) and pediatric advanced life support (PALS) as appropriate to patient population served in PACU phase I

    l. If departmentally feasible, cross training in preoperative area, OR, and/or PACU phase I

  3. Appropriate number of professional nursing staff

    a. PACU phase II: two competent personnel, one of whom is an RN competent in phase II postanesthesia nursing, are present whenever a patient is receiving phase II level of care.

    b. ASPAN defines "present" as being in the particular place where patient is receiving care.

  4. Staffing ratios

    a. Class 1:3—one nurse to three patients

      (1) Over 5 years of age, within one half hour of procedure or discharge from phase I level of care

      (2) Five years of age and under, within one half hour of procedure or discharge from phase I level of care with family present

    b. Class 1:2—one nurse to two patients

      (1) Five years of age and under without family or support staff present

      (2) Initial admission of patient postprocedure

    c. Class 1:1—one nurse to one patient

      (1) Unstable patient of any age requiring transfer

C. Scope of care

  1. PACU phase II

    a. Is level of care versus specific location

    b. Is care based on patient condition versus time

  2. The professional perianesthesia nursing roles during phase II focus on preparing the patient, family, and significant other for care in the home, phase III level of care, or an extended care environment.

II. Concepts of care

    A. RPP

        1. Definition: Involves rapid assessment and progression of patient through phase I PACU

        2. Conditions

           a. Progression based on patient condition versus time

           b. May be safely implemented in both

               (1) Inpatient setting

               (2) Outpatient setting

        3. Pros of RPP

           a. Provides holistic postanesthesia nursing care in phase I PACU by rapidly assessing patients in shorter time intervals, for example

               (1) Every 5 or 10 minutes

               (2) Over 15 to 25 minutes

           b. Until patient meets established discharge criteria for phase I PACU

           c. Earlier discharge reduces phase I PACU costs.

           d. Reduced total length of stay

           e. Aggressive nursing care based on needs of patient

               (1) Biopsychosocial

               (2) Emotional

               (3) Spiritual

        4. Cons of RPP

           a. Costly because patient still spends a limited time in phase I

           b. Depends on presence of motivated and proactive nursing staff who

               (1) Promote wellness concept

               (2) Efficiently deliver nursing care

    B. PACU phase I bypass (fast-tracking)

        1. Definition: Involves direct admission of general, regional, monitored anesthesia care (MAC), or local anesthesia patient from OR to phase II PACU

        2. Components of fast-tracking

           a. Appropriate patient selection

               (1) Patient is candidate for same-day surgery.

               (2) Health status is American Society of Anesthesiologists (ASA) physical status I or II

               (3) Patient is motivated for progressive continuum of care.

               (4) Patient's condition is deemed physiologically and psychosocially appropriate.

               (5) Competent caregiver is available following discharge.

           b. Preoperative education of patient and family

               (1) Begins in surgeon's office, continues through preadmission visit and preoperative phone call

               (2) Presents realistic expectations about

                    (a) Fast-tracking recovery process

                    (b) Possible need to aggressively manage postoperative pain prior to discharge

                    (c) Avoids perception of patient being "rushed out"

           c. Appropriate selection and management of anesthetic agents

               (1) Agents with rapid onset and short half-life with relatively few side effects, for example

                    (a) Propofol

                    (b) Desflurane

                    (c) Sevoflurane

                    (d) Mivacurium

                (2) Preemptive analgesic and antiemetic administration

               (3) Bispectral index of electroencephalogram

                    (a) Allows anesthesia to be maintained at lighter plane

        (b) Allows faster recovery

        (c) Fewer postanesthesia side effects

  d. Assessment criteria to evaluate patient readiness in bypassing phase I at end of surgical procedure

    (1) ASPAN discharge assessment: Phase I (Box 56-1)

    (2) Prior to transfer of patient from OR directly to PACU phase II

  e. Patient care should meet

    (1) American Society of Anesthesiologists (ASA) standards for postanesthesia care

    (2) ASPAN standards of care

  f. Discharge criteria from the department includes

    (1) Orientation

    (2) Pain

    (3) Nausea and vomiting

    (4) Surgical bleeding

    (5) Circulation and sensation

    (6) Vital signs

    (7) Ambulation

    (8) Oral intake

    (9) Voiding

  g. Monitoring and reporting patient outcomes

    (1) Incorporate monitoring and reporting of patient outcomes into PACU performance improvement process.

    (2) Reporting patient outcomes

        (a) Patient satisfaction

        (b) Medical and nursing care

        (c) Readmission to PACU phase I or to hospital

3. Not all patients are candidates for bypass of PACU phase I. Reasons for going to PACU phase I include

  a. Nursing care

    (1) Offers constant vigilance

    (2) Focuses on preventing complications

■ BOX 56-1
■ **DISCHARGE ASSESSMENT: PHASE I**

Data collected and documented to evaluate the patient's status for discharge include, but are not limited to:

1. Airway patency, respiratory function, and oxygen saturation
2. Stability of vital signs
3. Hypothermia resolved
4. Level of consciousness and muscular strength
5. Adequate pain control
6. Mobility
7. Patency of tubes, catheters, drains, intravenous lines
8. Skin color and condition
9. Condition of dressing and/or surgical site
10. Intake and output
11. Comfort
12. Anxiety
13. Child-parent and patient–significant others interaction
14. Numerical score, if used

From American Society of PeriAnesthesia Nurses, *2002 Standards of Perianesthesia Nursing Practice*, Cherry Hill, NJ: American Society of PeriAnesthesia Nurses, 2002, p 20.

   b. Patient safety needs
     (1) Optimal environment to avert harm caused by
       (a) Dysphoria, agitation
       (b) Physiologic conditions (e.g. pain, hypoxemia)
       (c) Developmentally challenged patients
     (2) Focus on safely moving patient to next level of care.
   c. Continuous monitoring
     (1) Preexisting morbidity may require additional monitoring.
       (a) Intraoperative electrocardiogram (ECG) changes
       (b) Inability to maintain acceptable Sao_2
   d. Complications
     (1) Untoward intraoperative event requires additional monitoring.
       (a) Bleeding
       (b) Myocardial infarction
       (c) Pulmonary embolism
     (2) Other concerns, for example
       (a) Hypothermia
       (b) Shivering
       (c) Resolved laryngospasm
   e. Hemodynamics
     (1) Hypertension caused by
       (a) Use of cocaine spray
       (b) Pain
       (c) Anxiety
     (2) Hypotension caused by
       (a) Inadequate fluid replacement
       (b) Blood loss
   f. Comfort care
     (1) Need for aggressive pharmacologic intervention, for example
       (a) Management of acute pain
       (b) Management of postoperative nausea and vomiting (PONV)
       (c) Other conditions
   g. Respiratory care
     (1) Need for supplemental oxygen for
       (a) New onset respiratory distress
       (b) Inadequate respiratory effort because of lingering sedation, age, obesity, for example
       (c) Preexisting health conditions (e.g., sleep apnea)
   h. Extremes of age
     (1) Infants routinely transfer to PACU phase I
       (a) Unstable condition can occur quickly.
       (b) Response time is critical.
     (2) Some children can bypass PACU phase I when appropriate.
       (a) Older than 7 years
       (b) ASA status I or II
       (c) Surgery lasts <90 minutes.
       (d) Meet established criteria specific to age group
     (3) Advantages
       (a) Minimizes parent-child separation
       (b) Reduces anxiety
       (c) Increases satisfaction
     (4) Elderly at greater risk for untoward events after general or regional anesthesia
       (a) Have more comorbidities
       (b) Have many physiologic changes affecting all systems
       (c) Evaluate appropriateness of bypassing PACU phase I by considering
         (i) Type of anesthesia administered
         (ii) Type of procedure performed

      i. Economic issues

         (1) Should never be a determining factor for bypassing PACU phase I

  4. Conditions to be met for fast-tracking

     a. Patient must meet all PACU phase I discharge criteria in the OR before being discharged directly to PACU phase II.

     b. Requires astute assessment by all parties involved

        (1) Anesthesia provider

        (2) Circulator

        (3) Receiving phase II perianesthesia nurse

     c. May be conducted only in the ambulatory setting

        (1) Patient receiving general or regional anesthesia should never bypass PACU phase I and be admitted directly to floor in inpatient setting.

  5. Pros of PACU phase I bypass

     a. Cost savings

        (1) PACU phase I care eliminated

        (2) Overall decreased length of stay

     b. Most patients feel better faster and want to be discharged earlier.

  6. Cons of PACU phase I bypass

     a. Focus is short-term, nonacute care for the purpose of

        (1) Discharge teaching

        (2) Reuniting patient with caregiver; therefore

     b. Patients should not require

        (1) Continuous monitoring

        (2) Aggressive pain or nausea management

     c. PACU phase II nurses may not have critical care skills needed to recognize and manage emergency situations.

III. Phase II patient assessment

  A. Transfer of patient to phase II

    1. Receiving nurse determines that the admission is appropriate to phase II.

    2. Transferring and receiving nurses cooperate in settling patient safely.

    3. Phase I discharge report (from OR circulating nurse or phase I nurse, as appropriate) includes

     a. Patient's name

     b. Procedure

     c. Type of anesthetic

     d. Discharge vital signs

       (1) Blood pressure

       (2) Temperature

       (3) Pulse

       (4) Respirations

       (5) Oxygen saturation

     e. Condition of dressings

     f. Circulatory and neurological checks

       (1) Following spinal or epidural anesthetic

       (2) Following surgery on an extremity

     f. Comfort

       (1) Level of pain

       (2) Presence of nausea

     g. Medications given

       (1) Analgesics

       (2) Antiemetics

       (3) Others (e.g., antibiotics)

     h. Intake

       (1) Intravenous (IV)

       (2) Blood and blood products

       (3) Oral

    i. Output
       (1) Urine
       (2) Emesis
       (3) Drains
    j. Preoperative comorbidities
       (1) Identify condition.
       (2) Generally under control?
       (3) Problematic during this surgical experience?
    k. Complications
       (1) Intraoperative
       (2) In PACU phase I
    l. Numerical score if used
    m. Special needs, deficits, challenges
       (1) Prosthetic devices
       (2) Sensory deficits
       (3) Language barrier
    n. Family and significant other
       (1) Waiting
       (2) To contact
    o. Known transportation arrangements
B. Initial assessment: Phase II
   1. Integrate data received at transfer of care.
   2. Assess
    a. Vital signs and share with transferring nurse
       (1) Blood pressure
       (2) Temperature
       (3) Pulse and rhythm
       (4) Respirations and respiratory effort
       (5) Oxygen saturation
    b. Level of consciousness
       (1) Drowsy
       (2) Responsive with stimulation
       (3) Spontaneously responsive
       (4) Alert and anxious for discharge
    c. Position of patient
       (1) Recumbent
       (2) Sitting
       (3) Elevation of extremity
    d. Patient safety needs
       (1) Stretcher positioned low to floor
       (2) Wheels of stretcher, wheelchair, or recliner locked
       (3) Call light within easy reach
    e. Condition and color of skin
       (1) Generalized
          (a) Pink or normal for patient
          (b) Cyanotic
          (c) Rash or hives
          (d) Broken skin
       (2) Operative site or extremity
          (a) Pink or normal for patient
          (b) Dark
          (c) White or light
    f. Neurovascular assessment as applicable
       (1) Capillary return in extremity
          (a) In <3 seconds
          (b) Within 3-5 seconds
          (c) Longer than 5 seconds

  (2) Sensation in extremity
   (a) Identify dermatome for spinal and epidural anesthetic.
   (b) Normal
   (c) Tingly
   (d) Numb
 g. Condition of dressings, drains, tubes as applicable
  (1) Dressings
   (a) Type of drainage
   (b) Color
   (c) Amount
   (d) Location
  (2) Tubes and drains
   (a) Type
   (b) Location
   (c) Patency
    (i) Color
    (ii) Amount
 h. Muscular response and strength and mobility status if applicable
  (1) Movement
   (a) Identify dermatome for spinal and epidural anesthetic.
   (b) Spontaneously
   (c) On command
   (d) None
  (2) Strength
   (a) Strong
   (b) Weak
   (c) None
 i. Fluid therapy
  (1) Location of lines
  (2) Condition of IV site
   (a) Normal
   (b) Red, tender
   (c) Infiltrated
  (3) Fluid infusing
   (a) Type
   (b) Amount
 j. Comfort level
  (1) Physical
   (a) Pain
    (i) Absent
    (ii) Present
     [a] Location
     [b] Pain scale indicator if used
   (b) Nausea
    (i) Absent
    (ii) Present
   (c) Environmental
    (i) Temperature
    (ii) Noise
    (iii) Light
  (2) Emotional
   (a) Calm
   (b) Anxious
   (c) Upset
   (d) Worried and distraught
  (3) Behavioral manifestation
   (a) Body language

         (b) Conversation
         (c) Activity
    k. Numerical score if used
  3. Care planning
    a. Stability of vital signs
      (1) Cardiovascular status
      (2) Respiratory status
    b. Progression to ambulation or approaching preoperative status
    c. Provision of adequate analgesia
    d. Prevention or aggressive treatment of nausea and vomiting
    e. Provision for nutrition and fluid status
    f. Observation of operative site
      (1) Associated symptoms of complications
    g. Psychosocial support
      (1) Speedy reunion with family and significant other
    h. Educational needs
C. Ongoing assessment and management: Phase II
  1. Monitor, maintain, and/or improve respiratory function.
    a. Encourage coughing, deep breathing as appropriate.
    b. Identify any respiratory changes.
      (1) Notify appropriate physician.
      (2) Provide appropriate follow-up care.
    c. Reassess condition.
  2. Monitor, maintain, and/or improve circulatory function.
    a. Monitor circulatory status as appropriate.
    b. Identify any circulatory changes.
      (1) Notify appropriate physician.
      (2) Provide appropriate follow-up care.
    c. Reassess condition.
  3. Promote and maintain effective pain management.
    a. Assess for presence and severity of pain.
    b. Medicate as necessary.
    c. Provide other comfort measures.
      (1) Reposition for comfort.
      (2) Elevate as appropriate.
      (3) Ice as ordered.
      (4) Distraction techniques
    d. Reassess effectiveness of comfort measures.
  4. Administer medication as ordered.
    a. Reassess condition.
    b. Document results.
  5. Promote and maintain physical and emotional comfort.
    a. Physical
      (1) Management of
        (a) Pain
        (b) Nausea and vomiting
        (c) Hunger and thirst
        (d) Bladder urgency
      (2) Environmental
        (a) Temperature
        (b) Light
        (c) Noise
        (d) Odors
    b. Emotional
      (1) Presence of family and significant other
      (2) Positive reinforcement
      (3) Privacy

      (4) Respect

      (5) Questions answered

6. Monitor surgical or procedural site.

    a. Continue procedure-specific care.

    b. Assess for changes.

      (1) Notify appropriate physician.

      (2) Provide appropriate follow-up care.

    c. Reassess condition.

7. Promote patient safety.

    a. Ambulate slowly with gradual progression.

      (1) Dangle at side of bed before standing.

      (2) Sit in recliner.

      (3) Ambulate.

    b. Precautions for ambulating patients

      (1) Sufficient number of assistants based on patient size and ability to ambulate

      (2) Nonslip shoes or slippers

      (3) Gait training with crutches or walker as ordered

    c. Environmental hazards eliminated

      (1) Wet floors

      (2) Obstacles on floor

    d. Refreshments within close range and easy reach

8. Encourage fluids by mouth as indicated.

    a. Safety measures

      (1) Ascertain presence of gag and swallow reflexes.

      (2) Have patients sit upright prior to taking fluids.

      (3) Begin with water or ice.

        (a) Least likely to cause lung damage if aspirated

      (4) Progress slowly to other fluids.

        (a) Some products prompt nausea and vomiting.

          (i) Dairy products

          (ii) Coffee

          (iii) Citrus juice

        (b) Room temperature liquids preferable to hot or cold

      (5) Follow with bland food.

        (a) Crackers

        (b) Dry toast

    b. Predominant determinants of PONV

      (1) Predisposition to nausea and vomiting

        (a) History of motion sickness

        (b) Previous experience with PONV

      (2) Appropriate prophylactic therapy

        (a) Histamine blockers

        (b) Prokinetic agents

        (c) Antiemetics

        (d) Bland food postoperatively

      (3) Psychological expectations

        (a) Self-fulfilling prophecy

        (b) Encourage patient to expect nausea-free recovery.

9. Progress to preprocedure level of mobility as appropriate.

    a. Ambulate slowly with gradual progression.

      (1) Dangle at side of bed before standing.

      (2) Sit in recliner.

      (3) Ambulate.

    b. Precautions for ambulating patients

      (1) Sufficient number of assistants based on patient size and ability to ambulate

        (2) Nonslip shoes or slippers

        (3) Gait training with crutches or walker as ordered

    c. Environmental hazards eliminated

        (1) Wet floors

        (2) Obstacles on floor

10. Discuss provisions for discharge other than to home as indicated.

    a. Refer to Chapters 57, 60.

    b. Determine need to transfer to another department prior to discharge home.

        (1) Physical therapy

        (2) Oncology for chemotherapy treatment

        (3) Radiology for radiation treatment

        (4) Dialysis unit

    c. Determine any discharge option arrangements made or needed.

    d. Discuss if arrangements made in advance.

        (1) Home health follow-up

        (2) Twenty-three hour observation

        (3) Short stay units

        (4) Hospital self-care

        (5) Hospital hotel or motel

            (a) Obtain phone number.

        (6) Package plans

        (7) Recovery center

    e. Determine appropriate follow-up.

        (1) Type

        (2) Time frame

        (3) Confirm correct address and phone number.

11. If returning home, review discharge planning with patient, family, responsible adult.

    a. Refer to Chapters 57, 58.

    b. Confirm appropriate caregiver available to stay with patient following discharge.

    c. Confirm safe, acceptable transportation arrangements.

    d. Confirm preparation of home environment.

        (1) Accessibility of necessary items if mobility is compromised.

            (a) Pillows

            (b) Ice bags

            (c) Phone

            (d) Phone numbers

            (e) Medications

            (f) Emesis receptacle

            (g) Tissue

        (2) Provisions for meals

        (3) Bathroom accessibility

        (4) Securing postoperative medical supplies

            (a) Crutches, walker, cane

            (b) Braces, slings

            (c) Continuous passive motion devices

            (d) Dressings

            (e) Sunglasses

        (5) Removing obstacles

            (a) Throw rugs

            (b) Cords

            (c) Excess furniture

    e. Discharge instruction content should address

        (1) Medications

            (a) Name

       (b) Type, purpose, side effects

       (c) Dose

       (d) Take with or without food, type of fluids

       (e) When next dose due

       (f) No alcohol for 24 hours

    (2) Activity restrictions

       (a) Limitations

       (b) Expectations

       (c) No driving for 24 hours or until approved by physician

       (d) Avoid signing legal documents for 24 hours.

    (3) Diet

       (a) Caution against heavy, spicy food on day of surgery.

       (b) Increase oral liquids.

       (c) Progress diet as instructed.

       (d) If nauseated, avoid causative food.

    (4) Care of surgical site

       (a) Amount and type of expected drainage

       (b) Care, replacement, removal of dressings

       (c) When and how to bathe and shower

    (5) Surgical and anesthesia side effects

       (a) Headache

       (b) Fatigue

       (c) Muscle soreness and weakness

       (d) Sore throat

    (6) Possible complications and symptoms

       (a) Bleeding in excess of anticipated amount

       (b) Swelling at surgical site

       (c) Change in circulation of affected extremity

       (d) Change in sensation of affected extremity

       (e) Fever

    (7) Postoperative treatment and tests to be done

       (a) Postoperative procedures

       (b) Exercises

       (c) Date, time, location of follow-up tests and treatments

    (8) Access to postdischarge and emergency care

       (a) Phone number of patient's physician

       (b) Phone number of ambulatory surgery department and hours of operation

       (c) Phone number of emergency care facility

    (9) Follow-up appointment with physician

       (a) Date, time, location

  f. Instructional process

    (1) Have patient and caregiver read material as appropriate.

    (2) Nurse reviews material with patient and caregiver.

    (3) Nurse clarifies information with patient and caregiver.

    (4) Nurse answers questions for patient and caregiver.

    (5) Nurse demonstrates techniques for patient and caregiver.

    (6) Nurse gets return demonstration from patient and caregiver as appropriate.

  g. Provide written discharge instructions.

  h. Call prescriptions to chosen pharmacy if patient desires.

  i. Determine appropriate follow-up.

    (1) Type

    (2) Time frame

    (3) Confirm correct address and phone number.

D. Discharge assessment: Phase II

  1. Intent is adequate recovery from anesthesia, not from surgical procedure.

2. Assessment includes
   a. Adequate respiratory function
      (1) Return of preanesthesia respiratory status
          (a) No symptoms of upper airway compromise
              (i) Wheezing
              (ii) Snoring
              (iii) Stridor
              (iv) Labored breathing
              (v) Crowing
      (2) Preexisting pulmonary conditions
          (a) Specific physician's evaluation and discharge order as
              appropriate for
              (i) Asthma
              (ii) Emphysema
              (iii) Ventilator dependence
          (b) No acute exacerbation of preexisting disease present at discharge
          (c) Comparison of preoperative and postoperative SaO_2 levels
   b. Stability of vital signs
      (1) Stable for predetermined time according to policy and procedure;
          check
          (a) On admission to phase II
          (b) Prior to discharge
          (c) As indicated by patient need
          (d) According to facility procedure
      (2) Blood pressure
          (a) Compare with preoperative and intraoperative levels.
          (b) Compare with preadmission visit or physician's office values if
              available.
          (c) Readings 20% of preoperative value
      (3) Pulse
          (a) Regular rate and rhythm
          (b) Reflect preoperative status
   c. Hypothermia resolved
      (1) Minimum temperature will be 36° C (96.8° F) or core prior to
          discharge.
      (2) Patient describes an acceptable level of warmth.
      (3) Signs and symptoms of hypothermia absent
          (a) Shivering
          (b) Piloerection
          (c) Cold extremities
      (4) Patient or caregiver describes methods of maintaining normothermia
          at home.
   d. Level of consciousness and muscular strength
      (1) Acceptable level of sedation at discharge is elusive.
      (2) Return to preoperative level of orientation.
          (a) Person, place, time
          (b) Aware of and assistance with transfer from surgical facility to
              home environment
      (3) If patients remain sleepy
          (a) Sleepiness does not necessarily constitute contraindication to
              being home if patient not left alone
          (b) Responsible adult willing to fulfill caregiver duties.
      (4) Assess strength.
          (a) Consistent with preoperative level
          (b) If weakness, assess possible causes.
              (i) Infiltration of local anesthetic or nerve block
              (ii) Effects of other anesthetic agents

        (iii) Preexisting condition

        (iv) Accident or injury

e. Ability to ambulate consistent with baseline and procedural limitations

    (1) Assess motor integrity of all extremities.

    (2) If Romberg test used to identify longer recovery period, positive test characterized by

        (a) Loss of sense of position

        (b) Loss of balance when standing upright with feet together and eyes closed

    (3) Absence of dizziness or faintness

    (4) Postspinal and postepidural anesthesia requires

        (a) Return of sensation and strength

        (b) Proprioception (sense of position of legs and feet)

    (5) Exceptions

        (a) Local infiltration of analgesic

        (b) Therapeutic nerve block for analgesia

f. Ability to swallow

    (1) All protective airway reflexes present

        (a) Swallow

        (b) Cough

        (c) Gag

    (2) Following manipulation of or administration of topical anesthesia to upper airway

        (a) Patient demonstrates ability to swallow.

        (b) If ordered, NPO for several hours

           (i) Specific time parameters to observe before drinking

          (ii) Begin with water.

         (iii) Avoid talking while drinking.

         (iv) Concentrate on swallowing.

g. Minimal nausea and vomiting

    (1) Ensure good hydration with IV fluids prior to discharge.

    (2) Reinforce comfort measures.

        (a) Limit heavy or spicy foods.

        (b) Remain recumbent until nausea subsides.

        (c) Avoid rapid position changes.

        (d) Base oral intake on desire to eat and drink.

h. Skin color and condition

    (1) Check color consistent with or better than preoperative condition.

        (a) Normal

        (b) Pale

        (c) Flushed

        (d) Mottled

    (2) Check capillary refill consistent with or better than preoperative timing.

    (3) Check skin for absence of injury.

        (a) Abrasions

        (b) Burns

        (c) Tears

        (d) Bruises

i. Condition of surgical site

    (1) No active bleeding

    (2) Observe dressings or surgical site for

        (a) Increased girth

        (b) Distention

        (c) Swelling

        (d) Vaginal flow and hematuria

        (e) Frequent swallowing

(3) Observe for
  (a) Tachycardia
  (b) Hypotension
j. Adequate pain control
  (1) Unrealistic to expect every patient to be pain-free at discharge
  (2) Have patient compare current pain level with stated preoperative expectations.
  (3) Infiltration with local anesthetic at operative site results in greater comfort.
    (a) Caution against increased activity.
    (b) Advise initiation of oral analgesics as local anesthetic wears off.
  (4) Pain should be controlled with oral analgesics.
  (5) Parenteral analgesia may be necessary.
    (a) If patient expected to have higher level of discomfort at home
    (b) Goal is comfort without excessive sedation.
    (c) Ensure presence of responsible caregiver.
k. Adequate neurovascular status of operative extremity
  (1) Assess circulatory status.
    (a) Pulses
    (b) Color
    (c) Temperature
  (2) Assess sensory integrity; consider presence of
    (a) Local anesthetic infiltration
    (b) Nerve block
l. Ability to void as indicated
  (1) Requirements vary among facilities.
  (2) To avoid complications at home, should void prior to discharge if potentially complicating conditions present
    (a) Prostatic hypertrophy, diagnosed or undiagnosed
    (b) Inadequate hydration
    (c) Primary kidney disease
    (d) Certain surgical procedures
      (i) Inguinal herniorrhaphy
      (ii) Rectal and pelvic procedures
      (iii) Urinary procedures because of potential for hematuria
    (e) Spinal and epidural anesthesia
      (i) Voiding indicates end of effects of sympathetic blockade.
      (ii) Voiding indicates adequate vasomotor function for maintaining normotension when standing and walking.
m. Physical, emotional, psychological factors
  (1) Patient may express vague complaints.
    (a) May find difficulty explaining
    (b) Slow the discharge process and avoid potential complications at home.
  (2) Avoid perception of "rushing" the patient.
    (a) Patient will perceive care as substandard even if of highest quality.
    (b) Have patient and responsible adult verbalize readiness for discharge.
  (3) Emotional responses following surgery vary.
    (a) May be individual reaction
    (b) May be response to surgical outcome
      (i) Biopsy result
      (ii) Extensive alteration in body image
      (iii) Relief at receiving positive report
    (c) Individual behavioral responses
      (i) May question behavior while awakening
      (ii) May experience pleasant or unpleasant dreams
      (iii) May experience confusion

    n. Patient and home care provider understand discharge instructions.

        (1) Answer any additional questions.

        (2) Provide and clarify any additional information.

    o. Written discharge instructions given to patient and accompanying responsible adult

        (1) Place in a safe, accessible location.

        (2) If appropriate, make available to patient when alert.

    p. Verify arrangements for safe transportation home.

    q. Confirm additional resource to contact if any problems arise.

    r. The professional perianesthesia nurse will complete a discharge follow-up to assess and evaluate patient status.

        (1) Refer to Chapter 59.

IV. Patient discharge issues

  A. General discharge guidelines established by national accrediting organizations

    1. Joint Commission for Accreditation of Healthcare Organizations (JCAHO) Ambulatory Care Accreditation Services

    2. Accreditation Association of Ambulatory Health Care (AAAHC)

  B. General discharge guidelines established by professional organizations

    1. ASA

    2. American Society of PeriAnesthesia Nurses (ASPAN)

  C. Each ambulatory facility must establish written protocol for discharge.

    1. Should specify discharge criteria

    2. Provides a foundation for practice decisions

    3. Should serve as a standard of care

V. Documentation of care

  A. Challenging because of

    1. High volume

    2. Rapid turnover of patients

  B. Documentation format must

    1. Be accurate

    2. Be comprehensive

    3. Be user friendly

    4. Provide for a smooth progression of care

  C. May incorporate a combination of

    1. Relatively standard assessments by checking off, filling in, or circling items

    2. Checklists

    3. Scoring systems

    4. Narrative notes to address specific issues for individual patients

BIBLIOGRAPHY

1. Burden N: Fast-tracking children postoperatively. *Perianesth Ambul Surg Nurs Update* 9:65-66, 2001.

2. Aldrete JA: Modifications to the postanesthesia score for use in ambulatory surgery. *J PeriAnesth Nurs* 13:148-55, 1998.

3. American Society of Anesthesiologists (ASA): Guidelines for postoperative care. Available at http://www.asahq.org/publicationsAndServices/standards/Postanesth.pdf. Accessed on December 1, 2002.

4. Apfelbaum JL, Walawander CA, Grasela TH, et al: Eliminating intensive postoperative care in same-day surgery patients using short-acting anesthetics. *Anesthesiology* 97:66-74, 2002.

5. *ASPAN Standards of Perianesthesia Nursing Practice.* Cherry Hill, NJ: American Society of PeriAnesthesia Nurses, 2000.

6. Barnes S: The state of ambulatory surgery and perianesthesia nursing. *J PeriAnesth Nurs* 16:347-352, 2001.

7. Barnes S, O'Brien D: Considering bypass of phase I PACU? *J PeriAnesth Nurs* 17:193-195, 2002.

8. Chung F, Mezei G: Adverse outcomes in ambulatory anesthesia: What can we improve? *Ambul Surg* 8:73-78, 2000.

9. DeFazio Quinn DM, editor: *Ambulatory surgery.* Philadelphia: WB Saunders, 1997.

10. Duncan PG, Shandro J, Bachand R, et al: A pilot study of recovery room bypass

("fast-track protocol") in a community hospital. *Can J Anaesth* 48:630-636, 2001.

11. Joint Commission on Accreditation of Healthcare Organizations (JCAHO): Standards clarification. Accessed at http://www.jcaho.org on December 1, 2002.

12. Joshi GP, Twersky RS: Fast tracking in ambulatory surgery. *Ambul Surg* 8:185-190, 2000.

13. Kovac AL: The difficult postoperative patient with nausea and/or vomiting. *Curr Rev PeriAnesth Nurse* 19:25-36, 1997.

14. Lauro HV, Berman LS: Cutting-edge pediatric anesthesia for the outpatient. *Same Day Surg Rep* Suppl, May 2002.

15. Lichtor JL, Alessi R, Lane BS: Sleep tendency as a measure of recovery after drugs used for ambulatory surgery. *Anesthesiology* 96:878-883, 2002.

16. Mamaril M: Fast-tracking the postanesthesia patient: The pros and cons. *J PeriAnesth Nurs* 15:89-93, 2000.

17. Marley RA, Moline BM: Patient discharge issues. In Burden N, DeFazio Quinn DM, O'Brien D, et al, editors: *Ambulatory surgical nursing*, ed 2. Philadelphia: WB Saunders, 2000, pp 504-526.

18. Mecca RS: Safety in the post anesthesia care unit, part I: Clinical safety. *Curr Rev Perianesth Nurse* 23:247-259, 2001.

19. Meeker MH, Rothrock JC, editors: *Alexander's care of the patient in surgery*, ed 11. St Louis: Mosby, 1999.

20. Pandit SK: Ambulatory anesthesia and surgery in America: A historical background and recent innovations. *J PeriAnesth Nurs* 14:270-274, 1999.

21. Patterson P: "Fast tracking" of patients through PACU: Is it safe? *OR Manager* 14:1, 8-9, 1998.

22. Patterson P: Discharge criteria: Are they keeping up with practices? *OR Manager* 15:1, 17, 19, 1999.

23. Saar LM: Use of a modified postanesthesia recovery score in phases II perianesthesia period of ambulatory surgery patients. *J PeriAnesth Nurs* 16:82-89, 2001.

24. Smith S: Progressive postanesthesia care: Phase II recovery. In Burden N, DeFazio Quinn DM, O'Brien D, et al, editors: *Ambulatory surgical nursing*, ed 2. Philadelphia: WB Saunders, 2002, pp 477-503.

25. Swearingen PL, Ross DG, editors: *Manual of medical-surgical nursing care: Nursing interventions and collaborative management*, ed 4. St Louis: Mosby, 1999.

26. Tessler MJ, Mitmaker L, Wahba RM, et al: Patient flow in the post anesthesia care unit: An observational study. *Can J Anaesth* 46:348-351, 1999.

27. Wallin E, Lundgren P, Ulander K, et al: Does age, gender or educational background affect patient satisfaction with short stay surgery? *Ambul Surg* 8:79-88, 2000.

28. Watkins AC, White PF: Fast-tracking after ambulatory surgery. *J PeriAnesth Nurs* 16:379-387, 2001.

29. White PF: What is new in ambulatory anesthesia? *Curr Rev Perianesth Nurse* 21:150-160, 1999.

30. White PF: What is new in ambulatory anesthesia? *Curr Rev Nurse Anesth* 22:77-88, 1999.

31. Williams BA, Kentor ML, Williams JP, et al: PACU bypass after outpatient knee surgery is associated with fewer unplanned hospital admissions but more phase II nursing interventions. *Anesthesiology* 97:981-988, 2002.

32. Wilson GWD: One institution's perspective on fast tracking same-day surgery patients: Post anesthesia care unit bypass. *Semin Periop Nurs* 10:29-32, 2001.

33. Yellen E, Davis GC: Patient satisfaction in ambulatory surgery. *AORN J* 74:483-486, 489-494, 496-498, 2001.

57 Patient Discharge Education in the Phase II Setting

PAMELA M. DARK

OBJECTIVES

At the conclusion of this chapter the reader will be able to:

1. Utilize the nursing process in providing patient and family education (assessment, nursing diagnosis, planning, intervention, and evaluation).

2. Review JCAHO (Joint Commission on Accreditation of Health Care Organizations) patient education standards.

3. Identify patient's, family's, and significant other's education needs preoperatively and postoperatively.

4. Identify patient's, family's, and significant other's learning deficits.

5. Develop the patient's, family's, and significant other's education plan based on learning deficits and needs.

6. Define education needed for the preoperative and postoperative patient, family, and significant other.

7. Determine effectiveness of education provided to patient, family, and significant other preoperatively and postoperatively.

8. Define documentation standards for patient, family's, and significant other's education.

I. Review of Joint Commission on Accreditation of Health Care Organizations (JCAHO) patient education standards
   A. "The goal of the patient and family education function is to improve patient health outcomes by promoting healthy behavior and involving the patient in care and care decisions" (JCAHO).[10]
   B. Expectations
      1. Provide the patient and family or significant other with information that will enhance their knowledge and the skills necessary to promote recovery and improve function.
      2. The patient receives education and training as appropriate to the care and services provided by the hospital specific to the patient's
         a. Assessed needs
         b. Abilities and learning preferences
         c. Readiness to learn (JCAHO Standard PF.3)
      3. Consider barriers in education assessment.
         a. Cultural
         b. Religious
         c. Physical
         d. Cognitive limitations
         e. Language
         f. Financial
      4. Educate patients about the safe and effective use of
         a. Their medications according to their needs
         b. Equipment and supplies and means of obtaining them

  5. Counsel patients as to foods and diets appropriate to illness as well as possible food-drug interactions.
  6. Provide patients leaving a facility with information on obtaining follow-up care and accessing community resources.[4]
  7. Provide patients with education about pain and pain management as part of treatment.
  8. Provide patients with information about their responsibilities in their care, including self-care activities.
      a. Patients have been identified as having responsibilities as well as rights.
  9. Provide discharge instructions that contain information about
      a. Diet
      b. Activity
      c. Medications
      d. Follow-up care and plan
      e. Contact number if the patient has questions
      f. Documentation of education is provided to patient and family in
          (1) Verbal form
          (2) Written form
  10. Provide patients with information about available resources that will facilitate habilitation or rehabilitation.
  11. Promote the patient education process among appropriate staff and disciplines that are providing care or services.
  12. Care is planned for and coordinated by the facility providing the patient services.
  13. Patient's rights information emphasizes the importance of educating patients regarding ongoing health care requirements following discharge.
  14. ASPAN standards state: "Reinforce discharge planning with patient and family or accompanying responsible adult as appropriate; provide written discharge instructions" (ASPAN 2002 Standards of Perianesthesia Nursing Practice, p. 31).[1]

II. Assessment
  A. Identify patient's, family's, and significant other's education needs.
      1. Preoperatively
      2. Postoperatively
  B. Utilize information collected through the
      1. Needs assessment (see Chapter 4)
      2. Health history
      3. Patient's, family's, and significant other's interview.
  C. Determine patient's preferred methods of learning (see Chapter 4 for more information).
  D. Consider the patient's, family's, and significant other's understanding of the surgical or invasive procedure and the process.
  E. Evaluate
      1. Health beliefs
      2. Practices
      3. Economic factors
      4. Cultural factors
  F. Determine patient support system.
  G. Determine
      1. Readiness to learn
      2. Motivation
      3. Reading level (see Chapter 4)
  H. Determine home care and postoperative education needs based on
      1. Patient learning and knowledge deficits
      2. Method of anesthesia
      3. Procedure
          a. Learning needs and deficits are determined by
              (1) Anticipated diet

(2) Activity

(3) Potential emergency conditions

(4) Dressing and wound care

(5) Medications—prescribed for postoperative period

(6) Routine daily medications

(7) Follow-up care

(8) Home care requirements

(9) Typical recovery progression

III. Nursing diagnosis

A. Identify patient's, family's, and significant other's learning deficits.

1. Learning needs can be designated in two ways.[2]

a. Patient's, family's, and significant other's primary concerns or problems

b. As the etiology of a nursing diagnosis associated with the patient's, family's, and significant other's response to health alterations or dysfunction

c. Nursing diagnosis from North American Nursing Diagnostic Association (NANDA) may be utilized and may be defined as

(1) Knowledge deficit: deficiency in cognitive knowledge or psychomotor skills concerning the condition or treatment plan, or information-seeking behaviors[2]

(2) Health-seeking behavior: the state in which an individual in stable health actively seeks ways to alter personal health habits and/or the environment in order to move toward a higher level of wellness[2]

(3) If the knowledge deficit is considered the etiology, then the nursing diagnosis will be identified as the "risk for..." (risk for infection...)

d. Examples of nursing diagnosis may include the following[3]:

(1) Altered skin integrity related to (R/T) surgical wound

(2) Potential for infection at surgical site

(3) Alterations in comfort—pain

(4) Alterations in comfort—nausea and vomiting

(5) Self-care deficit

(6) Actual or perceived loss of privacy or dignity

(7) Risk of hemorrhage

(8) Anxiety R/T fear of home care without nursing support, separation from family, potential diagnosis, for example

(9) Potential for injury R/T faintness, weakness, fatigue, prolonged regional block, altered sensory perception

(10) Altered thought processes and/or memory loss R/T sedation and anesthesia

(11) Ineffective airway clearance

(12) Potential for aspiration

(13) Ineffective breathing patterns, respiratory depression R/T sedation, anesthesia, positioning, pain, increased respiratory secretions, vomiting, or untoward reactions to medications or local anesthetics

(14) Potential alteration in tissue perfusion, cardiovascular instability; note: the NANDA approved nursing diagnosis implies a teaching-learning need

e. Outcome goals, nursing interventions, and resources determined as part of the patient discharge education plan may be R/T the preceding examples or other identified problems.

(1) Education provided must address the outcome goals, nursing interventions, and so forth, to provide consistency and safe care.

IV. Planning

A. Develop the patient's, family's, and significant other's education plans based on learning deficits and needs.

1. Formulate the teaching plan and modify to the patient's, family's, and significant other's needs.[3]
   a. Be conscious of sensory or language barriers.
   b. Include an overview of what will occur throughout the process.
      (1) Address the preparation phase.
      (2) Visitation policy–phase I and II recovery areas
      (3) Location of family and responsible adult waiting area
      (4) What to bring to the facility, how to dress
      (5) Leave valuables and jewelry at home.
      (6) Length of time in each phase of the perioperative period—what to expect in each area
      (7) Personnel who will be involved in and providing care
      (8) Environmental descriptions, such as sights, sounds, smells, equipment, and uniforms
      (9) Opportunity for questions R/T the perioperative experience
      (10) Use of preoperative medications (if applicable) and management of postoperative pain and nausea
      (11) How the patient will feel and look after surgery
      (12) Postoperative activity, activity limitations, and exercise recommendations and requirements
      (13) Discharge criteria
      (14) Appropriate follow-up care, and care services—home health, rehabilitation therapies, for example
      (15) Anesthesia-related precautions and expectations
   c. Plan education based on age appropriate considerations and/or special needs.
      (1) Be cognizant of cultural and social concerns.
      (2) Determine caregiver needs and abilities.
   d. Determine teaching priorities.[3]
      (1) Plan with patient, family, and significant other.
      (2) Patient will generally be more focused on high-priority needs and concerns.
   e. Set learning objectives—formally and informally
      (1) Formally—determine desired outcomes for nursing diagnosis and procedure.
      (2) Informally—based on assessed needs that may not be typical concerns or issues
      (3) Objectives will indicate specific behaviors that are desired, reflect observable measurable activity, include criteria specifying time by which learning should have occurred.
      (4) Determine when postoperative education will occur—may occur preoperatively and then be reinforced postoperatively
   f. Select content to be taught.
      (1) Ensure that information provided is accurate, current, based on specific learning objectives, adjusted for learner's age, culture, and ability.
      (2) Consistent with information the physician has provided regarding the procedure
      (3) Meets the time constraints, learning ability, and level of the patient (see Chapter 4)
   g. Select the teaching strategies to be utilized (Box 57-1).
      (1) Should be suited to individual, material to be learned, and to the teacher
      (2) Address areas causing anxiety promptly—anxiety and concerns impair concentration.
      (3) Teach the basics before proceeding to variations or adjustments.
      (4) Schedule time for review of content and determine issues that may need additional clarification.

■ BOX 57-1
■ **SELECTED TEACHING STRATEGIES**

Strategy	Major Type of Learning
Explanation or description (e.g., lecture)	Cognitive
One-to-one discussion	Affective, cognitive
Answering questions	Cognitive
Demonstration	Psychomotor
Discovery	Cognitive, affective
Group discussions	Affective, cognitive
Practice	Psychomotor
Printed and audiovisual materials	Cognitive
Role-playing	Affective, cognitive
Modeling	Affective, psychomotor
Computer-assisted learning programs	Affective, psychomotor, cognitive

From Berman AJ, Burke K, Erb G,. Kozier B: *Fundamentals of nursing: Concepts, process, and practice,* ed 6. Upper Saddle River, NJ: Prentice Hall Health, 2000, p 472.

    h. Discharge planning begins with initial contacts and preoperative assessment and evaluation.
        (1) Adequate preparation preoperatively results in a more positive perioperative experience for the patient, family, and significant other. "Anxiety levels are decreased, increased understanding of what to expect and improved level of satisfaction will result" (Burden,[3] p. 355).
  2. Identify patient discharge education materials.
    a. Base planning of materials on "need to know versus nice to know"
    b. Generic information and procedure-specific information
    c. Large print size—12 point font or larger
        (1) Sans serif or serif fonts (Arial, Tahoma, etc.)
    d. Readability of fifth grade level or less (various readability programs are available, for example, Simple Measure of Gobbledygook [SMOG] index, RIGHTwriter, Grammatique, Suitability Assessment of Materials [SAM]; readability formulas are also available in at least 12 languages) allows information to be more easily understood. Most individuals will read at four to five grade levels less than last formally completed grade level, unless they are reading technical journal type materials routinely.
        (1) Evaluate color contrast between ink and paper—avoid blues and greens for geriatric patients.
        (2) Simple sentences instead of complex sentence structures—short sentences
        (3) Limit number of three syllable words—increases reading level.
        (4) Use familiar words, not medical terminology.
        (5) Use active voice, not passive voice.
        (6) Limit number of components and facts in each paragraph.
        (7) Limit to two pages or less.
        (8) Layout should be easy to read—pleasant format that provides adequate "white space."
    e. Materials should be reviewed on a predetermined schedule—every one to two years.
    f. Avoid duplication and distribution of copies of copies—keep a master.
    g. Content should be developed through research from
        (1) Physician interview
        (2) Current literature
        (3) Standards of practice—regulatory agencies, medical associations, nursing and medical textbooks, and so forth

> **h.** Personalize instructions as necessary, based on patient's and family's needs.

V. Interventions

A. Define education needed for the preoperative and postoperative patient, family, and significant other.

  1. Education can be formal or informal.

  a. Encourage and facilitate learning—assess patient's understanding of process, information, and so forth.

  b. Assist patient, family, and significant other in verbalization of concerns, questions, and so forth.

  c. Build on knowledge that patient, family, or significant other has at that point in time.

  d. Skillful use of questions can reveal knowledge base and deficits.

  e. Provide education based on information indicated in planning section.

  2. Methods

  a. Written instructions, pamphlets, brochures, verbal, classes, return demonstration, and so forth

  3. Successful teaching techniques[3]

  a. Maintaining eye contact

  b. Providing a quiet, distraction-free environment

  c. Providing only necessary information

  d. Requesting feedback

  e. Using short sentences, simple words, and a conversational voice tone

  f. Using visual aids

  g. Progressing in the order that the information will be utilized

  h. Using familiar words and phrases

  i. Showing respect for the learner

  4. Preoperative education

  a. Process of what will occur—starts with initial contact with patient or in physician office

  b. Procedural information

  c. Postoperative issues, care, and expectations

  d. Anesthesia precautions

  5. Postoperative education—key points for standard discharge instructions[3]

  a. Medications

    (1) Name, purpose, dosage schedule for each medication; emphasize importance of following directions on label

    (2) Resume medications taken prior to surgery per physician's order and instructions.

    (3) Pain medication as prescribed—what medications to avoid, frequency, duration

    (4) Additional pain medication orders—what to do if problems occur

    (5) Take pain medication with food and so forth.

    (6) Review side effects of medication.

    (7) Take with other medications or alone.

    (8) Caution against taking additional acetaminophen and so forth.

    (9) Indicate on discharge instruction sheet when next dose of prescribed medication is due (pain medication, antibiotics, etc.).

  b. Activity restrictions

    (1) Take it easy for the remainder of the day or for the next 24 hours—dizziness and drowsiness are to be expected.

    (2) No driving for 24 hours or as long as regularly taking opioids or sedatives

      (a) Surgeon may restrict for longer time period.

      (b) Dependent on procedure

    (3) Do not consume any alcoholic beverages, including beer, for 24 hours or while taking pain medications.

    (4) Do not make any important personal or business decisions for 24 hours.

    (5) Be in the care of a responsible adult for 24 hours.

    (6) Specifics about lifting and so forth should be included as part of procedure-specific instructions.

c. Diet and elimination

    (1) Any specific restrictions; for example, start with liquids, progress as tolerated

    (2) If no restrictions needed, instruct to progress to a regular diet as tolerated.

    (3) Foods to avoid—spicy, fatty, heavy foods on day of surgery

    (4) Precautions if history of reflux or gastroesophageal reflux disease (GERD)

    (5) Avoidance of foods or liquids that might increase or potentiate nausea and vomiting

    (6) Use of laxatives, stool softeners based on opioids and/or procedure

    (7) Voiding—by when and what to do if unable to

d. Surgical and anesthesia side effects

    (1) Explain common side effects of dizziness and drowsiness.

    (2) Identify potential problems—nausea, vomiting, myalgia, bleeding, pain, sore throat, for example.

    (3) Delineate anticipated problems—pain, bleeding, for example.

e. Hygiene

    (1) Dependent on procedure, dressings, and so forth, when patient can shower or bath

    (2) How to protect dressings or incision

f. Possible complications and symptoms

    (1) Pertinent signs and symptoms that could indicate postoperative complications

    (2) Fever of >38.3° C or 101° F

    (3) Breathing problems

    (4) Bleeding problems—dressing saturated with continually increasing amount of blood; be specific for the surgery

    (5) Pain not relieved by pain medication

    (6) Urinary retention or inability to urinate within defined time frame

    (7) Continual nausea and vomiting

    (8) Extreme swelling or redness around surgical wound, drainage that has changed to yellow or green, or increased pain

    (9) Persistent, atypical pain

g. Treatments and tests

    (1) Procedures that the patient or responsible adult is expected to perform (dressing changes, warm compresses, ice packs, etc.)

    (2) Complete list of supplies needed

    (3) Date, time, and location of follow-up tests if ordered

    (4) Postoperative follow-up care—time, physician phone number, necessity of calling to make appointment, for example

    (5) Crutches, incentive spirometer, antiembolic stockings, emptying of drains, catheters, and so forth

h. Operative site and wound care

    (1) Instructions for appropriate care

    (2) Incision care

    (3) Preventing infection

    (4) Dressing changes

    (5) Drains

    (6) Sexual activity—clarify physician's instructions if appropriate.

    (7) Swelling, numbness, or tingling of affected extremity

    (8) Ice, elevation as appropriate or ordered

      i. Emergency care—when to go, where to go, whom to contact
        (1) Go to nearest emergency department if problems occur.
        (2) Avoid use of urgent care facilities for postoperative concerns.
   6. Anesthesia precautions
     a. General anesthesia concerns
       (1) Impairment of psychomotor and cognitive skills
     b. Sedatives
     c. Opioids
     d. Sensory blocks (regional blocks—spinal, epidural, plexus blocks, etc.)
       (1) Return of motor function prior to sensory function—need for careful positioning and protection
       (2) Signs and symptoms that should be reported
     e. IV catheter site observation and care if needed
   7. Transcultural considerations[2]
     a. Obtain teaching materials in language of patient and family if possible.
       (1) Required by law to provide materials for cultural group that is 5% or greater of the general population
     b. Use visual aids to communicate meaning.
       (1) Pictures, charts, or diagrams
     c. Use concrete instead of abstract words.
       (1) Simple language
       (2) Present only one idea at a time.
     d. Allow time for questions.
     e. Avoid the use of medical terminology or health care language.
     f. Validate brief information in writing if having difficulty understanding patient's, family's, or significant other's pronunciations.
     g. Use humor cautiously.
     h. Do not use slang words or colloquialisms.
     i. Do not assume that a patient and family who nods, uses eye contact, or smiles is indicating an understanding of what is being taught.
     j. Invite and encourage questions during teaching.
       (1) Avoid asking negative questions.
       (2) In some cultures expressing a need or confusion may be perceived as inappropriate or rude.
     k. Be cautious when explaining procedures or functions R/T personal areas of the body.
       (1) May be appropriate to have a nurse of the same sex do the teaching
       (2) Be aware of need to have family member or interpreter of same sex present when giving instructions.
     l. Include the family in planning and teaching.
     m. Consider the patient's, family's, and significant other's time orientations.
       (1) May be present-oriented—less concerned with schedules
     n. Identify cultural health practices and beliefs.
VI. Evaluation
  A. Determine effectiveness of education provided to patient, family, and significant other preoperatively and postoperatively.
   1. Evaluation is an ongoing and final process when determining what has been learned.
   2. Learning is measured against the predetermined learning objectives.[2]
   3. Evaluation can occur using a variety of methods.
     a. Direct observation of behavior—return demonstration
     b. Oral questioning
     c. Self-reports and self-monitoring
     d. Postoperative phone call
     e. Patient satisfaction surveys
     f. Feedback from physicians

4. Evaluate teaching.
   a. It is important for nurses to evaluate own teaching and content of teaching programs.[2]
      (1) Consider timing, teaching strategies, amount of information, whether teaching was helpful, and so forth.
   b. Patients, families, and significant others should be given opportunity to evaluate learning experiences.
      (1) Feedback questionnaires
      (2) Patient satisfaction surveys
      (3) Postoperative phone call contacts
   c. Forgetting is normal and should be anticipated.
      (1) Increases with level of anxiety and so forth

VII. Documentation
   A. Define documentation standards for patient's, family's, and significant other's education.[11]
      1. Document information provided to patient, family, and significant other.
         a. Preoperative instructions
         b. Postoperative instructions
            (1) Procedure specific information—what to expect, activity R/T procedure, pain, general care, and when to call the doctor
            (2) Information R/T anesthesia, diet, medications, activity, special instructions
            (3) Indicate to whom education was given (who will be caring for patient).
            (4) Follow-up contact information—phone number and who will be receiving information (patient, parent, or significant other—adhere to Health Insurance Portability and Accountability Act [HIPAA] guidelines)
            (5) Discharge orders for treatments, medications, nutrition, and activity
            (6) How and whom to contact in case of emergency
            (7) Specific instruction sheets provided
            (8) Method of discharge instruction—verbal, written, return demonstration, for example
            (9) Time of follow-up medical appointments
            (10) Provide copy of written instructions—follow facility policy.
         c. Physician's specific verbal instructions that vary from routine
         d. Patient's response to instructions provided
         e. Nurse's assessment of patient's, family's, and significant other's understanding of postoperative instructions
         f. Any specific instructions and requests from the patient for confidentiality that vary from the norm
         g. Instructions should be signed by nurse and person to whom they were delivered—family or significant other
            (1) If instructions given preoperatively, patient can sign if necessary—should only be for procedure-specific information.
            (2) Anesthesia and medication information should be given to family or significant other and signed for by this individual.

BIBLIOGRAPHY

1. *2002 Standards of Perianesthesia Nursing Practice.* Cherry Hill, NJ: American Society of PeriAnesthesia Nurses, 2002.
2. Berman AJ, Burke K, Erb G,. et al: *Fundamentals of nursing: Concepts, process, and practice,* ed 6. Upper Saddle River, NJ: Prentice Hall Health, 2000.
3. Burden, N: *Ambulatory surgical nursing,* ed 2. Philadelphia: WB Saunders, 2000.
4. Canobbio MM: Mosby's handbook of patient teaching, ed 2. St Louis: Mosby, 2000.
5. DeFazio Quinn DM, American Society of PeriAnesthesia Nurses: *Ambulatory surgical*

nursing core curriculum. Philadelphia: WB Saunders, 1999.

6. Doak CC, Doak LG, Root JH: *Teaching patients with low literacy skills,* ed 2. Philadelphia: Lippincott, 1996.

7. Intermountain Health Care, Urban Central Region Hospitals Education Department: Patient family education: Process for creating a patient education handout. (draft). Salt Lake City: Intermountain Health Care, June 2003.

8. Intermountain Health Care, Urban Central Region Hospitals Quality Resource Department: Commitments: Assessment of patients. Salt Lake City: Intermountain Health Care, April 2002.

9. Intermountain Health Care, Urban Central Region Hospitals Quality Resource Department: Fact sheets: Patient education. Salt Lake City: Intermountain Health Care, May 2003.

10. JCAHO: *Comprehensive accreditation manual for hospitals.* Oakbrook, IL: Author, 2003.

11. *Surefire documentation: How, what, and when nurses need to document.* St Louis: Mosby, 1999.

58 Discharge Planning: Home and Phase III

LOIS SCHICK

OBJECTIVES

At the conclusion of this chapter the reader will be able to:

1. Describe the best times for planning for patient's discharge.

2. Identify appropriate discharge instructions that should be provided to the patient.

3. Describe guidelines for discharging the ambulatory surgical patient.

I. Discharge planning
  A. Definition
    1. Individualize discharge plan to meet specific patient needs.
       (1) Patient transferred to long-term care facility
       (2) Ambulatory surgical patient needs
       (3) Ensure implementation of cost containment strategies.
       (4) Implement measures to improve patient outcomes.
  B. Process includes (nursing process)
    1. Identification
    2. Assessment
    3. Goal setting
    4. Planning
    5. Implementation
    6. Coordination
    7. Evaluation
  C. Initially takes the form of patient assessment
  D. Primary goal for ambulatory patient—in a minimal period of time patient will be
    1. "Home ready" ("fit for discharge")
    2. Safely discharged
    3. Able to return to "preprocedure" level of function
  E. Planning should start as soon as possible.
    1. Starts at the time patient is scheduled for the procedure or hospital admission
    2. Is discussed at the time of the preadmission visit
       a. Comprehensive nursing history is key tool in discharge planning.
       b. Are there support systems conducive to home management?
       c. Identification and resolution of physiological home care problems
          (1) Physical barriers that impede normal activities of daily living
              (a) Ability to shower
              (b) Ability to "get around" in home environment (stairs, tub, etc.)
          (2) Equipment needed (crutches, canes, wheelchair, continuous passive machine)
          (3) Supplies needed (dressings, medications, etc.)
    3. Review and reinforce plan in preoperative holding unit.
       a. Obtain comprehensive nursing history (if not done previously) to include
          (1) Personal coping deficits
          (2) Family and community support (or lack of)

(3) Geographic isolation

(4) Physical limitations

4. Planning discussed in phase II with patient and responsible adult prior to discharge

    a. Is the recovery of cognitive and psychomotor function sufficient to manage postoperative care?

F. Discharge planning addresses

    1. Safe home environment

    2. Availability of responsible adult caregiver

    3. Safe transportation home

G. Guidelines for discharging ambulatory surgery patients include

    1. Institutional guidelines

        a. Detailed process developed (in conjunction with nursing and anesthesia)

            (1) Protocols

            (2) Policies

            (3) Collaborative practices

    2. Responsible practitioner's name recorded on the patient record

    3. Discharge criteria (see Box 58-1) (Refer to Chapters 35 and 37 for examples of criteria based scoring systems.)

H. Responsible adult available to

    1. Assist patient with activities of daily living

    2. Ensure patient complies with postoperative instructions

    3. Ensure medications and special supplies are available

    4. Monitor patient's progress

I. Postoperative and follow-up care instructions are given to patient and care provider.

    1. Reviewed with patient and caregiver

        a. Reviewed verbally with hard copy (written) provided

        b. Nurse ensures patient or caregiver able to reiterate instructions (ensures patient and caregiver understanding).

    2. Written copy provided

        a. Written at fifth grade level

        b. Large print especially for visually impaired

        c. Emergency contact information provided in writing (physician's office and emergency contact)

    3. Place copy of instructions in patient's medical record.

    4. See Box 58-2 for education points to cover on instruction sheets.

J. Freestanding facilities have written transfer agreement with nearby hospitals in the event hospitalization for more definitive or prolonged care becomes necessary.

    1. Unplanned medical emergencies (cardiac, respiratory, etc.)

    2. More extensive surgery required

    3. Hemorrhage

    4. Dehiscence

    5. Persistent pain

    6. Unrelenting nausea and vomiting

■ BOX 58-1
■ **DISCHARGE CRITERIA**

Vital signs (circulation: blood pressure, pulse, respirations, oxygen saturations, temperature)	Level of consciousness
	Activity level (ambulation)
Comfort level (pain, nausea, oral analgesics)	Instructions
Surgical site (dressings)	Support of responsible adult
Nourishment	Ability to urinate if appropriate
Hydration	

■ BOX 58-2
■ **EDUCATION POINTS FOR DISCHARGE INSTRUCTIONS**

Medications
Note the name, purpose, and dosage schedule for each medication; emphasize the importance of following the directions on the label.
The patient should resume medications taken before surgery per the physician's order.
If pain medication is not prescribed, nonprescription, nonaspirin analgesics (e.g., acetaminophen, ibuprofen) may be effective for mild aches and pains.
Additional pain medication may be ordered by the physician after surgery. The patient should take these medications as directed, preferably with food to prevent gastrointestinal upset.

Activity Restrictions
Advise the patient to take it easy for the remainder of the day after surgery. Dizziness or drowsiness is not unusual following surgery and anesthesia.
For the next 24 hours, the patient should not:
Drive a vehicle or operate machinery or power tools.
Consume alcohol, including beer.
Make important personal or business decisions or sign important documents.
Activity level: In specific behavioral terms (e.g., do not lift objects heavier than 20 lbs), describe any limitation of activities.

Diet
Explain any dietary restrictions or instructions.
If no dietary restriction exists, instruct the patient to progress as tolerated to a regular diet.

Surgical and Anesthesia Side Effects
Anticipated sequelae of surgery (e.g., bleeding and pain) should be delineated.
Common side effects associated with anesthesia include dizziness, drowsiness, myalgia, nausea and vomiting, or sore throat.

Possible Complications and Symptoms
Instruct the patient and responsible adult in pertinent signs and symptoms that could be indicative of postoperative complications.
The patient should call the responsible physician if he or she develops:
Fever > 38.3° C (101° F)
Persistent, atypical pain
Pain not relieved by medication
Bleeding or unexpected drainage from the wound that does not stop
Extreme redness or swelling around the incision site or drainage of pus
Urinary retention
Continual nausea or vomiting

Treatment and Tests
Procedures that the patient or responsible adult is expected to perform (e.g., dressing changes or the application of warm moist compresses) should be described in detail.
A complete list of necessary supplies should be included.
If any postoperative tests are to be conducted, instructions as to the date, time, test location, and any previsit preparation should be listed.

Access to Postdischarge Care
Note the telephone number of the responsible and available physician.
Include the telephone number of the ambulatory center and the hours of operation.
Note also the name, address, and the telephone number of the appropriate emergency care facility.

Follow-up Care (See Chapter 59)
Identify the date, time, and location of the patient's scheduled return visit to the clinic or surgeon.

From Marley R, Moline B: Patient discharge issues. In Burden N, Quinn D, O'Brien D, et al, editors: *Ambulatory surgical nursing.* Philadelphia: WB Saunders, 2000.

K. Some patients require more sophisticated discharge planning (may require admission to rehabilitation facility).
  1. Severe multiple injuries, especially head injuries
  2. Elderly patients with limited ability to care for self
  3. Patients with significant disabilities and functional impairment
  4. Patients with advanced malignancy
  5. Patients with one or more significant socioeconomic difficulty
    a. Homeless
    b. History of substance abuse
    c. Acquired immune deficiency syndrome (AIDS)
L. Checklist for patient to discuss with health care provider
  1. Diet
    a. Are there any special dietary restrictions that should be followed?
  2. Activities of daily living
    a. How soon before I can resume driving and other routine activities?
      (1) Housework
      (2) Lawn care
      (3) Sexual activity
    b. When can I resume exercise and other rigorous activity?
    c. How soon before I can go back to work?
    d. Who will help until normal activities can be resumed?
  3. Wound
    a. What are special instructions regarding incisional care?
  4. Pain
    a. How long should I expect pain?
    b. Do I have pain medicines available?
  5. Follow-up
    a. Is there any kind of follow-up therapy to this surgery?
    b. When am I scheduled for a follow-up visit with the surgeon?
  6. Emergency contact
    a. In what instances should I contact my physician or nurse?
    b. What are the emergency contact numbers I should be aware of?
M. Research studies on discharge planning
  1. Show mixed results
    a. Reduction in hospital length of stay was seen.
    b. Reduction in readmission to hospitals
    c. Increase in patient satisfaction
    d. No evidence that health care costs were reduced
  2. Discharge planning programs are implemented in different ways.

BIBLIOGRAPHY

1. Cramer C: Ambulatory surgery: Nursing considerations. In *Current reviews for perianesthesia nurses.* Miami, FL: Current Reviews, 1987, pp 174-180.
2. Fakhry S, Rutherford E, Sheldon G: Postoperative management. In *ACS surgery principles and practices.* Elmwood Park, NJ: WebMD, 2002, pp 1625-1646.
3. Hospital discharge planning: Helping family caregivers through the process. New York: National Alliance for Caregiving and the United Hospital Fund of New York. Available at http://www.caregiving.org/ Discharge%20Planner_final.pdf. Accessed on January 6, 2003.
4. Marley R, Moline B: Patient discharge issues. In Burden N, Quinn D, O'Brien D, et al, editors: *Ambulatory surgical nursing.* Philadelphia: WB Saunders, 2000.
5. Parkes J, Shepperd S: Discharge planning from hospital to home. In *Hot topics of the month,* April 2002. Melbourne, Australia: Cochrane Collaboration Consumer Network, 2002.
6. University of Utah Health Sciences Center. Surgical care: Discharge planning. Available at http://uuhsc.utah.edu/healthinfo/adult/ surgery/discharge.htm. Accessed on January 6, 2003.
7. Zaglaniczny K, Akee J: *Clinical guide to pediatric anesthesia.* Philadelphia: WB Saunders, 1999.

59 Home Support Network

JUDITH E. ONTIVEROS

OBJECTIVES

1. **At the conclusion of this chapter the reader will be able to:**

2. Describe the professional nurse's role as patient educator.

3. Define the role of the ambulatory surgery nurse as it relates to discharge and follow-up home care.

4. Identify discharge criteria for the ambulatory surgery patient and the facets of continuing care postdischarge.

5. Describe alternative sources of care after discharge.

6. Explain the unique aspects of home care and instructions for the pediatric patient.

7. Identify strategies to help the geriatric patient have a successful ambulatory surgery experience.

8. State the role of the home health nurse and/or agencies and the use of technology in ambulatory postoperative home care.

I. Describe the professional nurse's role of patient educator as it relates to clinical outcomes in the home support network
   A. A successful patient outcome in the home care setting has its roots in the teaching the patient and responsible adult caregiver receive starting with the preoperative visit.
      1. Enhances patient autonomy by empowering the receiver of knowledge
      2. Increases confidence in the patient's self-care
      3. Decreases complications[27]
   B. Education in health maintenance and promotion is an expectation of the patient.
      1. Patients expect nurses to answer health care questions knowledgeably.
      2. The education process is grounded in the caring relation that is established between the nurse and patient.
         a. Person-nurse-carer and the person-patient-cared-for
         b. The relationship is collaborative, bound by caring and mutual respect.
         c. Nurses share and impart knowledge based on the assessed needs of the patient.[38]
      3. Resultant benefits to institution
         a. Improves patient outcomes
         b. Reduces costs
            (1) Every dollar spent on patient education results in a savings of three to four dollars.[46]
         c. Improves patient compliance
         d. Increases customer satisfaction[27]
         e. Inadequate preparation results in anxiety, pain, dissatisfaction with care, and may result in a visit to the Emergency Department for follow-up care.[14]
II. Definition of ambulatory surgery patient and the role of the ambulatory surgery nurse
   A. The ambulatory patient is "one who does not require hospital inpatient care" (Ferguson and Kaplan[18]).

1. Surgery may be done in
   a. A hospital-based outpatient service
   b. A freestanding ambulatory surgery center
   c. A physician's or dentist's office[33]
2. Patients may experience a very simple or very complex procedure because of
   a. The advancement of technology
   b. Medications
   c. Types of procedures[10]
3. The patients have progressed from the American Society of Anesthesiologists (ASA) Classification of I or II to III and IV, indicating that the patient may be medically compromised with coexisting morbidities.
4. After a period of recovery time from surgery and anesthesia in the phase I and phase II PACU, the patient is expected to be
   a. Hemodynamically stable
   b. Alert and oriented
   c. Experiencing manageable pain
   d. Having minimal nausea and vomiting
   e. Voiding
   f. Able to walk and travel to his or her home after treatment
5. Patients are discharged soon after surgery and anesthesia with the intention of having their postoperative care provided by either themselves and/or the family or significant other.
   a. More responsibility is given to the patient for aftercare.
      (1) Aseptic techniques for wound care
      (2) Vital sign stability
      (3) Assessment of neurovascular competency of extremities, grafts, and so forth
      (4) Adequate pain management[10]
6. Anesthesia is tailored for a rapid discharge.
   a. The use of premedication is often eliminated to prevent a prolonged stay.
   b. Anesthesia techniques and medications provide for a quick induction, with a shorter duration of action and fewer side effects on the central nervous system (somnolence and nausea and vomiting) and vital signs[13,20]
7. The following are needs of the ambulatory surgery patient that the nurse should discover in the assessment process and take steps to meet.
   a. Access to medical care after discharge
   b. Information on the perioperative experience and aftercare
   c. Fear of being discharged too soon
   d. Questions on how the surgical process will affect their overall health
   e. Postsurgical cares such as pain management, complications from the surgery, resuming activities, and going back to work
   f. Feelings of not being in control during the surgical experience[10]
B. Greater patient satisfaction is achieved with ambulatory surgery.
   1. There are fewer disruptions of normal daily activities.
      a. Important for both the pediatric and elderly patient[10]
      b. Quicker recovery time
   2. There is less separation from family and significant others.
   3. There is less time away from work and worry of financial outlay.
   4. Most men prefer to go home knowing they will, in most cases, be cared for.[14]
C. The patient and the family are active participants in the patient's plan of care along with the interdisciplinary team of the surgeon, the primary physician, the office staff, and the ambulatory surgery nurse.
   1. The patient assumes responsibility for his or her own care, including arranging for reliable adult support during the first 24 hours postsurgery.

2. Education is an integral part of the ambulatory surgery process, geared toward the ultimate outcome of a successful postdischarge experience.
   a. Continuous process, begins preoperatively and continues through discharge and the follow-up phone contact
   b. Facilitates the preparation needed to meet the postoperative needs of the patient
      (1) Preparation of home environment
      (2) Equipment, supplies, medication
      (3) Comfortable safe, clean environment
      (4) Appropriate food and beverages[10]
3. Discharge instructions
   a. Contain information on how the patient and family monitor untoward symptoms
   b. Teach the patient and family when to seek additional advice
   c. List telephone numbers of the physician and hospital emergency department
4. For the non-English-speaking or disabled (e.g., blind or hearing impaired) patient, instruction must be given in the patient's native language to ensure understanding.
   a. The Americans with Disabilities Act of 1991 mandates that facilities provide interpreters for the sensory deprived patient (available at www.usdoj.gov/ert/ada/pubs/ada.txt).
   b. The interpreter needs to be available at the time when the physician or nurse is communicating with the patient.
      (1) If the center has a large number of non–English-speaking patients, the discharge instructions should be printed in patient's language.
      (2) A family member is not a preferred translator because of patient confidentiality issues and the patient's hesitancy to say things in front of family members.
      (3) An interpreter in the facility is imperative if there is no family to interpret in the patient's language.
      (4) An interpreter should be of the same sex as the patient if possible.
      (5) Interpreter services may be obtained through ATT Language Line, 1-800-752-6096, if no other is available.
D. Financial considerations may affect the ambulatory patient.
   1. Third party payers may determine the types of surgical procedures that are done on an outpatient basis.
      a. More complex procedures are done with advances in technologies.
      b. Patients may need additional care beyond the ambulatory care provision because of the complexity of the surgery.
      c. Referrals need to be made to home health agencies for follow-up care.
   2. Specific guidelines need to be followed for funding from private insurance and government agencies.
   3. Access to care for those without insurance
      a. Up-front cash payments may keep some from obtaining needed surgical intervention.
         (1) Alternative methods for health care financing need to be explored.
E. The role of the ambulatory surgery nurse "provides comprehensive and intense nursing care, emotional support, and patient education".[9]
   1. Uses the nursing process to manage the patient's care
      a. Assessment is one of the most important phases in the perioperative experience.
         (1) Dynamically assesses the patient including needed education and home care follow-up
         (2) Key for a positive surgical outcome
         (3) Collaborates with the patient to meet needs expressed both for surgery and home care[17]

      c. Analyzes types of problems the patient may encounter at home

      d. Plans and implements an effective course of education to alleviate such problems

      e. Implements the discharge and home plan before the procedure begins

      f. Evaluates care with the postoperative phone call

   2. Provides focused nursing interventions on a continuum of care

      a. Education given on all facets of the surgical experience

         (1) Preoperative

         (2) Intraoperative

         (3) Postoperative

         (4) Discharge instructions

         (5) Education of caregivers

      b. Prepares the patient for surgery and discharge

      c. Cares for the patient—preoperatively, intraoperatively, postoperatively, and postdischarge through the follow-up phone call

      d. Provides psychologic encouragement

      e. Promotes patient satisfaction

   3. Manages the patient environment to minimize costs[28]

   4. Is technologically literate—promotes education and care through the Internet

      a. When the nurse is perceived as being computer literate, the patient views the nurse as being competent.[45]

      b. Provides information regarding patient education Web sites that are medically sound, including the hospital Web site

         (1) Facility Web site may contain

            (a) Standard preoperative instructions

            (b) Procedure-specific discharge sheets

            (c) Emergency contact numbers

            (d) General information and guide to hospital or facility services

      c. If computers are available on site, is able to guide patients and family in use of these hospital bay stations to access the Internet for education on procedures, pain management, expectations postsurgery and postdischarge

  F. Follows through with discharge plans

   1. Refers care to outside agencies if appropriate

   2. Postoperative phone call made day after surgery

  G. Evaluates ability of patient and caregiver in providing postoperative care.[9]

III. Discharge to home care

  A. Discharge planning begins when the patient's surgery is scheduled.[17]

   1. Proper assessment and evaluation are the keys to successful discharge and home care.

   2. Joint Commission for Accreditation of Healthcare Organizations (JCAHO) allows authorized personnel to discharge patients when discharge criteria have been established and are met by the patient.

   3. Discharge criteria should be based on outcome criteria following the nursing process and include the following but are not limited to

      a. Orders from physician or anesthesiologist

      b. Stable vital signs

      c. No respiratory depression

      d. Oriented to time, person, place

      e. Minimal nausea and vomiting

      f. Minimal or controllable pain

      g. No bleeding or excessive drainage

      h. Able to void as related to procedure

      i. Able to ambulate commensurate with preoperative status

      j. Able to take fluids orally, as appropriate

      k. Responsible adult escort

      l. Written discharge instructions

B. Continuing care
   1. Patient is educated preoperatively and during course of care that he or she should not plan to resume normal activities immediately after surgery.
      a. Effects of medication impair judgment; no important decisions for 24 hours following surgery
      b. No driving for 24 hours following surgery
      c. No alcohol for 24 hours following surgery
   2. Discharge instructions should be based on outcome criteria and include the following, but are not limited to
      a. Diet including management of nausea and vomiting
      b. Activity restrictions
      c. Wound care
      d. Possible complications
      e. Preexisting health care issues and management
      f. Medications
      g. Effective pain management
      h. Follow-up care: including doctor's visits, who to call in an emergency or if additional help is needed
   3. Verbal instructions given to the patient and family with a written copy to be sent home
      a. Written copy is signed and kept as a part of the chart.
      b. Medical record should contain documentation that instructions were given and understood.
   4. Return demonstration of care may be needed from patient or caregivers if care involves a physical activity associated with the procedure.
   5. Legal considerations—recurrent excuses for not seeking treatment postoperatively
      a. Patient did not know what to look for.
      b. Patient did not know the significance of the symptoms experienced.
      c. Patient did not know what to do or whom to contact.
   6. Medication instructions should be explicitly explained.
      a. Reasons for noncompliance are
         (1) Patient did not know when to take the medication.
         (2) Patient did not know when not to take the medication.
         (3) Patient did not know when to stop taking the medication.
      b. Nurse should reinforce physician's teachings.
      c. Instructions for taking medications should be written on discharge instruction sheet.
C. Accessibility to emergency care
   1. Preadmission discharge planning
      a. Discharge-related procedure that needs to be planned for preoperatively
      b. Presence of a responsible adult to assist the patient home, receive patient's discharge instructions, and summon help if needed
      c. If there is a significant risk that the patient cannot reach the emergency facility, then discharge should be delayed.
   2. Factors to be considered include
      a. The operative procedure
      b. The patient's general health
      c. Risk factors that are determined preoperatively
      d. Patient's present status
      e. Accessibility of emergency facilities in the event of a complication
D. Patient satisfaction follow-up (see Chapter 60)
IV. The pediatric ambulatory patient (see Chapter 13 for more information)
   A. Over 60% of surgeries performed on children are done on an outpatient basis.[21]
   B. Triad of care is established that includes the nurse, the child, and the family.
      1. The majority of children are treated from a wellness perspective.
      2. The family is seen as an integral part of the perianesthesia process.
         a. The parents are the child's greatest emotional support.

3. Normal physical and psychologic parameters must be understood and any deviation readily recognized.
   a. Nursing assessment includes
      (1) Patient's physical condition
      (2) Developmental levels
      (3) Behaviors
      (4) Learning readiness—verbal and nonverbal clues
   b. Parents help to interpret clues and behaviors that are exhibited by the child.
4. The plan of care is developed by the nurse with the parents and the child.
   a. Parents learn the disease process, know about the surgical procedure, and participate in the postoperative care.
      (1) By participating in the care in facility, the parent learns to care for the child, do procedures necessary, and feel comfortable dealing with the child.
   b. The child learns about the process and his or her care through curiosity and a desire to remain in control.[22]

C. Postoperative home care starts with the preoperative visit.
   1. Patient and family are interviewed to gather data, educate, and to provide emotional support to the child and to the family.
   2. Education on the entire surgical experience is given.
      a. Family actively involved in the care
      b. Family helped to accomplish tasks
   3. Care the parent will provide is given in detail.
      a. Verbally discussed with parents or caregiver
      b. Procedure-specific handouts given
         (1) Serves as a reference when the family is home
         (2) Includes care points that need to be stressed
         (3) Includes complications to watch for
         (4) Includes telephone numbers to call (physician or hospital emergency department) to report untoward symptoms
   4. Education and emotional support help to dispel the fear a parent may have in caring for the child at home.[22]

D. Common complications seen at home
   1. Nausea and vomiting
      a. More common with tonsillectomy and adenoidectomy, strabismus surgery, and orchiopexy
      b. Twice as common in surgeries lasting over 20 minutes
      c. More common in children above 3 years of age
      d. Prevention during surgery with good fluid replacement and low dosages of droperidol
      e. Parents cautioned to provide adequate liquids and call if child cannot retain fluids for a period of time
   2. Pain
      a. Pain is underrecognized in children.
      b. Children deserve to have their pain recognized and dealt with in a wholesome and acceptable manner.
         (1) Parents and child actively involved in assessing and managing pain
      c. Level of pain should allow the child to be active, cooperative.
      d. Pain medications should exhibit few side effects on the child.
         (1) Parents should know side effects of the medication.
         (2) Report to the physician any untoward effects or if pain is not relieved.
         (3) Parents taught how to give medications and what schedule to follow.
      e. Teach parents to use nonpharmacologic methods of pain control.
         (1) Music, play, distraction
         (2) Favorite toys, blanket, pacifier
   3. Sleepiness, cough, sore throat, hoarseness, croup, and fever

E. Transportation home
   1. Availability of responsible adult
   2. Two adults ideal for infant or small child; one can tend to child during ride home.
   3. Child should adequately be restrained in appropriate car seat or seat belt; not held by adult.
   4. Community resources can be arranged if help is needed.
F. Home care
   1. Follow-up phone call helpful the evening of surgery and within 24 hours.
      a. Inquire of
         (1) Any complications
         (2) Feeding, drinking, voiding
         (3) Pain
      b. Specific questions regarding the patient's condition are required for different procedures.
         (1) Tonsillectomy
            (a) Bleeding, nausea, vomiting, fluid intake
         (2) Hernia
            (a) Nausea, vomiting, taut abdomen, unrelieved pain
         (3) Orthopedic procedures
            (a) Color, warmth, movement (of extremity if in cast)
            (b) In-home nursing visit reserved for complicated, high-technology cases
            (c) Telephone support is usually sufficient.
V. The geriatric ambulatory surgery patient (see Chapter 16 for more information)
   A. The geriatric population, 65 years and older, is the fastest growing age group in the United States.
      1. This age group will double its size between the years 1990 to 2030.
      2. The 100 year olds and older are the fastest growing group within the elderly population.
   B. The health care industry will see major changes in the age group of patients for whom it is caring.
      1. Fifty percent of persons 60 and older will require surgery before they die.
         a. Forty to fifty percent of ambulatory surgery population is over 65.
      2. The elderly patient is being treated with surgery more aggressively than in the past.
      3. Out of one million surgeries done on the elderly in an outpatient setting, only 1.6% had to return to the hospital.[13]
      4. Cataract surgery has proven to be one safest surgeries of all surgeries done on outpatient basis.
   C. Proper postoperative home care is one of the most important factors in the good outcome of ambulatory surgery for the geriatric patient.
      1. Risk of surgical intervention is reduced by careful preoperative evaluation, planning, and education.
         a. Study of elderly women showed that plan fell short of the need because of the complexities of the care needed at home.[26]
         b. Assessment of physiologic functioning and chronic illness is done to plan the care of the elderly patient through the entire surgical phase.
         c. Evaluate psychosocial and educational needs.
            (1) Look beyond basic physical and medical needs.
            (2) Will alleviate many fears, risks, and complications
            (3) The patient may be concerned about a spouse, a pet, or a parent for whom he or she is the caregiver is caring.
      2. Barriers to successful home care for the elderly
         a. Communication breakdowns between patient, office, and hospital staff
            (1) Difficulty in collating preoperative tests results

      (2) Special needs of the elderly patient not communicated to outpatient facility

   b. Poor follow-up from private physician

   c. Long intervals between scheduling of surgery and follow-up on referrals to needed agencies, case managers, social workers

   d. Difficulty in getting prescriptions filled

   e. Preoperative teaching difficult because of time constraints

   f. Misconceptions of nurses may preclude necessary home care arrangements being made

      (1) The elderly should assume more responsibility in making arrangements for their care.

      (2) Lack of a caregiver—7% have no one to give care at home.

      (3) Effects of surgery are temporary and will quickly dissipate, negating the need for home care follow-up.

   g. Discharge instructions are too general—need to be more case specific for the elderly patient.[40]

D. Assessment of the patient begins in the preoperative interview.

   1. Activities of daily living (ADLs) are a good assessment tool to evaluate the extent of home care that the elderly patient will need.

      a. A relatively active, healthy 70 year old will need less care and concern than a 70-year-old bedridden patient with concomitant disease.

      b. Co-existing disease increases the risks.

      c. Polypharmacy needs careful investigation.[17]

   2. Assessment must include the evaluation of the home caregiver for

      a. Reliability

      b. Physical capability

      c. Emotional maturity

   3. Support services can be arranged in advance if needed.

      a. Social worker

      b. Home health care

      c. Visiting nurse

      d. Transportation

   4. The discharge plan

      a. The discharge planner or case manager may be needed to help with the patient's concerns.

      b. Preoperative discharge planning can evaluate whether the patient needs home nursing care postoperatively.

      c. Family members should be included in the preoperative education session on how they can and reinforce the postoperative care.

   5. Successful outcome of ambulatory surgery help for the elderly depends on

      a. Elective versus emergency surgery

      b. Optimum physical condition

      c. Thorough preoperative assessment

      d. Close intraoperative and postoperative monitoring

      e. Preventive measures to decrease any complications

E. Discharge instructions

   1. Education should be done in a nonhurried manner.

      a. Patient needs extra time to assimilate information.

      b. Quiet atmosphere can help patient focus attention on what is being presented.

      c. Preoperative teaching can effectively be done in the home by home health nurses.

         (1) Teaching done in the patient's home makes the patient more receptive to the instruction.

         (2) Familiarity with surroundings reinforces learning.

   2. Instructions need to be written.

      a. Large type may be needed.

      b. Colored paper (yellow or tan) will make instructions easier to read.

      c. Gives patient sense of control

         (1) Patient can refer to instructions that are easily understood.

         (2) Self-esteem is reinforced as patient does not need to ask for help.

   3. Instructions for hearing-impaired or sight-impaired

      a. Special provisions may need to be made.

      b. Braille standardized instructions or audiotapes for the sight impaired

      c. Sign interpretation for the hearing impaired

VI. Home health care nursing and use of technology

  A. Definition

   1. The health care team of today is charged with working to provide a process from admission to discharge and home care that is seamless, safe, and outcome oriented.[6]

      a. The patient is linked to many facets of health care through computers, satellite systems, optical fibers, and the telephone.

      b. Interactive web sites provide virtual tours of facilities and patient education.

      c. Many facilities communicate via email.

         (1) Appointments verified

         (2) Standard greetings sent

         (3) Postoperative surveys

         (4) Even follow-up care done via email[41]

      d. Diagnostic and monitoring services are provided over the Internet.[1]

      e. Clinical resource roles developed to provide support for sophisticated surgeries and procedures; resources available on-line

         (1) Decreases patient anxiety

         (2) Patients and family feel prepared, supported, and comforted.

         (3) Stress over home care decreases when patients feel prepared to carry on.

         (4) Innovative Web site regarding ambulatory surgery[12]

      f. Japan has provided public nursing care insurance.

         (1) Ten thousand homes connected to television phone

         (2) Nurse sees and assess patient via picture phone.

         (3) Service provided to those 65 or older[42]

      g. Home nursing care expanded in New Zealand because of increases in surgery[15]

      h. Timely education via the Internet affects clinical outcomes of care.

         (1) Pain reduced by being able to access pain management information after returning home

         (2) Fifty-two percent reported availability of Internet use[47]

   2. Provision of health care services specifically designed to meet the individual needs of the patient; services are provided in the patient's place of residence

      a. Promotes and maintains health

      b. Maximizes level of independence

      c. Emphasizes focus on wellness

      d. Services planned, coordinated, and made available through home health care emergencies

  B. Levels of care

   1. Concentrated or intensive services

      a. For those needing hospitalization

      b. Coordination of services under professional supervision allows the patient to be treated at home.

   2. Intermediate services

      a. Convalescent and rehabilitation—type of care

      b. Less concentrated type of care provided

      c. Personal care

      d. Environmental supportive social services
   3. Basic or maintenance services
      a. Long-term care needs
      b. Prevents or postpones hospital care
      c. Personal and supportive environmental care
      d. Social services
      e. Condition stable—periodic monitoring only
C. Role of the nurse in home health care—all encompassing
   1. To teach the family to care for the patient; including, but not limited to
      a. Changes in patient condition—infections
      b. Medications—use, times to be given, and side effects
      c. Skin care—prevent skin breakdowns.
      d. Nutrition—good nutrition program to promote healing of surgical wounds
      e. Elimination—changes that might occur in bowel movements from pain medications
      f. Mobilization and dressing the patient
      g. Wound dressing changes
      h. Safety of the patient
   2. Assessments
      a. Patient's physical assessment
      b. Assessment of the family and caregiver
         (1) Family dynamics—possible or anticipated changes
         (2) Type of relationships in the family
         (3) Educational and cultural backgrounds
            (a) Education affects the patient's ability to read, listen, and follow directions.
            (b) Attitude toward health and illness may be related to cultural background.
      c. Assessment of the community is a part of gathering resources for the patient.
   3. Support
      a. Link to physician and health care services
         (1) Physical and occupational therapies
         (2) Community resources
            (a) Meals on Wheels
            (b) Visitors
            (c) Senior centers
            (d) Home care social worker can be link to community resources for the patient.
         (3) Home health aide
            (a) Gives personal care to the patient
            (b) Reinforces care given by other health care workers
            (c) Reports changes in patient condition to other health care professionals
         (4) Arrange for equipment needed during convalescence.
         (5) Refer patient to organizations that can help with financial considerations if needed.
            (a) Red Cross
            (b) American Cancer Society
            (c) Multiple Sclerosis Society
            (d) Muscular Dystrophy Association
            (e) St. Vincent de Paul Society
            (f) United Way
      b. Support of decisions made by family regarding patient
   4. Performance of specific skills in connection with the patient's condition
      a. Involvement of the family in these skills reinforces teaching and connection to the patient.

   D. Complexity of procedures performed under ambulatory surgery is expanded.
     1. Procedures performed may include but are not limited to
       a. Vaginal hysterectomy
       b. Mastectomy
       c. Anterior cruciate ligament repair
       d. Endoscopic abdominal surgery
         (1) Salpingooothecectomy
         (2) Cholecystectomy
         (3) Appendectomy
         (4) Hysterectomy
         (5) Nephrectomy
         (6) Nephrolithotomy
  E. Clinical care maps and/or clinical care paths help to keep the nurse and the patient from deviating in the plan of care.
     1. The clinical pathway is a standardized, multidisciplinary, time-based plan of care.
       a. Identifies the patient care process
       b. Monitors patient progress to outcome
       c. Specific goals and clinical outcomes are listed.
     2. A clinical care map is adapted to a patient care guide.
       a. Results in compliance with regimens and satisfaction with care
       b. Results from a well-organized educational plan to meet the needs of short-stay surgical patients.
         (1) Empowers the patients by building self confidence
         (2) Describes what they can expect to experience in the perioperative period
         (3) Offers realistic management strategies for home self-care
         (4) Produces less anxiety, lower postoperative pain levels, fewer complications, and quicker recoveries
       c. Topics addressed
         (1) Management of pain, nausea, care of incisions
         (2) Dietary and activity needs
         (3) Signs and symptoms of infections
         (4) Resources for questions or concerns
       d. Patient and family education are integrated at every step of the clinical care map to teach patients about the treatment plan and expected outcomes.
       e. Additional material included to personalize to each patient
     3. Patients feel confident in managing their home care.[8,23]
  F. Plan of care—outpatient vaginal hysterectomy
     1. Careful preoperative screening according to selected criteria
       a. Decision involves patient and family agreement.
       b. Requires active participation by family
     2. Detailed education on the surgical experience
     3. Postoperative care map is followed for phase I and phase II recovery.
     4. Discharge criteria are met.
       a. Hematocrit remains constant.
       b. Ambulates successfully
       c. Voids
       d. Tolerates clear liquids
       e. Average length of stay is 9.5 hours.
       f. Transportation home
         (1) Private transportation
         (2) Ambulance with a registered nurse
       g. Home health care follow-up
         (1) Protocols differ per institution.
           (a) Registered nurse remains in attendance for 48 hours.
           (b) Intravenous (IV) fluids, narcotics, IV antibiotics are available.
           (c) Visit by home health nurse on postoperative days one and two.

(2) Detailed postoperative instructions given

(3) Role of nurse

    (a) Physical assessment

    (b) History since discharge—observing for possible complications

    (c) Blood drawn each day

    (d) Progress reported to physician or hospital-based protocol nurse

(4) Surgeon maintains contact via telephone

(5) Extended follow-up

    (a) Physician office visit at 2 and 6 weeks

(6) Outcome

    (a) Patient satisfaction expressed

    (b) Favorable outcome based on good education and support system

  5. Plan of care—anterior cruciate ligament repair

    a. Protocol of care established between the physician's office, visiting nurse association, and the hospital.

    (1) Preoperative instructions and education received

        (a) Receive standard preoperative instructions from hospital admission nurse

        (b) Instructed by hospital physical therapist on postoperative exercises and use of continuous passive motion (CPM) machine

    (2) Home care follow-up

        (a) Visits day of surgery and first postoperative day

        (b) Administers intramuscular (IM) injection of ketorolac each day

        (c) Assesses patient including neuroassessment of affected limb

        (d) Teaches and reinforces teaching on dressing care, exercises, CPM machine, self-assessment of involved leg, crutch walking

        (e) Physician visit 7-10 days postoperative and then every 2 weeks for 3 months

  6. Patient care guide for laparoscopic cholecystectomy (Figure 59-1)

    a. Care map developed to be read at the eighth grade level

    b. Map covers the day before surgery up to 2 weeks postsurgery.

    c. Topics covered include

    (1) People who will be part of the care team

    (2) Treatments involved with the plan of care

    (3) Diet

    (4) Activity

    (5) Caring for the incision

    (6) Whom to call for questions or concerns

    d. Detailed specific instructions given for each of the five time frames covered

    e. Part of the overall patient and family education plan

    f. Can be personalized for the individual patient

    g. Result in positive patient outcomes and reduced costs[8]

VII. Summary

  A. Outpatient surgery will continue to grow as a result of

    1. Advanced surgical technology

    2. Less invasive procedures

    3. Safer and quicker-acting anesthetic agents

    4. A high degree of patient satisfaction

  B. The outcome for a successful experience depends on thorough and detailed education.

    1. Preoperative

    2. During the facility stay

    3. Postoperative

  C. The use of the Internet for monitoring, communication, and education will increase the effectiveness and comfort of the public with outpatient surgery.

YOUR GALLBLADDER OPERATION (Laparoscopic Cholecystectomy)

	THE DAY BEFORE YOUR OPERATION	THE DAY OF YOUR OPERATION	ONE-SIX DAYS AFTER YOUR OPERATION	ONE WEEK AFTER YOUR OPERATION	TWO WEEKS AFTER YOUR OPERATION
People You Will Meet	• Nurse • X-ray & laboratory workers • Anesthesia nurse	• Nurses • Technicians • Doctors	• Nurses • Doctors	• Keep your appointment with your doctor.	• Keep your appointment with your doctor.
Your Treatments	• Blood work • X-ray	• Blood pressure • Temperature • A tube (IV) will be put in your hand or arm. • A shot may be given to help you relax. • Your doctor may let you go home in the evening, if you are able.	• You may go home the day after your operation if you are able to eat and drink and if your pain is less.	• Blood pressure • Temperature • Your stitches or staples may be removed by the doctor or nurse.	• Your doctor will look at your incisions, check your temperature and blood pressure.
Your Diet	• Do not eat or drink after midnight.	• No food or drink until after your operation.	• Eat light, low-fat meals. • Drink a lot of fluids. • Eat normal meals after the 1st day as you can.	• Normal food and drink. • If any foods cause constipation or diarrhea, do not eat them.	• Normal food and drink.
Your Activity	• Go to bed early the night before your operation.	• Cough and take deep breaths after your operation. • You may get up and walk to the bathroom with help 2 to 3 hours after you wake up.	• Rest a lot. • Do not lift anything over 5 pounds. • Do not drive. • Walk as much as you are able.	• Rest for short periods during the day. • You may be able to drive. • Walking is good for you. • Your doctor may let you go back to work, if you do not have to lift.	• Rest when you are tired. • Your doctor may let you go back to work.
How to Care For Your Incisions		• Big bandaids will be over your incisions. • You may take medicines for pain.	• Take your bandaids off the 2nd day after your operation. • You can take a shower on the 2nd day. • You may need to take your pain medicine.	• You may still need medicine for pain. • Keep your incisions clean and dry. • You can cover your incisions with bandaids if you want.	• Your incisions should be healed. There may be some soreness.
Who to Call For Any Questions or Concerns You Have	• Call the Day Surgery Center at (704) 326-3898 or your doctor.	• Ask your doctor or nurse.	• A nurse from the hospital will call you the day after you go home. You can ask questions then or call your doctor.	• Call your doctor for any concerns or if: - you have a fever (100° or more) or chills - there is fluid or drainage from your incisions - there is more pain or redness at an incision.	• Call your doctor if you have any questions or if you are having any problems.

FIGURE 59-1 ■ Clinical care map (Courtesy of Catawba Memorial Hospital, Hickory, NC.) (From Bumgarner SD, Evans ML: Clinical caremap for the ambulatory laparoscopic cholecystectomy patient. *J PeriAnesth Nurs* 14(1):12-16, 1999.)

D. Home health resources are enabling major surgeries to be done on an outpatient basis.
  1. Preoperative discharge planning
  2. Home health nursing
  3. Home health aides, physical therapist, occupational therapist
  4. Community resources can be utilized for
     a. Equipment needs
     b. Meals
     c. Socialization
     d. Financial help

BIBLIOGRAPHY

1. Anonymous: Advances in technology, demographics driving increased revenues in home health care market. *Health Ind Today* 63(7):16-17, 2000.
2. Anonymous. Report shows increase in postoperative recovery care. *AORN J* 72(6): 1075, 2000.
3. Anonymous: Studies on postop pain in ambulatory surgery. *OR Manager* 16(9):34, 2000.
4. Bailey C: Education for home care providers. *J Obstet Gynecol Neonatal Nurs* 23(8):724-729, 1994.
5. Baker B, Fillion B, Davitt K, et al: Ambulatory surgical clinical pathway. *J PeriAnesth Nurs* 14(1):2-11, 1999.
6. Barnes S: The state of ambulatory surgery and perianesthesia nursing. *J PeriAnesth Nurs* 16(6):347-352, 2001.
7. Bran DF, Spellman JR, Summitt RL: Outpatient vaginal hysterectomy as a new trend in gynecology. *AORN J* 62(5):810-814, 1995.
8. Bumgarner SD, Evans ML: Clinical caremap for the ambulatory laparoscopic cholecystectomy patient. *J PeriAnesth Nurs* 14(1):12-16, 1999.
9. Burden N: Nursing care of the ambulatory surgical patient. In Burden N, editor: *Ambulatory surgical nursing,* ed 2. Philadelphia: WB Saunders. 2000, pp 333-345.
10. Burden N: The specialty of ambulatory surgery. In Burden N, editor: *Ambulatory surgical nursing,* ed 2. Philadelphia: WB Saunders. 2000, pp 3-21.
11. Chung F. Analgesia: Morphine relieves postoperative pain best when administered intraoperatively. *Pain Cent Nerv Syst Week,* January 20, 2001, 2002, p 5.
12. Collettee CL, Costa MJ, Guglielmi CI: Ambulatory surgery approach fosters excellence in patient-centered care and a better workplace. *AORN J* 70(1):115-119, 1999.
13. Condor B: Surgical recovery in the express lane: Trends. *Los Angeles Times,* October 15, 2001; p S4.
14. Costa MJ: The lived perioperative experience of ambulatory surgery patients. *AORN J* 74(6):874-881, 2001.
15. Demand for services increasing. *The Press* (Canterbury, New Zealand). November 17, 1999; p 47.
16. Drew J: Testing the need for a follow-up visit after child day surgery. *Nurs Stand (AWH)* 10(10):38-43, 1995.
17. Dunn D: Preoperative assessment criteria and patient teaching for ambulatory surgery patients. *J PeriAnesth Nurs* 13(5):274-291, 1998.
18. Ferguson LK, Kaplan L: *Surgery of the ambulatory patient.* Philadelphia: Lippincott, 1966.
19. Fosko SW, Stecher JC: The role of home health nursing: A dermatologic case study. *Dermatol Nurs* 7(3):185-187, 1995.
20. Fromm CG, Metzler DJ: Preparing your older patient for surgery. *RN* 56(1):38-43, 1993.
21. Hannallah RS, Epstein BS: The pediatric patient. In Wetchler BV, editor: *Anesthesia for ambulatory surgery,* ed 2. Philadelphia: Lippincott, 1991, pp 131-195.
22. Ireland D. Pediatric patients and their families. In Burden N, editor: *Ambulatory surgical nursing,* ed 2. Philadelphia: WB Saunders, 2000, pp 613-642.
23. Irizarry JM, Graham MH, Cordts PR: Use of a critical pathway to move laparoscopic cholecystectomy to the ambulatory surgery arena. *Mil Med* 164(7):531, 1999.
24. Jeffries E: One-day mastectomy. *Home Healthc Nurse* 15(1):30-40, 1997.
25. Kirkpatrick L, Kleinbeck SVM: Surgery trends change nursing care: Operating room nurses share new procedures that will affect home healthcare. *Home Healthc Nurse* 9(6):13-20, 1991.
26. LeClere CM, Wells DL, Craig D, et al: Falling short of the mark: Tales of life after hospital discharge. *Clin Nurse Res* 11(3):242-263, 2002.
27. Marcum J, Ridenour M, Shaff G, et al: A study of the professional nurses' perceptions of patient education. *J Contin Educ Nurs* 33(3):112, 2002.
28. Marley RA, Moline BM: Patient discharge from the ambulatory setting. *J PeriAnesth Nurs* 11(1):39-49, 1996.

29. McCorkle R, Nuamah I, Strumpf N, et al: A specialized home care intervention improves survival among older post-surgical cancer patients. *J Am Geriatr Soc* 48(12):1707-1713, 2000.

30. Meeker MH, Rothrock JC: *Alexander's care of the patient in surgery.* St Louis: Mosby, 1995.

31. Moline B: Pain management in the ambulatory surgical population. *J PeriAnesth Nurs* 16(6):388-397, 2001.

32. Neal JN: Outpatient ACL surgery: The role of the home health nurse. *Orthop Nurs* 15(4):9-13, 1996.

33. Pandit S: Ambulatory anesthesia and surgery in America: A historical background and recent innovations. *J PeriAnesth Nurs* 14(5):270-274, 1999.

34. Redmond MC: Extensions of care: Phase III recovery. In Burden N, editor: *Ambulatory surgical nursing,* ed 2. Philadelphia: WB Saunders, 2000, pp 527-549.

35. Redmond MC: Phase III recovery: Referral options in postoperative discharge planning. *J PeriAnesth Nurs* 9(6):353-356, 1994.

36. Redmond MC: Using home health agencies to meet patient needs in Phase III recovery. *J PeriAnesth Nurs* 10(1):21-26, 1995.

37. Reichert A: Postoperative nursing care contributions to symptom distress and functional status after ambulatory surgery. *AORN J* 69(3):670, 1999.

38. Sanford RC: Caring through relation and dialogue: A nursing perspective for patient education. *Adv Nurs Sci* 22(3):1-15, 2000.

39. Singleton RJ, Rudkin GE, Osborne GA, et al: Laparoscopic cholecystectomy as a day surgery procedure. *Anaesth Intensive Care* 24(2):231-236, 1996.

40. Tappen RM, Muzic J, Kennedy P: Preoperative assessment and discharge planning for older adults undergoing ambulatory surgery. *AORN J* 73(2):464-474, 2001.

41. Thilo J: Ambulatory surgery and the Internet. *Inside Ambul Care,* September 1999.

42. Tomen to begin home nursing service via TV phone. *Kyodo World News Service,* August 11, 1999.

43. Whedon MA, Sabin P, et al: Practice corner: What do you do to expedite discharge after surgery? *Oncol Nurs Forum* 22(1):147-150, 1995.

44. Williams G: Preoperative preparation of the ambulatory surgery patient. In Burden N, editor: *Ambulatory surgical nursing,* editor: Philadelphia: WB Saunders, 2000, pp 346-361.

45. Yellen E, Davis G: Patient satisfaction in ambulatory surgery. *AORN J* 74(4):483-498, 2001.

46. Bartlett EE: Cost benefit analysis of patient education. *Pat Ed Counsel* 26(2):87-91, 1995.

47. Goldsmith D, Safran C: Using the Web to reduce postoperative pain following ambulatory surgery. *Proc AMIA Symp* 780-784, 1999.

60 Postprocedure Follow-up

JUDITH E. ONTIVEROS AND LOIS SCHICK

OBJECTIVES

At the conclusion of this chapter the reader will be able to:

1. List postprocedure follow-up techniques.

2. Identify information obtained from patients after discharge from the facility.

3. Describe educational information obtained when making postprocedure telephone calls.

I. Postprocedure follow-up
  A. Communication with patient and family
    1. When decision is made that a procedure is needed
    2. Preassessment testing and teaching period
    3. Immediate preoperative or preprocedure period
    4. Postprocedure
      a. Phase I
      b. Phase II
    5. Discharge home or to phase III site
    6. Follow-up care
      a. To assess patient status
      b. To evaluate if patient's recovery is progressing normally
  B. Means of follow-up
    1. Telephone calls
      a. Hospital or ambulatory surgery center initiated
      b. Patient initiated
    2. Written surveys
  C. Postprocedure phone call
    1. A call is placed to the patient 24-48 hours after discharge.
    2. Additional attempt made on subsequent day if patient is not reached
    3. Facility policy dictates how many noncontact calls are required.
      a. Until patient reached
      b. Limit to two or three calls (facility policy)
      c. Additional callbacks if problems uncovered (facility policy)
    4. Assignment of calls
      a. Primary care approach—each nurse calls the patient he or she cared for.
      b. Shared duty—any nurse calls during the day during down time.
      c. Assigned duty—one nurse responsible to do the calls
      d. Call center does all the calls (staffed 16-24 hours a day).
    5. Primary focus is to
      a. Evaluate the patient's general condition
        (1) Answer specific questions
        (2) Identify actual or potential problems
      b. Provide discharged patient means to communicate with facility
      c. Clarify and reinforce discharge instructions
      d. Provide reassurance and positive reinforcement

      e. Refer patient to the surgeon for concerns, or the nurse may call the physician with care recommendations if appropriate

      f. Convey ongoing interest in the patient and family (facility's caring attitude)

6. Provide opportunity to assess appropriateness and efficacy of referrals to other services
   a. Provide opportunity to gather information on patient satisfaction
      (1) Quality improvement data
      (2) Make changes to better improve patient care provided

7. Document call in patient's record (see sample record, Figure 60-1).
   a. Note patient's statement of progress.
   b. Note any problems that are occurring.
      (1) Untoward signs or symptoms must be recorded accurately.
      (2) If a problem is identified, the nurse has a duty to act on it in a timely manner.
   c. Note referrals given to physician or other source for follow-up care.
   d. Provide feedback to peers and co-workers on patient's comments.

8. Questions may be asked of the patient to determine satisfaction and the effectiveness of patient care at the facility.

9. Provide a positive marketing effect for the facility.

10. Provide a completion point of the ambulatory care service that was provided by the facility.
    a. Nurse gains sense of satisfaction in job completed.
    b. Chart is completed with the follow-up documentation.
    c. Demonstrate compliance with accrediting bodies and community standards.
    d. Legal aspects
       (1) Potential liabilities addressed as soon as possible
       (2) May avert potential lawsuit by early corrective action

D. Follow-up call information initiated at preoperative visit (Box 60-1)
   1. Patient is informed that postoperative call will be made and verification made of the following:
      a. Accurate telephone number
      b. Place where the patient will be staying
      c. Privacy compliance issues
         (1) Not to call at work
         (2) Not to divulge to family members who is calling
         (3) Best time to call
      d. The Health Insurance Portability and Accountability Act (HIPAA) requires that facilities must give notice to patients of privacy practices at each facility (available at www.hhs.gov/ocr/hipaa).

■ BOX 60-1
■ **SAMPLE QUESTIONS FOR FOLLOW-UP PHONE CALL**

> Do you have any problems relating to your procedure?
> Is your pain controlled?
> What level of pain are you experiencing (scale of 0-10)?
> Have you taken any pain medications?
> Did you receive verbal and written instructions?
> Did you understand the instructions given?
> How did you find your stay on the unit?
> How could we improve the service we provide?
> Is there anything we could have done to make your stay better?
> Allow questions to arise naturally in the conversation and respond accordingly.

To Be Completed By Patient	Or	To Be Completed by RN After Discussing with Patient (if patient unable to sign)

We may be contacting you.

Preferred contact phone #: _____

May we leave a message on your answering machine/voice mail: ☐ Yes   ☐ No

May we leave a message with the person answering the phone?   ☐ Yes   ☐ No

Patient Signature _____ Date _____

We may be contacting the patient.

Preferred contact phone #: _____

Patient agrees we may leave message on answering machine/voice mail: ☐ Yes   ☐ No

Patient agrees we may leave message with the person answering the phone: ☐ Yes   ☐ No

RN Signature _____ Date_____

To Be Completed By Clinical Staff

☐ Verify phone number

Outpatient Post-Procedure:

Procedure: _____

Type of Anesthesia: _____

Anesthesiologist: _____

Problems in PACU: _____

Minutes in PACU: _____

Medical Imaging Post-Procedure:

Procedure: _____

Date of Procedure: _____

Radiologist Performing
Procedure: _____

1. Attempted Contacts:

Attempt # 1
Date/Time: _____ Initials: _____
☐ Contacted   ☐ Phone Busy
☐ Left Message   ☐ No Answer
☐ Other _____

Attempt # 2
Date/Time: _____ Initials: _____
☐ Contacted   ☐ Phone Busy
☐ Left Message   ☐ No Answer
☐ Other _____

2. Information from: ☐ Patient _____(name)   ☐ Other _____ (specify)

3. Assessment of Patient's CURRENT STATUS:

Discomfort/Pain   ☐ No   ☐ Yes   _____ Pain Score _____

Nausea/Vomiting   ☐ No   ☐ Yes   _____

Drainage/Bleeding   ☐ No   ☐ Yes   ☐ NA   _____

Fever   ☐ No   ☐ Yes   _____

CMS (if extremity)   ☐ Normal   ☐ Abnormal   ☐ NA   _____

Able to care for current needs   ☐ No   ☐ Yes

Need to call MD or ER since procedure/discharge   ☐ No   ☐ Yes

4. Is there anything we could have done to make your stay better?   ☐ No   ☐ Yes _____

_____

5. Please rate your overall post-operative experience on a scale of 1 to 5 (when 1 = poor and 5 = excellent) _____

6. Intervention - Action resulting from follow-up call: ☐ None
   ☐ Supportive listening/teaching   _____
   ☐ Review of appointments   _____
   ☐ Review of medications   _____
   ☐ Review of treatments   _____
   ☐ Referral to: ☐ Physician   ☐ Other _____

Additional teaching/comments:

Interviewer's Name:

Exempla
HEALTHCARE
LUTHERAN MEDICAL CENTER

Post-Procedure Telephone Nursing Evaluation

EL-FR-NR-1165-0803

PATIENT INFORMATION

FIGURE 60-1 ■ Sample follow-up phone call form.

    E. Second postoperative call
       1. Made several weeks after surgery
       2. Pursue issues of infection control, long-term recovery issues.
          a. Return to work
          b. Level of activity
          c. Personal expectations and actual experience
          d. Complications and resolution
    F. Call used as quality improvement tool
       1. Information gained is studied and compiled to change practices if needed.
       2. Data used to increase patient satisfaction
    G. Feedback questionnaire (see Figure 60-1) may be given to the patient at discharge or mailed at a later date; feedback provided may include but is not limited to
       1. Service received
       2. Postoperative complications
       3. Education—did patients receive enough information regarding their surgical experience or procedure and how to care for themselves?
       4. Would they return to the facility?
       5. Provides an opportunity for additional comments or questions
       6. Prepaid envelope or folded postcards (to ensure privacy) have better return rate.

BIBLIOGRAPHY

1. Barnes S: Not a social event: The follow-up phone call. *J PeriAnesth Nurs.* 15(4):253-255, 2000.
2. Burden N: Follow-up after discharge. In Burden N, editor: *Ambulatory surgical nursing,* ed 1. Philadelphia: WB Saunders. 1993, pp 372-380.
3. Drain C: *Perianesthesia nursing: A critical care approach,* ed 4. Philadelphia: WB Saunders, 2003, pp 624-625.
4. Exempla Healthcare Lutheran Medical Center. Post procedure telephone nursing evaluation form. Denver: Exempla Healthcare Lutheran Medical Center, 2003.
5. Heseltine K, Edington F. A day surgery postoperative telephone call line. *Nurs Stand* 13:(9):39-43, 1998.
6. Tappen RM, Muzic J, Kennedy P: Preoperative assessment and discharge planning for older adults undergoing ambulatory surgery. *AORN J* 73(2):464-474, 2001.
7. Yellen E, Davis G: Patient satisfaction in ambulatory surgery. *AORN J* 74(4):483-498, 2001.

61 Phase III Settings

LOIS SCHICK

OBJECTIVES

At the conclusion of this chapter the reader will be able to:

1. Define phase III nursing.

2. List four settings where phase III nursing care is provided.

3. Identify the nurse's role in phase III settings.

I. Phase III
   A. Definition
      1. Extended postoperative period after discharge from phase I or phase II of a
         a. Hospital-based facility
         b. Freestanding ambulatory surgery center (ASC)
      2. Phase III may be referred to as
         a. An extended care unit
         b. A 23-hour observation unit
         c. An interventional observation unit
         d. A short-stay unit
         e. A self-care unit
      3. Nursing care may be provided to an
         a. Extended medical patient
         b. Extended surgical patient
         c. Extended procedural patient
      4. Surgery patients sent to phase III include those who
         a. Lack a "social support" system
         b. Home environment will not support care.
         c. Patient requires complex postoperative care.
         d. Patient exhibits personal coping difficulties.
         e. Patient elects to self-pay for services provided in phase III.
      5. Length of stay (LOS) may be 8 to 72 hours.
      6. Outpatient to observation status requires
         a. Physician declares as a medical necessity.
         b. The medical necessity is documented in the physician's orders.
      7. Not qualifying for outpatient to observation status unless there is documentation that the patient's condition is unstable are
         a. Late surgery
         b. Diagnostic testing
         c. Outpatient therapy and procedure
      8. PACU phase III
         a. Focuses on providing ongoing care or extended observation and intervention for
            (1) Persistent nausea and vomiting
            (2) Disabling pain not controlled with oral medication
            (3) Possible postsurgical occurrences
         b. Interventions directed toward
            (1) Preparing patient for self-care
            (2) Preparing patient for care by family and significant other

  c. Nurse: Patient ratio should be no greater than 1:5 because of patient mix.
   (1) Patient awaiting transportation home
   (2) Patient requiring minimal to no care being given
   (3) Patient who requires extensive observation and interventions

B. Ongoing assessments, interventions, and documentation
 1. Identify patient with name family uses.
 2. Assess, maintain, and/or improve respiratory function.
 3. Assess, maintain, and/or improve circulatory function.
 4. Promote and maintain physical and emotional comfort.
 5. Assess and monitor surgical or procedure site.
 6. Interpret and document data obtained during assessment.
 7. Administer medications as ordered or necessary, and record results.
  a. Analgesics
  b. Antiemetics
  c. Antibiotics
  d. Patient's prescription drugs
 8. Health Insurance Portability and Accountability Act (HIPAA)
  a. Provide maximum degree of privacy.
  b. Provide for safety.
  b. Provide for confidentiality of information and records.
 9. Encourage nourishment.
 10. Progressive ambulation.
 11. Monitor elimination patterns.
 12. Reinforce discharge planning with
  a. Patient
  b. Family or accompanying responsible adult
  c. Written home care instructions
 13. Provide follow-up for extended care as indicated.
  a. Phone call
  b. Postcard
 14. Concur on prearrangements for safe transport home.
 15. Provide additional resource to contact if problems arise.

C. Desired patient outcomes
 1. Identify untoward or unexpected symptoms
  a. Report to surgeon
  b. Seek emergency medical assistance
 2. Comply with postoperative instructions for self-care
  a. Enact physical and pharmacologic interventions to decrease pain
  b. Take prescription medications appropriately
  c. Provide required self-care as the result of surgery or procedure
  d. Identify foods and beverages that will decrease nausea and vomiting
  e. Eat, drink, and retain nourishment
 3. Perform self-care in relation to abilities
 4. Maintain normal bowel habits
  a. Increase oral fluids
  b. Increase activity
  c. High-fiber foods
 5. Display appropriate orientation to surroundings
 6. Avoid self-injury
 7. Demonstrate safe ambulation
  a. Proper use of assistive devices
   (1) Crutches
   (2) Canes
 8. Verbalize and/or demonstrate appropriate understanding and preparation for home care needs
 9. Accept assistance transporting home
 10. Verbalize understanding of consequences of actions or choices

    D. Supplies and equipment
       1. Determined need by facility based on
         a. Patient population
         b. Level of care provided
II. Phase III settings
   A. Ultimate goals
      1. Facilitate recovery in safe, monitored manner
      2. Reduce patient and family anxiety
      3. Control health care costs
      4. Facilitate return to preoperative state of functioning
   B. Hospital
      1. Twenty-three hour observation unit
        a. Medically warranted stay
        b. Allows physician to order additional tests
        c. Observes response to treatment
        d. Provides new treatment to patient
        e. Observes for potential complications
          (1) Bleeding
          (2) Pain
          (3) Nausea and vomiting
      2. Short-stay unit
        a. Nurse-staffed unit that provides
          (1) General nursing care
          (2) Comfort measures
          (3) Medication
          (4) Observation
      3. Self-care unit
        a. Prepaid out of pocket charges if insurances do not cover
        b. Emergency assistance available
        c. Usually 24 hours only
   C. Ambulatory surgery centers
      1. Observation unit in ambulatory surgery center (ASC)
      2. Recovery centers
        a. Short-stay center that houses healthy people
        b. Around-the-clock service
        c. Emphasis on
          (1) Wellness
          (2) Preparation for discharge
        d. Length of stay 23-72 hours
        e. Procedures that may go to a recovery center include but are not limited to
          (1) Joint, tendon, and ligament reconstructions
          (2) General surgery
            (a) Cholecystectomy
            (b) Hemorrhoidectomy
            (c) Mastectomy
            (d) Laparoscopic abdominal surgeries
          (3) Extensive plastic surgeries
          (4) Podiatric procedures
          (5) Ear, nose, and throat (ENT)
      3. Home health care
        a. Hospital provided
        b. Interdependent agency
        c. Visiting Nurse Association (VNA)
   D. Others
      1. Hotels and motels
        a. Healthy patient requiring extended nursing care
        b. Room available at reduced rate

          c. Provide transportation

          d. Provide special diet needed

     2. Bed and breakfast type facility

     3. Home health care

          a. VNA

          b. Hospital home care agency

  E. A recent report (2000) showed an increase in the number of recovery centers.

     1. Thirty-five states have some form of a recovery center.

          a. Fifty percent of these are in California, Indiana, Texas, and Colorado.

          b. Some state laws that limit the duration of care given to ambulatory patients have dampened widespread growth.

     2. Most are self-pay but some preferred provider organization (PPO) plans have increased payments from 19% to 28 %,

     3. General surgery admits showed the largest increase from 9% to 14%.

     4. Orthopedic cases dropped from 36% to 29%.[4]

III. Nurse's role in phase III

  A. Assessment, intervention, and documentation as previously described in this chapter

  B. Cross train in home health care.

  C. Teaching

     1. Assist and instruct responsible adult in role as

          a. Caregiver

              (1) Assistive care

                  (a) Dressing changes

                  (b) Range of motion

                  (c) To bathroom

                  (d) To ambulate

              (2) Appropriate positions

              (3) Use of ice or heat

              (4) Extremity checks if applicable

              (5) Back rubs and massage

              (6) Coughing and deep breathing

              (7) Splinting an abdominal incision

              (8) Nutrition and hydration

              (9) Pain management

                  (a) Prescribed medication

                  (b) Over-the-counter if appropriate

                  (c) Complimentary techniques

              (10) Safety

          b. Troubleshooter

              (1) Identifies problems

              (2) Staff provides phone numbers for assistance

          c. Cheerleader

              (1) Reinforces discharge instructions

              (2) Provides encouragement

              (3) Encourages compliance

  D. Post–follow-up with patients

     1. Telephone calls

     2. Surveys

  E. Knowledge of recovery referral options

     1. Medicare and Medicaid guidelines

     2. Other sources of information include

          a. Social Services

          b. Home health

          c. Business office

  F. Follow-up arrangements made (see Chapter 60)

BIBLIOGRAPHY

1. American Society of PeriAnesthesia Nurses: *ASPAN 2002 standards of perianesthesia nursing practice*. Cherry Hill, NJ: American Society of PeriAnesthesia Nurses, 2002.
2. Donovan M: Strategic/functional planning for short stay care and observational services. Presented at the Outpatient Care Institute on November 5-6, 1998, Atlanta, GA.
3. DeFazio Quinn D: Perianesthesia nursing as a specialty. In Drain CB: *Perianesthesia nursing: A critical care approach*, ed 4. St Louis: Elsevier, 2003.
4. Federated Ambulatory Surgery Association: Press release: Recovery care study. Alexandria, VA: Federated Ambulatory Surgery Association, August 15, 2000. *AORN J* 72(6):1075, 2000.
5. Marley R, Moline B: Patient discharge issues. In Burden N, DeFazio Quinn D, O'Brien D, et al, editors: *Ambulatory surgical nursing*, ed 2. Philadelphia: WB Saunders, 2000, pp 504-526.
6. Marley R, Swanson J: Patient care after discharge from the ASC. *J PeriAnesth Nurs* 16(6):399-419, 2000.
7. Redmond M: Extensions of care: Phase III recovery. In Burden N, DeFazio Quinn D, O'Brien D, et al, editors: *Ambulatory surgical nursing*, ed 2. Philadelphia: WB Saunders, 2000, pp 504-526.
8. Redmond M: Phase III Recovery: Referral options in postoperative discharge planning. *J PeriAnesth Nurs* 9(6):353-356, 1994.
9. Texas Medical Foundation: Outpatient observation frequently asked questions. Available on http://tmf.org/pepp/outpatientobfaq.html. Accessed on 7/17/03.

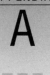

A Certification of Perianesthesia Nurses: The CPAN® and CAPA® Certification Programs

BONNIE NIEBUHR

Please note: For the most up to date information about the Certified Post Anesthesia (CPAN) Nurse and Certified Ambulatory Perianesthesia (CAPA) Nurse certification programs, contact American Board of Perianesthesia Nursing Certification (ABPANC) directly at 800-6ABPANC, email abpanc@proexam.org, or visit the website at http://www.cpancapa.org.

I. Sponsorship of CPAN and CAPA certification programs
 A. The American Board of Perianesthesia Nursing Certification, Inc., a not-for-profit corporation established in 1985, is responsible for providing specialty nursing certification programs for Registered Nurses caring for perianesthesia patients.
 B. ABPANC's vision is that "recognizing and respecting the unequaled excellence in the mark of the CPAN and CAPA credentials, perianesthesia nurses will seek it, managers will require it, employers will support it and the public will demand it".[1]
 C. ABPANC's activities are focused on achieving its mission of "assuring a certification process for perianesthesia nurses that validates the achievement of knowledge gained through professional education and experience, ultimately promoting quality patient care".[1] ABPANC's mission is driven by its commitment to
  1. Professional practice
  2. Advocating the value of certification to health care decision makers and the public
  3. The administration of valid, reliable, and fair certification programs
  4. Ongoing collaboration with the American Society of PeriAnesthesia Nurses (ASPAN), other specialty organizations, and key stakeholder groups; and
  5. Evolving psychometric and technological advances in testing
 D. ABPANC contracts with a nationally recognized testing company, Professional Examination Service (PES), to assist in the development of each examination and to administer the examinations at test sites worldwide.
II. Certification of perianesthesia nurses
 A. ABPANC offered the CPAN certification examination for the first time in 1986. Given the changing health care environment and the emerging trend of outpatient surgery, ABPANC began to investigate the need for a separate certification examination related to ambulatory nursing in 1991. The first CAPA examination related to this emerging specialty area was given in 1994.
III. Definition of certification
 A. Certification, as defined and adopted by the former National Specialty Nursing Certifying Organization (unpublished minutes, March 1984) and as used by ABPANC, is "the process by which a nongovernmental agency

validates, based upon predetermined standards, an individual nurse's qualifications and knowledge for practice in a defined functional or clinical area of nursing."

    B. State licensure, on the other hand, provides the legal authority for an individual to practice professional nursing.

    C. Private voluntary certification, as sponsored by ABPANC, reflects achievement of a standard *beyond licensure* for specialty nursing practice.

    D. Achievement of CPAN and/or CAPA certification status is indicative of the knowledge and experience necessary to practice in a particular specialty—in this case, perianesthesia nursing.

IV. CPAN and CAPA certification credentials

    A. The CPAN and CAPA credentials, granted to qualified Registered Nurses by ABPANC, are federally registered service marks.

    B. The initials CPAN stand for Certified Post Anesthesia Nurse and the initials CAPA stand for Certified Ambulatory Perianesthesia Nurse.

    C. Registered Nurses who have not achieved CPAN and/or CAPA certification status, or whose certification statuses have lapsed, are not authorized to use these credentials.

V. Eligibility requirements[1]

    A. Current, unrestricted RN licensure in the United States or any of its territories that use the National Council Licensure Examination (NCLEX) as the basis for determining RN licensure

    B. A minimum of 1800 hours of direct perianesthesia clinical experience, as an RN, during the past 2 years prior to application

        1. Nurses working as staff nurses, managers, educators, or researchers in the perianesthesia specialty are eligible for certification.

    C. Submission of an application, all required documentation of eligibility, and payment of fees

    D. Successful completion of either the CPAN or CAPA certification examination.

    E. Additional eligibility requirements may be adopted by ABPANC at its sole discretion, from time to time. Any such requirements will be designed to establish, for the purposes of CPAN and CAPA certification, the adequacy of a candidate's knowledge and experience in caring for the perianesthesia patient.

VI. Description of CPAN and CAPA examinations

    A. Each examination consists of 150 multiple-choice questions.

    B. Candidates may take up to 3 hours to complete the examinations.

    C. Candidates are tested on their ability to recall facts or understand principles, to relate two or more facts to a situation or analyze a group of facts, and to synthesize information and evaluate situations, in order to choose a correct course of action.

VII. Basis for examinations: a role delineation study (study of practice)

    A. The CPAN and CAPA examinations are based on the results of a role delineation study, or study of practice, conducted every 5-7 years to ensure that examination content remains relevant and current to the specialty.

    B. A variety of methods may be employed to gather data, the findings of which are reflected in newly designed or revised test blueprints.

    C. As of the publication date of this book, the most recent study of practice, conducted from 1999-2000 is described in the June 2001 issue of the *Journal of PeriAnesthesia Nursing.*[4]

VIII. Examination blueprints

    A. Based on the findings of the aforementioned study, both the CPAN and CAPA examination blueprints are organized according to four domains (or categories) of perianesthesia patients needs.

        1. Physiological needs

        2. Behavioral and cognitive needs

        3. Safety needs

        4. Advocacy needs

    B. Perianesthesia nurses will be tested on the knowledge required to meet specific patient needs listed under each domain.

    C. For example, a physiological need of all perianesthesia patients is stability of the respiratory system/patency of airway. Related knowledge required to meet that need includes physical assessment techniques and airway management.

    D. Given the differences in the time spent meeting patient needs in the four domains, the percentage of examination content for each domain differs depending on whether the candidate takes the CPAN or CAPA examination.

    E. For the most current examination blueprints that list specific patient needs and the knowledge required to meet these needs, please contact ABPANC directly or refer to its Web site at http://www.cpancapa.org.

IX. Determining which certification examination is most relevant to a candidate's practice

    A. Each candidate decides which examination is most relevant to his or her practice, based on patient needs and the amount of time patients spend in the specific phases described by the Perianesthesia Continuum of Care, as defined in ASPAN's Scope of Practice, Perianesthesia Nursing.[3]

    B. Regardless of the setting in which practice occurs, if most of a candidate's time is spent caring for patients in phase I, the CPAN examination is most relevant. If most of a candidate's time is spent caring for patients in the preanesthesia phase, phase II, and/or phase III, the CAPA examination is most relevant.

X. Studying for the CPAN and/or CAPA certification examinations

    A. A partial listing of publications that may be helpful study materials is found in the *Certification Handbook and Application*, obtained from ABPANC.

    B. After carefully reviewing the relevant examination blueprint and identifying individual learning needs, examination candidates should identify additional references, resources, and study opportunities that will meet their individual study needs.

    C. Helpful test-taking strategies are also described in a chapter of this publication.

XI. The application process

    A. To apply for a CPAN or CAPA certification examination, obtain a *Certification Handbook and Application* from ABPANC.

    B. Read the *Handbook* thoroughly, and note the date for upcoming examination administrations as well as registration deadlines.

    C. The application and all required documentation must be submitted by the postmark deadline.

XII. Examination administration and scoring

    A. Candidates are issued an admission ticket by PES to gain admittance to the test site.

    B. Read the ticket carefully and report at the time indicated on the ticket. Candidates arriving late risk the possibility of not being admitted.

    C. Specific information regarding test administration and the scoring process is contained in the *Candidate Handbook and Application*.

XIII. Certification period

    A. To ensure that certified nurses possess the most up-to-date knowledge and have recent and current experience, CPAN and/or CAPA certification status is granted for a period of 3 years and must be renewed.

    B. To renew credentials, CPAN and CAPA certified nurses must meet certain RN licensure and clinical practice eligibility requirements and either successfully complete the examination *or* earn contact hours related to continual learning.[1]

    C. For specific information about the Recertification Program, contact ABPANC directly. ABPANC is the source for the most current information about perianesthesia nursing certification!

    D. To contact ABPANC directly, call 800-6ABPANC, write 475 Riverside Drive, Sixth Floor, New York, New York 10115-0089, email abpanc@proexam.org, or visit the Web site at http://www.cpancapa.org.

BIBLIOGRAPHY

1. American Board of Perianesthesia Nursing Certification: *Certification handbook and application.* New York: American Board of Perianesthesia Nursing Certification, 2001.

2. American Board of Perianesthesia Nursing Certification: *Recertification Handbook: ABPANC's guide to CPAN and CAPA recertification.* New York: American Board of Perianesthesia Nursing Certification, 2001.

3. American Society of PeriAnesthesia Nurses: *ASPAN standards of perianesthesia nursing practice.* Cherry Hill, NJ: American Society of PeriAnesthesia Nurses, 2000.

4. Niebuhr B, Muenzen P: A study of perianesthesia nursing practice: The foundation for newly revised CPAN and CAPA certification examinations. *J PeriAnesth Nurs* 6(3):163-173, 2001.

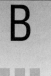 Certification Concepts and Testing Strategies

KATHLYN CARLSON

I. Certification concepts

  A. Purposes: commitment to professional nursing practice

    1. Validate a nurse's mastery of the core knowledge of the perianesthesia nursing specialty

      a. Nationally recognized credential of expertise

      b. Based on nationally established standards and scope of practice

      c. Knowledge gained through professional education and experience

      d. Maintaining credential requires nurse to regularly refresh and update learning.

      e. Offered by a nongovernmental agency, the American Board of Perianesthesia Nursing Certification (ABPANC)

    2. Promote quality care and safety for patients receiving anesthesia, sedation, and/or analgesia

      a. Reflect a nurse's own commitment to clinical and professional excellence

      b. Demonstrate a nurse's ongoing responsibility for educational growth

      c. Status measure for competitive recruitment and retention of expert, experienced nurses

      d. Market to consumers that nurses have achieved a level of knowledge and experience in the specialty to deliver patient care

    3. Personal and professional gratification and confidence

      a. Achieve a professional credential beyond licensure

      b. Personal choice to be the "best I can be"

      c. Inspire others by modeling achievement, leading, and mentoring

II. Certification examination: development and construction

  A. Role delineation study (RDS)

    1. Blueprint for examination development

      a. Study of the elements comprising a specialty nursing practice

        (1) Analyzes or defines areas *(domains)* unique to a specialty

          (a) Establishes boundaries or scope of the perianesthesia nurse's role

          (b) Most recent RDS describes *(delineates)* needs of the perianesthesia patient.

        (2) Identifies specific knowledge, tasks, and skills *(core competencies)* relevant to nursing practice in the specialty

          (a) Facts, procedures, purposes, data interpretation, proficiencies needed for perianesthesia nursing practice

        (3) Ensures each examination tests only the relevant, current concepts of perianesthesia practice

        (4) Conducted every 5-7 years to capture evolving characteristics of perianesthesia practice

        (5) Most recently conducted from 1999-2000 with nurses in current perianesthesia practice

        (6) Represents the spectrum of perianesthesia practice settings

          (a) Selected from an array of national geographic areas

      b. *Separate* RDS conducted for the CPAN and CAPA exams

        (1) Patient need identified as "fundamental reason" to certify nurses

      (2) Many common patient needs *regardless* of setting in which care occurs and other patient needs unique to care setting

      (3) Care settings include office, procedural areas, ambulatory surgery settings, inpatient units.

2. RDS *validates* domains accurately represent perianesthesia patient needs and nursing knowledge required to meet these needs. The 1999-2000 RDS validated needs as

    a. *Physiological*: organ system stability, assessment, comfort

    b. *Behavioral* and *cognitive*: communication, respect, support, education

    c. *Safety*: standards of care, discharge planning, freedom from harm

    d. *Advocacy*: accuracy, documentation, privacy, culture, ethics, legalities

3. RDS ranks *(weighs)* key competencies required of expert perianesthesia nurses to address patient needs.

    a. *Empathic care*: accepts patient need; then comforts, educates, supports

    b. Uses *standards of excellence*: works to improve quality, performance

    c. *Advocates* for patient and family: offers solutions, involves others

    d. *Initiative*: identifies obstacles, problems, seeks resolution, opportunity

    e. *Shows interpersonal understanding:* complex understanding of others' feelings, concerns

4. RDS verified continued need for both CPAN and CAPA examinations.

    a. Most salient needs in each domain identified, weighted for emphasis

    b. Validation process confirms the importance of each domain.

      (1) Considers the importance of each task, knowledge, or skill and potential outcomes if a specific knowledge or skill is not mastered

      (2) Focuses on the candidate who meets minimum qualifications for certification

    c. Examination questions designed to measure the candidate's knowledge required to meet patient care needs identified by the RDS

      (1) CPAN: physiologic needs and nursing knowledge weighted more heavily, therefore receive greater emphasis in examination

        (a) Psychological needs 65% of examination questions

        (b) Behavioral and cognitive needs 10% of examination questions

        (c) Safety needs 15% of examination questions

        (d) Advocacy needs 10% of examination questions

      (2) CAPA: cognitive, behavioral, psychological needs and required nursing knowledge weighted more heavily and therefore greater emphasis

        (a) Physiological needs 45% of examination questions

        (b) Behavioral and cognitive needs 30% of examination questions

        (c) Safety needs 15% of examination questions

        (d) Advocacy needs 10% of examination questions

    d. Total of 150 questions per examination with 3 hours to compete

    e. Examination revised annually

2. Item development: items (examination questions) are

    a. Written by

      (1) Certified perianesthesia nurses (CAPAs and CPANs)

      (2) Workshop participants working with mentors

      (3) Members of ABPANC committees or the Board of Directors

    b. Critiqued by ABPANC committee members and directors to ensure item is

      (1) Practice based, logical, and applies to the established patient care needs identified in the RDS

      (2) Focused on a relevant, not obscure, critical knowledge or skill the perianesthesia nurse must know for competent practice

      (3) National, not regional, in scope

      (4) Grammatically correct, clearly phrased, and presented in correct format

      (5) Specified answer is indeed correct.

      (6) Each distractor is absolutely *in*correct.

(7) Referenced to a source in current literature

(8) Revised, often more than once, then reviewed and revised again

(9) Assigned a level of difficulty: the cognitive skill needed to answer

   c. Accepted into the ABPANC item bank: a question storehouse

    (1) Secure, central location to house items for a future examination

    (2) Contains approximately 1000 items

    (3) *Separate* item banks for CAPA and CPAN exams

    (4) Maintained at Professional Examination Services, New York (PES)

    (5) Regularly reviewed by ABPANC to reassess relevance of specific items

  3. Examination construction: blending the questions

    a. Validated role delineation (RDS), the examination "blueprint," specifies the percentage of items from each patient need that appears on the CPAN or CAPA examination.

    b. ABPANC examination committee reviews each draft of an examination to consider the mix of questions selected by the computer, item readability, content accuracy, and grammar.

    c. Minimum passing score determined according to a criterion-referenced system

    d. PES compiles statistics and critiques each examination item's performance.

III. Examination questions—a critical-thinking approach to an examination item

  A. Level of difficulty: cognitive requirements to answer the question

    1. Level I: Knowledge and comprehension

     a. Recall of facts

     b. Understand principles

    2. Level II: Application and analysis

     a. Relate two or more facts to a situation.

     b. Analyze a group of facts.

    3. Level III: Synthesis and evaluation

     a. Analyze and evaluate facts to recommend action.

     b. Use facts to evaluate or resolve a situation.

    4. Aim to develop "higher level" questions for certification exams.

     a. Level II or III for most examination questions

     b. Better assessment of candidate's ability to apply knowledge

  B. Multiple-choice questions: applied reasoning with careful phrasing (see Table B-1)

    1. *Scenario*: may be inserted before a set of questions to provide background for a question and "set the clinical stage"

     a. Provides details: age, health, type of anesthetic, surgery, setting

     b. Candidate can imagine this situation when reading stem. *Example:* Twenty minutes after PACU admission following a knee arthroscopy with repair of a torn anterior cruciate ligament (ACL), Mr. Hobble Weakly's pulse oximeter reads 90%. He is alert, rates his pain as a 6 (scale 0-10) and blood pressure is 106/76 with heart rate 96 beats per minute in a sinus rhythm.

    2. *Stem*: sentence that begins the test item

     a. Poses a problem to solve

     b. Written as a question or incomplete phrase

     c. Find word hints: notice phrasing and use of key words (modifiers), such as *except, most likely, always, never, least*

     d. Modifiers tend to make a statement false.

    3. *Distractor*: three absolutely incorrect choices to complete stem

     a. Read critically: are you asked to plan, prioritize, evaluate outcomes, or determine best or worst intervention?

     b. Next, use reason to eliminate unlikely, implausible options.

     c. Turn the response around: what would make the statement absolutely true...or false?

     d. Answer of a well-crafted item should not obviously "stand out" among the distractors.

■ TABLE B-1
■ ■ **Critical Reasoning: Deriving the Item's Most Correct Answer**

Item 153	
Stem	*Patient education priorities for Ms. I. P. Sorely following her extracorporeal shockwave lithotripsy (ESWL) focus primarily on the importance of*
Distractors × 3 and correct answer × 1	A. Hematuria prevention B. Limited oral fluids C. Antibiotic complications D. Forced hydration
Reasoning process	To reason an answer to this item, the CAPA candidate must understand the ESWL procedure and the principles of postoperative care. Distractors in item 153 are plausible and could fit Ms. Sorely, *except*
Re: distractor A	Hematuria is a likely and expected result following Ms. Sorely's procedure; teaching her can't *prevent* mild hematuria, though she does need to report overt bleeding. Decision: *Choice "A" is probably incorrect.*
Re: distractor B	The nurse must know that Ms. Sorely has to force, not limit, fluids postoperatively; since she will return home, the nurse will teach and document I. P.'s tolerance of oral fluids. Decision: *Choice "B" opposes appropriate postoperative care after ESWL and is clearly incorrect.*
Re: distractor C	Ms. Sorely does need to learn about reportable side effects related to her antibiotic. The nurse includes this information with her discharge instructions, though perhaps with less emphasis than for a "primary" educational focus as asked in the stem. Decision: *Choice "C" is a plausible, but probably not so high priority as choice "D."*
Re: distractor D	To purge stone fragments from her kidneys after ESWL, Ms. I. P. Sorely requires at least 2000 ml of fluid each day. Fluids also help prevent infection, colic, and possible ureteral reobstruction. The CAPA candidate knows that, of all the distractors given in the item, noncompliance with forced hydration has the greatest risk of negative postoperative outcomes. Hydration becomes a primary educational priority for nurses because of the high medical priority after ESWL. Decision: *Choice D is the most correct of these distractors.*

    4. *Answer*: the *only* absolutely correct response to complete stem
        a. Continue to reason critically the most correct response.
        b. Reconsider the rationales used to eliminate other distractors (as in preceding choices a, b, and c).
        c. Ask again: does this option make the most sense in practice?
            (1) Does your intuition agree?
IV. Prepare for success: Planning to learn
    A. Self-assessment
        1. Attitude: Who am I? Why do I want to certify?
            a. Identify your motivation to certify.
            b. View as an educational opportunity, not an imposed requirement.
        2. Know your style. Appraise study habits and testing approach: be honest.
            a. Distractible or focused?
            b. Prefer independent or group study?
            c. Need a review course to refresh ideas?
            d. Anxious or calm?
            e. Prior success with multiple-choice examination style?
            f. Personality: How do I cope with test stress?
        3. Create a support system to manage your time and maximize fun!
            a. Affirmations for reassurance

  b. Helpful resources: family, friends, and colleagues
   (1) Ask to assume details of daily life so you can attend study groups, classes.
   (2) Shield interruptions by phone, family.
  c. Adopt a *positive* outlook: view examination as a *learning opportunity*, pass or not!
  d. Rely on ABPANC resources.
   (1) Connect with a Certification Coach.
   (2) Adopt a *Testing Teddy* as your cuddly study companion.
   (3) Consult published certification tips published in the American Society of PeriAnesthesia Nurses' (ASPAN's) *Breathline*.
 B. Examination preparation: let the blueprint be your guide.
  1. Set study priorities and implement a plan: prepare for 6-12 weeks before examination.
   a. Review the blueprint for the CPAN or CAPA examination to guide your study.
    (1) Outlines perianesthesia practice in the postanesthesia or ambulatory setting
    (2) Focuses on patient care needs
    (3) Specifies nursing knowledge required to meet patient care need
   b. Identify your clinical strengths: honestly ask, "What *do* I know?"
    (1) List content and knowledge about which you feel *most* confident.
    (2) Know your knowledge gaps: identify your less "secure" concepts.
    (3) Sample or create pretests
    (4) Discuss clinical practice and patient needs with other nurses.
   c. Choose specific areas on which to focus your study.
    (1) Concentrate first on your knowledge deficits.
    (2) Set long-term and short-term study goals.
    (3) Determine essential *"must know"* content: scope of practice, patient care needs, ASPAN standards of care.
    (4) Purchase or borrow review texts, scan journals, search literature for newest medications and practices.
     (a) ASPAN-sponsored publications and videos
     (b) Anesthesia-specific texts, particularly for a broad topic overview
     (c) Journals, particularly *Journal of PeriAnesthesia Nursing*, detail specific care for specific patient care needs or clinical issues.
    (5) Register for an ASPAN perianesthesia certification review course.
  2. Planned preparation: Your learning timeline
   a. *Schedule regular study-session* on your calendar.
    (1) Assign dates to study each topic.
    (2) Honor the blocked in time. No excuses!
   b. Study material in manageable chunks.
    (1) Learn and understand clinical and patient care principles.
     (a) For example: fluid concepts today, electrolytes next week
     (b) Imagine: relate relevant facts to clinical situations.
    (2) Develop long-term memory: create your personal database.
     (a) Accumulate tidbits of knowledge.
     (b) Levels of understanding develop over time.
     (c) Celebrate an "aha" moment when concepts come together in your thoughts and you confidently explain a situation.
   c. Consciously apply high-level critical thinking to clinical situations.
    (1) Borrow from your clinical practice situations to create questions, stories, and scenarios.
    (2) Brainstorm possible answers about the story, both sensible and nonsensical. Imagine:
     (a) "Why is this man restless?"
     (b) "How does this drug work?"

      (c) "What are the nurse's priorities?"

      (d) "Can I explain the physiology?"

  (3) Repeat a pretest and smile when you improve your score.

  (4) Periodically quiz yourself on difficult content.

  (5) Ask for and listen to verbal reinforcement by peers about your new knowledge.

  (6) During a quiet second between patients, quickly recall memory cues about a patient situation, jot thoughts, or consult your flash cards.

  (7) Practice nursing with newfound confidence.

d. Create a study group for support and interactive review.

  (1) Invite co-workers and/or colleagues in your ASPAN component.

  (2) Assign topics for each member to present.

      (a) Facilitates discussions and questions

      (b) Dialogue and debate clinical issues

      (c) Write your own items for scrutiny with your study group.

  (3) One nurse's knowledge strength may be another's clinical weakness.

  (4) Identify a "study-buddy" in your group if this "fits" your style.

  (5) Tap the expertise of educators, clinicians, certified colleagues, physicians.

  (6) Write 10 examination items, then reason answers with your study group.

e. Simulate situations.

  (1) Mentally create a picture of a situation or clinical syndrome.

      (a) Role-play asthmatic breathing.

      (b) Envision osmosis in hyperglycemic serum.

      (c) Imagine how a patient looks with inadequately reversed muscle relaxant: review physiology and nursing interventions.

      (d) Draw the electrocardiogram associated with a potassium of 6.6 mEq/L.

  (2) Practice listening to breath sounds on the cat's chest.

  (3) Demonstrate phase I care of a patient with a regional arm block.

  (4) Write cue (flash) cards about care considerations after spinal anesthesia.

  (5) Write a lesson plan for age-appropriate discharge educations for a 5-year-old.

  (6) Compare and contrast assessments and interventions to treat septic and hypovolemic shock.

  (7) Infuse humor for fun and memory.

      (a) Sing a memorable acronym to remember cranial nerves.

      (b) Clap rhythms of heart sounds.

      (c) Set electrolyte imbalances into limerick form.

f. Plan time to rest, reflect, and monitor your progress.

  (1) Relax: ideas gel, concepts connect, new questions arise.

  (2) Involve your body senses to reinforce learning.

      (a) Use your voice: teach a concept while walking through the park with a friend, who need not comprehend.

      (b) Mentally rehearse an approach to a patient need while changing your scrubs in the locker room.

      (c) Pretend a squirming youngster is a "wild" patient: brainstorm why, then how you can promote calm.

      (d) Demonstrate home care for a wound drain to your pet.

  (3) Near the end of your study timeline, test yourself with ABPANC practice exams to learn item analysis.

  (4) Refocus on examination blueprint to reconsider minor details. Ponder again "What do I *really* need to know?"

  (5) Notice your progress...and celebrate.

  (6) Quit studying! Rest before the test.

       g. *Never* cram!

         (1) Only creates a "mishmash" of unrelated, jumbled facts in your brain

         (2) Saturates short-term memory

         (3) Unproductive: you're less likely to recall on command.

  C. Certification day: time to show your stuff!

    1. Plan ahead, then show up early, rested, relaxed, prepared.

      a. Rehearse: wear a confident, positive manner.

        (1) Imagine success: see your name followed by CPAN or CAPA.

        (2) Eat breakfast, sleep well, and dress for success.

          (a) Comfortable clothes, in layers to accommodate varied room temperatures.

          (b) Show your colors: wear positive, optimistic reds, yellows, bright pink.

          (c) Avoid drugs (alcohol, excess caffeine, sugar).

        (3) Drive or walk to test site before test day; locate parking.

        (4) Assemble required materials for easy access on examination day.

          (a) *Photo* identification

          (b) *Examination Admission Ticket* (EAT!)

          (c) Several #2 soft-lead pencils

          (d) Your concentration

        (5) Rehearse your breathing and muscle relaxation techniques to reduce tension during the examination.

    2. Examination realities

      a. Remember mild anxiety is a benefit: increases focus, performance, and concentration.

      b. *Listen* to proctor's instructions and *read* directions carefully.

      c. Remember your affirmations...you can do this!

      d. Concentrate; ignore room distractions.

      e. Take periodic deep breaths.

      f. Focus: you have mastered this examination content.

        (1) Read each item carefully.

        (2) Do not rush—you have 3 hours.

        (3) Keep the pace: Plan 30-45 seconds per question.

          (a) Less for memory recall items

          (b) More for detailed analytic items

    3. Taking the test

      a. Read *carefully*: use systematic approach to reason each question.

        (1) Look for hints in stem: circle key words, phrases, clues to highlight ideas.

        (2) Rule out obviously incorrect, bizarre, or professionally inappropriate options.

          (a) Read *every* choice, even if you feel certain one is correct.

          (b) Determine whether *each* choice (distractor) is true or false.

          (c) Two distractors with overlapping or similar meanings are often *both* incorrect.

          (d) Ponder which answer emphasizes the same concept as the stem.

          (e) Remember: there is *only one* absolutely correct answer.

        (3) Less specific, more general statements are more likely to be false.

        (4) Apply the nursing process and nursing practice models.

        (5) Use context to identify best answers.

        (6) Rule out bizarre or professionally inappropriate options.

        (7) Do not "read in" any unstated meaning.

          (a) Interpret question at face value.

          (b) Answer only with information provided.

      b. Jot notes or memory cues in test booklet—it is acceptable.

      c. Answer every question: *guess* when uncertain of answers—there is no penalty.

      d. Trust your intuition—it is often correct.

4. Review your examination: accuracy counts.
   a. Correlate each item number on test with the correct number on answer form. *If you skipped an item to answer later, be sure you also skipped a space on answer sheet so every correct answer aligns with the correct item number*
   b. Continue this cross-check through entire examination.
   c. *Completely* erase stray marks.
   d. Review *all* your answers.
   e. Change answers when logically appropriate.
      (1) One often selects a correct response on second look.
      (2) May improve test result
5. Congratulations! Market yourself.
   a. Announce your certified self in a letter to your employer.
   b. Wear your certification pin.
   c. Create and distribute business cards using your certification credential.
   d. Mount your framed certification certificate on your office wall at home or at work.
   e. Add your CPAN or CAPA credential when charting.
   f. Introduce yourself as a "board certified nurse" and expect to explain the meaning of certification to your patients, customers.
   g. Send a press release.
   h. Offer your certified self as a mentor and certification coach to other candidates.
   i. Become an ABPANC item writer.

BIBLIOGRAPHY

1. American Association of Critical Care Nurses: New data reveals nurse certification key component of patient safety and recruitment and retention programs, 2002. Available at http://www.aacn.org/AACN/mrkt.nsf/vwdoc/CertWhitePaper?opendocume Accessed on January 3, 2003.
2. American Board of Perianesthesia Nursing Certification (ABPANC): *Certification handbook and application: ABPANC's guide to CPAN and CAPA certification*. New York: Professional Examination Service, 2002.
3. American Board of Perianesthesia Nursing: *Study tips for nurses seeking perianesthesia certification*. New York: American Board of Perianesthesia Nursing, 2002.
4. American Board of Perianesthesia Nursing: Role delineation study, 2002. Available at http://www.cpancapa.org/rolef.html. Accessed on January 3, 2003.
5. American Board of Perianesthesia Nursing: CPAN and CAPA certification: The future is now! *Breathline* 23(1, 2):5, 11, 2003.
6. American Society of Perianesthesia Nurses: Standards of perianesthesia nursing practice 2002. Cherry Hill, NJ: American Society of PeriAnesthesia Nurses, 2002.
7. Carlson K: *Certification review for perianesthesia nurses*. Philadelphia: WB Saunders, 1995.
8. Chase S: Test-taking strategies. In Silvestri LA, editor: *Saunders comprehensive review for NCLEX RN*. Philadelphia. WB Saunders, 1999, pp 19-23.
9. Litwack L: Test-taking techniques. *J Post Anesth Nurs* 10(5):277-227, 1995.
10. Mullen, CA: Strategies for success: Preparing for the certification examination. *J PeriAnesth Nurs* 11(5):324-329, 1996.
11. Niebuhr BS, Muenzen P: A study of perianesthesia nursing practice: The foundation for newly revised CPAN and CAPA certification examinations. *J PeriAnesth Nurs* 16(3):163-173, 2001.

Credits

As discussed in the Preface, this text is a combination of two previous ASPAN core curriculums. Several of the features have been reprinted from the previous two texts. For referencing purposes and to give appropriate credit, below is a listing of those reprinted features and their original sources.

The following features in this edition are reprinted from DeFazio Quinn DM: *ASPAN Ambulatory surgical nursing core curriculum.* Philadelphia: WB Saunders, 1999. Each one is listed under its feature number in this text and is followed by the page number on which it can be found in the 1999 core curriculum.

Table 12-2, Personality traits associated with Freud's first three stages of psychosexual development, p 236
Table 13-2, Communication with the child in the perioperative setting, p 262
Box 15-1, Developmental issues as related to ambulatory surgery, p 310
Table 15-1, Physiologic responses to hypothalamic stimulation, pp 316-317
Table 18-1, Developmental issues as related to ambulatory surgery, p 69
Table 18-2, Abnormalities in cranial nerve function, p 73
Table 18-3, Endocrine imbalances, p 77
Table 23-1, Signs and symptoms of electrolyte imbalance, p 69
Table 23-2, Abnormalities in cranial nerve function, p 73
Table 23-3, Endocrine imbalances, p 77
Box 24-2, Regulators of fluid and electrolyte equilibrium, p 216
Box 24-3, Symptoms associated with chemical and fluid imbalances, p 217
Table 24-1, Clinical indicators for preanesthetic laboratory assessment, p 211
Table 24-2, Primary electrolytes of the ECF and ICF, pp 213-214
Table 25-1, Carbonic acid regulation of acid-base balance, p 216
Box 34-1, Hematology: normal laboratory values, p 221
Box 34-2, Sickle cell anemia: predisposed by heredity, p 223
Table 35-2, Antiemetics, pp 124-125
Figure 35-1, Multiple pathways to and from the emetic center, p 122
Figure 43-6, Parathyroid glands, p 480
Box 45-1, Key patient educational outcomes, p 562
Box 48-1, Key patient educational outcomes, p 597
Box 53-1, Key patient educational outcomes, p 705
Box B-1, Critical reasoning: deriving the item's most correct answer, p 764

The following features in this edition are reprinted from Litwack K (ed): *ASPAN Core curriculum for perianesthesia nursing practice,* edition 4. Philadelphia: WB Saunders, 1999. Each one is listed under its feature number in this text and is followed by the page number on which it can be found in the 1999 core curriculum.

Box 16-2, Nursing diagnosis, p 67
Table 26-2, Classification of nerve fibers, p 128
Figure 26-3, Neuromuscular junction, p 101
Figure 26-4, Nondepolarizing muscle relaxants compete with acetylcholine for skeletal muscle receptor site, p 102
Figure 26-5, Paralysis with succinylcholine: initiation of skeletal muscle response, p 113
Figure 30-1, Phlebostatic axis, p 702

Index

Page numbers followed by f indicate figures; t, tables; b, boxes.

SCANDALOUS RISKS

SUSAN HOWATCH was born in Surrey in 1940. After taking a degree in law she emigrated to America where she married, had a daughter and embarked on her career as a writer. In 1976 she left America and lived in the Republic of Ireland for four years before returning to England. The idea for the *Starbridge* novels was conceived in Salisbury, where her flat overlooked the Cathedral, but *Scandalous Risks* was written at her home near Westminster Abbey in London.

From the reviews:

'Rich in human interest, sex, scandal, moral crises and a good deal of humour, it is a book to keep you hooked throughout'
Sunday Times

'Howatch writes thrillers of the heart and mind . . . everything in a Howatch novel cuts close to the bone and is of vital concern'
New Woman

'A mesmerising storyteller' *Daily Telegraph*

'One of the most original novelists writing today' *Cosmopolitan*

By Susan Howatch

The Dark Shore
The Waiting Sands
Call in the Night
The Shrouded Walls
April's Grave
The Devil on Lammas Night
Cashelmara
Penmarric
The Rich Are Different
Sins of the Fathers
The Wheel of Fortune

The Starbridge Novels

Glittering Images
Glamorous Powers
Ultimate Prizes
Scandalous Risks
Mystical Paths
Absolute Truths

The St Benet's Novels

The Wonder Worker
The High Flyer
The Heartbreaker

Susan Howatch

———◆———

SCANDALOUS

RISKS

HARPER

Harper

HarperCollins*Publishers*
77–85 Fulham Palace Road,
Hammersmith, London W6 8JB

www.harpercollins.co.uk

This paperback edition 2009
1

First published in Great Britain by
William Collins Sons & Co. Ltd 1990,
then in paperback by Fontana 1991
and by HarperCollins*Publishers* 1993

Copyright © Leaftree Ltd 1990

The Author asserts the moral right to
be identified as the author of this work

A catalogue record for this book is
available from the British Library

ISBN: 978 0 00 649690 8

Set in Galliard

Printed and bound in Great Britain by
Clays Ltd, St Ives plc

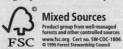

Mixed Sources
Product group from well-managed
forests and other controlled sources
www.fsc.org Cert no. SW-COC-1806
© 1996 Forest Stewardship Council

CONTENTS

PART ONE

THE GARDEN

'For the true radical is not the man who wants to root out the
tares from the wheat so as to make the Church perfect: it is only
too easy on these lines to reform the Church into a walled garden.
The true radical is the man who continually subjects the Church
. . . to the claims of God in the increasingly non-religious world
which the Church exists to serve.'

JOHN A. T. ROBINSON
Suffragan Bishop of Woolwich 1959–1969
Honest to God

ONE

'We all need, more than anything else, to love and be loved.'

JOHN A. T. ROBINSON
Suffragan Bishop of Woolwich 1959–1969
Writing about *Honest to God* in the
Sunday Mirror, 7th April 1963

I

I never meant to return to the scene of my great disaster. But one day, after yet another wasted weekend among alcoholic adulterers, I took a wrong turn on the motorway and saw the sign to Starbridge. Immediately I tried to escape. I drove up the next slip-road, but as I crossed the bridge to complete the U-turn I made the mistake of glancing south, and there, far away in the gap between the hills, I saw the spire of the Cathedral.

1988 dissolved into 1963. I glimpsed again my Garden of Eden, and as I hesitated at the wheel of my car, the rope of memory yanked me forward into the past. I forgot the U-turn, I forgot the motorway, I forgot my wasted weekend. On I drove to Starbridge along that well-remembered road which snaked between the hills before slithering to the floor of the valley, and ahead, appearing and disappearing with each twist of the road like some hypnotic mirage, the Cathedral grew steadily larger in the limpid summer light.

The city stood in the heart of the valley, but it was the Cathedral, eerie in its extreme beauty, which dominated the landscape, and as I stared at the spire I saw again that vanished world where the Beatles still had short hair, and skirts were yet to rise far above the knee and the senior men of the Church of England still dressed in archaic uniforms. Then as I remembered the Church in those last innocent days before the phrase 'permissive society' had been invented, I thought not only of those scandalous risks taken by Bishop John Robinson when he had written his best seller *Honest to God*, but of the scandalous risks taken by my Mr Dean as he had run his Cathedral and dallied with disaster and indulged in his dangerous dreams.

I reached the outskirts of the city.

It was very old. The Romans had built their city Starovinium on the site formerly occupied by the British tribe the Starobrigantes; the Anglo-Saxons had converted Starovinium into Starbrigga, a landmark in King Alfred's Wessex; the Normans had recorded the town as Starbrige in Domesday Book, and Starbrige it had remained until the author of an eighteenth-century guidebook had fabricated the legend that the name was derived from the Norman bridge across the River Star. Starbridge then acquired its modern spelling, but the link with its remote origins lingered on in the Bishop's official designation. In theory married to his diocese, he was entitled to use 'Staro' as his surname whenever he wrote his signature. I had no idea who the current bishop of Starbridge was, but I could remember the bishop of twenty-five years ago as clearly as I could remember the Cathedral's dean.

I drove into the city but it was not as I had known it. Starbridge had been raped in the later years of the 1960s, like so many other dignified county towns. The new housing estates now stretched to the cemetery; there was a bypass, a shocking aberration on concrete stilts – how my Mr Dean would have hated that! – and in the oldest part of the town I found a one-way traffic system so baffling that I had to circle the market-place three times before I could find my way out. Then I got lost in the network of streets I had known so well, the streets around St Martin's-in-Cripplegate. Butchers' Alley was a pedestrian precinct; Chasuble Lane was blocked by a NO ENTRY sign. Completely confused I fled down Mitre Street only to find a hideous multi-storey car-park leering at me as I flashed by Marks and Spencer's, but ahead I could see the traffic lights of Eternity Street and with relief I realised that the past was finally at hand. Seconds later, still swearing and sweating after my excursion in the maze, I was driving through the arched gateway into the Cathedral Close.

At once the constable on duty flagged me down. I was told that no parking was available unless I was calling on diocesan business or visiting a resident. I almost declared: 'I've come to see the Dean!' but somehow I hauled myself back to 1988, produced a five-pound note and said instead: 'Would this do?' The constable was deeply shocked. He said: 'I'm afraid not, madam,' and in rage I retired to the multi-storey car-park, but I felt cheered to learn that even now, in the heart of Mrs Thatcher's England, there were still some things which were not for sale.

I left my Mercedes sulking by a down-market Ford and emerged from the car-park into a street which ran down to the Crusader Hotel. I was progressing at last. The Crusader faced St Anne's Gate, the pedestrian entrance to the Cathedral precinct, and a minute later I was entering the huge walled enclosure of the Close.

The Cathedral rose from the lawn of the churchyard like a vast cliff towering upwards from a beach. The building still had the power to bring me gasping to a halt, but no sooner had I told myself that nothing had altered than I realised the place was awash with tourists. The Japanese, the Americans, the Germans, the French – all were on parade with their cameras and their guides, and amidst the flotillas of foreigners the English drifted idly, grey-haired ladies on outings, hikers with backpacks, even a bunch of teenage bores with beer cans, their ghetto-blasters silenced by the Constable of the Close. I was just marvelling at the diversity of these superfluous people when I became aware that they were united by their behaviour: they were all constantly looking up, and at last I looked up too; I looked beyond the slim windows, beyond the gargoyles, beyond the roof of the nave to the great cross which marked the summit of the spire.

That at least was unchanged.

But soon I felt the crowds were oppressive, and in the hope of escaping from them I tried to enter the Cathedral. The main doors of the west front were closed. So was the door in the north porch. Between the hours of ten and five, I discovered, all tourists were channelled through a side-door by the cloisters where turnstiles heralded a request for money. 'It's only a voluntary contribution, of course,' said the dragon on duty at the cash-register. I flung her the five-pound note which the constable had refused. In shock she gabbled her thanks but I ignored her and stalked into the Cathedral.

It was infested with tourists. They swarmed and buzzed and hummed and clattered. Official guides droned. Cameras flashed illicitly. In horror I fled down the side-aisle of the nave and re-entered the cloisters by the door in the south transept, but even in that secluded quadrangle it proved impossible for me to be alone with my memories. A bevy of matrons declared that everything was 'awesome' and 'wondrous' and far better than that cathedral they had seen yesterday or was it the day before. Elbowing my way past them I tried to find the wooden seat where my Mr Dean and I had sat so often, but it had been removed. Tears stung my eyes. I felt I was engaged in an exercise of overpowering futility. My Garden of Eden had been ploughed under. Here I stood, in one of the greatest cathedrals in England, and it was no more than a Disneyland theme-park. God was absent. There was no whiff of holiness, no whisper of religion and not even a clergyman in sight.

But then I saw my clergyman. I glanced down the north colonnade at the moment that he entered the cloisters by the transept door. It was not my Mr Dean; he was long dead. It was the man I had labelled my Talisman. He recurred in my life. I thought of him as a portent, sometimes heralding disaster but often merely signifying change. Some years had elapsed since we had last met, but now here he was again, a tall thin man some five or six years my junior with straight brown hair and a strong-boned face. He was no longer wearing glasses but I recognised him at once. He had more trouble recognising me. I saw him look in my direction, glance away, then stop to look back. The tourists swarmed between us, but as he moved forward they automatically stepped aside to make way for him.

'Venetia?' he said amazed, and at once as I saw myself through his eyes I realised how odd my presence must have seemed. It was surely not often that a raddled wreck of a society woman was washed up on such a beautiful but polluted shore.

'Hullo, soothsayer!' I said, instinctively assuming a synthetic gaiety, although why I attempted to deceive him about my state of mind I have no idea. I should have realised that the passing years would only have heightened his intuitive powers.

'This place is worse than Piccadilly Circus,' he said, ignoring my pathetic attempt to be debonair. 'Want to be rescued?'

'Passionately.'

'Follow me.'

With an unutterable relief I hurried after him as he led the way around the quadrangle. The door on the south side was marked PRIVATE but my Talisman, that human amulet who could achieve extraordinary results, ignored the sign and drew me into the stonemasons' yard beyond the wall. Various workmen, engaged in the unending task of restoring the Cathedral's fabric, were moving among the blocks of stone, but no one queried our presence. My companion's clerical collar was no doubt sufficient to rebuff any thought of a challenge. On the far side of the yard we reached a second door. This one was marked CHOIR SCHOOL ONLY, but once again my Talisman, ignoring the sign, led me through the doorway into another world.

'It's the garden of the old episcopal palace,' he said. 'Ever been here?'

'No.' The palace had been ceded to the Choir School after the war, and by the time I had started moving among the ecclesiastical élite of Starbridge, the Bishop had lived in the house known as the South Canonry on the other side of the Close.

I suddenly realised there were no other human beings in sight. A silence broken only by bird-song enveloped us. The garden shimmered bewitchingly in the hot bright light.

'Where are all the choirboys?' I said, hardly able to believe such peace was not in imminent danger of destruction.

'On holiday. Relax,' said my Talisman, and led the way past

13

a shrubbery to a newly-mown lawn which stretched to the river. Weeping willows trailed their branches in the water, and beyond the far bank meadows strewn with buttercups unfolded towards the hazy blue outline of the hills which surrounded the valley. The only building in sight was a farmhouse a mile away. Although we stood in the heart of Starbridge, nothing had changed on this flank of the city where the river looped around the mound on which the Cathedral stood. The water-meadows had been preserved as common land since the Middle Ages and protected in recent years by the National Trust.

As we sat down on a weathered bench by the water I said: 'How clever of you to bring me to a place where the past survives intact!'

'You were looking for the past?'

'God knows what I was looking for.'

'The past can survive in many forms,' said my companion, 'and unlike this beautiful view, not all those forms are benign.'

'Quite. Hence the massive fees commanded by psycho-analysts.'

'There are other liberators.'

'Don't you mean con-men?'

'No, con-men can't open the prison gates once the past has become a jail.'

'No magic wand?'

'No magic password.'

'And what, may I ask, is the magic password of the true liberator?'

'"Forgive".'

The conversation ceased but the river glided on, the brilliant light glittering so fiercely on the water that my eyes began to ache. Looking away I saw that my right hand was gripping the arm of the seat. The paint on my fingernails was the colour of blood, and suddenly I saw myself as someone who had long suffered a debilitating haemorrhage but had abandoned all hope of a cure.

'You're wasting your time,' I said. 'I'm beyond liberation. Run away and liberate someone else.' And then before I could

14

stop myself I was exclaiming in despair: 'I wish I'd never come back to this place! Usually I never even think of that bloody, *bloody* year —'

'Which year?'

'1963, but I don't want to talk about it.'

'That was the year of *Honest to God*, wasn't it? I remember it well — and I remember you too, full of *joie de vivre* —'

'Oh yes, that was me, oozing *joie de vivre* from every pore —'

'So what went wrong?'

There was another silence before I answered: 'Well, you see . . .' But I was unable to finish the sentence. Then I said: 'Well, to put the matter in a nutshell . . .' But again I had to stop. It was only after yet another silence that I heard myself say in a voice devoid of emotion as I confessed the emotion I could never forget: 'Well, the trouble was . . . I became so very, very fond of my darling Mr Dean.'

II

My Mr Dean had been christened Norman Neville and during the course of his career he had possessed various clerical titles, but I shall refer to him throughout this narrative by his surname, Aysgarth, because it was the one designation which never changed. He had left the name Norman behind in infancy when his mother decided to call him Neville, and he had left the name Neville behind in the 1940s when his ghastly second wife insisted on addressing him as Stephen; she had declared that the name Neville had been ruined by the unfortunate Mr Chamberlain, and that only a pure, noble, serious name such as Stephen could ever be good enough for the man she intended to marry. It had apparently never occurred to her that these dreary adjectives hardly did her husband justice, but Aysgarth, whose tolerance of his wife's peculiarities bordered on the masochistic, had raised no objection to this despotic rechristening, and after his second marriage in 1945 the number of people who knew him as Neville had steadily declined.

'If any woman tried to alter *my* name I'd put her in her place pretty damned quickly, I assure you!' my father declared once to my mother when I was growing up, although in fact Aysgarth's Christian name was irrelevant to him. My father was old-fashioned enough to call all men outside our family by their sur-names, so although he and Aysgarth were close friends the relationship sounded more formal than it was. For years after their first meeting Aysgarth had addressed my father as 'my Lord' or 'Lord Flaxton', but in 1957 after Aysgarth received his great preferment my father had said to him: 'Time to dispense with the title – address me as Flaxton in future.' This invitation, so condescendingly delivered, was intended – and received – as a compliment. Indeed Aysgarth, who was the son of a failed York-shire draper, was so overcome that he blushed like a schoolboy.

'Dear Mr Aysgarth!' mused my mother long ago in the 1940s when I was still a child. 'Not quite a gentleman, of course, but *such* a charming way with him at dinner-parties!'

My father and I first met Aysgarth on the same day in 1946. I was nine, my father was fifty-five and Aysgarth, then the Archdeacon of Starbridge, was forty-four. I had been sent home early from school after throwing an inkpot at some detestable girl who had called my father a 'barmy peer'. I hated this local hell-hole and longed for a governess, but my father, whose idealism forced him to subscribe to the view that patricians should make efforts to mix with the plebeians, was resolute in sending all his daughters to school. The schools were private; my mother would certainly have balked at the prospect of her daughters being sacrificed on the altar of state education, so I never met the so-called 'lower orders', only the infamous middle classes who, I quickly learnt, considered it their mission in life to 'take snooty, la-di-da pigs down a peg or two.' If the middle classes hadn't been so busy conquering the world for England in the nineteenth century I doubt if the upper classes would have survived into the twentieth.

'You did quite right to throw the inkpot!' said my father after I had defended my behaviour by telling him how he had been abused. 'One can't take insults lying down – I've no patience with Christians who waffle on about turning the other cheek!'

'And talking of Christians,' said my mother before my father could give his well-worn performance as an agnostic lion rampant, 'don't forget the Archdeacon's calling on you this afternoon.'

'What's an archdeacon?' I said, delighted that my father had supported me over the inkpot and anxious to retain his attention.

'Look it up in the dictionary.' He glanced at his watch, set me firmly aside and walked out.

I was skulking sulkily in the hall five minutes later when the doorbell rang and I decided to play the butler. I opened the front door. In the porch stood a short, broad-shouldered man who was dressed in a uniform which suggested an eccentric chauffeur. He had brown hair, rather bushy, and the kind of alert expression which one so often sees on the faces of gun-dogs. His eyes were a vivid blue.

'All chauffeurs should go to the back entrance,' I said, speaking grandly to conceal how unnerved I was by this curious apparition in gaiters.

'I'm not a chauffeur – I'm an archdeacon,' he said smiling at me, and asked my name. To put him to the test I answered poker-faced: 'Vanilla,' but he surmounted the challenge with ease. 'How very charming and original!' he exclaimed, not batting an eyelid, and told me I reminded him of Alice in Wonderland.

I was hardly able to believe that any adult could be so agreeable. 'If I'm Alice,' I said, testing him again to make sure I was not mistaken, 'who are you?'

'If you're Alice, I think I'd like to be Lewis Carroll,' said my future Mr Dean, exuding the charm which was to win my mother's approval, and that was the moment when I knew for certain that he was my favourite kind of person, bright and sharp, quick and tough, yet kind enough to have time for a plain little girl with ink-stained fingers and an insufferable air of grandeur.

My father's reaction to Aysgarth was startlingly similar to

17

mine. 'I like that man,' he kept saying afterwards. 'I *like* him.' He sounded amazed. Hitherto he had regarded all clergymen as the victims of an intellectual aberration.

'You'll never believe this,' said my mother that evening on the telephone to my elder brother in London, 'but your father's fallen violently in love with a clergyman – no, not the local parson who's gone round the bend! Your father complained about the parson to the Bishop, and the Bishop sent the Archdeacon to investigate, and it's the *Archdeacon* who's won your father's heart. Your father's even saying he's seen the Virgin Birth in a new light – he's dreadfully unsettled, poor dear.'

This evidently alarmed my brother very much. Outraged squawks emerged from the telephone.

However the truth was that my father was neither suffering from the onset of senility nor undergoing a religious conversion. He was merely having to upgrade his opinion of clergymen because Aysgarth, an Oxford graduate, was one of those rare beings, my father's intellectual equal. A clergyman who had won a first in theology could be dismissed; theology was not a subject which my father took seriously. But a clergyman who had been at Balliol, my father's own college, and taken a first in Greats, that Olympian academic prize which even my father had had to toil to achieve – there indeed was a clergyman who defied dismissal.

'I've come to the conclusion that Mr Aysgarth's a great blessing,' said my mother to me later. 'Clever men like your papa become bored if they don't have other clever men to talk to, so perhaps now he's discovered Mr Aysgarth he won't be such a crosspatch whenever he's obliged to leave London and spend time at Flaxton Hall.'

I said: 'If I read Greats up at Oxford, would Papa like me better?'

'Darling, what a thing to say! Papa adores you – look how he stood up for you about the inkpot! Papa and I love all our children,' said my mother vaguely, wandering away from me to attend to her plants in the conservatory, 'and you're a very lucky little girl to belong to such a happy family.'

I stood alone, staring after her, and wished I could be one of the exotic plants to which she paid so much devoted attention.

III

Aysgarth had a brother, who taught classics at a minor public school in Sussex, and a sister, who lived in the south London suburbs, but these siblings were rarely mentioned; he was fond of them but they had no place in the world he had carved out for himself since he had entered the Church. He had decided to be a clergyman when he was up at Oxford on his scholarship. This had been a brave decision, since he had had no money and no influential clerical connections, but Aysgarth was capable of great daring and possessed the iron nerves of a successful gambler.

'Aysgarth may look the soul of propriety in his clerical uniform,' my father remarked once to my mother, 'but by God, he takes scandalous risks!' My father often talked riskily, particularly when he succumbed to the childish urge to shock people he disliked, but in fact he lived a very conventional life for a man of his class. If he had been Aysgarth, obliged to make his own way in the world, he would have played safe, using the Oxford scholarship to follow an academic career. To enter the Church, where salaries were risible and worldly success for any self-made man was unlikely, would have struck my father as being reckless to the point of lunacy. Outwardly opposed to Christianity but inwardly attracted to the aspects which coincided with his own old-fashioned, sentimental liberal humanism, he was enthralled by the madcap idealism which seemed to him to characterise Aysgarth's choice of a profession.

'It was such a courageous step to take, Aysgarth!'

'Nonsense! God called me to serve Him in the Church, so that was that. One doesn't argue with God.'

'But your intellect – surely you were obliged to give rational consideration to –'

'What could be more rational than the decision to use my

gifts in a way which would most clearly manifest my moral and intellectual convictions?'

My father was silent. Unable to risk believing in knowledge which his arrogant intellect deemed unknowable, he was speechless when confronted by Aysgarth's act of faith. No rhetoric from an evangelist could have dented my father's agnosticism, but Aysgarth, never speaking of Christianity unless my father raised the subject, presented the most powerful apologetic merely by revealing his life story. My father was baffled but respectful, disapproving yet filled with admiration.

'But how did you have the nerve to marry when you were still a curate? Wasn't that an absolutely scandalous risk for a penniless young man to take?'

'I'd been engaged for seven years – wouldn't it have been even more of a scandalous risk if I'd waited a day longer?' retorted Aysgarth, and added to my mother as if he knew he could rely on her sympathy: 'I regarded my first wife as the great prize which lay waiting for me at the end of my early struggles to get on in the world.'

'So romantic!' sighed my mother predictably.

'Mr Aysgarth,' I said, fascinated by his unembarrassed reference earlier in the conversation to the Deity whom my family felt it bad taste to discuss, 'did God tell you to marry, just as He told you to be a clergyman?'

'Be quiet, Venetia, and don't interrupt,' said my father irritably. 'Sophie, why isn't that child in bed?'

But my Mr Dean – my Mr Archdeacon as he was then – merely winked at me and said: 'We might talk about God one day, Vanilla, if you've nothing better to do,' and when both my parents demanded to know why he was addressing me as if I were an ice-cream, I realised with gratitude that he had diverted them from all thought of my bedtime.

According to various people who could remember her, Aysgarth's first wife had been beautiful, intelligent, charming, religious and utterly devoted to her husband and children. Aysgarth seldom mentioned her but once when he said: 'Grace was much too good for me,' he sounded so abrupt that I realised any question about her would have exacerbated a grief which was still capable of being painfully recalled. The marriage had produced five children, four boys and a girl, Primrose, who was my age. The children were all either brilliantly clever or remarkably good-looking or, as in the case of Christian and Norman, both. James, the third son, was good-looking but not clever, and Alexander, the youngest, was clever but not good-looking. Primrose, who had a face like a horse, was brilliant and I became close friends with her, but I shall return to the subject of Primrose later.

Then in 1942 when Christian, the eldest, was fifteen and Alexander was little more than a baby, the first Mrs Aysgarth died and my Mr Archdeacon became entangled with the appalling creature who was to become his second wife. She was a society girl, famed for her eccentricities. Everyone declared that no woman could have been less suitable for a clergyman, but Aysgarth, bold as ever, ignored this judgement and lured his *femme fatale* to the altar soon after the end of the war. Everyone then proclaimed that the marriage would never last and he would be ruined, but 'everyone', for once, was wrong.

A year after the marriage came the vital meeting with my family. 'All clergymen with balls should be encouraged!' pronounced my father, and proceeded to throw his weight about at Westminster in an effort to win preferment for his new friend. Having devoted many years of his life to politics in the House of Lords my father was not without influence, and the Church of England, under the control of the Crown, was always vulnerable to the meddling of the Crown's servants in the Lords and Commons. Usually the Church succeeded in going its own way without too much trouble, but although on ecclesiastical matters the Prime Minister took care to listen to the leading churchmen, he was not obliged to act on their advice. This situation occasionally reduced eminent clerics to apoplectic frenzy and led to chilly relations between Church and State.

Into this delicate constitutional minefield my father now charged, but fortunately it proved unnecessary for him to charge too hard because Aysgarth was well qualified for a choice promotion; he had been appointed archdeacon at an unusually early age after winning the attention of the famous Bishop Jardine who had romped around Starbridge in the 1930s. Jardine had retired before the war in order to swill port in Oxfordshire, and without a powerful benefactor a self-made man such as Aysgarth might well have languished in the provinces for the rest of his career, but he did have an excellent curriculum vitae and my father did have the urge to play God. In consequence Aysgarth's transfer to London, where his talents could be fully displayed to the people who mattered, was hardly a big surprise.

'If you're an agnostic,' I said to my father at one stage of his campaign, 'why are you getting so mixed up with the Church?'

'The Church of England,' said my father grandly, 'belongs to all Englishmen, even unbelievers. It's a national institution which for moral reasons deserves to be encouraged, and never forget, Venetia, that although I'm an agnostic and even, in moments of despair, an atheist, I remain always an exceedingly moral man. This means, *inter alia,* that I consider it my absolute moral duty to ensure that the Church is run by the very best men available.'

'So it's all right for me to be interested in the Church, is it?'

'Yes, but never forget that the existence of God can't be scientifically proved.'

'Can the non-existence of God be scientifically proved?' I enquired with interest, but my father merely told me to run away and play.

Aysgarth was still too young to be considered for a bishopric or a deanery, and when it was agreed by the Church authorities that a little London grooming was necessary in order to eliminate all trace of his modest background, a benign Prime Minister offered him a canonry at Westminster Abbey – although not the canonry attached to St Margaret's church where so many society weddings took place. (This disappointed my mother, who was busy marrying off her eldest daughter at the time.) The canon's house in Little Cloister had been badly damaged by a bomb during the war, but by 1946 it had been repaired and soon Aysgarth's frightful second wife had turned the place into a nouveau-riche imitation of a mansion in Mayfair.

I must name this woman. She had been christened Diana Dorothea but her acquaintances, even my father who shied away from Christian names, all referred to her as Dido despite the fact that they might be socially obliged to address her as 'Mrs Aysgarth'. She was small, slim and smart; she dressed in a bold, striking style. Numerous falls from horses (the result of a mania for hunting) had bashed her face about so that she was ugly, but possibly she would have been ugly anyway. She always said exactly what she thought, a habit which regularly left a trail of devastation in her wake, and her wit – overrated, in my opinion – was as famous as her tactlessness. 'Dido can always make me laugh,' said my Mr Dean – my Canon, as he had now become. He was amazingly patient with her, always serene even when she was crashing around being monstrous, and his reward was her undisguised adoration. 'Of course I could have married anyone,' she declared carelessly once, 'so wasn't it too, too sweet of God to keep me single until I'd met darling Stephen?'

'Is any further proof needed,' muttered Primrose, 'to demonstrate that God moves in mysterious ways?'

Primrose hated her stepmother.

'Really, Primrose . . .' Those syllables always heralded some intolerable remark. 'Really, Primrose, I can't understand why you don't invest in some padded bras. I certainly would if I was unfortunate enough to have your figure . . .' 'Really, Primrose, we must do something about your clothes! No wonder no man asks you out when you look like someone from a DP camp . . .' 'Really, Primrose, you must try not to be so possessive with your father – possessiveness, I've always thought, is inevitably the product of a low, limited little nature . . .'

'If she were my stepmother,' I said to Primrose after witnessing one of these verbal assaults, 'I'd murder her.'

'Only the thought of the gallows deters me,' said Primrose, but in fact it was her love for her father that drove her to endure Dido.

Aysgarth wound up fathering five children in his second

marriage, but three died either before or shortly after birth and only a boy and a girl survived. Elizabeth was a little monster, just like her mother, but Philip was placid and gentle with an affectionate nature. Not even Primrose could object to little Pip, but she had a very jaundiced opinion of Elizabeth who would scramble up on to her father's knees, fling her arms around his neck and demand his attention at every opportunity. Aysgarth complicated the situation by being far too indulgent with her, but Aysgarth was incapable of being anything but indulgent with little girls.

My father had naively thought that once Aysgarth was ensconced in the vital Westminster canonry peace would reign until the inevitable major preferment materialised, but before long Aysgarth's reckless streak got the better of him and he was again taking scandalous risks. Having run a large archdeaconry he quickly became bored with his canonry, and as soon as he had mastered the intricacies of Abbey politics he decided to seek new worlds to conquer in his spare time. He then got mixed up with Bishop Bell of Chichester, a remarkable but controversial celebrity who was always tinkering with international brotherhood and ecumenism and other idealistic notions which the more earthbound politicians at Westminster dubbed 'hogwash'. The most dangerous fact about Bishop Bell, however, was not that he peddled hogwash from the episcopal bench in the House of Lords, but that he was loathed by Mr Churchill, and as the Labour Government tottered in slow motion towards defeat, it became increasingly obvious that Mr Churchill would again become Prime Minister.

'Think of your future, Aysgarth!' implored my father. 'It's death to get on the wrong side of these politicians!'

'Then I must die!' said Aysgarth cheerfully. 'I refuse to be an ecclesiastical poodle.'

'But if you want to be a bishop or a dean –'

'All I want is to serve God. Nothing else matters.'

My father groaned and buried his face in his hands.

'What's the difference between a bishop and a dean?' I demanded, taking advantage of his speechlessness to plunge into the conversation, and Aysgarth answered: 'A dean is the man in charge of a cathedral. A bishop is the man in charge of a diocese, which is like a county – a large area which contains in addition to the cathedral a number of churches all with their own parishes. A bishop has a special throne, his *cathedra*, in the cathedral and sometimes he goes there to worship, but often he's looking after his flock by attending services all over the diocese.'

'It's as if the bishop's the chairman of the board of a group of companies,' said my father morosely, 'and the dean is the managing director of the largest company. Aysgarth, how I wish you'd never got involved with that POW camp on Starbury Plain during the war! I can quite see how useful you are to Bell when he needs someone to liaise with the German churches, but if you want to avoid antagonising Churchill you've got no choice: you must wash your hands of all those damned Huns without delay.'

'I'm a disciple of Jesus Christ, not Pontius Pilate!' said Aysgarth laughing. 'Don't talk to me of washing hands!' And when my father finally laughed too, I thought what a hero Aysgarth was, unintimidated by my formidable father, unintimidated by the even more formidable Mr Churchill, and determined, like the star of a Hollywood western, to stand up for what he believed to be right.

However, real life is far less predictable than a Hollywood western, and contrary to what my father had supposed, Aysgarth's work with the Germans failed to result in a lethal confrontation with Mr Churchill as the clock struck high noon. Bishop Bell was undergoing that metamorphosis which time so often works on people once judged controversial, and in the 1950s he became so hallowed that any hand-picked confederate of his could hardly fail to acquire a sheen of distinction. With Bell's patronage Aysgarth became renowned as an expert on Anglo-German church relations. He formed the Anglo-German Churchmen's Society; he raised funds to enable German refugees in England to train for the priesthood; he kept in touch with the numerous German POWs to whom he had once ministered in the Starbridge diocese. Like Bell, Aysgarth had been uncompromisingly opposed to Nazism, but he saw his post-war work with the Germans as a chance to exercise a Christian ministry of reconciliation, and in the end it was this ministry, not his canonry at Westminster, which in the eyes of the senior churchmen made him very much more than just a youthful ex-archdeacon from the provinces.

'It was a terrible risk to mess around with all those damned Huns,' said my father, 'but he's got away with it.' And indeed Aysgarth's failure, once he turned fifty, to receive his big preferment lay not in the fact that he had aligned himself with the pro-German Bishop Bell; it lay in the fact that he had a disastrous wife.

Dido prided herself on being a successful hostess. Her dinner-parties were patronised by an astonishing range of distinguished guests who enjoyed her eccentric remarks, but clerical wives are hardly supposed to toss off letters to the newspapers on controversial issues or make withering remarks about the Mothers' Union during an interview with a women's magazine. The press were rapidly enthralled with appalling results. Dido stopped giving interviews but could seldom resist a tart comment on any matter of public interest. ('What do you think of the conquest of Everest, Mrs Aysgarth?' 'Thank God someone's finally done it – I'm bored to death with the wretched molehill!' 'Do you believe in capital punishment, Mrs Aysgarth?' 'Certainly! Flog 'em and hang 'em – and why not crucify 'em too? What was good enough for Our Lord ought to be good enough for mass-murderers!' 'What do you think of the Suez crisis, Mrs Aysgarth?' 'The Archbishop of Canterbury should declare that the entire disaster is a Moslem plot to humiliate a Christian country, and all the soldiers going to the Canal should wear crosses, like the Crusaders!')

'Aysgarth will never receive preferment now,' said my father in deepest gloom after the Suez comment had been plastered over William Hickey's Diary in the *Daily Express*. 'How could that woman ever be a bishop's wife? She'd outrage everyone in no time.'

Hating to abandon hope I said: 'Could he still be a dean?'

'Perhaps in one of the minor cathedrals a long way from London.'

'Dido will never leave London except for Canterbury or York,' said my mother dryly, but she was wrong. Late in 1956 after the Suez crisis had reached its catastrophic conclusion, Dido gave birth to her fifth and final child, a stillborn boy, and promptly lapsed into a nervous breakdown. From time to time in the past she had suffered from nervous exhaustion, but this episode was so severe that she was completely disabled. She had to spend a month in an establishment which was tactfully referred to as a convalescent home, and even when she emerged she could do no more than lie in bed in a darkened room.

'I think she fancies herself as Camille,' said Primrose. 'I'm just waiting for the first little consumptive cough.'

'Maybe she'll commit suicide,' I suggested.

'Not a hope. That sort never does. Too damn selfish.'

The day after this conversation Aysgarth turned up on the doorstep of our London home in Lord North Street, a stone's throw from Westminster Abbey and the Houses of Parliament. My mother was out at a charity coffee-party, my father was downstairs in his study and I was lolling on the sofa in the first-floor drawing-room as I reread *Middlemarch*. By this time I was almost twenty and had recently returned with relief to England after enduring weeks of exile with family friends in Florence.

When I heard the doorbell I laid aside my book and padded out on to the landing. In the hall below me the butler had just opened the front door and Aysgarth was saying: 'Lord Flaxton's expecting me,' but from the tone of his voice I realised I should abstain from cascading down the stairs to offer him an exuberant welcome. I paused, keeping well back from the banisters. Then as soon as the hall was empty I sped noiselessly down the staircase and pressed my ear to the door of my father's study.

'. . . and since you've always taken such an interest in my career,' I heard Aysgarth say, 'I thought you should be the first to know that I have to leave London. There's no choice. Dido's health demands it.'

My father at once became apoplectic with horror. I too was horrified but I did rouse myself sufficiently to check that my eavesdropping was unobserved. Fortunately a gossipy drone rising from the basement indicated that the servants had paused for elevenses. With confidence I returned my ear to the panel.

'. . . and now that I've spoken to the psychiatrist,' Aysgarth was saying, 'I can clearly see that she needs to make a completely fresh start somewhere else. The tragedy is that back in 1946 she so desperately wanted to come to London because she felt that here she could play a major part in advancing my career. The present situation – and of course we all know my career's ground to a halt – is very hard for her to bear.'

'Quite. But nonetheless –'

'The death of the baby was the last straw. Dido now feels she's a failure at everything she undertakes in this city, and she's convinced that she has no chance of happiness until she leaves it.'

'But Aysgarth,' said my father, trying to mask his despair by assuming a truly phenomenal gentleness, 'that's all very well for Dido, but what about you?'

'I couldn't live with myself unless I'd done everything in my power to make Dido feel successful and happy.'

There was a silence while my father and I boggled at this extraordinary statement. I was too young then to feel anything but a massive outrage that he should be acquiescing without complaint in the wrecking of his career, and it was only years later that I realised this was my first glimpse of the mystery which lay at the heart of his marriage.

'It's clear to me that I'm not meant to move any further up the ecclesiastical ladder,' said Aysgarth at last when my father remained silent, 'and I accept that. I confess I'd be happy to stay on in London and devote myself to my German interests, but obviously it's time for my life to take a new turn.'

My father managed to say in a voice devoid of emotion: 'I'll see what I can do about a Crown appointment.'

'That's more than good of you, but quite honestly I think you'd be wasting your time if you tried to pull strings in Downing Street. I'm sure I must have the letters "W.I." against my name in the clerical files.'

'"W.I."?'

'"Wife Impossible".'

'Ah.' There was a pause. Obviously my father was so appalled that he needed several seconds to frame his next question. It was: 'Surely Bell can do something for you?'

'Unfortunately no canonry's likely to fall vacant at Chichester at the moment, and apart from Chichester Bell's influence is mostly abroad – which is no use to me, since Dido couldn't possibly cope with the stress of living in a foreign country. I'll talk to Bell, of course, but –'

'If he can't produce anything suitable, Aysgarth, I believe your best bet would be to go straight to the top and talk to the Archbishop of Canterbury.'

'He's been implacably opposed to Dido ever since she criticised the hat Mrs Fisher wore at the Coronation.'

'Oh God, I'd forgotten that disaster! All right, pass over Fisher. What about the Bishop of London?'

'He's fairly new and I still don't know him well.'

'In that case you must approach his predecessor. Dr Wand's not dead yet, is he?'

'No, but I have a fatal knack of alienating Anglo-Catholics.'

'Then your Dean at Westminster –'

'He's been cool towards me for some time. I've been paying too much attention to my international concerns and not giving enough time to the Abbey.'

'But there must be someone who can rescue you!' said my father outraged. 'I thought Christians were supposed to be famous for their brotherly love!'

Aysgarth somehow produced a laugh but before he could reply my father said suddenly: 'What about your old diocese? Can you approach the Bishop of Starbridge?'

'He's another man I don't know well. You're forgetting that I left Starbridge before he was appointed.'

'But *I* know him,' said my father, who was one of the largest landowners in the Starbridge diocese. 'He's a dry old stick but we're on good terms. Just you leave this to me, Aysgarth, and I'll see what I can do . . .

IV

Neither my father nor Aysgarth hoped for more than a canonry, and both of them were aware how unlikely it was that any choice position would fall vacant at the right moment, but within twenty-four hours of their secret conference the Dean of Starbridge suffered a stroke and it was clear he would be obliged to retire. At once my father plunged into action. The deanery was a Crown appointment, but my father, undeterred by the thought of those hideous letters 'W.I.' in Aysgarth's file, started swamping the Prime Minister's clerical advisers with claret at the Athenaeum. He was helped by having an eligible candidate to promote: Aysgarth knew Starbridge well from his years as Archdeacon, and as a first-class administrator he was more than capable of running one of the greatest cathedrals in England. My father beavered away optimistically only to be appalled when the Prime Minister admitted to him during a chance encounter at the Palace of Westminster that since the deanery was such an important appointment he intended to let Archbishop Fisher have the last word.

'Oh my God!' I said in despair when my father broke the news. By this time I had insinuated myself into the crisis so successfully that my father was taking the unprecedented step of treating me as his confidante. 'Mrs Fisher's Coronation hat!'

'If Aysgarth fails to get that deanery,' said my father, 'just because Dido made a catty remark about a hat –'

'We can't let it happen, Papa, we simply can't – Fisher must be tamed.' It was now 1957 and the entire summer stretched before us. 'Is he interested in racing?' I demanded feverishly. 'We could offer him our box at Ascot. Or what about tennis? We could offer him our debenture seats for the Wimbledon fortnight. Or cricket – you could invite him to the Pavilion at Lords –'

'My dear girl, Fisher's hardly the man to be swayed by mere frivolities!'

'Then what's his ruling passion in life?'

'Canon law.'

The problem seemed insuperable.

After a pause during which we racked our brains for inspiration I asked: 'Who, technically, has the power to overrule the Archbishop of Canterbury?'

'The Queen and God. I mean, the Queen. I really can't start believing in God at my age –'

'Never mind God, let's concentrate on the Queen. Why don't you pull a string at the Palace?'

'What string? I don't have a string – you know very well that I've never been the courtier type!'

'Now look here, Papa: are you a peer of the realm or aren't you?'

'I'm beginning to feel like the inhabitant of a lunatic asylum. Venetia, the Queen would only refer the matter back to the Prime Minister, and since we already know Macmillan's determined to pass the buck to Fisher –'

'Then we've just got to conquer that Archbishop. Let's think again. He's an ex-headmaster, isn't he? If you were to invite him to dinner with the headmaster of Eton and throw in the Bishop of Starbridge for good measure –'

'This has all come to pass because back in 1945 Aysgarth married that bloody woman!' exclaimed my father, finally giving way to his rage. 'Why on earth did he marry her? That's what I'd like to know! Why on earth did he do it?'

It was a question I was to ask myself many times in the years to come.

V

Our fevered plotting resulted in my father's decision to give a little all-male dinner-party at the House of Lords. This made me very cross as I had planned to charm the Archbishop by begging him to tell me all about his life as headmaster of Repton, but my father merely said: 'Women should keep out of this sort of business. Why don't you start training for a decent job instead of loafing around smoking those disgusting cigarettes and reading George Eliot? If you'd gone up to Oxford –'

'What good's Oxford to me when all public school Englishmen run fifty miles from any woman who's mad enough to disclose she has a brain bigger than a pea?'

'There's more to life than the opposite sex!'

'It's easy for you to say that – you're tottering towards your sixty-sixth birthday!'

'Tottering? I never totter – how dare you accuse me of senility!'

'If you can spend your time making monstrous statements, why shouldn't I follow your example?'

My father and I had this kind of row with monotonous regularity; I had long since discovered that this was an infallible way of gaining his attention. The rows had now become stylised. After the ritual door-slamming my long-suffering mother was permitted to play the peacemaker and bring us together again.

However on this occasion events failed to follow their usual course because before my mother could intervene my father took the unprecedented step of initiating the reconciliation. He did it by pretending the row had never happened. When I returned to the house after a furious walk around St James's Park he immediately surged out of his study to waylay me.

'Guess what's happened!'

'The Archbishop's dropped dead.'

'My God, that's close! But no, unfortunately the dead man's not Fisher. It's the Bishop of Starbridge.'

I was appalled. 'Our best ally!'

'Our only hope! I feel ready to cut my throat.'

'Well, pass me the razor when you've finished with it.'

We decided we had to be fortified by sherry. My mother was

out, attending a meeting of the WVS. In the distance Big Ben was striking noon.

'What the devil do I do now?' said my father as we subsided with our glasses on the drawing-room sofa. 'I can't face Fisher without Staro on hand to make his speech about how well Aysgarth ran the archdeaconry back in the 'forties. In Fisher's eyes I'm just a non-church-goer. I was absolutely relying on Staro to wheel on the big ecclesiastical guns.'

'Personally,' I said, 'I think it's time God intervened.'

'Don't talk to me of God! What a bungler He is – if He exists – collecting Staro at exactly the wrong moment! If Aysgarth ever gets that deanery now it'll be nothing short of a miracle, and since I don't believe in miracles and since I strongly suspect that God is an anthropomorphic fantasy conjured up by mankind's imagination –'

The doorbell rang.

'Damn it,' muttered my father. 'Why didn't I tell Pond I wasn't at home to callers?'

We waited. Eventually the butler plodded upstairs to announce: 'Canon Aysgarth's here, my Lord.'

'Oh, for heaven's sake show him up!' said my father crossly. 'You know I'm always at home to Mr Aysgarth!'

Pond retired. My father was just pouring some sherry into a third glass when Aysgarth walked into the room.

'Sit down, my dear fellow,' said my father, 'and have a drink. I assume you've heard the disastrous news.'

'Abandon your sherry!' said Aysgarth. 'Send for the champagne!'

We gaped at him. His eyes sparkled. His smile was radiant. He was euphoric.

In amazement my father exclaimed: 'What on earth's happened?'

'Fisher summoned me to Lambeth Palace this morning. He said: "Let's forget all the nonsense those women stirred up. We can't let the Church suffer in 1957 just because my wife wore a certain hat in 1953."'

My father and I both gasped but Aysgarth, now speaking

very rapidly, gave us no chance to interrupt him. '"Starbridge is suddenly without either a bishop or a dean," said Fisher, "and both the Cathedral and the diocese have problems which need solving urgently by the best men available –"'

'My God!' said my father.

'My God!' said my voice at exactly the same moment. I had a vague picture of an anthropomorphic deity smiling smugly in a nest of clouds.

'He offered me the deanery,' said Aysgarth. 'By that time, of course, I was almost unconscious with amazement, but I did somehow manage to open my mouth and say "thank you".'

For a moment my father was silent, and when he was finally able to speak he could produce only a Latin tag. It was an emotional: *'Fiat justitia!'*

Aysgarth tried to reply and failed. Mutely they shook hands. Englishmen really are extraordinary in their ruthless pursuit of the stiff upper lip. If those men had belonged to any other race they would no doubt have slobbered happily over each other for some time.

'Venetia,' said my father at last, somehow achieving a casual tone, 'ring the bell and we'll ask Pond to conjure up the Veuve Clicquot.'

But I ignored him. Taking advantage of the fact that women were permitted to be demonstrative in exceptional circumstances, I exclaimed to Aysgarth for the first time in my life: 'My darling Mr Dean!' and impulsively slipped my arms around his neck to give him a kiss.

'Really, Venetia!' said my father annoyed. 'Young women can't run around giving unsolicited hugs to clergymen! What a way to behave!'

But my Mr Dean said: 'If there were more unsolicited hugs in the world a clergyman's lot would be a happier one!' And to me he added simply, 'Thank you, Venetia. God bless you.'

In ecstasy I rang the bell for champagne.

TWO

---◆◆◆---

'We need to be accepted as persons, as whole persons, for
our own sake.'

JOHN A. T. ROBINSON
Suffragan Bishop of Woolwich 1959–1969
Writing about *Honest to God* in the
Sunday Mirror, 7th April 1963

I

Aysgarth drank quite a bit. Not quite a lot. But quite a bit.
There's a difference. 'Quite a lot' means serious drinking twice
a day. 'Quite a bit' means serious drinking occasionally and
moderate drinking in between. Aysgarth was apparently the
kind of drinker who seldom touched alcohol during the day but
who regularly had a couple of whiskies at six o'clock. If he went
to a dinner-party later he would then drink a glass of sherry
before the meal, a couple of glasses of wine with the food and
a hefty measure of port once the cloth was drawn. This was by
no means considered a remarkable consumption in the political
circles in which my father moved, and probably the upper
reaches of London ecclesiastical society also regarded such
drinking habits as far from excessive, yet by 1957 my father was
afraid a rumour might circulate that Aysgarth was a secret
drinker.

'He keeps his bottle of whisky behind the Oxford Dictionary
in his study!' my father said scandalised to my mother after this
eccentricity had been innocently revealed to him. 'What a risk
to take! He's paying lip-service, of course, to the tradition that
clergymen shouldn't indulge in spirits, but what are the servants
going to think when they discover the clandestine bottle? He'd
do better to keep it openly on the sideboard!'

'Since Mr Aysgarth hasn't had a lifetime's experience of

35

dealing with servants,' said my mother delicately, 'perhaps he thinks they won't find out about the bottle.'

'I disillusioned him, I assure you, but he didn't turn a hair. "I'm not a drunk and my conscience is clear!" he declared, not believing a word I said, and he even had the nerve to add: "*Honi soit qui mal y pense*!" He's quite incorrigible.'

My father also disapproved of Aysgarth's occasional trick of drinking too fast. On that day in 1957 as we celebrated the offer of the Starbridge deanery, he downed three glasses of champagne in a series of thirsty gulps and sighed as if longing for more. It was not offered to him. 'Fancy drinking champagne like that!' said my father shocked to me afterwards. 'No breeding, of course. Not brought up to drink champagne properly.'

I opened my mouth to remind him of his blue-blooded friends who regularly consumed champagne as if it were lemonade, but then I decided not to argue. I was in too good a mood. Instead I merely proffered the opinion that Aysgarth was more than entitled to a quick swill after enduring his wife's nervous breakdown and the agonising worry over his future.

I was still savouring my relief that the crisis had ended when I learnt that a new cloud had dawned on the ecclesiastical horizon. Calling on us the next day Aysgarth confessed his fear that an old adversary of his might be appointed bishop of Starbridge.

It was six o'clock. (Aysgarth always timed his visits to coincide with the possibility of refreshment.) My mother was attending a committee meeting of the Royal Society of Rose-Growers. Once again my father and I joined forces to support our harassed cleric.

'Have a whisky, my dear fellow,' said my father kindly. 'We'll pretend you're not wearing your clerical collar and can drink spirits with a clear conscience. Who's this monster who might be offered the bishopric?'

'Oh, he's no monster!' said Aysgarth hastily, sinking into the nearest armchair as my father added soda-water to a shot of scotch. 'He's just someone I'd be happy never to meet again.'

'Your sworn enemy!' I said, reading between the Christian lines.

'Don't be facetious, Venetia,' said my father. 'This is serious. Do you have no power of veto, Aysgarth? Surely the Dean and Chapter are always consulted about the appointment of a new bishop?'

'Unofficially, yes, but officially we have to take the card we're dealt – and bearing in mind the fact that I've only just won the deanery by the skin of my teeth I'm hardly in a position to raise even an informal objection to this man.'

'But who on earth is he, for God's sake?'

'The rumour bouncing off the walls of Church House,' said Aysgarth after a huge gulp of whisky, 'is that Charles Ashworth's been approached for the job.'

'Oh, him! In that case you've nothing to worry about. He'll never take it.'

'I know he's already turned down two bishoprics, but this could be the one bishopric he's unable to refuse. He'd rank alongside the bishops of London, Durham and Winchester – there'd be a seat available immediately in the House of Lords – he'd be only ninety minutes by train from the centres of power in the capital – and as if all these advantages weren't sufficient to seduce him, he'd have the challenge of pulling the Theological College together, and he's an expert on theological education.'

'I've never heard of this man,' I said. 'Where's he been hiding himself? What's he like?'

'Oh, he's the most charming fellow!' said my father with enthusiasm. 'Very keen on cricket. A first-class brain. And he's got a nice little wife too, really a *very* nice little wife, one of those little women who listen so beautifully that they always make a man feel ten feet tall –'

'The Reverend Dr Charles Ashworth,' said Aysgarth, ignoring this sentimental drivel as he responded to my demand for information, 'is Lyttelton Professor of Divinity at Cambridge and a Canon of Cambridge Cathedral.'

'So what's wrong with him?'

37

'Nothing. We're just temperamentally incompatible and theologically in different camps.'

'Maybe he'll turn down the job after all!' I said brightly after we had all observed a moment of heavy silence. 'Why did he turn down the previous bishoprics?'

My father commented: 'Being a bishop isn't every clergyman's idea of heaven,' and Aysgarth said: 'Ashworth preferred life in his academic ivory tower.' However as soon as this statement had been made he modified it by adding rapidly: 'No, I shouldn't say that. Ashworth came down from his ivory tower in 'thirty-nine when he volunteered to be an army chaplain. That was something I never did. Then he was a prisoner of war for three years. I never had to endure that either. After the war he did return to academic life but not, I'm sure, because he wanted to escape from the world. He must have felt genuinely called to resume his career of writing and teaching, and I'm sure this call is why he's turned down the previous bishoprics.'

'So why should his call now change?'

'Because the offer's alluring enough to make him wonder if God might have other plans for him.'

'Let's get this quite straight, Aysgarth,' said my father, always anxious to eliminate God from any conversation. 'Have you actually had a row with this man or is this just a case of polite mutual antipathy?'

'In 1946,' said Aysgarth, 'we had such a row that he smashed his glass in the fireplace and stormed out of the room.'

'Impossible!' said my father, balking at the thought of a clergyman behaving like a Cossack. 'Ashworth's such a charmer! What on earth was the row about?'

'The theology of redemption and the theology of the Incarnation.'

'Impossible!' said my father again. 'Two highly intelligent men going berserk over *theology* – of all subjects! No, no, Aysgarth, I refuse to believe it, you must be romancing!'

'I assure you I'm not – although to be fair to Ashworth,' said Aysgarth with an effort, 'I should explain that at the time he was obviously still suffering from his experiences as a POW.'

Unable to restrain my curiosity I asked: 'What exactly do you mean when you talk about the theology of redemption and the theology of the Incarnation?' but my father at once cried imperiously: 'Stop!' and held up his hand. 'I refuse to allow theology to be discussed in my drawing-room,' he declared. 'I value my collection of glasses too highly. Now Aysgarth, I'm sure you're worrying unnecessarily. Ashworth's not going to bear you a grudge just because you once drove him to behave like a hooligan during some bizarre tiff, and besides, you're now both such distinguished Christian gentlemen! If you do indeed wind up living in the same cathedral close, then of course you'll both have no trouble drawing a veil over the past and being civil to each other.'

'Of course,' said Aysgarth blandly, but he downed the rest of his scotch as if he still needed to drown his dread.

II

The appointments were eventually announced within a week of each other in *The Times*. Ashworth did accept the bishopric, although it was whispered on the Athenaeum's grapevine that he nearly expired with the strain of making up his mind.

'I think I must now give a little men-only dinner-party for him and Aysgarth at the House of Lords,' said my father busily to my mother. 'It might be helpful in breaking the ice if they met again in a plain, simple setting without a crucifix in sight.'

'Anything less plain and simple than that baroque bastion of privilege would be hard to imagine,' I said, furious at this new attempt to relegate me to the side-lines, 'and why do you always want to exclude women from your dinner-parties?'

'Don't speak to your father in that tone of voice, please, Venetia,' said my mother casually without pausing to glance aside from the flowers she was arranging. 'Ranulph, you needn't be afraid to hold the dinner-party here; Dido won't come. When I telephoned yesterday to enquire how she was, her companion said she was still accepting no invitations.'

'And besides,' I said, turning over a page of *Punch*, 'if you stick to your misogynist principles, you won't be able to ogle that "nice little wife" of Professor Ashworth's at the dinner-party.'

'Nice little wife?' echoed my mother, sufficiently startled to forget her flower arrangement and face us. 'Well, I've only met her a couple of times at dinner-parties, but I thought she was tough as nails, the sort of chairwoman who would say to her committee: "I'm so glad we're all in agreement," and then effortlessly impose her views on the dissenting majority!'

'For God's sake let's have both Ashworths to dinner as soon as possible,' I said, tossing *Punch* aside. 'I can't wait.'

The dinner took place a fortnight later.

III

My mother invited Primrose to accompany her father to the dinner-party, and she also extended an invitation to Aysgarth's third son, James, who was stationed with his regiment in London. Any young man in the Guards who can look dashing on horseback in a glamorous uniform will always be popular with mothers of unmarried daughters, but twenty-four-year-old males with the cultural limitations of a mollusc have never struck me as being in the least amusing.

'I wish you'd invited Christian and Norman as well as James,' I grumbled, but my mother said she had to avoid swamping the Ashworths with Aysgarths. The Ashworths did have two teenage sons but at the time of the dinner-party Charley was doing his National Service and Michael was away at school.

I regretted being deprived of Christian; like every girl I knew I had gone through a phase of being madly in love with Aysgarth's eldest son, and although I had by this time recovered from my secret and wholly unreciprocated passion for this masculine phenomenon who looked like a film star and talked like a genius, a secret hankering for him lingered on.

Meanwhile, as I hankered in vain for Christian's presence at the dinner-party, my mother was obliged to add to the guest-list my brother Harold, an amiable nonentity, and his wife Amanda, an expensive clothes-horse. They were in London on holiday but would eventually return to Turkey where Harold had a job shuffling papers at the British Embassy and the clothes-horse fulfilled her vocation to be ornamental. Their combined IQ was low enough to lay a pall over any dinner-party, and to make matters worse my other brother – the one who on his good days could be described as no genius but no fool – had to speak in an important debate, a commitment which excluded him from the guest-list. Oliver, the Member of Parliament for Flaxfield, was also married to an expensive clothes-horse, but unlike Harold's ornament, this one had reproduced. She had two small boys who made a lot of noise and occasionally smelled. My three sisters, all of whom had manufactured quiet, dull, odourless daughters, were united in being very catty about Oliver's lively sons.

My eldest sister, Henrietta, lived in Wiltshire; she had married a wealthy landowner and life was all tweeds and gun-dogs interspersed with the occasional hunt ball. My second sister, Arabella, had married a wealthy industrialist and now divided her time between London, Rome and her villa at Juan-les-Pins. My third sister, Sylvia, had been unable to marry anyone wealthy, but fortunately her husband was clever at earning a living on the Stock Exchange so they lived in a chic mews house in Chelsea where Sylvia read glossy magazines and tended her plants and told the au pair how to bring up the baby. My mother disapproved of the fact that Sylvia did no charity work. Henrietta toiled ceaselessly for the Red Cross and even Arabella gave charity balls for UNICEF whenever she could remember which country she was living in, but Sylvia, dreaming away among her plants, was too shy to do more than donate clothes to the local church.

I was mildly fond of Sylvia. She was the sister closest to me in age, but since we were so different there had been no jealousy, no fights. Having nothing in common we had inevitably drifted apart after her marriage, but whenever I felt life was intolerable I would head for her mews and sob on her sofa. Sylvia would ply me with instant coffee and chocolate digestive biscuits – an unimaginative response, perhaps, but there are worse ways of showing affection.

All my sisters were good-looking and Arabella was sexy. Henrietta could have been sexy but was too busy falling in love with gun-dogs to bother. Sylvia could have been sexy too but her husband liked her to look demurely chaste so she did. They all spoke in sporano voices with the affected upper-class accent which in those days was beginning to die out. I was a contralto and I had taken care to speak with a standard BBC accent ever since I had been teased by the middle-class fiends at my vile country preparatory school for 'speaking la-di-da'. My sisters had escaped this experience. They had attended an upper-class establishment in London before being shovelled off to an equally upper-class boarding school, but in 1945 my parents were able to reclaim Flaxton Hall, which had been requisitioned during the war, and they were both anxious to spend time in the country while they reorganised their home. I was then eight, too old for kindergarten, too young to be shovelled off to boarding school. Daily incarceration at the hell-hole at Flaxfield, three miles from our home at Flaxton Pauncefoot, proved inevitable.

Possibly it was this torturous educational experience which set me apart from my sisters, but it seemed to me I had always been the odd one out.

'That child gets plainer every time I see her,' said Horrible Henrietta once to Absolutely-the-Bottom Arabella when they rolled home from Benenden for the school holidays. 'Those broad shoulders are almost a deformity – she's going to wind up looking exactly like a man.'

'Maybe she's changing sex. That would explain the tomboyish behaviour and the gruff voice . . .'

'Mama, can't something be done about Venetia's eyebrows? She's beginning to look like an ape . . .'

'Mama, have you ever thought of shaving Venetia's head and giving her a wig? That frightful hair really does call for drastic measures . . .'

My mother, who was fundamentally a nice-natured woman

whenever she wasn't worshipping her plants, did her best to stamp on this offensive behaviour, but the attacks only surfaced in a more feline form when I reached adolescence.

'Can't someone encourage poor darling Venetia to take an interest in clothes? Of course I know we can't all look like a fashion-plate in *Vogue*, but . . .'

'Venetia, my sweet, you simply can't wear that shade of lipstick or people will think you're a transvestite from 1930s' Berlin . . .'

Even my brothers lapsed into brutality occasionally.

'Oliver, you've got to help me find a young man for Venetia –'

'Oh God, Mama, don't ask me!'

'Harold, do explain to Venetia how ill-advised it is for a young girl to talk about philosophy at dinner-parties – she simply takes no notice when I tell her it's so dreadfully showy and peculiar –'

'Certainly, Mama. Now look here, Venetia old girl – and remember I speak purely out of fraternal affection – your average man doesn't like clever women unless they're real sizzlers, and since you'll never be a real sizzler . . .'

'Poor Venetia!' said Absolutely-the-Bottom Arabella to Horrible Henrietta when she knew quite well I was within earshot. 'No sex appeal.'

'Well!' said my father with a sigh of relief once his third daughter was married. 'Now I can sit back and relax! I don't have to worry about Venetia, do I? She'll never be a *femme fatale*.'

'. . . and I can't tell you how glad I am,' I overheard my mother confiding to her best friend, 'that Venetia will inevitably have a quieter life than the others. When I think of all I went through with Arabella – not to mention Henrietta – and even dearest Sylvia was capable of being a little too fast occasionally . . .'

I remembered that remark as I dressed for dinner on the night of the Aysgarth-Ashworth reunion, and wished I could be a sizzler so fast that no one would see me for dust. I slid into my best dress, which was an interesting shade of mud, but unfortunately I had put on weight with the result that the material immediately wrinkled over my midriff when I dragged up the zip. I tried my second-best dress. The zip got stuck. My third-best dress, which had a loose-fitting waist, was wearable but hopelessly out of fashion and my fourth-best dress transformed me into a sausage again. In rage I returned to number three in the hope that I could divert attention from its unfashionable lines by swathing myself in jewellery.

'Darling, you look like a Christmas tree!' exclaimed my mother aghast as she glanced into the room to inspect my progress. 'Do take off those frightful bracelets – and what on earth is Aunt Maud's diamond hatpin doing in your hair?'

I sank down on the bed as the door closed. Then in despair I tore away all the jewellery and began to wallop my impossible hair with a brush. Eventually I heard the guests arriving, and after a long interval Harold was dispatched to drag me into the fray.

'Come along, old girl – everyone's thinking you must have got locked in the lavatory!'

Loathing the entire world and wishing myself a thousand miles away I followed him downstairs. The sound of animated conversation drifted towards us from the drawing-room, and as I pictured everyone looking matchlessly elegant I had to fight the urge to run screaming through the streets to Sylvia's house in Chelsea.

'Here she is!' chirped idiotic Harold as I finally made my entrance.

All heads swivelled to gaze at my dead dress and diabolical hair. I had a fleeting impression of an unknown couple regarding me with mild astonishment, but just as I was wondering if it were possible to die of humiliation, my Mr Dean exclaimed warmly: 'My dear Venetia, how very delightful you look!' and he held out his hands to me with a smile.

IV

It was Aysgarth's kindness which first attracted me to Christianity; the contrast between his attitude and the callous remarks of the non-believers in my family was so great that I felt the explanation could only be theological. It was small wonder that I hero-worshipped him from an early age, but I must make it clear that I was never in love with him. Such a possibility was inconceivable, first because he was a married clergyman, a creature permanently unavailable for a grand passion, and second because he was over fifty years old and therefore incapable of being classed by my youthful brain as an object of sexual desire. Moreover Aysgarth had become considerably plainer since I had first met him in 1946. By the time of the Ashworth dinner-party eleven years later his springy brown hair was smoother, straighter and a shop-soiled shade of white, while his deeply-lined face was marred by pouches under the eyes. He was also much heavier, not repulsively fat but markedly four-square. 'Aysgarth's built like a peasant,' my father remarked once, not meaning to be unkind but unable to abstain from that insensitive frankness which can be such an unfortunate trait of the aristocracy.

However after Aysgarth's heroic kindness to me at the beginning of that dinner-party, I would hardly have cared if he had been built like an elephant, and as soon as Primrose and I had the chance for a quick word I said to her enviously: 'You're so damned lucky to have a father like that.'

'Isn't he wonderful? All other men seem so dreary in comparison.'

Immediately I felt annoyed with myself for giving her the opportunity to drool; once Primrose started flaunting her Elektra complex she was nauseous. 'Professor Ashworth doesn't look too bad,' I said in the hope of diverting her. 'In fact I'd say he was rather well preserved for a man of his age.'

After my embarrassing entry into the room my mother had cursorily introduced me to the Ashworths, but afterwards the Professor had been buttonholed by Harold while Mrs Ashworth had been cornered by my fascinated father so I had had no opportunity to converse with them. I now paused to inspect the Professor with care. He was a tall man who had kept his figure; I learned later that he had excelled at games in his youth and still possessed a single-figure handicap as a golfer. Middle age had given him a receding hairline, but his curly dark hair was streaked in just the right places with just the right shade of glamorous silver. He had brown eyes, a straight nose, a firm jaw with a cleft chin, and deep lines about his strong mouth. These lines, which immediately suggested past suffering, reminded me he had once been a prisoner of war.

I opened my mouth to remark to Primrose how rare it was to encounter a handsome cleric, but at that moment we were interrupted by James, Aysgarth's soldier son, and I was obliged to endure a lot of jolly talk about nothing. Nevertheless I kept an eye on the Professor. He was gliding around, displaying a formidable social technique as he talked to everyone in turn. From various syllables which reached my ears I gathered he was even able to talk to Harold's clothes-horse about fashion.

Eventually Primrose was unable to resist abandoning me to move to her father's side, jolly James decided to take a hand in passing around the canapés (our butler Pond was most put out) and I was just pretending to inspect my mother's somewhat constipated flower arrangement when the future Bishop of Starbridge materialised at my elbow and said with such a polished charm that I even thought for a moment that he was genuinely interested in me: 'I hear you've been visiting Florence. It's a beautiful city, isn't it?'

'Possibly,' I said, determined not to simper at him merely because he was one of the most distinguished churchmen in England, 'but I don't like Abroad.'

'In that case I assume you're glad to be home!'

'Not specially, but don't let's waste time talking about me, Professor. I'm not a bit interesting, although it's very kind of you to pretend that I am. Why don't you tell me all about you?'

I had pierced the cast-iron professional charm. 'Ah, so you're a listener!' he exclaimed with a seemingly genuine amusement. 'How delightful!'

Mrs Ashworth, slender and sleek in a black dress, chose that moment to interrupt us. My first impression had been that she was much younger than her husband, but now I saw that she was probably his contemporary; her neck had that crêpe-like look which afflicts women past the menopause, but she was so immaculately made up that one barely noticed the tell-tale signs of age. Her dark hair was swept back from her forehead and drawn into a bun at the nape of her neck. Her rimless spectacles gave her a chaste, schoolmistressy look which was curiously at odds with the wicked little dress which clung to her svelte figure, and at once I decided she was far more interesting than her husband. The Professor seemed a very typical product of the best public schools and universities, but Mrs Ashworth, whom I found impossible to place against any definitive background, didn't seem typical of anything.

She was saying lightly to her husband: 'Vamping young girls again, darling?'

'Indeed I am – I've just discovered Miss Flaxton's a listener.'

'Ah, a *femme fatale!*' said Mrs Ashworth, regarding me with a friendly interest as I mentally reeled at her choice of phrase. 'How clever of you, Miss Flaxton! Men adore good listeners – they have a great need to pour out their hearts regularly to sympathetic women.'

'I do it all the time myself,' said the Professor, effortlessly debonair. 'Apart from golf it's my favourite hobby.'

'How very intriguing that sounds!' said Aysgarth, sailing into our midst with his champagne glass clasped tightly in his hand. 'Am I allowed to ask what this hobby is or should I preserve a discreet silence?'

There was a small but awkward pause during which I was the only one who laughed – a fact which startled me because although the remark could have been classed as risqué it could hardly have been described as offensive. Yet both Ashworths were as motionless as if Aysgarth had made some error of taste, and Aysgarth himself immediately began to behave as if he had committed a *faux pas*. 'Sorry,' he mumbled. 'Bad joke. Silly of me.'

The Professor made a lightning recovery. 'No, no!' he said, smooth as glass. 'I was merely startled because you seemed to materialise out of nowhere!'

47

'Just thought I'd seize the chance for a quick word before we all go in to dinner –'

'Of course – I was thinking only a moment ago that I'd talked to everyone in the room except you –'

'Seems ages since we last met –'

'Yes, it's certainly a long time –'

'Oxford 'fifty-two, wasn't it?' said Aysgarth, having regained his equilibrium with the aid of a large swig of champagne. 'That weekend when we were both guests of the Master of Balliol.'

'No, you've seen Charles since then,' said Mrs Ashworth. 'We met in London when we all helped the Dean of Westminster recover from the Coronation.'

'So we did! I'd quite forgotten . . . I'm sorry, I can't quite remember – dear me, I'm beginning to sound like an amnesiac – but did I ever call you Lyle?'

'I really have no idea,' said Mrs Ashworth, as if such a feat of memory was well beyond her capabilities, 'but please do in future. Did I ever call you Neville?'

'Neville!' I exclaimed. 'But no one calls him Neville nowadays – he's always Stephen!'

'Ah,' said Mrs Ashworth, 'but you see, I met him before the war when Bishop Jardine appointed him Archdeacon of Starbridge. I was Mrs Jardine's companion at the time.'

Much intrigued I said: 'But how romantic that you should now be returning in such style to the house where you were once a mere companion!'

'It would indeed be romantic if it were true, but the Jardines lived in the old episcopal palace which is now the Choir School, whereas Charles and I will be living – thank goodness! – in the South Canonry. I wouldn't have wanted to return to the palace,' said Mrs Ashworth serenely. 'Too many –' She hesitated but for no more than a second '– poignant memories.'

Aysgarth said: 'Do you regret the loss of the palace, Ashworth?' but the Professor replied promptly: 'Not in the least – and my dear fellow, if you're going to call my wife Lyle, I really don't see why you should now fight shy of calling me Charles! I

48

only hope I have your permission to call you Stephen in the interesting times which I'm sure lie ahead for us all.'

Aysgarth at once became almost inarticulate with a shyness which I suspected was triggered not only by his social inferiority complex, but by his gratitude that Ashworth should be making such a marked effort to be friendly. He could only manage to say: 'Yes. Stephen. Fine. Please do,' and toss off the remains of his champagne.

Appearing in contrast wholly relaxed Ashworth observed: 'It really is most remarkable that our careers should have coincided like this – in fact, if you knew how often Lyle and I have been telling ourselves recently that God moves in mysterious ways –'

'Darling,' said Mrs Ashworth, 'if you quote that ghastly cliché once more I shall be tempted to strangle you with your brand-new pectoral cross.'

'More champagne anyone?' enquired jolly James, still playing the butler.

His father at once held out his glass. '"Well, I don't mind if I do, sir!" as Colonel Chinstrap used to say on *ITMA* –'

'Oh, how I adored *ITMA*!' said my mother, drifting over to us and eyeing her constipated flower arrangement as if she had suddenly realised it needed a laxative. 'Venetia, can you pass around the cigarettes? Pond seems to have disappeared in a huff for some reason . . .'

'That bishop-to-be is going to look simply too heavenly in gaiters,' Harold's clothes-horse was drawling as she demolished her third dry martini.

'Can someone stop young James playing the butler?' muttered my father. 'Pond's taken violent umbrage.'

'. . . and what I absolutely can't understand,' idiotic Harold was burbling in a corner, 'is how Pater, who can't bear going to church and has always said "Boo!" to God, has got himself mixed up with these high-powered clerical wallahs.'

'He'll probably wind up taking the sacrament on his death-bed,' said Primrose, 'like Lord Marchmain in *Brideshead*.'

'*Brideshead*?' said Harold. 'Where's that?'

'I'm damned hungry,' said my father to my mother. 'Are they all dead drunk in the kitchen?'

'Dinner is served, my Lord!' thundered Pond reproachfully from the doorway, and with relief we all descended to the dining-room.

V

The next evening Aysgarth called at six o'clock with a note of thanks and a bunch of carnations for my mother, but found only me at home. My mother had travelled down to Flaxton Pauncefoot that morning and my father was attending a Lords' debate on education. Harold and the clothes-horse had not yet returned from a day at the races.

When Pond showed Aysgarth into the drawing-room I was reading Professor Ashworth's latest book, *St Augustine and the Pelagian Heresy: the Origins of His Theology Concerning God's Grace*, which I had borrowed from the library. The Professor wrote in a cool, lucid prose which created an impression of scholarly detachment and yet succeeded in being surprisingly readable – but perhaps that was because he was writing of St Augustine's fight to master his sex drive, a fight which was to have immense repercussions both for Christianity and for the bluff heretic Pelagius who had said (more or less) that man could jolly well pull himself up by his own bootstraps and conquer sin not by God's grace but by will-power and a stiff upper lip.

Pelagius, it is hardly necessary to add, had been a Briton.

'Oh, I've read that book,' said Aysgarth as we settled down for a delectable discussion of the dinner-party. 'I thought it very bad. Like St Augustine Charles's twin obsessions are heresy and sex. Apparently up at Cambridge all his divinity undergraduates refer to him as Anti-Sex Ashworth.'

'How extraordinary! He seemed quite normal.'

'No, no – rabid against fornication and adultery. Such a mistake! In my opinion there are far worse sins than the sexual errors, and – whoops! Here's Pond with the drinks.'

Pond deposited the sherry and whisky decanters, the soda-siphon and a suitable selection of glasses on the side-table and waited for orders, but I waved him away.

'Help yourself, Mr Dean.'

'Well, perhaps a little soupçon of sherry –'

'Oh, go on – have a whisky! You don't want to go down in history as Anti-Alcohol Aysgarth!'

'That possibility,' said my Mr Dean, helping himself to a modest measure of scotch, 'is so remote that I don't think we need consider it seriously. And I must guard my tongue about Charles, who was certainly more than civil to me last night – even though I nearly shocked him to death with my opening remark –'

'But only a second before you arrived Mrs Ashworth had been teasing him about vamping young girls! I don't think you shocked him at all – he was just taken aback because you slunk up behind him and –'

'– hit him over the head with a *double entendre*! I must have been mad.'

'I thought you were sensational. And so was Mrs Ashworth, making that little black dress look like a hundred-guinea model from Harrods just by wearing one piece of jewellery – and choosing rimless spectacles instead of glasses with distracting frames – and dyeing her hair so cunningly that no man would ever dream it had been touched up –'

'*Dyeing her hair*? But no clergyman's wife would ever do that!'

'Yes, I expect that's what the Professor thinks too whenever he's not busy conquering everyone in sight by exuding that synthetic charm of his. But tell me: who *is* Mrs Ashworth? Where did she come from? And how did the two of them meet?'

'Ah!' said Aysgarth, settling down cosily for a gossip. 'Now that's quite a story . . .'

VI

Apparently Mrs Ashworth had grown up in a remote Norfolk parish where her great-uncle had been the vicar; her parents had died young. This clerical background had enabled her to obtain the post of companion to Bishop Jardine's wife when Jardine himself, rocketing racily up the Church's ladder of preferment, had been appointed Dean of Radbury in the 'twenties. Five years later in 1932 he had become the Bishop of Starbridge. In 1937, the young Charles Ashworth, already a doctor of divinity, had decided to visit Starbridge to do some research in the Cathedral Library, and since he was the protégé of Archbishop Lang he had been invited to stay at the episcopal palace. Crossing the threshold he had fallen instantly and violently in love with Mrs Jardine's companion.

Since Mrs Jardine had been an ineffectual woman who had relied on her companion to run the palace for her, this *coup de foudre* had caused chaos, but Ashworth, much to the Bishop's fury, had refused to be deflected from his romantic charge to the altar.

'The whole trouble was,' said Aysgarth, 'that Lyle's departure was a bereavement for the Jardines as well as a crippling inconvenience. They were a childless couple who'd come to regard her as a daughter, and they'd reached the stage where they couldn't imagine life without her.'

'Presumably they were all reconciled later?'

'Oh yes, but back in 1937 – '

' – the Jardine dragon had to be vanquished before St George could carry away the maiden on his shining white horse!'

'As a matter of fact whether he was a saint and she was a maiden was hotly debated later when the two of them produced a baby only seven months after the wedding, but since the infant was very small and delicate, just as a premature baby should be, everyone eventually agreed that the maiden's purity had been unsullied prior to her marriage.'

'Rather tricky to be a clergyman,' I said, 'and produce a baby a shade too fast.'

'Most embarrassing for poor Charles! However I never had any serious doubt that he'd behaved himself – he was always too ambitious to do anything else.' As an afterthought he added: 'He was married before – his first wife was killed in a car crash

– but although he was a widower for some time before he met Lyle you can be sure he kept himself in order. The first thing a successful young clergyman learns to acquire, if he wants to continue as a success, is an immaculate self-control in dealing with women.'

'At least nowadays clergymen can get married, which is more than poor St Augustine could – although actually I don't understand why St Augustine couldn't marry. Why did he have to be celibate?'

'Well, in the days of the Early Church . . .'

We embarked on a fascinating conversation about the origins of clerical celibacy, and Aysgarth promised to lend me his copy of St Augustine's *Confessions*.

'My dear Venetia,' he sighed at last as he finished his whisky and rose reluctantly to his feet, 'how very much I enjoy talking to you!'

I smiled radiantly at him and felt like a sizzler.

VII

I should perhaps make it clear that contrary to the impression I may have created while describing the turning point of his career, I did not see Aysgarth often. He led a busy life at Westminster, and I was often away. After leaving boarding school I had been obliged to endure periods of exile in Switzerland and Italy, and even when I returned to England I often sneaked down to Flaxton Pauncefoot in order to escape from the ghastly London social events where I was either ignored or treated as a freak. Life drifted on. I had no idea what I wanted to do. My métier seemed to consist of sipping drinks, smoking cigarettes and reading books. There was no calling, no summons from God written in the sky in letters of fire, and increasingly often it seemed to me that my career as an adult was incapable of beginning so long as I remained condemned to the sidelines of life by my unfortunate looks and my embarrassing intellectual inclinations.

Sometimes I gave way to despair. Supposing I had to suffer the ultimate horror of not marrying? Then I would be 'poor old Venetia', that pathetic freak, till my dying day. The prospect was intolerable. My depression deepened. My parents found me increasingly difficult, and soon after the Aysgarth-Ashworth dinner-party they decided that something would have to be done.

It was unusual for my parents to stage a joint attack. My mother preferred to leave the bombastic behaviour to my father and take refuge in the conservatory, but on this occasion she was apparently desperate enough to decide that I was more important than her plants.

'We just thought we'd have a little word, darling,' she said soothingly after we had all assembled for battle in the drawing-room of our house in Lord North Street. 'Your father's actually quite worried about you.'

'Worried?' said my father, bristling with rage. 'I'm not worried, I'm livid! I shouldn't have to deal with a recalcitrant daughter at my age – it's bad for my blood pressure.'

'You should have thought of that,' I said tartly, 'before you frolicked around with Mama in Venice in 1936.'

'*Frolicked?* What a damn silly word – makes me sound like a bloody pansy!'

'Oh, do stop screaming at each other!' begged my mother, fanning herself lightly with the latest edition of *Homes and Gardens*. 'What happened in 'thirty-six is quite irrelevant – except that here you are, Venetia, and we have to help you make the best of your life – which means we simply must insist that you now stop frivolling and –'

'Frivolling?' I mimicked. 'What a damn silly word! Makes me sound like a bloody butterfly!'

'Oh my God,' said my mother, taking refuge in *Homes and Gardens*.

'Just because you happen to be reading St Augustine's *Confessions*,' said my father, storming into the attack, 'you needn't think you're not frittering away your time – and I must say, I think Aysgarth should have asked my permission before he lent you that book. Parts of it are most unsuitable for an unmarried young woman.'

'If you mean that incident in the public baths when Augustine was fourteen –'

'What a lovely picture of a cyclamen!' murmured my mother, gazing enrapt at a page of her magazine.

'If you'd gone up to Oxford,' said my father to me, 'as I wanted you to, you wouldn't be lying around sipping gin at odd hours, smoking those disgusting cigarettes and reading about fourteen-year-old boys in public baths!'

'If I'd gone up to Oxford,' I said, 'I'd be studying the work of Greek pederasts, ordering champagne by the case and damn well *looking* at fourteen-year-old boys in public baths!'

'Now look here, you two,' said my mother, reluctantly tossing her magazine aside, 'this won't do. Ranulph, you must try not to get so upset. Venetia, you must stop talking like a divorcée in an attempt to shock him – and you must try to remember that since he watched his own father die of drink and his brother die of – well, we won't mention what he died of – your father has an absolute horror of the havoc wealth can cause among people who lack the self-discipline to lead worthwhile, productive lives. The truth is that people like us, who are privileged, should never forget that privileges are always accompanied by responsibilities. We have a moral duty to devote our wealth and our time to worthy causes and live what the lower orders can see is a decent upright life.'

'Hear, hear!' bellowed my father.

'I'm sure you think that was a dreadfully old-fashioned speech,' pursued my mother, encouraged by this roar of approval to sound uncharacteristically forceful, 'but believe me, it's neither smart nor clever to be an effete member of the aristocracy. You *must* be occupied in some acceptable manner, and fortunately for you, since you live today and not yesterday, that means you can train for an interesting job. I do understand, I promise you, why you chose not to go up to Oxford; being a blue-stocking isn't every woman's dream of happiness. But since you've rejected an academic life you must choose some other career to pursue while you fill in your time before getting married. After all, even Arabella had a job arranging flowers in a hotel! I know she wound up in a muddle with that Italian waiter, but –'

'I don't want to arrange flowers in a hotel.'

'Well, perhaps if you were to take a nice cordon bleu cookery course at Winkfield –'

'I don't want to take a nice cordon bleu cookery course at Winkfield.'

'You don't want to do anything,' said my father. 'It's an absolute waste of a first-class brain. Awful. Tragic. It makes me want to –'

'Ranulph,' said my mother, 'don't undo all my good work, there's a pet. Venetia –'

'I think I'd like to be a clergyman.'

'Darling, do be serious!'

'All right, all right, I'll take a secretarial course! At least that'll be better than arranging bloody flowers!'

'I can't stand it when women swear,' said my father. 'Kindly curb your language this instant.'

'You may have spent a lot of your life declaring in the name of your liberal idealism that men and woman should be treated equally,' I said, 'but I've never met a man who was so reluctant to practise what he preached! If you really believed in sexual equality you'd sit back and let me say "bloody" just as often as you do!'

'I give up,' said my mother. 'I'm off to the conservatory.'

'And I'm off to the Athenaeum,' said my father. 'I simply daren't stay here and risk a stroke any longer.'

'How typical!' I scoffed. 'The champion of equality once again takes refuge in an all-male club!'

'Bloody impertinence!' roared my father.

'Bloody hypocrite!' I shouted back, and stormed out, slamming the door.

VIII

If I had been living in the 'sixties I might then have left home and shared a flat with cronies; I might have taken to drink or drugs (or both) and chased after pop singers, or I might have opened a boutique or become a feminist or floated off to Nepal to find a guru. But I was living in the 'fifties, that last gasp of the era which had begun in those lost years before the war, and in those days nice young girls 'just didn't do that kind of thing', as the characters in *Hedda Gabler* say. (*Hedda Gabler* was one of Aysgarth's favourite plays; he adored that clever doomed sizzler of a heroine.)

It was also a fact that in between the acrimonious rows my life at home was much too comfortable to abandon in a fit of pique. My parents, exercising a policy of benign neglect, were usually at pains to avoid breathing down my neck, ordering me about and preaching nauseous sermons about setting an example to the lower orders. I was waited on hand and foot, well fed and well housed. In short, I had sufficient incentives to postpone a great rebellion, and besides, like Hedda Gabler, I shied away from any idea of not conforming to convention. If I flounced around being a rebel I knew I would only earn the comment: 'Poor old Venetia – pathetic as ever!' and wind up even worse off than I already was.

So after that row with my parents in 1957 I did not rush immediately upstairs to pack my bags. I gritted my teeth and faced what I saw as the cold hard facts of life: no longer could I sit around sipping gin, smoking cigarettes and soaking up the sexy reminiscences of St Augustine. The day of reckoning for my refusal to go up to Oxford was at hand, and just like any other (usually middle-class) girl who considered that the hobbies of flower-arranging and playing with food were far beneath her, I had to embark on a secretarial training.

However as I reflected that night on my capitulation to parental bullying, I thought I could face my reorganised future without too much grief; a secretarial course could well be my passport to what I thought of as Real Life, the world beyond my mother's gardens and my father's clubs, a world in which people actually lived – swilling and swearing, fighting and fornicating – instead of merely existing bloodlessly in charity committee meetings or in cloud-cuckoo-lands such as the Athenaeum and the House of Lords.

I decided to go to Mrs Hoster's Secretarial College because Primrose had attended a course there while I had been fighting off death by boredom in Switzerland and Italy. Like me, Primrose had been encouraged by her school to try for a place at Oxford, but she had convinced me that an Oxford education was the one thing we both had to avoid if we were to have any hope of experiencing Real Life in the future.

'Christian told me frankly it would reduce my chance of marrying to nil,' she had confided, 'and there's no doubt spinsters are always regarded with contempt. Besides, how on earth could I go up to Oxford and leave poor Father all alone with Dido? He'd go mad if he didn't have me to talk to whenever she was driving him round the bend.' Primrose had never been away from home. She had attended St Paul's Girls School in London while I had been incarcerated at Cheltenham Ladies' College, and I had always secretly resented the fact that her father had considered her indispensable while mine had been willing to consign me to an institution.

Although Primrose was anxious to marry eventually, just as a successful woman should, she never seemed to mind having no boyfriends. Instead she channelled her gregarious inclinations towards forming a circle of female friends whom her brothers condescendingly referred to as 'the Gang'. Some of the Gang had been at school with her, some had been débutantes with us in 1955 and some had been her classmates at Mrs Hoster's. Aysgarth adored us all. Dido used to refer to us as 'Stephen's Little Harem' and look indulgent. 'Name your favourite of the day!' we would tease him as he sat beaming on the sofa and we lounged on the carpet at his feet, but he would sigh: 'I can't decide! It's as if you were asking a chocolate addict to select from a row of equally luscious peppermint creams!'

When the Aysgarths moved to Starbridge in 1957, it was thought the Gang might drift apart, but Starbridge was an easy journey by train from London and the core of the Gang kept in touch. Abandoning all thought of a secretarial career in London, Primrose landed a job at the diocesan office on Eternity Street, and in order to avoid constant clashes with Dido she had her own flatlet in the Deanery's former stables. Time ticked on. I completed my secretarial training and drifted through a series of jobs in art galleries and antique shops and publishing houses. Then with the dawn of the new decade the Gang at last began to disintegrate. Penny and Sally got married, Belinda joined the Wrens, Tootsie became an actress and was expelled from the Gang for Conduct Unbecoming, Midge dropped out to grow daffodils in the Scilly Isles, and by 1963 only I was left in 'Stephen's Little Harem' – 'The last peppermint cream left in the box!' as my chocolate-loving Mr Dean put it so saucily, much to his wife's annoyance.

'You really should make more effort to get married, Venetia,' she said soon afterwards. 'In the game of life women who don't marry are inevitably regarded as such amateurs, and you wouldn't want people to look down on you pityingly, would you, my dear? That's one thing a clever girl can never endure.'

I could have withstood that woman better if she had been merely mad and bad. But it was her talent for disembowelling her victims with the knife of truth which made her so thoroughly dangerous to know.

It was 1963. The innocent days were almost over, and in the early spring, just after John Robinson, the suffragan bishop of Woolwich, published the book which was to shake the Church of England to its foundations, the foundations of my own world were at last rocked by the earthquake of change. Exasperated by my failure to stay in any job longer than a year, my father went to great trouble to obtain a post for me at the Liberal Party's headquarters. I handed in my notice a week later.

'How dare you do this to me!' shouted my father, who was now seventy-two and even less capable of managing a recalcitrant daughter.

'My dear Papa, I'm the victim, not you! I was the one who actually had to work at that ghastly place!'

'Well, if you think you can loaf around under my roof doing nothing for the next six months –'

'Nothing would induce me to loaf around under your roof a day longer!' I said, almost twenty-six years old and finally summoning the strength to burst out of my luxurious prison. 'I'm off to Starbridge to meditate on God and contemplate Eternity – which is exactly what you ought to be doing at your age!'

And having delivered myself of this speech, which could be guaranteed to infuriate any humanist past endurance, I embarked on my journey into adventure.

THREE

—◆◆—

'But now "God" is news!'

JOHN A. T. ROBINSON
Suffragan Bishop of Woolwich 1959–1969
Writing about *Honest to God* in the
Sunday Mirror, 7th April 1963

I

At Waterloo Station I encountered Charley Ashworth, the Bishop's elder son, whom I had occasionally met in Starbridge during my visits to the Aysgarths. He was a year my junior, small, chatty and bumptious. It was generally agreed that the bumptiousness masked an inferiority complex which had arisen because he was plain while his brother Michael was handsome. After completing his National Service Charley had gone up to Cambridge, where he had taken a first in divinity, and in 1961 he had entered a theological college, also in Cambridge, to learn how to be a clergyman. This exercise, which hardly seemed compatible with his pugnacious personality, was still going on.

'Good heavens – Venetia!' he exclaimed, speeding towards me with a suitcase in one hand and a copy of Bishop Robinson's *Honest to God* in the other. 'What are you doing here?' He made it sound as if I were trespassing.

'Just admiring the view from platform twelve.' I had set down my bags in order to rest my wrists; I never managed to travel light. Around us throbbed the echoing noise and mouldy smell of a mighty station. I had been gazing at the inert train nearby and trying to decide which end would have the best chance of offering me a solitary journey.

'But I'd heard you were running the Liberal Party!' Charley was protesting as I realised my hopes of solitude had been dashed.

'I decided I wasn't political.'

'Good for you! Personally I think women should keep out of politics.'

'And what do you think they should keep in?'

'The home, of course.' He heaved open the door of the nearest carriage and flung out his hand generously towards the interior as if he were offering a child a treat. 'In you go!'

'Could you deal with my bags?' I said. 'We girls are such delicate little flowers that we have to rely on strong brave boys like you to help us whenever we're not sitting at home being plastic dolls.'

'Very funny!' said Charley good-humouredly, my sarcasm quite lost on him, and without complaint turned his attention to my bulging suitcases.

'How are you getting on with *Honest to God*?' I enquired as he tossed his book on to the seat.

'Oh, have you heard of it?'

'I can read, you know. OUR IMAGE OF GOD MUST GO, SAYS BISHOP –'

'That article in the *Observer* was a disgrace!'

'Did you think so? I adored it – such fun when a Church of England bishop declares to all and sundry that he doesn't believe in God!'

'But that's not what Robinson's saying at all –'

'That's what laymen think he's saying.'

'And that's exactly why the book's a disgrace! It's so bad for laymen. My father says that Robinson's being thoroughly irresponsible as well as intellectually slipshod, and I agree with him,' said Charley, exuding outraged virtue as he heaved my bags up on to the rack. 'My father and I always agree on everything.' Closing the carriage door he pulled down the window and began to scan the platform.

'Tedious for you,' I said. 'My father and I are in perpetual disagreement. Life's just one long glorious row.' But Charley, leaning out of the window, was too absorbed in some private anxiety to reply.

'Bother the infant,' he said at last, glancing at his watch. 'He's cutting it very fine.'

'What infant's this?'

'I doubt if you'd know him – he's only twenty. He's supposed to be staying tonight with us at the South Canonry.' Again he hung out of the window in an agony of suspense but a moment later he was bawling 'Hey!' in relief and wildly waving his arm.

A tall, pale youth, earnest and bespectacled, appeared at the door and was hustled into the carriage. He wore very clean jeans and a spotless blue shirt with a black leather jacket. All he was carrying was a duffle-bag. 'Sorry I'm late,' he said. 'I got lost on the underground.' Unaware that Charley and I knew each other he wasted no time looking at me but removed his glasses and began to polish them with an exquisitely ironed white handkerchief. In the distance the guard's whistle blew and after a preliminary jerk the train began to glide out of the station.

'Venetia,' Charley said, remembering his manners, 'this is Nicholas Darrow. Nick, this is the Honourable Venetia Flaxton.'

'I find it more comfortable these days to drop the Honourable,' I said. 'Hullo, Nick.'

Replacing his spectacles he looked me straight in the eyes and at once I felt as if I stood in a plunging lift. 'Hi,' he said politely without smiling. His eyes were an unnaturally clear shade of grey.

'Have we met before?' said my voice. I sounded as unnerved as I felt, but I knew that the obvious explanation for my loss of poise – sexual bewitchment – was quite wrong. He was a plain young man. Yet somehow he contrived to be compulsively watchable.

'No, we haven't met,' he was answering tranquilly, opening his duffle-bag and pulling out a book. It was *Honest to God.*

'Nick's father was principal of the Starbridge Theological College back in the 'forties,' Charley said. 'Maybe Nick's jogging your memory of him.'

'No, that's impossible. I wasn't involved in Starbridge ecclesiastical circles until the Aysgarths moved to the Deanery in 'fifty-seven.'

Charley obviously decided to dismiss my confusion as a mere feminine vagary. 'Nick's reading divinity up at Cambridge just as I did,' he said, 'and – good heavens, Nick, so you've bought *Honest to God*! What's your verdict so far?'

'Peculiar. Can it really be possible to reach the rank of bishop and know nothing about the English mystics?'

'Maybe he can't connect with them,' I said. 'I certainly can't. I think Julian of Norwich's description of Christ's blood is absolutely revolting and borders on the pathological.'

The grave grey eyes were again turned in my direction and again I wondered why his mysterious magnetism should seem familiar.

'Well, of course it's very hard for a layman to approach these apparently morbid touches from the right angle,' Charley was saying with such condescension that I wanted to slap him, 'but if one takes the time to study the mystics with the necessary spiritual seriousness –'

'You're a church-goer,' said Nick suddenly to me.

'Now and then, yes.'

'But you're not a communicant.'

'I watch occasionally.' I was still trying to work out how he had made these deductions when Charley exclaimed in delight: 'In college we debate about people like you! You're from the fringes – the shadowy penumbra surrounding the hard core of church membership!'

'I most certainly am not!' I said, concealing my fury behind a voice of ice. 'I've been christened and confirmed – I'm just as much a member of the Church of England as you are!'

'But if you're not a regular communicant –'

'I've never been able to understand why chewing a bit of artificial bread and sipping some perfectly ghastly wine should confer the right to adopt a holier-than-thou attitude to one's fellow-Christians.'

'Shall I give you my best lecture on the sacraments?' said

Charley, allowing a sarcastic tone of voice to enhance his nauseous air of condescension.

'No, read *Honest to God* and shut up. It's narrow-minded, arrogant believers like you who give the Church a bad name.'

Charley flushed. His pale brown eyes seemed to blaze with golden sparks. His wide mouth hardened into a furious line. 'If all so-called believers were a little more devout, we might have more chance of beating back sin!'

'Who wants to beat back sin?' I said. 'I'm mad about it myself.' And opening my bag I casually pulled out the famous unexpurgated Penguin edition of *Lady Chatterley's Lover*.

That closed the conversation.

The train thundered on towards Starbridge.

II

'Sorry,' said Charley to me an hour later. 'I didn't mean to offend you. Since you don't come from a religious family, it's very praiseworthy that you go to church at all.'

'Oh, my father's devoted to religion,' I said. 'He just has trouble believing in God.'

'So he didn't mind you being baptised and confirmed?'

'Mind! He insisted on it! In his opinion all loyal English people ought to go through the initiation rites of the Church of England – it's part of our tribal heritage, like learning about King Alfred burning the cakes and memorising the patriotic speeches from *Henry V* and singing "Land of Hope and Glory" at the last night of The Proms.'

'This is most interesting, isn't it, Nick?' said Charley. 'When one comes from a religious home one doesn't realise what extraordinary attitudes flourish elsewhere.'

'What's so extraordinary about them?' I said. 'Isn't the main purpose of our glorious Church to reassure us all that God is without doubt an Englishman?'

'You're teasing me!' said Charley. But he sounded uncertain. I suddenly became aware that Nick was gazing at me. I had intercepted his gaze more than once during our hour of silence, and as I caught him in the act yet again I demanded: 'Why do you keep staring at me as if I'm an animal at the zoo?'

He lowered his gaze and shifted uncomfortably in his seat. 'Sorry.' His voice was almost inaudible. 'It's the aura.'

'Nick's a psychic,' said Charley serenely as my jaw sagged. 'That's how he knew you were a church-goer but not a communicant.'

'No, it wasn't!' said Nick angrily. 'Her knowledge of Dame Julian suggested she was interested enough in Christianity to be a church-goer, and her repulsion towards the description of Christ's blood suggested she was unlikely to take part in any symbolic ritual involving it. The deduction I made was completely rational and involved no psychic powers whatsoever!'

'Okay, but you can't deny you're a psychic – think what a whizz you were at Pelmanism!'

'Shut up, I don't want to talk about it.'

'I always thought it was such a shame when your father stopped you telling fortunes –'

'*Shut up*, Charley!' Jumping to his feet the youth heaved open the door into the corridor and stalked out in a rage.

'It's not my day, is it? said Charley with a sigh. 'Why do I always put people's backs up? I can't understand it. I only want to be sociable and friendly.'

Leaving him brooding with touching innocence on his abrasive personality I prowled down the corridor to the buffet where I found Nick slumped at a table and sipping Coca-Cola. After buying some liquid which British Rail had the nerve to market as coffee I sat down opposite him.

'Now look here,' I said sternly, trying to take advantage of my years of seniority. 'You've made a disturbing statement and I want an explanation. What's the matter with my aura? Is it exuding gloom and doom?'

He failed to smile. He was a very serious young man. 'No, turbulence,' he said. 'You must be very unhappy. You look so self-assured in your expensive clothes, and you talk so carelessly as if you hadn't a worry in the world, but underneath you're throbbing with pain.'

'Supposing I were to tell you that you're dead wrong?'

'I don't see how I can be. As soon as you mentioned your revulsion towards Dame Julian's description of Christ's blood I sensed *your* blood, spattered all over your psyche, and I knew you were in pain.'

I boggled but recovered. 'Here,' I said, shoving my hand palm upwards across the table. 'Read that and tell me more.'

'I don't do that sort of thing nowadays.' But he glanced at my palm as if he found the temptation hard to resist. 'Anyway I'm not trained in palmistry. I just hold the hand and wait for the knowledge.'

I grabbed his fingers and intertwined them with mine. 'Okay, talk. You owe it to me,' I added fiercely as he still hesitated. 'You can't just make gruesome statements and go no further! It's unfair and irresponsible.'

Sullenly he untwined our fingers, set my hand back on the table and placed his palm over mine. There followed a long silence during which he remained expressionless.

'My God!' I said, suddenly overwhelmed by fright. 'Am I going to die?'

'Oh no,' he said. 'You're going to live.' And for one long moment he stared at me appalled before blundering out of the buffet in confusion.

III

I caught up with him just before he reached the carriage. 'What the hell did you see?'

'Nothing. I just don't like meddling with psychic emanations, that's all, and I promised my father I wouldn't do it. If I seem upset it's because I'm angry that I've broken my word to him.' Diving into the carriage he collapsed in a heap on the seat.

Charley, who had been dipping into my copy of *Lady Chatterley's Lover*, hastily shoved it aside but I paid him no attention.

I remained in the corridor and stared out of the window at the smooth hills of the Starbridge diocese. The train was now hurtling towards our journey's end.

'Nick and I are down here for Easter, of course,' said Charley, appearing beside me as the train slowed to a crawl on the outskirts of the city. 'Nick stayed on after the end of term to begin the swot for his exams, and I delayed my return to Starbridge in order to make a retreat with the Fordite monks in London . . . Are you staying with the Aysgarths or are you heading for home?'

'The former.' As the train lurched over a set of points on its approach to the station I stepped back into the carriage and said abruptly to Nick: 'Are we going to meet again?'

'Oh yes. And again. And again. And again.'

'What a terrifying prospect!'

'No, it's okay, you don't have to worry. I'm benign.'

'I see,' I said. 'A recurring phenomenon which ought to be entirely harmless. Like Halley's Comet.'

Finally I saw him smile. I noticed that he had good teeth, very even, and that when his mouth was relaxed he lost the air of solemnity conjured up by his spectacles. Again my memory was jogged, and as it occurred to me that he was as watchable as a gifted actor I at last solved the riddle of his familiarity. 'Wait a minute,' I said. 'Are you any relation of Martin Darrow, the actor?'

'He's my half-brother.'

I relaxed. Although I'm not averse to paranormal puzzles I much prefer mysteries that are capable of a rational explanation. 'My mother's mad on him,' I said agreeably, 'never misses an episode of his comedy series, stays glued to the TV. But surely he must be at least thirty years older than you are?'

'My father had a rather peculiar private life.'

'Come on, chaps!' exclaimed Charley, plunging bossily back into the carriage as the train finally halted at the platform. 'Get a move on! Nick, as you've only got a duffle-bag, could you give Venetia a hand with her suitcases?'

I stepped down on to the platform accompanied by my

psychic porter. The sun was shining and far away in the distance beyond the train, beyond the railway yard, beyond the roofs of the mean little villas which flanked the tracks, I saw the slim straight spire of the Cathedral.

Blazing with energy Charley bounded ahead and by the time Nick and I emerged from the station he was bouncing towards the episcopal car, a black Rover, as Mrs Ashworth emerged from the driver's seat. I knew now, six years after our first meeting, that she was the same age as Aysgarth, but on that day she looked more like forty-five than sixty-one. It was not only her slender figure which made her seem youthful but the smooth straight hair coiled simply in a bun; an elderly woman who has the guts to flout fashion by refusing a permanent wave really does deserve to look a long way from the geriatric ward.

Ever since our first meeting when she had boldly identified me as a *femme fatale* despite the massive evidence to the contrary, I had secretly labelled her my heroine and now, once again, my admiration for her was renewed. She was wearing a pale lilac-coloured raincoat, unbuttoned to reveal a straight grey skirt and a sky-blue blouse – unremarkable clothes, but on her they looked as if they had arrived by special messenger that morning from Paris. Her navy shoes, so different from the old ladies' 'support' footwear which my mother favoured, were notable for the elegance of their stiletto heels. Mrs Ashworth might have turned sixty, but this boring fact had evidently long since been dismissed by her as trivial. Her triumph over the ravages of time was superb.

'Hullo, Nicholas!' she exclaimed warmly after she had given Charley a peck on the cheek, but I knew she was much more interested in me. 'Venetia – what a surprise! I saw Dido Aysgarth earlier today but she didn't mention they were expecting you at the Deanery.'

'They're not expecting me. To be quite honest, Mrs Ashworth, I'm not exactly sure why I'm here. I'm a bit *bouleversée* at the moment.'

'How exciting! Come and have tea. I've got a prayer-group turning up later and there's a visiting American bishop who comes and goes like the Cheshire cat's smile, but at the moment I'm absolutely free.'

My spirits rose, and accepting her invitation with gratitude I slid into the back seat of the Bishop's Rover.

IV

The South Canonry, where the Ashworths lived, was an early Georgian house far smaller than the old episcopal palace but still too large for a modestly-paid executive with a wife and two adult sons. The garden consisted almost entirely of labour-saving lawns; full-time gardeners were no longer an episcopal perk, and the Ashworths were aided only by a man who came once a week to civilise the lawns with a motor-mower. Mrs Ashworth hated gardening and kept no plants in the house. I always found the bare, uncluttered look in her home immensely appealing.

As I was almost the same age as Charley I had been invited to the house occasionally in the past along with various Aysgarths and other young people in the diocese, but the visits had been infrequent and I had never come to know the Ashworths well. Neither had my parents. My father respected the Bishop's intellect but found Ashworth was fundamentally unsympathetic to his sentimental, old-fashioned brand of humanism. Whereas Aysgarth was tolerant of agnostics Ashworth seemed hard put to conceal his opinion that agnosticism was an intellectual defect – and there were other differences too, as we all discovered over the years, between the Bishop and the Dean. Aysgarth was gregarious with an apparently inexhaustible supply of good humour, whereas Ashworth, behind his cast-iron charm, was a very private, very serious man. Laymen like my father dubbed Ashworth 'churchy' – that sinister pejorative adjective so dreaded by clerics – but Aysgarth was unhesitatingly labelled 'one of us'. Ashworth, isolated to some degree by the eminence of his office, was held to resemble Kipling's cat who walked by himself; his close friends had been left behind in Cambridge in

1957, and perhaps this was one of the reasons why he was so close to his wife. It was widely observed how well attuned they were to each other. They seemed to generate that special harmony which one finds more often among childless couples, the harmony of two people who find each other entirely sufficient for their emotional needs.

Considering that the marriage was successful, people found it immensely interesting that the two sons should have undergone such obvious problems: Charley had run away from home when he was eighteen while later Michael had been thrown out of medical school. However, these embarrassing episodes now belonged to the past. Charley had been rescued, sorted out and replaced on the rails of conformity, while Michael had been steered into the employment of the BBC with happy results. Why Charley should have run away from home no one had any idea, but Michael's hedonistic behaviour was universally attributed to a desire to rebel against his father's puritanical views on sin.

'There's a screw loose in that family somewhere,' Dido would say darkly, 'you mark my words.'

The irony of this statement was that Aysgarth had the biggest possible screw loose in his family – Dido herself – yet all his children were turning out wonderfully well. This fact must have been very galling to the Ashworths as they struggled to surmount their problems at the South Canonry.

When I arrived at the house that afternoon I was immediately soothed by its well-oiled serenity. The drawing-room was notably dust-free and arranged with a tidiness which was meticulous but not oppressive. A superb tea was waiting to be served. The telephone rang regularly but was silenced almost at once by the Bishop's secretary in her lair by the front door. Dr Ashworth himself was out, fulfilling an official engagement, but if he had been present he too would have been running smoothly, just like the house. I could remember him appearing during my past visits and saying to his wife: 'What did I do with that memo on the World Council of Churches?' or: 'Whatever happened to that letter from the Archbishop?' or: 'What on

71

earth's the name of that clergyman at Butterwood All Saints?' and Mrs Ashworth, indestructibly composed, would always know all the answers.

After tea Charley went upstairs to unpack, Nick wandered outside to tune into the right nature-vibes – or whatever psychics do in gardens – and Mrs Ashworth took me upstairs to her private sitting-room. Unlike my mother's boudoir at Flaxton Hall there were no dreary antiques, no ghastly oil-paintings of long-dead ancestors, no boring photographs of babies and no vegetation in sight. The air smelt celestially pure. On the walls hung some black-and-white prints of Cambridge and a watercolour of the Norfolk Broads. The only framed photograph on the chimney-piece showed her husband as an army chaplain during the war.

'Sit down,' said Mrs Ashworth, closing the door. 'Now that we've got rid of the men we can relax. Cigarette?'

'I do like this room,' I said, accepting the cigarette and sinking into a comfortable armchair. 'It's all you, isn't it? Everything's your choice. All my life I've had to put up with revolting inherited furniture and now I've finally reached the point where I'm determined to have a place of my own.'

'Splendid! All young people need to express themselves through their surroundings. You should have seen Michael's room when he went through his Brigitte Bardot phase!'

'I bet Charley puts up all the right pictures,' I said, not daring to ask what the Bishop had thought of the Bardot pin-ups.

'Fortunately Charley only has space on his walls for books. My former employer Bishop Jardine left Charley his entire theological library – no doubt because Charley always said he wanted to be a clergyman when he grew up . . . But let's get back to you. So you're seeking a room of your own! But why seek it in Starbridge?'

'I'm not sure that I will – I've only drifted down here because I've got a standing invitation to use the Put-U-Up sofa in Primrose's flat. I'm such a drifter, Mrs Ashworth! I despise myself for drifting but I don't seem able to stop. It's as if I'm marking time, waiting for my life to begin, but nothing ever happens.'

'When will you consider that your life's begun? At the altar?'

I was grateful for her swift grasp of my dilemma. 'Well, I know marriage shouldn't be the be-all and end-all of a woman's life, but –'

'It certainly was before the war. Perhaps this is a case where "the more things change the more they remain the same".'

'I think it must be. As I see it, I really do have to get married in order to live the kind of life I'd enjoy, but here I am, almost twenty-six, and I'm beginning to think: supposing I never marry, never win respect and status, never stop drifting – I could wind up wasting my entire life.'

'A nightmarish prospect.'

'Terrifying. And then I start to feel desperate – *desperate*, Mrs Ashworth, I can't tell you how desperate I feel sometimes – and now I'm convinced I've got to act, got to get out of this rut –'

'Well, it sounds to me as if you're making progress at last! You're looking for a place where you can express your real self; you've embarked on an odyssey of self-discovery . . . Do you have to worry about money?'

'No, I've got a hefty income because I came into money from both my godmothers when I was twenty-one. Maybe that's part of the problem? If I were penniless –'

' – you'd hate it. I did. Now let's consider your situation carefully –'

'I don't have a situation, Mrs Ashworth, I just have a non-event.' The words suddenly began to stream out of my mouth. 'I want to live – I mean *live* – I want to swill gin and chat about philosophy with a gang of brilliant people and smooch with handsome men and dance till dawn and burn the candle at both ends, but all I get are boring nine-to-five jobs, social events where I'm an embarrassing failure, no love-life and evenings spent swilling gin on my own while listening to Radio Luxemburg. I've never had a boyfriend. I did belong to a gang of clever people but they were all girls. Here I am, bursting to join in the Great Party of Life yet confined to the margins by my utter lack of sex appeal, and it's awful, Mrs Ashworth, absolutely *awful*, so utterly vile and unfair –'

'But anyone,' said Mrs Ashworth, 'can have sex appeal. It's simply an attitude of mind.'

I stared at her. She gave me a sphinx-like smile. Enrapt I tried to speak but failed.

'It's all a question of confidence,' said my heroine, flicking ash from her cigarette casually into the nearby tray, 'and in your case it would be confidence in your appearance. You want to be able to walk into a room and think: I'm glamour personified – how lucky all those men are to see me!'

'But I'm not beautiful!'

'Neither was Cleopatra.'

'Yes, but she was Queen of Egypt –'

'– and she made the most of it. That's what you have to do too – make the most of your assets. Stand up for a moment.'

I stood up.

'Revolve.'

I revolved.

'Yes,' said Mrs Ashworth tranquilly, waving her cigarette to indicate I could sit down again, 'it's all very simple. Wear plain, tailored clothes which emphasise your waist and hips. Never wear flat shoes even though you happen to be tallish. Favour V-necks to distract the masculine eye from your shoulders and take care not to stoop – that only makes the shoulders more noticeable. And grow your hair.'

'Grow it? But Mrs Ashworth, I'll turn into a sort of yak!'

'Nonsense, men adore the Pre-Raphaelite look. Oh, and go to a beauty salon and get advice on make-up. You have the most beautiful eyes. Make them a focal point.'

'But do you really think that if I do all this –'

'That's just the beginning. Then you must plot how to get in with a crowd of clever, interesting people by exploiting a clever, interesting person who's already known to you. How about Christian Aysgarth? You can't be much younger than his wife.'

'Well, yes, I do know Christian and Katie, but –'

'Splendid! They're your passport to your new life. Don't

linger in dull old Starbridge. Seek that room you want in Oxford and wangle your way into Christian's set.'

'But Christian just sees me as one of Primrose's gang of virgin spinsters!'

'He won't when you arrive in Oxford flaunting glamorous eye make-up and Pre-Raphaelite hair. I think that you and Primrose,' said Mrs Ashworth, careful in her choice of words, 'may have reached the parting of the ways.' Before I could comment she was adding with regret: 'I wish I could invite you to stay tonight, but thanks to Nicholas and our visiting American bishop, we've got a full house.'

I said with curiosity: 'What's Nick's connection with your family?'

'His father and Charles have known each other for many years, and since Jon Darrow's now very old Charles likes to keep a paternal eye on Nicholas to make sure he's all right.'

'Isn't there a mother?'

'She died. There's a half-brother in London –'

'The actor.'

'That's right – and there was a half-sister, but she's dead now too and Nicholas never had much in common with her children.'

'He's very . . .' I tried to find the right word but could only produce a banality '. . . unusual.'

'Yes, isn't he? Sometimes I think he needs a substitute mother, but I never feel my maternal instinct can stretch far enough to take him on – although I must say, my maternal instinct seems to have stretched out of sight during this conversation! I seem to have forgotten I'm a bishop's wife. Instead of advising you to vamp the intellectuals of Oxford I should be telling you to get a job at the diocesan office and help me with my charity work in your spare time!'

I laughed but before I could reply the front door banged far away in the hall. 'That'll be either Charles or our American bishop,' said Mrs Ashworth, rising to her feet, 'and let's hope it's Charles. I do like Americans, but all that sunny-natured purring's so exhausting.'

'Darling!' shouted the Bishop downstairs.

'Coo-ee!' called Mrs Ashworth with relief, and added indulgently to me: 'Isn't he funny? He so often arrives home and shouts: "Darling!" like that. It's as if he has no idea what to do next and is waiting for instructions.'

In walked the Bishop, looking like a film star in a costume melodrama. The old episcopal uniform of apron, gaiters and frock-coat, so suitable for the eighteenth-century bishops who had had to ride around their dioceses on horseback, was finally giving way to more modern attire, but for his official engagement that afternoon Dr Ashworth had decided to be conservative, and he looked well in his swashbuckling uniform. He was two years older than Aysgarth, but like his wife he appeared younger – not much younger, perhaps, but he could still have passed for a man on the right side of sixty.

'How are your parents?' he said to me agreeably after the greetings had been exchanged.

'Seething. I've just left home and embarked on a new life.'

He gave me his charming smile but it failed to reach the corners of his eyes. Perhaps he was trying to decide whether I could be classified as 'wayward' or 'lost' or even 'fallen'. Smoothly he fell back on his erudition. 'This sounds like a case of *metanoia*!' he remarked. 'By which I mean –'

'I know what it means. The Dean told me. It's a turning away from one's old life and the beginning of a new one.'

'In Christ,' said the Bishop casually, as if correcting an undergraduate who had made an error in a tutorial. 'I hope the Dean didn't forget to mention Christ, but these liberal-radicals nowadays seem to be capable of anything.' He turned to his wife and added: 'I lost count of the times I was asked about *Honest to God* this afternoon. People were deeply upset. It's a pity Robinson wasn't there to see the results of his ill-informed, half-baked radicalism.'

'I thought Robinson was supposed to be a conservative,' I said. 'After all, he wasn't invited to contribute to *Soundings*, was he?'

The Bishop looked startled. 'Who's been talking to you of *Soundings*?'

'The Dean was very enthusiastic when the book was published.'

'I'd have more confidence in Stephen's bold espousal of the views contained in these controversial books if I knew he was a trained theologian,' said Dr Ashworth. 'However, as we all know, he read Greats, not Theology, when he was up at Oxford.'

'But since he's been a clergyman for almost forty years,' I said, 'don't you think he might have picked up a little theology somewhere along the way?'

The Bishop was clearly not accustomed to being answered back by a young female who had never even been to a university. Possibly he was unaccustomed to being answered back by anyone. He took a moment to recover from the shock but then said suavely enough: 'Good point! But perhaps I might draw a parallel here with the legal profession. Barristers and solicitors are all qualified lawyers, but when a knotty legal problem arises the solicitors refer the matter to the barristers, the experts, in order to obtain the best advice.'

'Well, I'm afraid I must now leave you to your expertise,' I said politely, rising to my feet, 'and descend from the mountain top of the South Canonry to the valley of the Deanery.' I turned to my hostess. 'Thanks so much for the tea and sympathy, Mrs Ashworth.'

'Drop in again soon,' said my heroine with a smile, 'and if there's anything I can do, just let me know.'

'Yes indeed,' said the Bishop, suddenly becoming pastoral. 'If there's anything we can do –'

'I'll see you out, Venetia,' said his wife, and led the way downstairs to the hall. As she opened the front door she added: 'You won't want to lug your suitcases to the Deanery – I'll ask Charley to bring them over later in the car.'

I thanked her before saying anxiously: 'I do hope I didn't upset the Bishop when I answered back.'

'My dear, he was enthralled! Such a delightful change for him to meet someone who doesn't treat him as a sacred object on a pedestal.' She looked at me thoughtfully with her cool dark eyes before musing: 'Maybe you've been concentrating on the wrong age-group; very few young men have the self-assurance or the *savoir-faire* to cope with clever women. Try looking for something intelligent, well-educated and pushing forty.'

'It'll be either married or peculiar.'

'Not necessarily . . . Didn't I hear a rumour once that Eddie Hoffenberg was rather smitten with you?'

'Oh, for heaven's sake, Mrs Ashworth – I'd rather die a virgin spinster!'

Mrs Ashworth merely smiled her enigmatic smile and said: 'Do keep in touch.'

I drifted away down the drive towards the Deanery.

V

Eddie Hoffenberg emerged from the Deanery just as I approached the front door, so there was no possibility of avoiding him. My father had once referred to him as 'Aysgarth's poodle – that bloody Hun,' but my father, who had lost his best friends in the First War, was notorious for his anti-German sentiment. Other people, less outspoken than my father, were content to regard Eddie with a polite antipathy. 'It's my cross,' Eddie would say with gloomy relish, and sometimes he would even add: 'Suffering is good for the soul.'

'It's clergymen like Eddie Hoffenberg,' I had said once to Primrose, 'who make Christianity look like an exercise in masochism.'

'It's Germans like Eddie Hoffenberg,' said Primrose, 'who encourage the belief that we were doing them a favour by trying to kill them in the war.'

However although there was no denying that Eddie was a German, he was hardly typical of Hitler's so-called master race, and the fact that he had eventually acquired British citizenship marked him out as a very unusual German indeed. He was tall, bald and bespectacled; his faintly Semitic cast of features had caused him to be bullied by Aryan monsters in the Nazi army, but since he had no Jewish blood in him, this experience had provided him with additional evidence that he was doomed to special suffering. Fortunately his army career had been brief. In 1944 at the age of twenty he had been captured by the British in Normandy, imported to England and dumped in a prison camp on Starbury Plain. Two weeks later Aysgarth, then Archdeacon of Starbridge, had paid a pastoral visit to the camp and naturally Eddie had been quite unable to resist the opportunity to moan to him about how awful life was.

It was not difficult to understand why Eddie had chosen to adopt Aysgarth as a hero, but it was far harder to understand why Aysgarth had chosen to return Eddie's devotion. 'Aysgarth has five sons,' my father remarked once to my mother. 'Why should he want to play the father to a Teutonic disaster who's perpetually encased in gloom?' My mother had no answer, but Primrose eventually produced an explanation. 'Eddie changed Father's life,' she told me. 'It was Eddie who wrote to Bishop Bell and said how wonderful Father was with the POWs, and since that letter led to Father's vital friendship with Bell, Father can't help being sentimental about Eddie and regarding him as a mascot.'

Eddie came from Dresden, which had been devastated by fire-bombing in 1945. None of his family had survived. After the war he had quickly reached the decision that he had to begin a new life elsewhere, and when he thought of the one friend he still possessed he sought Aysgarth's help. Aysgarth encouraged him to be a clergyman. Eddie had been a Lutheran once, but that was in the old, vanished life. Once Aysgarth had extracted the necessary money from the new Anglo-German Churchmen's Fellowship, Eddie began his studies at the Starbridge Theological College and spent his holidays with the Aysgarths in London.

Ordination as a clergyman of the Church of England followed and a curacy was squeezed out of a Westminster parish. (A German was lucky to get any job in Westminster, but the Bishop of London caved in after Aysgarth and Bell staged a joint assault.) When Aysgarth became Dean of Starbridge he at once approached the new bishop on Eddie's behalf, and Dr Ashworth, striving to exercise a Christian spirit after his own years as a POW, proved unwilling to make any move which could be construed as anti-German. Possibly he also saw the chance of unloading his current diocesan problem, a seedy Starbridge parish in the area of the city known as Langley Bottom where there was a run-down Victorian monster of a church, an equally run-down Victorian monster of a vicarage and a working-class congregation of twenty.

Eddie the masochist embraced this challenge with zest. Having been trained at the Starbridge Theological College in its Ango-Catholic heyday under Nick's father Jonathan Darrow, he had no hesitation in resorting to the most florid ritualism (traditionally popular among the religious members of the working classes), and before long the parish was rising from the dead. Consolidating his success Eddie slaved on, organising clubs, running Bible classes, raising money. The parishioners, who had at first regarded him with suspicion, came to the conclusion they preferred the attentions of a foreigner, even a German foreigner, to the ministrations of some toffee-nosed English gentleman who had been educated at a public school. (The plebs are such dreadful snobs.) Eddie flourished. The parish boomed. The Bishop was both amazed and admiring. When a residentiary canonry at last fell vacant at the Cathedral, he had no objection to Aysgarth's suggestion that Eddie's talents should now be employed in a more elevated sphere, and so Eddie became a canon, working hard at his Chapter duties and beavering away on various diocesan committees. He had arrived. Franz Eduard Hoffenberg, that pathetic young German prisoner of war, had been transformed into a pillar of the English ecclesiastical establishment. All he now had to do was live happily ever after.

Of course being Eddie he remained gloomy but it was impossible for him to dispute that his life was now very comfortable. He had a snug little house in the Close, a surrogate family, the Aysgarths, a reasonable income and a pleasant amount of prestige. No one was surprised when he made a success of the canonry. Discarding without difficulty the Anglo-Catholic trappings which he had used to conquer Langley Bottom, he fitted easily into the Cathedral's middle-of-the-road pattern of worship. In theological matters he was more conservative than his hero, but like Aysgarth he was an idealist prone to talk soppily about the brotherhood of man when he had downed a couple of drinks. His odd, ungainly, pear-shaped figure was always carefully dressed. He observed English customs rigorously, even declaring how devoted he was to Walls' pork sausages and Dickens when we all knew he must be hankering for *bratwürst* and Goethe. Priding himself on his mastery of slang he spoke English almost flawlessly except when he began to ponder on the mystery of suffering. Those were the occasions when I thought he was a joke. Otherwise I just thought he was a thundering bore.

As we encountered each other outside the Deanery that afternoon I inwardly recoiled but nevertheless achieved a passable smile.

'Hi Eddie,' I said and automatically added: 'How are you?' but that was a mistake. One never asked Eddie how he was. He was all too likely to reply in excruciating detail.

'Well, as a matter of fact my back's playing me up again,' he began, 'but I've found this wonderful osteopath who –'

'Super! Is the Dean in?'

'Yes, but we're just off to evensong. I say, Venetia, I had no idea you were about to visit the Aysgarths!'

'Ah well, ignorance is bliss, as the saying goes . . .' I was trying to edge past him but his bulk was blocking the way. The Deanery, a rambling medieval concoction enhanced by Georgian meddling, had no formal drive up to the front door; instead a pebbled lane at the side of the house led to the old stables, while a flagstone path flanked with lavender bushes led through the front garden. Eddie was planted on the flagstones and I was trying to slink past the lavender.

'Are you here for long?' Eddie was enquiring, apparently unaware of my attempts at circumnavigation.

'No, I'm heading for Oxford.'

The front door swung wide. 'Venetia!' cried Aysgarth in delight. 'What a marvellous surprise!'

'Mr Dean!' I said as my spirits soared, and firmly pushing my way past Eddie I clasped Aysgarth's outstretched hand.

'Must see you!' I hissed. 'Top secret!'

His bright blue eyes at once became brighter and bluer. He loved being conspiratorial with young women. 'You go on ahead,' he called to Eddie. 'I'll catch you up.'

'We're late already, Stephen –'

'I'll run all the way to the vestry!' said Aysgarth lightly, and with reluctance Eddie sloped off through the front gate.

Wasting no time I said: 'I've left home and I need advice. Any chance of a quick word without half the Close breathing down our necks?'

'Meet me in the cloisters after evensong.'

'Wonderful! Thanks so much . . . In that case I might as well go to evensong, mightn't I?'

'Why not?' said the Dean amused. 'It would help to pass the time!'

As it occurred to me that Dr Ashworth would have responded far more coolly to my lukewarm attitude to worship I exclaimed: 'How glad I am you're not the Bishop! I've just been hobnobbing with him at the South Canonry.'

'How on earth did you end up there?'

'I got mixed up with Charley on the train. Mr Dean, what do you think of *Honest to God*?'

'Superb! Quite splendid! A breath of fresh air sweeping through the Church of England!'

'Yes, I thought it probably was. The Bishop's decided it's absolutely the bottom.'

'The trouble with Charles,' said Aysgarth as we left the garden, crossed Canonry Drive and entered the churchyard of the Cathedral, 'is that he was trained as a theologian. Such a pity! A theologian's approach to religion is nearly always much too cerebral and he inevitably becomes cut off from ordinary believers.'

'But isn't this book supposed to be bad for ordinary believers?'

'Rubbish! It's the best thing that's happened to them for years. Robinson's realised that the ordinary believers are waiting for a new comprehensible interpretation of Christianity which will relate to the lives they're living right now in the 1960s – they're not waiting for cerebral restatements by theologians in their dead, dry, alienating academic language!'

'But if the book's too radical –'

'Nothing could be too radical! Let's have this New Reformation Robinson talks about! Let's have this New Morality! Now that we're finally emerging from the long shadow of the war and shedding the millstone of the Empire, we need to celebrate our psychological liberation by making everything new – so why not start by flinging religion into the melting-pot, as Robinson suggests, and recasting our beliefs in a bold, creative dynamic style that's thoroughly attuned to our day and age?'

I began to feel excited – insofar as one can ever feel excited about a subject such as theology. I was, in fact, very much in the mood for revolution and I deeply fancied the thought of an iconoclastic assault on any part of the established order. 'Long live Bishop John Robinson!' I declared, making Aysgarth laugh, and we quickened our pace across the sward to the Cathedral.

VII

At the north porch we parted, Aysgarth walking on to the Dean's door, the special entrance for the clergy, and I wandering through the porch into the nave. A sidesman showed me to a seat in the choir. This was not an unusual favour to bestow prior to a weekday service when few laymen would be present, but nevertheless it made me feel privileged.

The Cathedral was quiet. By that time the tourists had left and it had reverted to the inhabitants of Starbridge, most of whom preferred to admire it loyally from afar. However the congregation did eventually mount to thirty. I sat gazing up at the vaulted ceiling and trying to think noble thoughts, but I was pondering on Mrs Ashworth's advice about eye make-up when the organ marked the beginning of the service.

I liked the weekday choral evensong. It required no effort apart from kneeling down and standing up at regular intervals, and there was no sermon either to stretch the brain or induce rigor mortis. The choirboys sang in their unearthly voices; the vicars-choral bayed with authority; the vergers marched around providing touches of ceremonial; the clergy lolled meditatively in their stalls. I thought it was all so luxuriously restful, like a hot bath garnished with an expensive perfume, and as I watched the sun slant through the great west window I thought how clever God was to have invented the Church of England, that national monument dedicated to purveying religion in such an exquisitely civilised form.

Aysgarth was looking untidy as usual. His shop-soiled white hair always seemed to need trimming. Wearing a dignified expression he rose to his feet to read the lessons, while in the intervals Eddie, crammed into his canon's stall at the other end of the choir, intoned the versicles and recited the prayers. I was always surprised by how well Eddie did this, but no doubt Aysgarth had trained him not to sound as if he was fathoms deep in depression. Aysgarth himself read the lessons beautifully in his deep, resonant voice. In fact I was so busy thinking how well he read that I forgot to listen to what he was reading. Appalled by my lack of concentration I was on the point of making a new attempt to focus my mind on the service when I saw Nick Darrow staring at me from the opposite side of the choir. I supposed I had been too busy thinking about eye make-up to notice him earlier.

As soon as our glances met he looked away but I went on watching him and wondering if he was destined to be my lucky mascot. But mascot seemed the wrong word to describe someone like Nick. It was too cosy, too banal. For Nick Darrow I needed a word which implied magic, extraordinary happenings, paranormal phenomena –

'Ah-ah-ah-men!' sang the choir, winding up the service.

The organ trilled and fell silent for a moment before embarking on a fugue. Everyone hauled themselves to their feet. The choir tripped out jauntily, mission accomplished, and the clergy followed, looking inscrutable. Aysgarth never once glanced in my direction.

Wandering towards the transept I found Nick had fallen into step beside me.

'Ah!' I said, finally grasping the word I wanted. 'It's my Talisman! I shouldn't be surprised to see you again, should I, but why are you on your own?'

'Charley's busy with his father.'

'Mrs Ashworth was telling me about yours. I hear he's very old.'

'Yes, but he's okay.'

'How old is "old" exactly?'

'He'll be eighty-three in May. But he's okay.'

'*Compos mentis?*'

'Yep.'

'Super! I often think my father's mad as a hatter. Is your father able to do much?'

'Yep. He prays.'

'Ah. All the time?'

'No, he does see people occasionally.'

'He sounds like a hermit!'

'He is a hermit. But he doesn't mind me being with him because we don't have to talk.'

I suddenly realised I was gazing at him as if he were a creature from another planet. 'How restful!' I said, not sure what to say. 'My father's the very reverse of a silent hermit!'

'He might become one later. My father only became a recluse after my mother died.' He turned abruptly towards the nave. 'So long.'

'When are we due to meet again?'

He shrugged and walked away.

I gazed after him in fascination. Then heaving open the massive door in the south transept I passed at last into the cloisters.

VIII

In the centre of the quadrangle lay the lawn beneath which in previous centuries the eminent men of Starbridge had been buried, and overshadowing this ancient graveyard an enormous cedar tree towered above the roof of the colonnade. There was a faint breeze. The cedar's dark upper branches were stirring against the pale, limpid sky.

I was still gazing at this tranquil scene when the door creaked behind me and Aysgarth slipped out of the transept. Unlike Dr Ashworth he had entirely rejected the archaic uniform of a senior churchman, but perhaps that was less because he wanted to be modern than because his thickset figure was unsuited to fancy dress. On that evening he was wearing a black suit, slightly crumpled, and the black clerical 'stock' which was worn over an ordinary shirt and secured by ties at the back beneath the jacket. He had no pectoral cross; he belonged to the generation of Protestant churchmen who thought such papist adornment pardonable only when adopted by bishops. His hair, perhaps disarranged when he had removed his surplice after the service, swooped wildly over his ears in undisciplined wings and bumped against the back of his stiff white clerical collar. He looked like an eccentric scientist who has just made an important discovery.

'Let's go and sit on Lady Mary Calthrop-Ponsonby!' he suggested blithely as I moved to meet him.

'I *beg* your pardon, Mr Dean?'

With a laugh he led the way to a wooden seat on the northwestern corner of the lawn, and as I drew closer I saw that the back of the seat bore a brass plaque inscribed: 'In memory of Lady Mary Calthrop-Ponsonby, 12th February 1857–8th November 1941. "FIGHT THE GOOD FIGHT WITH ALL THY MIGHT."'

'Three cheers for Lady Mary,' I said as we sat down, and told him how I had decided to abandon London in search of a new life. '. . . and I've now reached the point where I'm trying to decide what to do next,' I concluded. 'Mrs Ashworth thinks I should go to Oxford, park myself on Christian and Katie and wangle my way into their set, but I'm not sure I have the nerve to exploit them so brazenly.'

'I don't see why you shouldn't stay with Christian and Katie for a few days while you decide if Oxford has anything to offer you, but I can't quite see why Lyle is pointing you in that direction.'

'She thinks I'd enjoy mixing with an intellectual *jeunesse dorée*.'

'On the contrary I think you'd soon be bored stiff with all those academics.'

'Would I? Are you sure? I just feel that if only I could get in with the right set –'

'In my experience right sets tend to be much too fast.'

'When one's been crawling along like a tortoise, Mr Dean, the idea of pace begins to seem attractive.'

He laughed. 'Was London really that bad?'

'Yes, it really was. I've been a failure there. Don't just tell me to go back and try again.'

'Very well, let's be more imaginative. This could be a great opportunity for you, Venetia! A fresh start is always a great opportunity, but you should remember that happiness isn't ultimately dependent on getting in with the right set; it's about serving God by using your God-given gifts in the best possible way.'

'I only seem to have a God-given gift for drifting in and out of boring jobs.'

'It's obvious that you haven't yet found your métier, and in my opinion pondering on the right métier, not choosing which city to live in, should actually be your number one concern at the moment. You need to escape to somewhere very quiet and very remote for a few days so that you can ponder in peace and see your situation in perspective . . . Come on holiday with me after Easter!'

I nearly fell off Lady Mary. 'What a breathtaking suggestion!'

He laughed again before adding: 'Dido's not coming but Eddie's accompanying me and Primrose is joining us twenty-four hours later. Come up on the Wednesday after Easter with Primrose!'

'Where's "up"?'

'The Outer Hebrides.'

'*Is* there an Outer Hebrides?'

'Apparently. The new Earl of Starmouth has very kindly lent me his hunting-lodge on Harris.'

'Don't Elizabeth and Pip want to go?'

'Dido's taking them to her sister in Leicestershire where they'll ride horses with her and be blissfully happy.'

'*Chacun à son goût*,' I said. 'Personally I'd rather live it up in a Caledonian Shangri-La.'

'My sentiments exactly!' said Aysgarth, and as he smiled I suddenly wondered if he, like me, was seizing the chance to escape from intractable private problems.

FOUR

'What is most real to you? What matters most for you? Is it money and what money can buy? I doubt it, deep down. For you know that you "can't take it with you". And seldom does it bring real happiness. Is it love? That's a good deal nearer, because it has to do with persons, not things.'

JOHN A. T. ROBINSON
Suffragan Bishop of Woolwich 1959–1969
Writing about *Honest to God* in the
Sunday Mirror, 7th April 1963.

I

After staying the night in Primrose's flat, I caught a train the next morning to my country home at Flaxton Pauncefoot, a village which lay ten miles from the port of Starmouth in the south of the diocese. Here I sorted out some appropriate clothes for the holiday, selected a couple of books and dumped my current stock of dirty laundry on the housekeeper who returned it, faultlessly washed and ironed, that evening. Nowadays there are very few advantages in being a member of the aristocracy, but at least one never has to worry about laundries. Nor does one have to waste time shopping for food or sweating over a hot stove. I said to the housekeeper: 'I'd like baked beans on toast with a poached egg on top, and tell Pardoe to look out a half-bottle of that nice St Julien, the one with the picture of the purple vineyard on it.' That solved the problem of dinner.

Afterwards, greatly fortified, I phoned my mother to inform her I would be heading for the Hebrides, retired to the blue drawing-room where the television set lurked behind a fire-screen, and watched the latest episode of the comedy series *Down at the Surgery* in which two doctors have their virtue constantly assailed by a stream of diverse nymphomaniacs. The elder doctor was played by Martin Darrow with a professional deftness which prompted me to giggle so hard that I dropped cigarette ash all over the floor. He was far better looking than his young half-brother, but nevertheless I was conscious of the strong resemblance between them. I wondered idly what their father, the ancient hermit, thought of his elder son's career as a television star.

The next morning I extracted my red MG from the stables, heaved my bags into the back and returned to Primrose's flat. I had remembered it was Sunday but somehow I managed to arrive too late to attend matins, so taking advantage of the spring sunshine I lounged on the seat in the Deanery's garden as I waited for everyone to return from the Cathedral. Unfortunately Primrose and the Dean stayed on for the sung Communion service. I should have remembered that possibility and removed myself, but I was still lolling in the sunshine when Dido turned up to torpedo me.

'So there you are, Venetia! Primrose was under the impression you'd be back in time for matins. I do think you might have telephoned to say you'd be late, but then that's the upper classes, isn't it, my dear, always expecting the entire world to fall into step beside them, and personally I've always been devoutly thankful that I was merely the daughter of a self-made Scottish millionaire and irredeemably nouveau riche because at least I was taught consideration for others from the cradle. Now –' She paused for breath as she parked herself purposefully on the bench beside me '– I'm so glad I've got the chance for a word alone with you, because I think it's time that an intelligent, *honest* older woman – and as you know, my dear, I always pride myself on my candour – I think it's time,' said Dido, without even pausing for breath after this parenthesis, 'that I gave you a piece of sensible and I hope not unaffectionate advice – because of course I'm very fond of you, Venetia, just as Stephen is, although I do see all your little faults and foibles *rather* more clearly than he does, because darling Stephen's so noble that he always sees the best in everyone, whereas I, being a realist –

and I'm always being complimented on my realism – I, being a realist,' said Dido, battling her way out of the jungle of this monstrous sentence, 'take a much more pessimistic view of humanity, and having been a rich young girl myself I know all about the pitfalls waiting to ensnare rich young girls who drift around without any proper *direction* – which brings me to what I want to say.'

I raised an eyebrow and looked hopeful.

'What you have to do, my dear, is not simply to drift hither and thither like a piece of flotsam – or is it jetsam? – on the sea of life while you dabble in antiques and publishing or sidle off on little holidays to the Hebrides with an elderly clergyman who really should have known better than to invite you – although, of course, I do understand that darling Stephen, so soft-hearted, only wanted to be kind – but I'm afraid he didn't stop to think, did he, that suggesting a holiday was actually only offering you a way of escaping from your problems, and what you really have to do, Venetia my dear, is not to *escape* from your problems but to *face* them. To put matters absolutely candidly, if you can't find a husband you must find a suitably worthy cause to which you can devote your energies, and quite honestly – and I know it's unfashionable to say this, but since I always believe in calling a spade a spade –'

I raised the other eyebrow and looked even more hopeful.

'– I think you need to find God. I began my search for God when I was about your age – it was after my favourite sister died – and once I'd started I was always so cross with myself that I'd never started before because religion's so absolutely fascinating and I can't understand why it's not taught properly in schools, especially when they go to such lengths to teach useless things like algebra and hockey. Anyway, once I'd started looking for God I met Stephen and lived happily ever after, and I think the same sort of thing might happen to you if only you could stop being so self-centred. As it happens I know the most wonderful clergyman in London who specialises in spiritual direction, and I'm quite certain that if I were to ring him up and tell him about you –'

'How terribly kind of you, Mrs Aysgarth, but I'm afraid I've absolutely had it with London.'

'Oh, that won't last, you'll go back, you're a London person. Now my dear, I do hope you're not thinking that darling Stephen will give you spiritual direction in the Hebrides, because Stephen's not at all spiritual on holiday, he just likes to sit around eating and drinking and reading detective stories, and I honestly think he'd be most put out if you started chatting to him about God. Anyway, Stephen really can't start giving spiritual direction to young girls, even here in Starbridge, because he's much too busy running the Cathedral and keeping the Chapter from murdering each other, and even if he wasn't much too busy he prefers to exercise his pastoral skills these days among men – and usually German men, as Eddie Hoffenberg will be the first to tell you. And talking of Eddie, I do think you might be kinder to him, he's *such* a nice man and he's had such awful tragedies in his life and he just doesn't deserve to have you and Primrose poking fun at him behind his back. God only knows what the two of you will get up to in the Hebrides – I can just see you egging each other on and smirking in corners – and in fact to be quite candid and to cut a long story short, I think this holiday is a thoroughly bad idea for all concerned. Why don't you and Primrose run off to Cornwall and leave those two clergymen to recharge their spiritual batteries in peace?'

'I don't think Primrose would care for that idea at all, Mrs Aysgarth.'

'Oh, Primrose! If that girl were to spend a little less time doting on her father and a little more time being nice to Maurice Tait her life would be vastly improved – and so, God knows, would mine! In fact in my opinion you'd be doing us all the biggest possible favour, Venetia my dear, if you lured Primrose away to – no, not Cornwall, too unoriginal, how about the French Riviera? Take her to your sister's villa at Juan-les-Pins!'

'I don't like the French Riviera.'

'Well, you certainly won't like the Hebrides. Dr Johnson thought it was quite awful, he told Boswell so.'

'I don't like Dr Johnson.'

'Venetia dear, don't you think you're being just the teensiest bit negative?'

'I'm sorry, Mrs Aysgarth. It really is so kind of you to worry about my spiritual welfare, and I'll think very carefully about everything you've said, I promise.'

We looked at each other. Her hard dark eyes bore a sharp, shrewd, sceptical expression, and although I tried to exude a docile respect I knew she was not deceived. Rising to her feet abruptly she said: 'I must see about lunch. Why don't you come indoors and have a chat with Elizabeth? She always feels so hurt when you and Primrose go out of your way to ignore her.'

Smiling meekly but seething with rage I followed her into the house to talk to her daughter.

II

Primrose usually ate her meals in her flat, but for Sunday lunch, that sacred British institution, she joined her family in the Deanery dining-room, and on that Sunday before Easter I sat with her at the long table. As usual on such occasions, a crowd turned up. In addition to Dido's two children – not only Elizabeth, who was now a precocious fourteen, but little Pip, who was a nine-year-old pupil at the Choir School – there was a female called Miss Carp, known within the family as Polly (in memory of Polycarp, a bishop of the Early Church); she kept the household running while Dido poked her nose into everyone else's business, popped up to London to patronise Harrods and pampered herself with the occasional attack of nervous exhaustion, a condition which Primrose described as 'sheer bloodyminded self-indulgence'. There had been a succession of au pair girls who had looked after the children, but these creatures had been dispensed with once Pip had begun his career at the Choir School.

The other guests at lunch that day consisted of Aysgarth's second son by his first marriage, Norman, who lectured in law at King's College, London, Norman's wife Cynthia who always looked as if she might sleep with everyone in sight but probably never did (although my sister Arabella always said Cynthia was the vainest, most sex-mad girl she ever met – and coming from Absolutely-the-Bottom Arabella that was really something), Aysgarth's third son James, the jolly Guardsman who was so good at talking about nothing, James's girlfriend, whose name I failed to catch although it was probably Tracy or Marilyn or something non-U, Aysgarth's fourth and final son by his first marriage, Alexander, known as Sandy, who was doing postgraduate work up at Oxford, a chum of Sandy's called Boodle (I never found out his real name either), two elderly female cousins of Dido's from Edinburgh who appeared to be quite overwhelmed by all the English, Primrose, me and – inevitably – Aysgarth's most devoted hanger-on, Eddie Hoffenberg. The two people whom I most wanted to see – Aysgarth's eldest son Christian and his wife – were conspicuous by their absence.

'They were here last weekend,' xplained Primrose.

All Aysgarth's children visited their home regularly and all appeared to get on well with their father who was unfailingly benevolent to them. The contrast with my own family could hardly have been more marked. My elder brother Harold was too stupid to hold my father's attention for long, and although my brother Oliver was no fool – no genius but no fool – he too was uninterested in intellectual matters. Henrietta, Arabella and Sylvia could only be regarded by my father as pretty little playthings. I drove him up the wall. In consequence family gatherings were notable for my father's impatience and irritability, my mother's valiant efforts to pour oil on troubled waters, and my siblings muttering to one another in corners that 'Pater' really was getting a bit much and Mama had to be some kind of saint to stand him and only a liberal supply of champagne could save everyone from going completely and utterly bonkers.

At the Aysgarths' lunch that day everyone talked animatedly, Dido inflicting her usual outrageous monologues on her defenceless cousins – with occasional asides to Eddie Hoffenberg who took seriously his Christian obligation to be charitable –

Norman commenting on some judge named Denning (this was just before the Profumo affair made Denning famous), Cynthia describing the work of some besotted artist who yearned to paint her portrait, James saying: 'Really? How splendid!' at intervals, Sandy and Boodle arguing over the finer points of Plato's Dialogue on the Soul, Elizabeth throwing out the information that actually she was an Aristotelian and that Plato simply rang no bells for her at all, Primrose arguing that the whole trouble with the Roman Church was that St Thomas Aquinas had based his *Summa* on Aristotle's philosophy, and my Mr Dean chipping in to observe that the world was always divided into Aristotelians and Platonists, and wasn't the treacle tart absolutely first-class. In the midst of all these stimulating verbal fireworks, little Pip, who was sitting thoughtfully on my left, turned to me and said: 'Do you like the Beatles, Venetia?'

'They're a little young for me, Pip, but I liked "Love Me Do".'

'I think they're fab,' said Pip. 'Much better than Plato or Aristotle.'

One of the most attractive aspects of life with the Aysgarths was the wide range of the topics discussed. I doubt if my parents and siblings had heard of the Beatles in the spring of 'sixty-three.

Later in the drawing-room I had an interesting talk about politics with Norman but Cynthia became jealous and winkled him away from me. By this time the Dean had shut himself in his study for his post-prandial snooze, but Eddie Hoffenberg was still hovering as if eager to tell me about his osteopath, so I slipped away to take refuge in Primrose's flat. Primrose herself had departed after lunch with her boyfriend Maurice Tait, one of the vicars-choral who sang tenor in the Cathedral choir and taught at the Choir School. In fact she cared little for Tait (a damp, limp individual whose hobbies were stamp-collecting and supporting the Bible Reading Fellowship) but she liked to keep him around so that she could talk about 'my boyfriend' and look worldly. I didn't despise her for this. I wouldn't have minded a neutral escort myself, if only to silence the fiends who muttered: 'Poor old Venetia!' behind my back, but no limp, damp individual had presented himself for acquisition. I didn't count Eddie, of course. Not only was his Wagnerian gloom intolerable but he was so ugly that if I had accepted him as an escort the fiends would merely have gone on muttering: 'Poor old Venetia!'

I also had to face the fact – an unpalatable one for my ego – that Eddie had never actually tried to do more than trap me in corners and talk about his health. He had never invited me to his house on my own or suggested a visit to the cinema – or even invited me for a walk on a Sunday afternoon. Tait always took Primrose for a walk down by the water-meadows after he had lunched with his mother. Primrose would sigh beforehand and say what a bore these walks were, but I suspected that if Tait had failed to appear one Sunday she would have been very cross indeed.

The rest of the day passed most agreeably, providing a tantalising glimpse of what fun life could be when one was accepted by a group of congenial people; at least at the Aysgarths' house I was never left out in the cold. After tea we all played croquet and I beat everyone except Boodle. There was much laughter as we languished on the lawn. Then having completed my odyssey among the croquet hoops I ate baked beans on toast with Primrose in her flat and we discussed Life, a ritual which involved reviewing the day's events, pulling everyone to pieces, putting a few favoured individuals together again and tossing the rest on the scrap-heap. This was fun. Primrose had her faults (priggishness, intolerance, intellectual snobbishness) but she was witty and seldom bored me. I only became bored when she was either talking soppily about her father or droning drearily about her work at the diocesan office on Eternity Street. Every time she began a sentence with the words 'The Archdeacon and I', my teeth automatically gritted themselves, so when at ten o'clock that evening the dread words tripped off her tongue I waited until she had finished her sentence and then immediately asked if I could have a bath. Half an hour later I was stretched out on the Put-U-Up sofa, now transformed into a bed, and tuning into Radio Luxemburg on my transistor.

'Good heavens, Vinnie!' exclaimed Primrose, appearing crossly in curlers as I was smoking a final cigarette and wriggling my toes in time to Elvis Presley. 'You're not still listening to that drivel, are you? I can't understand why you're so keen on pop music!'

'No, you wouldn't. You're not fundamentally interested in sex.'

'Honestly, Venetia! What a thing to say!' She flounced back to her bedroom.

Elvis quivered on vibrantly. As I stubbed out my cigarette I wondered – not for the first time – if anyone would ever invite me to have sexual intercourse, but it seemed like a forlorn hope. Switching off the transistor I pulled the bed-clothes over my head and allowed myself to shed a single furious tear of despair.

III

Easter was the following weekend. In the interval I loafed, smoked and vegetated, unwilling to think deeply about the future and telling myself I needed a few days of absolute rest in order to recuperate from the horrors of London life. I did toy with the idea of reading *Honest to God* but the desire to escape from my problems by being intellectually mindless was so strong that I could only reread Primrose's childhood collection of Chalet School books.

Finally I was roused from my torpor by the spectacle of Easter in a great cathedral. I avoided the Good Friday services but attended matins on Sunday morning and was rewarded when Aysgarth preached a most interesting sermon about how Christianity was all set to undergo a dynamic resurrection, recast and restated for the modern age. The Bishop, who was ensconced in his *cathedra* at one end of the choir, spent much time gazing up at the east window as if he were wondering how it could possibly be cleaned.

The next day Aysgarth was obliged to supervise the conclusion of the special services, but on Tuesday he was free to depart for the Hebrides; he and Eddie planned to drive to Heathrow airport and leave the car in the long-term car-park. At half-past eight that morning after Primrose had departed for her office I wandered across the courtyard of the stables to say goodbye to him, but no sooner had I entered the house by the side-door than I heard Dido's voice, throbbing with emotion, in the hall. Automatically I stopped dead. I was still well out of sight beyond the stairs.

'. . . I'm sorry, I'm sorry, I absolutely *swore* I wouldn't break down like this, but I do so wish you were coming to Leicester-shire – I know horses bore you, but you could read quietly in the library and –'

'Darling –'

'– and at least you'd be *there*. I just think it's so sad for Elizabeth and Pip that we're never together on our own as a family –'

'But that's not true!'

'Not on our *own*, Stephen – there's always someone from your first marriage there – all right, we won't talk of Primrose, but it just seems so wrong that we're not going to be together –'

'But when Lord Starmouth offered me the lodge the first thing I did was ask you to come with me!'

'How could I when I'm ill every time I try to go in a plane?'

'I was quite prepared to go overland, but since you were adamant that nothing would induce you to go to the Hebrides –'

'I thought you'd back down and come to Leicestershire. I never dreamed you'd run off instead with Primrose and Eddie and – my God! – Venetia –'

'What's wrong with Venetia? Isn't she Primrose's best friend and the daughter of one of my own oldest friends?'

'I don't give a damn who she is, that girl's sly, not to be trusted, a trouble-maker –'

'My dearest, I really don't think this conversation does you justice –'

'Oh, I'm sorry, I'm sorry, it's just that I feel so depressed, so alone, so utterly *abandoned* –'

There was a silence. I guessed he had been driven to silence her with an embrace. Pressing my back against the wall of the passage I held my breath and waited until at last she said tearfully: 'How I hate separations!'

'I'll write every day.'

'If only there was a phone at this stupid place –'

'I'll try and phone from the nearest village.'

'Promise?'

'Of course I promise.'

'Oh Stephen . . .' Another silence elapsed before Aysgarth said abruptly: 'Here's Eddie with the car. Quick, take my handkerchief and dry your eyes – where are the children?'

'I don't know . . . Elizabeth! Pip! Your father's leaving!'

At once I slipped silently away.

IV

Primrose and I began our journey north twenty-four hours later after the day-long diocesan conference of the Young Christians for Peace, an event which Primrose had helped to organise and which apparently could not take place without her. Primrose had always been an enthusiastic organiser. She had acquired the taste for power when she had become a Girl Guide leader, and since then the local branches of the Student Christian Movement, the Bible Reading Fellowship, the Missions to Africa Fund and the Inter-Faith League had all benefited from her efficient interference.

'You really ought to get interested in some worthwhile cause, Venetia!' she exclaimed as she returned, flushed with triumph, from her conference. 'If I were to do nothing but read dated schoolgirl books, watch television and listen to Radio Lux., I'd go mad in no time!'

I refrained from argument; I was all for a quiet life, and since I was a guest in her flat I had a moral obligation to be docile, but I realised then that Mrs Ashworth had been correct in deducing that Primrose and I had reached the parting of the ways.

Meanwhile we had to go on holiday together. Driving to Heathrow in my MG we caught a late-morning flight to Glasgow and arrived in the town of Stornoway, the capital of the Outer Hebrides, in the middle of the afternoon. Although it was the largest settlement on the island of Lewis and Harris, the town was small and the airport was primitive. On stepping out of the little plane I felt a soft damp wind on my cheek. A vast vista of white clouds and green treeless wastes stretched before me, but when I had an immediate impression not of desolation but of peace I realised my mood of torpor was at last beginning to dissolve.

'There's Eddie,' said Primrose.

Eddie's ungainly figure was clad in the English holiday uniform of grey trousers, a casual shirt and a tweed jacket, but he still managed to look like a foreigner; the uniform was much too well-tailored. He was driving a hired car, a faded white Morris which had seen better days but which bucketed along the narrow roads with surprising spirit. Lewis, I realised as I stared out of the window later at Harris, was the tame, domesticated part of the island. Harris was all bare hills and sinister peat-bogs and glowering little lakes with hardly a croft in sight. Yet I was intrigued. It seemed light years away from London, and beyond the village of Tarbert we appeared to leave civilisation behind completely. A single-track road adorned with the occasional hardy weed wound through brutal hills. Now and then the sea was visible as a lurid strip of midnight blue. Squalls of rain swooped down from the hills and swept away along the coast. Rainbows appeared fleetingly during improbable bursts of sunshine. The car groaned but battled on. I began to be excited.

'Is there really anything at the end of this road, Eddie?'

'Wait and see!' He pulled the car round a hairpin bend, and a second later Primrose and I were both exclaiming in wonder. Before us lay a small bay, shaped like a crescent moon and fringed with pale sand. Overlooking this idyllic seascape stood an Edwardian house, not too big but solid and well-proportioned. Beyond a walled garden the brown-green moors, dotted with rocks, rose towards mountains capped by cloud.

'Just like *Wuthering Heights*!' remarked Primrose. 'True romantic isolation! All we need now is Heathcliff.'

The front door opened as if on cue, and the Dean of Starbridge stepped out into the porch to welcome us.

V

Despite its remoteness the house turned out to be very comfortable, in that plain tasteful style that always costs a lot of money, and this comfort was enhanced by a married couple who did all the boring things such as cooking, shopping, cleaning and keeping the peat fires burning. At that time of the year in the far north the weather was still cold, particularly in the evenings, but having spent so much of my life at Flaxton Hall, where the heating was either non-existent or modest, I took the chill in my stride. In contrast, wretched Eddie was soon complaining of rheumatic twinges and saying that whenever he was in pain he was convinced he was going to die young.

'In that case,' said Primrose, 'please do die now and save us from listening to any more of your moans,' but at that point Aysgarth intervened, reminding Eddie lightly that life had been much worse in the POW camp on Starbury Plain and begging Primrose not to encourage anyone to die because it would be so annoying to have to cut short the holiday.

Our days in the wilderness began with breakfast at nine. Eddie then walked to the village and collected the specially ordered copy of *The Times*; on his return he studied it for twenty minutes. Another brisk trot followed, this time up and down the beach, but finally he allowed himself to relax in the morning-room with *The Brothers Karamazov*.

In contrast Aysgarth followed quite a different pattern of activity. After breakfast he sat in the drawing-room for a while and gazed at the sea. Then he dipped into one of his newly-purchased paperbacks (all detective stories) and read a few pages. More sea-gazing followed but at last he roused himself sufficiently to pen a letter to his wife. ('The daily chore,' commented Primrose to me once in a grim aside.) By the time the letter was finished Eddie had returned from the village but Aysgarth refused to read the newspaper in detail after Eddie had discarded it; he merely glanced at the headlines and tried to do the crossword. Despite his intellect he was very bad at crosswords, almost as bad as he was at bridge, and had to be helped by Primrose and me. The completion of the puzzle took at least twice as long as it should have done because we all spent so much time laughing, but once the last letter had been pencilled in Aysgarth invariably announced with regret: 'I suppose I ought to take some exercise.' He then staggered outside, inhaled deeply a few times and staggered back indoors again. As soon as the clock in the hall chimed twelve he declared it was time for drinks. Eddie, who preferred to abstain from alcohol till the evening, remained in the morning-room with *The Brothers Karamazov* but Aysgarth and I would swill champagne while Primrose toyed with her customary glass of dry sherry.

At some time during the morning Primrose and I would have been out, either scrambling along the rocky coast or following the path up into the stark wild hills. It rained regularly, but since we always wore macks and sou'westers the weather was never a serious inconvenience. Besides, the rain never lasted long. When the sun did shine we continually marvelled at the colours around us: the sea was a sapphire blue, the waves bright white, the sands dark cream, the moors green-brown mixed with ash-grey rock. Primrose took numerous photographs while I tried to impress the scenes on my memory and wished I could paint. Often as we scrambled along the low cliffs we saw seals playing near the beach, and several times in the hills we glimpsed deer. There were never any people. As the days passed my sense of peace increased until I even began to wish I could have been one of those ancient Celtic saints, dedicated to a solitary life in a remote and beautiful place in order to worship God. At least I would have been spared the rat-race in London and the hell of attending the Great Party of Life as a wallflower.

After lunch every day Aysgarth retired for 'forty winks', which usually lasted half an hour, Primrose and I read *The Times* and

Eddie wrote letters. Then at three o'clock we departed with a picnic tea for an outing in the car. All over the long island we rambled; on two consecutive days we stopped on the road to Leverburgh at a point above the vast sands which stretched across the bay towards the distant range of blue mountains, and twice we visited the remote church at Rodel on the southernmost tip of Harris. Then I, who was so very bad at worship and so very reluctant to be 'churchy', found myself thinking of Jesus Christ, living thousands of miles away in another culture in another millennium, writing nothing, completing his life's work in three years, a failure by worldly standards, dying an ignoble death – yet still alive in the little church at Rodel on the remotest edge of Europe, still alive for his millions upon millions of followers worldwide, not a despised, rejected failure any more but acknowledged even by non-Christians as one of the greatest men who had ever lived, etched deep on the consciousness of humanity and expressing his mysterious message of regeneration in that most enigmatic of all symbols, the cross.

'What are you thinking about, Venetia?' said that pest Eddie, ruining my rare moment of feeling religious as I stood staring at the church.

'Elvis Presley,' I said to shut him up. Eddie loathed pop music.

By then I was missing my daily dose of the pops on Radio Luxemburg which seemed to be unobtainable in the Hebrides; perhaps the weather conditions were unfavourable – or perhaps Luxemburg was merely too far away. The BBC in those days devoted little time to musical trivia so my deprivation was severe, but on the other hand there was little time to tune into the wireless. When we returned from our picnic the moment had arrived for a gin-and-tonic for me, whisky for the men and another glass of sherry for Primrose. During dinner we sampled a claret or a white burgundy – or possibly, depending on the menu, both; Aysgarth was taking seriously his absent host's invitation that we should help ourselves to his well-stocked cellar. After dinner we played bridge or, if we were feeling frivolous, vingt-et-un. Conversation, spiked by all the drink, sparkled. Even Eddie shuddered with mirth occasionally.

'Father,' said Primrose late one evening after Eddie had scooped the pool of matchsticks at vingt-et-un and Aysgarth had suggested a nightcap of brandy, 'isn't this holiday turning into a distinctly Bacchanalian orgy?'

'I hope so!' said Aysgarth amused.

'So do I!' I said at once. 'Primrose, these poor clergymen spend months on end being saintly and strait-laced – why on earth shouldn't they let their hair down on holiday?'

That idiotic Eddie was unable to resist sighing: '"Eat, drink and be merry for tomorrow we die."'

'Well, I'm not dying yet!' declared Aysgarth robustly. 'I've still got a lot of living to do!'

A chord twanged in my memory. '"I've gotta – *whole* lotta living to do!"' I sang, imitating Presley. '"*Whole* lotta loving to do – and there's-uh no one-uh who I'd rather do it-uh with-uh than you – COME ON, BABY!"'

'*Venetia!*' exclaimed Eddie, appalled by the vulgarity, his eyes almost popping out of his head.

'*Venetia!*' cried Primrose scandalised, casting an embarrassed glance at her father.

'What a splendid song!' said my Mr Dean naughtily, unable to resist the urge to shock them still further. 'Does it come from the repertoire of those young men Pip likes so much?'

'The Beatles? No, it's an Elvis Presley number.'

'Ah, Mr Presley! The Bishop thinks his records ought to be banned – which inevitably means they're first-class fun. "Charles," I said to him after I'd supported the publication of *Lady Chatterley's Lover*, "the real obscenity in our culture isn't sex. It's violence." But of course he refused to agree. Funny how Charles takes such a dark view of sex – it's as if he can never forget some very profound sexual sin which affected him personally in some quite unforgettable way.'

'Isn't the most likely explanation,' said Eddie, who had had a good deal to drink, 'that he had a strong sex drive in his youth and that he was constantly afraid of giving way to temptation?'

'I don't know why you throw in the phrase "in his youth",

Eddie!' said Aysgarth more naughtily than ever. 'Why shouldn't he still have a strong sex drive even now he's past sixty?'

Eddie went pink. Primrose stood up and said brightly: 'Who's for cocoa?'

'I thought we were all going to have a nightcap of brandy,' I said. 'Go on, Mr Dean! Do you think the Bishop and Mrs Bishop go in for Lady-Chatterley-style high jinks at the South Canonry?'

'VENETIA!' chorused the horrified voices of Canon Hoffenberg and Miss P. Aysgarth, Girl Guide leader.

The Dean could barely speak for laughing but managed to gasp: 'Eddie, why don't you keep Primrose company while she goes in search of cocoa? Venetia and I are going to discuss D. H. Lawrence!'

'This is all your fault, Vinnie,' said Primrose exasperated. 'If you hadn't mentioned Elvis Presley –'

'I'd very much like to hear this Mr Presley,' said Aysgarth. 'Could we tune into Radio Luxemburg on that radiogram in the morning-room?'

'Not a hope, Mr Dean – unless the reception's a great deal better tonight than it's been so far.'

'Eddie,' said Primrose, 'let's leave them to their decadence.'

Eddie said drunkenly: 'We draw the line at rock-'n'-roll, Stephen!' and stalked after her.

'Snob!' I shouted after him before adding to Aysgarth: 'The mystery about that radiogram is that there appear to be no records to go with it. Wouldn't you think that the Earl's teenage daughters would keep a supply of old favourites here to wile away the rainy days?'

'Let's have a search!' exclaimed Aysgarth, leaping to his feet.

'Tally-ho!' I cried, leading the charge into the hall. Then I stopped. 'But it's no good searching the morning-room,' I said, 'because I've already done that. I've searched the drawing-room too. Perhaps the attics –'

'What about that cupboard over there under the stairs?'

We bowled over to the cupboard and I dived inside.

'There's probably a light,' said Aysgarth as I floundered in the darkness. 'Thank heavens this place has a generator and we don't have to rely on candles . . . ah, well done!'

I had found the light switch and was now surveying a jungle of mackintoshes, wellington boots and bric-à-brac which stretched far back below the stairs. Ploughing forward I nearly disembowelled myself with a fishing-rod. 'Bloody hell,' I muttered before I remembered the Church. 'Whoops! Sorry, Mr Dean —'

'Oh, did you speak? I didn't hear a word.'

The old pet! I adored him. Heaving aside a battalion of boots I struck gold in the form of six cases, all designed to carry records. 'Eureka!' I shouted, ripping open the first case of twelve-inch LPs, but found only the Beethoven symphonies with a dash of 'Swan Lake'. Attacking the second case I glimpsed the word 'Wagner' and slammed shut the lid with a shudder.

'Any luck?' called Aysgarth excited.

'Hang on.' I opened the third case — and there, miraculously, was Presley, glittering in gold lamé and slouched in a pose to launch a thousand screams. 'Whoopee!' I yelled and staggered backwards past the macks and wellies with the record-case clasped to my bosom.

'Jiminy cricket!' said Aysgarth awed as I showed him the picture on the sleeve.

'Just you wait, Mr Dean! This is the kind of stuff guaranteed to make the Bishop pass out in the pulpit!'

We plunged into the morning-room where I crammed the LP on to the turntable. Then I hesitated, holding the arm above the revolving disc as I tried to select the most suitable track. I didn't want to bludgeon him into a coma with 'Heartbreak Hotel'. A milder introduction seemed called for. Finally the decision was made, and the next moment Presley — Presley before he became decadent and bloated and corrupt — the young, unspoilt, unsurpassable Elvis Presley began to belt out 'You're Right, I'm Left, She's Gone'.

VI

'This is wonderful!' cried the Dean. 'Wonderful!' And as I lifted the needle from the groove at the end of the track he exclaimed: 'It makes me want to catch up with all the fun I missed out on in my youth!'

'Was your youth really so drab?'

'Drab! That's an understatement. Primitive Methodists, no money, working day in, day out, in order to get on – why, the most thrilling moment of my youth consisted of a forbidden visit to the cinema where I watched Clara Bow oozing "It" as I sank my teeth into a sinful peppermint cream! Never mind, those times are gone now – and how glad I am that I've lived to see the dawn of a new era! Class barriers collapsing, sexual inhibitions being overcome –'

'Good old Elvis! Want to hear some more?'

'I want to hear everything! Play that song you were singing at dinner!'

I rummaged around and found it. 'Okay, Mr Dean!' I cried. 'Off we go!'

The beat began to pound. Presley began to celebrate the joy of life. And suddenly Aysgarth rose to his feet.

'Isn't it great?' I shouted, turning up the volume, but he merely cried enthralled: 'Let's dance!'

I kicked off my shoes, we grabbed each other's hands, he drew me to the centre of the floor. And there, as Elvis Presley sang his heart out and the boards vibrated beneath our feet, I danced with the Dean of Starbridge to the beat of rock-'n'-roll.

VII

As the final chord throbbed and we clutched each other, breathless with laughter, I saw that Primrose and Eddie were standing appalled in the doorway.

'Honestly!' said Primrose as I abruptly switched off the radiogram. 'I've never seen anything quite so undignified in all my life!'

'My dear,' said her father, 'you mustn't be so serious that you forget how to have fun.'

At once Primrose turned her back on us and stalked off across the hall.

'Leave her to me, Stephen,' said Eddie. 'You go on having fun.' And he too withdrew, closing the door behind him.

'That's the nicest thing Eddie's done in a month of Sundays,' I said. 'But why on earth is Prim being so idiotic?'

'I'm afraid she realised I was cross with her.'

'*Cross?* That wasn't being cross! You should hear my father when he roars like a lion – that's what being cross is all about!'

'But Primrose is particularly dependent on me for my love and approval. Ever since her mother died –'

'But her mother's been dead for over twenty years – isn't it time Primrose grew up? God knows, I never thought I'd hear myself say this but sometimes when I see this so-called "dependence" on you I really feel quite sorry for Dido.'

He merely regarded me with grave blue eyes and said nothing.

A panic-stricken remorse assailed me. 'Sorry,' I mumbled, furious with myself for plunging around in his family problems like an elephant cavorting among eggshells. 'Tight as an owl. Rude as hell. Forget I spoke.'

'My dear Venetia, there's no need for you to apologise!' he said at once, sloughing off both my tactlessness and his problems as if they were supremely unimportant. 'Let's be tight as owls together and go on having the time of our lives!' And as he stretched out his hands to me again I was suddenly transported to the very centre of life.

My world turned itself inside out. In a split second of blinding clarity I saw him at last not as the family friend who was always so kind to me, but as the irresistible stranger whose personality, by some great miracle, uniquely complemented my own. My loneliness was annihilated; my despair exploded into a euphoric hope. Knowing I had to withdraw at once before my emotion could utterly overwhelm me, I blundered across the hall to the cloakroom, sagged in tears against the door and mutely contemplated the vastness of my discovery.

VIII

'Venetia?'

'Just a sec.' I pulled the plug of the lavatory and emerged dry-eyed into the hall. As I saw the anxious expression on his face I realised he thought I was suffering from the effects of too much to drink, but although I opened my mouth to reassure him no words came. I was speechless because his entire appearance had changed. His white hair now seemed not shop-soiled but creamily distinguished. His forehead had assumed exactly the right height and breadth to enhance this impression of distinction and his nose, formerly large, had become exquisitely and nobly Roman. The lines on his face no longer suggested antiquity but the power of a fascinating and formidable character. His eyes, radiantly blue and steamily bright, made me feel weak at the knees, while his thin mouth, which turned down slightly at the corners, no longer seemed tough in repose but overpoweringly sultry; I felt weaker at the knees than ever. In fact when he smiled I felt so demolished by his sheer sexual glamour that I actually had to sink down on the hall chest. I had forgotten he was sixty-one. Or, to be accurate, I had not forgotten but the fact no longer had any meaning for me. He could have been twenty-one, forty-one or eighty-one. Such a trivial fact was of no importance. All that mattered was that he was the man I wanted to go to bed with that very night and marry the very next morning.

I suddenly realised he was speaking again. He was saying: 'How about some black coffee?' and my voice was replying without a second's hesitation: 'I think I'd prefer a very large Rémy Martin.'

He laughed. Then reassured that I was no longer expiring from an excess of alcohol, he vanished into the dining-room to raid the sideboard.

'What happened?' he enquired with curiosity as he returned with two brandies and sat down beside me on the hall chest. 'Were you overwhelmed by Mr Presley?'

'No, by *joie de vivre* – and by you, Mr Dean,' I said, somehow keeping my voice casual. 'You must be the trendiest dean in Christendom!'

He laughed in delight, and I saw then that his attitude towards me was quite unchanged; untouched by any emotional earthquake he was merely savouring the concluding moments of an entertaining evening. 'I always regard it as a very great blessing that Pip was born when I was fifty-two,' he said. 'He keeps me young in outlook.'

Primrose chose that moment to return to the hall. 'Sorry,' she said. 'I didn't mean to be such a kill-joy, but I genuinely can't stand that sort of music.'

Aysgarth gave her a kiss to signal that her apology was accepted and asked: 'Where's Eddie?'

'In the drawing-room. He started talking about the decadence of pop music and then before I could stop him he was holding forth on the decadence of Berlin in the 'thirties. I walked out when he began to ruminate on the nature of evil.'

'I'd better go and rescue him.'

'Why not just hit him over the head with *The Brothers Karamazov*? I nearly did.'

They wandered off together to save Eddie from his turgid metaphysics. Knocking back the rest of my brandy I reeled upstairs to my room and passed out in a stupor of alcohol, ecstasy and rampant sexual desire.

FIVE

❖

'The universe, like a human being, is not built merely to a mathematical formula. It's only love that gives you the deepest clue to it.'

JOHN A. T. ROBINSON
Suffragan Bishop of Woolwich 1959–1969
Writing about *Honest to God* in the
Sunday Mirror, 7th April 1963

I

The next day was Sunday and Aysgarth had earlier mentioned that he would be celebrating Communion in the dining-room at eight. Since Eddie and Primrose would inevitably attend the service I had decided I should make the effort to join them, but when Primrose woke me I realised, as my hang-over hit me between the eyes, that my virtuous decision would have to be revoked.

'There's something so wonderfully moral about alcohol,' observed Primrose as I pulled the bed-clothes over my head with a groan. 'Punishment always follows excess.'

I could have murdered her, but by that time I was too enrapt with my memories of the previous evening to bother. She departed unscathed and immediately the door closed I sat up, ready for Day One of my new life. I tossed off the necessary potion to soothe my liver. Then I flung back the curtains and exclaimed: 'A celestial day has dawned for Venetia Flaxton!' Outside it was raining, but who cared? The view, wreathed in shifting mist, seemed more romantic than ever. Sliding back into bed I lit a cigarette, hummed a verse of Presley's 'I Need Your Love Tonight' and prepared for a delicious hour of meditating on the object of my desire.

It was immediately obvious that I could never speak of my love. Since nothing could come of my grand passion there could be no conceivable point in disclosing my feelings, and besides, there was no one in whom I could confide – except Mrs Ashworth, but I could hardly babble to the wife of a bishop about my new-found adulterous lust for a dean.

Having reached this conclusion I perceived a second obvious truth: not only would I have to keep my mouth shut but I would have to rise to great thespian heights to conceal my secret. No one must ever guess the truth because no one would ever understand the height and breadth and depth of my well-nigh incinerating desire. I pictured my siblings sniggering: 'Poor old Venetia! A crush on an elderly clergyman – whatever will she think of next?' And as for Primrose . . . but no, the mind boggled. I had to carry the precious secret to my grave, but I could accept this necessity because I was so happy. I had been granted the power to love; nothing else mattered, and indeed to have wanted more would have been disgustingly greedy. Since it was quite impossible that Aysgarth could fall in love with me it was pointless to hope that my passion might be reciprocated, but I would be blissfully content with his continuing avuncular friendship, and so long as I could live near him, see him regularly and have the occasional little chat about God or Eternity or whatever else might interest him, my life would be indescribably rich and fulfilling.

So be it. I would still die *virgo intacta*, but having experienced passion on a cosmic scale I could at least tell myself that my years in the world hadn't been a complete waste of time.

With a sigh I stretched myself luxuriously and decided I was in paradise.

II

My next task was to choose what to wear for Day One of my new life, but all my clothes now seemed so dreary, no more than a drab mass of browns, beiges and moss-greens. Then I remembered the red sweater which I had bought on impulse when I had visited Marks and Spencer's to replenish my stock of underwear; I had just had a row with my father and was feeling aggressive, but now the scarlet seemed to symbolise not aggression but passion. I selected the sweater and eyed a pair of earth-coloured slacks. Did I dare wear trousers on a Sunday? Yes. I was in the mood to take a scandalous risk. My mother had brainwashed me into thinking slacks were vulgar on any day of the week, but I had long since realised they suited me. I have longish legs and not too much padding around the hips. It was true that I was usually at least seven pounds overweight, but we can't all be the Duchess of Windsor.

I brushed my horrible hair and clipped it severely behind my ears to curb its tendency to billow around my head in a frizz. Then I slapped on some powder and went wild with the mascara which normally I reserved for evenings. My mother believed only fallen women wore eye make-up during the day, but Mrs Ashworth had confirmed my suspicion that this piece of folklore was out of date. I tried to recall whether Mrs Ashworth herself wore eye make-up but the memory eluded me. Dressing the part of a bishop's wife, Mrs Ashworth was the kind of clever woman who would spend half an hour making herself up to look as if she was not made up at all.

Did I wear lipstick? No. Lipstick was going out of favour. The 'look' consisted of emphasising the eyes and hair. Jewellery? No, quite inappropriate for a Sunday morning in the Hebrides, and anyway I had decided to emulate Mrs Ashworth's uncluttered simplicity of style. Was I ready? Yes. For anything. Forgetting my liver, which was still feeling a trifle battle-scarred, I sailed downstairs for breakfast just as the clock in the hall chimed nine.

They were all seated at the dining-room table. Primrose was pouring herself some coffee, Eddie was spooning sugar on his porridge and Aysgarth was buttering a slice of toast. Immediately in my imagination six trumpets blasted a triumphant fanfare while drums rolled and cymbals clashed.

'Mr Dean!' I exclaimed with a radiant smile. 'Do please forgive me for missing Communion but I was prostrated!'

'Maybe you should be prostrated more often!' retorted Aysgarth, much amused. 'You look remarkably well!'

'Sheer mind over matter! As soon as I had willed myself to leap out of bed and sing the "Ode to Joy", I felt simply too wonderful to be true . . . Eddie, why are you goggling as if you'd swallowed an octopus?'

Eddie stammered with an uncharacteristically marked German accent: 'You look tremendous, Venetia!'

'I *am* tremendous,' I said, helping myself to eggs and bacon from the sideboard. 'What else is new?'

Aysgarth started to laugh and when I glanced at him over my shoulder he gave me one of his saucy winks which meant, as I well knew, absolutely nothing.

I nearly passed out. Then winking back at him, as befitted a platonic friend of many years standing, I prepared to toy in ecstasy with a hearty breakfast.

III

'Why are you made-up to the nines and behaving as if you'd just quaffed an entire bottle of champagne?' demanded Primrose baffled as we set out in the rain for our morning walk.

'It's the after-effects of listening to Elvis.' I then realised it was time to act the part of my old nonchalant self, but before I could say anything else Primrose was confiding: 'I think Eddie's terribly smitten – I've never before seen him turn such a strangulated shade of puce!'

'Oh, people are always saying Eddie fancies me, but I don't believe a word of it! He never makes anything which could be remotely described as a pass.'

'Probably too frightened. After all, if you're as ugly as Eddie, you'd be afraid that any girl you approached would simply shriek: "Dracula!" and run screaming in the opposite direction.'

'True. I wonder if he's ever done it.'

'Approached a girl?'

'No, had sex.'

'Honestly, Venetia, why have you suddenly developed this appallingly one-track mind?'

'As a matter of fact Eddie doesn't strike me as being unsophisticated about sex – look at that cunning remark he made about Bishop Ashworth's sex-phobia.'

'Imagine doing it with Eddie!' said Primrose shuddering.

'Imagine doing it with your Maurice Tait!'

'Maurice is actually rather good-looking when he takes off his glasses –'

'Yes, but would he remain good-looking if he took off anything else? God, what a bloody peculiar thing sex is! Do you suppose your father still does it with Dido?'

'Don't be obscene!'

'Yes, I'm sorry, that *was* a bit far-fetched –'

'Of course all that stopped years ago!'

'You mean they have separate bedrooms?' I knew my Mr Dean was languishing in a ghastly marriage, and I knew it was impossible that he should love the middle-aged gorgon whom I had overheard nagging him so mercilessly, but I saw no harm in establishing beyond doubt that the marriage was entirely nominal.

'They've had separate bedrooms almost from the start,' said Primrose, wrinkling her nose in distaste. 'That was because of her insomnia. But the separate bedrooms didn't stop her getting pregnant five times.'

This was not exactly the news I wanted to hear. 'In that case why do you think they've stopped having sex?'

'The doctor told her after number five was born that she mustn't have any more children.'

'So what? I can't see that proves anything, the state of contraception being what it is –'

'I'm quite sure,' said Primrose firmly, 'that an eminent cleric of the Church of England would never engage in anything so sordid as contraception.'

'But perhaps contraception's no longer required. If the old hag's had the change of life –'

'I don't think she has. I know she's forty-eight and ought to be absolutely over the hill but she still gets monthly migraines when she has to lie in a darkened room and pretend she's dying.'

'In that case you're right and your father must be entirely frustrated.'

'He's more likely to be faint with relief! Surely once a man gets past sixty he just wants to go to bed with a good book?'

But I thought of my Mr Dean regretting his repressed youth, and although I was sure he would recoil from copulating with Dido I did wonder how content he was with his enforced chastity.

'He should never have married her,' Primrose was saying, reverting to a well-worn theme. 'Well, he never would have married her if she hadn't ensnared him when he was still mad with grief after Mother's death.'

I was, of course, familiar with the Primrose Aysgarth version of history, and out of delicacy I had never tried to debate it with her, but I was well aware that other people saw her father's past in a different light and now for the first time I was sufficiently intrigued to throw tact to the winds.

'Primrose, two and a half years elapsed between your mother's death and his marriage to Dido! He couldn't have been mad all the time!'

'Dido kept him mad by chasing him so hard that he had no chance to recover his equilibrium.'

'But I've heard it said that he himself was the one who did the chasing —'

'That was simply a rumour Dido put into circulation in order to boost her ego. The truth was she sank her talons into him when he was vulnerable and then clawed away until he agreed to marry her.'

'But that makes your father sound absolutely feeble!'

'Nonsense! On the contrary it shows he was strong enough to marry out of compassion and tough enough to survive the inevitable disaster!'

'So are you saying he never loved Dido at all?'

'How could he have done? It was Mother he adored. He just saw Dido as a neurotic, pathetic failure and he was idealistic enough to think he could heal her by marriage. He acted, I assure you, not out of love but out of sheer nobility of soul.'

Elektra had spoken. I had no doubt I was supposed to swallow whole this theory which showed her father as a self-sacrificing saint, but I could not help but feel it raised more problems than it solved. There were plenty of neurotic women in the world; why had he allowed himself to be nailed by someone as dreadful as Dido? And why had he been driven to heal a neurotic woman anyway? And why had he felt it essential that the healing should take place within the framework of marriage when it must have been obvious that such a marriage could only prove disastrous? The more I considered the theory the more unsatisfactory it seemed; I could only conclude that Primrose had been carried away by her Elektra complex and that her father's second marriage was a mystery she had never even begun to unravel.

Idly I heard myself say: 'Bearing in mind the fact that your father must often have been vilely unhappy with the gorgon, do you think he's ever looked at anyone else?'

'Good heavens, no!' Primrose was genuinely appalled. 'Of course, I know one does occasionally hear about vicars who let the side down, but *Father* – the former Archdeacon of Starbridge – a Canon of Westminster – and now the Dean of one of the greatest cathedrals in England –'

'Sorry, forget I spoke.'

'I know he talks racily sometimes, but underneath all that he's quite exceptionally serious and devout! In fact you can be one hundred per cent certain that ever since he took his ordination vows not a single adulterous thought has ever crossed his mind.'

Yet again Elektra had spoken, but this time I was prepared to accept the pronouncement without question; it chimed with everything I knew about my heroic Mr Dean. I sighed, but I had never seriously thought that my grand passion had a hope of being consummated.

I vowed never to entertain such a futile thought again.

IV

'Venetia,' said Eddie that evening as we waited for the others to join us in the drawing-room for cocktails.

'Uh-huh?' I was flicking through the pages of one of the bound volumes of *Punch*, thoughtfully provided by the Earl of Starmouth to ward off any television withdrawal symptoms among his guests.

'Instead of going for a walk with Primrose tomorrow morning, would you come for a walk with me?'

I somehow restrained myself from exclaiming: 'Good God!' Turning another page of *Punch* I enquired: 'Down to the village to pick up *The Times*?'

'No, later. Are you playing for time while you think of an excuse to refuse?'

'Oh Eddie, don't look so mournful!'

'How am I supposed to look when you respond to my invitation with such a lack of enthusiasm?'

I felt caddish. Poor old Eddie! Why should I make him miserable when I myself was in such ecstasy? I resolved to be benign. 'Okay,' I said, closing the volume. 'Let's go for a walk tomorrow morning. But how do you suggest I get rid of Primrose? She'll want to come too.'

'I'd thought of that. I'll ask Stephen to suggest she keeps him company. She'll never refuse a request from her father.'

This plan struck me as both simple and efficient. I thought: trust a German to plot like a machine! And in alarm I wondered if I had given the machine an oiling I would later regret. However a second later I had dismissed this suspicion as ridiculous. Eddie was hardly going to do more than talk about his osteopath, and besides . . . one could always rely on a clergyman to bust a gut to preserve the proprieties.

V

At eleven o'clock the next morning we set off along the path which wound around the hillside at the back of the house and led into a long empty valley. The sun was shining. Huge clouds scudded across a pale sky. Stretching into the distance ahead of us the moors suggested both loneliness and freedom.

'It's a pity Wordsworth never had a go at this landscape,' I remarked after we had been walking for some minutes in a silence which had become increasingly oppressive. 'Plenty of scope for nature-mysticism.'

'Gerard Manley Hopkins would have come closer to catching the atmosphere, I think. He'd have been starker and grittier.'

'Don't you find Hopkins a bit difficult? Since English isn't your native tongue –'

'Like Stephen I enjoy a challenge.'

Delighted to have the opportunity to talk about Aysgarth I said: 'I suppose a self-made man like the Dean has to face continual challenges.'

'It was certainly a challenge for him to make his way in the world after his father died bankrupt. He was lucky to have that uncle who egged him on.'

'What uncle?'

'Oh, has he never mentioned him to you? But no, he wouldn't have bothered – Stephen never seems to talk about his extreme past nowadays . . . Well, he had this uncle who used to egg him on by urging: "You've got to go chasing the prizes!" and the result was –'

'He married Dido. What a booby-prize!'

'Dido has immense wit and charm,' said Eddie reproachfully.

'Oh God, I'm talking to a Dido fan! I'm sorry, I quite forgot – temporary aberration –'

'She's always been very kind to me. Of course she has her problems –'

'Well done, Eddie, a superb example of a British understatement!'

'– but she's in a tough situation, isn't she? Thanks to Primrose she never has much chance to be on her own with her husband and children.'

'I agree the Primrose situation is impossible,' I conceded with reluctance. 'Prim really ought to move right away from the Deanery – it's no good camping on the doorstep in that flatlet, it's much too close and she and Dido still wind up screaming at each other most of the time.'

'The person I feel sorry for is Stephen, caught in the middle, but sometimes I feel he exacerbates the problem by never taking a firm line.'

'Maybe taking the line of least resistance is the only way he can survive being married to Dido.'

'I hardly think the marriage is that bad! He married her because she amused him – and I think she still does. He likes that smart life she provides, all the dinner-parties and the socialising – and why shouldn't he? After that poverty-stricken early life, isn't it only natural that he should now favour a little luxury and glamour?'

'Eddie, are you seriously trying to tell me they're well suited?'

'An attraction of opposites is by no means always a recipe for disaster. I think their personalities complement each other, hers so volatile, his so calm –'

'It's curious how we're all different people to different people,' I interrupted, finally losing the patience to keep listening to this earnest opinion which struck me as being almost bizarrely wide of the mark. 'Dido's obviously one person to you, another to me and Primrose and yet a third to the Dean.'

'Stephen would say the apparent diversity is an illusion. "It's all a unity!" he would say. "It's all one!" One of Stephen's most marked theological traits is that he believes in unity, not duality, and that's why he gets so irritated with neo-orthodox men like the Bishop who employ the principles of dialectic to –'

'Oh God, Eddie, we're not going to discuss theology, are we?'

'I thought you liked it! I can remember you listening enrapt to Stephen when he talked about *Soundings*!'

'Well, I'm one person for the Dean,' I said, 'and I'm quite another for you. Let's go back to Gerard Manley Hopkins.'

Eddie immediately began to discuss Hopkins' miserable life as a Roman Catholic priest.

We trudged drearily on across the moor.

VI

'Primrose mentioned that you were thinking of looking for a flat in Oxford,' said Eddie as finally, to my profound relief, we returned within sight of the lodge. By that time I was so exhausted by our literary discussion that I feared I might fall into a coma at any moment. 'When will you be leaving Starbridge?'

'I'm not leaving. I've changed my mind.'

Eddie halted. I wandered on but eventually paused to wait for him. Beyond the house the dark, restless sea was swirling over the arc of sand.

'You're going to stay on in Starbridge?' He sounded stupefied.

'Yes, I'll start looking for a job when I get back. Any objections?'

'No. No, of course not. No, I was just so surprised – I thought Starbridge would be much too provincial for a sophisticated girl like you.'

'I feel I need a complete change.'

'I see . . . But that's tremendous! I'm so happy, I –' He somehow pulled himself together sufficiently to add in a casual voice: 'Perhaps we could go to the theatre together sometime.'

'Oh, is that old dump still operating?'

'It's no dump nowadays, I assure you! Last autumn there was an Ibsen season – and after Christmas they did an exceptionally good production of *Lady Windermere's Fan* – and this summer they'll be trying out a revival of one of the Noël Coward plays before it opens in London. I forget the title, but Martin Darrow will be playing the lead.'

'In that case you can accompany me as I stampede through the streets to the theatre. I'm getting rather keen on the Darrow family.'

I had made Eddie's day, his week, his month and possibly his entire year, but as we moved on once more along the path I began to regret my decision to be kind to him.

The road to hell, as we all know, is paved with good intentions.

VII

It seemed a great irony that now I at last had a man panting for my attention I could hardly have cared less, but I supposed I could at least regard this conquest as gratifying to my ego. Having reflected that my triumph would have been far more gratifying if Eddie had not been physically repulsive and mentally exhausting, I was inclined to conclude that I could have done without such a perverse development in my private life, but then I wondered if Eddie might have his uses as a smoke-screen. The thought of him playing Romeo certainly diverted Primrose.

'Did he jump on you?'

'Don't be absurd! There's no doubt he's a trifle smitten, but I'm sure he prefers to worship from afar.'

'He might get bolder now he's broken the ice!'

'Not Eddie! No true masochist could pass up such a splendid chance to languish in frustration,' I declared, and putting all thought of Eddie aside I began to make plans for my future.

I had already decided to look for a flat which was as near the Close as possible, but I knew it might take time to find the right place and meanwhile my need to escape from Primrose was urgent. I was terrified that she might soon see past the smoke-screen created by Eddie and sense I had been invading her territory.

I debated whether to beat a temporary retreat to Flaxton Pauncefoot, but that was miles away and besides, I had no wish for my parents to assume my will to be independent was wavering. To visit home, pick up my car and sort out my clothes was acceptable, but to roost at Flaxton Hall for days would create an impression of pusillanimity. Plainly I had to stay somewhere in Starbridge while I hunted for a flat, but where could I go? Primrose would be baffled and suspicious if I decamped abruptly to a hotel. I did know several of the inhabitants of the other houses in the Close, but I could think of no one – apart from Mrs Ashworth – whom I could ask to put me up for more than a couple of nights, and the South Canonry, like Primrose's flat, was highly unsuitable for me in my present state; I could hardly live in close proximity to the Bishop while I was harbouring torrid thoughts about the Dean.

I was still wrestling with this apparently insoluble problem when Aysgarth, reading his daily letter from his wife, paused to observe to Primrose: 'Dido may be in Leicestershire, but she's still tuned in to the Cathedral Close grapevine. Apparently Marina Markhampton's in Starbridge. She's looking after the Chantry while her grandparents are visiting the south of France.'

Marina Markhampton was the youngest child of a wealthy gentleman of leisure who had married an equally wealthy wife and divided his time between Newmarket, where he kept racehorses, Monte Carlo, where he gambled away the money the horses won, and Camlott Edge in Dorset where the Markhamptons had their ancestral home; in the hope of avoiding death duties his father, Sir William, had already ceded him the family estate.

Long ago in the 1930s Sir William's wife Enid had been a devoted fan of that legendary bishop of Starbridge, the portswilling Dr Alex Jardine, and she had never forgotten her amusing visits to the episcopal palace in those golden days before the war. Accordingly when her husband ceded the family estate to his son, Lady Markhampton had succumbed to a bout of nostalgia and demanded to spend her declining years in the Cathedral Close. The Chantry, a little six-bedroomed gem on Choristers' Green, happened to be vacant, and after a new lease had been extracted from the Dean and Chapter, Sir William and Lady Markhampton had lived there in bliss until one sad day in the 1950s when a burst pipe had ruined the priceless carpets. The Markhamptons had been in Cannes at the time and the naughty housekeeper had gone AWOL to some seaside resort in the north. As a result of this grisly experience, which had destroyed not only her carpets but her faith in housekeepers, Lady Markhampton had recruited her unmarried sister to house-sit when necessary, but the sister had recently died and now it appeared that Marina had accepted the invitation to replace her.

This was odd; Marina was not the sort of girl one pictured house-sitting in a provincial city. She was younger than I was, no more than twenty-one, and in addition to being beautiful and popular she had jet-setting tendencies. In the past I had occasionally encountered her at ghastly parties where I had been a wallflower and she had been pursued incessantly by panting young men. My brother Oliver said that the great debate about Marina Markhampton centred on whether she was *virgo intacta*. Apparently no debate was needed to establish the fact that she was the biggest cock-tease in town.

Having long since decided that Marina was someone who could never interest me, I now found myself revising my judgement. The Chantry would be wonderfully convenient. Choristers' Green, a square of lawn where the choristers had played before the Choir School had moved to the palace, lay at the north end of Canonry Drive, not far from the spot where the Deanery faced the west front of the Cathedral. Could I possibly cultivate this repulsive society stunner and wangle a bed while I looked for a flat? Before my days of ecstasy I would have dismissed the question as outrageous, but now, wafting along on my tidal wave of euphoria, I merely thought: hell, what have I got to lose?

I began to plot my cultivation of Marina Markhampton.

VIII

On the last day of our holiday Primrose was felled by a malevolent attack of menstruation and decided to spend the morning in bed. I was delighted; her absence meant that at long last I had the opportunity to talk to Aysgarth on his own. Keen to make amends to her father for her kill-joy behaviour over Elvis she had insisted on joining us for our next record-session – with the result that I had soon replaced all the records in the hall cupboard. I could hardly go wild with the Dean while Primrose was supervising us like a schoolmistress. Aysgarth, I suspected, understood my feelings perfectly but said nothing for fear of upsetting his daughter. She really was the most colossal bore.

On that final morning at the lodge I waited until Eddie had trekked off to retrieve *The Times* and then headed for the drawing-room where Aysgarth was contemplating the sea. 'Do you want to be alone, Mr Dean?' I said tactfully. 'Or can I sit with you and think beautiful thoughts?'

'What a good example you'd set me – yes, sit down at once! I was just plotting how I could murder Canon Fitzgerald and frame the Bishop for the crime.'

'Are they driving you round the bend?'

'It's a wonder that I haven't grabbed a crozier from the sacristy and committed mayhem long since! What with the Cathedral staff and the Chapter and the Greater Chapter all brawling away –'

The Chapter consisted of the three Residentiary Canons, Fitzgerald, Dalton and Eddie, who all lived in the Close and helped the Dean run the Cathedral. The Greater Chapter consisted of the Prebendaries, or Honorary Canons, who were sprinkled through the diocese, many, though not all, with their own parishes to run. The title of prebendary was bestowed on the clergymen who had given exceptional service to the diocese.

'– and then that Archdeacon's always buzzing around like a wasp –'

The Archdeacon was the Bishop's henchman. The diocese was divided into two archdeaconries, and the Archdeacon of Starbridge, though not directly concerned with the running of the Cathedral, kept an eye on it from the diocesan office on Eternity Street.

'– and all the time the Bishop's breathing fire about the coach-park –'

'What coach-park?'

'I want to allocate that broad strip on the edge of Palace Lane to coaches. We really must cater for all these modern pilgrims, but of course Charles takes the snobbish line and says all vulgar charabancs must be left beyond the walls of the Close.'

'How unchristian!'

'Yes, isn't it? One day, I swear, I'll lose my temper and remind him that Jesus didn't go to public school – and talking of education, I've succeeded in locking horns with the Archdeacon over the Theological College.'

'How on earth did you get drawn into that?'

'The Principal is a prebendary of the Cathedral and he's been asking my advice about the college finances, but every time I try to teach the bursar how to add two and two, someone tips off the Archdeacon who immediately accuses me of interference –'

'I'd murder the whole lot of them, if I were you, Mr Dean. Why confine yourself to Canon Fitzgerald?'

'Why indeed?' said Aysgarth laughing, and then exclaimed impulsively: 'How far away all that bickering seems, how unimportant! This holiday's done me so much good. I only wish I could stay here longer.'

'So do I. It's hard to believe that tomorrow –'

'– I'll be back fighting the Bishop over the coach-park. But whatever happens I mustn't give way to the temptation to have a row with Charles over *Honest to God*. That really would be the last straw.'

'I'm getting so interested in *Honest to God*!' I said. 'Could you possibly explain it to me sometime?'

He reached out and playfully patted my hand. So close did I come to swooning as the result of this wholly asexual gesture of affection that I only dimly heard him say: 'Eddie could probably explain the theological background better than I can. The three theologians Robinson extols are all German.'

I was still trying to utter the words: 'Forget Eddie!' when Primrose staggered downstairs to spoil our fun. I might have known she would stuff herself with aspirin and stage a spectacular recovery.

It occurred to me for the first time that it was going to be very difficult to see Aysgarth on his own after our return to Starbridge. A possessive daughter, a clinging wife, a time-consuming Cathedral, a waspish Archdeacon, a truculent Bishop and hordes of modern pilgrims were hardly going to leave much time for delicious little meetings *à deux*.

A faint shadow began to fall across my euphoria.

IX

When we arrived at Heathrow airport on the following afternoon we found Dido lying in wait for us. Aysgarth was pounced on, pawed and peppered with tearful kisses – 'Disgusting!' muttered Primrose. 'What a way to behave in public!' – and I had to try not to look as if I had unexpectedly encountered a full complement of the Spanish Inquisition. Even though I had no doubt that he had engineered their separate holidays in order to preserve his sanity, I hardly welcomed the reminder that he was legally yoked to a doting gorgon.

After Dido had flicked away her tears with a flap of her lace handkerchief, she found time to say brightly: 'How pale you are, Primrose! Such a pity there's no sun in the Hebrides,' and to me she added: 'I'm so glad you didn't die of boredom, but my dear, you look extremely liverish – you should take a strong dose of salts as soon as you get home.'

A chauffeur-driven limousine was waiting outside the terminal; Dido liked to make extravagant gestures with her private income. After Aysgarth had been whisked away, Eddie, Primrose and I rattled off in a bone-shaking bus to the long-term car-park. Depression crawled across my consciousness like a tarantula on the march. As I drove out of London all I could think was: that bloody Dido.

However in Starbridge I recovered my equilibrium, and by the time Primrose and I had dined off baked beans and Spam followed by tinned Ambrosia rice pudding, I had realised that since there was no hope of my passion being reciprocated it hardly mattered that Aysgarth had a wife. My destiny was to burn with unrequited love, and with a sigh of ecstasy I once more consigned myself to the flames.

We had returned on a Thursday, just over a week after our departure. The next morning I waited till Primrose had gone to work and then I strolled up Canonry Drive to Choristers' Green. The Chantry was wedged between a handsome Georgian house, formerly the Choir School but now a museum, and a dainty, early Victorian cottage; one of the best features of the Close was that its houses were all different and yet in their diversity they achieved a satisfying harmony. Studying the Chantry with care I noted that the curtains were still drawn across one of the bedroom windows. I moved on.

Five minutes later in Mitre Street I visited Boots, where I bought a few essential items such as toothpaste, and consulted a very well-informed girl at the cosmetics counter about eye make-up. Various experiments followed as I confirmed my suspicion that mere mascara was not enough to produce the glamour to which I now aspired, but eventually I emerged transformed and retired to a tea-shop called The Copper Kettle where I drank coffee and read the *Daily Mail*. More time passed. Then I padded back to the Close and once more eyed the Chantry. The bedroom curtains were now drawn back. For another minute I prowled around Choristers' Green in an agony of indecision, but at last I marched up to the Chantry and rang the bell.

'Is Miss Markhampton at home?' I said when the housekeeper opened the door. 'I'm Miss Flaxton.'

'*Flaxton?*' cried a disembodied voice in the distance.

'Hi, Marina – it's Venetia! Any chance of saying "Welcome to Starbridge" or are you in the bath?'

'No, in shock! My God, Vinnie, what on earth are you doing in this gorgeous dump?' said Marina Markhampton, appearing at the top of the stairs in a white silk dressing-gown which looked as if it had been personally hand-stitched by Dior, and glided down to meet me as if I were one of her oldest friends.

SIX

'"It's love that makes the world go round." That's what all
Christians have always said.'

JOHN A. T. ROBINSON
Suffragan Bishop of Woolwich 1959–1969
Writing about *Honest to God* in the
Sunday Mirror, 7th April 1963

I

She was shorter than I was, about five foot four, and had thick,
smooth, natural blonde hair which cascaded to her shoulders as
gracefully as if it had been arranged a minute earlier by some
genius of a hairdresser. Beneath their heavy lids her eyes were
a lazy, limpid blue. The cats-about-town used to say that her
bone structure was reminiscent of a prize sheep, but in fact like
many beautiful women her face was striking in its originality.
She wore no make-up but looked radiant. If I had been feeling
less nervous I might well have succumbed to the jealousy
exhibited by all the cats-about-town.

'Let's have some coffee,' she said after we had chatted about
nothing for a couple of minutes. 'Take a pew while I snap my
fingers at the slave.'

Still marvelling at my unexpectedly warm reception I sank
gratefully on to the drawing-room sofa.

'It really is heavenly to see a familiar face,' said Marina,
wandering back into the room with a packet of chocolate
biscuits. 'Everyone in the Close appears to be either nine or
ninety or simply impossible. Where are all the amusing people
of our age?'

'In London, I suppose.' I accepted a biscuit. 'Which reminds
me, Marina –'

'You want to know why I'm here, making sure the housekeeper doesn't sidle off to Blackpool amidst a salvo of bursting pipes. Well, it just so happened that I was being absolutely *persecuted* in London by two men at once, and the last straw came when my boss tried to play the "Moonlight" sonata all over my left thigh.'

'How hackneyed.'

'Exactly what I thought. I was doing some temporary work – nothing strenuous, just answering the phone and pouring the champagne in one of those little art galleries in St James's – and after the sonata I thought hell, I've simply got to claw my way out of this *seething* sexual cesspit, I'll house-sit for Granny, gaze at the Cathedral and think pure thoughts about eternal life – but I've now reached the stage where quite frankly eternal life is wearing a bit thin, so I've decided to give an Orgy to resurrect this dump from the dead.'

'Give a what?'

'An Orgy – with a capital O. Wouldn't it be madly way-out to dance semi-nude on the Cathedral lawn in the moonlight? Even better than last year during a May ball up at Cambridge when I wound up punting semi-nude on the Cam . . . But how frightful, I'm talking all about my boring old self – how are *you*?'

'Also in flight from the cesspits of London. I've just been on holiday in the Hebrides.'

'The Hebrides?' said Marina intrigued as the housekeeper arrived with coffee. 'How original! What inspired you to go there?'

'The Dean invited me. He'd been lent the Starmouths' hunting-lodge, and –'

'Oh yes, you're in cahoots with the Aysgarths, aren't you? I went out with James Aysgarth a couple of times in London when I was a deb – he's rather a dear but not terribly bright and I do like something with a high IQ. Norman Aysgarth's super but he's guarded night and day by Cynthia the Siren – who's actually quite fun when there are no men around –'

'I suppose the Aysgarth closest to you in age is Sandy. His IQ's high enough –'

'Yes, but he's got no sex appeal. However the best Aysgarth, the *crème de la crème* of the Aysgarths, the Aysgarth I'm simply passionate about is –'

'Christian,' I said. 'Welcome to the club. How do you get on with his wife?'

'Oh, I'm passionate about Katie too! In fact I was just deciding that they've simply got to be the guests of honour at my Orgy. And I shall invite Perry Palmer and Robert Welbeck and Katie's brother Simon – oh, and super old Norman too, I must have Norman because he's so like Christian, and that means Cynthia the Siren will have to come, but that's okay, I don't mind Cynthia. I shan't invite Sandy, though, because he's dull, and I shan't invite James because I'm not having anyone from the Guards. I've just about had it with all those Guardsmen trying to rape me in corners whenever they're not trying to rape each other.'

'One must draw the line somewhere.'

'Exactly. And I'm not inviting any floozies either – except Cynthia, and Cynthia'll be fine so long as no one tries to rape Norman – and no one will because my friends Holly and Emma-Louise are both so stylish, so absolutely trustworthy, and I do think it's important, don't you, to have girlfriends you can *trust*. I don't know what I'd do without Holly and Emma-Louise to soothe me whenever I've been pounced on by some wild-eyed Romeo – which reminds me, I'm going to invite Michael Ashworth, the Bishop's son. He's a real pouncer de luxe, but he deserves an invitation because of his first-class sex appeal.'

'How about Charley?'

'That ghastly prig? No fear!'

'By the way, is it true that Michael got kicked out of medical school for pouncing?'

'My dear, no nurse escaped.'

'You mean he actually –'

'– broke every bed in sight. One of Emma-Louise's dearest friends is a nurse, and she told Emma-Louise –'

A long session of gossip followed.

'You don't happen to know why Charley Ashworth ran away from home when he was eighteen, do you?' I was tempted to ask eventually, much impressed by Marina's wide-ranging knowledge of our acquaintances.

'He inherited three thousand theology books from Granny's pal, dear old Bishop Jardine, and the shock sent him temporarily round the bend.'

'But seriously, Marina –'

'Oh, I expect it was just a fit of adolescent pique. I know heaps of people who ran away from home for a weekend just to underline the fact that they were no longer in rompers. I did it myself as a matter of fact – flew off to Rome to see a performance of *Aida* in the Baths of Caracalla, cadged a lift on Banger Marsden's private plane . . . Do you know Banger?'

'Not exactly –'

'He was on his way to Naples, but after he'd dropped me off in Rome I linked up with Holly's brother – queer as a coot, absolutely safe – and off we toddled to *Aida*.'

'But what on earth did your parents think?'

'Oh, my father doesn't think at all – he gave all that up years ago. And my mother just said: "*Darling!*" in despair as usual and began to paint another picture. Parents needn't be difficult, you know. It's all a matter of being kind but firm.'

'Every time I try to be firm with my father he roars like a lion!'

'How exhausting! No wonder you've left London, although I must say, I do think you'd find Rome more amusing than Starbridge. You're obviously rather soignée nowadays, the sort of person who's been around.'

'Well, by the time one's twenty-six, I suppose one *has* seen more or less everything –'

'Oh, of course!' She gazed at me with respect. 'Yes, I can see that I completely misjudged you in the past – I thought you were a churchy bluestocking like Primrose Aysgarth, the sort of person who's hopelessly square, yet now you're obviously a real trendsetter – imagine going to the Hebrides instead of to the boring old Riviera! I suppose the Hebrides will be the next "in" place.'

'The beaches were, I have to admit, quite stunning –'

'I bet. I say, I *am* glad you've wafted into my life just at the very moment when I need the assistance of someone really cool and with-it! Will you help me organise my Orgy?'

'Love to. Thanks.'

'Where are you hanging out?'

'At the Deanery, but as a matter of fact, Marina, I've just had a brainstorm: there isn't enough room in Primrose's pad to swing a cat, so –' I took a deep breath '– is it at all possible – and of course you must be quite honest and say no straight away if the idea appals you –'

'If I'm on my own a day longer in this place I'll go crazy. How soon can you move in?'

I wanted to shout 'Whoopee!' in triumph but instead I said carelessly, as befitted the coolest of trendsetters: 'Today?' and produced what I hoped was a grateful but sophisticated smile.

II

'In my opinion,' said Marina some hours later, 'the best parties are the ones attended by a carefully-picked handful of people, most of whom are known to one another. Those débutante balls with a cast of thousands were too dreary for words, weren't they?'

'Absolutely the bottom.' I had rejoined her at four o'clock that afternoon after making a quick trip to Flaxton Pauncefoot to deposit my laundry and pick up some clean clothes. We were now drinking Earl Grey tea and nibbling slices of that delicious walnut cake from Fuller's. In between nibbles Marina chewed the end of her pencil as she contemplated her notepad and meditated on her guest list.

'I want to have between eight and twelve of my favourite people – my basic coterie – plus between four to six outsiders – the wild-cards, as it were, in the pack,' she was saying, 'but accommodation could be a problem. We can't have too many bodies stacked up here or the slave might have hysterics and phone Granny in Monte Carlo.'

'I'm sure we could devise a passable sardine arrangement for the girls. Then the Aysgarth crowd can cram themselves into the Deanery, and if Michael Ashworth comes that opens up the beds at the South Canonry –'

'The Bishop might have apoplexy at the thought of condoning an orgy.'

'Well, of course we promote this to the older generation as just supper for a few friends with music afterwards.'

'Oh, I see you know all the right moves!' said Marina. 'Okay, assuming we neutralise Anti-Sex Ashworth, I think we've solved the accommodation problem –'

'If we're exploiting the beds at the South Canonry I don't see how you can invite Michael and not that prig Charley.'

'Easy. Michael's in London but Charley will be in Cambridge by the time we give the Orgy, and Cambridge is so far away, almost in *terra incognita*, isn't it practically in the North Sea? No, we can't possibly ask anyone to trek down here from Cambridge – although ... I say, I tell you who I'd like to invite! I was introduced to him last year during that May ball when I wound up punting semi-nude on the Cam. He's reading *divinity* – of all subjects! – and he's not good-looking, all glasses and bones and mousey hair, but there's something about him which is absolutely mesmerising –'

'Does he by any chance tell fortunes?'

'*Does he tell fortunes!* I'll say he does. "The Church is in your future," he says, holding my hand so hard I nearly pass out. "I see you moving in the shadow of a great cathedral!"'

'You're making this up, Marina!'

'No, I swear it – as soon as Granny asked me to house-sit, I remembered Nicky Darrow's prophecy! Listen, we simply must get hold of him – do you know if the new term's started up at Cambridge? Maybe he's still at home with the Holy One.'

'The *who*?'

'Nicky's father's a holy hermit who lives in a wood and eats nothing but Communion wafers. He's about a hundred years old and very wise, like the Delphic Oracle, and people come from all over England to see him, but very few make it into the holy presence because he's guarded day and night by his disciples, a savage band of Anglo-Catholic monks who –'

'Marina, this couldn't come within a hundred light-years of being true!'

'My dear, it's *gospel*. Old Mr Darrow – or is it "Father" Darrow – or is it possibly even "Saint" Darrow –'

'No, that's too much, I balk at sainthood –'

'Well, saint or no saint he's in tune with the music of the spheres and has a hotline to God. Honestly! No kidding!'

'Talking of God,' I said, glancing at my watch and scrambling to my feet, 'it's time I popped over to the Cathedral for evensong.'

'Heavens above, Vinnie, you're not religious, are you?'

'Oh no!' I said. 'But I like to pay my respects to God every now and then as a safety measure. After all, since the non-existence of God can't be scientifically proved, it seems only sensible to allow for the fact that He could be around.' And leaving her boggling at my canny behaviour, I glided across Choristers' Green towards the Cathedral.

III

After feasting my eyes on Aysgarth for half an hour I sped out of the Cathedral before Eddie could waylay me and headed for Primrose's flat. When I had removed my possessions earlier I had left a note of explanation, but nevertheless I thought I should call to smooth any feathers which might have been ruffled by my defection. On my arrival I found that Primrose had just returned from the diocesan office and was relaxing with the current edition of the *Church Gazette*.

'. . . so don't take offence, Prim, because I really do think I'd be an ogre of exploitation if I cluttered up your space a day longer – I simply must give you back your privacy . . .'

Touched by such high-minded consideration, Primrose said how understanding I was and we parted good friends. My next task was to work out how I could avoid inviting her to the Orgy. The last person I wanted to see there was Primrose, looking down her nose as I launched myself into my new life as a member of Marina Markhampton's 'basic coterie'.

'Marina,' I said as soon as I returned to the Chantry, 'what the hell am I going to do about Primrose? I don't want to invite her to the Orgy but I don't see how I can ditch her. We've been friends too long.'

'Has she a boyfriend whom we could coax to whisk her off to a champagne supper on the night in question?'

'Maurice Tait couldn't whisk off anything.'

'Trust Primrose to fancy a non-whisker! But don't worry, we'll invite them both and make sure they're so appalled that they leave early. A basic coterie bash soon separates the wheat from the chaff – which reminds me, talking of the wheat, we must pick the rest of the wild-cards. I've chosen Nicky Darrow. Who do you fancy?'

I tried to look as if I were considering vast numbers of eligible males. 'All the really interesting people are abroad,' I mused mendaciously. 'I'll leave the selecting to you.'

'Okay, I'll give Dinkie Kauffman a whirl – she's an American girl who worked with me at the art gallery. Then I'll ask Christian to bring an interesting man – oh, and why don't we ask Michael Ashworth to produce a trendy male from the BBC?'

'But that means three out of the four wild-cards will be men!'

'So what? All the more fun for us girls!'

'Ah yes,' I said, feeling that my mask of sophistication had slipped. 'Silly of me.'

'So much for the guests,' said Marina, scribbling busily on her notepad. 'Now perhaps we should consider the really vital matter of drink. What shall we order?'

'Champagne, naturally,' I said. 'How about Veuve Clicquot 'fifty-five?'

My mask of sophistication was instantly restored. 'How marvellous!' said Marina admiringly. 'You're a wine expert!' And I allowed myself a deprecating smile as I modestly examined my fingernails.

We were just trying to calculate the number of bottles which would be required when the telephone rang.

Marina picked up the receiver. 'The Orgy Planning Office – may I help you?' she droned in the manner of a secretarial zombie, and then a second later her entire demeanour changed. 'Christian!' she exclaimed. 'So you got my message . . .' And as she talked on, telling him about her plans, it suddenly dawned on me not only that she was in love with him but that the unsupervised stay in a beautiful house, the placing of herself against the ravishing backdrop of the Cathedral, the exact nature of the social event which would inevitably lure him from Oxford – all had been planned long before she had left London. It seemed I had met yet another slave to a one-sided grand passion.

No wonder we had discovered we were soul-mates.

IV

Christian Aysgarth was at that time nearly thirty-six and had been married for six years to the granddaughter of a former Earl of Starmouth, the ninth earl who had so interested himself in the affairs of the Church earlier in the century and whose wife – his second wife, Katie's grandmother – had prided herself on her collection of distinguished clerical acquaintances; like Marina's grandmother she had been one of swashbuckling Bishop Jardine's 'Lovely Ladies', happily married aristocratic women who could offer him a devoted platonic friendship in those fabled days before the war when bishops had apparently had no trouble combining a worldly glamour with the indestructible virtue required by their office.

Aysgarth – my Mr Dean – had been Jardine's protégé. Inevitably he had gravitated into Lady Starmouth's benevolent orbit, but although Christian could remember being introduced to her during his adolescence, he had not met her granddaughter Katherine until he was twenty-six, down from Oxford with his double first and poised to be a 'deb's delight', one of those eligible young males who were invited to adorn the débutante balls. Christian had been educated at Winchester and Balliol; he appeared every inch the gentleman, but nevertheless Lady Starmouth could probably never quite forget that his grandfather had been a draper. Katie, of course, only cared that Christian was tall, dark, handsome, brilliant and charming, an extraordinary specimen of masculine perfection, but like the rest of us who yearned for Christian she was obliged to yearn in vain – until he decided that the right wife could be a useful acquisition.

Katie was without doubt the right wife, perfectly equipped to play the heroine in the great romance which his life now demanded. Intelligent but not intellectual, beautiful, rich, well-connected and well-bred, she was acquired in 1957. By that time the Starmouths had forgotten the grandfather who had been a draper. Christian had won such distinction up at Oxford that his pedigree had ceased to be important, and besides, his father had just been appointed Dean of Starbridge. The Aysgarths, as my father remarked at the time, had finally arrived.

My description of Christian may seem a trifle barbed but I have no wish to present him as a cardboard cut-out character, all surface and no depth, like the hero of a bad romantic novel. Let me now add that although he often seemed too perfect to be true, he was capable of exercising an unexpectedly cruel wit; he could also be arrogant and selfish. Katie adored him even when he was being monstrous, and I always thought this was a mistake. It might have been better if she had occasionally screamed abuse at him and slapped his face; it could have made the marriage more intriguing. However it was generally agreed that the marriage was a success, and although Christian never seemed much interested in the two little girls it had produced this may have been because he was not a demonstrative man and seemed to be repelled by any display of emotion. (On reflection perhaps Katie was right not to scream abuse at him and slap his face.)

Sometimes I wondered if he ever felt nervous because there was so little left for him to achieve. After leaving Winchester, where he had been a scholar, he had completed two suitably heroic years of National Service before going up to Oxford to read Greats. Having won his brilliant first he had then read Theology with equal success, but had afterwards refused to proceed to a theological college to train as a clergyman. No reason was ever given. 'He just told Father he wasn't called to serve God in the Church,' Primrose had told me at the time.

'But didn't your father want to know why?'

'Oh, he could never have asked. Father finds it difficult to talk to his sons – and the boys find it equally difficult to talk to him.' Primrose had then paused as if searching for the appropriate words before adding obscurely: 'I'm all right; Father has different standards for girls. I don't have to win scholarships or "get on" in a first-class career because Father thinks I'm perfect just as I am. But it's much harder for the boys to be perfect. They live in terror of disappointing him.'

'But why does he expect you all to be perfect?' I had said baffled. My father never expected his children to be anything but trouble.

'He sees us all as prizes – ultimate prizes – prizes awarded him by God – and of course those sort of prizes could never be other than perfect.'

'But nobody's perfect, Primrose!'

'No, but Father's such an idealist and he loves us all so much so naturally we don't want to let him down. That's why the boys always do their best to hide their problems from him; they couldn't bear him to be upset.'

'But that means they must all lead a double life – the perfect life on the surface and the imperfect life underneath!'

'No, the boys all lead a single life; they simply bowdlerise their reports of it to Father. If anyone leads a double life it's Father himself, living as the dynamic dean and the harassed husband. Probably the only way he can survive that awful woman is to divide himself into two in order to escape from her regularly.'

I was to recall this conversation more than once in 1963, but I first recalled it on that April evening at the Chantry when I realised Marina was in love with Christian; I started to wonder if he too, like his father, was living a divided life. There was no denying his dynamic career at Oxford. Following up the medieval interests which he had acquired during his theological studies he was now coasting along towards the inevitable chair in medieval studies or medieval philosophy – or whatever the crucial professorship was in his rarefied field of endeavour. He had written two acclaimed books, both about the effect of Aristotle's influence on the medieval Church, and he was now working on a study of Averroes, the Arab philosopher. But how far did this distinguished career satisfy him? And how content was he with his apparently idyllic marriage? I had no idea, but the thought of Marina, hoving to on the horizon like some latter-day Helen of Troy, was vaguely worrying.

I have described Christian at length not merely because he was to be the star guest at the Orgy, but because it would have been obvious to someone more mature than I was then that the Aysgarth family was far more convoluted than was apparent during the jolly Sunday lunches which I occasionally attended at the Deanery. However, contrary to the sophisticated image I was so busily promoting to Marina, my experience of the world was still very limited.

The date of the Orgy depended on the state of Christian's engagement diary, but a blank space was uncovered beside Saturday, the eighteenth of May, and Christian said it would be a relief to escape briefly from Oxford while the undergraduates, tortured by examinations, were threatening to commit suicide en masse. Marina then spent much time worrying that her chosen guests might have other engagements, but in the end the Coterie proved quite unable to resist the magic combination of the Cathedral Close, Marina Markhampton and countless cases of Veuve Clicquot. In London imaginative excuses were produced to soothe various jilted hostesses. Only Nick Darrow in Cambridge said he was too busy with exams to accept the invitation, but Marina found out by chance from Michael Ashworth that Nick was planning to sneak back to the Starbridge diocese that weekend to see his father; apparently

St Darrow was about to celebrate his eighty-third birthday. Immediately Marine badgered Nick with a series of winning little notes until he wrote back and said he might be able to look in on the party for a short time after all.

'Imagine playing hard to get when one's only twenty,' said Marina acidly. 'He'll be a terror when he grows up.'

'Maybe he genuinely doesn't want to come but doesn't have the experience to shake you off gracefully.'

'But *everyone* wants to come to this party!' protested Marina outraged. 'Everyone always wants to come to *all* my parties!'

'Maybe he's too young to know that.'

I was somewhat perturbed by the guests' diverse ages, but Marina insisted that mixing age-groups created no problems for the Coterie. 'Christian always likes to be with younger people,' she said. 'He missed so much fun when he was young because he had to study so hard, and now he says he'll be making up for lost time until he's at least forty. Anyway, apart from little Nicky, who's clearly very juvenile, the youngest man present will be Michael Ashworth and since he always carries on like a roué of thirty instead of an innocent of twenty-three, he'll fit in perfectly. The ages of the unmarried girls don't count, of course, so long as everyone's under twenty-eight. I've noticed that once unmarried girls get to that fatal age they become so nervous of winding up on the spinsters' scrap-heap that they set every man's teeth on edge.'

I absorbed this information in silence as I realised that only two years separated me from the scrap-heap, but soon I was able to blot out this nightmare by ordering champagne by the case and arranging for the best firm of caterers in Starbridge to provide a sumptuous buffet supper. I did occasionally spare a thought for that sordid subject, money, but Marina was sublimely confident that her grandmother would foot the bills.

'Granny told me to have a lovely time while I was here,' she said, 'so I may as well take her at her word.'

'Marina, I rather doubt that when Lady Markhampton made arrangements for you to buy food and drink on tick, she visualised you ordering umpteen cases of champagne.'

'Well, if she gets cross Daddy can toss her a couple of hundred guineas next Christmas.'

I decided to stop worrying about Lady Markhampton's potential cardiac arrest and start worrying about what on earth I was going to wear.

In those days one still dressed formally for parties – unless one was a student at some redbrick university or a freak at art school – so although Marina mused on the possibility of wearing nothing but a leopardskin bikini she was quick enough to whip a masterpiece of *haute couture* out of her wardrobe when the discussion became serious. As usual I looked frightful in all my evening dresses. Starbridge, typically provincial, was only good for tweeds and twin sets. Making a quick dash to London I avoided Knightsbridge, where the snooty shop assistants made me feel like one of the Ugly Sisters in *Cinderella*, and waded through that Lethe of plebeian consumerism, Oxford Street. Since no one I knew ever went there except to buy underwear at Marks and Spencer's, I felt I could sink into a liberating anonymity and forget my inferiority complex.

I was just wandering past Richards – or was it C&A? – and thinking how grim life must be for the 'lower orders', obliged through lack of money to buy their clothes in cheap shops, when I saw a greenish-golden slinky creation in the window and knew immediately that I was being offered the opportunity to convert myself into a sex symbol. I sped across the threshold. The little assistant was charming and deferential. (Why *do* the upper classes confine themselves to ghastly, expensive shops? Why don't we *all* invade Richards and C&A?) The dress, which would have cost some astronomical sum in Bond Street, was mine at the drop of a ten-pound note. Then having saved myself so much money I decided I should celebrate my success by having a little flutter at Fortnum's. They do roast beef so well in the main restaurant, and a woman can lunch there on her own without being regarded as a freak.

At Waterloo Station I finally bought a copy of *Honest to God* but on the train I fell asleep before I had even reached page two. A half-bottle of Nuits St Georges is probably not the ideal prelude to any serious study of theology.

When I awoke an hour later the guest-list for the Orgy was revolving in my mind, just as it so often did in those days in response to my eager anticipation. At the top of the list stood Christian and Katie, who would be leaving their two little girls behind with the au pair in order to make the lightning trip to Starbridge. Then came our second married couple, Christian's brother Norman, the barrister who lectured in law at London University, and man-eating Cynthia who had kept Norman from an academic appointment in Oxford by insisting that she was unable to live in the provinces. Their one child was also to be left at home, but unfortunately this always had to happen as there was something wrong with him; he was looked after by a full-time nurse. Whenever I saw Cynthia preening herself before the mirror in an ecstasy of vanity, I always reminded myself that she had a tragedy at the centre of her life and that allowances had to be made for her.

Chief among the unmarried guests was Peregrine Palmer, who had been at Winchester with Christian and who was reputed to have some secret job in the Foreign Office. (The word 'spy' was never mentioned but everyone knew he spoke Russian.) Following Perry on the list was Katie's brother Simon, a handsome slab who was supposed to be 'something in the City' – a euphemism which described the paid idleness of various upper-class males who were too brainless to do more than play polo – and after Simon came Robert Welbeck, who had been up at Oxford with Marina's brother Douglas some years ago and who was now employed by a merchant bank. The ranks of the bachelors were then boosted by Michael Ashworth, the Bishop's younger son, now learning to be a television producer after his hedonistic romps at medical school.

Next came the two girls who were due to join forces with Marina and me to keep the bachelors amused: Emma-Louise Hanson had become friends with Marina during their débutante days, and Holly Carr had been at school with Marina at Downe House. I don't think either girl did much. Holly was a cordon bleu cook and occasionally whipped up a chic boardroom lunch. Emma-Louise was supposed to be a secretary but was usually unemployed in order to attend to her social life.

These girls completed the list of the Coterie members. There followed the 'wild-cards', chosen to add spice to the party. Dinkie Kauffman, Marina's American friend from the art gallery, sounded promising; she was reputed to look like Jane Russell and talk like Philip Marlowe. Nick Darrow was too young to be seriously amusing but could nonetheless be relied upon to produce stimulating vibes. Don Latham, Michael's friend from the BBC, was an unknown quantity but since Michael had enthusiastically described him as 'outta sight' one could hope for something original to materialise. Whom Christian intended to bring we had no idea, since he refused to tell us, but I was prepared to share Marina's confidence that this 'Mr X' would be fascinating.

At the bottom of the guest-list lurked Primrose and that drip Tait, but Marina and I had long since hatched a foolproof scheme for their speedy disposal.

I sighed, excitement pushing aside the inertia that so often follows an afternoon snooze, and at that moment realised that *Honest to God* was still lying in my lap. On an impulse I opened the book at random and read: 'The words of St Augustine, "Love God and do what you like", were never safe. But they constitute the heart of Christian prayer – as they do of Christian conduct.'

So Bishop Robinson was dusting off those highly ambiguous words of St Augustine! No wonder Bishop Ashworth was having apoplexy at the South Canonry. Love God and do what you like. That seemed to imply . . . although of course St Augustine hadn't meant . . . or had he? No, of course not. But what a potentially stupendous slogan for the sizzling 1960s!

Racing back to the Cathedral for evensong I prepared to love God and dote on the Dean.

V

By this time I had discovered that if one is violently in love the desire to talk constantly about the object of one's passion is very strong. I considered I was successfully maintaining a languid façade, but although I suppressed the urge to betray myself by addled chatter, Marina soon noticed my regular attendance at the Cathedral and finally I could no longer write off this behaviour as a metaphysical safety measure. In the belief that a half-truth is often more convincing than an outright lie I responded to her growing suspicion that I was a religious fanatic by confessing: 'Well, the truth is I'm so fond of the Dean that I simply can't bear to disappoint him by not showing up regularly for services – he's been so kind to me ever since I was nine years old.'

Marina was quite satisfied by this sentimental explanation but afterwards, with superhuman self-restraint, I confined myself to attending evensong no more than three times a week and entering the Cathedral on Sunday only for matins. By loitering near the vestry after the service I often managed to bump into Aysgarth, but such golden moments were not guaranteed and indeed it would have looked odd if I had been perpetually encountering him. Soon I began to feel somewhat starved of his presence, but starvation, as anyone on a strict diet knows, can initially induce a powerful sense of well-being.

I was certainly overflowing with well-being when I returned to the Chantry after my quick trip to London and showed an admiring Marina my new dress. I was just rummaging in my bag for the receipt – of course Marina had refused to believe the dress had only cost ten pounds – when *Honest to God* fell out. At once Marina spotted the naked man on the cover and shrieked: 'Super – pornography!'

'Down, Fido, down! It's a best seller, available over the counter!'

'But what's it about?'

'God. He's the new "in" thing. Everyone's mad about Him.'

'Help! Maybe I should read a page or two. I'm actually quite keen on God, deep down, but the Church is so dreadfully square, isn't it?'

'No more!' I cried, brandishing *Honest to God* in triumph. 'Bishop Robinson's making it trendy! He says that the heart of Christian conduct is loving God and then doing what you like!'

'No! You mean –'

'Of course. So long as you love God, everything's okay,' I said, wondering idly if St Augustine was turning far away in his unknown grave, and having poured myself into my new dress I began to practise various sultry poses in front of the looking-glass.

VI

I remember the Orgy, that innocent affair; if it had been a real orgy we would have called it a party – or possibly, later in the 'sixties, a happening. How long ago it all seems now as I look back from the 1980s! It's hard to remember the exact quality of that lost era, but in 1963 if one was under thirty one lived in a world of untarnished dreams and ideals, unpolluted gaiety and adventure. Except for nicotine and alcohol drugs were seldom encountered – and who needed pot when one could get high on vintage Veuve Clicquot? Drugs were for riff-raff in those days, and we were the opposite of riff-raff; we were the *jeunesse dorée*, gathered by Marina Markhampton to celebrate life with style in ravishing surroundings, not to 'turn on and drop out' in some sordid urban squat. Looking back at that magical evening I can see us all with such painful clarity, sophisticated yet innocent, fast but not corrupt – and above all so mercifully blind to that terrible time ahead when the enchanting *communitas*, the group spirit, of the early 'sixties fell apart and terminated in chaos.

'To the future!' cried Christian Aysgarth, raising his first glass of champagne, and at once my heart missed a beat because he was so attractive, his shining career seemingly stretching ahead of him into the distance, and when he spoke, his wife Katie gazed up at him as soulfully as if they were newly-weds while Marina, completing the triangle which I was later to find so mysterious, flung her arms around his neck and exclaimed what heaven it was to see him again. At that point Perry Palmer, Christian's old schoolfriend, said dryly: 'You really should be a Moslem, Christian, in order to accommodate all these doting women in a respectable style!' whereupon Marina retorted: 'Don't be a bitch, Perry!' and Christian drawled: 'I'd like to see my bank manager's face if I were to tell him I intended to keep four wives!' Then Katie commented with unflawed serenity: 'Think of the fun I could have gossiping with the other three whenever you were away!' and when they began to debate harems I lost the thread of the conversation until suddenly Christian caught my eye across the room as I held court with Norman Aysgarth and Robert Welbeck; I heard him declare: 'If I have a harem I'm going to have Vinnie in it!' and when he winked at me I was reminded of his father.

I turned over the LP of Floyd Cramer, who had played the piano on so many of the Presley records, and as the party gathered speed time became displaced, just as it so often does when vintage champagne flows freely, and the exact sequence of events is now muddled in my memory, but I can recall wandering past the sofa some time later – had the buffet disappeared? No, there was still plenty left – and I can remember changing the record again – we were on Cliff Richard by that time, but no, it couldn't have been Cliff because Marina didn't like him, so perhaps it was Adam Faith – or could it conceivably have been Eden Kane? – anyway, the record-player was drooling in the corner, but not too noisily, we didn't want to drown the conversation – and as I said, I was wandering past the sofa where Michael Ashworth was trying to grope two girls at once – I can't think who they were now, but I'm sure one was the American girl Dinkie Kauffman, who had a cleavage reminiscent of the Grand Canyon, while the other girl might have been Emma-Louise – and as I said, I was wandering past the sofa when I bumped into Katie's brother Simon, the handsome slab, who said: 'Whoa there!' as if I was a horse – he always talked to women as if they were horses – and I had only just managed to stagger out of his way when I came face to face with Christian's friend Perry Palmer, who looked so ordinary, medium height, medium build, medium brown hair, medium plain face, but was supposed to be something rather extraordinary in the Foreign Office – although nobody knew for sure – and Perry lived in London at *Albany*, which was very grand and I couldn't help wondering how he'd wangled a flat there – a set, I mean, they call them sets in Albany – but perhaps the Foreign Office had some special pull.

Anyway, Perry said to me: 'You seem to be the only intelligent girl here – you're the only one who's not swooning over Christian,' and I said to him as I refilled our glasses: 'Don't worry, darling – I'm not in love with him!' – which was a most peculiar thing to say, but fortunately Perry laughed and answered: 'Didn't I say you were intelligent?' and it occurred to me that he was really rather entertaining and perhaps not a homosexual after all – although after the Burgess and Maclean scandal one could never be quite sure about anyone in that line – and certainly no one knew for certain that Perry was a homosexual, just as no one knew for certain he was a spy – in fact Marina said he was a eunuch, although when I asked her if she'd inspected his genitals she had to confess she hadn't – which just goes to show that no one ever tells the truth about sex, not really, it's all wishful thinking and fantasy tricked out with little flashes of romantic illusion.

'No one tells the truth about sex,' I said to Perry in the kind of voice one uses to proclaim a profound truth after a couple of tankards of Veuve Clicquot – and Buddy Holly was playing on the gramophone which was strange because I could have sworn I put on Del Shannon – but Perry had been collared by Don Latham, the pal Michael Ashworth had brought down from the trendy division of dear old Auntie BBC, and I found myself facing Christian's wild-card, the mysterious Mr X. And now I must go back to the beginning of the party when Floyd Cramer was playing the piano, because I have to record that when Christian walked in with Mr X I couldn't believe it, I just *couldn't believe it*, because Mr X turned out to be Eddie Hoffenberg – Eddie of all people! – and as soon as I could get Christian to myself – no mean feat – I hissed: 'Chrissie, how dare you bring that Teutonic masochist!' Christian always hated being called anything but Christian, so he knew how cross I was, but to my fury he just laughed and said: 'Eddie's one of the most interesting men I know – and I'm perpetually in his debt because he keeps Father happy by chatting about the Church. That's more than I can ever be bothered to do.' And then he was snapped up by Marina before I could reply. I wanted to snap him back, but at that moment – it was still the Floyd Cramer era of the party – Primrose arrived with that drip Tait so Marina and I had to put our anti-Prim programme into action.

I shovelled some champagne down Primrose as quickly as possible while Marina replaced Floyd Cramer with Elvis Presley. Primrose turned pink, and when she was no more than halfway through her first glass – Elvis was panting 'I Got Stung' – she said to me: 'It's such a nuisance about this prior engagement but I'm afraid we simply have to go, don't we, Maurice?' Then Tait, who was goggling at Dinkie's cleavage, said obediently: 'Yes, I suppose we do,' but I thought nonetheless that he looked wistful as he was led firmly away by Miss P. Aysgarth, Girl Guide leader, and as I detected in him an embryonic inclination to lust after an exposed bosom I realised he was not quite the damp squib I had always thought he was.

'You look sensational, Venetia!' said Eddie, cornering me as soon as Primrose had departed with Tait in tow, and I was aware of Marina swapping Elvis for Jim Reeves now that our mission had been accomplished.

'You don't look so bad yourself, Canon,' I said kindly, casting a vague glance at his well-cut suit and daringly striped shirt, and then I managed to escape from him by circulating with a plate of hors d'oeuvres. However instead of moping against a wall and wondering why he had come, Eddie circulated too, chatting away brightly to Norman's wife, man-eating Cynthia, who enjoyed talking to anything in trousers, even if it did look like Eddie, and then he had a long session with Marina's schoolfriend Holly Carr – Holly was nice, I liked her better than Dinkie or Emma-Louise – and finally as Christian, the beau of the ball, beckoned Eddie to his side I realised dimly that Eddie was being a social success – which seemed so unlikely that I had to have another glass of champagne to recover from the shock.

Then after I had declared to Perry Palmer that no one ever told the truth about sex – and now I'm jumping forward again and Buddy Holly was singing 'Peggy Sue' – or was it 'That'll Be The Day'? – I found myself confronting Eddie again and he was saying urgently: 'I *must* talk to you,' which seemed sinister, so I said to play for time: 'You're in a peculiar state, Eddie – what's the matter?' and he was just beginning to tell me when Michael Ashworth, who had finished his double grope on the sofa, slid his arm around my waist and purred: 'Hullo, Gorgeous – how's life among the coronets?' That Michael was smooth enough to play host to a brigade of skates.

'Much the same as life among the mitres, I expect,' I retorted, but Michael begged: '*Please!* Can't we leave the Church out of this?' – which made me realise what a problem it must be if one's father's known as Anti-Sex Ashworth and one's brother's famous as the biggest prig in town.

'But I'm mad about the Church!' I protested to Michael. 'Wildly, passionately mad about it!' And at that moment, as if on cue, the Church entered the room in the form of a divinity undergraduate – Marina's personal wild-card, hours late, floated into the party on a magic carpet of psychic vibrations and stared appalled at the riotous scene that confronted him.

'NICKY!' screamed Marina, halting in the act of dishing out chocolate mousse from the buffet. 'You angel – you've arrived!'

'Who's this?' I heard Dinkie say intrigued.

I said: 'It's my Talisman,' but for some reason no one, not even Dinkie, took any notice of me. Then I realised this was because I had spoken the words in a whisper. Possibly it might be time to think about black coffee, but first of all I had to have a little more champagne to neutralise the shock brought on by the appearance of my very own Halley's Comet.

'Have a drink, Nick!' I cried, waving a bottle in his direction.

'Thanks,' he said. 'Just half a glass. I can't stay long. Sorry I'm late.'

'I suppose you were treading your mystical paths so hard that you didn't notice the time!' said Marina, radiating indulgent charm.

'No, to be honest I just forgot about the party altogether.' He accepted the full glass I offered him and looked hopefully at a dish of sausage-rolls. 'Can I have one of those, please?'

'You *forgot*?' echoed Marina, hardly knowing whether to be amazed or outraged.

'Isn't he original?' I said, trying to galvanise her into displaying a sense of humour. 'I bet no one's ever forgotten one of your parties before!'

There was much laughter and Marina sensibly decided to pass off the incredible *faux pas* as a joke. 'Ladies and gentlemen!' she declared to her guests. 'This is the Coterie's soothsayer-in-residence – Nicholas Darrow!'

Nick gave her a most unfriendly look and devoured his sausage-roll in an agony of embarrassment.

'Brother of Martin Darrow the actor!' trilled Marina.

'Really?' exclaimed Holly.

'Gee whiz!' drawled Dinkie.

'Way out!' breathed Emma-Louise.

'Idiot!' I muttered to Marina. 'For God's sake put on another record and give the poor child a chance to merge with the crowd.' I turned back to my Talisman. I felt I wanted to protect him. 'Come over here, Nick,' I said briskly, 'and take no notice of all those asinine females. Do you know any of the Aysgarths? This is Christian – and his wife Katie –' To my relief Elvis began to warble 'It's Now or Never' and the Orgy picked up speed again as everyone finished boggling at the Infant Phenomenon.

The Aysgarths were kind to him but he was very shy and clearly out of his social depth. I wondered if he was embarrassed because he was casually dressed – I realised then that even the Oxbridge undergraduates had begun to display sartorial informality at parties – but after a while I came to the conclusion that he was oblivious of his blue shirt and jeans. It seemed far more likely that he hated parties and only attended them because someone had told him he ought to be more sociable. I was just wondering how I could alleviate his misery when he was kidnapped by Michael Ashworth, who knew him well, and borne off to amuse Dinkie and Emma-Louise.

I said to Christian: 'We've got to save little Nicky from being mauled to pieces by those voracious floozies and then reassembled by Marina to perform parlour-tricks. Do something brilliant – instantly.'

At once Christian rose to the challenge.

VII

He set down his glass. He swept to the record-player. He plucked the needle from the groove. Then adapting the famous Shakespearean technique for grabbing the attention of a crowd he declaimed: 'Friends! Revellers! Companions! Lend me your ears!' And as soon as the raucous conversation ceased he declared: 'It's time to propose a toast. Norman – draw back the curtains! And Perry – turn off the lights!'

The curtains skimmed on their rails, the switches clicked – and there beyond the window towered the Cathedral, floodlit and fantastic, a miracle of light erupting from the darkness, a stone vision that stunned the eye. I was not unfamiliar with this extraordinary sight, but at that moment the drama of the occasion was such that I felt as if I were seeing the nocturnal Cathedral for the first time. Like everyone else in the room I gasped, and suddenly the Orgy seemed trivial. I was reminded of Platonic philosophy. I had thought that reality had lain in the room around me, but that had been merely the shadow of the substance, and I now saw that ultimate reality, eternal and unchanging, lay elsewhere, beyond the pane.

'To Starbridge!' said Christian, raising his glass. 'And to the Cathedral!'

There was a reverent silence as we all drank to the vision before our eyes, and then Dinkie – or was it Emma-Louise? – no, it was Dinkie, I remember the American accent – said: 'Wouldn't it be just wonderful to go up on that roof and dance in the light of the moon?' and Katie's brother Simon shouted: 'Whoopee!' in the manner of John Peel calling 'View halloo!' but Robert Welbeck said more rationally: 'How could we ever get in?' Then Christian said to Norman: 'Shall we nip down to the Deanery and filch the key from Father's study?' but Eddie interposed suddenly: 'No need – I've got a key.'

Dinkie's idle wish was at once brought out of the world of dreams and revealed as a practical possibility. Marina exclaimed gratefully to Eddie: 'I'm *so* glad you came to my Orgy!' and Michael Ashworth (who I had just realised was very drunk) carolled: 'A canon in the hand is worth a bishop in the bush!' but this clouded attempt at wit was greeted with howls from Dinkie and Emma-Louise, who pulled him down on the sofa and sat on him to keep him in order. Meanwhile Perry Palmer had switched on the lights again and Nick Darrow, who had been surreptitiously stuffing the last of the sausage-rolls into his pocket under cover of darkness, was saying politely to Marina: 'I'm afraid I have to go now.'

'But you can't!' wailed Marina. 'I absolutely forbid it. Come up on the Cathedral roof and tell fortunes!'

'Sorry, I've got to get home to my father.' He thanked her formally for the party and turned away as if there was no more to be said. At once Marina started to wail again but when Christian said lightly: 'Where's my hostess with the mostest?' Nick was forgotten. I was just feeling grateful to Christian for preventing Marina from behaving like a spoilt child when I realised that Nick had paused by the door as if there was something he had forgotten. Then, very slowly, he turned to face me.

Around us everyone was shrieking and laughing again, but Nick and I seemed to be wrapped in a mysterious silence. Automatically we moved towards each other, and as we met in the centre of the room he said in a low, urgent voice: 'Don't go to the Cathedral.'

I stared, but before I could speak he had vanished, bolting from the room as if he had embarrassed himself.

So the Coterie's 'soothsayer-in-residence' had been unable to resist delivering an enigmatic warning! Too radiant with Veuve Clicquot to be other than vastly entertained, I murmured indulgently: 'Bless his little cotton socks!' (a favourite idiotic phrase of the time) and prepared for the assault on the Cathedral.

VIII

'I'll have to run home and pick up the key,' Eddie was saying to Christian, 'but I'll meet you all by the Dean's door of the Cathedral in five minutes.'

'Fine. I'll whip these Goths and Vandals into something that resembles a civilised order.'

Eddie disappeared. Christian clapped his hands to recall everyone's attention and said laconically: 'Let's keep the decibels low or the Constable of the Close will arrive frothing at the mouth. Are we ready?'

We weren't. The girls had to cover up their bare shoulders to protect themselves from the May night and various people found they had to go to the lavatory, but finally we all streamed out of the house across Choristers' Green and crossed the North Walk to the Cathedral churchyard.

I glanced at my watch. The time was almost eleven; Nick would only just have had time to escape from the Close before the Constable shut the gates for the night. I tried to picture my Talisman returning to his father, but I found I could not quite imagine the ancient St Darrow who lived in a wood on Communion wafers, and meanwhile we were all gliding and giggling across the sward, the girls' dresses glinting and the men's shirt-fronts gleaming in the darkness. Michael and Dinkie, prancing in front of the floodlights, began to jive silently together and vast shadows were cast on the huge walls ahead of us. In the distance the houses of the Close were almost all in darkness. The silence was profound.

'Here's Eddie,' breathed Marina, who was holding Christian's hand. 'Isn't he a pet?'

'I didn't know orang-outangs could be classified as pets,' I said tartly, whereupon Robert Welbeck, the merchant banker who had been up at Oxford with Marina's brother, linked his arm through mine, declared he worshipped glamour-girls who reminded him of Humphrey Bogart films and demanded to know why we had never met at a party in London.

'We did,' I said, 'but you were too busy worshipping elsewhere to prostrate yourself at my feet.'

At that moment, which must have been eleven o'clock precisely, a time-switch flipped in the bowels of the Cathedral and all the floodlights went out.

Once again we gasped at the sight which met our eyes. The harsh glare of electricity was replaced by the soft glow of the moon. A delicate pale light bathed the ancient houses of the Close and conjured up images of the idyllic settings of countless fairy-tales, while the sward of the churchyard, shining eerily around us, suggested a magic garden full of lost echoes from the past. The black mountain of the Cathedral's north wall seemed to vibrate as if it were part of a huge animal – in fact so strong was this impression of life that I actually touched the stones as if I expected them to pulse beneath my fingers but of course the wall was cool, dank and still.

'What a sight!' I heard Perry say in awe as he stood hand in hand with Katie Aysgarth, while Norman, quoting from Macaulay with the confidence of a Winchester scholar, murmured: '"Such night in England ne'er had been, nor e'er again shall be."' Michael then tried to croon Presley's 'Such a Night' but his pal Don Latham managed to cuff him while the girls – Dinkie and Emma-Louise but not Holly, who was spellbound – hissed: 'Shhh!'

'No sacrilege, please, chaps,' said Christian casually as Eddie unlocked the Dean's door, and Marina whispered to him: 'It's a holy place, isn't it?'

'Well, what did you expect?' I muttered, irritated by this banal chatter which was marring the Cathedral's colossal vibes. 'Brighton Pier on a bank holiday?'

'Hang on a minute,' Eddie was saying, opening the door and switching on his torch. 'I have to turn off the alarm before it summons the entire Starbridge police force and all three fire engines.' He disappeared but returned in less than a minute to announce: 'All clear!'

Drunken but awe-struck we tiptoed into the huge dark interior beyond.

IX

'I won't switch on any lights,' said Eddie, 'or someone might see us and summon the Constable in panic, but I've brought two torches so if I lead the way –'

'Marina and I will bring up the rear and provide extra light,' said Christian. 'Well done, Eddie.'

We set off in a hushed crocodile, crossing the Cathedral to the door at the tip of the south transept; the stairs beyond led not only to the tower below the spire but to the roof of the nave. Vast columns rose around us and disappeared into blackness. Long windows languished in the moonlight. Eerily the echo of our footfalls rebounded from the invisible ceiling. No one spoke until Eddie said, opening the door: 'I think I can risk the light on the stairs – the windows overlook the cloisters, not the Close,' and he flicked on the switch.

It was curious how the arrival of artificial light made us all relax. We staggered up the twisting staircase, various people making idiotic remarks, but once I paused to look down on the moonlit quadrangle of the cloisters and when I saw the seat donated by Lady Mary Calthrop-Ponsonby, I yearned for my Mr Dean. In fact suddenly I was so overpowered by the wish that he could be with me that I had to lean for support against the wall.

'Get a move on, Vinnie,' said Katie's brother Simon, addressing me as a horse as usual. I could have murdered him.

We reached the roof of the nave. I saw a dark velvet sky suffused with a pure white light. Below me the bishop's palace, now the Choir School, rose in a flurry of Victorian gothic towers and turrets from its long garden, and beyond the silver gleam of the river the meadows, enchanted pastures, stretched to the distant mass of the hills. The sight was so beautiful that tears stung my eyes and again I found myself wishing with passion: if only he could be here!

Someone paused beside me. I looked up. It was Christian.

'Incomparable, isn't it?' he said.

'Stunning.' The adjective seemed so inadequate that I wished I had remained silent.

'You're looking rather stunning yourself,' Christian remarked idly. 'In fact I've never seen you look better. Is the obvious explanation the true one?'

'What's the obvious explanation?'

'Are you in love?'

'Oh, good heavens!' I said languidly, but then in a moment of bravado I cast aside the mask of nonchalance and retorted: 'Well, as a matter of fact yes, I am – but not with you, I promise!'

'And now, of course, I long to seduce you on the spot!'

Robert Welbeck, who had somehow become separated from me during the long haul up to the roof, chose that moment to lurch into us. 'Venetia reminds me of Lauren Bacall,' he said to Christian. 'Venetia, any time you want me to play Humphrey Bogart –'

'Sweet of you, darling,' I said, 'but I wouldn't dream of stopping you running off to Casablanca with Ingrid Bergman.'

'Save your energy, Robert!' advised Christian amused. 'Venetia's in love with someone else.'

'Oh God, why am I always last past the post in the race for the glamour-girls?'

Perry Palmer said behind him: 'Let me give you a lesson in racing! Venetia, when you're next in London, have a drink with me at Albany and I'll show you my very curious Japanese prints.'

'Fabulous – name the day!' I said promptly, and Christian laughed.

Marina, slinking up to our group, said with a commendably genuine affection: 'What a *femme fatale* you are, Vinnie, luring these three gorgeous creatures into your net!' I suppose that if one has absolute confidence in one's ability to be the belle of every ball, one can afford to be generous, but I still admired Marina for not unsheathing her claws. My sister Arabella would have been scratching away furiously by that time.

In gratitude I said to Marina: 'They're all yours, Helen of Troy. I'm off to the other side of the roof to contemplate eternity.' I felt quite faint with euphoria. I had been called a glamour-girl – twice – and openly acknowledged as a *femme fatale*. My life as a social outcast was over. I had moved from the sidelines of life to the centre at last. I was madly in love. The world lay at my feet. I was in paradise.

At the west end of the roof I looked back and saw that Katie had joined the group I had abandoned. Christian was slipping his arm around her waist – and Marina perhaps found that too hard to watch; she was moving away, and although Perry held out his hand to her she ignored him. Robert Welbeck, in search of another glamour-girl, was prowling purposefully towards Dinkie, but Dinkie, in an unexpected twist, began to snog with the BBC's Don Latham. Norman and man-eating Cynthia were already locked in a voracious marital embrace as Cynthia settled down to her customary picnic, and out of the corner of my eye I saw Simon the horse-lover jump on Emma-Louise with such gusto that I could almost hear him thinking: tally-ho! Meanwhile Robert, balked of Dinkie, had sensibly decided to settle for that nice girl Holly Carr, and Marina, as if to show Christian she could survive well enough without him, was marching towards me with her head held high. But when she passed the door which led to the stairs Michael ambushed her and she surrendered with relief. Trust Michael Ashworth, I reflected not unamused, to wind up smooching with the belle of the ball.

Drifting away from them I reached the north side of the Cathedral and paused to stare at the city beyond the walls of the Close. At that point I could no longer see my companions, who were all on the south side; the vaulted roof of the nave towered between us as I stood on the north walkway and leaned against the parapet. I sighed, savouring my solitude, and gazing over the city I prepared to abandon myself to the most delicious luxury of dreaming about the man I loved.

A footfall sounded behind me. My solitude shattered. Too late I realised I was trapped. Then as a shadow fell across the parapet beside me the dreaded voice said hoarsely: 'Venetia!' and Eddie Hoffenberg moved in for the kill.

X

'Venetia, I must talk to you!'

'Oh God, Eddie, not now!'

'Yes, now, I must speak, I must – Venetia, you're the most tremendous girl I've ever met but I've never dared say so because I know you think I'm so ugly and I know how your father hates Germans –'

'Eddie, this is sheer masochism!'

'No, it isn't, it's sheer courage at last! Venetia, as soon as I saw you tonight I thought you were so beautiful, so radiant, so heroic –'

'Heroic? That makes me sound like a twenty-stone Wagnerian opera singer!'

'I'm sorry, heroic's the wrong word, I'm in such a state that my English has broken down –'

'Well, run away and mend it.'

'Venetia –'

'I'm sorry, I know I'm being beastly, but I simply can't cope –'

'You don't have to cope. Just say you'll marry me. Venetia, I adore you, I'm demented with passion, I dream of you night and day –'

I tried to run away. He grabbed me. I shrieked: 'Let me go!' and struggled violently, but his awful, flapping, great wet mouth descended on mine in a nightmare of revolting intimacy. I lashed out blindly with my foot. He recoiled with a yelp.

Slapping him I wrenched myself free and dashed around the roof. All the snoggers looked up startled as I crashed by. Flinging wide the door I shot down the stairs and hurtled into the shadowy splendour of the transept. Moonlight was now pouring into the nave. Great sobs tore at my throat but somehow I managed to blunder across the transept and grope my way through the darkness of the northern aisle to the Dean's door. At last my fingers closed on the handle. I heaved the door open, I staggered outside – and I cannoned straight into a man who was about to enter the Cathedral.

But before I could even draw breath to scream he was grasping me reassuringly. 'It's all right!' he said at high speed. 'It's all right, it's all right – it's only me!'

I cried: 'Oh, Mr Dean!' and with all my defences utterly destroyed I collapsed sobbing against his chest.

XI

'Oh, Mr Dean!' I cried again, controlling my sobs but not my desolation as he continued to clasp me firmly. 'Why is life always so bloody unfair, why am I always getting kicked in the teeth, why does every attempt I make to be successful wind up in failure – no, don't tell me I'm so lucky, so rich, so privileged, don't talk to me about the starving millions in India, I don't want to know about the starving millions in India, I need all my strength to survive my own starvation, because what's the point of being rich and privileged if you're not loved, and I've never been loved, never, no one's ever really understood but I've been so lonely, I've felt as if I've been locked up in a prison on the edge of life, and I've tried and tried to escape – and then tonight I really thought I'd done it, I thought I'd made it to freedom at last, and I was so happy, being accepted by a group of my sort of people, and it was all so wonderful, so perfect – and so beautiful up there on the roof – and I didn't even mind when everyone paired off and started snogging because I didn't actually want to smooch with anyone, it was enough that everyone accepted me as one of their set, and I was just thinking it was the happiest night of my entire life – except for that unforgettable night in the Hebrides, of course, when we danced to Elvis Presley – and in fact I was just wishing you could have been there on the roof with me when that *oaf* Eddie Hoffenberg crashed in and staged this ghastly love-scene which ended in his proposing marriage and slobbering all over me – and oh God, it was *foul* and worse still, *farcical*, I felt any audience would have passed out laughing because the scene was so bathetic – and although I didn't mean to be unkind to him, I was, I was beastly because it was just such a nightmare being slobbered over by someone who's physically repulsive, and I know you're thinking I should be grateful to be loved by anyone, even Eddie, but I'm not grateful, I'm not, I just want to scream with despair because no *real* man has ever found me attractive and I'm sure now no *real* man ever will, and I'm sorry, I do realise I shouldn't mind so much, but I do mind, Mr Dean, I mind terribly because it seems so wrong that I should have so much love and no *real* man to give it to –'

Eddie burst panting through the door in an agony of anxiety and remorse.

XII

'Venetia, I – good heavens, Stephen!' He shied away in shock.

'Hullo, Eddie,' said Aysgarth, very casual. 'Having fun?'

'My God!' The expletive, forbidden for a clergyman, revealed the depth of Eddie's horror. 'Has the Bishop been looking out of his bedroom window at the South Canonry?'

'No, fortunately for you I was telephoned by a star-gazing master at the Choir School.'

'Stephen, I'm so sorry, I – I can't think why I let them all in, but it was just such a wonderful party and –'

'Quite. Now get them all out before the Bishop steams up here to defrock us both.'

'Yes, Stephen. Yes, of course. Yes, straight away. Venetia –'

'Oh, don't you worry about Venetia,' said Aysgarth. 'I'll take care of her.'

'Yes,' said Eddie. 'Yes. All right. Thanks.' He stumbled back into the Cathedral and we listened to the sound of his footsteps as they receded into the distance.

At last the silence was absolute. It was too dark for me to see Aysgarth's face as we both stood in the shadow of the north wall. I could only wait in an agony of shame for him to pass judgement on my disgusting emotional outburst, but just as I was thinking hysterically that I could bear the silence no longer, he said in a tone of voice he had never used to me before: 'My dearest Venetia,' and then I knew he had moved through the looking-glass to join me in an utterly different world.

PART TWO

———◆◆◆———

THE SERPENT

'For nothing can of itself always be labelled as "wrong". One cannot, for instance, start from the position "sex relations before marriage" or "divorce" are wrong or sinful in themselves. They may be in 99 cases or even 100 cases out of 100, but they are not intrinsically so, for the only intrinsic evil is lack of love.'

JOHN A. T. ROBINSON
Suffragan Bishop of Woolwich 1959–1969
Honest to God

ONE

I

'My dearest Venetia,' said Aysgarth, setting aside the past, transforming the present and redesigning the future, 'it does indeed seem very unfair that you should have to endure such unhappiness, but never think there isn't at least one person who understands exactly how you feel and who cares deeply what happens to you.'

I tried to reply but speech proved impossible. I was now crying soundlessly, the tears streaming down my cheeks. Without thinking I rubbed my eyes with my hand, and then remembered – too late – that I was wearing eye make-up. Without doubt my face was now a mess. My tears welled faster than ever.

Then he gripped my hands. As he said: 'I'll take you back to the Chantry,' I was acutely aware that his fingers were very strong and very hot. They clasped mine so hard that I quite literally reeled, stumbling off balance, turning my ankle and snapping the heel of my shoe.

'Oh God –'

'It's all right, I've got you.' He gathered me in his arms. I almost passed out.

'Sorry – tight as an owl – can't seem to keep upright –'

'Never mind, at least one of us is resolutely vertical!'

We laughed. My tears had stopped. The possibility of recovering my equilibrium no longer seemed fantastic.

'What's happened to your shoe?' he was saying.

'Accidental death.' I stepped out of both shoes and he promptly released me in order to pick them up. I was now the same height as he was, and suddenly he seemed much closer.

Carrying my shoes in one hand he clasped my fingers again with the other and we began to walk out of the shadow of the Cathedral. The ground beneath my feet was cool and damp but of course I was walking on air so I barely noticed. With my free hand I tried to wipe the smudged eye make-up from my cheekbones. We said nothing. His fingers seemed hotter and stronger than ever.

We crossed the North Walk, we crossed Choristers' Green, we crossed the little lane which ran past the Chantry's front gate. The moonlight seemed blindingly white, and when we turned at last to face each other I could clearly see the downward curve of his sultry mouth. The expression in his eyes was inscrutable.

All he said was: 'I think Lady Mary Calthrop-Ponsonby requests the pleasure of our company after evensong tomorrow.'

I nodded. He handed me my shoes. I took them and opened the gate.

'Are you all right now?'

'Oh yes,' I said. 'Very much so.'

We smiled at each other. Then he began to walk briskly away towards the Deanery.

II

The Orgy rolled on till dawn, but I barely noticed. I repaired my make-up, slipped into another pair of shoes, smoked a cigarette and savoured my euphoria. Eventually the Coterie floated back to the Chantry but to my relief there was no sign of Eddie.

'Gone home to do penance for permitting an orgy on consecrated ground,' said Christian, giving me a penetrating look. 'I must see Father tomorrow and claim full responsibility . . . Are you all right, Venetia?'

Before I could reply Marina cornered me. 'Darling, do tell! Did Eddie try and rape you? What was going on? Why did you rush off the roof like a bat out of hell?'

'Eddie always drives me mad,' I said with a yawn. 'He just drove me madder than usual, that's all.' And then driven by the urge to escape I tottered upstairs and passed out. God knows what happened as the Orgy drew to a close, but probably not very much. It was, after all, 1963, not that anarchic year 1968 and certainly not the year afterwards when everyone bucketed around burbling: ''Sixty-nine is divine!' What a bore social life became – which is no doubt why I look back on Marina's Orgy with such uncharacteristically heavy nostalgia.

The next morning I rose early, my hang-over soon negated by a potent combination of Alka-Seltzer and euphoria, and wondered if I was feeling energetic enough to buy a newspaper, but in the end I merely lay on my bed and thought of Aysgarth. At noon Marina appeared, looking fragile. Dinkie, Emma-Louise and Holly remained stacked in the spare-room for another hour but eventually they too emerged, looking vanquished by Veuve Clicquot. I had to be careful not to appear too hale and hearty when I eventually gave them a lift to the station.

Time crawled on. The housekeeper and the charwoman, both heavily tipped, finished cleaning up the mess. At three o'clock I picked a flower and meditated on the ravishing symmetry of its petals. The sun shone. The birds sang. Drinking some tea I gazed in rapture at the Cathedral.

Sunday evensong was at four o'clock, and never in my life had a church service seemed more meaningful. I listened to every note sung by the choir, every word of the prayers and lessons. Phrase after phrase of the Collects, the Magnificat – even the Nunc Dimittis – seemed impregnated with a new and glorious meaning. As I tried not to look too often at Aysgarth I resolved recklessly to ignore the risk of being dubbed a religious maniac and to attend evensong every day. Let everyone think I was experiencing a religious conversion! Why not? Other people experienced religious conversions. It happened all the time. Indeed perhaps I really was experiencing a religious conversion: I certainly felt God had decided to take some notice of me at last, and if God was now playing an active role in my life, surely I had a moral duty to be as devout as possible in order to express my gratitude?

I had just reached this virtuous conclusion when the service ended. The hour had come. Slipping away along the transept I heaved open the great door into the cloisters and skimmed down the north colonnade towards Lady Mary's seat on the edge of the lawn.

III

Birds were singing in the cedar tree. The sky had clouded over, though the air was still warm, and the colonnades were empty save for two tourists who were examining memorial tablets. Sitting on Lady Mary I watched them inch their way around the quadrangle. They were on the point of disappearing through the door into the nave when Aysgarth finally emerged from the transept.

He was looking exceptionally smart. His hair had been combed. He was wearing a well-pressed suit and highly polished shoes. His brisk, authoritative walk created an impression of power and confidence. He exuded a subtle air of distinction. As I repressed my desire to rush headlong into his arms a voice in my head was whispering in awe: this is the Dean of Starbridge, *the Dean of Starbridge*, and the Dean of Starbridge at present wants to see me more than anyone else in the world.

'Sorry to be so long,' he said, rapidly covering the last yards that separated us. 'I was buttonholed by the Bishop in the vestry. That row over the coach-park is still going on.'

'Are you winning?'

'Of course!' He smiled radiantly. Then he sat down, positioning himself so that his right thigh was at least six inches from my left, and folded his hands primly in his lap. 'So!' he said, giving me a hot look with his steamy blue eyes. 'How are you today?'

'Indescribably better.' I too smiled radiantly, but he did not see me. He was too busy taking a quick look around the cloisters to make sure we were alone.

'Good.' Reassured of our solitude he relaxed but for some reason refused to look at me. I supposed he wanted to ensure that the scene remained dignified and civilised. At once I resolved to be indestructibly nonchalant to signal to him that I was aware of his great eminence, that I understood his wish to remain unemotional in a public place and that I was not the kind of woman who indulged in embarrassing scenes.

'Have you heard from Eddie?' he said idly, flicking a speck of dust from his cuff.

'A pathetic little note of apology was pushed through the letter-box this morning. I felt lower than the lowliest worm.'

'You can't help it if you don't love him.' He gazed at the cedar tree as if it had developed an immense fascination for him. 'And talking of love –' He clasped his hands together tightly '– Christian said you told him last night that you were keen on someone else. He wondered if the man might be Marina's brother, since that would explain your rather unlikely new friendship with Marina herself, and this seemed to me to be a plausible theory.'

I managed to say: 'Believe me, I'm not dying of unrequited love for Douglas Markhampton.' I had suddenly realised that despite the hints I had dropped in my impassioned monologue he was still so unsure of my feelings that he felt driven to proceed with extreme caution. I wanted to shout: 'It's you, *you*, YOU!' but of course I said nothing. I merely continued to loll on Lady Mary as if I hadn't a care in the world.

Meanwhile Aysgarth was savouring his relief that I was uninterested in Douglas Markhampton. As I watched, his clasped hands parted and his thick strong fingers uncurled themselves until they were resting lightly on his thighs. Then he said: 'I don't see why you should die of unrequited love for anyone. Love should always be reciprocated in some form or another. It's too precious to waste.'

'You mean,' I said, wilfully obtuse in an effort to preserve my nonchalance, 'I should somehow reciprocate Eddie's grand passion?'

'Oh, love can't be made to order, of course,' said Aysgarth hastily. 'All you can do there, I'm afraid, is be kind.'

'I've certainly no wish to be unkind.' I was watching his fingers curling and uncurling on his thighs. 'But surely when people are plunging around in a sex-frenzy they're not interested in mere kindness?'

'Sex, I agree,' said Aysgarth primly to the cedar tree, 'presents enormous problems, but in the end it's love, not sex, that makes the world go round. I don't mean to denigrate sex, of course; God made the world and it was good, as the Bible says, and this means that sex is fundamentally good too, but love doesn't always require a sexual expression. Indeed love can transcend sex altogether.'

'Honestly, Mr Dean, I think Eddie's a long way from transcending sex!'

'He needs time to cool off, but perhaps later some form of friendship might be possible for you both. Of course there are those who declare that a true, loving friendship which transcends sex is impossible for any normal man or woman,' said Aysgarth, interlocking his fingers again. 'They say that in the garden of life sex is always the serpent lurking in the undergrowth to corrupt Beauty and Truth and Goodness, but I reject that kind of cynical, pessimistic view of the world. Even a serpent can be tamed and domesticated because with love nothing's impossible. In *Honest to God* Bishop Robinson says –'

'I've simply got to read this masterpiece!' I exclaimed, recklessly casting aside my nonchalance. 'So far I've only read him quoting St Augustine's slogan: "Love God and do what you like."'

'Ah yes, but laymen so often misunderstand that command –'

'It doesn't mean, does it, that you can jump into bed with

whoever you like just so long as you turn up in church on Sunday?'

'Hardly!' He had at last relaxed; I thanked God for theology. 'It means that if you love God – which is the purest, noblest sort of love – you should be able to love your fellow-men in the same way and then the love will both protect you from sin and steer you into the paths of righteousness. "Love God and do what you will" thus becomes "Love God and you'll automatically do the right thing" – and Robinson's relating that principle to what the Germans call *Situationethik*: he's saying that in moral dilemmas there are no hard and fast rules and that each situation should be regarded as unique; he's saying that love – the best kind of love – should be the only guiding light in seeking a resolution of moral problems.'

'So love – the best kind of love – is the highest reality we can know?'

'Certainly, and it's there that we find God. God is Love – and Love, as Robinson points out so truthfully, can be found within the best human relationships. Therefore a truly loving relationship, whatever the context, can never be wrong.'

'But supposing two people love each other,' I said, 'and one happens to be married to someone else?'

'Adultery,' said Aysgarth, smoothing the material of his trousers over his thighs with strong sensual movements of his fingers, 'is prima facie wrong. That we all know. But if, for example, a married man found himself in a *truly* loving relationship with a woman who was not his wife, there would be no adultery because he would love that woman enough to abstain from any behaviour which was morally wrong.' Suddenly, quite without warning, he swivelled to face me and our thighs brushed. At once we gave galvanic starts and he glanced hastily around the colonnades, but we were still unobserved and a second later he was saying in his most urgent voice:

'Love's one of the ultimate prizes of life so it must never be torn up and chucked away. An illicit love must be transformed; a licit love must be exalted. Christians have always laid such emphasis on love. Tertullian tells us that in the days of the Early

171

Church the pagans used to say: "See how those Christians love one another!" Love's the key-note in Christianity, and Robinson's emphasising that fact in order to bring Christianity up to date so that it can speak afresh to modern man. God isn't out there in space, says Robinson, He's here, He's within the world, He's the very ground of our being. "See how those Christians *love* one another!" says Tertullian, quoting the pagans. Christianity conquered that pagan world – and why? Because it was a religion based on love, the best kind of love, the love everyone needs in order to thrive and become whole. Sometimes it's possible for that love to have a sexual context, sometimes it isn't, but as I said just now, it's love, not sex, that makes the world go round. You told me last night how starved you were without love, and now I want more than anything else in the world to bring that starvation to an end. *"See how those Christians love one another!"* God's in every truly loving relationship. He's here now, with us.'

He stopped abruptly and there was a pause before he exclaimed with an awkward laugh: 'What a sermon! Forgive me – I didn't mean to behave as if I were in the pulpit.' To my amazement he even began to blush, smoothing back his hair in an agony of embarrassment and staring furiously at his shoes as if he feared he had made a fool of himself.

'My darling Mr Dean,' I said, so touched by this wholly unexpected vulnerability that my eyes filled with tears, 'you can preach to me as often as you wish for as long as you like, and I hope it'll be *very* often and for *very* long.'

He finally dared to look at me again. Then overwhelmed by the unspoken message which must have been emanating from every line of my face, he dared to believe the unbelievable. Automatically he grabbed my hand and tried to speak but no words came. I found I was tongue-tied too. We could only sit clutching each other, my left hand locked in his right, but at last he managed to say: 'You're a wonderful girl – and if Eddie's the only man under forty who can see that, I despair of the younger generation.'

'Who cares about the younger generation?' I retorted, so racked by the urge to fling myself into his arms that I hardly knew what I was saying. 'I certainly don't!'

He smiled. Then suddenly he began to radiate confidence. 'If I write to you,' he said, 'will you write back?'

'Instantly. But Mr Dean, don't tell me that our new friendship is to be solely confined to letters!'

'Perish the thought! But it won't be easy for us to meet on our own, and —'

He broke off. Far away in the north-east corner of the cloisters the transept door had closed with a thud and the next moment footsteps were ringing out in the colonnade. My view of the intruder was hidden by the pillars but Aysgarth, dropping my hand as if it had scalded him, signalled that danger was at hand. At once I assumed my most languid expression and pretended to examine a fingernail.

'Yes, well, to return to my earlier remarks,' said Aysgarth as if we were engaged in an earnest intellectual discussion, 'Bishop Robinson has studied the work of three German theologians, Tillich, Bultmann and — oh hullo, Charles! I thought you'd gone home.'

Looking unexpectedly modern in a grey suit, the Bishop glided to a halt by Lady Mary. To indicate his episcopal rank he was wearing a purple stock and pectoral cross, but he seemed less intimidating without his old-fashioned uniform and I was surprised when I realised I was nervous.

'As a matter of fact I did set off for home,' he was saying in response to Aysgarth's remark, 'but then I remembered I wanted to look up a reference for a sermon. I've just paid a quick visit to the library.'

There was a pause during which Aysgarth and I somehow restrained ourselves from staring in horror at the library windows which faced us above the east colonnade. Indeed I was still gazing at the Bishop as if driven to memorise every line on his face when he added in his pleasantest voice: 'Did you enjoy your party last night, Venetia?'

'Oh, enormously!' I said, producing my best friendly smile

as my heart began to thump. 'I'm so glad Michael was able to come!'

'It was nice of you to invite him,' said the Bishop, smooth as glass. 'I was talking to someone at the Choir School this morning, and he seemed to think the party was really rather exceptional.'

Aysgarth at once cleared his throat and made a great business of examining his watch. 'Good heavens, look at the time! Venetia my dear –'

'Yes, of course, Mr Dean,' I said swiftly. 'I'm sure you've got a thousand and one things to do. Thanks so much for sparing the time to talk to me about Bishop Robinson.'

'How much longer will you be staying at the Chantry, Venetia?' said Dr Ashworth suddenly as Aysgarth rose to his feet.

'Until Lady Markhampton returns in ten days' time.'

'And then, I assume, you'll be heading back to London?'

'No.' I was acutely aware of Aysgarth pausing, unable to resist the temptation to listen to my reply. 'I'm going to get a flat.'

'Here?' said the Bishop surprised. 'In Starbridge? Does this mean you've been offered some exceptional secretarial post?'

'No, although naturally I hope –'

'Oh, you'll need an interesting job or you'll soon be very bored! There's not much in provincial old Starbridge, is there, Stephen, to keep a sophisticated young woman like Venetia amused!'

'I think Venetia might want rather more from life, Charles,' said Aysgarth equably, 'than mere sophisticated entertainment. Perhaps you could find her a job at the diocesan office?'

'Perhaps I could. If that's what she wants.' With his most charming smile he added to me: 'Come and see us again at the South Canonry! I'll ask my wife to phone you and fix a date.' And before I could do more than murmur a conventional word of thanks he had gone, striding away from us without a backward glance and disappearing through the door which led into the churchyard.

'Glory!' I muttered. 'Do you think he looked out of the library window and saw us holding hands?'

'Why shouldn't we hold hands?' retorted Aysgarth. 'Aren't we old friends? *Honi soit qui mal y pense!*'

'But –'

'Personally I'm more worried about the star-gazing master at the Choir School who's apparently been unable to resist bleating to Charles about last night's rooftop revels. That could have a very adverse effect on the coach-park struggle.'

'It could?'

'Yes, Charles could say to me: "If you can't stop your own family running riot with their friends in the Cathedral, how can I trust you to control the occupants of ten coaches parked simultaneously in Palace Lane?"'

'Honestly, Mr Dean, I can't think how you keep so sane amidst all these brawls and back-stabbings –'

'I've simply no time to go mad – which reminds me, I must dash home because a dozen people are coming for drinks. But when am I going to see you again?'

'I could attend Communion tomorrow. That would set the Bishop's mind at rest.'

'I'd stop worrying about Charles, if I were you.'

'But if he looked out of the window just now –'

'I'm sure he didn't. The last thing any dedicated academic does in a library is look out of a window.'

'All the same it might be politic if –'

'My darling, you mustn't attend Communion merely to re-assure the Bishop! That wouldn't be right.'

After I had recovered from the delicious shock of being addressed as 'my darling' I managed to mumble: 'I want to attend Communion to try to be a better Christian. If Christianity's all about finding God in loving relationships, then I want to be a far better Christian than I've ever been before.'

This pleased him. He gave my hand an approving squeeze before saying: 'Stay on in St Anselm's chapel after the service tomorrow and I'll slip back from the vestry to meet you.' In a burst of enthusiasm he added: 'I can't tell you how much I enjoy talking to you – your destiny is obviously to be my Egeria!'

'The name rings a bell but I can't quite –'

'She was a great listener.' He clasped both my hands as we faced each other. I had remembered to wear flat shoes so I was the perfect height to gaze into his eyes.

'St Anselm's chapel,' he managed to say after an emotional silence. 'Tomorrow morning at eight.'

I nodded, once more beyond speech, and we went our separate ways.

IV

I staggered back to the Chantry where I found Marina reclining on the sofa in a dusty-pink negligée and indulging in one of her lengthy phone conversations; the faint squeak of a voice (male) was audible as I drifted past the receiver. When the squeak ceased Marina said: 'Michael, how wonderful! I'd adore it,' and stopped caressing a strand of her blonde hair in order to wave at me buoyantly. I deduced the Bishop's son was trying to line her up for another pounce. Vaguely I wondered if the Bishop himself had ever pounced around in his youth, but the thought of Dr Ashworth behaving in a manner which could be described as sexually seamy was quite inconceivable.

The next thing I knew I was in my room and collapsing in a heap on my bed. I was in a stupor of ecstasy. The Dean of Starbridge – *the Dean of Starbridge* – had said I was wonderful. In other words – and I had to rephrase this sentence in order to savour its extraordinary content to the full – a brilliant, successful, attractive man had expressed a genuine admiration for me. Perhaps he even loved me, although of course I knew it would be unwise to assume this without further evidence that his feelings ran deeper than mere compassionate affection – and of course I knew I had no right to expect so much. But nevertheless he had said I was 'wonderful' and called me 'my darling'. How intoxicating! I could still barely grasp the dimensions of my changed universe; I felt I could only gaze in amazement at the cosmic vista which had unfolded before my eyes.

Finding a sheet of writing-paper I printed: 'N. N. Aysgarth. Norman Neville Aysgarth. Neville Aysgarth. Stephen Aysgarth.' So many designations! For good measure I added all the titles he had had during his career. 'The Reverend N. N. Aysgarth.' (That described him when he had been a vicar.) 'The Venerable N. N. Aysgarth.' (That covered the years as Archdeacon.) 'The Reverend Canon N. N. Aysgarth.' (That dealt with Westminster Abbey.) 'The Very Reverend the Dean of Starbridge' –

The Dean of Starbridge! And *me*! Carefully I drew a little heart, pierced it with a delicately etched arrow and wrote VENETIA at one end and NNA at the other. Never before had so trivial a doodle afforded me such immense satisfaction, and as I contemplated those magic initials my excitement reached new heights. Never mind that he had a wife. Never mind that he was a clergyman, a fact which prohibited anything so unspiritual as a full-scale adulterous love-affair. At least – thanks to Bishop Robinson – we could indulge in a high-minded love, a romantic self-denial and countless erotic meetings . . . However, it seemed unlikely that the Bishop of Woolwich had openly advocated eroticism when he had outlined his scheme for a new morality based on the noblest form of love. Picking up my copy of *Honest to God*, which had somehow become buried beneath the latest James Bond novel, the current copy of *New Musical Express* and *Lady Chatterley's Lover*, I opened the book and scanned the chapter on ethics. A heading announced: 'Nothing Prescribed – Except Love.' What a prescription! Enthralled I read on:

'This position, foreshadowed thirty years ago in Emil Brunner's great book *The Divine Imperative*, is given its most consistent statement I know in an article by Professor Joseph Fletcher in the *Harvard Divinity Bulletin*, entitled "The New Look in Christian Ethics". "Christian Ethics," he says, "is not a scheme of codified conduct. It is a purposive effort to relate love to a world of relativities through a casuistry obedient to . . ."'

I lost interest. It was really amazing how those theologians could make even a subject like love seem boring. Tossing the book aside I paused only to burn my fevered jottings in the ash-tray and then I began to dream of a future in which nothing was prescribed except love.

V

The Bishop was absent from Communion the next morning, but I knew that only Anglo-Catholics were in the habit of attending 'mass', as they called it, every day. Aysgarth, being Low-Church by inclination, privately considered it quite unnecessary to attend Communion except on Sundays and special Holy Days, but since the Bishop always turned up at least twice during the week Aysgarth too, not to be outdone, appeared with a similar regularity in St Anselm's chapel for the weekday services of matins at seventhirty and Communion at eight. This spiritual one-upmanship would have been amusing if it had not reflected the antipathy between the two men, but in view of their strained relationship the situation could only seem unfortunate. I felt sorry for my Mr Dean being burdened with a bishop he disliked, and I felt wary of Dr Ashworth who I suspected might well harbour a ruthless streak behind his steel-plated charm. The desire to keep on the right side of such a formidable figure was strong, and I was sorry that I had no opportunity that morning to impress him by my presence at Communion.

I was also disappointed that the celebrant was not the Dean himself but the current canon-in-residence, Fitzgerald; Aysgarth merely assisted him. (Fortunately there was no sign of Eddie.) I did try to follow the service carefully in my Prayer-book, but I was feeling so exalted that I continually lost my place and had a hard time keeping up with the other members of the small congregation, the retired clergy and withered old women who seemed to fill up so many nooks and crannies in the Cathedral

Close. I must have been the youngest person present by at least thirty years.

I had never felt entirely comfortable with the Communion service. It had always conjured up for me images of cannibalism, and I had been accustomed to justifying my repulsion by arguing that we can't all find certain symbols equally meaningful. However, I was now so transformed by my new universe that I discovered even my attitude to Communion had changed. How could I have found that beautiful symbolism repulsive? How very far astray I must have been – in fact, how had I even dared to call myself a Christian? I resolved to turn over a new leaf. When my turn came to approach the altar-rail I remembered my confirmation classes, took the sacrament reverently and sank to my knees to pray as soon as I returned to my seat.

A shaft of sunlight penetrated the chapel and emphasised the delicate lines of the vaulted ceiling. Love, Truth, Beauty – the absolute values – all were present, Love represented by Aysgarth, Truth by the service which pointed to Christ, Beauty in the architecture of the chapel. How futile the Orgy seemed in retrospect, how meaningless and trivial! Eating too much, drinking too much, running around after men and thinking of nothing but sex – what an intolerable waste of time such pursuits were when there was this other world waiting to be explored! I could now clearly see that this other world was the true reality. Everything else was mere illusion.

I was still pondering on these radical thoughts when the service ended; Fitzgerald and Aysgarth padded off behind the verger to the vestry and all the old dears in the congregation tottered home to breakfast. I waited, watching the sunlight and mentally reciting religious poetry. I was just skimming through Blake's 'Jerusalem' and had reached the line: 'Bring me my arrows of desire!' when Aysgarth slipped back into the chapel.

'We'll go to the library,' he said as I sprang to my feet. 'The Librarian's never there before nine-thirty so we'll have the place to ourselves.'

'Let's hope the Bishop isn't about to look up another reference!'

He laughed and we left the chapel together. There were two cleaning women at work, one flicking a duster in the nave and the other pushing a droning Hoover over the carpet by the high altar, but no one else was in sight as we crossed the transept to the door which opened on to the library staircase. On the landing above the first flight, the stairs continued upwards to the gallery which encircled the nave, but Aysgarth ignored them, advanced to the double doors ahead of us and produced a key. The door swung wide. We entered the library.

It was a long room, very old, with a vaulted ceiling and that special musty smell of ancient paper and antiquated leather. Books lined the walls and beyond the Librarian's table I saw the chained manuscripts, treasures so precious that the pre-Reformation canons had tethered them to the reading-desks. On the west side of the room the long thin windows looked across the lawn of the cloisters to the wooden seat donated by Lady Mary.

'Have you been here before?' Aysgarth was saying as he closed the door.

'When you first became Dean you gave me and my parents a guided tour.'

'So I did! But did I show you the cat?'

'Cat?'

'He's a doodle in our most famous manuscript, one of the earliest copies of St Anselm's *Prayers and Meditations*. The first Bishop of Starbridge somehow managed to extort it from the monks at Canterbury.' Moving to one of the chained treasures he opened the manuscript at a place which was already marked, and when I drew closer I saw illuminated capital letters, lines of pale brown unreadable script and, in the left margin, an exquisite little painting of a cat with a mouse in his mouth.

'He's been under discussion lately,' said Aysgarth as I exclaimed in admiration. 'I want to have coloured picture-postcards of him made to sell in the Cathedral shop, but I've met with opposition in Chapter. Fitzgerald said Puss-in-Boots here was neither a pertinent nor a reverent representation of St Anselm's mighty work, and Dalton agreed with him.'

'Honestly, Mr Dean, how square – and how stupid!'

'My darling, you can't go on calling me Mr Dean when we're alone together! Call me Stephen.'

I said at once: 'Oh no. Not Stephen. That's *her* name for you.'

There was a silence. He looked away and lightly fingered the edge of the manuscript. My heart gave a massive thud.

'And anyway,' I added rapidly, 'don't you think it would be a mistake if I got into the habit of calling you by your Christian name? Supposing I slipped up in public. Primrose would say: "Oh Venetia, why are you suddenly addressing Father as if he were someone of our generation?" And your wife would immediately deduce –'

'We mustn't talk of my wife,' said Aysgarth. 'The morality of the situation demands that we never discuss her.'

With an enormous effort I managed to avoid a second deadly silence. In my most casual voice I said: 'Okay, fine. If that's the way the cookie crumbles, so be it.'

At once he laughed in delight and the tension vanished. 'What a marvellous phrase!' he exclaimed. 'Where did it come from?'

'It's one of Dinkie's gems. She's an American pal of Marina's and was one of the guests at the Orgy.'

'I want to hear about this Orgy!' said Aysgarth, reaching out to clasp my hands. 'Let's sit down on the window-seat and luxuriate in a long gossip!'

'How exciting that sounds, Mr Dean!'

'Neville – please! I insist! It'll be such a change to become Neville again – but wait a minute, which Neville am I? I've been several Nevilles in my time.'

'Well, now you can be a new one, specially for me.'

I had spoken flippantly but I had enthralled him. 'A new Neville!' he exclaimed, and gazed at me as if I had opened some indescribably alluring Pandora's box. Then tightening his grasp on my hands he declared buoyantly: 'What a stimulating prospect – and now stimulate me further by telling me all about the Orgy!'

I laughed, unable to resist his high spirits, and firmly setting

aside the queasiness which had assailed me when he had refused
to discuss his wife, I began to describe the revels of Marina's
Coterie.

VI

Half an hour later at a quarter past nine someone, thinking the
double doors were locked, inserted a key and tried to walk in.

'Quick!' whispered Aysgarth, 'Puss-in-Boots!'

We raced silently to the reading-desk and by the time the
Librarian had worked out that the doors were already unlocked
we were gazing in rapture at the little painted cat.

'And the truth is,' said Aysgarth in ringing tones, 'the scribe
almost certainly got bored with copying the manuscript, and –
oh hullo, Gilbert! You're early this morning!'

'I have to leave early this evening to go to the dentist.' The
Librarian, a faded little wisp of a man wearing horn-rimmed
spectacles and a suit which smelt of mothballs, was looking
anxiously at me as if he feared he ought to remember who I
was.

'Venetia, this is Mr Pryce,' said Aysgarth. 'Gilbert – Miss
Flaxton. I was just showing her our famous cat.'

'Oh, I see,' said the Librarian in the voice of one who was
obviously baffled.

'Well, thank you so much, Mr Dean,' I said. 'I mustn't take
up any more of your valuable time.'

'Not at all. I'll just escort you downstairs –'

'Oh, please don't trouble –'

'It's no trouble whatsoever!'

We escaped.

'That was bad luck,' muttered Aysgarth on the stairs. 'Let's
step into the cloisters for a moment. He won't see us if we stay
beneath the library in the east colonnade.'

Seconds later we were gazing across the lawn to Lady Mary.

'Before we part,' Aysgarth was saying, 'we really must solve
the problem of where we can meet without the Bishop, all three

residentiary Canons and the entire Cathedral staff tripping over us with remorseless regularity.'

'There's an obvious solution,' I said at once. 'My time at the Chantry's running out, and when I get a flat –'

'Oh, I could never visit you there.'

I was stunned. 'You couldn't?'

'No, much too dangerous. I'm well-known in Starbridge, my visits might be noted, and besides . . . We have to remember that serpent, the one who's gliding alongside us in our beautiful garden and wearing a collar and leash like a well-behaved pet. If I really love you – and of course I do – I've no option but to keep that serpent under control.'

'But if you can't come to my flat –'

'How I wish you could come to the Deanery as my secretary! But I don't see how I can fire dear old Miss Trotman. She's served under three deans, and . . . dear me, how improper that sounds!' He began to shake with laughter.

'But I don't see how I could possibly accept a job as your secretary . . .' I started to giggle. His laughter was very infectious.

'No, you couldn't. I'm fantasising. Now let me see –'

'Do you have a day off?'

'Certainly! Clergymen who work twenty-four hours a day seven days a week always wind up being no use to anyone.'

'Well, in that case –'

'– we'll meet on Wednesday afternoons. Why don't I take you for a drive? Usually on Wednesdays I just eat a big lunch, quaff a bottle of wine and snooze the afternoon away, but now's obviously the time for radical reform!'

'But won't it seem odd if you revolutionise your day off so violently?'

'I'll say the doctor's advised me to lose weight by eating light lunches, cutting back on the drink and going on little excursions once a week!' He was excited. His eyes sparkled. He gave me a radiant smile. 'Why don't we meet outside the Staro Arms at two next Wednesday?'

'Fine, but how do I communicate with you if something ghastly happens and I can't make it?'

'Ring the Deanery and say to whoever answers the phone: "Please tell the Dean that Lady Mary wishes to speak to him about the memorial tablet."'

'If only Lady Mary knew how useful she was being to us! Or at least . . . Good heavens, Mr Dean, we don't really think, do we, that Lady Mary's watching us from her own personal cloud in heaven?'

He laughed. 'My dear, Christians no longer believe in the three-decker universe with heaven above the clouds, hell below the ground and the world in between! In the opening chapters of *Honest to God* –'

'I *must* read that book –'

'I'll tell you more about it on Wednesday.'

Briefly our hands clasped. Above us the sky was a brilliant, cloudless blue, and as euphoria gripped me again I forgot about sex and marriage and all those other popular hobbies that human beings rated so highly. I remembered only that I was standing in the heart of a mighty cathedral, one of the greatest cathedrals ever built, while beside me stood its master, one of the most powerful churchmen in England, a man who had treated me as if I were truly exceptional and declared that he loved me. What more could I possibly want? Nothing. Indeed so great was my happiness that to have asked for more, I felt, could only have damned me as a monster of greed.

Skimming back to the Chantry I resolved to tackle *Honest to God* without delay.

VII

Marina was on the phone as usual. I heard her voice as soon as I entered the house, and glancing into the drawing-room I saw she was lounging on the sofa, the telephone receiver tucked casually between her left shoulder and ear as she varnished her nails. She was wearing skin-tight white trousers and a turquoise shirt and looked like an actress in one of those Hollywood films where Rock Hudson is always chasing Doris Day across massive sets with minimal results.

'But Don, of course I'm not interested in Michael!' she was saying. 'Dinner? Well, perhaps when I'm back in London, but I may be going to stay in Oxford, so . . .'

I left her driving poor Don Latham round the bend, filched a glass of milk from the kitchen and retired to my room to wrestle once more with *Honest to God*. I had just read the sentence: 'But he could use it to the spiritually sophisticated at Corinth with no consciousness that he must "demythologise" if he were to make it acceptable,' and I had just realised I had no idea either who 'he' was or what 'it' could possibly mean, when Marina, fresh from her telephonic dalliance, wafted into my room.

'I've now heard from everyone except Christian,' she said fretfully. 'I can't think why he doesn't ring.'

'Marina,' I said in my kindest voice, 'if Christian were free to chase you as everyone else does, would you still be so anxious for him to phone?'

'But Christian's not like everyone else,' she said earnestly. 'He's special.'

'In some ways, certainly. But perhaps not in others. Does he still love Katie, do you think?'

'He adores her. So do I. And she adores us – in fact we all adore each other, it's so blissful, so perfect – and so miraculous too that I've at last found a man who only wants to offer me a pure romantic love! If all the other men only knew how fed up to the back teeth I get with their pawing and pouncing and groping –'

The telephone rang. 'Christian!' shrieked Marina and pounded away to her grandmother's bedroom to take the call on the extension.

I closed *Honest to God* and decided that Marina was either very ingenuous or else raving mad. What did Christian and Katie really think of this unsought third dimension to their marital life? Perhaps they thought Marina was a colossal bore but were too kind to say so. Surely any normal, happily married young couple would fight shy of an entanglement which converted them into two sides of an eternal triangle? Moreover although Marina might be happy with her pure romantic love, it seemed unlikely that Christian would be so easily sastisfied; most men took one look at Marina and were overpowered by lust. Why wasn't Christian slavering at her feet? And why wasn't Katie offering her a poisoned chalice instead of an affectionate friendship? I was quite prepared to believe that idyllic eternal triangles could exist (usually in France) between very sophisticated middle-aged people who by their past sexual excesses had become anaesthetised to the primeval pangs of jealousy, but this triangle between a young Oxford don and two charming, well-brought-up young Englishwomen could only make the mind boggle.

I was still allowing my cynicism free rein when I remembered that I too was a member of an eternal triangle – although of course my triangle was straightforward with no mystery about it whatsoever. Dido was mad and bad. My Mr Dean was privately sick and tired of her. The marriage was a mere formality. These facts had become obvious to me over the years and had been confirmed by my holiday in the Hebrides.

But the next moment I was recalling the queasiness which had assailed me that morning when Aysgarth had refused to talk about Dido. I knew the obvious explanation for his resolute silence was that as a devout Christian he was morally bound not to speak ill of his wife, but I knew too, as I looked back upon the incident with a cool, analytical eye, that I had wondered for a split second whether he might still care for her. I had dismissed the notion at once as preposterous, but that, I now saw, had been a mere reflex action, the fobbing off of an unpalatable possibility. Supposing the marriage was a little more complicated than I had always assumed it was? Even though they no longer had sex he might still wish to keep silent not, as I had blithely supposed, out of Christian duty, but out of a genuine affection. And as in my memory I heard Eddie say: 'He married her because she amused him – and I think she still does,' I was aware of the queasiness sliding back into the pit of my stomach.

Dimly I became aware that I was no longer alone in my bedroom. Marina had returned and was saying exasperated:

'Hey, wake up, Vinnie! Have you gone deaf? The call's for you!'

'Ah.' I stood up automatically and then realised I had no idea what she was talking about. 'How was Christian?' I said, trying to conceal my confusion.

'It wasn't Christian. *The call's for you!*'

The information finally registered. 'Sorry!' I said, trying to look intelligent, but I still felt as dazed as if I had been slammed on the head – or as if Aysgarth's sedate little serpent, gliding along on his leash, had reared up to hiss straight in my face.

Outwardly casual but inwardly shattered by the twin demons of jealousy and doubt, I drifted past Marina to the telephone and discovered that my caller was none other than the Bishop's wife, Lyle Ashworth.

TWO

'Brought up with the bells of Canterbury ringing in his
ears, never doubting what he believes to be the essential
truth of Christianity, [Robinson] has been led to ask some
radical questions about his faith . . . No question can be
too radical, but one must ask whether the questions are
rightly put, as well as whether they are rightly answered,
and still more whether the answers are not incomplete.'

JOHN LAWRENCE
The Honest to God Debate
ed. DAVID L. EDWARDS

I

'Mrs Ashworth – what a surprise!' I exclaimed, somehow pulling
myself together. 'How nice of you to phone!'

'I meant to phone long ago,' said my heroine apologetically,
'but social events multiplied at just the wrong moment and then
to cap it all Charles, poor love, had to do his stint of reading
the prayers in the House of Lords – which always puts him in
such a bad mood because if he travels up to London daily the
journey exhausts him and if he stays up in town he gets cross
thinking of the work he could be doing at home. Anyway he's
recovered now, I'm glad to say, and we were wondering if by
any chance you were free to have dinner with us tonight.'

I was so intrigued by this glimpse of a rough edge to Dr
Ashworth's glass-smooth episcopal life that I was at last diverted
from jealous speculation about Dido. I said promptly: 'I'd love
to come, Mrs Ashworth! Thanks so much.'

'Splendid! Seven-thirty for dinner at eight? We'll look forward
to seeing you,' said Mrs Ashworth, perfectly sincere but now
exuding the deft social manner of a successful 'Mrs Bishop', and
with her mission accomplished she set down the receiver.

II

By the time I returned to my room I could clearly see that my queasy plunge into the pit of doubt was an emotional vagary, perhaps some form of psychological reaction to my previous unflawed euphoria. It was, of course, quite inconceivable that my Mr Dean could still care for the monster. A saintly toleration would be the most a woman like that could ever expect from her husband – who, out of sheer chivalrous good taste, would never complain about her to the woman he loved. How could I ever have succumbed to that degrading pang of jealousy? Only by first allowing myself to flirt with the notion that in an eternal triangle all might not be quite as it seemed, but I was sure now that I knew exactly where reality lay. I had him to myself; Dido was irrelevant; the serpent was under control again.

Feeling infinitely better I began to plan what I should wear that evening at the South Canonry.

III

I dressed with care in a plain green linen dress with cream-coloured accessories (belt, Italian shoes, bag, all matching) and spent half an hour applying my make-up in the hope that Mrs Ashworth would be impressed by my progress in making the best of myself. My horrible hair was at that 'in-between' stage, not short enough to be tidy, not long enough to be spectacular, but I curbed its yak-like tendencies by shoving it into a French roll and spearing it with an interesting metal object, somewhat like a miniature rake, which I had bought at Boots. Deciding that I could have looked better but that I could also have looked infinitely worse, I tottered off on my high heels to the South Canonry.

Mrs Ashworth was wearing a severely tailored navy-blue dress with a touch of white at the lapels, no jewellery and her sphinx-like smile. Her smooth, flawlessly dyed hair was immaculate and her creamy skin was a perfect example of subtle make-up. Only the unusually dark shade of her nylons hinted that she might need to cover up varicose veins, but otherwise her appearance, as always, constituted a triumph of art over age.

It was she herself who answered my ring at the front door. The episcopal cook-housekeeper, charwoman and secretary all lived out and had gone home before my arrival; the chaplain and the lay-chaplain had retired to their cottages nearby; the Bishop and Mrs Bishop were now free to pretend they were just like any other well-to-do elderly couple with two grown sons and a pleasant home in the provinces.

'How well you look, Venetia!' said my heroine, regarding me with approval. 'Positively glowing – and how clever of you to choose cream accessories for that smart dress!'

My spirits soared. I felt as if I had been awarded high marks in a vital examination.

In the drawing-room the Bishop, evidently enjoying a day off, was wandering around in a dark suit, which seemed to shout SAVILE ROW from every seam, a snow-white shirt and a dark tie adorned with a motif which I (through lack of acquaintance with Cambridge University, perhaps) failed to recognize. I suddenly realised Dr Ashworth must have a private income. He looked much too glossy to be maintained on a clerical salary, even a clerical salary of episcopal dimensions, and his wife's clothes too had the kind of simplicity which can only be achieved by a generous expenditure.

'Venetia! How nice to see you!' As he exuded his famous charm it was impossible to imagine him sulking about the chore of reading the prayers in the House of Lords, and suddenly I was more acutely aware than I had ever been of the gap existing between a private individual and his public persona. 'I'm so glad you were able to come at such short notice,' he was saying. 'May I pay you the compliment of saying how delightful you look?'

'Yes, please!' I said, thinking how odd it was that the Bishop's distinguished good-looks should leave me unmoved while the Dean could reduce me to pulp by a mere twitch of his sultry mouth.

'Drink, Venetia?' said Mrs Ashworth.

I requested a gin-and-tonic. Both the Ashworths were drinking sherry.

'I bumped into your father the other day in the House of Lords,' said the Bishop, pouring out an austere measure of gin. 'He very kindly gave me dinner.'

I tried not to look too surprised. My father, loyal to Aysgarth, was not in the habit of showering Dr Ashworth with impromptu hospitality at Westminster.

'He asked after you, of course,' said the Bishop, creating a lavish waterfall of tonic before handing me my glass, 'and I felt rather guilty that I couldn't give him more news.'

'But I've written my parents a line every week since I've been at the Chantry!'

'Yes, he said he was grateful to know you were still alive but he was anxious for more details.'

'Parents are so inquisitive,' said Mrs Ashworth casually, offering me a cigarette. 'They simply can't help themselves. Michael says it's a terrible failing.'

'Oh, but my parents aren't normally inquisitive at all!' I said, very suspicious now of my father's uncharacteristic behaviour and wondering in alarm if he was on the brink of interfering in my affairs. 'As I'm the youngest of six, they'd exhausted their capacity for being inquisitive long before I was born.'

'Heavens, Lyle!' said the Bishop, giving me a light for my cigarette. 'Where would we be now if we'd had six children?'

'In the grave,' said Mrs Ashworth, exercising a deadpan humour, and added without a pause: 'Charles did his best to reassure your father, Venetia. I don't think you need worry too much.'

'Perhaps not, but I'd better pour a little oil on the troubled waters.' Obviously my father, having concluded I was drifting along aimlessly as usual, was revving himself up to intervene on a grand scale. 'I'll ring my mother. I suppose I should have phoned before but I was waiting until I had some interesting news to impart.'

'Maybe I can provide it!' said Dr Ashworth, finally sitting

down. 'I was very struck by your disclosure yesterday that you're looking for a job in Starbridge. Would you by any chance be interested in working for me on a part-time basis?'

I nearly dropped my glass.

'Charles is anxious to write a book,' said Mrs Ashworth, following on from her husband with such effortless fluency that I was reminded of a pair of acrobats pirouetting together on the high wire, 'and since his secretary's seriously overworked he feels he can't ask her to take on such a substantial new project.'

'I'd pay the top rate, of course,' the Bishop chimed in with such perfect timing that I even began to wonder if the dialogue had been rehearsed. However, I came to the conclusion that it was not the dialogue but the stylish marital double-act which had been rehearsed, time and again, in the past whenever the Bishop and his wife had worked together on a scheme dear to both their hearts. 'I can't say for certain how long the job would last,' Dr Ashworth was adding, 'but I'd estimate a minimum of three months.'

'How very exciting!' I said, finally finding my tongue. 'Am I allowed to ask what the book will be about?'

'I intend to demolish *Honest to God* by John Robinson, the Bishop of Woolwich.'

I nearly dropped my glass again.

'Charles adores demolition work,' said his wife serenely. 'His first book demolished the Arian heresy. He's never looked back since.'

'Super!' I said. It seemed the safest banality to utter.

'The biggest difficulty about this job from your point of view,' resumed the Bishop, conveying moderate anxiety by a slight furrowing of the brow, 'is that as I'll be dictating the book in my spare time your hours will be somewhat irregular, but my wife tells me you dislike the conventional nine-to-five routine so perhaps you'll take this snag in your stride. It would be easier if I could dictate into a dictaphone, but I've never been able to establish a satisfactory working relationship with a machine.'

'So like a clergyman!' murmured his wife. 'Always has to have an audience when he holds forth.'

'Nonsense!' said the Bishop good-humouredly. 'The truth is machines encourage verbosity, whereas if one talks to human beings one has to stick to the point or else they fall asleep. I shall depend very much on the quality of your reaction,' he added to me with a smile, 'in order to gauge how accurately I'm hitting the nail on the head.'

'Robinson's supposed to be writing for the intelligent layman, benign to the Church and interested in theology,' said Mrs Ashworth, 'and Charles wants to do the same. Then he remembered you'd heard of *Soundings* and knew the meaning of *metanoia*, so –'

'– so I realised you'd be ideal for the job,' said the Bishop, turning on the full force of his charm as the Ashworth double-act pirouetted gracefully to its finale on the high wire. 'Do say you'll take it on!'

I had a quick think. At least episcopal employment would stop my father barging into my new life and accusing me of drifting. And the job would without doubt give me the best possible reason for remaining in Starbridge; any embryonic suspicions would be instantly annihilated. I had a brief vision of Aysgarth, listening with avid amusement as I recounted every detail of the Bishop's fulminations against *Honest to God*, and the next moment my mind was made up. Returning Dr Ashworth's smile I said with sincerity: 'Thanks so much, Bishop – I'm immensely flattered. When would you like me to start work?'

IV

The Bishop declared he wanted to start work as soon as possible but was then reminded gently by his wife of his numerous engagements for the coming week. Finally we agreed that I would present myself at the South Canonry on the following Monday at nine o'clock; since he took his day off on Mondays he would have the leisure to make an early start, but on Tuesdays, Wednesdays, Thursdays and Fridays he would be obliged to postpone me until five and might even be obliged to cancel me altogether if he had a long afternoon engagement. At these set times he would dictate for an hour and afterwards I could type up my notes whenever I wished. What kind of a typewriter would I like? He would hire any machine I fancied. He quite realised that a smart London secretary would expect only the best equipment.

'I'd like an IBM Electric,' I said, deciding to play up to this glamorous image he was imposing on me. In 1963 only the most favoured super-secretaries in London were blessed with this great dream-machine. 'But I don't know whether you'd be able to hire one in Starbridge.'

The Bishop said he was sure the biggest office equipment firm would be delighted to track down an IBM Electric especially for him. What a treat it would be to have a secretary who was young and up to date! He would have to take care that Miss Peabody didn't become jealous; he foresaw he was going to wind up delectably pampered.

'Yes, darling,' said Mrs Ashworth, 'but before you get carried away by your luscious masculine pipe-dream, try pampering Venetia by offering her another drink.'

I surrendered my glass with relief. I had in fact been feeling thirsty for some time.

'You must order all the stationery you need from Paige's in Chasuble Lane,' said the Bishop to me as he flashed the gin bottle at my glass and again drowned the result ruthlessly with tonic. 'Miss Peabody will give you a letter of authorisation. Incidentally, thinking of Miss Peabody, I hope I don't dictate too fast for you. She sometimes has trouble keeping up with me.'

'I have a certificate for a hundred and forty words a minute,' I said reassuringly, playing the super-secretary for all I was worth, but in fact God only knew what my shorthand speed was by that time. It was some years since I had sweated blood scribbling hieroglyphics at a breakneck pace in the classroom, and I had never bothered to sweat much blood since.

'A hundred and forty words a minute!' marvelled the Bishop.

'A real Rolls-Royce of a secretary! I doubt if Miss Peabody can even reach ninety.'

'Well, darling,' said Mrs Ashworth, rising to her feet, 'if you'll excuse me I'll leave you for a moment with your Rolls-Royce while I toss off a few miracles in the kitchen.'

Immediately the Bishop began to ask me about my past jobs. His sympathetic interest was very appealing and I had no doubt he was sincere, in the sense that he genuinely wanted to find out more about me, but nevertheless I found it quite impossible to tell whether this desire sprang from a detached curiosity or a Christian concern or a mixture of the two. I came to the conclusion that he was fundamentally unreadable. His professional persona was so strong that he resembled a book cast in bronze.

However, no sooner had I reached this sinister conclusion than his elder son telephoned from Cambridge and at once the Bishop's manner changed. The professional charm and well-oiled pastoral skills were discarded. The suave prelate vanished. In his place appeared a friendly father, relaxed, affable and unaffected. Evidently with Charley the Bishop could be himself.

'Can't wait to see you again, old chap,' he said at the end of the conversation. 'There'll be so much to talk about.'

I tried to imagine either of my parents saying such words to me but my imagination was unequal to the challenge. I could only comment lamely after the Bishop had replaced the receiver: 'I suppose that since Charley's going into the Church you have a lot in common with him.'

'That's true,' said Dr Ashworth with unexpected simplicity. 'I'm so lucky to have Charley. He's a very great blessing to me.' And then as he looked past me I glanced over my shoulder and saw Mrs Ashworth was standing in the doorway.

'So that was Charley,' she said, moving back into the room to join us. 'I was hoping it was Michael.' She smiled at me. 'Michael's like you,' she said. 'Saddled with elderly parents whom he finds incurably "square".'

'My dear Lyle!' exclaimed the Bishop, effortlessly concealing himself again behind the mask of his formidable charm. 'I'm sure Michael would remain devoted to us even if we were hexagonal! How are the miracles going in the kitchen?'

'All performed. "Dinner, my Lord," as the butlers used to say to bishops in the old days, "is served."'

I knocked back my gin-flavoured tonic and wondered anxiously if there would be wine to accompany the meal.

V

To my relief the Bishop offered me a decent claret to accompany the delicious boeuf bourguignon which, so Mrs Ashworth told me without shame, had been produced earlier by the cook-housekeeper. There were fresh vegetables and some crusty French bread. I had been indifferent to food since the onset of my grand passion, but landing a job with the Bishop had made me hungry and I now settled down to indulge in the sin of gluttony with the necessary civilised restraint.

The conversation soon began to bounce along at a brisk pace. I found myself engaged in discussing John Freeman's television programme *Face to Face*, speculating about the play based on C. P. Snow's *The Masters* (due to open in London at the end of the month), debating how far *Lord of the Flies* reflected the truth about British schoolboys, damning the architecture of the new Guildford Cathedral, analysing the brand of existentialism currently being purveyed by Jean-Paul Sartre and reflecting on Dr Ashworth's assertion that theologians should fight the impulse to hitch their wagons to the philosophy which was currently in favour among the intelligentsia.

'If I may repeat the immortal opinion held by Dean Inge,' concluded Dr Ashworth, 'he who marries the spirit of the age will quickly find himself a widower.'

'So you don't approve of Dr Robinson embracing Tillich's existentialism?' I enquired boldly, remembering a comment made by Eddie in the Hebrides. By this time I had downed two glasses of claret and staged a fighting recovery from my ethereal gin-and-tonics.

'A bishop who is apparently ignorant of various basic theological concepts – who misuses, for instance, the word "supernatural" – is most unlikely to grasp the complexities of a theologian like Tillich. What Robinson has done is to pluck some quotations from the Tillich canon and declare them to be in some way magically relevant to the 1960s. But that's not serious scholarship. That's journalism.'

'But I thought Dr Robinson *was* a serious scholar!'

'He's done some sound work on the New Testament,' conceded Dr Ashworth graciously, 'but in writing *Honest to God* he's moved right out of his depth.'

'The moral of the whole story,' said Mrs Ashworth, 'is never read avant-garde theology when you're confined to bed, as Robinson was, with a slipped disc; it can produce a fatal craving to write a scandalous book. More vegetables, Venetia?'

'No, thanks. But Bishop, surely Robinson's right to try to restate Christianity for modern man?'

'Who *is* this modern man Robinson keeps talking about?' said the Bishop. 'And more interesting still, why is Robinson so obsessed with him? In my opinion he feels obliged to make amends for his privileged clerical background by being sentimental about the unchurched masses, but if he'd actually grown up among the unchurched masses – as I did, coming not from the Cathedral Close at Canterbury but from Surrey's outstandingly secular "Stockbrokers' Belt" – he'd regard them far more realistically, I assure you.'

'But are you saying modern man doesn't exist?' I pursued, determined not to be diverted by speculation about Dr Robinson's psychology. By this time my tongue was almost hanging out for a third glass of claret.

'Modern times exist,' said the Bishop, replacing the stopper in the claret decanter, 'but modern man, I fear, remains his ancient, sinful self. Darling, is there pudding or do we graduate straight to cheese?'

'There's a rather extraordinary syllabub. Are you brave enough to sample it, Venetia?'

I said I was feeling brave enough for anything, and for a while the conversation veered towards cookery, but eventually as I dug into some Stilton and pined – fruitlessly – for a glass of port, I was able to return to the Bishop's subtle attempt to undermine Robinson's credibility.

'Dr Ashworth, is it really your thesis that the driving force behind the writing of *Honest to God* was Robinson's inverted ecclesiastical snobbery?'

'Not entirely, of course,' the Bishop had to admit, 'but I think I'm making a valid comment on the origins of his compulsion to slate the Church, pander to atheists and attempt to redesign God to suit some mythical variety of *homo sapiens* which he's pleased to describe as "modern man". I'm afraid his current antics only remind me of those young people who rebel against their conventional middle-class families by becoming rabid Marxists.'

'Heavens, I hope Michael doesn't go red!' said Mrs Ashworth, much struck by this parallel. 'That really would be the last straw.'

'My dear,' said the Bishop, 'this family may be middle-class, but I don't think I'd call it conventional.'

'Surely no one who's entitled to be addressed as "my Lord Bishop" can seriously continue to consider himself middle-class,' I said, reluctantly abandoning all hope of a glass of port.

'Oh, that's just window-dressing,' said the Bishop airily. 'Just part of my current worldly trappings. It doesn't alter my basic ingredients at all.'

'Darling, you sound like a recipe in need of a good cook,' said Mrs Ashworth, 'but I'm going to leave you to simmer on the stove while I whisk Venetia away to my sitting-room. Give me a shout if you need stirring.'

We withdrew first to the kitchen, where coffee had percolated for us. Apparently the Bishop never drank coffee in the evening, but Mrs Ashworth produced two large mugs, each adorned with a painting of the Cathedral, and we prepared to overdose on caffeine. I liked the idea of drinking post-prandial coffee out of mugs; the rejection of the conventional demi-tasse struck me as being both pragmatic and adventurous.

'I wanted to talk to you on your own anyway,' Mrs Ashworth was saying as we settled ourselves in her plant-less, flower-less sitting-room, 'but I also felt I had to remove you before Charles lost control and embarked on another *Honest to God* sermon. What on earth did clergymen talk about before that book appeared? I honestly find it hard to remember.'

'Have you read it, Mrs Ashworth?'

'Yes – in bed, so that Charles could nudge me whenever I dozed off.'

'Thank heavens – I thought I was the only one who found it tough going!'

'I think a lot of laymen find it tough going but nobody dares say so.'

We smiled at each other. After the effort of sustaining such an intellectual conversation at the dinner-table without benefit of a substantial infusion of alcohol, I was finding it a relief to relax with my sympathetic hostess.

'Have a chocolate,' said Mrs Ashworth, opening a box of Cadbury's Milk Tray, 'and tell me everything. How are you getting on with that charming little glamour-puss Marina Markhampton?'

'Amazingly well,' I said, selecting an orange cream. 'You mightn't think it, but she's not the usual cat-about-town at all. She puts a high value on friendship with girls and she's not stupid.'

'I think Michael's wishing she could put a higher value on friendship with men!'

'I bet he does! He's madly attractive,' I added generously, 'although of course much too young for me.'

Mrs Ashworth smiled and said: 'What did you think of the other men at the party?'

'Oh, they were all fabulous, Mrs Ashworth – except for Katie's brother Simon who insists on treating women as if they were horses.'

'All whips and lumps of sugar?'

'All slaps on the rump and hearty laughter. I reeled with relief into the orbit of Christian's Winchester chum Perry Palmer who lives at Albany and keeps curious Japanese prints in a room he refuses to specify.'

'Sounds more intriguing. Is Perry the one who's attracted you?'

I sipped my coffee and said: 'What makes you think I'm attracted by anyone?'

'Oh, my dear! A little while ago this interesting but dowdy girl tells me with deep gloom that she's on the sidelines of life because no man has ever found her attractive. Tonight this same interesting girl, now transformed into a radiant young woman coruscating with charm and glamour, appears in my drawing-room and inspires my normally level-headed husband to burble about secretarial Rolls-Royces! Of course I'm just a clergyman's wife,' said Mrs Ashworth, as if she were the unworldly partner of an innocent curate in some country parish far from the fleshpots of Mammon, 'but it does occur even to me, in my ancient respectability, that this particular Rolls-Royce is currently running on some very high-quality petrol indeed. But I don't want to pry. Would you rather talk of something else?'

'Not before I've thanked you for all those compliments! And I really am very excited about being the Bishop's Rolls-Royce. May I ask . . . was it you who suggested the idea to him?'

'No, he thought of it all by himself,' said Mrs Ashworth, as if the Bishop were an exceptionally clever small child. 'I simply egged him on. By the way, have you found a flat yet?'

'No, I must have a blitz on the estate agents tomorrow.'

'Well, before you start blitzing perhaps you'd like to consider an idea of mine. Do you know Archdeacon Lindsay?'

'Only by reputation. Primrose is mad about him.'

'Then you'll probably know that the Archdeaconry of Starbridge is attached to the benefice of St Martin's-in-Cripplegate – which means, among other things, that the Lindsays live in the centre of Starbridge at St Martin's vicarage. At the bottom of the vicarage garden are the old stables, and on the first floor of these stables there's currently a vacant flat.

The building has its own entrance on Butchers' Alley, so you wouldn't have to worry about Mr and Mrs Archdeacon spying on all your comings and goings, and on the ground floor, which Mr Lindsay uses as a garage, I'm sure there'd be room for your car. Michael was telling me that you have this snazzy little MG –'

'And I was worried about finding parking once I'd left the Close! Mrs Ashworth, you're a genius. How big is this place?'

'Small bedroom, large living-room, kitchen and bathroom. The previous archdeacon had the flat made to house his mother-in-law, who was an awful old fusspot, so I'd imagine it's reasonably comfortable.'

'It's quite obviously paradise. How do I get an appointment to view?'

'Shall I phone Mrs Lindsay now? She's a nice woman, I think you'll like her – and she's trying so hard to marry off her four daughters that I guarantee she'll be much too busy to breathe down your neck.'

'The ideal landlady presiding over the ideal flat where I shall live while I work at the ideal job! Do you realise, Mrs Ashworth, that you and your husband have just redesigned to perfection my entire life in Starbridge?' I said, radiant with gratitude, and it was only when she gave her sphinx-like smile that it occurred to me to wonder why she and the Bishop had decided to take so much trouble over a young woman they hardly knew.

THREE

'God, Tillich was saying, is not a projection "out there", an Other beyond the skies, of whose existence we have to convince ourselves, but the Ground of our very being . . .'

'For assertions about God are in the last analysis assertions about Love – about the ultimate ground and meaning of personal relationships.'

JOHN A. T. ROBINSON
Suffragan Bishop of Woolwich 1959–1969
Honest to God

I

When I arrived back at the Chantry I stumbled across a large envelope which was lying on the hall floor by the front door. It was marked: 'The Hon. Venetia Flaxton', and in one corner Aysgarth had printed 'BY HAND'.

'Coo-ee!' shouted Marina, who was watching television in the drawing-room. 'How was Anti-Sex Ashworth?'

'Thundering about the sinfulness of man!'

The telephone rang. As I hesitated in the hall with the envelope in my hands I heard Marina say: 'Robert! What a lovely surprise! I was afraid you might be Michael or Don . . .'

I sped upstairs, shut myself in my room, ripped open the envelope and pulled out the contents. In addition to the May issue of the Cathedral magazine there were two letters. The first read: 'My dear Venetia, I was delighted to see you at Holy Communion this morning, and I thought you might like to see the latest edition of our magazine. My leading article, dealing with the importance of art in connection with religion, may remind you of my recent attempt to have the beautiful painting of the cat in the St Anselm manuscript made available to a wider public in the form of a picture-postcard. In sending you my blessings, I remain your affectionate friend, N.N.A.'

The second letter read: 'My darling Venetia – my Egeria! – I felt I must write and tell you how wonderful it was to see you this morning – I could have murdered that old stick Gilbert for tottering into the library just as your narrative describing the Orgy was becoming delectably racy! How I wish *I* could have gone to a party like that when I was young, but I never did, not even up at Oxford; I was the wrong class, didn't know the right people, had no money, etc., etc., and anyway I had to work so hard to "get on" that I could ill afford to take time off for pleasure. Never mind, I can now enjoy youthful orgies vicariously, through you!

'You looked quite ravishing in your party gown – and equally ravishing in that striped frock you were wearing this morning, and how I managed to avoid "pouncing" on you (as you would say) in the manner of young Michael Ashworth as we stood side by side gazing at Puss-in-Boots I can't imagine. Incidentally I was quite shocked by your description of Michael, and I'm sure none of *my* boys would ever carry on in that tasteless fashion. I'm sure – indeed I hope! – they've done some hard chasing in their time, but young drunks who "grope" (as you put it) in public are most definitely not amusing, and I've always impressed on my boys – though by example, not by sermons, I hasten to add – that women should be put on pedestals and reverenced.

'Dear me, how strait-laced that sounds! And as you know I'm not a bit strait-laced, I pride myself on my liberal outlook, but although I passionately believe that sexual love is good and right, I utterly disapprove of behaviour which is self-centred and lacking in respect for the opposite sex – and thus uncivilised to the point of vulgarity. Someone once remarked that the biggest argument against immorality is that it's in such bad taste. (Could this have been Oscar Wilde? But no, Wilde would surely have turned the comment inside out and declared: "The biggest argument against immorality is that it's in such *good* taste!") Of course the remark about bad taste is an exaggeration, but there's an element of truth in it because man was made to reach for the stars, not to roll around in the mud – and now we're definitely in Wilde's territory; do you remember that line from *Lady Windermere's Fan*: "We're all in the gutter but some of us are looking up at the stars"? Maybe I'll preach on that theme soon and stress that we should *all* be star-gazing. How I'd love to see the Bishop's face if I took Oscar Wilde for my text!

'I'm enclosing the Cathedral magazine because I need an excuse for delivering this missive by hand – and I also enclose a fake letter for you to show Marina in case she sees me pop the envelope through the letter-box. I intend to entrust my letters to the post in future, but I was so bursting to communicate with you that I thought I must just take one little risk! Now darling, remember your promise and write back *instantly*. Our rendezvous on Wednesday afternoon is still (as I write this) forty-two hours away and I can't wait till then to hear from you. Much, *much* love, NEVILLE.'

II

'My darling Mr Dean,' I wrote later after Marina had retired yawning to bed, 'I adored both your letters, even the fake one, and thought your article about art was fabulous. Do keep on with your crusade to get Puss-in-Boots on a postcard!

'So glad you wanted to pounce on me in the library – I bet your pounces are everything pounces should be (private and paradisical) and not ghastly plunges made in an alcoholic fog (public and pukeworthy). But I'm not sure I really want to be put on a pedestal and reverenced – unless, of course, the reverence came in the form of regular dusting of the most stimulating variety.

'But before you produce your duster, "get a load of this!" (as Dinkie would say). There have been sensational goings-on at the South Canonry where I've just dined off an extraordinary syllabub and a measure of claret so small that all I could do was inhale it. That famous double-act, Dr and Mrs A., kidnapped Yours Truly, and as the result of my incarceration beneath the episcopal roof I'm on the point of winding up in the Archdeacon's lap! I'm also on the point of winding up on the episcopal pay-roll, as my Lord Bishop has bribed me to work for him by offering me an immense salary and an IBM dream-machine.

'He vows – wait for it! – to demolish the divine Dr Robinson in a new book (to be dictated at odd hours to the Hon. V. Flaxton, super-secretary) and his wife implies this will be his biggest demolition job since he took an axe to the Arian heresy in his gilded youth. He's a little nervous of his secretary, an item called Peabody (I didn't dare ask how many bishops she'd served under!) but he fancies he can get away with taking me on as a luxury and he's already referring to me as a secretarial Rolls-Royce.

'This letter, designed to form part of a lurid best-seller entitled *How to Get On in the Church of England: a Guide for Single Girls under Thirty*, comes to you with best love from your devoted EGERIA. PS. Why on *earth* have I been so suddenly marked out for this extraordinary episcopal attention? Did Dr A. play Peeping Tom after all as we sat on Lady Mary? Could he conceivably regard me as a "lost girl" who has to be "redeemed"? (I seem to remember that Gladstone underwent similar behavioural problems when he kept bringing prostitutes home to tea.) Any light you can throw on this bizarre situation would be greatly appreciated.'

The next morning, on my journey to the newsagent's shop beyond St Anne's Gate to buy the *Daily Mail*, I dropped the letter in the pillar-box on the North Walk and had the satisfaction of knowing it would catch the first post. To my amazement it reached the Deanery by the second post that morning. (The post then was not nearly so bad as it is now, but even in 1963 such extraordinary speed was a notable occurrence.) Aysgarth wrote back that afternoon, and the following morning, the day of our rendezvous, I was ripping open the envelope.

'My darling Venetia,' I read, 'I'm truly appalled by this

episcopal skulduggery which is driving you into the Archdeacon's lap – does Mrs Lindsay know you intend to use this singularly unattractive archidiaconal feature as a resting-place? – and I'm *very worried indeed* about this "dream-machine" you mentioned. It sounds exceedingly improper. The initials IBM are, of course, quite unknown to me since clergymen should have better things to do with their time than read articles in *The Times* about American corporations, but in my opinion all single girls under thirty who aspire to "get on" in the Church of England should regard such questionable modern devices, labelled IBM or otherwise, with suspicion.

'My Lord Bishop's daring in risking the wrath of Miss Peabody is second only to his nerve in engaging my Egeria to string his pearls of wisdom – or, as would seem more likely, his fake pearls of folly. If he were to spend more time reconstructing the Christian faith for our day and age, as our hero Robinson is doing, and less time demolishing what he's pleased to call heresy, the level of church attendance in the diocese of Starbridge might conceivably rise from its present all-time low! My dearest, must you really indulge in esoteric rites with your dream-machine in the company of this over-educated reactionary? How can I save you from such a sinister fate at the South Canonry, and how, for goodness' sake, can I prevent you winding up in the Archdeacon's lap? This letter comes to you with best love from your devoted but deeply concerned MR DEAN, now to be addressed by you (*please!*) as NEVILLE.

'PS. No need to worry about the Ashworths. To me the explanation of the unprecedented benevolence is simple: (1) The Bishop's reached the age when he'd far rather dictate his rubbish to a gorgeous young creature like you than to a hideous old hag like Peabody; (2) Mrs Bishop has reached the age when she wants to compensate herself for her absent sons by acquiring a substitute daughter; and (3) they may well be engaged in a conspiracy to capture you as a girlfriend – perhaps even as a wife – for Charley, whose continuing lack of interest in girls would be enough to worry any parents who want a normal life for their son.

'PPS. As soon as we meet in the courtyard of the Staro Arms I shall demand an explanation of the Archdeacon's lap! *Longing* to see you, N.'

III

'I thought this moment would never come!' said Aysgarth as I scrambled into the front seat of his dusty Humber that afternoon. 'My darling, you're looking like a Pre-Raphaelite Guinevere, radiating mysterious allure, and how Lyle Ashworth dares to leave you alone with a sex-obsessed bishop and a dream-machine I can't think. What's the news from the Archdeacon's lap?'

The Humber had halted seconds earlier in the courtyard of Starbridge's oldest hotel, a former medieval hostelry rumoured to have been patronised by Chaucer. No native of Starbridge seriously believed this fable, but it made fine fodder for the tourists and had spawned a cottage industry which produced cheap mugs adorned with pictures of Chaucer fondling a quill pen.

As Aysgarth enquired about the Archdeacon's lap he spun the car into a three-point turn and with an anguished squeal of tires the Humber shot out of the courtyard into Eternity Street. I had long suspected that Aysgarth was a racing-driver *manqué*; whenever he was behind the wheel of a car he seemed to be celebrating an escape from his life as an eminent churchman. That afternoon he was wearing an ancient pair of grey flannel trousers, a faded blue shirt which was stretched tightly across his midriff, no tie and a shabby tweed jacket which looked as if it had been rescued from a jumble sale. His white hair was bedraggled, suggesting that he had repeatedly run his fingers through it in a fever of romantic impatience, and as he smiled at me he revealed his square, raffish teeth, proved indisputably genuine by the fact that they were out of alignment. (I suspected the Bishop possessed dentures; his teeth were far too even to be true.) As soon as I had entered the car I had been aware of a fascinating odour of cigarettes and Lux soap overlaid with a faint, tantalising whiff of whisky.

'My darling Mr Dean!' I exclaimed impulsively. 'How exciting you are! Just like an English version of James Cagney!'

He laughed and laughed. At the humpbacked bridge which spanned the river, the car swooped up and down so wildly that my stomach seemed to hit the soles of my feet, but all he gasped as I shrieked was: 'Isn't life fun?'

We drove on in ecstasy out of the city.

IV

'. . . so I'm all set to take up residence in the Archdeacon's lap next week,' I said, concluding my report on the flat in Butchers' Alley as the city rapidly vanished into the distance behind us. 'My own home at last! The moment I move in I shall put a rose between my teeth, open a bottle of champagne and loll naked on a tiger-skin rug beneath a poster of Elvis Presley!'

'I must lurk beneath the window with a periscope! Do you really have a tiger-skin rug?'

'No. I don't approve of skinning cats.'

'Neither do I. By the way, talking of cats,' said Aysgarth as the car roared down the valley towards the hills which marked the beginning of Starbury Plain, 'I was all set to fight for Puss-in-Boots again at yesterday's Chapter meeting, but I never got the chance. That fatuous ass Fitzgerald, who's long been seduced by the Parish and People Movement, started nagging me to make the Sung Communion the main service on Sunday mornings and call it a Eucharist, and by the time I'd beaten him off –'

'But isn't that just a High-Church fad?'

'Yes, but now we've got an Archbishop of Canterbury who runs around in a purple cassock instead of a decent pair of gaiters the Catholic wing of the Church of England thinks it can get away with anything.'

'No Popery!'

'Well, one mustn't be bigoted. Certainly as a liberal I favour ecumenism – unity for all Christians – even though it's no good expecting the Roman Catholics to do anything except kick us in the teeth. The first move towards unity will have to come from them.'

'So while you wait you amuse yourself by beating up the Anglo-Catholics whenever they get too Romish!'

He laughed. 'Oh, I can be charitable towards the Anglo-Catholics – with an effort! That's the point of the Church of England – Catholics and Protestants are united under one umbrella. But no one's going to catch *me* tinkering with the Communion service and destroying the basic pattern of Sunday worship in the name of some half-baked liturgical fashion which seduces every High-Churchman in sight! Low-Church by inclination I may be, having been brought up by evangelical Nonconformists, but in worship I've always tried to follow the Church of England's famous "Middle Way", the road between the extremes of Catholic and Protestant practice, and it's in the name of that "Middle Way" that I absolutely refuse to downgrade Sunday matins. "Over my dead body," I said to Fitzgerald –'

'What bad luck that you should be saddled with an Anglo-Catholic canon!'

'Oh, there'll be murder done in our Chapter meetings yet, I swear it! No good looking to the Bishop for support, of course; you've only got to mention the word "Eucharist" to him and he's off on some outstandingly boring dissertation on the Early Church –'

'But the Bishop's not an Anglo-Catholic, is he?'

'No, but he has Catholic leanings. He's keen on confession and retreats – and he's always saying that every clergyman should have a spiritual director –'

'Have you got one?'

'Certainly not! Using an intermediary in dealing with God is a very Catholic concept, and anyway my soul's my own business; I don't want some stranger messing around with it, and in my opinion agonising over one's spiritual life simply encourages

morbid introspection. God helps those who help themselves –
although of course,' said Aysgarth, becoming cautious as if he
had suddenly realised he was being too dogmatic, 'sometimes
in very difficult situations one's unable to help oneself. Then
one does indeed need the help of an older clergyman of great
spiritual wisdom. But usually such occasions are rare.' He
paused before adding: 'I used to talk to Bishop Bell occasionally
about various private problems. I've missed him since he died
in 'fifty-eight.'

'You don't feel tempted to unburden yourself to your current
father-in-God Bishop Ashworth?'

'What an appalling thought! No, I'll leave that sort of charade
to Fitzgerald. What a bishop! What a canon! Or as Cicero
would have said –'

'"*O tempora!*"' I quoted. '"*O mores!*"'

'My darling!' He turned his head to smile at me in delight
and the car nearly plunged into the ditch. I screamed lightly
but I was enjoying myself too much to care whether or not we
veered off the road. I was enthralled by his frank talk about the
Chapter, and I felt as privileged as if I had been listening to the
Prime Minister describing the private feuds of his publicly
united cabinet.

By this time we had left the main road and were zipping
along a country lane. A wandering cow bellowed in horror as
we shot past within inches of its flank. The occasional pot-hole
tested the durability of the back axle. The car panted uphill with
all the zest of a bloodhound pounding across wide open spaces.
We were now climbing on to Starbury Plain, and as we left the
trees of the valley behind, the bare hills began to level out
around us to form a vast, undulating plain.

'Can't you get rid of Fitzgerald, Mr Dean?'

'No cause, I assure you, is dearer to my heart, but unfortunately removal isn't so easy . . . Darling, do stop calling me "Mr
Dean" now that we're alone together! I – heavens above, here's
the car-park! I nearly missed it.'

The brakes squealed, the tires screeched and the car behind
us gave a blast on the horn. Cutting our speed violently in a

few hair-raising seconds, Aysgarth swung the Humber off the road into the parking area laid out by the National Trust when it had acquired the acres surrounding the famous ancient monument, Starbury Ring. This megalithic stone circle, reached by a twenty-minute walk along a bridle-path, was fortunately unpopular with the majority of modern tourists, most of whom preferred to avoid exercise. On that afternoon there were no coaches in the parking area and only a couple of cars. No one was in sight. The cars' occupants had all disappeared over the brow of the hill on their way to the Ring.

'What shall we do?' said Aysgarth, switching off the engine. 'Walk or luxuriate?'

'Oh, luxuriate – much more fun!' I said at once, remembering that he too, like most tourists, shied away from exercise.

He sighed and gazed without enthusiasm at the bridle-path. 'I really should walk,' he said. 'It would be good for me.'

'It would be even better for you if you relaxed here in the car and told me all about *Honest to God!*'

He laughed and quoted: '"I can resist everything except temptation!"' Then he reached out and clasped my hand.

V

But in fact he resisted temptation well. Apart from clasping and squeezing my hands he attempted no other torrid activity; he seemed far more interested in indulging in stimulating conversation. At the end of our interlude he sighed: 'This has been such fun – what a pity we can't stay longer!' And he gave me a peck on the cheek. Back in Starbridge he dropped me in Eternity Street so that we could return separately to the Close, blew me a kiss, breathed some passionate parting words and disappeared in a cloud of exhaust fumes.

Staring after him I tried to work out why I felt not merely disappointed but confused.

'My darling Neville,' I wrote that night at the Chantry. 'It was marvellous to see you today without everyone breathing down our necks, and many thanks for explaining the first part of *Honest to God*.'

I paused. I was sitting at the table in the dining-room and across the hall in the drawing-room Marina was engaged in a telephone conversation with Katie Aysgarth. Christian had finally sent Marina a note of thanks for the Orgy and she had used this communication as an excuse to ring him up, but Katie had soon followed her husband to the phone, and as I listened I realised Marina was being invited to Oxford as soon as Lady Markhampton had returned home. Marina's expressions of gratitude were numerous and ecstatic; she appeared to give no thought to the masculine groans which would erupt when she cancelled her London dates, and soon she was gossiping away to Katie on the theme of how awful all men were except Christian. I was now more convinced than ever that their eternal triangle was very odd indeed.

Meanwhile that other odd person, Perry Palmer, had phoned me to confess that the curious Japanese prints were a fiction but that he would be delighted to show me instead another great curiosity, his full coal-cellar, whenever I returned to London; it was an old joke among Christian's friends that Perry, whose set in Albany had hardly been altered since Victorian days, had absent-mindedly ordered a vast quantity of coal for his fireplaces shortly before London had been declared a smokeless zone. Amused by the flaunting of this legendary museum-piece I promised to phone him when I was next up in town; I had already decided that Perry could replace Eddie as my smoke-screen, deflecting the world's attention from the real object of my passion.

The thought of the object of my passion prompted me to turn back to my letter. 'Of course Robinson's absolutely right,' I wrote fluently. 'We can't go on thinking of God as an old man in the sky who made a space-trip to Bethlehem two thousand years ago, dressed up as Christ, and left the universe untended. Much better to chuck away all those obsolete old myths and throw the whole Christian tradition in the melting-pot in order to recast the faith in terms that are intelligible to the secular mid-twentieth century! That's exactly what people of my generation want. We want to move forward from our parents' world, the world the war rendered obsolete, and create a world that's *new*. No more dead wood, no more hidebound tradition that's meaningless, no more risible fairy-tales. Everything must be hard, cool, clear and unsentimental.

'So no more talk of God as an old man in the sky who carries on like some irascible father-figure! People of my generation have quite enough trouble with their fathers without wanting a father-figure God! I think it was quite brilliant of Paul Tillich to say instead that God is the "Ground of our being", and I think it's even more brilliant of Robinson to pick up this definition and develop it. To think of God as being present throughout the whole world, present in some mysterious way deep down inside us, is much more meaningful than thinking of him as "out there", high up in some corner of the universe that the scientists can never quite find. How clever of Robinson to see that the concept of depth has so much more meaning for us today – after all the talk of "depth psychology" – than the concept of height!

'Next time we meet you must move on from Tillich and tell me about those other German theologians Robinson likes so much. I want to hear more about Bonhoeffer's "religionless Christianity" and Bultmann's "demythologising". (Does Bultmann really say that the only thing that matters is the message? How modern that sounds! Do you suppose he's ever worked in an advertising agency?)

'It's agonising to think we have to wait a whole week to resume such a riveting conversation – please write SOON to ease my torment! Lashings of love, EGERIA.'

I had just tucked this letter in an envelope and was sealing the flap when Marina arrived in high spirits after her stimulating phone call. 'Writing to the mysterious Mr X?' she said. 'I told

Christian just now that I suspected you were on the brink of a mad affair with Perry, but Christian just said: "Whoever the lucky man is, it certainly isn't my friend Peregrine" – which rather suggests, doesn't it, that he knows something about Perry that we don't. I wonder what went on when they were at school together . . . Do they swim in the nude at Winchester?'

'I should think they do a lot of things in the nude at Winchester.'

'I was wondering about Perry's possible lack of genitalia.'

'Perhaps all – or nothing, as the case may be – will be revealed to me when I inspect his coal-cellar.'

'But seriously, Vinnie, who *is* this secret man in your life?'

'Jesus Christ. Everyone and no one. God – who's to be found in loving relationships. God's the Ground of Our Being. He's not up there in the sky – he's down here, deep down inside every one of us –'

'Darling, have you been hitting the gin?'

The telephone rang. Marina flitted away to answer it but flitted back to report: 'It's churchy old Primrose – are you in or out?'

'Oh God! I'd better be in, but what a bore.' Still clutching my unaddressed envelope I slunk to the phone. 'Primrose! How thrilling to hear from you – how's life with the Archdeacon?'

'Well, that's just it,' said Primrose, very cool. 'The Archdeacon and I were just going over the minutes of the last meeting of the diocesan Board of Finance when he happened to mention –'

Mr Lindsay had revealed I was about to move into his lap and work for the Bishop.

'Oh, didn't I tell you?' I said glibly. 'Really, I'm getting so old that I'm forgetting what I said to who!'

'Rubbish!' said Primrose. 'You've simply dropped me with such a bang that everyone in Starbridge must be deafened. Now look here, Venetia. Is it anything I've said? Because if I've done something to offend you, I want to know so that I can put things right. You're my best friend, and –'

'Oh, Primrose . . .' I felt a complete heel. 'No, it's nothing you've done, I promise –'

'Then I simply can't understand what you see in Marina Markhampton. She's so absolutely trivial, not worthy of someone with your brains. You're not having some ghastly lesbian affair with her, are you?'

'Honestly, Primrose! What a suggestion!'

'Dido says she's sure Marina's a lesbian.'

'I'm surprised to find you listening to Dido!'

'Dido's very shrewd about who's carrying on with who. For instance, do you remember that alto-tenor with the long blond hair who sang in the Cathedral choir last year? Tommy Fitzgerald said Father ought to make the alto-tenor cut his hair to disguise the fact that he was obviously queer as a coot, but Dido just looked Fitzgerald straight in the eyes and said: "My dear, he only pretends he's queer because he wants to cover up the fact that he's having an affair with the organist's wife." The alto-tenor ran off with her a week later. Fitzgerald was livid – not with the alto-tenor, of course, but with Dido for being right.'

'Well, if Dido thinks I'm having a lesbian wing-ding with Marina –'

'I didn't say Dido thinks that. Dido just thinks Marina's a lesbian. Dido's only comment on *you* is: "If dear Venetia's lingering in Starbridge just for the thrill of working for the Bishop, I'd be very much surprised."'

There was a silence.

'Hullo? Venetia?'

'Sorry, just trying to figure out what on earth Dido's getting at. Does she think I'm about to run off with the new alto-tenor?'

'Well, there's a rumour going around that you're madly in love –'

'Oh, my God! I make one drunken joke to Christian and for some perverse reason he chooses to broadcast it as gospel truth to all and sundry! There's no one, Prim, honestly – except perhaps Perry Palmer. He's just invited me to see his coal-cellar.'

'Perry's a eunuch.'

'Have you cast-iron evidence of that fact?'

'Well, no, but ... I say, Venetia, you haven't finally discovered a mad passion for Eddie, have you?'

'Don't be revolting! Look, come and see me on Monday after I've moved into the Archdeacon's flat, and we'll knock back a bottle of champagne together to celebrate my acquisition of the new pad.'

'I'll bring a bottle of sherry,' said Primrose. 'If I drink more than two glasses of champagne I get a headache.'

'Oh, for God's sake, Prim, you drink your two glasses and I'll toss off the rest! You talk like an old maid sometimes!'

There was a pause. Then: 'Sorry,' I mumbled. 'I didn't mean that. How's Maurice Tait?'

'Very well, thank you,' said Primrose politely. 'What time shall I come on Monday?'

'Oh, just roll along when you've finished work. It'll be fabulous to meet again!'

'Fabulous,' said Primrose.

We said goodbye and hung up.

VII

After the conversation I spent several unpleasant seconds thinking of Dido's talent for discerning who was sleeping with whom, but then I dismissed her from my mind by recalling that in fact I was sleeping with no one and that there was no logical reason why she should regard me with suspicion. My episcopal job, socially glamorous and intellectually stimulating, was quite sufficient to justify my stay in Starbridge to all but the neurotically suspicious.

I then remembered that I had not yet summoned the energy to inform my parents of my great coup in landing a job with the Bishop, and it occurred to me that before they, like Dido, succumbed to the neurotic suspicion that I was on the brink of behaving like a decadent member of the aristocracy, I should pen the required letter without delay. Accordingly, having returned to my writing-case in the dining-room, I found a fresh sheet of paper and wrote: 'Dear Mama, I've rented a flat (12 Butchers' Alley) and intend to live in Starbridge for at least three months as from next Monday, in order to help Bishop Ashworth write his new book. My landlord is Archdeacon Lindsay. I don't anticipate being in London in the immediate future, but I might look in at Pauncefoot some time if you happen to be around. Meanwhile please try and stop Papa rampaging around the House of Lords, collaring prelates and badgering them with questions about me. I hope you and your plants are thriving. Love, VENETIA.' I spent five minutes trying to decide whether to provide my new telephone number but finally wrote it down as a postscript. I had realised that if one of my parents died I would feel guilty if the survivor was unable to contact me immediately.

'Writing letters again?' said Marina, nursing a cup of hot chocolate as she drifted into the room to say good-night. 'You write more letters than any girl I've ever met.'

'Just keeping the parents happy.' I began to address the envelope.

'Oh, parents!' said Marina. She spoke as if referring to a rare species of animal which only existed on the far side of the globe. On an impulse she sat down opposite me at the table and gave her hot chocolate a stir. 'I've trained my mother never to expect a letter from me, but if you can keep your parents at bay with letters, maybe I've made a mistake. That weekly phone call I have to make is really a fearful bind.'

I had by this time had ample experience of the weekly Markhampton phone call. Marina would sigh and moan beforehand, but the conversations with her mother always sounded happy enough. 'Why don't you try talking to your father occasionally?' I said, folding the sheet of writing-paper in half. 'It might provide a welcome variation in the routine.'

'Oh, my father barely talks at all,' said Marina. 'Not to me anyway.'

'What bliss.' I began to slip the letter into the envelope and the silence that followed was broken only by the rustle of paper, but at last Marina said nonchalantly, so nonchalantly that I hardly realised what she was saying: 'Well, I don't care. What the hell? He's not my real father anyway.'

My tongue halted in its progress down the envelope's flap. Then I completed the lick and very carefully pressed down the seal. 'No?' I murmured so vaguely that I sounded as if I were barely concentrating on the conversation. 'I don't think I knew that.'

'Oh, good. Sometimes one imagines the whole world's twittering about it behind one's back, so it's nice to know you weren't keeping quiet out of an urge to be tactful . . . I never quite know what you're thinking, Venetia. You're a bit of a mystery in some ways.'

'Well, at the moment my thoughts are utterly predictable and completely mundane. I was wondering when you found out about this tiresome little kink in the family tree.'

I had struck the right casual note. As she relaxed, stirring her hot chocolate, I realised she wanted neither sympathy nor a prurient curiosity but a detached interest which bordered on the clinical. All emotion had to be kept ruthlessly at bay.

'It happened last year,' she said. 'I was at that restaurant off Berkeley Square – you know the one, all fish and dim lighting – and someone in the party said to me: "Of course your real father's the art critic Walter Forrest, isn't he?" and I said: "Of course, who else?" and then I didn't hear anything for five minutes – at which point I had to rush to the lavatory to be sick.'

'I hope there wasn't some quizzy dragon on duty.'

'I don't know what was on duty. All I remember now is the revolting pink carpet. Anyway, after that I decided to ask my mother about Walter Forrest – I was actually rather excited to think I'd been fathered by something intelligent – so eventually I cornered Mummy in her studio. She was painting the most sensational picture, lots of naked legs and pubic hair and stray breasts floating all over the place, and I don't think she really wanted to be interrupted but I stood my ground and said: "So I'm Walter Forrest's bastard – how thrilling!" For a moment she just went on mixing her paints. Then she said: "Don't worry, darling, Daddy and I both adore you and Walter's never been in the least interested in children. I'd forget all about him, if I were you." I asked why I hadn't been told and she just said: "I honestly didn't think it would make you happy." I tried to explain that I felt a bit of a fool since obviously everyone knew except me, but she never batted an eyelid. "Oh no!" she said. "No one knows anything for certain, but you do have a great look of Walter and of course it's well known that among our sort of people the last child in the family is often a cuckoo in the nest." Then she went on painting. I wanted to ask her more but then I realised I had to find a lavatory and vomit again . . . Well, I mean, the scene really was rather pukeworthy, wasn't it?'

'Terribly dreary,' I said. 'What a drag.' I suddenly realised I was creasing my mother's envelope at one corner with small, furtive movements of my fingers.

'Sorry to waffle on about something so sordid,' said Marina, taking a sip of her hot chocolate. 'I've never told any of my other girlfriends, but perhaps I was lured on this time because you're so much more soignée than they are. For instance, I'm sure you know all about what goes on among our sort of people, and anyway you're the last child in a family yourself, aren't you? I suppose I knew subconsciously that you'd understand.'

'Uh-huh.' I smoothed the crease out of the envelope. 'Did you ever confront Walter Forrest?'

'Why do you think I got that job in the art gallery? When he turned up at one of the exhibitions, I marched straight up to him and said: "I'm Marina, Alice Markhampton's daughter." And he said: "Oh yes? It's years since I've seen Alice. I hope she's well." Then he turned his back on me and began to talk to someone else.'

'Brute. I'd have clobbered him.'

'It *was* a bit much, wasn't it? Oh, how I hated all men at that moment, *hated* them – in fact I still do sometimes, it comes over me in waves . . . although never when I'm with Christian, of course.'

'I like Christian,' I said. 'I always have. But I don't know what goes on there.'

'Then I'll tell you. He's good and decent and kind. That's why I love him. On that ghastly evening at the restaurant after I'd vomited in the pink-carpeted lavatory, it was Christian who took care of me. I couldn't tell him what was wrong and he didn't ask. He just got a taxi and brought me home and we drank tea together while he held my hand and told me all about how awful life was in the Middle Ages. Wasn't that nice of him? By the time he'd finished I'd almost forgotten how awful London was in 1962.'

'Good old Christian,' I said. 'Does he ever kiss you?'

'Oh, just the occasional peck on the cheek. But he holds hands beautifully.'

'You don't think he might ever try and do more?'

'Why should he?' said Marina, finishing her hot chocolate. 'He's got Katie.' She stood up. 'I'd better totter off to bed before my eyes close. Thanks so much for listening, Vinnie. I hope I didn't bore you.'

But I was unable to reply. My entire world had suddenly gone pitch black. Horror had paralysed every muscle in my body.

'Venetia?'

In the nick of time the instinct to dissimulate in order to survive came to my rescue and will-power triumphed over paralysis. I managed to say casually: 'Sorry. Still thinking of Christian. No, of course you didn't bore me, Marina.'

'You won't tell anyone about Walter Forrest, will you?'

'Never.'

She smiled gratefully and wandered away.

VIII

I had already tortured myself with the notion that Aysgarth's silence on the subject of Dido might indicate he still retained a trace of asexual affection for her, but the possibility that now assailed me was infinitely more pulverising. Later, sleep proved impossible. I was quite unable to forget Christian, able to indulge in a chaste romantic friendship with Marina because his sexual appetite was satisfied by his wife. Their triangle now seemed uncomplicated; I felt I could understand not only Katie's serenity and Christian's restraint but the ambivalence towards men which made Marina no threat to either of them at the profoundest level of their relationship.

But my own triangle, previously so straightforward, was now distorted by doubt.

I tried to pull myself together. No matter what Christian was doing with Katie, it was unthinkable that my Mr Dean might still be having sex with Dido.

So why was I thinking the unthinkable?

At two o'clock I went downstairs and mixed myself a whisky-and-soda, a drink I normally avoided because it had a soporific effect on me, but twenty minutes later my eyelids showed no inclination to droop. I began to pace around the drawing-room.

If I refused to believe that my Mr Dean was continuing to have sexual intercourse with his wife, what were the implications? I tried to survey the facts with detachment. Of course our grand passion was as yet at an early stage, but I could not deny I had been puzzled by his failure to express his feelings more hotly in the car-park of Starbury Ring. But perhaps he had been shy. I had not forgotten his unexpected shyness on Lady Mary when we had met after the Orgy. On the other hand, he had appeared to be unafflicted by shyness in the car-park. So if he wasn't having sex with his wife and if he wasn't overwhelmed by his inhibitions, what was the explanation for the marked absence of passion which had left me feeling bewildered and dissatisfied?

I toyed with the appalling possibility of impotence, but discarded it. It was true that Aysgarth was sixty-one but plenty of men skipped around at that age and he had often boasted he had the constitution of an ox. Certainly I could never remember him being ill. While eavesdropping long ago on a conversation of Arabella's I had gleaned the information that impotence could be caused by indulging too heavily in alcohol, but surely an ox-like constitution could absorb generous doses of alcohol without disastrous side-effects? And anyway, Aysgarth had always seemed to have this risky pastime well in control.

I applied myself afresh to the mystery. Then suddenly I realised I had quite overlooked the fact that he had powerful moral reasons for restraining himself with me. I hadn't exactly forgotten that he was a clergyman, but I had been so carried away by my desire for a strong physical response from him that I had reacted like an ignorant layman and underestimated the spiritual force of his beliefs. The most obvious solution to the mystery of his non-passionate behaviour, as I now realised, was that he was being compulsively high-minded and noble.

It was also time I remembered that clergymen had no choice but to be high-minded and noble; that was what was expected of them and if they frolicked around committing adultery they were defrocked – although that, of course, only applied if they committed the ultimate sin of being found out. How often did clergymen stray from the moral path? It was bound to happen occasionally, since they were human beings and not robots, but I doubted that it happened often, and I found it hard to believe it happened to anyone who got beyond the rank of vicar. A clergyman able enough to progress to the upper reaches of his profession would be able enough to know how to ensure his survival. Aysgarth had evidently worked out (with the aid of Bishop Robinson) that he could allow himself a warm, flirtatious friendship with me, but his moral beliefs, which I had no doubt were strong, and his instinct for survival, which I had no doubt was well developed, would ensure he carried the affair no further.

That all made sense. And that indeed was the situation I had been prepared to accept after the Orgy when, riding high on a tidal wave of euphoria, I had decided it would be greedy to want more than a chaste romantic friendship. But no matter how valid these rational deductions were, they didn't tell me what I was to do now that greed had triumphed – and they didn't tell me either what Aysgarth was currently doing about sex. According to Arabella, men had to have sexual intercourse of some kind regularly (unless, I assumed, they were like Perry Palmer – and no one knew for sure about Perry anyway) but I had apparently argued myself into believing Aysgarth was at present a complete sexual abstainer. Was this abstinence possible? Was it likely? Arabella would without doubt have answered no to both questions, but Arabella had never been mixed up with a high-minded clergyman. I thought abstinence was possible but I had a terrible feeling it was not very likely – and if Aysgarth was keeping me at a chaste distance, there was only one other woman to whom he was likely to turn for sexual satisfaction.

I had a second whisky-and-soda.

I then tried to tell myself that I didn't care what he was doing about sex so long as he loved me, but I knew this assertion bore no relation to reality. I did care. I cared passionately. I didn't want to share him with anyone. I wanted him all to myself. In fact, as I could now acknowledge, recklessly embracing my mounting greed, I wanted to be his mistress. Marriage, unfortunately, was out of the question, since I could never ruin his career by involving him in a divorce, but I was sure that a consummated grand passion would at least give me peace of mind; never again did I want to swill whisky and pace the floor in the early hours of the morning while I tormented myself with revolting thoughts about his relationship with that appalling woman.

Of course it was impossible that he should still be sleeping with her. But I could see I had to make it more than impossible; I had to make it inconceivable.

Then alongside me in the world of allegory, the demure little serpent, gliding along on his leash, slipped his collar at last and slithered away beyond my control into the garden.

FOUR

'[Bishop Robinson's] attempt to be honest to God is so dishonest to the God of, for example, Athanasius or the fourth century Cappadocian writers or of Thomas Aquinas, let alone Augustine, or again, to the God of the author of the *Cloud of Unknowing* or, say, to the God who is worshipped in and through the shape of the Orthodox Liturgy, that it is clearly high time that we were confronted by an explosive reminder of the need to "get our theism right."'

DAVID JENKINS
The Honest to God Debate
ed. DAVID L. EDWARDS

I

'Let me tell you what I plan to do,' said the Bishop, resplendent in his old-fashioned uniform, his episcopal ring glinting in the light as he toyed with his pectoral cross.

It was Monday, the first day of my new job, and we were closeted together in the South Canonry's morning-room which had been turned into an office for me. My hired IBM Electric typewriter gleamed on its table by the window. I myself was arranged nearby in the classic secretarial position, one leg crossed over the other and my shorthand notebook resting on my uppermost knee. I wore an austere white blouse and a black skirt and looked (I hoped) vaguely religious, as befitted an office serf in attendance on a prelate. My horrible hair, now growing wildly towards a Pre-Raphaelite length after its tiresome 'in-between' stage, was scraped off my face and stuffed into a sort of net which I had speared with another interesting metal object from Boots. I could feel the hair weighing on the nape of my neck like an enormous doughnut as I held my pencil lightly above the blank page.

'First of all,' said the Bishop, lounging elegantly against the chimney-piece, 'I shall simply be dictating random observations. These may seem quite disconnected. Then after I've studied these opening remarks on paper I shall arrange them under various headings so that they form an outline of the book. It's possible that I might keep Robinson's structure of God, Christ, worship, ethics and so on, but his writing is so emotional, his theology so vapid and his conclusions so wild that I fear any attempt to mimic his structure can only have unfortunate results. However, we shall see. Now Venetia, do stop me if I go too fast. When I'm in full theological spate I tend to get carried away.'

'Yes, Bishop.' I felt as if I were attending some famous general who was surveying the battlefield before a world-shattering military engagement.

'Very well, off we go. Number one: the Bishop of Woolwich, whose fame hitherto has rested on his New Testament scholarship, has with great courage ventured into fresh woods and pastures new. Unfortunately he has chosen to plunge into the woods of doctrine and the pastures of ethics. Since it is clear that his grounding in both is slender – to put it kindly – his brave little book cannot in truth be described as a work of scholarly importance. It would be more accurate, I think, as well as more charitable to classify this latest addition to the Robinson *oeuvre* – that's O-E-U-U –'

'*Oeuvre*. I've got it, Bishop.'

'– latest addition to the Robinson *oeuvre* as a devotional work. Dr Robinson is clearly devoted to God, to Jesus Christ and to the Christian religion. This is admirable. The only trouble is that his God is not the Christian God, his Jesus is not, as the doctrine of the Church upholds, God incarnate, and his Christian religion is merely an exotic amalgamation of various Christian heresies which have long since been discredited. End of paragraph. Can you read that back to me, please?'

I read it back.

'By Jove, you're good!' said the Bishop. 'Well done. All right, on we go. Number two: Dr Robinson is zealous in proclaiming that the metaphor of height, so long used in descriptions of God can no longer be meaningful to – quote – modern man – unquote. He insists that we can abolish the metaphor by speaking of God as something which exists "deep down" in every individual, and he validates this proposition by declaring that it will be more easily understood by "modern man" because of his familiarity with the concept of depth psychology. However, since all talk of God can only be in terms of symbols, depth is just as much a metaphor as height. In the name of depth psychology – which is probably only fully understood by a very small number of so-called modern men – Dr Robinson has fatally limited the doctrine of God by abolishing the concept of transcendence. Note: I shall deal later with his wholly inadequate attempt to give transcendence a new definition.

'New paragraph. Number three: the Bishop appears to have fallen wildly in love with the writings of three German theologians: Rudolf Bultmann, Dietrich Bonhoeffer and Paul Tillich. The latter has described God as "the Ground of our being", an appellation which the Bishop seems to find peculiarly intoxicating. Wrenching this phrase from the context of Tillich's interesting though questionable existentialist theology, Dr Robinson expands his depth metaphor to declare that since God is the Ground of our being we can find Him, regardless of whether we go to church or not, by gazing down into our inmost depths. This, of course, as any student of the Early Church will know, was the attitude of the philosopher Valentinus in the second century – see my book *Valentinus, Scourge of Orthodoxy*, published by Cambridge University Press in 1954. In other words,' said the Bishop with a gleam in his eye, 'what we have here is a brand new version of the heresy of the Christian Gnostics who nearly destroyed the Church in the first centuries after Christ. Venetia, Gnostic is spelt –'

'G–N–O–S–T–I–C.'

'This is wonderful!' said the Bishop. 'You're the first secretary I've met who could spell Gnostic! But I mustn't forget, must I, that I'm writing for lesser laymen who won't know what that word means, so I think I'd better now dictate a paragraph on the Gnostics – or shall I leave it till later? No, let's strike while the iron's hot. Before I go on to enquire why Robinson, in his passion for the work of German theologians, has chosen to fall in love with Bultmann, Bonhoeffer and Tillich instead of with Barth and Niebuhr, I shall just pause to demolish the heresy of Christian Gnosticism.'

Dr Ashworth was enjoying himself hugely. Feeling quite overwhelmed by the devastating confidence of his scholarly authority I began to feel far more confused than I had ever anticipated.

II

When I arrived back at the Chantry for a sandwich lunch I found a letter had arrived for me by the second post. 'My darling,' I read, 'I must see you – can't wait till Wednesday to find out what went on at the South Canonry during your first encounter with the dream-machine! Lady Mary post-evensong Monday? Hope this catches you before you move into the Archdeacon's lap. In great haste, all love, N.'

This was very satisfactory, and I phoned Primrose at the diocesan office to postpone our house-warming drink. Then I gathered up my possessions, said a genuinely fond farewell to Marina and bucketed away in my MG to my new flat overlooking Butchers' Alley.

III

About half a dozen tourists were wandering around the cloisters as I took possession of Lady Mary, but there was no sign of any member of the Cathedral staff. It was a clouded evening and after a wet morning Lady Mary was somewhat damp. Adjusting my raincoat carefully under my bottom I resigned myself to rheumatism and waited.

'Phew!' said Aysgarth, hurrying up to me five minutes later.

'Sorry about the delay but I got mixed up with one of the vergers who reports a sinister smell emanating from St Anselm's chapel – there's been a recurring drainage problem there ever since my predecessor Dean Carter built a lavatory on the cheap at the back of the sacristy. What a life! But my darling, don't keep me in suspense – what happened at the South Canonry?'

'The Bishop demolished the Gnostic heresy.'

'Oh good heavens, not that old rubbish again!'

'You may laugh, but it was pretty powerful stuff! Is there any possibility he might wind up Archbishop of Canterbury?'

'No, he wasted too much time turning down those earlier bishoprics in order to write about Church history – and talking of Church history, what on earth's the Gnostic heresy got to go with poor old John Robinson?'

'Well, apparently there was a Christian Gnostic called Valentinus –'

'Never heard of him. No, wait a minute –'

'The Bishop – Ashworth not Robinson – wrote a book –'

'So he did, yes, I do dimly remember skimming through a review years ago, but what's the point in raking up people like Valentinus who lived in a completely different world and whose thought-forms in consequence are wholly irrelevant to the 1960s?'

'Dr Ashworth seems to operate on the theory that the more things change the more they remain the same. He thinks that when Robinson substitutes the depth metaphor for the height metaphor he's just as much a heretic as Valentinus was.'

'What utter nonsense! To say that God is the Ground of our being and that we can find him by looking deep into our consciousness is entirely consonant with the Bible. Think of the quotation: "The kingdom of God is within you!"'

'Ah yes, of course. Yes, I see. But how amazingly complicated theology becomes once you scratch below the surface –'

'That's exactly why it has to be kept simple for laymen and expressed in fresh up-to-date terms which are instantly meaningful to them. God is within the world and God is love; therefore God is to be found in one's deepest, most loving relationships. That's how one translates the technical term "the immanence of God" for modern man.'

'Yes, I see. Gosh, thanks for reasserting Robinson's thesis for me – I was beginning to feel quite –' I broke off as I saw that drip Maurice Tait trickling down the colonnade towards our corner of the lawn.

'Oh hullo, Mr Dean – hullo, Venetia –'

'Hullo, Maurice!' said Aysgarth. 'I caught Venetia meditating here and we've somehow wound up discussing heresy. Am I seeing you at the Deanery for dinner tonight?'

'No, that's tomorrow. Tonight Primrose and I have our Bible study group.'

'Ah yes, of course. I remember now.' He waited till Tait had trickled away before adding under his breath, 'We really mustn't meet here too often. It's too public.'

'Never mind, the day after tomorrow's Wednesday, and –'

'– and you can bring me the latest report on the Bishop's heresy hunt!' He gave me a sparkling smile. 'Two o'clock at the Staro Arms?'

'Can't wait!'

We parted with a torrid squeeze of the hands.

IV

'. . . and the truth is,' said the Bishop, pausing in his prowls around the morning-room to adjust one of the buttons on his gaiters, 'that if one denies God's transcendence by reducing Him to some all-pervasive presence within the world, one sails in very dangerous waters indeed. God is Love, says Dr Robinson – correctly. But he writes as if what he really believes is that Love is God, a pagan concept resulting – at its best – in the notion that God is scattered throughout the world in a sentimental *esprit de corps*, and – at its worst – in the notion that God can be evoked by orgiastic sexual rites. The reduction, dilution and downright perversion of the doctrine of the immanence of God in this manner should not be countenanced by any responsible Christian theologian. To indulge in such slipshod thinking,' said the Bishop, the gleam returning to his eye, 'is to succumb to the age-old heresy of pantheism.'

He prowled on, glossy, distinguished and formidable, around the austere morning-room of the South Canonry. 'Dr Robinson declares,' resumed Dr Ashworth dreamily, pausing by the window to gaze into the far distance, 'that he is not a pantheist, but this declaration, I fear, cannot alter the fact that much of what he says is pure pantheism. God is much greater, more infinitely Other, more mysteriously transcendent than Dr Robinson's puny vision of a disseminated love ethic can ever suggest, and no matter how often the Bishop claims to be preaching panentheism –'

'Hang on,' I said. 'You've finally floored me. Pan–'

'Pan*en*theism. That's what pantheists claim to believe when they're trying to pass their belief off as orthodox. Perhaps I'd better dictate a note explaining –'

The Bishop demolished the heresy of pantheism.

V

'Charles has wilfully misunderstood Robinson,' said Aysgarth as his car roared around a rural corner at fifty miles an hour on Wednesday afternoon. 'Robinson clearly rejects pantheism and there's no reason why he shouldn't support panentheism, the theory that the world is only part of God. Charles is getting all steamed up because he thinks Robinson's abolished God's transcendence, but in fact he hasn't abolished it at all; he's simply redefined it. He says the transcendent is the Beyond in our midst.'

'But what on earth does that mean?'

'It relates to the numinous, those moments when one becomes aware that there's something greater than ourselves all around us. It's a well-documented anthropological phenomenon.'

'Oh, I see. But –'

'If you ask me, Charles just isn't in touch with the ordinary worshipper in the pew. Modern man wants to be told in plain language what God's like and where he can find Him.'

'Does he?' I said, as we took another corner too fast and an oncoming car hooted at us. 'It seems to me that all modern man wants to know is: one, what can God do for me; two, why should I bother to believe in Him when I'm doing very nicely, thank you; and three, what are the odds on life after death?'

'Oh yes, yes, yes!' said Aysgarth indulgently, slamming the car into a lower gear in order to roar up a steep hill. 'All people who are undeveloped spiritually get stuck on those sort of questions, but that's only because they've got completely the wrong idea about God and think of Him as a tyrannical old man up in the sky. Once you show them that God is the Ground of their being and that He can be found in loving relationships, then their whole self-centred, self-seeking perspective on life will change and the way will be paved for spiritual progress.'

'Ah!' I said intelligently, but in fact I was no longer thinking of God. I was much too busy watching Aysgarth, much too occupied with fantasies about his short, thick, sexy fingers as they idly caressed the wheel.

VI

'Should we make amends for last Wednesday's sloth and walk up to the Ring?' he suggested reluctantly when he parked the car ten minutes later.

'No, it looks like rain – let's play safe and stay here,' I said at once, and he laughed as he switched off the engine.

After we had spent some time gossiping about a variety of subjects, he told me about his latest problem, a dispute over a modern sculpture which he had commissioned for the Cathedral churchyard. I was always surprised by Aysgarth's interest in art, but apparently his impoverishment as a London schoolboy had prompted many retreats on wet winter weekends to the picture galleries where no charge was made for admission, and years later when he had become a dean his interest in art, long dormant, had revived. Many deans believed they had a duty to reflect the art of their times in their cathedrals, and Aysgarth had soon decided he was called to leave an aesthetic mark on Starbridge.

He had started by commissioning a stained-glass window from the Frenchman Chagall (then almost unknown in England except by the cognoscenti) and when this had been received with startled enthusiasm, he had formed his ambition to acquire a modern sculpture. However, photographs of the semi-completed work had now been greeted with horror by Fitzgerald and Dalton, and even Eddie, the Chapter's third canon, had been dubious.

'But what's wrong with this great work of art?' I demanded.

'Nothing – it's "fab", as Pip would say!' Aysgarth became enthusiastic. 'It's red, white and blue, and consists of a match-stick type of man rising up a climbing-frame from an open box of cigars. The climbing-frame represents the spiritual life and the seven cigars represent the temptations of the material world – although of course they're not really cigars; they're a purely abstract representation of the seven deadly sins. Harriet's calling the work "Modern Man in Search of God".'

'Who's Harriet?'

'The sculptress. Harriet March, the widow of Captain Donald March who was killed on Everest. Surely you've heard of her?'

'Trust you to have a beautiful girlfriend panting to offer you a symbolic representation of the seven deadly sins!'

'My darling!' said Aysgarth, greatly entertained. 'So long as I have you, the beautiful Harriet can pant in vain!'

'Quite right – why bother with symbolic representations when you can have the real thing?' I retorted, and as he laughed, my right hand, which had apparently acquired a will of its own, came gently to rest on his left thigh.

I heard his sharp intake of breath and saw his mouth curve downwards in its sultriest line as the laughter died. The next moment he had grabbed my left shoulder with his right hand and was wrenching me closer to him. I was startled to discover that a passionate embrace in the front seat of a car requires a considerable degree of bodily contortion. It always looks so easy in films.

But if the embrace was passionate, the kiss was not. After grazing my cheek with his lips he stopped short of my mouth.

'No, no, no,' he said abruptly, slumping back behind the wheel. 'That won't do at all.' He shoved open the door. 'Let's walk up to the Ring.'

'Do we have time?'

Glancing at his watch he grimaced and pulled the door shut. 'No.' Glowering through the windscreen at the bare sensuous lines of the landscape he gripped the steering-wheel so hard that the brown age-spots on the back of his hands stood out starkly against the pale skin.

A long silence ensued.

Eventually I felt driven to mutter: 'Sorry. My fault,' but he answered in his curtest voice: 'Don't be absurd.'

As we continued to sit in the car a gust of wind hurled some drops of rain at the windscreen, and I was about to venture a comment on our wisdom in avoiding a walk when he said suddenly, not looking at me: 'If it's anyone's fault it's mine for permitting this friendship, but I can't believe it's wrong. I've been granted a unique opportunity to practise what I preach, and what I believe in is the primacy of love; I believe that if you really love someone you'll love them enough not to damage them in any way. One must be self-denying, not selfish; protective, not destructive; reaching up always towards the light, not stooping to grovel in the dark. And when our friendship's over – when you marry a man of your own generation who's utterly right for you – then I want you to be able to look back without regret and think with affection: *there* was a man who really loved me.'

'My darling Mr Dean –'

'Neville. Of course, being only human, I do find myself wishing . . . But that's no good, is it? One can drive oneself mad by wishing. What is, is. One must accept it and do the best one can, serving God according to one's conscience – and it would go against my conscience to destroy what we've found

233

together. It's a sin to destroy love, a *sin*. A genuinely loving relationship such as this . . . well, Robinson says it all, doesn't he? Let the conservative churchmen thunder away about absolute moral rules that can never be altered! The only ethic that matters is to act with love and compassion.' Reaching out blindly he turned the key in the ignition but the engine stalled. He was in such a state that he could only stare afterwards at the dashboard as if he had forgotten how to drive.

Hesitantly my voice said: 'Neville, this may seem a very silly question in the light of all you've just said, but . . . well, if you love me –'

'If!' He looked at me as if amazed that I should be so tentative. 'Of course I love you!'

'So does that mean . . . that's to say, do you . . . oh God, I can't quite put this into words –'

'Do I what?'

'Have other romantic friendships. I mean, do I have to share you with anyone else? I mean –'

He was appalled. 'My darling, you're the most marvellous girl in the world and I love you so much I hardly know what to do with myself – how could I look at anyone else?'

'Oh, Neville –' I broke off, sick with relief, but then doubt smote me again. 'But if there's no one else,' said my voice rapidly, 'what do you do about . . . oh God, I'm sorry to be so ignorant and unspiritual, but . . . well, unless a man's called to celibacy, doesn't he go mad unless he has sex regularly?'

There was a pause. For a split second his eyes went blank but then the next moment he was responding in the way I had least expected: he laughed.

'So that's the reason for my Chapter's erratic behaviour!' he exclaimed amused. 'Maybe I could solve my entire problems as Dean by prescribing mass-fornication!"

'But seriously, Neville –'

'Seriously, my dear, not only can the sexual drive vary enormously from individual to individual but it can also vary enormously within each individual. There are no hard and fast rules, I assure you, about the sexual behaviour of human beings.' And he added helpfully: 'Take my Chapter, for example. Fitzgerald professes to be called to celibacy. He's probably a repressed homosexual, but whatever he is it's plain that sex is low on his list of interests. Dalton's a widower who would like to marry again. I suspect he's becoming fed up with his enforced celibacy, but on the other hand he seems to get by all right – he usually manages to present an equable façade. Eddie's probably got the strongest sex drive of the lot, but unfortunately he has problems which have so far prevented him marrying. Possibly his enforced celibacy exacerbates his tendency towards hypochondria and morbid introspection, but one can't be certain; maybe an active sex life would in fact make very little difference to the neurotic side of his personality. The point to note, of course, is that none of my three celibate canons is either raving or dying from lack of sex, and contrary to all the male moanings you may have heard, no one has ever yet expired from chastity.'

I felt sick with relief again. Obviously he was implying that it was possible for him to do without sex.

Or was he? I remembered that split second when his eyes had gone blank. But probably the blankness had reflected a mere bourgeois *frisson* arising from the fact that an unmarried girl had asked him a blunt sexual question.

'Gosh, Neville, thanks for talking so frankly – you must be thinking me a complete ignoramus, but –'

'My darling, I'd be rather shocked if you weren't!'

Yes, that, of course, was a typically bourgeois response and the split-second blankness of the eyes was now explained. At last I could relax. Without doubt he was undergoing a period of chastity, unwilling to sleep with the neurotic wife who was too paralysed by her fear of pregnancy to want to sleep with him.

I resolved to think no more of Dido.

VII

I was just manicuring my nails on the following afternoon and thinking that I might potter along to the South Canonry to do a little typing, when the front doorbell rang at the foot of the stairs which led up to my flat. Marina had gone to Oxford and Primrose would almost certainly be at work in Eternity Street. I decided it was probably my landlady, Mrs Lindsay – or possibly one of her four jolly-hockey-sticks daughters with whom I had nothing in common. I was still trying to devise a plan which would enable me to repel their friendly overtures without being rude, but fortunately I suspected that they already regarded me as an aloof freak and were anxious to leave me alone.

With reluctance I descended the stairs and opened the front door.

'Ah, there you are, my dear,' said Dido, streaming past me across the threshold and skimming up the stairs. 'I'm sure you don't mind if I come in, do you, but I was just passing down Butchers' Alley on my way to Mitre Street to buy a wedding present for that dreadfully plain daughter of Mrs Pinn – such a mercy some man wants to marry her, it just shows one should never give up hope – when I remembered you, tucked away in the Lindsays' flat above their garage – and my dear, I must tell you that a couple were burnt to death in a flat over a garage only the other day when the car underneath them blew up, I read it in *The Times* so it must be true. However, you're not going to be here for long, are you, so I doubt if you'll be burnt to death, but nevertheless you should be very careful of exhaust fumes and always keep your window open.

'Anyway, my dear, Maurice Tait came to dinner the other night and mentioned that he'd seen you loitering with Stephen in the cloisters and I thought: Venetia! How dreadful, I've quite forgotten her – and I'm famous for remembering all my acquaintances, from the Bishop right down to that poor Cathedral cleaner with the cleft palate – so *immediately* I said to Stephen: "Darling," I said, "we must have Venetia to dinner – it's ages since she's been here!" and Stephen looked pleased because he's so fond of you, Venetia dear, along with Harriet March and half a dozen other young women – Stephen always has to have his little harem! – and as my entire life is devoted to making Stephen happy I'm all for encouraging these harmless friendships by including the girls in my guest-lists – why, I even post his letters to his female correspondents when I find them lying on the hall table! I've never been able to understand wives who can't take a generous, tolerant attitude to all their husbands' friends, and indeed, as I've so often told Primrose, I'm firmly convinced that possessiveness is the mark of an inferior nature – good heavens, look at this! What a dingy little room, no light, and the carpet needs replacing and what a pity the walls are such a sickly shade of cream, but never mind, at least you must be saving money as the Lindsays would surely never dare charge much for such a run-down little garret.

'Now, Venetia my dear, I've been examining my diary, and it's a *little* difficult to slip you in at present, but how about the Saturday after next, eight o'clock for eight-thirty? I shan't invite Eddie, I know things are delicate there – and never let it be said that I'm not a supremely tactful hostess – but I'll try to lure Perry down from London for the weekend.

'Well, I really must rush off to Mitre Street, but it's been lovely to see you and I'm glad you've at least got some sort of a roof over your head – although if you'll take my advice you'll remove those vulgar posters from the walls and put up something more dignified. After all, we mustn't forget, must we, that you're now nearer thirty than twenty and really too old to behave like a teenager over Elvis Presley. Well, goodbye, my dear, it'll be lovely to see you on Saturday week, I'm so glad you're working for the Bishop, living on top of the Archdeacon and having little chats after evensong with the Dean – I mean, it's all so terribly *seemly*, isn't it, and I'm sure it's such a relief for your parents who must have been wondering where on earth you were going to drift to next – no, don't worry, don't bother to come down, I'll see myself out . . .'

She flew away like the evil witch in a fairy-tale.

VIII

I was literally shaking with rage. Collapsing on the sofa in my beautiful flat, the first home I had ever had of my very own, I stared in the dim light, which I found so restful, at my glorious posters of Elvis celebrating the joy of life. The posters, offset by the rich, Cornish-cream shade of the walls, looked stunningly vivid, an inspired stroke of off-beat interior decoration. The threadbare brown carpet, so arrestingly different from all the priceless rugs I had had to endure in my parents' houses, blended perfectly with the Cornish-cream paint and the flowery, yellow-green pattern of the curtains. My record-player sat snugly in a corner. My current selection of books, ranging from *Honest to God* to *Lady Chatterley's Lover*, stood proudly on a shelf. There was not a plant in sight. The room was MINE, and I loved it fiercely.

I spent some time wishing that Dido would fall under a bus in Mitre Street, but eventually my rage was superseded by fright. That drip Maurice Tait! I might have known he'd go bleating to Dido that he'd seen me loitering with Aysgarth on Lady Mary. But on the other hand, why shouldn't I loiter occasionally with Aysgarth after evensong? Considering my long acquaintance with him, most people would judge my behaviour unremarkable, and surely Dido couldn't be thinking . . . But God alone knew what Dido thought. And when a woman was as neurotic as she was, what did her thoughts matter anyway?

But the more I recalled her words, the more uneasy I became. That reference to Harriet March had been unwelcome. And did Dido really post her husband's letters to a variety of youthful lady-friends? That sounded like fantasy – or perhaps a memory of the days when Aysgarth had occasionally penned a line to members of Primrose's 'Gang', now defunct. Aysgarth had told me plainly that he loved me too much to look at anyone else. So why was I experiencing these twinges of anxiety? Of course Harriet March was a woman of exceptional charm and glamour, but my Mr Dean only had one day off a week and the vital afternoon away from home was spent with me. That was undeniable. I supposed he was in correspondence with her about the sculpture, but nonetheless I was sure no letter to her ever began 'My darling'. So much for Harriet March.

I relaxed but I felt worn out. I had had no idea jealousy could be so exhausting. 'Possessiveness is the mark of an inferior nature,' Dido had said, but that statement was soaked in irony because she herself was possessiveness personified. I thought of the ghastly scene she had staged before Aysgarth had departed for the Hebrides, and suddenly, before I could stop myself, I was feeling uneasy again. Surely when a woman was as possessive as Dido she would want to possess the object of her adoration? But if she was frightened of conceiving . . . if she was neurotic enough to have what Dinkie called 'hang-ups' . . . No, sexual intercourse was out of the question and I had been mad to allow myself to be tormented by doubt again.

Concluding that her appalling visit had made me thoroughly overwrought, I pulled myself together and headed for the South Canonry to resume my typing.

IX

I decided not to describe Dido's visit in detail when I wrote to Aysgarth, but I did mention that she had called as the result of Tait's betrayal. Aysgarth was unperturbed; he wrote back that there was no need to worry about Tait's gaffe since Dido had not thought the episode in the least suspicious and was indeed genuinely remorseful that she had not invited me to dinner earlier. I doubted the remorse but was glad to be reminded that Dido often did have good intentions. I even saw that she had probably descended on my flat with no prior intention to reduce me to pulp and might even have thought she was doing me a favour by reminding me that I was nearer thirty than twenty. Dido's devotion to what she was pleased to describe as her 'candour' arose from the belief that one had a moral duty to help others towards self-improvement by pointing out their faults and mistakes. It was quite possible that in making her criticisms she had had only my welfare in mind.

Usually I managed to avoid mentioning Dido when I replied to Aysgarth's letters which soon began to arrive every day. Our correspondence ranged over a broad number of subjects – literature, art, current events, television, Church gossip – but before long I realised that what he enjoyed most was telling me about his work. It seemed to be a relief to him to complain not only about the bickering in Chapter but about the many minor crises which occurred regularly among the community of over a hundred people who worked at the Cathedral. When it dawned on me that he was very much alone, poised at the top of the Cathedral's organisational pyramid, I had a fresh insight into Eddie's role in his life. In the absence of a friendly relationship with the Bishop, Aysgarth relied heavily for support on the one Cathedral executive whom he could trust to be loyal under any circumstances.

'At least I can always rely on Eddie never to stab me in the back,' Aysgarth wrote, 'but nevertheless I feel I can never fully confide in him – and this isn't just because we've always had a relationship in which he pours out his troubles and I do the listening. It's because I feel that with men I have to "put up a front" – show no weakness, be tough, appear successful at all times. That's the result of my upbringing, when I was brow-beaten into "getting on" in the world, and attitudes acquired in childhood are sometimes not so easy to slough off in later life. Bearing this idiosyncrasy of mine in mind you'll be able to understand why it's such a luxury for me to have a female confidante; I can relax at last, stop "putting up a front", be myself – *my new self* – THE NEW NEVILLE! Darling, I can't tell you what a psychological liberation I experience not only when I see you but when I pick up the pen to write you a letter . . .'

I was just wishing yet again that Aysgarth's liberation would be less psychological and more physical when I received a communication from Eddie, the first I had received since his pathetic note apologising for his behaviour on the Cathedral roof. Having written a one-line reply to suggest that we treated the fiasco as if it had never happened, I had not expected to hear from him again, and I unfolded his new letter with considerable reluctance.

'Dear Venetia,' I read, 'I hope you didn't tear this up as soon as you saw my writing on the envelope. Let me say straight away that I won't refer to the episode on the cathedral roof again, but I wonder nevertheless if something of value might yet be salvaged from the débâcle. Stephen is always adamant in insisting that love should never be just chucked in the nearest wastepaper basket and forgotten, so perhaps my love could eventually be recycled in a more acceptable form. Certainly it's purely in the spirit of Platonic friendship that I write to remind you that Martin Darrow will be appearing soon in Coward's *Present Laughter* at the Starbridge Playhouse as part of a trial run in the provinces before the show opens in the West End. If you'd still like to see him, then I'd still like to take you. No fuss, no mess, I promise. Think it over. Yours, EDDIE.'

Feeling faintly nauseated I tossed off a note which read: 'Dear Eddie: Better not. It's a bit early yet, I think, to talk in terms of Platonic friendship.' I gritted my teeth before forcing myself to add: 'But maybe one day. Yours, VENETIA.'

Then I began to prepare for my next expedition to Starbury Plain with the Dean.

X

It was a wet afternoon so once again we failed to reach the Ring. We sat in the car and smoked and gossiped and laughed while he squeezed my hand in a dozen different ways amidst countless sultry looks and frequent observations about how wonderful I was. How I stopped myself plastering him with kisses I shall never know, but I had made up my mind that the affair should proceed at his own pace. My brush with his thigh last week had only upset him, and besides, never having been romantically involved with anyone before, I was in fact reluctant to take the lead in making advances; the thigh-brush had merely resulted from a mindless spontaneity. So although I was longing for a passionate kiss I endured without complaint the agonising frustration generated by the hand-squeezing, and told myself sternly that deep moral convictions in a clergyman could never be rapidly overcome.

I eventually received another peck on the cheek when we parted. Making an enormous effort I convinced myself I admired him more than ever for his devotion to the high ideals implicit in Robinson's New Morality, and made a new resolution to be patient.

XI

Three days later I went to dinner at the Deanery.

When I arrived I found to my dismay that I had been included in one of Dido's notorious 'little dinner-parties for sixteen', evenings of social carnage during which she threw together some ill-assorted guests, mixed them ruthlessly with her family and interrupted every conversation until everyone was either silenced or outraged. On that evening little Pip escaped the lethal frivolities; he was considered young enough to have an early supper and listen in tranquil bliss to Radio Luxemburg, but Dido's daughter Elizabeth was present, flexing her intellect and competing not unsuccessfully with her half-sister Primrose as the female brain-box of the family. But Elizabeth, even at fourteen, was far sexier than Primrose and batted her eyelashes precociously at some sixteen-year-old male infant who had been roped in to keep her amused.

The other guests consisted entirely of residents of the Close, the boring ones who enjoyed reading the obituaries in *The Times* and discussing who had just had a stroke. Evidently Dido was swiping a bunch of unwanted people off her party-list in one fell swoop. None of Aysgarth's sons by his first marriage was present, and there was no sign of Perry, who had obviously had the brains to elude Dido's attempt to kidnap him. The nadir of the dinner arrived when I caught the attention of a retired general who kept squeezing my knee under the table until I managed to tread on his toe. His wife said with mild interest: 'Is your gout troubling you again, dear?' as he turned purple and yelped with rage.

At the head of the table Aysgarth, looking serene, caressed his glass of claret but drank little. I never once caught him looking in my direction.

In the drawing-room after the meal he did manage to say to me pleasantly: 'And how's your new flat, Venetia?' but before I could tell him what he already knew the witch descended on her broomstick, slipped her arm through his and declared: 'Venetia's looking a trifle wan, don't you think, Stephen? But then working for the Bishop must be so exhausting – which reminds me, do tell Stephen, Venetia, what the Bishop's putting in his book because it's certain to be something about sex – we all know dear Charles can't think of anything else – and Stephen always adores it, don't you, my love, when the Bishop is simply too puritanical to be true.'

'Do I?' said Aysgarth vaguely, but he was smiling at her, his bright eyes crinkling at the corners, and she was leaning hard enough against him to ensure he slipped an arm around her waist to prop her up.

'Darling Stephen!' exclaimed Dido as I glanced at the ceiling, the fireplace, the door, the windows – at any object except her adoring dark eyes. 'Always so wonderfully discreet!'

I managed to say: 'If you'll excuse me for a moment . . .' Then I escaped, dived into the cloakroom and collapsed shuddering on the lavatory seat. Some time passed. Eventually I dragged myself back to the fray. Aysgarth had his arm around his daughter Elizabeth by this time and was talking to a couple so old I felt they ought to be dead. Meanwhile Primrose was chatting about the Girl Guides to some battle-axe whose sex was denoted only by a long skirt, and Dido was still swooping around on her invisible broomstick. As I re-entered the room I saw with dread that I had once again caught her attention.

'Venetia –' I braced myself for another pulverising assault

'— I'm so sorry I couldn't lure Perry here tonight but he was going sailing with a crowd of friends — did you know Perry kept a boat at Bosham? — and although he swore he was devastated to miss you, he couldn't alter his plans.'

'That's all right, Mrs Aysgarth. I can live without Perry.'

'Then who's the one you can't live without? I'm sure we're all agog to know! Christian said —'

'Christian got it wrong. There's no one in my life at present except God.'

'*God?*'

'Uh-huh. You told me to find Him. So I did.'

'You mean you've had a religious conversion?'

'Thanks to you, yes. I've just read Bishop Robinson's book.'

'Oh?' said Dido, and added in a not unfriendly voice: 'What did you think of it?'

'I was terribly impressed. It's wonderful to find a bishop who speaks for our day and age.'

'I think it's a load of codswallop,' said Dido, 'and I don't think he speaks for our day and age at all. How can anyone think that's a relevant book for modern man when the author never mentions what kind of world modern man has to live in? He spends enough time quoting Bonhoeffer and Tillich, but he never mentions that Bonhoeffer was hanged by the Nazis and Tillich was driven into exile. What does he have to tell us about sin and evil? Damn all! It's all airy-fairy liberal optimism about how God's really down here on earth, but Robinson, it seems, is firmly wedged up there in the clouds! Darling Stephen — who of course is quite the most romantic idealist who ever lived — may choose to fall in love with *Honest to God*, but that's only because he's so high-minded that he'd stagger through a sewer and still manage to keep his eyes on the stars.' As if allowing me time to digest this Wildean metaphor she turned aside to survey the progress of the party and bawled in a stage-whisper to her step-daughter: 'Primrose, do pass round the cigarettes!'

'Mrs Aysgarth,' I said, unable to help wondering where she had picked up this withering critique of Bishop Robinson, 'have you actually read *Honest to God*?'

'My dear, at a sitting! Doesn't everyone? I always like to keep up with Stephen's interests so that I can discuss them intelligently with him, and no matter how busy we are during the day, we always make time to meet at night for a cosy chat *à deux*. He comes to my bedroom and – Primrose dear! *Primrose!* My God, there's none so deaf as those that refuse to hear – excuse me a moment, Venetia.'

I looked wildly around for any object which might have contained alcohol but saw only coffee-pots.

'And as I was saying,' said Dido, swooping back after a mini-slanging match with Primrose who had refused to pass around the cigarettes, 'Stephen comes to my room every night and we talk about everything – really, I always feel so sorry for couples who say they can't communicate with each other because I'm convinced that communication is the secret of a really successful marriage – and having been married successfully for eighteen years I should know what I'm talking about. Indeed I honestly feel that where Stephen's concerned I'm practically psychic, but I suppose that's what happens when you know someone through and through – and God knows, no one knows Stephen as well as I do – except possibly Jon Darrow, but unfortunately he's senile now and sees no one, poor old man. Well, my dear, my duty as a hostess calls and I must run off and ask the General about his gout – but do help yourself to something from the decanters over there behind the Admiral. Perhaps a little Rémy Martin might be appropriate? Brandy's always so useful if one's feeling as peaky as one looks.'

She swooped away.

I drank two triple brandies. Then having made my escape I drove erratically back to my flat and lay awake in torment until dawn.

FIVE

'Chastity is the expression of charity – of caring, enough.
And this is the criterion for every form of behaviour, inside
marriage or out of it, in sexual ethics or in any other field.
For *nothing else* makes a thing right or wrong.'

JOHN A. T. ROBINSON
Suffragan Bishop of Woolwich 1959–1969
Honest to God

I

I overslept and missed not only the early service but Sunday
matins. I did rush to the Cathedral in time for the sung
Communion, but the Dean glided away afterwards without
once looking in my direction. In despair I retired to the cloisters
and waited on Lady Mary but no one came. I felt demented.

Back at the flat I wrote: 'Darling Neville, I really was rather
demolished by dinner last night. Any chance of seeing you
before Wednesday? All love, V.'

Then I returned to the Cathedral with the idea of leaving the
letter in the Dean's stall to await his arrival for evensong, but
the eagle-eyed Cathedral guides were everywhere and a stout
lady arranging flowers by the lectern made any attempt to sidle
unobserved to the stall impossible.

Stumbling home I tore up the letter and phoned the Deanery.
Dido answered.

I hung up and mixed myself a dry martini which would have
stopped even James Bond dead in his tracks. Then I slumped
down on the sofa beneath the Elvis posters and began to cry.

II

'. . . and when Bonhoeffer states that mankind has come of age,' dictated the Bishop, 'and implies that man – modern man – can get along without God, he is clearly flirting with nothing less than the Pelagian heresy. Or in other words, Dr Robinson follows Bonhoeffer on this point *at his peril*.

'However,' added Dr Ashworth kindly, stroking his pectoral cross as if it were a domestic pet, 'the Bishop tries hard to redeem himself by stressing the importance to modern man of Christ, and indeed his view of Jesus is not entirely without merit. His statement, for instance, that Christ is the window through which we see God is well in line with orthodox thinking. Nevertheless I fear that when he mocks the traditional concept of the Incarnation in various facetious sentences, he not only diminishes the doctrine of God; he puts himself squarely in line with those who followed Arius in the days of the Early Church. What we are dealing with here,' concluded Dr Ashworth, blissfully happy, 'is yet another resurgence in a brand-new form of an age-old challenge to orthodoxy.'

And he proceeded to demolish both the Pelagian and the Arian heresies.

III

'My darling, I'm desperately sorry – I got your letter yesterday, but I couldn't meet you on Lady Mary because – oh hullo, General! Fancy seeing you here!'

'Just had a spot of lunch, Dean.' The General gazed at me with his protuberant, gooseberry-coloured eyes as I paused by the open door of Aysgarth's car in the courtyard of the Staro Arms. 'Good afternoon, Miss Flaxton.'

'Good afternoon, General.' I slid uneasily into the passenger seat.

'Well, Venetia,' said Aysgarth. 'We mustn't keep Lady Mary waiting, must we?'

'It's so kind of you to give me a lift,' I said to him in ringing tones. The General was slightly deaf. 'I do hope I'm not taking you too far out of your way.'

'Were you in the dining-room, Miss Flaxton?' said the General, now exhibiting a marked curiosity. 'I didn't see you.'

'No, I was in the river-garden.'

Aysgarth said firmly: 'If you'll excuse us, General –'

'Of course, of course . . .'

As the car shot forward across the courtyard, Aysgarth muttered: 'We'll have to arrange a different rendezvous – we can't risk that old buffer seeing us again.'

'Never mind, we're finally alone together. That's all that matters.'

The car roared with a screech of the tires into Eternity Street and rocketed away towards the river and the suburbs.

IV

'My darling, why were you so upset in your letter? Why did you want to meet me last night on Lady Mary?'

'It was that dinner-party.'

'I knew you'd find it dull, but –'

'Dull! Do you think I simply wanted to whine that I was bored? I tell you it was vile – vile, vile, *vile!*'

He was very shocked. 'But what happened?'

'Let's wait till we get to the car-park. I can't possibly discuss this unless I have your full attention.'

In response he promptly trod on the brakes, pulled the car round the corner into a side-road and halted beneath the branches of a chestnut tree. We had crossed the river by that time and were in one of the quiet, dignified residential streets of the suburb called Parson's Mill.

Switching off the engine he demanded: 'What did Dido say?'

I tried without success to speak.

'You shouldn't take any notice of her,' he said. 'Just let all those words pour off you like water off a duck's back.'

'Unfortunately,' I said, 'her words aren't water and I'm no duck.' I stared fiercely out of the window at the flower-filled front garden of the nearest house as I added: 'I'm sorry – I know you don't want to talk about her –'

'I'll talk about her till the cows come home if that'll put things right. Tell me exactly what she said.'

'It wasn't so much what she said as what she implied.'

'And what was that?'

But I was silent. In the end all I could say was: 'I had this horrible feeling that she knows everything about us.'

'Impossible.'

'She said you discuss everything together –'

'Hardly! Do you think I tell her about my Wednesday excursions?'

'But what do you say to explain your absences?'

'Nothing. She's out playing bridge with her girlfriends. It's a regular four. Next week, when she's the hostess at the Deanery, I shall have to take a little more care when I slip out, but she'll be much too busy to notice me.'

'But if she suspects we meet, she'll watch you more closely and –'

'She suspects nothing. It sounds to me as if you've completely misread her. The trouble with reading Dido is that she shoots innumerable arrows at the target of truth and just because she scores a certain number of bull's-eyes one can easily be fooled into thinking not only that she hits the mark every time but that she knows much more than she actually does. Now listen to me and I'll set your mind at rest by explaining exactly what's going on. You're female, under thirty and congenial to me so Dido's going to be lukewarm towards you. Nothing new there, of course; that's been the situation for years and from Dido's point of view little has changed. But from your point of view everything's changed – which explains why you're now ultra-sensitive to every arrow Dido shoots from her bow. But what you should remember is that from Dido's point of view the only change in the situation is your mysterious decision to stay in Starbridge and live in a déclassé flat when you could be bobbing around London and living somewhere smart.'

'Exactly. Dido probably thinks –'

'No, she doesn't. I've pointed out that this is the 1960s and upper-class girls are no longer as hidebound by convention as they were twenty – even ten – years ago. You've always been intrigued by the ecclesiastical – what could be more natural than that you should be unable to say no when the Bishop, very flatteringly, offers you a job? And since you've finally made the break with your parents, what could be more natural than that you should rebel against your upbringing in a stately home by living in a small flat? Dido, I assure you, quite saw the logic of that argument, and as soon as you pushed your religious conversion claim on Saturday night she was fully prepared to concede that your continuing presence in Starbridge was no longer a mystery. She was actually very benign towards you, said how greatly you'd improved –'

'You discussed me, then,' I said, 'after the party.'

'Oh, we discussed everyone! We always have a post-mortem on our social events!'

'Yes. She did in fact say that you go to her bedroom every night for a cosy little chat.'

There was a silence while I stared fiercely at the flowers again, but at last I heard him say: 'Darling, you don't have to be jealous of Dido.'

'Why not?' I swung to face him. 'She's your wife, isn't she?'

'Yes, but . . .' Now it was his turn to stare at the flowers. Then he said: 'Try to understand. She's a sad person in many ways. She has many difficulties. She needs someone to look after her and I'm the one who's been called to do it. But all that has absolutely no bearing on the strength of my love for you.'

'You mean – what you're really saying is –'

'Dido's Stephen's responsibility,' he said. 'But neither of them has anything to do with us.'

I stared at him but he was smiling as if he had not compounded the mystery but elucidated it. 'Feeling better?' he said lightly. 'Shall we go on?'

I nodded. I felt I needed time to think. Reaching out he gave my hand a comforting squeeze and then started the engine to resume our journey.

V

'We really must walk up to the Ring today,' said Aysgarth, parking the Humber. 'I feel we need to be wary of too many delicious incarcerations in the car.'

We set off along the bridle-path which led upwards over the ridge, and soon vast views of the Plain began to unfold in every direction. Aysgarth's was the only car in the parking area, but ahead of us some hikers were moving steadily towards the brow of the hill.

'Are you all right?' he said, reaching for my hand. 'You're very quiet.'

'I was just thinking that although I've known you for so many years, I don't really know you at all. This Stephen whom you now talk of as a separate person – when did he come into being?'.

'1946.'

'But you married Dido in 1945 and I thought she'd always called you Stephen!'

'Yes, but it took me a while to grow into him, and I was still Neville in 1945. That was Neville Three,' he added placidly, apparently unaware that the conversation was in any way bizarre. 'Now, of course, I'm Neville Four.' Pausing for breath he turned to survey the landscape. The hill was steeper than it looked from the car-park. 'My goodness, what splendid views! he exclaimed. 'But I don't like the look of those black clouds over there.'

'Never mind the black clouds. Tell me about the first three Nevilles.'

Without a second's hesitation he said: 'Oh, they wouldn't interest you at all.'

'Everything about you interests me, Neville. I love you so I want to know you through and through.'

'My darling!' He gave me his sexiest smile. 'How very sweet you are, but I think we've wasted quite enough of our precious time together talking about matters which just aren't relevant to our wonderful love here and now in the summer of 'sixty-three. I want to talk about *you*! Tell me everything you've been doing – how's life at the South Canonry?'

I gave up and began to describe the Bishop's continuing demolition of heresy.

VI

'Charles has got it entirely wrong as usual,' said Aysgarth. 'He's misunderstood the Bonhoeffer dictum and he's perverted Robinson's views on the Incarnation. The truth is Robinson's remarks on Jesus clearly indicate – whoops! Here comes the rain! What an unjust reward for my virtuous attempt to exercise!'

Haring downhill hand in hand as the heavens opened, we reached the car and hurled ourselves inside.

'How out of training I am!' gasped Aysgarth as he subsided behind the steering-wheel. 'Darling, if I drop dead, abandon me at once, I implore you, and thumb a lift back to Starbridge. I'd hate to embarrass everyone by dying in scandalous circumstances . . . Good heavens, look at this!' he added as the rain began to pound more heavily than ever against the windscreen.

'There was a very erotic song in the hit parade some time ago,' I said, watching him smooth back his wet hair. 'It was called "The Day that the Rains Came."'

'Did it conjure up images of wet earth and steaming grass and people plunging naked through the undergrowth?'

'You're thinking of D. H. Lawrence!'

We laughed, and suddenly the expression in his eyes changed. For a moment I thought he would do no more than look at me, but I was wrong. He leant forward to kiss me on the mouth.

Then I ceased to hear the rain drumming on the roof, ceased to see the water streaming down the glass, ceased to think of anything except the man I wanted – and alongside us in the land of allegory the powerful, predatory serpent, no longer sedate and domesticated, surged forth from the undergrowth to encircle us both at last.

VII

'It can't be wrong,' said Aysgarth. 'I just don't believe it's wrong. Love makes everything right. It must do. It must.'

I was unable to reply. I was aware of a variety of physical reactions which I have no intention of describing in clinical detail, but my awareness was dim because I was almost unconscious with ecstasy. I could only stay glued to his wet shirt-front and pray not to weep with frustration when the embrace inevitably ended.

Then I heard him whisper: 'You're such a prize, Venetia, *such a prize*! So of course,' he added with a sigh as he finally released me, 'I must never win you.'

At first I thought I had misheard him. 'Never win me?'

'No, I must keep you perfect. All prizes are perfect, naturally, or they wouldn't be prizes, but winning them can be dangerous. One can win a prize, discover its imperfections and then realise one doesn't want it any more.'

I stared at him. Yet again he seemed quite unaware that the conversation had become bizarre. 'Are you implying,' I said incredulously, 'that if you won me you'd soon get bored and toss me aside?'

'No, I'm merely reminding myself that if I won you I'd be winning a flesh-and-blood person, not a fantasy, and we might well fail to live happily ever after – or in other words, I was reminding myself that chasing the prizes can lead one into a world of illusion. It's always vital that I remember that.'

'Neville, all this talk of prizes –'

'Yes, it's absurd, isn't it? It used to be a fixation of mine, the result of my impoverished youth and an uncle who urged me to go "chasing the prizes of life" in order to make the best of myself. But I've got a more balanced outlook on life now.' He fumbled in the pocket of his jacket and produced a packet of cigarettes. 'Shall we smoke?'

I waited until our cigarettes were alight before I said: 'Eddie mentioned that uncle of yours.'

'Uncle Willoughby – a marvellous old boy he was, took care of us all in the difficult days after my father died. No doubt it was because my life was so far from perfect then that I used to dream of perfection – to dream, as Uncle Willoughby would have put it, of the ultimate prizes: a perfect home, a perfect career, a perfect wife, perfect children –'

'But Neville,' I said, 'no one's really perfect, are they?' I was remembering Primrose telling me long ago of her brothers' unflagging efforts to acquire flawless masks.

'No, of course true perfection can't exist in this world,' he agreed willingly enough, 'but one should still dream of perfection, cherish ideals, aim for the finest prizes – goals, I mean –'

'There you go again!'

He laughed. 'I'm incorrigible, aren't I! Let's talk of something else.'

'No, I want to talk more about you.'

'But there's nothing to say! You know it all.'

'Do I? I know you were born in Yorkshire and that your father died bankrupt when you were seven. I know you and your brother were then boarded out in London in order to go to a good school while your mother's poor health forced her to live by the sea in Sussex with your sister. I know you won a scholarship to Oxford where you took a first in Greats and received your call to be a clergyman. I know you married at twenty-four and had five children. I know you were Rector of Willowmead, Archdeacon of Starbridge and a canon of Westminster. I know that after your first wife died you married again and had five more children, only two of whom survived. I know you're now Dean of Starbridge. Yes, it's quite true – I do know all about you. So why do I increasingly feel you're a complete stranger?'

'My darling, I can't imagine why you're so keen to wrap me in mystery! I'm just a Yorkshire draper's son who's made good. What could be more simple than that?'

'I'll tell you: all the Yorkshire drapers' sons who haven't made good. They're the simple ones. I now realise that you must be quite extraordinary and tremendously complex, but I don't see how I'm ever going to know you through and through when you resolutely refuse to talk about yourself.'

'But you understand me perfectly! You're so sympathetic, so intuitive, so clever, so –'

'Thank you, I hope I'm all those things, but –'

'You're all those things and much, much more,' he said, stubbing out his cigarette and switching on the ignition, 'so can't you see how unnecessary it is to delve into my utterly irrelevant past? Neville Four doesn't have a past, that's the truth of it. He just has this glorious present with you.'

I took the hint and pursued my cross-examination no further, but as the Humber descended from the hills into the valley, I began to wonder if I understood even less than I had imagined.

VIII

We were more than halfway to Starbridge before I summoned the nerve to ask: 'Neville, what exactly is your connection with Nicholas Darrow's father, that clergyman who ran the Theological College back in the 'forties?'

The car swerved slightly, but to my relief he seemed more astonished than annoyed by this new attempt to probe the past. 'Jon Darrow?' he exclaimed. 'Why on earth should you want to know about him?'

'I've been told he knows you through and through.'

At once he said sharply: 'Who said that?'

'I'm sorry, I really don't want to mention her name again, but –'

'Why in heaven's name should Dido have been talking to you about old Darrow?'

'Well, she was boasting about how well she knew you, and –'

'Ah, now I understand this new obsession of yours to know me through and through! Darling, you must stop seeing Dido as a rival – and you must stop believing every word she says. She doesn't know me well at all. She only knows Stephen.'

Dimly it occurred to me that in order to participate intelligently in these extraordinary conversations I needed a wisdom which I had not lived long enough to acquire.

'And who does Darrow know?' I said cautiously.

'The first three Nevilles.'

'Not Stephen?'

'No, I haven't seen much of the old pirate since Stephen evolved.' He tried to overtake the car in front, thought better of it and dropped back. The oncoming car hooted furiously as it skimmed past our wing-mirror.

'Why do you call the old boy a pirate?' I said when the sound of the horn had died away. 'I thought he was a holy hermit who lived in a wood on Communion wafers.'

Aysgarth laughed so hard that he nearly drove through a red light. We were now re-entering the suburb of Parson's Mill. 'It's really amazing,' he exclaimed, 'how myths form around that buccaneer! My dear, Father Jonathan Darrow is an eccentric Anglo-Catholic priest who used to perform charismatic wonders, flirt with scandal and make strong archdeacons weep. His years at the Theological College constituted his respectable phase. Before that he'd done more or less everything – he was even a monk in the Anglican Fordite Order during the 'twenties and 'thirties! Young Nicholas, of course, was fathered later. Martin the actor was fathered long before.'

'But is the old boy really living in a wood as a hermit?'

'I think it would be more accurate – though less amusing – to say he lives as a recluse twelve miles from Starbridge; he had a cottage built for him in the grounds of the Manor House which his second wife owned at Starrington Magna. She's dead now, I'm sorry to say – a nice woman she was, I liked her – and the Manor itself is run by a religious community of about eight men and women who keep an eye on the old boy to make sure he's all right.'

'You mean he's capable of living alone in his cottage? Someone told me he was senile.'

'There was a rumour he was unhinged for a time by his wife's death, but I suspect the people who say he's senile are the people who can't imagine why anyone should want to live as a recluse.'

'But Neville,' I said as we approached the bridge over the river, 'how did this clerical eccentric, whom you don't seem to like much, come to know you so well?'

'Ah,' said Aysgarth. He paused. Then he said: 'Well, as a matter of fact he gave me a helping hand once. Very decent of him and I appreciated it. I was going through a bit of a spiritual crisis at the time.'

'You mean you'd lost your faith?'

'Good heavens, no!' said Aysgarth shocked. 'Who do you think I am – one of Graham Greene's whisky-priests? No, life just became a trifle awkward for a few days, that's all. However, I survived. I'm a born survivor,' said Aysgarth, hands resting lightly on the wheel as the car shot over the bridge, 'and so's that old pirate Jon Darrow. Incidentally, what do you think of that boy of his? I haven't seen him since he was a child.'

'He's a psychic. He gives the impression of never travelling without his crystal ball.'

'That sounds like a chip off the old block! There was some wild talk about how his father foresaw Pearl Harbor but I never believed a word of it. Dear old Darrow, he used to drive me mad when I was an archdeacon, but he was a great character. I shall feel sorry when he's finally called to meet his maker.'

That remark gave me a jolt. St Darrow, Nick had told me, was eighty-three. The old boy could be borne off by the angels at any minute. I had to act fast.

After parting from Aysgarth outside the Staro Arms amidst the usual torrid hand-squeezes and smouldering looks, I retired to my flat and tried to work out how I could gain access to this ancient recluse who had once known my Mr Dean so well.

From the telephone operator I obtained the number of Laud's College in Cambridge, but when I put through the call I was told term had ended. I then looked up the number of Starrington Manor where one of St Darrow's disciples managed to produce my Talisman after a three-minute hunt.

'Sorry to bother you, Nick,' I said, determined not to make Marina's mistake of drowning him in cloying enthusiasm, 'but I was hoping you could give me some advice about your brother. I've been invited to see *Present Laughter* and –' I paused with thespian skill to convey the impression that a casual thought had just drifted into my mind '– oh, by the way, I assume you'll be heading for the Starbridge Playhouse too some time that week?'

'On the Friday, yes.'

'Ah, I think Eddie – Eddie Hoffenberg, my escort – can only manage the Saturday, so I doubt if I'll see you, but I must just ask this: as I told you once, my mother's a huge Martin Darrow fan – would he think me a colossal bore if I went backstage and asked for his autograph for her?'

'Actors never mind being asked for autographs,' said Nick in a tone of voice which suggested he considered all actors far beneath him. It occurred to me then to wonder if he might be jealous of his handsome, successful brother.

'But do I have to mention your name in order to win admittance to the august presence?' I pursued, craftily signalling to him by my facetious tone that I too thought actors were a race apart.

'I shouldn't think so. But mention it if you like,' said Nick, picking up my signal and becoming gracious.

'Lovely, thanks so much. I say . . . will your father be going to see the play?'

'Yes.'

'How exciting for him! I hope he likes it. Older people often find Coward quite shocking, I believe.'

'My father isn't that sort of old person,' said Nick, becoming austere, 'and since my mother was a Coward fan, he's familiar with the text of *Present Laughter*.'

'Super! Okay, Nick, mustn't delay you any longer – see you around some time. 'Bye.'

I hung up, found pen and paper and wrote: 'Dear Eddie, After that mean-spirited, unchristian little note I sent in response to your last letter, am I allowed to change my mind about *Present Laughter*? I've decided I'd like to go, although for various reasons the only evening I can manage is the Friday. However, if you'd prefer not to escort me – indeed if you'd prefer to tear up this note and jump on it – I shall quite understand. Yours, VENETIA.'

I posted this missive five minutes later in the Chasuble Lane pillar-box. Then feeling confident that I would eventually come face to face with St Darrow, I congratulated myself on my Machiavellian skills and began to speculate again – fruitlessly – on the mysterious multiple personalities of my extraordinary Mr Dean.

X

An hour later I was just goggling at the television news (the Profumo scandal was now in full flower) and spooning baked beans into my mouth when the telephone rang. It was my mother, who had discovered that Martin Darrow was to appear at the Starbridge Playhouse. Enthralled by the thought of seeing her hero in the flesh she was already planning her visit to Flaxton Hall which could be used as a base for her assault on the theatre.

'. . . and I was wondering if we could go to *Present Laughter* together, darling,' she added. 'I'd so like to see your flat – perhaps we could have an egg or something before the play. Can you boil an egg yet?'

'Oh yes, but it's so messy – all that steam –'

'Well, never mind, a sandwich would do –'

'Will Papa be with you?'

'Oh no, he'd never go near anything by Coward. That's why I thought that perhaps you and I —'

'Mama, it's terribly unfortunate but I've just agreed to go to the play with Canon Hoffenberg. Could you arrange to go with one of your Starbridge pals instead? You could come here for a drink first, of course —'

'Canon Hoffenberg!'

'Yes, but don't tell Papa — he'll ring up and start bawling away about the damned Huns, and frankly I'm not in a mood to take it.'

'Oh, I know, darling, I know, so exhausting, and personally I've always rather liked Canon Hoffenberg —'

'Just let me know when you're coming, Mama, and I'll go out and buy some gin.'

'No, no, don't buy any gin — your father will be so relieved when I tell him with a clear conscience that you don't keep spirits in your flat. A glass of sherry would be quite sufficient for me.'

We parted amicably. Eyeing the gin bottle nearby I made a mental note to hide it in the airing cupboard before my mother arrived. Then I returned to the apparently endless television report on the Profumo scandal (distinguished married man ruined by ravishing young floozie) and began munching away once more on my baked beans.

XI

'Dear Venetia,' wrote Eddie in a letter which was delivered by hand, 'I've got two tickets for the front row of the circle for the Friday performance. I shall be having dinner first at that new restaurant, the Quill Pen, in Wheat Street and if you'd like to join me, just let me know. Otherwise I'll pick you up at your flat at 7.40. The restaurant column of the *Starbridge Weekly News* said that on the Quill Pen's wine-list there was a very bold sparkling Mosel (which one seldom encounters in this country), but perhaps you'd prefer champagne, which I've no doubt the

Quill Pen can also supply in abundance. Yours, EDDIE.'

I wrote back: 'Dear Eddie: Congratulations on the front row of the circle! I thought the best seats would already have been nabbed, but maybe the Cathedral clergy have a special pull at the box office. I'll drink anything that sparkles – in fact I'll drink anything – but I'm on a diet so I'll say no to the Quill Pen. See you at 7.40 as you suggest. Many thanks. Yours, VENETIA.'

Then I picked up Aysgarth's daily report, read it through yet again and wrote: 'My darling Neville, Thanks so much for your letter, but honestly, there's no need to work yourself into such a frenzy of remorse – it wasn't *your* fault that I was demolished at the Deanery! In fact I can see now (thanks to you) that I overreacted to all D's remarks and made a mountain out of a molehill, so really I can blame no one for the demolition but myself. Sorry I got so fixated on your past and tried to turn you into a mystery man. I'm sure you really are terribly simple and that I really am being terribly stupid. It's just that I find you so enthralling that I tend to go into an overheated feminine flat spin unless I understand every single thing you do. Such a drag for you! I promise to behave more rationally in future.

'Apart from my idiotic behaviour (as specified above) I adored every minute of our meeting, especially the bit where we stuck together so torridly that steam rose from our wet clothes. But I think you're right and we should change the rendezvous from the Staro Arms. How about the car-park of the Starbridge Playhouse? Which reminds me, I decided to make my peace with Eddie by agreeing to go with him to see *Present Laughter*. Eddie suggested this outing some time ago and I thought it might be a painless way of compensating him for my beastliness on the Cathedral roof. Then I shan't have to go out with him again.

'Darling, what a *bore* about Fitzgerald taking a phallic view of the sculpture's "box of cigars"! He must have a mind like a sink – in fact I'm really quite shocked. As for him saying that the sculpture displays no Christian message but only symbols of the old earth-mother type of religion, all I can say is that I think he's behaving like a Freudian case-book.

'*Longing* to see you again and *panting* for your next letter. By the way, I suppose it's a bit late in the day to start worrying, but are you sure it's safe for me to write as frankly as this? Wouldn't it be wiser if I addressed you as "Dear Mr Dean", signed off "love, Venetia", and cut out all references to generating steam? Whenever I think of the Profumo scandal (can't wait for the House of Commons debate!) I get very nervous of taking any potentially scandalous risk. Much, *much* love from your devoted EGERIA.'

Aysgarth wrote back by return: 'My darling, don't worry about our letters. I always get up early to put in an hour's work before breakfast, and D always has breakfast in bed as compensation for the fact that she seldom manages to sleep before three in the morning. My study, as you know, is next to the front door and I see the postman come up the garden path – usually around seven. There's absolutely no possibility that D would ever be up at that hour, and by the time the second post arrives Miss Trotman's here to pounce on it (though she would never, of course, open an envelope marked "Private and Confidential"). The only tricky time is on weekends but I'm very vigilant and D's really much too absorbed in her own affairs to bother to ambush the postman. All your letters I keep under lock and key, and the key itself is always in my pocket. So say whatever you wish when you write to me – there's no scandalous risk involved!

'As for John Profumo, I'm sorry for him, of course – I'd be sorry for any man who wrecked a successful career – but I fear my sympathy is limited. Any distinguished man who's fool enough to mess around with the demi-monde as represented by Christine Keeler is taking not merely a scandalous risk but a suicidal one.

'I've thought a lot about our last meeting (the steam in the front seat!) and I'm sure everything's all right. You have such a benign influence on me; I'm feeling more energetic, drinking less, losing weight – even praying better! (And like John Robinson I confess I always found schematic teaching about prayer rather a dead loss – there! I've never told anyone that before.) Robinson is right, of course, in saying that prayer shouldn't mean a withdrawal from the world but a wholly committed engagement with it. Praying is working, relating to other people and above all LOVING. How clearly I can see that now, and you're the one who's helped me to see it. So I'm sure our love is right, sent by God to help me become a better clergyman. The gifts of the Spirit, as the famous saying goes, can be recognised by their fruits.

'How very good of you to be so kind to poor old Eddie. I think this is admirable. Well done! I too shall be going to see *Present Laughter* but not until the Saturday – D plans to give a farewell party for the cast afterwards at the Deanery. I must say, I'm looking forward to comparing Martin Darrow's stage skills with his father's – that old ecclesiastical adventurer used to act like mad whenever he donned a cassock and glided around performing his Anglo-Catholic rituals! No wonder he spent seventeen years being a monk; the urge to dress up in medieval costume and play the holy man would have been far too delectable to resist, and as for his faith-healing phase later – when he tried to play Svengali, Rasputin and Our Lord Jesus Christ all rolled into one – well! Poor old Dr Ottershaw (Bishop of Starbridge 1937–1947) nearly had a heart-attack.

'If it hadn't been war-time Darrow would never have been recruited to teach at the Theological College, but the situation was desperate and he did have the right academic background. But look what his invasion produced! A perfectly respectable college, known for its middle-of-the-road churchmanship, was turned into a hotbed of Ango-Catholicism laced with periodic outbreaks of charismatic wonders! I admit the College became a huge success, but as soon as Darrow retired in 1950 it collapsed like a pricked balloon and became rather nasty. There was a terrible scandal in the 'fifties when . . . but no, I must be loyal to the Church and preserve a discreet silence! Charles Ashworth mopped up the mess when he became Bishop. I'll say this for Charles: he doesn't stand any nonsense when it comes to clerical behaviour which is really quite unacceptable.

'Must stop now, darling, but I send my best love as always,

N. PS. Let's have a quick tryst on Lady Mary – how about Sunday post evensong?'

Drinking a cup of black coffee I wondered how much longer I could tolerate a diet of occasional quick trysts on Lady Mary and a weekly steamy kiss on Starbury Plain.

XII

'And now,' said the Bishop, gorgeous in the yellow sports-shirt and snow-white slacks which he had elected to wear for his morning's round of golf, 'having demonstrated that Dr Robinson is ill-advised to ignore all the great mystics of the Church who throughout the centuries have withdrawn from the world in order to pray – having demonstrated, in other words, that prayer is *not* solely a matter of engaging with the world and exuding love from every pore – we will turn to assess what Dr Robinson is pleased to call the New Morality. We're going to examine the spectacle of a well-meaning, fatally idealistic middle-aged cleric who proposes to grapple with the increasing problem of sexual licence by tearing up all the old rules and merely urging people to love one another. What sort of a world, I ask myself, does the good Bishop think he's living in?'

Dr Ashworth paused, reaching upwards to stroke that domestic pet, his pectoral cross, but encountered instead only the glossy grey hairs which were exposed by the open neck of his sports-shirt; he had forgotten that the cross had been discarded for his round of golf. 'I'll have to rephrase all that later, of course,' he said to me. 'The tone is much too withering for publication, but while I'm getting my ideas down on paper I shan't bother to apply a coating of sugar. Now let me think. Ethics has many aspects and I'm not sure which one I should tackle first.' So absorbed was he in his thoughts that he was unaware of his wife opening the door of the morning-room. 'Shall we have sex straight away?' he mused to me as she peeped in. 'Or shall we save it for later?'

The point of my pencil snapped.

'Darling,' said Mrs Ashworth serenely from the threshold, 'that remark deserves to go straight into the *Oxford Dictionary of Quotations*.'

The Bishop gave a galvanic start and then, to his great credit, laughed with genuine amusement. I promptly giggled in sympathy and Mrs Ashworth produced her sphinx-like smile.

'Dear me!' exclaimed Dr Ashworth. 'What an extraordinary clanger! I really didn't think I was capable of such a performance –'

'" – as the bishop said to the actress,"' droned Mrs Ashworth, successfully giving the famous old joke another whirl.

This time no one made any attempt not to laugh, and it was some seconds before Mrs Ashworth managed to say: 'Charles, I came to tell you that your brother's on the phone. Can you possibly tear yourself away from Venetia to speak to him?'

'I'm sure Venetia would welcome a break from my inanities!' gasped Dr Ashworth, and disappeared, still laughing, to his study.

'If he's going to dictate about sex,' said Mrs Ashworth, 'you'd better have a drink. Gin-and-tonic?'

'I'd love one, but no – it might have a fatal effect on my shorthand.'

'In that case stay and have a drink afterwards. Since he switched you today from nine to five in order to trek over that awful golf course, I think the least I can do is provide a gin-and-tonic in compensation.'

I agreed to a drink at six. Dr Ashworth returned from his study but was soon recalled by another phone call which was promptly succeeded by a third.

'Sorry, Venetia,' he said afterwards, 'but I'm going to have to call off this session. The Archdeacon's coming round to discuss an emergency.'

Was I disappointed or was I relieved that the Bishop had been obliged to postpone his demolition of the New Morality? I had no idea. Then I realised that this was because I wanted to have no idea. For one long moment I saw myself marooned amidst an array of mirrors which tilted up and down so rapidly that I could no longer distinguish between reality and illusion in their shifting reflections, but then I pushed this unnerving image from my mind, pulled myself together and prepared to enjoy a drink with my heroine.

SIX

'The chapter on "The New Morality", for example, is particularly disquieting. One feels that a careful study of the troubles that befell St. Paul in Corinth ... would be profitable to the Bishop. It is likely that the Apostle would prove a far better guide than D. H. Lawrence, that devotee of a religion far older than Christianity and still one of its principal rivals.'

GLYN SIMON
The Honest to God Debate
ed. DAVID L. EDWARDS

I

'How's the love-life?' said Mrs Ashworth after we had been chatting for a while in her sitting-room.

'Promising. I may be going sailing soon with Perry Palmer. He keeps a boat at Bosham.'

'That's Christian's friend, isn't it – the young man you mentioned to me the other day?'

'Yes, that's the one.' I suddenly wondered if she had heard the rumour that Perry was a eunuch, but since the Aysgarths and the Ashworths had never lived in each other's pockets I felt there was a good chance the story had failed to reach the South Canonry.

'What does he do for a living?'

'No one knows for sure but he's reputed to be a spy.'

'How fashionable!'

'Oh, he's hardly the James Bond type –'

'Just as well, perhaps. Michael adores the James Bond novels,' added Mrs Ashworth as an afterthought, 'and Charles gets so cross, says they're decadent. Of course he's read them all.' Casually she flicked ash from her cigarette into the nearest tray.

'Well, congratulations on landing an old Wykehamist who lives in Albany and keeps a boat at Bosham! But why aren't you living up in London so that you can see him more often?'

'Oh, that wouldn't do at all, Mrs Ashworth!' I said glibly at once. 'He might think he was being chased. I've made up my mind to play this very cool.'

'How sensible,' said Mrs Ashworth, blowing some smoke languidly towards the ceiling.

I realised it was time I displayed some passion. 'Of course we do write a lot –'

'Write! I thought your generation only used the phone!'

'Well, naturally we phone each other as well –'

'It sounds as if you've got yourself very well organised,' said my heroine kindly. 'I'm so glad.'

Without warning I heard myself blurt out: 'Yes, I'm very lucky compared with Dinkie – that's Dinkie Kauffman, an American friend of Marina's. She's got herself mixed up with a married man, and it all sounds desperately frustrating because they can only meet once a week and since he won't go to her flat the meetings always have to take place in his car.'

'How intriguing. I've never before heard of a married man who wouldn't snap up the chance to go to his mistress's flat.'

'Oh, she's not his mistress, Mrs Ashworth! It's all rather peculiar. You see, he keeps insisting that he doesn't want an affair but he also swears he's madly in love with her – which is all so confusing to poor Dinkie who can't figure out what's really going on – and I couldn't figure it out either when she asked my advice.'

'Maybe he wants to do the right thing and marry her first. Is there a divorce in the offing?'

'Oh, there's no question of a divorce! And the wife could live for ever, according to Dinkie.'

'It sounds to me,' said Mrs Ashworth, 'as if Dinkie's wasting her time.'

'But Mrs Ashworth, surely an affair is always a strong possibility when two people are madly in love? I mean, *I* know, of course, that an affair would be morally wrong, but poor Dinkie

– who's not religious – is in such a state over her grand passion that she's nearly being driven mad by all this high-minded abstaining. She feels that if only she could have a little bit of bed now and then –'

'The trouble with grand passions is that the lovers are never content with just a little bit of bed now and then.'

'But half a loaf's better than none, surely? And she does absolutely accept that she can't marry him –'

'That's purely a temporary phenomenon, the result of lack of experience and wishful thinking. Once she was his mistress she'd soon start to wonder how long the wife was going to go on.'

'Dinkie already wishes the wife was dead, I know – and oh, Mrs Ashworth, the most ghastly part of the whole situation, the part that's driving Dinkie up the wall, is that she thinks he may still be sleeping with his wife. He says he's not – or rather, he implies he's not – I mean, he's never actually said to Dinkie: "I DO NOT SLEEP WITH MY WIFE", but he obviously wants to give the impression that he –'

'Of course. No married man in his right mind is going to say cheerfully to his potential mistress: "Oh, by the way, I'm still sleeping with the old girl, but you don't mind, do you?"'

'You mean . . . You think the likelihood is –'

'Oh yes. Have another gin.'

I accepted another gin. I had to concentrate very hard to make sure that my hand was steady when she returned my glass. Then I said evenly: 'I don't know how you can be so certain, Mrs Ashworth. Surely it's fairly common for couples who have been married for years not to sleep together? In fact I thought this was always the main reason why husbands strayed.'

'A straying husband would certainly indicate that the marriage has its difficulties, but those difficulties needn't necessarily be sexual. If this man's content to breathe passion over Dinkie but take the affair no further, I'd guess the marriage has its private compensations which aren't apparent to the outsider.'

'But surely there must be another explanation! If the man's a romantic – or an eccentric –'

'Oh, anything's possible, certainly. I suppose the next most likely explanation for his abstinence is that he's impotent: he'd get his thrills out of passionate kisses and he'd make some excuse – a moral objection to adultery would do nicely – to ensure he stayed out of the bedroom.'

'As a matter of fact, Dinkie says he *has* voiced a strong moral objection to adultery –'

'Ah well, there you are.'

'But Mrs Ashworth, couldn't he be genuinely held back by his moral beliefs?'

'My dear,' said Mrs Ashworth, 'I know it's quite wrong for a bishop's wife to be so cynical but at least I'm being entirely honest when I say that in my opinion a man in the grip of a grand passion can always work out a way to circumvent his moral beliefs. He'd still hold those particular beliefs, of course, but he'd decide his case wasn't covered by the rules. There's nothing like a grand passion for encouraging self-deception on an epic scale.'

'So you think that eventually he'll work his way around his moral beliefs and sleep with Dinkie after all?'

'Goodness only knows what he'll do, but tell Dinkie that if she paddles in the pool of adultery she could well wake up one morning and find that the waters have closed over her head. I knew a young woman once,' said Mrs Ashworth, sipping her gin, 'who got in a fearful mess with a married man – a very respectable married man – really most eminent – someone who had absolutely no hope of a divorce – and at first she thought she'd be satisfied with just a passionate kiss now and then but she wasn't, she wasn't satisfied at all, she was soon so jealous of the wife that she became bitter and miserable – even in the end unbalanced – yes, in the end she became quite mad, so mad that she was almost destroyed – *almost destroyed* – and even when by some undeserved miracle she was rescued by a good man who married her, she wasn't right, not for years, and that was so terrible for the husband . . . although I'm glad to say that in the end everything came right and they were happy. But at what cost! And after such suffering! It was an appalling case and I'll never forget it. Never.'

After a pause I managed to say: 'What happened to her married lover?'

'Oh, he was ruined, of course,' said Mrs Ashworth in the manner of a pathologist dictating a report from the morgue. 'He resigned his job. He never worked again. He died before his time of cancer.' And she ground out her cigarette in the ash-tray as if to symbolise the life that had been so inexorably extinguished.

There followed a silence which I was unable to break. Then she said with an effortless resumption of her relaxed, friendly manner: 'Charley's making a quick visit home this weekend – are you free for Sunday lunch? I'm sure he'd enjoy seeing you.'

'I don't think he would, Mrs Ashworth. When we met on the train before Easter we had rather a slanging match.'

'That sounds promising! Charley loves to be combative. Do come!'

Unable to think of an excuse more compelling than sheer incompatibility I gave way and accepted the invitation. Then feeling deeply disturbed I returned home and watched television without comprehension in the dusk.

II

At three o'clock in the morning I was finally able to think: he's undeniably healthy and so the likelihood is he's sexually unimpaired; therefore if he's not sleeping with his wife, the chances are that he'll eventually work his way around his moral convictions and wind up sleeping with me. Then I was able to doze off, but when I awoke four hours later my resolution to be patient withered in seconds and I felt overpowered by the longing to see him.

Recalling his spiritual timetable I realised he would be absent that morning from the early services in St Anselm's chapel so I made no effort to go to the Cathedral, but soon after nine I telephoned the Deanery.

Aysgarth's secretary Miss Trotman took the call.

'Good morning,' I said. 'Could you remind the Dean, please, that Lady Mary wishes to speak to him this evening about the memorial tablet? Thank you so much.' But as I hung up I realised I would now have to devise a new telephone message; Lady Mary could hardly go on wanting to speak to the Dean about a memorial tablet.

The difficulties of communication suddenly seemed intolerable. For a moment I sank deep into depression, but then pulling myself together I began to look forward to seeing him later in the cloisters.

III

He called back at noon. 'Can't talk now,' he said. 'Just wanted to say "message received". See you on Lady Mary after evensong,' and he hung up.

Some hours later I was just rising to my feet at the start of the service when I noticed that Dido was present in the congregation. She appeared unaware of me, but I found myself unable to stop looking at her and eventually, inevitably, our glances met. At once she gave me a bright smile. Not to be outdone I gave her a bright smile in return, but when I stared fiercely at the high altar afterwards I could only see the cross through a haze of tears. At the end of the service Aysgarth walked past without looking at me and Dido zipped across to the vestry door to wait for him.

Abandoning all hope of a tryst on Lady Mary I went home and drank three double-gins.

IV

'My darling,' wrote Aysgarth in a letter which caught the last post and arrived at my flat early on Wednesday morning. 'I'm devastated that I shan't be able to get to Lady Mary after all this evening – D, who hasn't been to evensong for ages, has just announced that she feels spiritual and knows she's being called to attend. (This is a very typical D remark and is probably more or less true, so you needn't worry that she suspects anything.) Thank God tomorrow's Wednesday and we can have plenty of time to talk. I'm just praying the Lady Mary signal doesn't indicate some dire emergency.

'Life certainly seems to be increasingly fraught on the ecclesiastical front, and Harriet March's magnificent sculpture is fast becoming too hot to handle. The traitor Fitzgerald, hatching a fiendish anti-sculpture conspiracy with all the reactionary philistines in Starbridge, has roped in Archdeacon Lindsay who now informs me that I have to seek a faculty (that's a form of ecclesiastical permission) before I install any structure in the Cathedral churchyard. Now, this would seem to be nonsense as deans are autonomous and neither their cathedrals nor their churchyards are subject to the Chancellor (chief legal eagle) of the diocese who sits in the Consistory Court and grants faculties. But Lindsay informs me that legally the magnificent sward which surrounds Starbridge Cathedral is not in fact a consecrated churchyard (used for burials) but unconsecrated curtilage (mere adjacent land), and all unconsecrated curtilages require a faculty before alteration. Again, this would appear to be rubbish, because although the sward is no longer used for burials it certainly was in the old days, but Lindsay declares that all the burials were irregular since under a Cathedral statute the only consecrated burial ground is the lawn of the cloisters.

'Well, of course it's easy to see what happened: once the cloisters' lawn was full up they started burying people out on the sward – and since no one in the old days would have dreamed of having themselves laid to rest in unconsecrated ground, this must mean that at some time or other the place was consecrated. I pointed this out to Lindsay, but he only said stuffily: "In the absence of evidence of consecration, the statute must prevail." That was more than I could take. "*Evidence?*" I said. "The evidence lies in the few tombstones you can still find embedded in the churchyard's turf! They prove consecration beyond any shadow of doubt!" But Lindsay dug in his toes, announced that the Chancellor would have to rule where the burden of proof lay, and stalked off.

'So the fight is on, and what I have to prove is that no one has power over that sward except me. I shall collar Gilbert (the Librarian) and get him (1) to look up the appropriate statute in the original Latin (Lindsay only has an English translation), and (2) if no mistake's been made in interpreting the statute, to start tracking down the inevitable later consecration. There *must* be a record of it somewhere! I just can't believe that any past Dean of Starbridge would be so unfamiliar with the Cathedral statutes as to permit burials on unconsecrated curtilage.

'I need hardly remind you that Lindsay is the Bishop's henchman and I need hardly add that this whole devious episcopal attempt to cut back my power makes me absolutely *furious*.

'To cap it all – as if I needed more trouble! – our guest preacher for Sunday matins has been knocked over by a motorbike so I'll have to deliver a sermon in his stead. Dalton's preaching at evensong, so I can't ask him, and Fitzgerald insists that he has to go to see his widowed mother that weekend. (*Typical!*) Eddie's volunteered, always the masochist, but I had to ask him to do an awful job only the other day (chairing the Cathedral guides' meeting – i.e. presiding over a mass manifestation of verbal diarrhoea) and I really can't always be exploiting poor Eddie.

'My darling, forgive this grim catalogue of debilitating anxieties – I can't tell you how I long to see you again, you're my life-line and I know that when I see you I'll be able to dredge up some new strength. Next week looks as if it'll be even more frightful than this week – three diocesan committee meetings, two big funerals and one of those stupefyingly dull special regimental services stuffed with field-marshals, generals and other prize asses, and mitigated only by a touch of royalty. D, needless to say, has long been planning the buffet-lunch for sixty, and has acquired a fantastically expensive new outfit in order to dazzle the Duke and Duchess. How I remain solvent God only knows, since even D's substantial private income can hardly be expected to stretch from here to eternity, but so far my bank manager hasn't cut me dead in Mitre Street.

'Occasionally, very occasionally I think how nice it would be not to have to worry about money, but I suppose I'm so used to living on a financial knife-edge that I'm now well past the sleepless-nights stage. One can get used to anything in the end, but oh, how *tired* I get of all the strain sometimes, how utterly fed up and exhausted – yet when I see you, so young, such fun, so full of life, then not only does my weariness vanish as if it had never existed but I can remember what it's like to be happy.

'Darling, I love you and I can't wait, *can't wait*, till tomorrow – 2.00 in the Playhouse car-park – do you think this time we'll finally make it to Starbury Ring? All my love, N.'

Refolding the letter I thought: he can't stand her; I'm the one he wants.

And all doubt was once more wiped from my mind.

V

'Starbury Ring!' I exclaimed. 'At last!'

We laughed and clutched each other, still breathless from our climb over the ridge from the car-park. Then we staggered forward in search of a suitable place to recover from our uncharacteristic exertion.

Starbury Ring, a mysterious circle of standing stones, was usually described as resembling Stonehenge, but I always thought it was more like Avebury; each stone stood by itself and no three had been placed together to form an arch. On that afternoon the sun shone strongly from a sky dotted with large white clouds, and the view to the horizon, usually misty, was as clear as if it had been drawn by a fine-nibbed pen. A few hikers were wandering around flapping their guidebooks, and there were one or two prone hippies soaking up the vibes, but as usual the site was underpopulated. Retreating into the shade of one of the stones we were easily able to tuck ourselves out of sight of our fellow-visitors.

'It's wonderfully phallic, isn't it?' I said, gazing at a tall slim stone nearby.

'Wonderfully!' he said smiling, and when he took me in his arms nothing mattered, neither the separations, nor the frustrations, nor the suspicions, nor the bewilderment, nor the anguish, nor the tears – nothing mattered except that we were together. I kissed him and hugged him and gasped when he rolled over on top of me and laughed when he rolled all the way over to the other side by mistake, and when he laughed too we clutched each other in an ecstasy of happiness and I heard him whisper: 'Isn't this fun?' But once he released me the fun was wiped out and the frustration was so agonising that my eyes filled with tears. Much humiliated by my weakness but determined not to make a nauseating exhibition of myself, I covered my face with my hands.

'My darling . . .' Realising how upset I was he tried to take me in his arms again, but at that moment some people walked past and I knew he immediately thought, just as I did, how appalling it would have been if one of those casual passers-by had been known to him.

I began to struggle to my feet. 'I can't stand this lack of privacy any longer. Let's go to my flat.'

Without a second's hesitation he said: 'I can't.'

'Oh yes, you could!' I said fiercely, demented enough to abandon my waiting game and hammer at the mystery of his abstinence. 'You'd take the slight risk involved, but you won't because you don't love me enough!'

'That's not true!' He seemed genuinely appalled.

'Then I don't understand anything here.' In exhaustion I slumped against the standing stone.

'But I've explained in great detail! If I don't come to your flat, it's not because I don't love you but because I love you too much to use you for my own selfish purposes when I'm quite unable to offer you marriage. According to John Robinson –'

'Dr Ashworth thinks John Robinson's up the creek.'

'Ah well!' said Aysgarth at once, all scorn. 'What else can you expect from a reactionary like Charles?'

The last shreds of my self-control were destroyed. Stepping forward until my face was only inches from his I said rapidly in a voice which shook with emotion: 'I like that Bishop. I admire him. I think he's a very clever man with a good sense of humour who talks a lot of sense. All those "Anti-Sex Ashworth" slurs are rubbish. I don't believe he's anti-sex at all. He's obviously got a happy, successful relationship with that wife of his – and she's *really* fabulous, so intelligent and sensible and sympathetic and unchurchy, in fact I think she's a truly *Christian* person. So who are you to criticise the Ashworths – you with your unhappy marriage and your neurotic wife who manages to drive everyone up the wall? Who are you to look down your nose at Charles Ashworth just because he has the brains and the training and the guts to swim against the John Robinson tide and stand up for what he believes to be right? Dr Ashworth's battling away in the *real* world and Mrs Ashworth's right there alongside him, but we don't live in the real world, neither of us does when we're together like this, it's all a fantasy, all just an unconsummated dream!'

If I had thought I would shock him into silence, I was wrong. Immediately he answered: 'You're the most real thing in my life. This *is* reality,' and as he kissed me I knew he was right; we were living in the real world, we truly were, and the Ashworths were just a dream couple I had idealised when I was in a disturbed state of mind. And in my sinister hall of mirrors all the glass abruptly tilted to reflect clear, dazzling images once more instead of a horrific assembly of distortions.

'My darling Mr Dean,' I whispered, the hated tears streaming down my face, 'forgive me, I didn't mean what I said, I didn't mean it –'

'It's all right,' he said gently, holding me close. 'I do understand. The Ashworths have been very kind to you – why shouldn't you stand up for them if you wish? That's admirable. But never think they have some God-given monopoly on reality because I'm just as capable, I assure you, of being absolutely down-to-earth and realistic.'

'Then Neville, what exactly's going on? I accept that your

religious beliefs are very strong and entirely genuine, but –'

'They are, yes. Do I need another reason for abstaining from adultery?'

'No, of course not, but –'

'I can't quite see why you're so anxious to shroud me in mystery all the time.'

'I suppose I'm afraid that you've got some sort of peculiar hang-up –'

'What on earth's a hang-up?'

'A psychological block which results in abnormal behaviour.'

'My darling, you're the one who seems to be behaving abnormally, suspecting me of lunatic tendencies! How could I hold down a top job in a major organisation unless I was exceptionally sane and well-balanced?'

'I'm not talking about sanity exactly. I'm talking about –'

'Why should you think I have one of these hang-up things?'

'Well, when you were talking about prizes –'

'Oh good heavens, I got that old *idée fixe* under control years ago! Now listen to me. Since you rate realism so highly I suggest you forget the fantastic explanations and focus on the rational thinking which buttresses the moral beliefs which you apparently find so implausible. The rational thinking goes like this: Dido's thirteen years younger than I am, and the odds are she'll outlive me. That means I can never offer you marriage, and in the end it'll be marriage you'll want. Moreover in a few years' time you won't want to be married to a man who's pushing seventy. You'll want to be married to a man of your own generation – and so, no doubt, you shall be. Some great paragon will come riding along on his white horse, and –'

'How loathsome! And even if you're right, why should that affect us now? While we wait for this big bore to arrive, why can't we –'

'Because if you got too involved with me, you'd never even see the great paragon, let alone recognise him as a potential husband.'

'Thank God – a merciful escape!'

'No, my dear, that wouldn't be a merciful escape. That would be a great tragedy – and I'd be responsible. I'd have destroyed your best chance of happiness and probably ruined your life.' He shuddered so violently that I at last realised how serious he was. 'To take a woman's love,' he said, 'and then to destroy her – no, I couldn't do that. I couldn't live with myself afterwards. It would destroy me too.'

'Oh darling, surely that sort of melodrama only happens in nineteenth-century novels!'

'You think so?' He turned away abruptly, and because he then had his back to me I barely heard him add: 'Women should be preserved from destroyers. Whatever I do I'm going to avoid putting you through hell.'

Before I could stop myself I said: 'Sometimes when you keep rejecting me like this I feel I'm in hell already.'

When he spun back to face me I saw he was appalled. 'My darling –' He broke off, then exclaimed in despair: 'Maybe I've got this all wrong and I should give you up.'

'Oh no!' I said at once. 'I'd be in a far worse hell if you did that!'

He gave me a long kiss before saying: 'I'll never give you up, never – at least, not until the great paragon rides out of the mist on his shining white horse!' And at last he managed to smile at me.

'But even then – supposing I were to marry just for the social convenience – couldn't we –'

'Oh, you aristocrats!' he said laughing. 'What a bunch of pagans you are!'

'But seriously, Neville –'

'My dear, I don't share my prizes, and besides . . . if you lose a prize it ceases to be a prize any more, doesn't it?'

'Here comes that *idée fixe* again –'

'Yes, but it's not an *idée fixe* any more, it's just a little quirk in my personality. My darling, if you married of course our friendship would have to end. It would be quite immoral if I cast any kind of a shadow over your married life, and anyway you must never, never marry just for convenience.'

'But if I can't marry you –'

'Don't let's think of the future,' he interrupted. 'Let's make it a taboo subject, like the past.' And as he began to kiss me again I knew that juxtaposed to us in the land of allegory the serpent was tightening the grip of his coils.

VI

'I've made a decision,' said the Bishop, sleek in his Savile Row suit, as he absent-mindedly moved his pectoral cross to the exact centre of his purple stock. 'I'm going to postpone my comments on the New Morality until I can gauge approximately how much space I can afford to give it. Otherwise I shall get carried away and dictate enough material to give my publishers heart failure at the thought of the production costs.'

'Okay, Bishop.' I could now clearly identify as relief the emotion which seeped through me as this new postponement was announced.

'I want to make a stab at the opening chapter,' Dr Ashworth was saying, 'but before I start, could you just make a note that the depth metaphor which Robinson finds so startlingly original has of course been used by the mystics for centuries? I think I ought to point out that it doesn't necessarily lead straight to Valentinus' Gnostic heresy.'

I scribbled away busily.

'Oh, and remind me to stress the role of the Devil in the propagation of heresy, would you? These starry-eyed liberal churchmen who peddle heretical theories are always so anxious to gloss over him.'

I somehow managed to scribble on without batting an eyelid.

'The Devil,' mused Dr Ashworth, 'is a symbol representing an aspect of absolute reality. He's not a mere fable which "modern man" can water down and redesign, and any churchman who gives the impression that the Devil's no longer important deserves a stern rap across the knuckles . . . All right, let's make a stab at the opening chapter. Are you ready? Good, then off we go. "Chapter One: The Doctrine of God" . . .'

VII

'My darling,' wrote Aysgarth, 'do please forgive me for upsetting you so much up at Starbury Ring. What I was really saying, as I believe you understood in the end, was that it's not merely preferable but *vital* that we should love each other in the right way. Then we'll both survive. The truth is I feel I've driven a very special bargain with God. If I keep our love within acceptable bounds it'll remain a blessing; it'll continue to give me the strength to survive what is at present a tough professional and domestic life, and it will even (as I mentioned to you before) inspire me to be a better clergyman. But if I let my love stray beyond the pale, God will withdraw his blessing and (as the old-fashioned churchmen used to thunder) the Devil will move in. Of course no one seriously believes in the Devil any more – he's just a childish image from a bygone era, like the picture of God as an old man in the sky – but one can "demythologise" the Devil by talking of him in psychological terms (alienation, dissociation) and literary metaphors (dereliction in the wasteland).

'My darling, I want to ensure your happiness, not drive you into the wasteland of a breakdown, and you're so special, so precious, so perfect, that I'm determined to put aside all my selfish desires in order to preserve you from harm.

'I suspect I'm now sounding turgid in my earnestness, so let me hastily move on to another subject. The Bishop at once springs to mind, and I must confess straight away how startled I was when you leapt so loyally to his defence! Charles has, of course, a superb intellect and is without doubt a most devout Christian, but he's a typical product of a privileged public school/Oxbridge background: all charm on top, all reactionary attitudes and snobbery and stab-you-in-the-back ruthlessness underneath. Perhaps it's because I'm just a Yorkshire draper's son, but the older I get the less patience I have with these pillars of the Establishment. It's all dinner at the Athenaeum and gossip at the House of Lords and let's-keep-everything-(especially-the-Church)-exactly-as-it-is. Well, time will deal with them all in due course! *Honest to God* is a watershed. In twenty-five years' time all the conservative elements in the Church will have been swept away and we'll be living with the triumph of liberalism in the form of a dynamic radical theology.

'As for Lyle Ashworth, I was even more startled that you should have adopted her as a heroine! She's not the sort of woman other women usually like. Men always get on with her all right, of course, (although personally I've never found her in the least attractive) and in fact I've sometimes wondered if she was faithful to Charles during those three years he spent as a prisoner of war. She used to slink around in a little black dress and very high-heeled shoes and look like a cross between Greta Garbo and Marlene Dietrich. However, that's all a long time ago now and I can't deny she's transformed herself into an irreproachably seemly "Mrs Bishop".

'Darling, I hardly know how I'm going to endure the agonising wait for our next meeting! I can't exaggerate how utterly renewed you make me feel; when I returned from our outing to the Ring I tossed off that Sunday sermon with no trouble at all and it's turned out to be a stunner. (Excuse the boasting but I wanted to leave you in no doubt of your amazingly beneficial effect on me!) Always remember that I'm PASSIONATE about you and that you're the most vital thing in my life. All my love, N.

'PS. (LATER) Fitzgerald has just denied he ever mentioned the sculpture's phallic cigars to the Archdeacon and says Lindsay's only concerned about the legal status of the church-yard. What a liar Fitzgerald is! Of course he's deliberately roped in the Bishop's henchman in order to involve Charles in the fight against the sculpture!

'PPS. (LATER STILL) Gilbert's just phoned after a fearful intellectual session in the library with a professor whose speciality is medieval Latin. There seems to be no doubt that the Cathedral statute only refers to the cloisters lawn as the Cathedral's consecrated burial ground. Gilbert says the reasoning behind this rather curious state of affairs almost certainly arose from the fact that while the Cathedral was being built, the deceased of Starbridge were buried at St Martin's-in-Cripplegate which in those days had a far more extensive burial ground than it has now. As you probably know, St Martin's church preceded the Cathedral; it was originally built for the spiritual benefit of the Cathedral workmen, and soon afterwards it became the parish church, replacing the Saxon round church which had been destroyed by fire. According to Gilbert's theory, the first bishop probably reckoned that the hoi-polloi could go on being buried at St Martin's while the Cathedral could be reserved for the nobs – and since the graveyard at St Martin's was already the official parish burial ground, he wouldn't even have had to issue an edict; all he would have needed to do was acquiesce in the status quo.

'So the evidence so far certainly supports Lindsay's claim that the Cathedral churchyard is unconsecrated curtilage, but I'm going to assure him that the hunt is now on in earnest for evidence of the later consecration which I feel sure must exist. That'll make Lindsay sweat blood! Meanwhile little Gilbert is almost hysterical with excitement and has plunged back into the library to comb the archives. Join the Church for an action-packed career liberally seasoned with suspense! But seriously – what a life . . .'

VIII

'I think it's terrific that you've chucked up your vapid society life in order to live in a small flat in a provincial town and work for a clergyman,' said my fiery contemporary Charley Ashworth, pale brown eyes almost golden as he regarded me with whole-hearted approval. 'I wouldn't have thought you had it in you.'

His mother groaned lightly, laying down her knife and fork in protest, but I was enjoying my food too much to follow her example. It was Sunday, and in accordance with Mrs Ashworth's invitation I had presented myself at the South Canonry for lunch. The roast beef was succulent. The Yorkshire pudding had already melted in my mouth. The roast potatoes and the peas were sublime enough to qualify the South Canonry for three stars in the *Guide Michelin*. Having recently suffered from a surfeit of solitary encounters with tins of baked beans, I had already decided that this perfectly cooked meal represented gourmet cuisine in its most triumphant form.

'What have I said now?' demanded Charley in response to his mother's quiet moan of despair.

'Darling, Venetia may not like to hear her respectable past described as a "vapid society life", nor may she be very happy to hear that you didn't think she had it in her to live differently. When are you ever going to learn that this mania of yours for being outspoken is often tactless, offensive and just plain wrong?'

'Come, Lyle, that's a bit stiff, isn't it?' said the Bishop good-humouredly, spearing his last slice of Yorkshire pudding. 'Charley's merely anxious to be truthful, and one should always seek to discern the truth, whatever the truth is.'

'Not if it means getting everything wrong and being downright rude,' said Mrs Ashworth.

'I don't get everything wrong!' said Charley indignantly. 'Of course we all make mistakes, but most of the time I think the truth's blindingly obvious.'

'That remark just shows you've reached the age of twenty-five without growing up,' I said, finally giving way to the urge to have a bash at his bumptiousness. 'Most of the time the truth's a complete mystery − in fact sometimes I think it's a miracle that anyone ever has an inkling about what's really going on.'

'Well spoken, Venetia!' said my heroine.

'Over to you, Charley!' said the Bishop, effortlessly neutralising the friction between his wife and son by adopting an amused, affectionate tone. 'How are you going to respond to that "palpable hit"?'

'Venetia has obviously been too greatly influenced by the philosophical idiocies of Berkeley,' retorted Charley, 'but I stand by the absolute values of Plato and hold that the fully real is fully knowable!'

'But surely,' I said, moving in for the kill with my verbal

rapier, 'Platonic philosophy has been exploded by the logical positivists?'

'Plato will be remembered when A. J. Ayer is forgotten!' said Charley, furiously parrying the blow. 'Logical positivism is just a temporary aberration from the truth, like the theology of John Robinson!'

'Rubbish!' I said, fighting bravely on although my rapier was now shuddering in my hand. 'In twenty-five years' time the conservative wing of the Church will be extinct and we'll be living with liberalism in the form of a dynamic radical theology!'

Charley snorted with contempt. His remarkable eyes seemed to blaze with golden sparks, and his wide, mobile mouth was set in a passionate snarl. He looked like an outraged Pekinese.

'In twenty-five years' time,' he declared, 'John Robinson will be a back number, radical theology will have reached a dead end and the Evangelicals will be on the march again to set the Church back on course after the mid-century decades of decadence and debility!'

'Phew!' said the Bishop. 'That was a real scorcher! Lyle, is there any more of that sensational Yorkshire pudding?'

My rapier had shattered. Aysgarth's bold prophecy was in shreds. Automatically I turned to the Bishop for the final word of authority. 'And you, Dr Ashworth,' I said, 'what do you think?'

'I think,' said the Bishop, 'that the gifts of the Spirit can be recognised by their fruits, and that "Truth", as the old saying goes, "is the Daughter of Time".'

'Seconds, Venetia?' I suddenly realised Mrs Ashworth was hovering at my elbow with a plate of sliced roast beef.

'No, thank you.' I felt unable to face another mouthful; the mere thought of food made me recoil.

'I hope I haven't upset you,' said Charley, dropping his abrasive manner as he saw my leaden expression. His naive concern was curiously appealing. 'It's so nice to talk to a girl who can actually talk back. I just love having a good slanging match.'

In the ensuing silence the Bishop tried to smother a smile,

Mrs Ashworth assumed her most inscrutable expression and Charley, who had turned red after paying me this extraordinary compliment, furiously attacked his last roast potato.

I came to the unexpected conclusion that although he was now too juvenile to take seriously he might well evolve into the most stimulating man. However, I could hardly afford to waste my energy visualising Charley in the 1970s; I needed all my strength to face the approaching treacle tart and custard.

It really was the most superb Sunday lunch.

IX

'. . . and grim news has emerged from the library,' wrote Aysgarth. 'Gilbert, twittering with horror, has unearthed some most unwanted evidence in the papers of Josiah Samuel Hawkyns, Bishop of Starbridge 1703–1716. Apparently the Cathedral statutes were lost during the Civil War – the clergy thought Cromwell might burn the library, so as many books and documents as possible were removed and hidden when the Roundheads were reported to be closing in on Royalist Starbridge. As it turned out, the Roundheads only rampaged through the Cathedral smashing up all the side-chapels, but the Bishop died of shock and later it was realised that no one knew where he had hidden the statutes. Cromwell hanged the Dean *en passant* and so Starbridge later had a new bishop and a new dean, neither of whom had any idea of the exact rules laid down for the governing of the Cathedral. Inevitably, within a generation, people were being buried on the sward in the belief that they were committing their mortal remains to consecrated ground.

'And now we come to Bishop Josiah Samuel Hawkyns. In 1707 he found the statutes hidden behind a secret panel in the dining-room of the old episcopal palace and to his delight he discovered – here we go! – that the Cathedral churchyard was not a consecrated burial ground in the power of the Dean and Chapter but unconsecrated curtilage to which he as bishop could stake a claim. Accordingly he dispossessed the Dean and Chapter, banned all future burials from the churchyard and used the sward for grazing his horses. Dean Augustus St John Merrivale is reported to have drunk three bottles of claret and died of apoplexy – and I'm not in the least surprised.

'However, unlike poor Augustus St J M, I shall somehow restrain myself from knocking back a vat of St Estèphe and survive to fight the next battle – which, of course, will now centre directly on the sculpture. I have to apply for a faculty in order to place it in the churchyard, and Charles, through Lindsay, is bound to oppose my application, but by heavens I'll get that faculty even if I have to extract it by shaking the Chancellor until his teeth rattle!

'Meanwhile Fitzgerald was seen by my spy Eddie lunching in the Quill Pen with the Archdeacon – the whole issue reeks of conspiracy, but I'll fight these philistines to the last ditch. Fitzgerald even had the nerve to say to me in Chapter that it was impossible for a phallic symbol to be aesthetically pleasing. "My dear Tommy," I said, "what could be more phallic than our unique and ravishing spire?" Fitzgerald went purple, as if I'd uttered a string of four-letter words, and Dalton said primly: "Isn't that going a little far, Stephen?" I'd like to shoot the pair of them – and the Bishop and the Archdeacon too!

'Talking of Charles, I'm now convinced the Ashworths want to marry you off to Charley, so I'm most relieved to hear you think he's too juvenile to take seriously. He has a volatile temperament, and volatile temperaments, as I know full well, can make married life very exhausting. However, despite this handicap I'm sure he's a good boy; I've always taken an interest in him ever since he told me when he was very small that he wanted to be a clergyman, but because Charles and I were never exactly the best of friends I haven't seen as much of either Charley or Michael as I might have done. My mentor Bishop Jardine (Lyle's former employer) was very partial to them both and even asked me on his deathbed to keep an eye on them while they were growing up, but that, of course, was when we thought Charles wouldn't come home from the war.

'You didn't tell me anything about your conversation during this culinary dream of a Sunday lunch, but I assume Charles was too busy demolishing roast beef to demolish heresy!

'Now, darling, as I've already told you this is the most frightful week for me, and although I thought I'd be able to escape on Wednesday afternoon as usual, the vast funeral allocated to Wednesday morning has acquired a sting in its tail in the form of a lunch for the most important mourners, and to my rage I shall be unable to get away. Thursday is this ghastly regimental service followed by a buffet-lunch for sixty. Friday afternoon would have been possible – the morning's no good as I shall be kidnapped by Miss Trotman for dictation – but now I have to go and see the Cathedral's solicitors about my application for a faculty. Saturday's useless as both James and Sandy are coming down for the weekend, while Sunday – ah yes! On Sunday I'm supposed to be worshipping God in the Cathedral! I knew there was something I wanted to do if only I could find the time! But seriously . . . what a life.

'All I can suggest is Lady Mary on Wednesday evening. Darling, I'm sorry, sorry, *sorry* to be so inaccessible, but I'll make it up to you on Wednesday week, I promise – if I'm not dead with frustration as the result of being unable to swamp you with kisses this week among all those superbly phallic standing stones. Write soon – only the thought of receiving your letters makes the prospect of this week bearable, all love, N.'

X

'. . . and that concludes my account of the drama of regiment and royalty,' wrote Aysgarth after describing Thursday's special service so wittily that I laughed out loud. 'Let me now pass to a different form of drama and remark how amazing it is that *Present Laughter* opens next week – time seems to have flown lately, although it now seems an eternity since I last saw you (I don't count our rendezvous yesterday on Lady Mary – that was just a crumb to keep me from starving). How I rely on your letters to ease the agony of waiting for next Wednesday – and talking of your letters, thank you so very much for the understanding you displayed when you commiserated with me about that **** Fitzgerald. As an eminent cleric I shouldn't even think this word, let alone hint at it in a letter to a lady, but since it's not a blasphemy and since I know you supported the use of four-letter words in *Lady Chatterley's Lover*, I think I can at least be permitted an explosion of asterisks! If *only* I could get Fitzgerald promoted out of the diocese! I'll have to renew my machinations at Church House.

'I'm toying with the idea of writing a survival manual for deans, and the chapter headings are forming effortlessly in my mind's eye. (1) How to survive your bishop. (2) How to box with your archdeacon. (3) How to kick a canon upstairs. (4) How to outwit a conspiracy to grab your churchyard. (5). . . .oh, the possibilities are endless! Isn't it amazing that the Church should give the impression to laymen of being a stagnant pool? What a masterly exercise in public relations! But no, on second thoughts, perhaps the image isn't so wide of the mark after all. Any biologist will tell you that a stagnant pond is always teeming with life – and that the life can take very unattractive forms. All my love, darling, longing, absolutely *longing* for Wednesday, N.

'PS. (LATER) Lindsay's just phoned to ask when I'm seeing Trumpet (senior partner in the Cathedral's firm of solicitors). "Tomorrow," I said, "and I'm sending the bill for the consultation to the diocesan office." There was a strangulated gasp. I waited for the thud which would indicate that his body had hit the floor, but he somehow kept upright and said in a voice which quivered with rage: "I think that's a somewhat inappropriate remark. The Chancellor will, of course, make an order later in respect of costs." Well, I couldn't resist it; that snooty upper-middle-class tone was like a red rag to a bull, and I wanted to scare him out of his wits. "Fine," I said, "but let me warn you that by the time I've won this case by fighting it through the Consistory Court to the Court of Arches and the

Privy Council – with the aid of the best ecclesiastical lawyers in London – the Chancellor's going to award me costs so large that you'll need a thumbscrew and a rack to extort the money from the parishes." Then I hung up and had a triple whisky to calm me down! Heaven only knows what Lindsay had, but I only wish it was three bottles of claret and apoplexy. The plot thickens! Be sure to tune in tomorrow for the next instalment of *The Aysgarths*, an everyday story of clerical folk . . .'

XI

'Neville,' I said on the following Wednesday after we had been embracing for some minutes in the car-park on Starbury Plain, 'don't you think the front seat of a car is entirely the wrong place to demonstrate one's white-hot passion? I always seem to wind up being much too intimate with the hand-brake.'

He laughed, resuming the embrace, but he soon became wedged, as before, between the seat and the steering-wheel. He kept the driver's seat placed well forward in order to accommodate his short legs and the result was that the wheel allowed him little room to manoeuvre. 'We must look on the front seats,' he said humorously, pausing for air, 'as a modern version of the chastity belt!'

'But I'm so tired of these contortions! Why don't we transfer to the back seat?'

'Passers-by might think –'

'I'm tired of passers-by. In fact I'm tired of this car-park. If you don't want to walk up to the Ring, let's go down to Chancton Wood and romp naked through the undergrowth!'

We both rocked with laughter at the ridiculous picture the proposal evoked. 'You, of course, have the figure for earnest, earthy Lawrentian romps!' he gasped at last. 'I'm keeping my clothes on!'

But he drove to Chancton Wood.

'I'm sorry,' I said after we had wound up far off the beaten track in a grove of beech trees, 'I know I've dragooned you here against your better judgement and you're probably wondering what on earth I'm going to suggest next, but I do accept that we can't "go all the way", as my American friend Dinkie would put it. I just got so tired of other people milling around us, that's all.'

'So did I. And there's been no dragooning. I drove here of my own free will.' Suddenly he exclaimed in despair: 'How little I can offer you! No wonder you became so angry up at the Ring two weeks ago – and no wonder you became so discontented today. I so much wish –' But he stopped.

At once I said: 'It's all right. You're utterly convinced it would be disastrous as well as morally wrong. I do understand.' But as I spoke my mouth was dry with excitement. It had occurred to me that his despair might drive him towards some form of capitulation.

'I know John Robinson's right,' he was saying unevenly. 'I know he is.' But the next moment he was scrambling away from me out of the car as if he were unable to endure the emotional dilemma which Dr Robinson had so serenely sketched.

Flinging open the passenger door I joined him as he slumped against the side of the car and shoved his hands deep into his pockets. His misery was evident in every line of his bowed head, drooping shoulders, downcast eyes and downturned mouth, and suddenly all my longings seemed intolerably immature and self-centred; I wanted only that he should be happy again, secure in his indestructible idealism.

'My darling Mr Dean,' I said, 'of course John Robinson's right! And I'm more than willing to cope with the demands of the New Morality. What I couldn't have coped with would have been some peculiar hang-up about being too terrified to win a prize in case you later found you didn't want it – or perhaps some peculiar mania for preserving women from destruction. Do you remember how you once wrote to me and said quaintly that women should be put on pedestals and reverenced? That really made me very nervous! But of course I can see now that you were just expressing your romantic idealism and your high moral principles. And they're the reason, aren't they, why you're unable to discuss your marriage. It's not because you're still sleeping with Dido, still emotionally involved with her. It really is because your high moral principles demand that you don't talk about her behind her back.'

He froze. 'You didn't seriously think –'

'Yes, I did, as a matter of fact. I was convinced that the only reason you were able to take a high moral line with me was because you were still sleeping with her.'

He was ashen. He opened his mouth, shut it again and ran his fingers wildly through his hair. At last he managed to say: 'I'm going to explode that theory once and for all,' and then he pulled me violently into his arms.

During the embrace that followed I became aware – as indeed I had been aware two weeks before at the Ring – that he was a long way from being impotent. He kissed me so hard my tongue hurt. Then without looking at the door of the car's back seat, he reached out and pulled down the handle.

XIII

'Of course,' he whispered, 'we won't go far. But I want to go far enough to prove . . . and it would be just such a luxury to . . .' Words finally failed him.

I said: 'I always did think it was the little luxuries that made life worthwhile,' and we both laughed, hugging each other.

Then he began to fumble clumsily with his trousers.

XIV

A long time later as we were lighting cigarettes he said in a low voice: 'Be honest with me – did you find all that unspeakably sordid?'

'*Sordid*? For God's sake, what kind of a Victorian middle-class chump do you think I am?'

'I'd have thought any girl, no matter what her class, might react adversely to an unfettered display of male carnality.'

'Unfettered display of . . .' I dissolved into helpless laughter. 'Darling, you're talking exactly like a character in one of the Victorian pornographic novels that Arabella found in Great-Uncle Frederick's library! But no, on second thoughts the seducer would have talked about his "member", not about his male carnality. Must you really be quite so bourgeois and old-fashioned?'

He winced. Instantly I was stricken. 'Oh darling, I'm sorry, I'm sorry –'

'I'm the wrong class, the wrong age, the wrong everything as far as you're concerned!' he cried in despair.

'So what? I'd love you even if you were a working-class navvy of ninety. Now stop worrying that I found that delicious groping sordid because the truth is I thought it was complete and utter bliss – in fact I'm quite sure the full sex act could only have been an anticlimax,' I added in my firmest voice, and as he smiled shyly – he even blushed – I had a glimpse of the passionate but strait-laced young man he must have been long ago in a remote era which I could not quite imagine.

I kissed him. 'Have I really shocked you so much?' I said amused. 'What happened to that bold, freewheeling dean who supported the publication of *Lady Chatterley's Lover* and who's now fighting tooth and nail for the right to install a box of phallic cigars in the Cathedral churchyard?'

To my relief he laughed and relaxed. 'He was temporarily elbowed aside by Neville One who was brought up by Primitive Methodists!'

'And when do Nevilles Two and Three make their appearance?'

'Never, they're dead. Good heavens, look at the time! My darling, I must drive back to Starbridge as fast as if I were Juan Fangio chasing the world championship!'

We rocketed out of Chancton Wood and roared down the main road to the city. I think I only screamed three times. At least we didn't kill anyone. As we soared over the river into Eternity Street I gasped: 'Don't forget to drop me by the Staro Arms!'

'No, can't stop – there's a hulking great monster pawing the back bumper –'

'Then turn into the Close!'

'No, someone might see us –' We shot off at a tangent towards the Market Place '– but don't worry, I'll go round by St Martin's and drop you at the top of Butchers' Alley.'

We zipped around the Market Place, dived up Wheat Street, zoomed down Barley Road and bounced to a halt in Chasuble Lane behind a parked van. 'Bother!' said Juan Fangio's impersonator with commendable control of his language, and gamely nosed the car around the van's right wing. Brakes screeched as a lorry coming the other way successfully avoided a head-on collision, and in the distance the screaming abuse of the appalled driver wafted towards us on the summer air. 'They really should make more one-way streets in this city,' said Aysgarth placidly, trying to reverse back behind the van but finding that the car following us was blocking his path. 'Now, I wonder what I ought to do next?'

'Perhaps I'd better nip out and vanish,' I said as an intrigued policeman began to cruise in our direction.

'That might be a good idea. Juan Fangio's temporarily stuck. Goodbye, darling – all my love – write soon . . .'

The last thing I heard as I headed for Butchers' Alley was the policeman saying genially: 'Well, well, well, Mr Dean! You seem to be causing a little bit of chaos here . . . ?'

I thought: that's the understatement of the century.

Then I fell into my flat, sank into a delicious hot bath and reflected that even though I might still die *virgo intacta* I at least knew all there was to know about orgasms.

XV

'I've brought you a plant,' said my mother an hour later as I opened the front door and found her standing with a nasty-looking potted object in her arms. Behind her the uniformed chauffeur languished at the wheel of the Daimler which was slumbering, with superb insolence, beneath a sign which declared NO PARKING. *Present Laughter* had opened that week at the Starbridge Playhouse, and my mother was now on her way to worship Martin Darrow. 'Plants are such nice house-warming presents, I always think,' she was adding, 'and that's a particularly superior one because it does well with little light – it occurred to me that if you overlooked a narrow street like Butchers' Alley the absence of light might create difficulties. All you need to do is water the plant until the soil is moist, *but not sodden*, and never let it stand in a pool.'

'Thanks so much, Mama . . . Sorry these stairs are so steep.'

'They're no steeper than the servants' stairs at Flaxton Hall . . . Oh, what a dear little attic! I like it *very* much – how charming! But I do think Mrs Lindsay might have put up more suitable pictures – it looks as if those teenage daughters of hers made the selection! Next time you're at the Hall, darling, do help yourself to a couple of old masters from the attics.'

'Yes, Mama. Sherry?'

'Lovely – yes, please! I must say, Venetia, you're looking very well, really most striking – and so much more dignified than Arabella who's suddenly gone ash-blonde and was photographed at Pompadour's (always a fatal sign) with Archie Blenham's ex-brother-in-law who's now on his third divorce. I don't *think* she's sleeping with him, but of course it's quite impossible to be sure.'

There was a pause. Then my voice said: 'I'm sorry, Mama, but could you just say that last sentence again?'

'I said I don't think she's sleeping with him but of course it's quite impossible to be sure. She absolutely swore to your father last week that she'd never committed adultery in her life – so sweet of her to want to protect him from unpleasantness! – but a woman with dyed ash-blonde hair is surely *capable de tout*. Oh, and by the way, darling, while I'm on the subject of your father, I do wish you'd drop him just a *tiny* line so that he stops complaining about being neglected. It would make my life so much easier – and talking of letters I must tell you that Enid Markhampton wrote the other day and said how delighted she was to meet you again when she returned to the Chantry – she said what a charming girl you'd become! There! Isn't that nice? I always believe in passing on "dew-drops". Apparently Marina had mentioned to her that you went regularly to the Cathedral – well, naturally I didn't tell your father because he would have worried that you might be "getting religion" and becoming un-balanced, but believe me, as the worn-out mother of four lively daughters, I was *delighted* to think of you surrounded by clergy-men and thinking noble thoughts! And talking of clergymen, how's that nice Canon Hoffenberg?'

I began to talk about Eddie and tried hard not to think of my Mr Dean in Chancton Wood.

XVI

Later when I was alone I thought: he still never said directly that he wasn't having sex with Dido, he still refused to consum-mate our affair, and he was still evasive about his past. We had appeared to progress in Chancton Wood but in fact the progression had been an illusion. Nothing had changed because none of the mysteries had been solved.

My mother's fatal words echoed in my ears. 'I don't think she's sleeping with him but of course it's quite impossible to be sure.' However in my case it was indeed possible to be sure. If my Mr Dean had looked me straight in the eyes and said: 'I don't have sex with my wife,' I would have believed him. But instead he had only said: 'I'm going to explode that theory,' as if a sexual blitzkrieg was more convincing than a clergyman's simple denial.

I mixed myself a dry martini and sat sipping it as the twilight thickened.

After a while a new truth dawned. I saw it had now been proved that moral convictions alone could not be responsible for his refusal to have full sexual intercourse with me, because if he could overcome those convictions sufficiently to ensure we were both sexually satisfied in Chancton Wood, there was no reason why he shouldn't satisfy us both in the conventional manner. What kind of a tortuous casuistry was responsible for his decision that one route to sexual satisfaction was permitted while another was taboo? It made no sense at all, but I now had a terrible suspicion that his behaviour was somehow connected – in the most intimate way imaginable – with Dido.

Yet I couldn't be certain. The rock-bottom truth was that I still had no idea what was going on in Aysgarth's mind, and that, of course, was why it was still so vital that I should succeed in milking Father Darrow for information.

In forty-eight hours' time I would come face to face with him in the Starbridge Playhouse.

But I had no idea how I could ever contrive to see him on his own.

XVII

'That's odd,' I said to Eddie in the front row of the circle on Friday evening. 'I know Nick Darrow's going to be here with his father, but I can't see them.'

'I didn't think Father Darrow went anywhere nowadays,' said Eddie, looking up from his programme in surprise.

'The opportunity to see his famous son tread the boards was obviously too potent to resist.' I cast a quick look around the circle again but there was still no sign of Nick. The Starbridge Playhouse, an art-deco lump built to replace a decayed Edwardian gem, was a miniature version of the palatial cinemas of the 1930s. The facilities it offered were excellent, a fact which explained why Starbridge was so often favoured by West End producers who wanted to try out their work in the provinces, and the audience, seated on only two levels, had been shamelessly pampered by the architect; in addition to the first-class acoustics and comfortable seats there was a bar on each floor. Nevertheless, in the perverse manner of human beings, the older inhabitants of Starbridge were united in pining for their rat- and rot-infested Edwardian gem and regarded the modern theatre as 'characterless'.

'Why are you so anxious to see Nick?' Eddie was asking curiously.

'He's my Talisman and whenever I see him something extra-ordinary happens. I met him in the spring and was whisked away to the Hebrides, I met him in May and was whirled into the Orgy –' But before I could say more the lights began to dim. Casting one last fruitless glance around the auditorium for the Darrows, I prayed fiercely that they were both present and then made up my mind not to let my acute anxiety ruin the play.

XVIII

Martin Darrow, seemingly tailor-made for the part of Gary Essendine, was given a rapturous welcome by the audience as soon as he made his entrance and with the aid of an able supporting cast transformed Coward's dated play into a sparkling entertainment for the 1960s. Taller than I had thought he would be but looking younger now that he was not subjected to television close-ups, he moved with effort-less grace around the stage, spoke his lines with masterly skill and somehow resisted the awful temptation to 'go over the top' once he had the audience in the palm of his hand.

'He's very good, isn't he?' said Eddie with genuine admiration as the curtain descended amidst thunderous applause for the first interval, but I was already saying: 'Excuse me – must find Nick,' and dashing up the gangway to the exit.

I hung around the foyer as people gushed out of the stalls, but no Darrow of any kind emerged.

'I should think the old man's staying put,' said Eddie as he joined me.

'Then they've got to be in the seats underneath the circle,' I muttered. 'There's nowhere else they can possibly be.' I charged into the auditorium and to my vast relief saw Nick straight away. He was sitting in a row near the back, and beside him was a very, very ancient item indeed, an apparition which displayed the almost translucent skin of extreme old age. I thought vaguely how good it was of him to come and was sure he was hating every moment of it. Poor old man! No doubt he wished he was tucked up in an armchair in front of the television. In panic I wondered if I had made a colossal mistake in believing that St Darrow could be a source of enlightenment; he looked much too old to be a source of anything, and perhaps Dido had been right in dismissing him as senile.

'Venetia!' Nick had risen to his feet and was gaping at me. 'I thought you were coming to the play tomorrow!'

'Change of plan!' I said brightly, moving down the row in front of him where all the seats had been temporarily vacated. 'And how's my Halley's Comet? Is something extraordinary just about to happen?'

Nick smiled and turned to his father. I heard him say: 'This is Venetia Flaxton.'

The very, very ancient item moved. It rose to a vast height, gave me an enigmatic, fascinating smile and offered me a thin, beautiful, elegant hand which achieved an astonishingly firm, positive, compelling grip. Grey eyes, immensely steady, looked not only at my face but deep into my soul. My jaw sagged. My eyes widened. I was speechless.

'How do you do, Miss Flaxton,' said Father Jonathan Darrow.

PART THREE

———◆◆———

THE GREAT POLLUTANT

'Where, one must ask, will the ravages of liberal theology end? The Devil and Hell went long ago; the position of the Blessed Virgin has been seriously undermined; God, who until last week was invulnerable, is now distinctly on the defensive. What will ultimately be left except a belief in the need for bishops, if only to give evidence in trials about obscenity and to talk to pop singers on television?'

T. E. UTLEY
The Honest to God Debate
ed. DAVID L. EDWARDS

'The fact that the old land-marks are disappearing is not something to be deplored. If we have the courage, it is something to be welcomed . . .'

JOHN A. T. ROBINSON
Suffragan Bishop of Woolwich 1959–1969
Honest to God

ONE

'. . . it seems to be assumed throughout [*Honest to God*]
that what "modern man" can or cannot believe is the test
of truth. Yet the problems of "modern man" are not always
as new as they are made out to be. Christianity is not
easy for the natural man to accept in any age. Nor is
mid-twentieth century man of necessity the type of the
future. In the next century man may be astonished at the
confidence of some of our disbeliefs.'

> JOHN LAWRENCE
> *The Honest to God Debate*
> ed. DAVID L. EDWARDS

I

Did I manage to utter the formal words of introduction as I
shook hands with Father Darrow? I have no idea. I was in a
trance. All I could think was that this was no pathetic old man
but a magic seer who could tell me everything I wanted to
know. Immediately the stakes in the complicated game I was
playing seemed to increase tenfold. Now it was not merely
important but vital that I should see him on his own.

'. . . and you know Canon Hoffenberg, don't you, Father?'
Nick was saying.

'We met when I attended the Theological College after the
war,' Eddie said. 'How nice to see you again, Father Darrow!
I hope you're well?'

'Well enough, thanks.' He smiled thinly as if he felt a man
deserved a more austere expression of good will than the fascinating greeting he had produced for me.

I finally managed to recover my poise. 'You must be so proud
of your son!' I said. 'I'm hoping to go backstage afterwards to
get his autograph for my mother.' And I added brightly to
Nick: 'Will you be going backstage too?'

Nick obviously felt such adulatory behaviour was far beneath him. 'No, we're meeting Martin at the Staro Arms.'

'What a coincidence!' I exclaimed wide-eyed. 'We'd planned to have a drink there, hadn't we, Eddie?'

'Oh yes!' said Eddie, playing up with unexpected resourcefulness. 'Perhaps you can get your autograph there instead, Venetia – it would save you fighting your way backstage!'

'What a brilliant idea! Although of course,' I added smoothly to Nick, 'we wouldn't want to intrude on any family reunion.'

'There'd be no intrusion,' said Father Darrow before Nick could speak. 'The reunion's already taken place.'

'And Martin's spending Sunday with us anyway,' said Nick, taking his cue from his father but not looking particularly enthralled at the prospect of seeing us later.

'Marvellous!' I said gaily, smiling at him. Then I stole a glance at Father Darrow. With shock I found he was looking straight at me and at once I was aware of the irrational conviction that he was reading my mind, skimming through it in the manner of someone obliged to absorb the main story of a newspaper in seconds. Again I felt as if I had plunged to the ground in a lift; I was reminded of my first meeting with Nick on the Starbridge train at Waterloo.

'Well!' said my voice with a dreadful false heartiness. 'We'll look forward to seeing you both later! Come along, Eddie.'

The next thing I knew I was reeling into the foyer.

'Shall I fight for a gin?' offered Eddie, eyeing the bar where a dense multitude was screaming in a haze of cigarette smoke.

'Please.' I felt I had to get rid of him in order to concentrate on my recovery.

He battled back with a couple of gin-and-tonics just as the bell rang to signal the end of the interval.

'Eddie, you're heroic.' I knocked back my drink. 'And thanks for playing along with my performance in the stalls.'

'Am I allowed to ask what's going on?'

'No. Just keep on being heroic.'

The bell started to ring again.

We returned to our seats in the circle.

II

'Is this my family I see before me?' mused Martin Darrow, half in and half out of the character of Gary Essendine as he made a grand entrance into the main reception room of the Staro Arms. 'It is! But who's the lovely lady with the tiger eyes, the Pre-Raphaelite locks and the exquisitely-dressed companion?'

Eddie boggled at this histrionic approach and I was aware of Nick fidgeting in an agony of embarrassment, but I sprang up, captivated by such uninhibited charm, and replied promptly: 'I'm Venetia Flaxton and this is Canon Eddie Hoffenberg of the Cathedral. Congratulations – we enjoyed your performance enormously!'

'Now if this were a Hollywood musical,' said Martin amused, 'a dozen singing waiters would immediately appear with champagne! Thank you, Venetia. How do you do, Canon. Well, in the absence of the singing waiters, what are we all going to drink?'

'The bar's closed,' said Nick austerely.

'Well, of course it is! This is spiritual downtown Starbridge, not wicked old Sunset Strip! But as I'm a resident I can still terrorise the lounge waiter. What would you like, Miss Tiger-Eyes?'

'I'd adore a brandy,' I said. 'Rémy Martin would do.'

'I'm mad about this girl,' said Martin. 'What a throwaway line! Like saying: "I'd adore a car – I think I could just about stand a Rolls-Royce!"'

We all laughed. Eddie settled for a whisky-and-soda, Nick for a Coca-Cola and the old man, after a fractional hesitation, requested a glass of port.

'. . . and my usual orange juice, please, Bill,' said Martin to the waiter as he offered me a cigarette. 'Now Dad, let's hear your verdict – were you appalled?'

'Not in the least,' said the old man serenely. 'It was a most entertaining and well-constructed play and I'm sure it was most difficult to write. It occurred to me that Mr Coward is probably underrated by the serious critics despite – or perhaps because of – his popular success.'

If I had had any lingering doubts about his mental faculties these shrewd remarks would have destroyed them. I was delighted by this tribute to Coward's craftsmanship, but before I could say so Nick muttered in an urgent voice to his father: 'What Martin wants to know is not what you thought of the play but what you thought of him.'

This amused Martin very much. 'You funny boy!' he exclaimed indulgently as if Nick were a child who had made a precocious remark. 'Do you really think Dad isn't aware of that?'

Nick shot him a furious look but the old man said in a soothing voice: 'He only wanted me to put you out of your suspense – and of course I should have congratulated you straight away, just as Miss Flaxton did. Most of the time I quite forgot you were Martin, and on the rare occasions when I did remember I was always so thankful that you weren't like Mr Essendine in real life.'

This was evidently the right thing to say. Martin laughed and commented to Eddie: 'There speaks the ex-monk and the priest!'

'Of course Gary Essendine was very naughty,' I said, 'but so were the girls. I loved it when Joanna said she'd lost her latch-key – I laughed like a drain.'

We were still deep in our discussion of the play when the drinks arrived, but as Martin raised his glass to me with a smile I summoned my nerve, produced my programme and asked him to autograph it for my mother.

'. . . and she's Lady Flaxton, not Mrs,' I added hastily after he had declared he would produce a personal dedication.

'I'm wild about the aristocracy,' said Martin, scribbling busily. 'I always think "All Men Are Equal" is quite the most boring lie ever invented.'

The conversation, sustained almost entirely by Eddie, Martin and me, continued to bowl along at a smart pace while I racked my brains to devise a scheme for separating Father Darrow from his family so that I could beg him for a private audience at a later date. Nick, out of his social depth again, gazed into his glass of Coke as if he were seeing mystical images in the depths, but was probably only longing to go home. The old man sat very still and said little but appeared quite content to sip his port and listen to us. However, as soon as I had swallowed my last mouthful of Rémy Martin he said to his younger son: 'We must be going – can you bring the car to the door?' and Nick jumped up with alacrity.

'I hope you won't be offended if I offer to pay for the drinks,' said Eddie to Martin. 'We actually came here with the intention of playing host – if the bar had been open –'

The futile argument began over who was to foot the bill. I write 'futile' because it was quite obvious that Martin intended to pay and equally obvious that Eddie could not bring himself to accept this generosity without making a lengthy protest.

I looked at Father Darrow and Father Darrow looked at me. We were still seated. Martin and Eddie were drifting, like boats turned loose from their moorings, towards the centre of the long, low-ceilinged room. Nick had by this time vanished to retrieve the car.

Father Darrow said quietly but distinctly: 'You want to see me, don't you?' and somehow I managed to utter the syllable: 'Yes.'

'Come to my cottage at Starrington Manor at eleven o'clock tomorrow morning.'

'Okay.' I could barely speak.

Martin, having won the argument, drifted back to attend to the aged parent. 'Want a hand, Dad?'

'No, thank you.' The old man rose carefully to his feet. Although he stooped he was still taller than either of his sons. Taking his time he moved across the room as if he were a great actor making a supremely dignified exit, and Eddie hurried ahead to hold the swing door open for him. Beyond the main entrance of the hotel Nick was waiting beside a small black car.

'I was glad to see you again, Canon,' said Father Darrow, offering Eddie his hand. 'May God bless you. And please remember me, if you will, to your friend the Dean.' Then he turned to me. 'Goodbye, Miss Flaxton.'

'Goodbye, Mr Darrow – Father Darrow, I mean,' I said, so jolted by his unexpected reference to Aysgarth that I made a mess of the farewell, but he smiled at me before disappearing into the night.

Afterwards as Eddie and I walked down Eternity Street I realised it was time I provided some explanation, no matter how fantastic, of my peculiar behaviour, so I said with fervour: 'Martin's fabulous, isn't he? Much better-looking than either Nick or the old man. I suppose he's on his third or fourth wife by this time and keeps a glamorous mistress in some thrillingly seamy place like Pimlico.'

Eddie heaved the windy sigh of the dedicated masochist. Too late it occurred to me that by pretending I had a crush on Martin I was being brutally tactless.

'Such a pity he's so old!' I said hastily. 'Of course I could never be really serious about anything over fifty.'

Eddie sighed again as if he had decided it would be more fun to disbelieve me. All he said was: 'I think I must make another appointment with my osteopath. My back's taken a turn for the worse.'

I could have slapped him.

In silence we walked on down Eternity Street.

III

Starrington Magna, a sprawling village which stood twelve miles from Starbridge, was surrounded by farms owned by wealthy London businessmen who liked to play in the country at weekends. However, Nick told me that Starrington Manor's Home Farm was run by a local man while the Community cared for the Manor's extensive grounds. The house itself, I discovered, was not a Georgian mansion like my home but a rambling old pile which reminded me of a gingerbread house designed by a talented cook. It sat placidly in the sunshine amidst daisy-strewn lawns and looked hospitable. I found it a marked but not unattractive contrast to the glacial symmetry and manicured swards of Flaxton Hall.

'It's most peculiar of Father to see you like this,' said Nick, leading me across the back lawn towards a wood. 'I can't understand it. He never sees women. In fact he seldom sees anyone. You must be careful not to stay more than ten minutes, and please don't stage an emotional scene because he wouldn't like it. He's too old now for all that sort of thing.'

'Who do you think you are?' I said. 'A Norland nanny, complete with pram and nappies?'

Nick said obstinately: 'He's got to be looked after.'

'I thought the Community did that.'

'Huh!' said Nick in contempt and fell silent.

Before we entered the wood we passed a long, tangled herbaceous border bright with blooms. I thought how my mother would have rushed to tidy it up and ruin it.

'I like this place,' I said impulsively. 'It's got a good atmosphere.'

Nick stopped mooching along like an overgrown James Dean and decided to be gracious. 'Father keeps the atmosphere clear,' he said mysteriously, 'and not even the Community can pollute it.'

'What's wrong with the Community?'

'Bunch of silly neurotics playing at the religious life. Father only keeps them around for my sake so that I don't have to worry about either him or the house when I'm away.'

Having entered the wood we were now following a well-marked path. The light, filtering through the leaves, was green and dim and cool.

'How did your father find these nut-cases?'

'They found him. Weak people are drawn to him because his psyche's so strong,' said Nick proudly, as if his father were an extra-sensory Tarzan. 'He started with a couple of ex-monks – Anglican Benedictines from the Fordite Order – who needed a home while they readjusted to life in the world. They eventually married but, thank God, haven't reproduced. Probably don't know how. Then we've got an ex-missionary, an ex-Naval chaplain, an ex-theological student and an ex-pop-singer, all with various terminal hang-ups. The pop singer's writing an opera about God.'

I was much intrigued, but before I could ask more questions the bushes parted on my left and I saw below me in a fairy-tale dell, framed by beautiful trees and magical shafts of sunlight, a vision of architectural perfection. It was a little chapel, exquisitely proportioned, a miniature variation on the classical themes expressed so sublimely by St Paul's church in Covent Garden.

'My God!' I said, stopping dead to gape in admiration.

'Nice, isn't it?' said Nick, now very friendly.

'Celestial. What's that ruin in the background?'

'A chantry destroyed by religious thugs at the time of the Reformation.'

Dreamily we wandered on down the path towards the glade on the floor of the dell. Birds sang. Beyond the intricate pattern of motionless green leaves the sky was a pure, misty blue. The sense of peace was overpowering.

On reaching the glade I noticed that beyond the chapel stood a little house with a slate roof and walls of golden stone. Flowers grew in the window-boxes which flanked the open front door, and a tough-looking tabby-cat, guarding the threshold, watched our approach with a knowing expression before disappearing nimbly into the interior.

Nick paused. 'I'll hang around out here,' he said, becoming bossy again. 'Father might need me. And remember: no more than ten minutes. I don't want him tired.'

'Anyone would think *you* were the parent here! Incidentally, why do you call him Father while Martin addresses him as Dad?'

'He doesn't like being called Dad but Martin doesn't know because Father never liked to tell him for fear of hurting his feelings.' Nick sounded pleased by this, as if he had scored in some important way over his famous half-brother.

I was about to say frankly: 'You Darrows are the oddest bunch!' when a shadow moved in the doorway and I realised that Father Darrow was now standing watching us, the tough tabby-cat curled neatly in his arms.

IV

'Come in, Miss Flaxton,' he said. 'Off you go, Nicholas.'

'But Father –'

'Quite unnecessary for you to stay, thank you.'

Reconverted into an overgrown James Dean, Nick slouched off across the glade with his fists shoved deep in his pockets.

'It's very difficult for Nicholas that I'm so old,' said Father Darrow, setting down the cat before ushering me across the threshold. 'Old people can seem so fragile to the young and he's become over-protective, but as you see, I'm quite capable of looking after myself.'

I stared around. The room was perhaps fifteen foot square and contained a bunk bed with drawers underneath, a small wardrobe, a table with two chairs, an easy chair with a footstool and numerous shelves of books on either side of a stone fireplace. There were no pictures, no photographs, only a crucifix hanging over the bed. Everywhere was fanatically tidy and spotlessly clean. The old man was spotlessly clean too, just like the room, and neat as a new pin. In contrast to the previous evening, when he had been dressed as a layman for his outing to the theatre, he had now chosen to appear as a clergyman; he wore a black suit, a black stock and a snow-white clerical collar. He also, unlike most ordinary Anglican clergymen, wore a small pectoral cross, representative, I supposed, of the Anglo-Catholic churchmanship which made him prefer to be addressed as 'Father' rather than 'Mr'. His beautiful hands gestured that I should sit down at the table. He offered me tea.

'Well, if it's not too much trouble . . .'

But the kettle had already been boiled in the little galley-kitchen. 'They were able to bring electricity to the cottage without much trouble,' he said, as if he felt obliged to explain the presence of modern conveniences. 'The main road runs close to here beyond the wall of the grounds. However, I chose not to have electric radiators. I prefer an open fire, even if it does mean a little extra work.'

The tabby-cat was washing its paws on the hearth but when Father Darrow sat down opposite me the animal padded over to us. The old man poured out the tea and nodded to the cat. Instantly it leapt into his lap and began to purr.

'It's very good of you to see me like this,' I said, watching his hands stroke the stripey fur, 'especially when you never see women.'

'What a nasty old misogynist that makes me sound!' He gave me his most fascinating smile. 'It's true that in the old days my ministry was to men, but that wasn't because I disliked women; it was because I liked women too well. However, at the advanced age of eighty-three . . . Well, nowadays I see just whom I want to see, that's the truth of it. Most people I don't want to see. Nothing to say. But occasionally I come across a person who screams silently: HELP! HELP! – and then, I assure you, I'm the most sociable creature you could imagine.'

I was entranced. 'You really heard me screaming for help?'

'A young woman,' said Father Darrow, 'attractive, delightful and obviously well-to-do, sits down at a table with four men. But she has no eyes for her escort, no eyes for the famous actor who's being so charming to her and no eyes for the young man who's too shy to be more than conventionally civil. Again and again she steals glances at this very decrepit old party who's quite clearly, as they say, "past it". And again and again, whenever the decrepit old party meets her fascinated gaze she looks away as if she's been caught in a fearful indiscretion. Now what can be the meaning of this curious behaviour? In addition it's clear that the young lady's in a state of profound agitation. She twists the strap of her bag; she drinks her brandy too fast; she talks with great style but little content. Adding two and two together I make an unlikely four: the young lady has heard about me and for some reason believes that I can ease her agitation. I take a gamble, I suggest an interview and she almost collapses with relief. So! Here you are, and all I now have to do is ask how I can help you.'

'Why, you fabulous old pet!' I cried, but then realised in embarrassment that this was hardly the most respectful way to address a clergyman. 'Sorry,' I muttered. 'Demented with relief. Slip of the tongue.'

But Father Darrow looked delighted that a young woman should be calling him a fabulous old pet, and as he smiled at me again he seemed so sympathetic, so kind and above all so immensely approachable that I felt I could talk to him without pause for hour after hour while I bared my soul for his inspection. Having been obliged in recent weeks to keep my own counsel and dissemble endlessly in order to preserve my great secret, I found that the impact of meeting someone to whom I could open my heart was so great that I had a wild desire to weep. But I controlled myself. No emotional scenes, Nick had said. I didn't want the old pet regretting his decision to give me an audience.

'Well, you see, it's like this,' I said, dry-eyed but not, unfortunately, very coherent. 'I seem to have got myself into rather a peculiar situation with a clergyman – I mean, don't get me wrong, I'm not his mistress, at least not exactly, but nevertheless . . . well, it's just rather a peculiar situation.' Gulping some air I tried not to panic.

'Oh, I'm very used to clergymen in peculiar situations,' said Father Darrow, mercifully unshocked and still exuding his bewitching sympathy from every pore. 'Have a little sip of tea.'

I had a little sip of tea. Then I managed to add: 'We're madly in love but it's all very confusing.'

'There's a wife, I daresay, in the background,' suggested Father Darrow helpfully, stroking the cat behind the ears.

'Yes, but we've both accepted that there can be no divorce.' Suddenly the words began to stream out of me. 'The real problem,' I said, 'is what sort of relationship we can have. You see, he believes – and he's terribly modern in his outlook – he believes there are no hard and fast rules any more when it comes to dealing with ethical situations; all you have to do is act with love – which sounds like an invitation to a sexual free-for-all but it's not. The catch is that you have to act with the very best

313

kind of love, pure and noble. So if a man loves a girl and says to himself: "Do I take her to bed?" the answer's not yes, it's no, because if he really loves her he won't want to use her to satisfy himself in that way.'

'This sounds like the New Morality outlined by Bishop Robinson in *Honest to God*.'

'So you know all about that!' I had thought an ancient recluse would hardly bother to keep abreast of modern theology. 'What do you think of it?'

'The important question is what *you* think of it.'

'I just don't know any more, I'm so confused. My clergyman, following the New Morality, says that even though he's married we're allowed a romantic friendship so long as we truly love each other, because so long as we *truly* love each other we'll be high-minded enough to abstain from anything that's wrong – wrong in the sense that it would hurt either us or other people. Well, that's fine, so heroic, but the trouble is, the deeper I get into this relationship the less sense that seems to make. I mean, if you love someone you do want to go to bed with them, you can't stop yourself, sex becomes like a tank, crushing all the noble thoughts into the dust.'

'You're saying that the gap between Dr Robinson's idealism and your experience of reality has now become intolerably wide. And what about our clergyman? Is he experiencing this gap too?'

'Yes, but . . . Honestly, Father Darrow, I just don't know what's going on in his mind. There's no doubt he's a deeply moral man – I mean, this is not, repeat *not*, your typical runaway vicar who periodically features in a *News of the World* scandal – but sometimes I think he's making the New Morality an excuse for not going further with me; I've begun to suspect he's held back not by his moral beliefs, genuine though they are, but by some sort of psychological block which arises out of his past.'

Father Darrow was deeply interested. 'Have you any idea what this could be?'

'In my worst moments I suspect it's all connected with his wife, and in my very worst moments I get obsessed with the thought that he's still sleeping with her, but the truth is I just don't know. All I do know is that occasionally he seems very mixed up – some of his conversations are really bizarre – yet at the same time he must be extremely sane and well-balanced.'

'What makes you so sure of that?'

'Well, I wasn't exaggerating a moment ago when I said he's not your typical runaway vicar. He's not a vicar at all. He's terribly distinguished, he's one of the most important men in the diocese, and he simply couldn't hold down such a job unless he was sanity personified.'

'Ah yes,' said Father Darrow, 'I see it all now.' He set down the cat. 'You wanted to see me because I know him well and you think I can unlock the mystery of his personality for you.'

'That's it.' I sagged with relief. 'His wife says you know more about him than anyone else except her, so I thought that if only you could explain him to me I'd at last be able to understand what's going on.'

'What's going on,' said Father Darrow, 'is adultery, Miss Flaxton.'

'Oh no!' I said at once. 'Didn't I make myself clear? We haven't had sex. I mean, we haven't had complete sex. I mean –'

'How often do you see this man?'

'Once a week on his afternoon off, when we go for a drive in his car, and sometimes we're able to see each other for a few minutes in between, but he writes every day and I write back so we're in close touch.'

'He likes your letters, does he?'

'Oh, he adores them! And he adores me – he says I'm the greatest prize he's ever encountered –'

'Yes, of course. He would. I recognise him now.'

I stared. 'You do?'

'Oh, he's quite unmistakable. Tell me, has he perhaps encouraged you to call him by another name, a name he doesn't normally use?'

Shock locked itself in a lump in my throat as the mounting strain of the interview finally took its toll on me. I was unable to speak.

'It's the Dean, isn't it?' said Father Darrow.

I covered my face with my hands and began to tremble.

V

'Don't be afraid,' said Father Darrow instantly. 'I'm sorry I sounded tough. Men often prefer compassion laced with toughness – it helps them maintain their self-control when such things are still important to them, but of course women aren't confined in that kind of emotional strait-jacket.'

'Too bad they're not,' I said. 'I can't stand either sex when they're slobbering all over the place. Disgusting.' I looked away as my eyes filled with tears.

'Let me pour you some more tea,' said Father Darrow.

'Oh, please don't now bend over backwards to be gentle and kind!' I said. 'That would finish me off altogether. Go on being tough. I'd prefer it.' A tear rolled down my cheek. Loathing myself for being so feeble I made a mighty effort, dashed the tear aside and commented with a meticulous logic: 'Since you recognised Aysgarth from the way he's conducting this affair, I can only assume that this has all happened before.'

Father Darrow only said: 'What name's he using now?'

'He's gone back to Neville.'

'No, he's gone on. This would be Neville Four.'

I suddenly realised I was terrified. I forgot my desire to cry. I could only stare at him transfixed as he so casually conjured up the vision of a Dr Jekyll accompanied by a gang of Mr Hydes, but at last I managed to stammer: 'Father Darrow, you've just got to explain – what in God's name is going on?'

'What's going on, as I've already told you, is adultery, Miss Flaxton.'

'Yes, yes, yes, but what's really going on?'

'That *is* what's really going on. That's reality. Aysgarth's psychology is in fact very unimportant in this context.'

'But –'

'You think that if you understand his psychology you'll be

able to discern where the affair is going and what you may reasonably expect from it in the way of emotional satisfaction. But Miss Flaxton, fortunately you don't need to know anything more about Aysgarth in order to make this crucial discernment. It's quite obvious that the situation's leading to catastrophe and that you should escape from it at once.'

I whispered: 'Catastrophe?'

'You both stand in very great danger.'

'You mean in danger of being found out?'

'No, in danger of spiritual destruction. Can't you feel the Devil caressing the hair at the nape of your neck?'

Instantly my neck prickled. In fact so powerful was the impact of his suggestion that my hand automatically sped to the nape of my neck to clamp down on the hairs which I felt sure were standing on end. Then reason reclaimed me. Withdrawing my hand I wiped my sweating palm on the skirt of my dress and said in fury: 'You can't frighten me like that! No one believes in the Devil any more!'

'Don't connive at your own destruction, Miss Flaxton. To pretend the Devil doesn't exist is to invite him to annex your soul.'

'But this is 1963! We don't believe in a three-decker universe any more! We don't believe in God as an old man up in the sky! We don't believe –'

'We don't believe the Devil is a charming little imp with horns. That's true. The symbol's outdated. But that doesn't mean the Devil doesn't exist, and that doesn't mean the 1960s can do without symbols in their attempt to express ultimate reality. Believe me, Miss Flaxton, there's nothing so very special about the 1960s – although future historians may well look back in wonder that so much was disbelieved so irrationally by so many.'

'But Bishop Robinson says –'

'The Bishop's reaching for new ways to speak about God, but two can play at that game – let me reach for a new way of speaking about the Devil. Forget the little imp with horns! Throw him in the melting-pot, as Dr Robinson would say! But now think of Hiroshima, Miss Flaxton. When the atomic bomb was dropped many were killed but some people did survive apparently unscathed. Yet they were not unscathed. They had been contaminated by a great pollutant. It was invisible, but it entered the flesh of those unfortunate victims and settled in their bones and is to this very day busy destroying them. That was a very great pollutant, Miss Flaxton, one of the greatest mankind has ever known. But there's another pollutant, the greatest pollutant of them all, and it attacks not men's bodies, like radioactivity, but their souls. The attack is launched through the human consciousness, which, as any psychiatrist will tell you, is a dense and often impenetrable mystery. Human consciousness is like a well, and into that well, through every little crack in the brickwork, the Great Pollutant will seep unless rigorous efforts are made to keep it out. But if no efforts are made or if the efforts made are too feeble to be effective, the shaft will be fatally contaminated; a scum will form upon the water and in the end the entire well will be rank and putrid. Then the well, that source of life, will be dead, and the Great Pollutant will have triumphed over the miracle that was once clear and shining and beautiful in God's sight.'

There was a silence. I smoothed the nape of my neck again with shaking fingers and stared blindly down at the table.

'You may think you stand in the light, Miss Flaxton, but it's a false light, and wherever the false light exists *it* will be there, the Great Pollutant, pouring darkness into the well of consciousness in order to lay waste the human soul.'

'But I love Neville! And since love is good —'

'As I said, you may think you stand in the light but the light is false. Now let me abandon the language of mysticism and talk directly of hard facts. I believe you when you say you love this man. But since he belongs to another woman, there's no place for your love to exist. This truth is symbolised, of course, by the fact that you can only meet for any considerable time in that transient object, his motor car. To create a place where your love can exist in any satisfactory way is in fact impossible, and indeed any attempt to create such a place is to dabble in the dangerous delusion that your love can bring you anything other than the most destructive suffering. I beg you, Miss Flaxton, face reality. Don't be beguiled by Aysgarth's fantasies – or by your own.'

'But I *am* trying to face reality! If you could only explain his psychology to me –'

'That's beyond my power. I'm a priest. I can't betray the secrets of the confessional.'

For a moment I was dumbfounded. Then I was furious with myself for not foreseeing this impasse, and my fury combined with my disappointment to form an overwhelming despair. Again I found myself struggling to suppress my tears.

'I'm very sorry,' said Father Darrow, 'but what I can and will do is list the facts which – unlike Aysgarth's psychology – are absolutely crucial here. One: Aysgarth is obviously living in a state of very great illusion. Two: this is probably, though not necessarily, generated by a desire to escape from profound problems either in his private life or in his professional life or in both. Three: because he's in such severe difficulties he needs spiritual counselling without delay. Four: you're in a position to wreck both his public and private life, and five: he's in a position to destroy you. That's reality, Miss Flaxton, and in consequence the only realistic advice I can possibly give you is to end the affair immediately.'

I sat shaking, shocked and shattered in my chair as the tears rolled silently down my cheeks.

'Now let me warn you against the pitfalls you'll be tempted to rush into as you automatically try to resist this advice,' said Father Darrow. 'One: don't write me off as a senile old codger who's forgotten what it's like to be in love. I was about Aysgarth's age when I fell violently in love with my second wife, who was then a woman not much older than you are now, and that's a memory that can never die. Two: don't write me off as an old-fashioned priest who's mindlessly committed to supporting a conventional moral line. My support is rational, not mindless, because conventional morals actually evolved to deal with realities; they weren't invented by a gang of old buffers who sat down one afternoon and decided to flex their imaginations in order to cause the greatest possible inconvenience to the greatest number of people – indeed if morals were invented in that way I wouldn't be interested in them; my business is entirely concerned with reality, not fantasy. Three: don't deceive yourself with the thought that Mrs Aysgarth might suddenly die. It's true any of us can die at any time, but if you spend your life waiting for her to die you'll wind up wanting to murder her – which will mean you've gone out of your mind. Four: don't deceive yourself with the thought that this marriage could break up. Clerical marriages do break up, sad to say, but this one won't. It's not in my power to say why he's bound to that wife of his, but believe me, he's tied with ropes of steel. Whether he's still intimate with her – a question you obviously find of deep interest – I have no idea, but in fact that's not important. All that's important is that by making love to you – in whatever sense – he's doing you nothing but harm.'

'But he's not! He couldn't! He's so good, so kind, so –' I choked on my words, lost control, started sobbing. 'He hasn't harmed me!' I shouted hysterically. 'He hasn't done anything to me!'

Father Darrow rose to his feet and said simply: 'Follow me.'

I stumbled after him as he led the way to a door on the other side of the room. When he opened the door I saw a bath, lavatory and basin beyond.

'Come along,' he ordered as I hesitated. 'Come here.'

I staggered over the threshold and instantly he gripped my shoulders and spun me to face the mirror over the basin.

'There,' he said. '*Look* what he's done to you.'

I stared into the glass. A bleary, blotched, blighted face, haggard with sleeplessness and drawn with grief, stared back. All my eye make-up had smudged. My chalk-white cheeks had a greenish tinge. Tears were everywhere.

Wrenching myself from Father Darrow's grip I hurtled back to the table and collapsed in a heap on my chair.

'And that's just the beginning,' said Father Darrow. 'That's just a little preview of the inexorable horrors to come. Now tell me –' unexpectedly his voice softened as he altered his approach '– are your parents alive?'

I nodded dumbly.

'Could you not go and visit them? They might be able to offer support to you in this very difficult time.'

'Well . . .'

'But perhaps they're not particularly sympathetic.'

'They're okay.' I groped on the floor for my bag and began a long search for a handkerchief. 'But they're old, you see, so old, and I couldn't bother them with my problems. It wouldn't be right.'

'How considerate. That sounds as if you're fond of them.'

'Oh yes,' I said, 'very fond.'

'Are you an only child?'

'No, I'm the last of six children.' Quite without warning my voice added dully: 'Sort of an accident, I expect.' I was astonished. It was as if my voice had acquired a will of its own.

'Oh yes?' said Father Darrow, exuding his bewitching sympathy again and mentally wrapping it around me as if it were a rug.

'Yes . . . At least, that's the impression one gets.'

'Does one?' said Father Darrow, metaphorically tucking me up in the rug and adjusting each fold to make sure I was cosy.

'Well,' said my voice, responding to the cosiness by becoming confidential, 'when I was conceived my parents were visiting Venice – which was a very peculiar thing for them to do as Papa hates Abroad – and since they were both over forty and since it's hard to imagine them being much interested in sex even when they were young, one can only suppose that Venice went to Mama's head with extraordinary results.'

'What about your father?'

'Oh, nothing goes to his head except Latin and Greek. I can just imagine him sulking in Venice while Mama yearned to have a fling with some gorgeous Venetian . . . In fact ever since I saw the film *Summer Madness* in which Katharine Hepburn falls in love with Rossano Brazzi in Venice, I've wondered . . .' But my voice trailed away.

321

'Yes?' said Father Darrow, very, very gentle now, his tough manner utterly abandoned. 'What have you wondered?'

'I've wondered if Mama had a similar fling . . . but I don't suppose she did.'

There was a silence. Father Darrow was uncannily still. I was reminded of a cat waiting with infinite patience and extreme cunning outside a promising mousehole.

'My friend Marina Markhampton's father isn't her father at all,' said my voice vaguely after a while. 'They say it happens quite often among our sort of people. But of course I don't really believe it happened in our family.'

Another silence fell. The cat continued to wait outside the mousehole and at last my voice remarked idly: 'My father's a frightful bore, but I'll say this for him: he always does his moral duty. He's taken a most conscientious interest in my welfare, and considering that I'm a freak, not like any of the others, and haven't even been able to get myself married, I think he's heroic to take any interest in me at all. In fact when we drive each other up the wall – which is most of the time – I almost wish he'd stop being so heroic and disown me altogether. But of course he never would. That wouldn't be doing his moral duty.'

I looked around the room. The cat was snoozing on the hearth. A clock was ticking somewhere, and on the wall above the bed the crucifix hung in shadow.

'My father's a very moral man,' said my voice. 'He's always crusading for some worthy, enlightened cause in the House of Lords – yet he's not demonstrative with people, only with causes. The last time he kissed me, for instance, was at my sister Sylvia's wedding – he kisses people at weddings for some reason – but that doesn't matter, does it? I don't mind him not slobbering over me. What I mind is being treated like a worthy cause which has to be hammered into shape. I don't want to be hammered into shape. I want to be me. But he doesn't see *me* at all, doesn't care, doesn't want to know, doesn't understand . . . Yet he's brilliantly clever – I don't want to give the impression he's a fool, and I don't want to give the impression he's a monster either. When he's in a good mood no one can be more charming and amusing – except his playmate Aysgarth, of course. But wait a minute – you don't know, do you? I was forgetting. Now this is *really* bizarre. Aysgarth and my father are devoted to each other, have been for years. Isn't it the most extraordinary coincidence that I should have fallen so violently in love with my father's best friend?'

'Extraordinary,' said Father Darrow without expression.

VI

At that point I noticed that my handkerchief was stained black with my ruined eye make-up and I asked his permission to retire to the bathroom for repairs. Glancing in the mirror again I had a fleeting vision of myself as a hag past fifty.

'Sorry I waffled on like that,' I said as I returned to the table and collapsed once more in my chair. 'I'm afraid I digressed from the main problem. If we can get back to Aysgarth –'

'I can well imagine him enjoying *Honest to God*.'

'Yes, he adores it, but on the other hand Bishop Ashworth thinks it's absolutely the bottom – which is so confusing, because they can't both be right, can they?'

Father Darrow merely smiled and said: 'They're creating a paradox but the real truth lies beyond.'

'And what's the real truth?'

'*Honest to God* is more than one book. It's one book for the Bishop, another for the Dean – and no doubt it's yet another for someone else. This has happened because the work is written with the most passionate emotion, and it's this emotion which is striking all the different chords in people's hearts as they watch a bishop, who is supposed to be all-knowing in spiritual matters, grappling with the faith like an ordinary pilgrim. Some people admire him for his honesty and humility but others cannot forgive him for it. Some commend his attempt to frame original opinions, but others merely despise him for his lack of scholarship. Poor Dr Robinson is a beleaguered man at present and deserves, if nothing else, our prayers.'

'But you, Father Darrow – where do *you* stand in the *Honest to God* debate?'

'Beyond it. I think that beyond all the words lies the Word which dwarfs them all. "In the beginning was the word . . ." How well do you know St John's Gospel? It's the greatest mystical tract ever written and deals, as mysticism always does, with matters which can't in truth be translated accurately into ordinary language at all. God is very much greater than a little book like *Honest to God*, Miss Flaxton, and *Honest to God* in fact reflects not God at all but twentieth-century man, bewildered and alienated, freed from witchcraft but enslaved by the dogmas of science, liberated by the Enlightenment but imprisoned by rationality, blessed with the power of improving his material world but knowing too that one push of a button could bring it all to an end. Dr Robinson is wrestling with the tragedy of modern man, and as a modern man himself he conducts his fight within the wrestling-ring of modern times, but the whole truth, of course, can never be confined to a mere wrestling-ring. Our bodies may be obliged to exist in such a confined environment, but our real selves,' said Father Darrow, regarding me with his clear grey eyes, 'are not confined by the prison of space and time.'

I suddenly realised, as I had a split-second vision of the vast mysteries which enfolded mankind, that he had folded up the Church of England into the size of a handkerchief and tucked it neatly away in his pocket. I said, groping for words: 'You're beyond all formal religious structures, aren't you, as well as being beyond all fashions in religious thought,' but he answered at once: 'Mysticism is certainly beyond fashions in religious thought, but all mystics need a formal religious framework in order to achieve a proper balance in their spiritual life.'

'And you've chosen Christianity.'

'No, Christ chose me. Are you too a Christian, Miss Flaxton, or are you merely an interested observer?'

'I'm a Christian, but no one did any choosing. It was simply dished out to me, like a British passport, because I was born in a certain time and a certain place.'

'Perhaps the choosing's now about to begin. Have you thought much about your faith?'

'Well, off and on, I suppose, the way one does occasionally . . . I mean, yes, I have, of course I have.' I hesitated but then said impulsively: 'It's all true, isn't it? It must be. St Paul talked to the eyewitnesses. You can't get around that. And then there's the transformed behaviour of the Apostles. You can't get around that either. Something happened, although we'll never know for sure what it was, and now we're sitting here talking together and the whole great circus of the Christian church is lumbering merrily on its way because two thousand years ago in an obscure Roman province a carpenter conducted an itinerant ministry, wrote nothing and was executed. That's so unlikely that one couldn't possibly believe it except that it happens to be true.'

Father Darrow smiled and commented: 'Tertullian said: "It must be believed, because it is absurd!"'

'My father says Tertullian was a fool. My father's got a psychological block about Christianity – he can't discuss it rationally at all.'

Father Darrow said: 'Go home and see your father. Talk to your mother. Perhaps she can act as a bridge between the two of you.'

'Why do you keep going on about my parents?'

'There's something there that needs healing, and once the healing's been achieved you may see your present situation in a different light.'

'But my father's not a problem at present! My real problem –'

'Tell Aysgarth,' said Father Darrow, 'that last night at the Staro Arms Jon Darrow sent his compliments to him and invited him to call any time at Starrington Manor. Now kneel down, please, and we'll pray that the power of the Holy Spirit may heal you of your sickness and grant you the strength to survive the times which lie ahead.'

I was a little startled by this suggestion and more than a little appalled by the implication that I was ill, but I told myself strength was well worth praying for and that I really did have a moral obligation to be polite to the old pet. Trying not to feel too self-conscious I knelt down, clasped my hands together and closed my eyes. He was silent for so long that I glanced up but when I saw his lips were moving I shut my eyes again and waited. Eventually he said a prayer aloud. I recognised it. It was one of the Collects which were recited at evensong.

'Lighten our darkness, we beseech thee, O Lord . . .'

I thought of the Great Pollutant, spreading through my life like a lethal poison, and I was just beginning to pray very earnestly indeed for an antidote when Father Darrow, quite without warning, laid his hands on my head and pressed down so strongly that I nearly collapsed. My mind went blank. I felt as if I had been given an electric shock, although of course that must have been an illusion created by the power of his personality. But the most shattering part of all was that I felt sexually excited. In fact I thought I was going to have an orgasm. For a moment I was transfixed, too appalled and repulsed to move, but as he himself faltered, knowing something had gone wrong, I ducked away from his hands, grabbed the rim of the table and hauled myself to my feet. I was shuddering from head to toe.

He said in great distress: 'My dear child, I –' but he was interrupted by a thunderous knocking at the door.

'It's all right, I'm okay, don't worry . . .' But I hardly knew what I was saying. The whole incident was so unspeakably sinister that I could only batten down my horror by pretending I was unscathed, but he barely heard my reassurance. He said stricken: 'Forgive me – I should have realised the state you'd be in as the result of your association with that man – I shouldn't have tried any healing which involved physical contact –' But again he was interrupted by a thunderous knocking on the door and this time Nick burst in without waiting for an invitation to enter.

His father was livid. 'Nicholas, go outside this instant!'

'But I only came back because –'

'OUT!' shouted the old man, now very distressed.

'No, wait!' I cried, seizing the chance to escape, and to Father Darrow I added at high speed: 'I've got to go now, thanks for seeing me, please don't worry, I'm all right, everything's fine, it doesn't matter.' I grabbed my bag and stumbled to the door.

'I only came back,' Nick said soothingly to his father, 'because I was sure you'd be getting tired and needing to be rescued.'

'Ah, Nicholas, Nicholas . . .' But the old man's anger was spent, and as I glanced back from the doorway I saw him sink down exhausted upon the nearest chair. 'Very well, take Miss Flaxton away.'

Nick promptly hustled me past the threshold and closed the front door. Since I was too shattered to speak and he was too furious, we walked in silence out of the dell, but when we finally emerged from the woods he said, still outraged: 'You shouldn't have seen him. His psychic judgement's not as sound as it used to be, that's the trouble. A year ago he'd never have dreamed of seeing a woman alone for a consultation which involved healing.'

'How did you know he –'

'I looked through the window. Of course I could see it had gone wrong. Imagine chucking up his golden rule like that at the age of eighty-three – what an absolutely idiotic risk for a clever old priest to take!'

'Oh, for God's sake, Nick, why shouldn't the fabulous old pet have some fun while there's still time?'

'You've simply no idea what I'm talking about.'

We stalked on without speaking across the daisy-studded lawn but when we at last reached my car he did manage to mutter apologetically: 'I'm sorry you're so upset.'

'How do you know I'm upset?'

'I can feel. If only I could help you . . . but I don't know how.'

'Some day, baby,' I said, mimicking Dinkie's New York twang. 'Some day. Now run off and play with your crystal ball.' By this time I was as exhausted as Father Darrow. Slumping into the driver's seat I drove raggedly away, but as I glanced in the mirror and saw Nick was still staring after me, I felt the nape of my neck tingle with fright again.

In horror I wondered if he had been not only spying at the window but eavesdropping at the door.

VII

I somehow succeeded in convincing myself that Nick would never have been so naughty as to eavesdrop; a quick glance through a window was pardonable, particularly since he had been worried about his father's stamina, but listening at the keyhole would have been impossible to justify under any circumstances. However, this conclusion only made his parting expression more sinister. He had looked as if he was watching me drive to my doom, but of course that statement was mere fanciful nonsense and indicated that the closing moments of the interview with Father Darrow had put me in a thoroughly neurotic frame of mind. Obviously it was now time to make a supreme effort, face the incident with all the calmness and rationality at my disposal, and defuse the horror by working out exactly what had happened.

I shuddered but pulled myself together. I had no doubt that Father Darrow had acted in good faith and had had no salacious designs on me whatsoever; the old pet wasn't an old monster. Yet sex had been present in that fiasco somehow and it hadn't been a normal kind of sex. It was as if the sex, dark and distorted, had been a mere marker, an indication that another far more dangerous force had been on the loose in that room, and suddenly I heard Father Darrow saying: 'I should have realised the state you'd be in as the result of your association with that man.' He had spoken as if my state, whatever that was, had adversely reacted with his psychic healing in the manner of two chemicals frothing and hissing when they were mixed in the same test-tube. It was as if Father Darrow had produced a clear, unpolluted essence, and I had produced —

I suddenly realised I was going to be sick. I had to stop the car so that I could vomit into the ditch which ran alongside the country lane, and afterwards I sat shivering for a long time in the driving-seat before I was able to light a cigarette.

But I could now put into words what had happened. Father Darrow had tried to cast out my polluted essence, but because his psychic judgement had been impaired (as Nick had put it) he had tackled the task in the wrong way. The exorcist had slipped up. Game, set and match to the –

But of course we didn't talk about the Devil, not now, not in 1963. And we didn't talk of polluted essences either, or psychic healing, or two chemicals snarling at each other in a test-tube as if they were people. I was going off my rocker. I had to calm down. Where was my intellect, my rationality, my comforting mid-twentieth-century scepticism? The paranormal was great fun, of course, but once one started taking it seriously one wound up in a loony-bin.

Everyone knew that.

The cigarette continued to shake in my hand.

I thought: what I need's a drink. So I stopped at the nearest pub and downed two gin-and-Frenches. That fixed me up. The world stopped looking as if it had been painted by Hieronymus Bosch and began to look like a landscape by Constable again. Very pretty country around Starbridge. Lovely part of the world.

As I drove on I thought: I just got overwrought. The old pet battered home the morality message with a hammer the size of a croquet mallet and destroyed my defences. Then I compounded my weak emotional state by drivelling on and on about my father, and finally I was so debilitated that when the old pet pressed me on the head I lit out in the craziest possible way. Not the old pet's fault, of course. It was a mere reflex action stemming from the fact that I'd recently discovered the joys of sex. Obviously any male touch at present had the power to send me bananas. All rather amusing really.

I stopped at the Staro Arms and had another couple of gin-and-Frenches, just to make sure I stayed madly amused and the world stayed like a Constable landscape. I decided I adored the Staro Arms. So picturesque. Such fun. Super.

Guiding my car with light-hearted flair through the streets to Butchers' Alley I reached my flat and after several attempts succeeded in fitting my latch-key in the lock. The front door swung open – and there on the mat lay a letter which had arrived in the second post.

At once all thought of the old pet was wiped from my mind. Riding high on my tidal wave of euphoria I ripped open the envelope and feverishly started to read.

VIII

'. . . and there was Charles,' wrote Aysgarth, 'dressed to kill in full episcopal uniform and playing the Boss with a capital B. "Sit down, please, Stephen," he says in the creamy voice prosecuting counsel use when they aim to destroy a leading witness for the defence. "Malcolm Lindsay's told me you're a trifle worried about the potential cost of your application for a faculty, and it occurred to me that both the diocese and the Cathedral could save money on legal bills if you and I got together for a little chat." Which, translated from Ashworth-speak, meant: "The Archdeacon's run screaming to me about your threat to bankrupt the diocese but I'm here to tell you that I'm not standing any nonsense over that blank-blank sculpture and you'd better pull yourself together pretty blank quick."

'Well, I sit myself down, very cool, calm and collected, and I cross one leg over the other so that I look wholly relaxed – these little gestures are very important in any power-struggle – and then Charles idly starts fingering his pectoral cross, underlining the fact that he's the Bishop – a cunning counter-play – and he even has the nerve to angle it so that it flashes in the sunlight. First round to him. Then he says: "I must be quite frank and tell you that the most extraordinary rumours have reached me about this sculpture. According to Tommy Fitzgerald it may well be a fine work of art, suitable for display in a museum, but in his opinion it's quite unsuitable for display in a churchyard. He says it'll cry out to be vandalised by the hooligan element in Starbridge's teenage population."

'This was certainly a new approach from the traitor Fitzgerald. I said, mild as milk: "Why does Tommy think it'll attract vandals?" and Charles answered: "He says part of the sculpture looks like a bunch of used condoms." To which I instantly replied: "I rather doubt if Tommy would know an unused condom if he saw one, let alone a used one." That hit the target all right. Second round to me. Charles said: "The fact that Tommy's been called to lead a celibate life doesn't automatically mean he has no knowledge of contraceptives." At once I riposted: "Well, if it doesn't mean that it certainly ought to." Third round to me. Charles said: "I can't help thinking that Tommy's sexual history is entirely irrelevant to this discussion, but while we're on the subject of sex perhaps this might be the moment to inform you of the rumour that you know Harriet March rather better than would be prudent for a man in your situation."

'That really jolted me. I managed to say: "That's a slander!" and Charles, I think, realised that I was speaking the truth. He said: "Yes, I was sure it was, but people have noted the fact that you've commissioned this work from a youthful and attractive woman, and they wonder what prompted you to select her." I answered reasonably enough: "The Cathedral can't afford Henry Moore. Mrs March was recommended to me by a friend at the Tate." Charles at once backed down on that subject (another round to me) but then plunged back into the attack. He said: "Very well, I accept that she's a reputable artist, but the fact remains that we can't have anything which can be mistaken for either condoms or male genitalia – or both – lying around in the Cathedral churchyard. Think of the inevitable blown-up photographs in the gutter press!"

'Sometimes I really do wonder about Charles. I'm very keen on sex, but it's never occurred to me to imagine blown-up photographs of those cigars – what a pornographic imagination he must have! However I refrained from any barbed remark and said politely: "I think it would set your mind at rest if you visited Mrs March's studio and saw the work as a whole instead of relying solely for information on photographs of isolated details." (I should explain that after I had the idea of commissioning Harriet, she produced some rough sketches so that the matter could be discussed by the Chapter, and everyone, even Fitzgerald, backed me in approving the commission. It was only when Harriet very kindly sent along some photos of the work in progress that Fitzgerald started getting hysterical.)

'Charles said coolly: "The photographs I was shown were very explicit," but of course he knew I was right in principle so he's agreed to visit Harriet's studio. The most ironic part about the whole brouhaha is that I honestly believe the sculpture will be a brilliant work of modern art. It's not as if I'm deliberately trying to be outrageous.

'Well, I won that particular skirmish but I can see there's an almighty battle approaching because Charles is obviously dead set against the sculpture and I don't think for one moment that this visit to the studio will change his mind. He'll try and strong-arm me into backing down – and if I were him I'd do it before my application for a faculty reaches the Consistory Court. He won't want the whole diocese twittering over the fact that the Bishop and the Dean are locked in mortal combat over a bunch of phallic cigars.

'My darling, I must just see you for a few minutes so that we can exchange views on *Present Laughter* – Lady Mary after Sunday evensong? (D's attending matins and won't turn up twice.) All my best, best love, N.'

I thought vaguely of Father Darrow talking of the Great Pollutant, but that seemed a mere fantasy from the realms of science fiction.

I began to count the hours that separated me from Lady Mary.

IX

'. . . and there, sitting beside Nick in the stalls, was this ancient sage, ghost-pale and quietly vibrating in time to the music of the spheres. I thought he was a fabulous old pet.'

'*Darrow?*' exclaimed Aysgarth, vastly amused. 'That ecclesiastical buccaneer?'

'I thought he was adorable. And afterwards at the Staro Arms –'

'– he asked to be remembered to me. Yes, Eddie told me that yesterday.'

'Oh, that was only half the message! While Eddie and Martin were haggling over the bill the old pet said to me: "Next time you're visiting your friends the Aysgarths, tell the Dean that Jon Darrow sends him an invitation to call at Starrington Manor at any time."'

Aysgarth looked startled. 'The sinister old magician! Why did he say that to you and not to Eddie?'

'It was only an afterthought –'

'The old pirate doesn't have afterthoughts. He has psychic intuitions – which of course I don't believe in.' But he looked rattled.

After a pause I said uncertainly: 'Will you go?'

'To see Darrow? Well, I suppose I might drop in around Christmas, just to be friendly.'

I suddenly started to feel confused. 'You won't go now?'

'Darling, I'm a very busy man and to tell the truth I just don't have time for him at present. Old pet indeed! However, I suppose I shouldn't be surprised you were mesmerised. The naughty old charlatan was always a dab hand at hypnosis.'

My heart began to beat rapidly. 'What do you mean?'

'Oh, those psychics are capable of hypnotising anyone – it's all part of the stock-in-trade! You remember I told you how he bounced around my archdeaconry trying to be Svengali, Rasputin and Our Lord Jesus Christ all rolled into one?'

'Yes, but –'

'He called it a ministry of healing. I called it a shameless use of hypnosis combined with an appalling psychic parlour-trick which he had the nerve to call the laying-on of hands. The whole episode ended scandalously, of course, but then that sort of sinister quackery always does.' Glancing at his watch he sprang to his feet. 'I must fly. Two o'clock on

Wednesday in the car-park of . . . shall we say the Crusader Hotel?'

'I'll be there.'

Turning his sexy mouth well down at the corners he gave me a smouldering look, told me he loved me and vanished.

After a while I realised the glass had tilted again in my hall of mirrors. Father Darrow was no longer a gifted sage whom Aysgarth in his guilt was trying to avoid. I had been deceived after succumbing to hypnosis, and the gifted sage was in reality a senile eccentric whom Aysgarth very sensibly wanted to forget.

Embracing this rational conclusion with profound relief, I was finally able to write the old pet off as a back number.

TWO

❖

'Bonhoeffer's theory, much admired by the Bishop of
Woolwich, that man has now "come of age" seems to me
a silly and unprofitable one ... Has man, having come of
age, ceased to be a sinner? Has he ceased to be limited and
mortal?'

R. P. C. HANSON
The Honest to God Debate
ed. DAVID L. EDWARDS

I

'My darling,' wrote Aysgarth later that week after another
scorching session in Chancton Wood. 'HORRORS! Jack
Ryder, who's the editor of the *Church Gazette*, rang me up
this morning and said the rumour's reached London that I'm
planning to install a machine for French-letters in the Cathedral
churchyard! I said: "I know I defended the publication of *Lady
Chatterley's Lover* but this accusation's ridiculous – and what's
more, you know it!" Jack brayed with laughter and said: "Okay,
spill the beans and I'll try to print a report which doesn't teeter
into pornography." So I explained that I was in the process of
applying for a faculty to install a work of art in the churchyard,
and then I dictated a dignified paragraph about how the Dean
and Chapter had commissioned from the celebrated sculptress
Harriet March a work entitled "Modern Man in Search of
God". Jack then demanded baffled: "But what's all that got to
do with condoms?" and I was at last able to declare roundly:
"Absolutely nothing!"

'I was just thinking that I'd successfully trounced the *Church
Gazette* when my spy there, a very nice young woman called
Flora MacBain who edits the Children's Column, rang to make
sure I'd remembered that Jack Ryder was bosom friends with

Charles Ashworth when they were up at Cambridge together in the 'twenties. "If you're not levelling with Jack he'll find out!" warned Flora, who was clearly reluctant to stop believing in the fable of the ecclesiastical condom dispenser. My first reaction was: Charles won't gossip about the cigars to any newshound, even if the hound's the distinguished editor of the *Church Gazette* and even if the hound's a Cambridge chum. Then I thought: wait a minute. Who else but Charles could have ensured that Jack Ryder was so well primed with the latest gossip from the Cathedral Close at Starbridge? And I realised that this was almost certainly the beginning of Charles' attempt to strong-arm me – he was using Jack to drive me into a corner.

'Five minutes later the phone rings. It's Charles. Could he possibly drop in at the Deanery? "Certainly – come over straight away!" I exclaim, radiating Christian hospitality. Then I mop the sweat from my brow, gird my loins for battle and somehow manage to abstain from swilling a triple whisky to calm my nerves.

'Finally in walks Charles in one of those show-off Savile Row suits that make him look like a tailor's dummy. However, I note that he's not in episcopal uniform (apart from the purple stock and pectoral cross) and I've already noted that he's calling on me instead of summoning me to the South Canonry. Deduction: he wants to soften me up before he tries to twist my arm out of its socket.

'"My dear fellow, have a sherry!" I say at once with a welcoming smile, but he declines. He's just heard, he says mildly, from Jack Ryder that the condom rumour's reached London and in his opinion it was imperative to act before the *News of the World* moved in for the kill. What did I propose to do?

'I said I couldn't see the need for immediate panic, since the *News of the World* reporters were hardly about to storm Harriet's studio, and I suggested that the best course was for Jack to run a piece to defuse Fleet Street's fire – a responsible article which stressed the symbolic meaning of every feature of the sculpture. Then Charles began to twist my arm. He said: "The gutter press aren't going to be deterred by any high-minded piece in the *Church Gazette*. As soon as this matter's aired in the Consistory Court, we're in for banner headlines."

'I took a deep breath, looked him straight in the eyes and declared: "Let me disabuse you of any notion that I'll withdraw my application for a faculty just because there's a possibility that this superb work of art might be mocked by a gang of Fleet Street philistines. It would be against my liberal principles to submit to such censorship."

'I thought I'd rocked him but he snapped back: "No one's asking you to submit to censorship. I'm merely asking you to exercise your common sense. Do you really want to make a laughing-stock of our Cathedral?"

'"It's *my* Cathedral," I said, "and in any other diocese in England it would be *my* churchyard. If you hadn't hit on the idea of raking up all that rubbish about unconsecrated curtilage, we wouldn't now be heading for the Consistory Court and banner headlines in the *News of the World*."

'"And if you hadn't commissioned a wholly unsuitable sculpture from an attractive young woman you met by chance at a party," said Charles, hitting well below the belt, "I wouldn't have been obliged to rake up the rubbish about unconsecrated curtilage in order to preserve the dignity of the Cathedral churchyard." Then before I could reply he stood up and added in his plummiest public-school voice: "I confess I find this conversation singularly unedifying so I shall now terminate it with the suggestion that we both pray for guidance." And off he stalked to the South Canonry.

'Very tricky. The awful part is that there's a lot of truth in what he says; Fleet Street could go to town over those cigars. I honestly didn't think anyone would take much notice of proceedings in a Church court, but maybe I wasn't thinking too clearly. It only needs some bright spark on the *Starbridge Weekly News* to flash the news to a London hack and then the whole tinder-box of Fleet Street will be ablaze – with the result that the Consistory Court will be turned into a circus and the sculpture will become as much a *cause célèbre* as *Lady Chatterley's Lover*. But what am I to do? As

I see it, I've no choice; I've got to defend good art from the onslaught of the philistines and I've got to oppose any attempt at censorship by arm-twisting. To back down at this point would be a craven act of cowardice and I refuse even to consider that such an option could be open to me.

'What maddens me most of all is to reflect that if that fatuous ass Fitzgerald hadn't gone around Starbridge bleating about used contraceptives, this whole disaster would never have happened! Sometimes I think that widowed mother of his really does have a lot to answer for . . .'

II

'My darling, I absolutely mustn't go any further –'

'Are you worried in case I get pregnant?'

'There's no question of me ever putting you in a position where you might get pregnant.'

'How can you say that when we're so obviously on the brink of –'

'But we're not. I'm reining myself in.' Drawing back from me he began to rearrange his clothes.

'Who's reining himself in?' I burst out, overpowered by my frustration. 'Neville One who was brought up by puritan Nonconformists? Nevilles Two and Three who are supposed to be dead? Stephen, who's supposed to be left at home with Dido? I know it can't be Neville Four – he loves me and wants to go on!'

'For heaven's sake!' he said irritably. 'Stop treating a mere metaphor as a concrete fact!'

'Your behaviour *is* a concrete fact, and I've come to suspect this whole mystery's somehow bound up with your multiple personality –'

'I have no multiple personality. What mystery?'

I ignored him. 'If Neville One can be subjugated,' I persisted recklessly, 'and Nevilles Two and Three are dead, then it must be Stephen who's holding you back – which in turn must mean that your behaviour's all connected with Dido. Look, Neville, just what the hell is your relationship with that woman?'

He got out, slammed the door so violently that the whole car shuddered, and strode off into the woods.

I stifled a sob. Then I hared after him.

III

'How dare you talk to me like that!' he shouted. 'How *dare* you!' His short, powerfully-built figure was now exuding an anger so violent that I recoiled from him in terror. Nothing had prepared me for such rage because never had I seen him so transformed. My Mr Dean had vanished and in his place stood a monster who looked murderous. I nearly fainted with fear.

Then the horror ended. The stranger vanished. My Mr Dean, white with fright, stammered: 'Forgive me, forgive me, forgive me –' and hugged me so tightly that I could hardly breathe. 'How could I have lost my temper like that?' he said appalled. 'And with you – the most precious thing in my whole life! How vile, how wicked, how –'

I sobbed no, no, no, it was all my fault and I'd never mention Dido again as long as I lived and please, *please* could he say he forgave me for making him so angry.

The dialogue eventually reached its foregone conclusion when we embraced, but afterwards he was unable to let the matter rest. He said urgently: 'That wasn't Neville Four. I promise you that wasn't Neville Four.'

'No, of course not.' I dried my eyes.

'That was Neville Two,' he said, fathoms deep in mystified anxiety, 'Neville Two when Neville Three was too weak to contain him. But how could he possibly have staged a resurrection?' Catching sight of my expression he added hastily: 'It's all right, you'll never see him again, I promise. Neville Four's reburied him and covered the grave with cement.'

Unable to frame anything which could resemble a reply, I clasped his hand and we walked slowly back to the car. Above us in the trees of Chancton Wood the beech leaves were a vivid, sunlit green.

When we were sitting in the car again he said rapidly: 'I'm under such stress at the moment. That's no excuse for what happened, of course, but at least it's an explanation for such a horrific failure of self-control.'

'Honestly, Neville, let's just forget it.'

'I can't. Supposing I'd hit you?'

'But you didn't.'

He seemed not to hear me. It was as if he were immersed in some private nightmare and was flailing around trying to wake up. 'I have this horror,' he said, gripping the steering-wheel, 'this absolute horror of hurting women. They have to be kept safe, cherished, put on pedestals, worshipped, preserved from destruction.' He was now gripping the wheel so hard his entire hands shone white. 'If I ever wound up destroying a woman I couldn't live with myself – I've told you that before, I've told you that I'm afraid of destroying you. And now I'll tell you that I'm afraid of destroying *her*. A wife must always be able to believe with confidence that there's one act her husband would never do with another woman. Then she won't be destroyed.'

After a while I managed to say: 'Darling, I do understand.'

But of course I didn't. I could now see the 'ropes of steel' that bound him to Dido and prevented him from consummating our affair, but where those ropes had been forged and how they had come to bind him I had no idea.

He remained, as before, a mystery.

IV

The phone rang as I was drinking a de luxe dry martini, smoking my umpteenth cigarette of the day and feeling light-headed with relief. I had just worked out that Aysgarth, terrified of destroying Dido with another pregnancy, could not possibly be having sex with her; the very thought of such destruction would be sufficient to render him instantly impotent.

'Hullo, darling,' said my mother as I answered the phone. 'It's me. How's the plant?'

'Oh, doing wonderfully well!' I had thrown out the corpse that morning.

'Do remember what I said about not watering it too much —'

'Yes, Mama. Any news?'

'Well, we're coming down to Pauncefoot the weekend after next — I have to judge the flowers at the village fête and your father's decided to come too, which is a good thing as he's been working so hard in London (*endless* committees) that I really feel it's time he had a rest. Anyway, darling, we'd love to see you — why don't you come for the weekend and bring some young people?'

'Will anyone else be there?'

'Only the Dean,' said my mother satisfied, and added as I nearly knocked over my martini: 'By a tremendous stroke of luck we discovered Dido was going to be away that weekend — she's taking the children to visit her sister in Leicestershire — so as soon as he heard the good news your father rang the Dean to issue the invitation.'

'Splendid — I'll cadge a lift. Is he arriving on Saturday morning?'

'No, Friday night. That'll give him a little extra time because he has to leave early on Sunday morning in order to get back for matins. We were hoping he could give the Cathedral a miss that weekend, but apparently that's not possible.'

'What a bore. Okay, Mama, expect me to turn up with him on Friday week.'

'You wouldn't like to bring a friend? Perhaps Primrose —'

'No, Primrose is fearfully busy at the moment,' I said, 'and as I've seen so little of you recently I'd rather come on my own.'

That pleased her. She asked after the Bishop, my work, the Lindsay family and my flat. Then she maundered on about Arabella's marital problems, but when I at last succeeded in terminating the call I yodelled: 'Yippee!' at the top of my voice and mixed myself another jumbo martini.

'. . . and it's certainly very exciting that we can be together for a weekend,' Aysgarth wrote, 'although I daresay your father will stick to me like glue. However, no doubt we can wangle some time together in your little sitting-room! Do you remember how we read Browning together there once when you were seventeen? You said (knowing everything, of course, just as one always does at that age) that Browning was hopelessly passé, but I persuaded you to change your mind! How my mother loved Browning's poetry. In some ways you remind me of her. She was an exceptionally clever, charming woman who – wait for it! – wrote the most delightful letters! I was her favourite. We always got on famously.

'But I shall hastily terminate that Freudian digression – how tiresome it is that nowadays a man can't even make an innocent remark about his mother without being suspected of all manner of complexes! – and pass on to my current ecclesiastical nightmare. A diocesan committee which will advise the Chancellor on the artistic merit and general suitability of the sculpture is now being assembled, but I've no faith that the members will do anything except fling up their hands in horror. Meanwhile I'm still recovering from the spectacle of my bishop throwing his weight around like a *mafioso*. But why should I be so shocked? Power-mania is an occupational hazard for big-time executives in large corporations, and no doubt I was being naive in supposing that a man who wears a flashy gold cross is somehow miraculously uncontaminated from all the seamier aspects of corporate life at the top. Fancy Charles trying to strong-arm me out of a hearing in the Consistory Court like that! Disgraceful.

'To further complicate my life – as if it needed further complications – a thoroughly ridiculous storm in a teacup has erupted and threatens to turn into a hurricane-force gale. Lady Bone-Pelham, widow of the very recently deceased Sir George Bone-Pelham who did something so secret in the war that nobody ever discovered what it was, telephoned me this morning to say that Sir George made a deal with my predecessor to ensure he'd be buried in the cloisters. The preposterous sum of £3,000 is reported to have changed hands. My predecessor Dean Carter, who is even now, no doubt, shaking hands with Sir George in some unimaginable realm of the hereafter, is not available for questioning but I'm prepared to bet heavy money that he'd never have taken a bribe. I explained to Lady Bone-Pelham that for hygienic reasons we no longer buried people within the Cathedral but I offered her space on the cloisters' wall for a memorial tablet and earnestly assured her that Sir George could be laid to rest in the very best part of the cemetery. "Over my dead body!" was Lady B-P's retort. Unable to cope with the thought of two Bone-Pelham corpses on my hands, I then told her I'd have to consult the Chapter. Eddie thinks she's almost certainly certifiable. Fitzgerald and Dalton, loyal to their former boss Dean Carter, are outraged by the bribery slur and say they don't even want to sanction a memorial tablet. But meanwhile how on earth do I convince a senile old lady that I can't dig up the cloisters' lawn to receive her distinguished husband? All my love, darling, from your demented but devoted N.'

VI

'Well, Venetia,' said my father a week later at Flaxton Hall, 'so you've finally deigned to visit us! You look, I may say, quite remarkably well, which is very perverse of you since young girls who storm off to lead independent lives are supposed to be rapidly wrecked by numerous unspeakable adventures . . . My dear Aysgarth, how delightful to see you again! What did you think of that article I sent you on Mithraism?'

Aysgarth and I had been unable to enjoy ourselves in Chancton Wood that week because he had been obliged to attend an important meeting, but fortified by the knowledge that we would be spending the weekend under the same roof we had faced the loss of our Wednesday outing with equanimity.

Leaving Starbridge on Friday afternoon in his car we had paused among the ruins of Flaxmundham Priory, but our hope of a romantic interlude had been terminated by a coachload of trippers. Undaunted, confident that there would be better opportunities later, we had pressed on to Flaxton Pauncefoot and had arrived at the Hall in time for tea.

'What a lot of weight you've lost, Mr Dean!' said my mother admiringly as soon as she saw him. This observation was true but although Aysgarth should now have appeared smart and streamlined he still contrived to look scruffy. On that day he wore his best suit and a new white shirt, but both were the wrong size for his new figure; moreover his tie was carelessly knotted and he had forgotten to have his shoes cleaned. In contrast my father, lounging around in his shabbiest country clothes, contrived to look not only distinguished but elegant. It was a great sartorial mystery.

Dinner was a success. Aysgarth's dinner-jacket was well worn and his trousers were a fraction too long, but he was in such sparkling form that I was sure no one cared that he looked as if he was wearing hired clothes. He and my father spent some time discussing the resemblance between the Kennedy brothers of America and the Gracchi brothers of Ancient Rome. (This conversation took place before either of the Kennedy assassinations, a fact which no doubt explains why I remember it as a prophetic debate.) I slung in a controversial comment now and then and enjoyed the conversation immensely. My mother made a valiant effort to conceal her boredom and was once allowed to murmur what fun it must be for the Americans to have a young couple in the White House, but everyone was much too busy arguing about the Gracchi to reply.

Eventually I was obliged to leave the men to their port and retire to the drawing-room where my mother droned on and on about Absolutely-the-Bottom Arabella and whether or not Sylvia was pregnant again. I yawned and flicked through *Country Life* and wished I could be swilling port with the men.

They joined us for coffee but afterwards my father was unable to resist the temptation to monopolise his favourite playmate and Aysgarth was borne away to the library for further delicious intellectual debate. I was so livid that I had to have a bath to calm myself down. Then I hung around my little sitting-room upstairs for hours but no one came. Finally I was once more in such a state of frustrated rage that I sneaked down to the dining-room to filch some brandy from the sideboard, but as I passed the library door and heard my father's animated voice I knew I could give up all hope of seeing Aysgarth that night. I fell asleep on my sitting-room sofa at one o'clock in the morning and woke in a filthy mood with a crick in my neck some time after four.

However my spirits revived at breakfast when my father said: 'It's a damn nuisance, Aysgarth, but I'll have to put in an appearance at the village fête this afternoon. Would you mind pottering around here on your own for a couple of hours?' and Aysgarth answered that he wouldn't mind in the least and perhaps Venetia could take him for a little stroll in the grounds.

I gave him a chaste smile and instantly began to wonder if against all the odds and despite all the hang-ups I could lure him from my sitting-room sofa to my bed in the room next door.

VII

It began to rain but I never noticed. It was Aysgarth who remarked: 'Why are village fêtes always so unlucky with the weather?' but I barely heard him because I was gripped with the hope that I might finally lose my virginity. We had started off sitting on my sofa with a battered volume of Browning but the book had soon fallen to the floor. So much for Browning. No buttons had been undone but I had slipped out of my shoes and we were just pausing while I began to undo his tie. He had one hand on my thigh, I remember – under my skirt, of course – and the other hand was playing sensuously with my hair.

Then the catastrophe happened.

Without warning the door swung open and my father walked into the room.

VIII

He stopped dead.

Fortunately the sofa faced the fireplace, not the door, so it was impossible for him to know that Aysgarth's hand was beneath my skirt. All he could see was Aysgarth stroking my hair – a gesture which could have been dismissed as a casual manifestation of affection – and I apparently fidgeting with Aysgarth's tie. This was certainly curious behaviour but not necessarily either suggestive or compromising. In fact in that appalling moment after my father's entrance I saw that the scene was not beyond redemption. All we had to do to survive the disaster was remain cool, behave casually and laugh off the apparent intimacy as mere asexual playfulness between old friends.

But Aysgarth leapt to his feet as if he had been caught *in flagrante*, and to my horror I saw him begin to blush.

My father quietly closed the door.

Still no one spoke. I was now so shattered that I could only act instinctively and my instinct was to protect Aysgarth by calling attention to myself. Slipping back into my shoes I wandered to the window, peered vaguely out at the rain and enquired: 'Was the fête washed out?'

'The diehards adjourned to the marquee but I thought I'd come home.' My father's voice was as idle and untroubled as my own. Pleasantly he added: 'You'll excuse us, Aysgarth, but I'd like a word with Venetia in private.'

'Yes, of course, my Lord,' said Aysgarth fatally, and walked out. He had not called my father 'my Lord' since the accession to the Deanery six years before.

The door closed again. I went on watching the teeming rain and at last I became aware that my father was watching it too. He was standing beside me with his hands in his pockets. We were about four feet apart.

'I wanted to have a word with you,' he said, 'about your mother's seventieth birthday next month. I've decided to give a little family dinner-party for her at Lord North Street. I did think of having it down here – much nicer to be in the country in August – but Harold and Amanda can only stop in London for twenty-four hours en route from Turkey to America. Apparently Harold has to go to Washington that weekend. I can't imagine why.'

'Curious.'

'Very. Anyway, the big question is: what will you children give her as a present? Oliver's organising the matter – you'd better have a word with him. There's been talk of a silver rose-bowl.'

'Super! Asprey's or Garrard's?'

'I doubt if Oliver's got that far yet. But the point's this, Venetia: make sure you're up in town on Saturday the twenty-fourth of August or I'll be very cross.'

'Wild horses wouldn't keep me away.'

'Good. By that time, of course,' said my father as we continued to gaze at the rain, 'you may well have become a little tired of Starbridge. The city has its charms, I quite see that, but when all's said and done . . . well, it really is a trifle provincial.'

I said nothing.

The rain drummed on and on against the long slim Georgian window.

'Nevertheless,' said my father mildly, 'I'm sure it's been an interesting interlude for you. I admit I was cross when you left home, but now I see it's been all for the best.'

After a moment I said cautiously: 'Oh?'

'Yes, I was stupid not to see that straight away. In fact I can see now I behaved very stupidly, throwing scenes and taking umbrage. Only the other day your mother called me a very stupid man and said I had only myself to blame if you didn't write to me.'

'Mama said that?'

'I can understand your surprise. That was, of course, most uncharacteristic behaviour on your mother's part as she's renowned for her placid nature and affectionate disposition. But the other day she spoke her mind. About you. Most interesting. Made me think a bit, I can tell you. Felt quite chastened afterwards.'

'Good heavens. How very remarkable.'

'Yes, wasn't it? "You stupid man!" she stormed at me. Me! *Stupid!* I nearly had apoplexy. Then I had to face the ghastly truth: she was right. I've been very, very stupid all my life about women. Never understood them. Closed book. My mother died young and I had no sisters. Eton – Oxford – all-male establishments . . . Emerged brilliantly accomplished and a complete fool. Most extraordinary paradox. Suppose it must happen quite often. Very hard for the wives, though. And the daughters.'

He began to roam around the room and after a moment he exclaimed: 'What a wonderful stroke of luck it was that your mother agreed to marry me! I wasn't even heir to the title then, just a younger son and so very stupid – how brave it was of her to take me on! I knew nothing about women, nothing at all. My father – all that drink – all those mistresses – disgusting! I was so ashamed . . . And then my brother dying of – well, I can't tell you what that was like, no words could describe the horror, particularly at the end when his brain rotted. So I always said to myself: bloody women, do without them, live like a monk. But then I met your mother, so comfortable, so ordinary, so nice-natured, so SAFE, and it occurred to me I was really very miserable living like a monk, so . . .

'How your mother put up with me I don't know. Miracle. Anyway, we wound up very happy and the boys came and then the girls and our family was complete. It was complete after Arabella, as a matter of fact – two boys and two girls, that was exactly what we wanted – but then Sylvia turned up unexpectedly. Not that I minded. I liked my girls, nice little bits of fluff, pat them on the head regularly, tell them how pretty they were – easy. But your mother was much put out by a fifth pregnancy and said afterwards: "*No more.*" Well, I quite understood. "Don't want any more," I said. "I'm quite happy.

Two sons and three little bits of fluff. Marvellous." But you know, Venetia, it wasn't so marvellous. In fact as time passed it really wasn't so marvellous at all.'

My father had paused by my writing-table and as I slowly turned to look at him I saw him start to fidget with the edge of the blotter. 'Of course,' he said, not looking at me, 'I was proud of my boys, fine little fellows, and I was devoted to my three bits of fluff, pretty little things, but as they all grew older none of them shared my interests and I still had no one to talk to. I didn't admit to myself that I was disappointed, but your mother knew, and when I finally went through an exceptionally glum patch – the forties can be a very depressing time – she said to me: "I can't stand you mooching around like this – take me somewhere beautiful like Venice for a holiday!" I said: "I don't like Abroad." That maddened her. "You beastly, selfish man, thinking of no one but yourself!" she cried. "What about me? I'd love to see Venice!" So off we went and at first I sulked but soon I found it all most interesting and in the end we had a whale of a time, the best time we'd had since our honeymoon, and when I returned to London I felt fit to burst with high spirits. And then . . .

'Well, you know what happened. I said aghast to your mother when she told me: "I'm dreadfully sorry – I know you didn't want any more," and she laughed and laughed – oh, how she laughed! Then she said: "You silly man, do you think I didn't plan it all right down to the special four-poster bed?"

'What a woman! I was so grateful to her and so excited and I kept thinking: this'll be the one, this'll be it, Latin and Greek prizes galore, intelligent conversation, the comfort of my old age. Then you came.

'Well, I was disappointed, wasn't I? I was such a very stupid man, and the stupidest part of all was that I didn't realise how stupid I was being. All I could see was that there you were, just like me, but the wrong sex. No good. First of all I wanted to write you off. Then I found I couldn't write you off, I couldn't bear it, it seemed such a waste, so I decided to overlook the fact that you were a girl, pretend you weren't, and push you towards the best possible education – you couldn't go to Eton but at least you could go up to Oxford and be a pseudo-boy following in my footsteps. And that, incidentally, was when I got interested in promoting the cause of higher education for women; what I was actually interested in was converting women into pseudo-boys.

'I never stopped to think, did I? I never stopped to say to myself: Venetia's not a pseudo-boy, she's a girl. Such a mistake, because as your mother pointed out to me the other day, you've always resented me for not accepting you as you are. Very wrong of me, not fair to you, but now, thanks to your mother screaming out all those home truths when I moaned about you not writing to me, I finally understand what's going on. You're a girl and you want to get married; you want to have a husband, children, a nice home, all that sort of thing. Not much good having brains if you wind up an old maid. The way of the world. Not the way things ought to be, perhaps, but when one gets down to the hard facts of life, that's the way things really are.

'So,' said my father, having mangled the top sheet of the blotter into a crumpled heap, 'I now hear from various reliable sources – your mother and her Starbridge grapevine – that Canon Hoffenberg has been paying his respects, and perhaps this is the moment when I should state unequivocally that I've recovered from the First and Second World Wars. Can't keep hating Germans for ever. The Christians always behave as if they have a monopoly on forgiveness, but they haven't – there are times when forgiveness is a moral duty for everyone, and although I'm not religious,' said my father, finally abandoning the writing-desk and wandering back to the window to inspect the rain, 'let no one say that I'm not a deeply moral man.'

He paused to gaze at the sodden garden before adding: 'I like Hoffenberg. Good brain. Pleasant fellow. Successful in his field. Nothing much to look at, of course, but then neither was your mother – by which I mean that if you're like me (and you are) you'll want to feel SAFE with a good companion, not tormented by a thorough bad lot. So what I'm saying is, Venetia, to put the matter in a nutshell, if you wanted to go ahead with Hoffenberg,

I wouldn't stand in your way, quite the reverse, I'd be very pleased. I shouldn't have been so prejudiced against him earlier, I can see that now. I should have said to myself: if Aysgarth rates him a capital fellow, he's got to be all right.'

There was a pause while he fingered the hem of the faded velvet curtain. Then he said vaguely: 'I worry about Aysgarth sometimes, stuck with that bloody awful wife. If he were a layman there'd be no difficulty; he'd keep a nice little bit of fluff somewhere and everyone would live happily ever after, but clergymen can't afford to keep little bits of fluff. Clergymen can't afford to keep anything except their heads. Very dangerous, losing your head if you're a clergyman. Aysgarth's a clever man, one of the cleverest men I've ever met, but unfortunately even clever men have their blind spots, as your mother knows all too well.' He hesitated. The rain continued to drum against the pane. Then as he peered down at the velvet hem in his hand I heard him say indistinctly: 'Sorry I've always been such a bloody fool, Venetia. Damn stupid. But I swear all I want now is your happiness. Remember that.'

In the long silence that followed he stopped inspecting the curtain and very slowly turned to face me, but when he saw the tears streaming down my face he was quick to act. He exclaimed surprised: 'Silly little thing! What's all that for?' and gathered me clumsily in his arms.

IX

Making an enormous effort I pulled myself together. There are some things which one just should not do in the presence of an elderly parent devoted to the art of maintaining a stiff upper lip, and my father was already intensely flustered. He was muttering: 'There, there!' and patting me gingerly on the back as if I were a baby suffering from a troublesome case of indigestion. His tweed jacket smelled of tobacco and mothballs and that vague aroma of sketchily-washed male which is so pervasive among Englishmen brought up in the days when bathrooms were uncomfortable ice-boxes. His body, ramrod stiff, exuded an agonised fright. He really was, as he had so bravely confessed, quite hopeless with women.

'So sorry,' I said at last, using the cuff of my cardigan to wipe my eyes. 'Slightly overcome. Temporary aberration. Nothing to worry about.'

We parted.

'You'd better go and wash your face,' said my father. 'It looks an awful mess and I don't like that black stuff around your eyes at all. Oh, and deal with Aysgarth, would you? I know the poor fellow can't help being a draper's son, but sometimes these self-made men really have no idea how to behave.'

'Leave him to me.'

The conversation closed. My father collapsed on the sofa to recover while I staggered away to the bathroom to wash my face. I spent some time re-applying my make-up. Then I went to Aysgarth's room and knocked on the door.

It flew open. 'Venetia –' He was distraught. His hair swooped wildly over his ears as if he had raked it over and over again with his fingers. His bright eyes were clouded with anxiety, anguish, even terror. He could barely speak.

'Yes, yes, yes,' I said soothingly, setting him aside so that I could slip into the room and close the door. 'It's all right. It never happened.'

He stared at me without comprehension.

'Just act as if it never happened,' I said patiently as if I were instructing a small child, 'and everything will be fine.'

'But I don't understand – what on earth did he say?'

'He rambled on about Mama's coming birthday and indulged in a long sentimental reminiscence about how wonderful she was.'

'But what did he say about me?'

'Oh, he implied you were wonderful too. He said you were one of the cleverest men he'd ever met.'

'But my dear Venetia –'

'Oh, can't you see it doesn't matter? You're his friend and

352

he'll stand by you! All you have to do now is chat about the classics to him as usual – and for God's sake stop calling him "my Lord".'

He stood there, as baffled as if I had spoken in a foreign language, and groped for the words to express his feelings. 'But if I'd been him – and if you'd been Primrose –'

'But that's the whole point,' I said exasperated. 'He's Ranulph Flaxton and I'm Venetia. We're different.'

Light finally dawned. 'Ah yes,' he said. 'Yes, I see.' And he looked around the room as if he were trying to work out how he had arrived there after his long, long journey from the small town in Yorkshire where his father had kept a shop.

'Here,' I said, trying to help him along. I picked up his hairbrush from the dresser. 'Tidy yourself up a bit. You look like an eccentric scientist.'

He accepted the brush without a word, smoothed his hair and straightened his tie.

'Fabulous!' I said encouragingly. 'Now off you go. We can't talk in private again this weekend, of course. Everything will have to wait.'

'But when I drive you back to Starbridge –'

'Oh, that's impossible now. I'll have to stay on and get the train back on Monday.'

Again he seemed nonplussed. 'But you'll still meet me,' he said painfully, 'on Wednesday?'

'Of course!'

'And you'll keep writing?'

'Reams. Oh Neville, do stop asking these idiotic questions! Just go and have a nice bright chat with my father about Livy or Plutarch or Xenophon or Tacitus or –'

He nodded and stumbled away.

X

I sat for a long time on the sofa in my sitting-room and stared at the unlit fireplace. Outside the rain eventually stopped. The room was very quiet. The serenity of Flaxton Hall enfolded me like a womb.

Having made the decision to skip tea I went out, wandering through the dank Italian garden and ploughing in my welling-ton boots along the muddy path which encircled the lake. From the far side I looked back at the Hall. Its ruthless Georgian symmetry seemed peculiarly satisfying, a dream from the brain of a classicist devoted to geometry, a vision from which all the mess and muddle of the world, all the anomalies and contradictions, had been magically eliminated. I suddenly realised how devoted I was to Georgian architecture and how partial I was to the classics. I began to wish I had gone up to Oxford after all.

Squelching back around the lake I reached the floral garden designed by my mother where huge blooms reeked and flashed in artificial chaos among vast curving borders. I was still faintly revolted by such horticultural excess, but now I could see how well that riotous extravaganza of colour complemented the austere lines of the house. I paused to stare at the Hall again. Some people would have said it was as repellant as the garden, as lifeless in its perfection as the over-manicured mausoleums which the National Trust propped up for tourists, but I knew it could never be lifeless for me. It was home. It was where I belonged, and when I thought of my little nest in Starbridge I could see that although it was wonderfully original the orig-inality would one day wear thin. Starbridge, as my father had said, was really just an interlude for me, and later when I was married I would have a large house of my own, another geometrical dream, with a huge garden, all lawns and trees, no flowers in sight, and there would be a lake, not necessarily an artificial lake designed by Capability Brown, but nevertheless a serene stretch of water where I could lie in a boat and gaze at the sky and think beautiful thoughts.

The best part about being married would be that I'd have the chance to achieve an idyllic life as a châtelaine. All the Coterie would roar down for weekends, and what fun we'd have, celebrating life with lashings of champagne! In fact I now realised I could hardly wait to acquire my own little corner of England because once I was a châtelaine with a husband to prove I was no pitiable freak I could become *me* at last, lying on a couch like Madame Récamier, smoking a cigar like George Sand, talking philosophy like George Eliot, tossing off witticisms like Dorothy Parker and hipping and thighing around like Mae West. I would be faithful to my husband, of course; it would be my moral duty to reward him as lavishly as possible for transforming me from a pathetic spinster into a married sizzler, but nevertheless I thought I might amuse myself – just occasionally – by dallying with a little bit of masculine fluff during my leisure hours . . .

Returning to the house as well as to earth after this mesmerising fantasy, I left my wellingtons in the flower-room, slipped back into my shoes and padded upstairs. On reaching my bedroom I found that a letter had been pushed under the door. It read:

'Darling, I'm so sorry about the mess. Your father's been wonderful, and we've just finished mulling over his new monograph on the Battle of Actium. He thinks it was entirely Cleopatra's fault that she and Antony were defeated but I think this view hardly does justice to Cleopatra – or indeed to young Octavian who, as history subsequently showed, was a far more formidable man than either of his rivals in the Triumvirate. I must say, it was pleasant to forget all about Harriet's sculpture – and Sir George Bone-Pelham's corpse! But I confess I remain rather bothered by the scene between you and your father. I can't visualise it at all. Surely *something* must have been said? I can't believe he would have condoned our new intimate friendship. I daresay I'm being very lower middle-class, but I just don't "get it", as the younger generation say. Do please explain! All my love, N.'

I wrote back: 'Darling Neville, You can't talk about your wife. And I can't talk about my father. Let's leave it like that, shall we? Masses of love, V. PS. Glad you survived the monograph on the Battle of Actium. Papa's such a bore about Cleopatra – I think he honestly believes all her troubles stemmed from the fact that she wasn't educated at Cheltenham Ladies' College.'

I shoved this note under his door and slipped away without attempting to talk to him.

Some people from Flaxfield joined us for dinner. Mr Wharton, an old friend of my father's, talked incessantly of politics, Mrs Wharton discussed gardening with my mother, and Margaret Wharton and I reminisced fitfully about the schooldays we had shared at Cheltenham. Halfway through the meal old Wharton remarked brightly that he had seen a book on sale at W. H. Smith's and it appeared to be about theology even though it had been placed among the best sellers; there was a naked man on the cover and the book had some sort of catchy title – had the Dean ever come across it?

I had a sudden glimpse of a vast, indifferent world which Dr Robinson's theological H-bomb had never reached, and it was then, as my imaginary mirrors tilted to reflect yet another reality, that I began to be fatally disorientated.

XI

In bed that night I asked myself which scenes represented reality and which scenes represented a dream. Then it occurred to me that all the scenes were real but that they took place in different worlds which existed alongside one another in parallel strips of time. All I had to do in order to sort myself out was to perceive which world I belonged in, but perception was no longer easy; I seemed to be living in more than one strip. I still thought that Starbridge was intensely real and that the interpretation of *Honest to God* was the most crucially important intellectual question of my life at that moment, but the other world was now equally real, the world of geometric houses and sensible marriages and agnostic indifference to theology, the world where my father, stupid man, had had the brains and the cunning and the sheer bloody guts to bare his soul and thus prove, without ever mentioning the word love, exactly how much I meant to him.

I thought: *that* was real.

But Aysgarth was real too, my darling Mr Dean, so vital, so amusing, so clever, so passionate, so adoring . . . and such a mystery. *He* refused to bare his soul, but what did his silence actually mean? Did it mean he didn't care for me sufficiently to be honest? Or did it mean he was so mixed up that he could find no words to express his secrets? How could I know? How could I ever know? All I knew was that I didn't want to give him up . . .

And that, I had no doubt, was the greatest reality of all.

XII

'My darling,' wrote Aysgarth early the next morning, 'you looked quite lovely at dinner last night, much the most attractive woman in the room. How amusing that Wharton had barely heard of *Honest to God*! But if he was abroad when it was published and reads only the secular press, all is at once explained. I was impressed by your father's summary of the book! I always feel he would have made a good theologian if only the tragedies which overtook his father and brother had not resulted in him rejecting God in order to come to terms with his pain.

'While on the subject of your father I must tell you that I shall not, of course, press you further about your interview with him; I can quite see this may well have been upsetting and best forgotten. But darling, when I refused to talk about Dido, it wasn't because I didn't want to share everything with you. I did. And I do. It's just that the subject is so awkward that words are hard to find.

'However, let me now make a big effort to "deliver my soul", as the Victorian preachers used to say. Actually I think it'll be easier in a letter because I can always tear it up and start again if I get in a muddle. Or if I can't immediately think of the right word I can sit and wait for it to come. So here goes – I shall tell you the whole truth about all the aspects of my past which you've found so baffling. Darling, believe me, I long to be completely honest with you.

'Let me start with the phenomenon which you call my "multiple personality". There is in fact only one personality, me, but I've gone through different phases. As you know, I've travelled a very long way in my life on an upward social curve, and like a motor car ascending a steep gradient I've periodically had to change gears. In other words, I've had to adjust my personality in order to keep pace with my changing circumstances, and I've mentally labelled each readjustment with a new name (Nevilles One, Two, Three, Four and Stephen). Some of these "personae" have been better integrated, as the psychologists say, than others, but rest assured that Neville Four is perfectly integrated and "the real me"! Neville One was an innocent – naive and shy. In contrast, Neville Two was a pushy, ambitious creation of whom I came to disapprove profoundly. Neville Three was my attempt to contain him, but the attempt was not altogether successful. Stephen, on the other hand, has been a good creation; he's without doubt my mature self, but he's always cost me a lot of effort to maintain. What's so wonderful about the emergence of Neville Four is that he's just as good as Stephen but he costs me no effort. That's why I feel I've uncovered my real self at last. I feel I've achieved a perfect inner harmony.

'Whenever I "change gears" – that is, move into a new "persona" – I like to forget all that's gone before. This is because adjustment to a new life is easier once one's wiped the slate clean. Also, to forget is a form of psychological survival. I had hard times in my youth after my father died bankrupt. My first marriage ended in the tragedy of Grace's death. My marriage with Dido began awkwardly and was only set right when I was reborn as Stephen. My life has in many ways been very difficult – although I don't want to turn this letter into a prolonged moan! Charles Raven, the hero of my younger days in the Church, used to say that until a man has been down into hell he's not fully mature, and I believe that to be true. It's part of the mystery of suffering. I know I'm fully mature, but sometime

I can't help reflecting what a price I've had to pay for that maturity.

'This must be where I talk about Dido.

'(LATER) I've just spent ten minutes writing nothing and now feel I must put down at least something, no matter how inadequate, in order to overcome my writer's block! Let me start by saying this: my first wife was so wonderful and so perfect that after she died I knew I had to marry her exact opposite. I couldn't have stood some lesser version of Grace, perpetually reminding me of what I'd lost. And I knew I had to remarry. I was well aware that I wasn't designed by God to be a Victorian hero chastely mourning his lost love for the rest of his life.

'I must also state that I felt very guilty about Grace's death. As you know, she died of pneumonia during a family holiday. We always took our family holiday in Devon, but that year I insisted on a change of plan and we went to the Lake District. It was a long way from our rented cottage to the shops and one morning Grace got soaked to the skin and a chill set in. It could never have happened in Devon where our cottage stood next to the village shop. So after she died, I felt responsible. It even seemed I'd destroyed her, although I concede this was taking an extreme view of what happened. However, gradually I conceived the idea not only of marrying her exact opposite but of marrying someone whom I could rescue, look after and keep safe – I saw it as a way of atoning for what I'd done.

'I thought of Dido straight away. I'd actually met her before Grace died, although of course we were mere social acquaintances then; there was no romance of any kind between us while Grace was still alive. When I eventually approached Dido she didn't want to marry me, but that only made me keener – I've always liked a challenge! I realised she had a lot of problems but that merely reinforced my conviction that I was being called to look after her, and later, when she did come to love me, my call seemed even clearer. Love is one of the ultimate prizes of life. One can't just tear it up and chuck it in the wastepaper basket. Once Dido had come to love me I knew I had to cherish her and preserve her from destruction. There was no choice. You don't argue with a call from God. You simply roll up your sleeves, get down to work and do the best you can.

'And I did. My reward has been not only Elizabeth and Pip, to whom I'm devoted, but the three children who died either shortly before or shortly after birth. These lost sons of mine I named Arthur (after my father), George (after Bishop Bell) and Aidan (after an elderly clergyman I deeply respected). Dido was never interested in choosing names for them and couldn't understand why I bothered, but to me the naming was important; it was an acknowledgement of their reality, perhaps even a symbol of thanksgiving for their very short existences, certainly a statement that they had been welcomed, not rejected, by their parents.

'At first Dido did accompany me to the cemetery to visit their grave, but once she had her living boy and girl she lost interest in the dead – whom she always saw, I'm afraid, as representing her failure to reproduce successfully – and now I go to the cemetery on my own. I've never lost interest in those children. They're very real to me, even though I may never speak of them. I see them all quite clearly. They're never tiresome or difficult as living children inevitably are sometimes; they're always happy, always bright, always perfect. When Arthur had his seventeenth birthday the other day I thought: how amazing that Arthur should be seventeen! And I could see him at once, looking like me but tall and slim like my father. But of course I can't talk about him to Dido. She'd think I was being morbid, but how can a shining dream be morbid? I love my shining dreams, my world of might-have-been.

'In novels dead babies always seem to draw a couple together, but that didn't happen in our case. Quite the reverse. But I try not to blame Dido too much for her attitude because she always found childbirth an ordeal and perhaps the births were traumas which ultimately she could only surmount by blocking out her most painful memories. I never wanted her to go on having children like that, but she had to have her boy and her girl. I overheard Primrose saying once to one of her Gang that Dido had to have five children in order to keep up with Grace, but that wasn't true. Dido didn't want Aidan at all because by then she already had Elizabeth and Pip; Aidan was an accident. But she wouldn't have an abortion, which was what the doctor recommended and which I certainly didn't oppose, since her life was in danger. I think possibly she wanted to die. She was in a very bad mental state at the time and afterwards she did have a severe breakdown. But at least she survived, thank God, and I didn't have to live with the knowledge that I'd destroyed her with that pregnancy. No more babies after that, of course. While they were doing the Caesarean they sorted out that problem. During the breakdown afterwards Dido used to sob for hours and say she'd been deprived of her femininity, but they didn't take anything out, they just tied something up. I explained that over and over again but she only went on sobbing. It was a very bad breakdown. I felt so sorry for her. She was so pitiful, so pathetic. Her life has in many ways been a tragic one.

'That's why I was so impatient with you when you seemed to be jealous of Dido earlier. If only you'd known! You have so much: your youth, your health, a good temperament free of neurosis, looks, brains, charm, a talent for getting on well with people instead of putting their backs up . . . And Dido has so little, just her children and – well, yes, she has me. Or rather, she has Stephen. But she doesn't have *me*, Neville Four. I belong entirely to you, and what goes on between Stephen and Dido just doesn't count, it's of no significance – why, it doesn't even happen! Everything important, everything that's *crucial* doesn't happen with Dido at all. Of that you can be quite certain.

'Well, there it is, darling – the plain, unvarnished truth at last. As you see, I'm at heart a very simple, honest person, but I admit I do sometimes have difficulty finding the words to explain myself, particularly if the explanations involve deep emotions. (When we meet, please don't ask about Arthur, George and Aidan unless I raise the subject first.)

'I suppose the earnest disciples of Freud and Jung would want to know all about my parents and my Uncle Willoughby, but I hardly feel that sort of ancient history's relevant to us now in 1963, and anyway an old codger's sentimental reminiscences about his extreme past could only be monumentally boring to anyone under thirty! Suffice it to say that my father, my mother and my uncle were all wonderful, all perfect, and they loved me as much as I loved them.

'And talking of love I shall now close this letter by telling you that you're the most miraculous thing that's ever happened to me and I hardly know how to wait until I can take you in my arms again. Be sure to write me a line as soon as you return to the Archdeacon's lap on Monday morning! My darling, I remain always – till the day I die – your most devoted and adoring N.'

XIII

'Darling Neville,' I wrote, 'Thanks so much for your marvellous letter – I can't tell you how much better I feel now that you've explained everything, all I can say is that I feel as if a vast load as big as six elephants has finally rolled off my mind. To be quite honest, I've been absolutely *torturing* myself about D. However, if nothing of crucial importance ever happens between you and her, then my torment is at an end and I can simply feel sorry for her. I'm sure you're right and she's pathetic. It must be awful to yearn to be a social success and yet wind up loathed by so many people. As you say, she's had a tragic life.

'I do think you overreacted a bit to your first wife's death – after all, it was hardly your fault that the heavens opened and she got soaked! However I quite understand that in the aftermath of such a catastrophe you would have been obsessed by the thought of women being destroyed and longed to do your share of conscientious preservation. I must be quite honest and say I don't think your behaviour was exactly *rational* – in fact if this were a book I'd find your explanation somewhat implausible – but real life is full of oddities and of course great tragedy does make people behave irrationally and succumb to various *idées fixes*.

'I promise not to speak a word about Arthur, George and

Aidan unless you mention them, but I must write, even if I can't say, that in my opinion you're quite entitled to your "shining dreams" and I don't think you're being morbid at all. I think it's admirable (not quite the right word, but I can't think of a better one) that you feel so deeply connected to them; it makes you seem so loving and compassionate, and in some strange way *wise* – you clearly know how to value and cherish things which other, lesser men might pass off as unimportant, and by loving those lost children you bring them to life. I feel I can picture Arthur exactly, looking just like you but elongated!

'Of course I understand completely now about your different "personae". "Persona" is the word for mask, isn't it, the mask an actor used to wear in a Greek play. Your identities are not really identities at all but different masks and underneath is the real you – whom I know as Neville Four. Being a self-made man, constantly obliged to remake your mask in order to keep up with your changing circumstances, must be very exhausting. But perhaps we're all self-made to some extent, all engaged periodically in "shifting gears" and remaking our masks. I know I remade Venetia's mask when I went to stay with Marina at the Chantry, and I believe I've remade it yet again with you – although in your company the mask is the real me, just as Neville Four is the real you. What an odd thing personality is. Was it you who told me that the Greeks and Romans had no word for "personality" in its modern sense? Or was it my father? I can't remember. I get confused between the two of you sometimes.

'Can't wait for Wednesday, darling – shall we chance the Crusader's car-park again? Lots and lots of love, V.'

XIV

'My darling,' wrote Aysgarth in reply, 'I fell upon your letter this morning like a starving man pouncing on a crust of bread, and devoured every crumb with a sensuous delight! I was also much touched by your kind, sensitive, understanding paragraph about Arthur, George and Aidan. It's such a psychological luxury to be able to share them with someone at last.

'Yes, you're quite right about "personality" being a modern concept. That's why people get in such a tangle with the creeds when they read that God is three persons in one – they fall into the heresy of tritheism (where are you, Bishop Ashworth!) and think that God is three separate individuals, whereas in fact the word person in that context means "persona", the mask. There's one person with three masks: the Idea (God), the manifestation of the Idea in a form comprehensible to man (Jesus) and the continuing influence of that Idea throughout the world (the Holy Spirit). But I must set aside theology and say how glad I am that you now understand about Stephen and the Nevilles – and about Dido too, of course. I do desperately want to be open and frank with you in every way.

'How I wish you could have travelled back to Starbridge with me on Sunday morning! Your presence would have given me some much needed extra strength to cope with the Bone-Pelham crisis, now billowing wildly out of control. No sooner had I finished presiding at matins when Eddie buttonholed me in the vestry with the truly appalling news that Lady B-P has produced a letter from Dean Carter acknowledging the receipt of the £3,000! But I *cannot* believe it of Carter. Neither can Fitzgerald, who says there must be an explanation and he'll interrogate Carter's widow in Budleigh Salterton. Meanwhile the undertakers are getting restless, Lady B-P is still hot against a burial in the cemetery, and her doctor (milked for information by Fitzgerald during a lavish lunch at the Quill Pen) says she's eccentric but not, in his opinion, certifiable. As I so often sigh to you: what a life! My darling, I long with an almost unbearable intensity to see you – yes, let's meet again at the Crusader. All my love, always and forever, N.'

XV

I browsed pleasurably among the sentences of this letter for some time. Then it dimly occurred to me that apart from the paragraph on the babies and the lines responding to my enquiry about the word 'personality' he had made no attempt to answer my letter in depth at all. I had thought he might respond to my very bald remarks about Dido and the distinctly critical note I had struck when commenting on the source of his *idée fixe*, but it seemed these were matters he preferred to gloss over. And why not? Surely there was no need for him to expand on the explanations which he kept saying he found so difficult.

It was at this point that Mrs Ashworth telephoned.

'Charles tells me you're coming in this afternoon at five,' she said after we had exchanged pleasantries, 'and I'm just phoning to say do stay on for a drink if you can. I've got a tea-party but with luck everyone will be gone by six.'

I accepted the invitation with alacrity.

'How are you?' she added in her kindest voice. 'It seems ages since we last met for a gossip.'

'Oh, I'm fine,' I said. 'Absolutely fine.'

But was I?

Unlocking my writing-case I retrieved the long letter Aysgarth had written earlier on Sunday morning before his departure from Flaxton Hall. Again I noted the reference to Dido's sterilisation, a fact which exploded my theory that he was abstaining from marital sex because he was afraid of destroying her with another pregnancy. Then I reached the part where he was mixing up his current 'personae' in such a way that he implied nothing ever happened with Dido. I read that passage over and over again until it no longer seemed a model of honest clarity but a convoluted masterpiece which was capable of more than one interpretation.

The glass shuddered again in my hall of mirrors.

I began to wonder if I was going mad.

THREE

'Having disposed of God as a separate Being or Person, Dr. Robinson is in difficulties over many Christian activities, including prayer. How does one pray to "ultimate reality"?'

ANONYMOUS
The Honest to God Debate
ed. DAVID L. EDWARDS

I

'Divert me,' said Mrs Ashworth, as we began to sip our gin-and-tonics, 'by telling me all about your glorious love-life. Mrs Lindsay said you were away last weekend – were you sailing at Bosham with your young man?'

'No, just checking up on my parents at Flaxton Pauncefoot. As a matter of fact the Perry romance has cooled – he seems to be more interested in boats than in girls.'

'Too bad! But I'm sure someone else will soon turn up now that you're looking so glamorous. By the way, how I envy you that thick, wavy hair! I'd have to spend half my life at the hairdresser's to get that effect.'

We talked about hair for a time. Mrs Ashworth revealed that she had her hair 'coloured' by the smartest salon in Starbridge. 'Clergymen's wives, of course, never have their hair "dyed",' she said with her deadpan humour. I expressed deep interest in the 'colouring' and said I was sure the Bishop had never guessed. Mrs Ashworth commented indulgently that men were so innocent sometimes. Sipping our gins we became steadily cosier.

'. . . and talking of men,' said Mrs Ashworth, 'what happened to the man who lured your poor friend Dinkie into that most unfortunate romance?'

'Oh, he's still dead keen on her,' I said, 'but I think she's recently come to realise it's a dead-end street.'

'Good. That must represent progress.'

'Does it? She still can't imagine ever giving him up.'

'Tell her to take a holiday – go back to America for a while, perhaps – so that she can see the situation from a fresh perspective.'

'That would be quite difficult. He depends on hearing from her every day, and –'

'How appalling! This sounds like a really dangerous situation – an emotional dependency which is fast swinging out of control. Has he opened his heart to Dinkie yet about his marriage?'

'Yes, but . . . to be quite frank, Mrs Ashworth, I don't think he's levelling with her. Dinkie believes every word he says, of course, but the more he writes to her that he wants to be absolutely honest –'

'If he's running two women at once I'd think he was lying to the back teeth. Living in two different worlds necessarily involves considerable verbal juggling.'

'I don't think he's living in two different worlds,' I said slowly. 'The three of them are all in the same world. But he's living as two separate people.'

'That's the most terrifying thing you've said yet,' said Mrs Ashworth at once. 'Tell Dinkie that a split personality leading a split-level life is big, big trouble.'

'You think he's mad?'

'Well, obviously Dinkie would realise if he was raving, so the short answer to that question must be no, but I do think he sounds spiritually, if not mentally, unbalanced. One has to be whole, not divided, in order to be spiritually healthy . . . Did Jon Darrow say that to me once? I can't remember. Maybe it was Charles.'

Automatically I said: 'I met Father Darrow the other evening at the Starbridge Playhouse.'

'Oh yes, *Present Laughter*. Amusing, wasn't it?'

'Tremendously . . . Mrs Ashworth, Father Darrow's rather weird, isn't he?'

367

'I don't think I'd use the word "weird". Unusual, perhaps. But he's very wise and good. Charles thinks the world of him.'

My voice said woodenly: 'He does?'

'Jon's been his spiritual director for over twenty-five years.'

After a pause I managed to say: 'So he's not a crank – not a charlatan?'

'Good heavens, no! He's a most distinguished man. Who's been telling you he's a charlatan?'

Far away in the hall the front door opened and the Bishop, true to his long-established custom, shouted: 'Darling!' as he returned to the house. After our session of dictation he had departed to visit his chaplain, who lived in a cottage nearby.

'Have another drink,' Mrs Ashworth said to me as he entered the room to join us, but I excused myself, feeling far too disturbed to prolong the conversation.

Then I stumbled back to my flat.

II

I poured out the gin and sat sipping it in the twilight as the clock of St Martin's-in-Cripplegate tolled the hour. The little flat was shadowed and still.

After a while I began to wonder if the Ground of my being was staging a conservation battle against the Great Pollutant.

No, I didn't. I wondered if God and the Devil were fighting for the possession of my soul.

Strange how much more chilling – how much more *real* – the battle seemed when described by the old terminology. One couldn't get very worked up about something called the Ground of one's being, that was the trouble. And how on earth did one pray to it?

I thought: someone should tell John Robinson that.

Eventually, after a lot of gin, I started to cry.

III

'Dear Eddie,' I wrote, 'What's cooking? I see you're the canon-in-residence for August, so I shall look forward to hearing you preach at matins next Sunday. Make sure you keep me awake! Yours, VENETIA.'

IV

'I thought we might have a change from Chancton Wood,' said Aysgarth as I slid into the passenger seat of his car the next day, 'so in a fit of inspiration I bought an Ordnance Survey map which marks every place of interest in the diocese and found an ancient monument called Castle Brigga not far from Starwater Abbey. I think it must be one of the old hill-forts built by the Starobrigantes – shall we go and have a look?'

We drove away out of the city.

'We're all in such a state over this Bone-Pelham crisis,' he was saying as the spire of the Cathedral receded into the distance behind us. 'Fitzgerald drives to Budleigh Salterton tomorrow to talk to Dean Carter's widow. I must say, Fitzgerald can be extraordinarily dynamic so long as the situation isn't connected with sex.'

'I thought everything was connected with sex.'

We laughed.

'My darling!' said Neville Four, who of course never slept with his wife, and reached out to put his left hand on my thigh.

But what had Stephen been getting up to with Dido?

V

The hill-fort, a vast mound ringed by two broad ditches, afforded plenty of seclusion. We settled ourselves in the shade of a clump of bushes conveniently placed in a hollow far from the path, and soon the glass in the hall of mirrors no longer reflected terrifying distortions but a clear radiant reality, the only reality that had any meaning. Eventually rain drove us back to the car, but by that time I felt nothing could mar my happiness. We lit cigarettes; then he entertained me by reminiscing about his days as a canon of Westminster Abbey when he had regularly prowled the corridors of Church House.

'. . . and the Archbishop came storming in saying: "If I were still a headmaster I'd cane him, I swear I would!" and of course all the time the lawyer who'd drafted the offending clause was hiding in the broom-cupboard! The secretaries, two nice old girls with grey hair and double chins, nearly had kittens on the spot. Well, someone lured Fisher away and we opened the cupboard and the lawyer keeled out like a corpse in a horror film –'

I laughed and laughed. Outside the car the world was grey with rain but I no longer noticed.

'– and someone shrieked: "Is there a doctor in the house?" and my friend Derek gasped: "My God, he's dead!" but the very next moment the corpse groaned: "Brandy!" and the old girls screamed: "He's alive!" So I skipped out across Dean's Yard, dived into my house in Little Cloister, shoved the brandy in a shopping bag, raced back to Church House – and bumped straight into the Archbishop who was about to leave for Lambeth . . .'

As I started laughing again I asked myself why I had written to Eddie but I no longer knew. I tried to recall my doubts and suspicions but found they no longer existed. All I knew was that I was in ecstasy and that I wanted the afternoon to last for ever.

'. . . and the net result was that we all polished off the brandy. The old girls were quite tiddly in the end . . . Heavens, look at the time! We must go.'

Without warning my laughter dissolved into tears of despair.

'Venetia – darling –' He was at once immensely distressed.

I got a grip on myself. 'Sorry,' said my voice. 'Temporary aberration. Bit of a strain, seeing you so seldom and for such a short time.' And suddenly, as the confusion began to pour back into my mind, I heard myself say rapidly: 'Neville, I'm beginning to think it might be a good idea if I went away for a while to

London – not permanently, of course, but I'm getting so muddled here and I feel I need the chance to –'

'For God's sake!' he said ashen, and as he spoke I knew – I just knew, I was wholly convinced – that he no longer had sex with his wife. 'Don't leave Starbridge! Please, Venetia, please – I absolutely rely on these meetings – the meetings and the letters – they keep me going, I don't know what I'd do without them – oh my darling, I love you so much, I adore you, I can't imagine how I ever existed without you, how could you ever think of leaving me even temporarily, I thought you loved me, I thought you understood –'

I collapsed in floods of tears again and swore I would never leave.

VI

'Dear Venetia,' wrote Eddie by return of post, 'I shall look forward to spotting you in the congregation next Sunday. My text will be: "Be not deceived; God is not mocked: for whatsoever a man soweth, that shall he also reap." I used to reflect often on that text when I was a POW in May 'forty-five. However, in my sermon I shall substitute the decadence sown by secular society for the devastation sown by Hitler. Yours, EDDIE. PS. Any chance of you dropping in for a drink some time this week? I've got a rather interesting bottle of Château Lafite which I've been saving for a rainy day.'

VII

'Dear Eddie, Passionate about the Château Lafite but this week's a bit difficult. Can we "take a rain-check", as Dinkie would say? Yours, VENETIA. PS. Marina tells me Dinkie's having a mad affair with Katie's brother Simon. I wouldn't have thought brainless hulks were in her line, but Americans are notorious for their lack of discrimination. PPS. Thanks for warning me about the extremely sinister text on which you intend to preach. I shall bring a hip-flask of brandy in case I feel faint with terror.'

VIII

'My darling,' wrote Aysgarth, 'I didn't sleep a wink all last night because I was so worried about you, and so far I've written three letters but torn them all up. Your distress appalled me. What can I do to put things right? It would kill me to give you up but I'd rather be dead than make you unhappy. One day, as I've said before, I *will* have to give you up; you'll meet someone of your own generation who'll make you the best possible husband – you may even meet this Great Paragon tomorrow, for all I know, but darling, make sure he *is* the Great Paragon because it would break my heart if you wasted yourself on someone who was unworthy of you.

'Forgive all this turgid agonising, but I fear you might be thinking me selfish, begging you to stay in Starbridge, and I'm anxious to demonstrate that I *am* capable of putting your welfare above my selfish longings. What I want more than anything else is for you to be happy. That's how I can face the knowledge that one day I shall have to cede you to the Great Paragon. However, meanwhile you're free, and until that terrible day when my great prize is irrevocably lost I feel I can't bear to part from you even temporarily. In fact I –

'(LATER) Fitzgerald's just rung up. The Widow Carter says she knows nothing of her late husband's financial affairs – she never even had a cheque-book until he died – but she does remember that their retirement bungalow in Budleigh Salterton cost £3,000 more than they could afford and that her husband was thrilled when he managed to get the money from somewhere.

'This is, of course, horrific and the potential for scandal is enough to give any Dean and Chapter a collective nervous breakdown. Imagine Carter, one of the premier deans in England, taking a bribe like that! Fitzgerald and Dalton still doggedly refuse to believe it. Eddie, always the optimist, says it can only be a matter of hours now before the tabloid press hear Lady Bone-Pelham shrieking that the Dean and Chapter have welshed on the deal to give her heroic husband the distinguished last resting-place he deserves. Meanwhile Sir George is still lying in state at the undertakers', and the undertakers themselves are getting very shirty indeed. I confess I'm sorely tempted to dig up a little patch of the Cloisters' lawn in order to bury Carter's iniquity along with Sir George's corpse, but if I start bending the rules all the nobs will want to be buried there and I'll have the Health Department trying to prosecute me for operating an insanitary establishment. (Or does this only apply to restaurants?) The whole thing's a nightmare.

'Must close, darling – I'll try not to be so selfish in future, I promise – I really do accept that I can't keep you for ever, but meanwhile let's not think of the future, let's blot it out, let's just live in the present, let's have our shining dream, because I love you more than words can ever express and the thought of living without you is absolutely, utterly and entirely UNBEARABLE. All my love, my darling, my angel, my adored one, for ever and ever, N.'

IX

'Dear Venetia, I'm extremely surprised to hear that Dinkie was having an affair with Simon. According to Perry Palmer, who invited me to Albany for a drink when I was visiting my London dentist last week, she's ended up as a scalp in Michael Ashworth's collection. Incidentally, Perry asked when you were coming to see his coal-cellar. Yours, EDDIE. PS. I'll try not to terrify you from the pulpit! Any chance of seeing you for a cup of coffee after matins? I think I can get out of the sung Communion by putting pressure on Tommy Fitzgerald – I substituted for him in May when he had to waltz off to wait upon his widowed mother. PPS. I shan't be missing Communion altogether on Sunday, of course – I'll be the celebrant at the early service. (I don't want you to think I'm lax!)'

X

'Dear Eddie, Having drained my hip-flask during your sermon, I shall without doubt require black coffee afterwards to revive me. Thanks. By the way, Perry's got it quite wrong and it was Emma-Louise who wound up as a scalp. She's now flirting hard with Robert Welbeck who, so Marina tells me, is dying of unrequited love for her (Marina). Marina herself, of course, is still welded to the frame of her asexual triangle with Christian and Katie and avoiding the furious pounces of Michael Ashworth who can't bear to think that such a gorgeous scalp might elude his collection. Just as an afterthought: do you think Perry's queer? I'm trying to decide whether the coal-cellar's worth a visit. Yours, VENETIA.'

XI

'Darling, *darling* Neville, I cried when I read your letter, wept for hours, because you were trying so hard to be noble when all I really deserved was a kick on the bottom for being so *cruel* as to talk as I did. Of course I'll never leave you, never – except later this month when I have to go up to town for my mother's seventieth birthday. No way out of that, I'm afraid, but don't worry – I'll come straight back to Starbridge. And again, don't worry – I don't want to marry anyone except you, and if you're never free, then I'll never marry. So please, *please* treat my silly remark about leaving as if it had never been uttered, and *do* stop talking about that repulsive Great Paragon, because I adore you, I couldn't live without you and there couldn't possibly be anyone else, not now, NOT EVER . . .'

XII

'This is amazingly good coffee, Eddie. Congratulations.'
  'It takes a foreigner to make decent coffee in England!

Well, tell me the worst – what did you think of the sermon?'

'Great fun. Can't wait to reap what I've sown.'

Eddie laughed. We were sitting in the drawing-room of his little house in the North Walk and beyond the bow window the Cathedral basked in the hot August sun. The room was carefully furnished with reproduction antiques, and the walls were lined with English sporting prints; all books were confined to the study across the hall. Eddie himself was still wearing his cassock and looked like a huge black pear.

'. . . and I simply must take this opportunity to tell you how grateful I am that you never treat me as a clergyman,' he was saying earnestly. 'After being continually addressed by the elderly inhabitants of the Close as "dear Canon" and viewed as if I were a stainless-steel robot, it's so refreshing to receive letters from someone who has no hesitation in writing about affairs and asexual triangles and pounces and queers –'

'That reminds me, do you think Perry's queer as a coot?'

'I find it quite impossible to tell. In fact I don't believe it's possible to know much about anyone's sex-life unless one happens to be a priest who hears confessions.'

I said vaguely: 'You don't hear confessions, do you, Eddie?' and was surprised when he said he did. 'I share the job with Tommy Fitzgerald,' he added. 'I'm not High-Church by inclination as Tommy is, but I had plenty of experience of the confessional when I was running my Anglo-Catholic parish at Langley Bottom.'

'Yes, I remember your triumph among the bells and smells. But Eddie, since confession isn't compulsory in the Church of England and since it's regarded by the majority as a High-Church fad, I'm amazed to hear the Dean allows such goings-on in his Cathedral!'

'Oh, *he'd* never hear anyone, of course! The very word "confession" makes him regress instantly to his Nonconformist upbringing!'

'Then who performed the impossible feat of persuading him to allow confessions?'

'The Bishop. Charles is the kind of priest who's difficult to classify: his churchmanship's middle-of-the-road, but he can preach like an Evangelical once he gets going on sin and he's as fervent about confessions as any Anglo-Catholic.'

'But how on earth did the Bishop force Aysgarth to –'

'Oh, the clash was resolved without too much trouble because Charles had Cathedral tradition on his side and Tommy was already there, willing to hear confessions. Stephen soon decided it would be prudent not to meddle too violently with the status quo – he'd only just been appointed Dean – and later he did come to see that the Cathedral, as the mother-church of the diocese, really does have to provide a confessor for the occasional penitent who turns up. But we've got another big churchmanship clash brewing, and this one won't be resolved so easily. Charles is in favour of experimenting with the idea of making the Eucharist the main service on Sunday morning, but Stephen just says: "Over my dead body."'

'What do you three canons say?'

'Nothing. We're far too busy praying for a resolution to our eternal problem.'

'What eternal problem?'

'How to prevent our Bishop and our Dean killing each other.'

'But good heavens, Eddie, are you saying these clashes go on all the time?'

'Oh, we live dangerously in this Cathedral Close! It's blood and thunder all the way! I hesitate to say this to you, Venetia – and perhaps I can only say it because I know you're as devoted to Stephen as I am – but he really does behave very foolishly sometimes.'

'What do you mean by "foolishly"?'

'Well, he's got this odd, reckless streak. He takes such risks.'

'Scandalous risks?'

'Potentially, yes.' Eddie hesitated but when I interposed: 'Go on, you can trust me,' he said: 'Let me give you an example of the most fearful crisis which has recently blown up as the result of a risk he took. He commissioned a sculpture for the Cathedral churchyard, and he did it without consulting the Chapter. Of course he quickly asked us for our approval, showed us some vague sketches and produced an impressive title for the work – "Modern Man In Search Of God" – but that didn't alter the fact that he was imposing his decision on us. Apparently he'd met this attractive young sculptress Harriet March – maybe you know her? – at one of Dido's Art Evenings, and she'd charmed him so much that he'd offered her the commission on the spot. But he knew nothing about her work, nothing at all! What a risk to take, what a potential scandal! However, fortunately for him the Tate were prepared to vouch for her so it seemed he'd brought off the gamble, although Tommy and Paul remained livid about the lack of consultation and Tommy made a very cutting remark about Stephen's penchant for young women – which, as you and I both know, is a perfectly harmless idiosyncrasy that he's been indulging in innocently for years. Anyway, just when we'd decided we'd all learn to love the sculpture, Mrs March sent some photographs of the work in progress and it was quite obvious that the masterpiece will be pornographic.'

'Help! Naked ladies?'

'Naked men – and only one portion of their anatomy is portrayed.'

'Glory!'

'Well, of course we can't possibly have it in the churchyard – the gutter-press would feast off the story for days and we'd be the laughing-stock of the Church of England. I realise that, Paul realises that, Tommy realises that, but thanks to Tommy playing his cards wrong and roping in the Archdeacon, Stephen's got locked in a power-struggle with the Bishop and that's absolutely FATAL. I tell you, Venetia, those two should never be living in the same cathedral close. They're not only theologically incompatible; they're temperamentally mismatched. Stephen can really only get on with cuddly, pliable old bishops like the late Dr Ottershaw back in the 'forties, but Charles is neither cuddly, nor pliable nor even particularly old. God knows where it'll all end . . . I say, Venetia, would you like a drink? It somehow seems to have turned into twelve o'clock. I've got rather an intriguing bottle of hock in the fridge –'

'Lovely. Thanks. But Eddie –' Automatically I followed him

into the kitchen '– this is horrific. I didn't quite realise – I mean, I had no idea –'

'No, of course not – how could you have known? I shouldn't really be telling you, but to be honest I'm just so worried that it's the most unutterable relief to confide in someone I can trust. I can't really discuss the situation with Paul and Tommy because I'm afraid of seeming disloyal to Stephen.'

'Well, you can trust me to the hilt and I swear I'll never think you're being disloyal. Supposing this ghastly mess does get splashed all over the worst front pages in Fleet Street? What would happen then?'

'Disaster. The Bishop would be down on us like a ton of bricks. He'd make a visitation.'

'What's that?'

'Well, it certainly wouldn't just be dropping in at the Cathedral for elevenses. What does the chairman of the board do when his biggest branch office goes off the rails? He turns up with the auditors and lawyers, tracks down the source of the catastrophe and sacks the man responsible.'

'My God.' I had to lean against the doorpost, but fortunately Eddie was unaware of the full dimensions of my horror; he was too busy extracting the cork from the bottle. 'But surely Ashworth can't fire Aysgarth!'

'No, he can't, not directly, because the deanery's a Crown appointment, but if a really serious mess is uncovered –' Eddie began to pour out the hock '– Charles will go to the Archbishop of Canterbury. There'd be no trial in the Church Courts, of course – much too scandalous – but Archbishop Ramsey, with the Crown, as it were, in the pocket of his purple cassock, would gently suggest a retirement with full pension rights on the grounds of ill health.'

I was speechless. It was only when we had returned with the wine to the drawing-room that I managed to say: 'Eddie, if you're deliberately piling on the gloom and doom in order to frighten me –'

'Let me cheer you up by saying that although the sculpture could turn into a fiasco big enough to warrant a visitation, the

Cathedral itself is still bowling along in an acceptable fashion – or in other words, I don't believe a visitation would turn up a mess serious enough to justify an appeal to the Archbishop.'

'Thank God!'

'But what really worries me,' said Eddie, barely listening, 'is that this is only the latest of a long series of clashes between the Bishop and the Dean, and now Charles could well have reached the point where he'd seize any opportunity to pull out the long knife. If he can't drive home a charge of mismanagement, he'll be itching to prove a charge of personal misconduct, and although Stephen may wriggle out of this present tight corner, where on earth will his gambler's streak lead him next? Thank goodness he's at least cut back on the drink recently. I can't even begin to describe the scandalous risks he's taken during his long love affair with the bottle . . . Hm, this hock's really very passable! Have a sip, Venetia.'

I sipped the hock. It tasted of nothing. When I replaced the glass on the table I was aware that my hand was trembling. 'Now you really are exaggerating, Eddie!' said my voice brightly. 'I know our Mr Dean drinks quite a bit, but –'

'*Quite a bit?* Sorry – excuse the heavy irony. But perhaps I'd better not say any more, it'd be a mistake, I'd regret it later –'

'Oh no,' I said. 'No, you tell me everything. Good for you to get it off your chest. And don't worry, I swear I'll never tell a soul.'

'Well, you won't believe half of what I say,' said Eddie, knocking back his hock. 'You simply won't believe it, but . . .'

He embarked on his revelations.

And then the horrors really began to unfold.

XIII

'He's been a heavy drinker for years,' said Eddie, 'and like many heavy drinkers he's skilled at covering it up, but every so often he goes over the top. Then we have to protect him – and we've all done it, even Tommy.'

'Over the top? You mean –'

'Drunk for services. Evensong's the worst. He probably starts drinking at lunch and then goes on. Whoever's canon-in-residence keeps an eye on him and if Stephen can't walk straight the canon volunteers to take the service on his own. As you know, we usually field at least two of the senior clergy at each evensong, one for the readings and one for the prayers and versicles, but it's a flexible arrangement and sometimes during the week the canon either copes on his own or gets one of the minor canons to assist him. However, if it's one of the months when the Dean himself is in residence, we three canons make very sure someone's always there to partner him and if necessary take over.'

'But surely he must know when he's drunk! How does he have the nerve to turn up?'

'Oh, he thinks he can get away with anything! It's actually very difficult to coax him not to take part in a service; the trick is to tell him he looks exhausted and say one's only too pleased to do him a favour when he's obviously been working so hard. You'd think he'd go in for absenteeism in a big way, but no, he's very conscientious about attendance. I think he believes that so long as he shows up he's got everything in control. Funnily enough for the past three months or so he really has seemed to have everything in control, although why he should suddenly be drinking less I've no idea. He hasn't been drunk at a service since before Easter. But the real horror story happened last Christmas. He turned up so drunk for the Midnight Eucharist that he passed out in the Dean's stall.'

I said: 'I don't believe it,' and drained my glass of hock.

'I told you that you wouldn't believe half of what I said.' He gave me a refill. 'The Bishop, thank God, was preaching. Stephen would never have made it to the pulpit.'

'The Bishop!' I was so appalled that I could barely speak. 'Are you trying to tell me that Aysgarth passed out at a service where the *Bishop* was present?'

'Yes, but we canons performed the most fantastic rescue act and I don't think Charles noticed anything. Before the service he was the last to enter the vestry, and as soon as he came in Paul buttonholed him and steered him away from Stephen while Tommy and I acted as a screen. Luckily there were masses of people milling around, not just the choir and the vergers but the retired clergy who help administer the sacrament at Christmas, so it wasn't so difficult to keep the Dean and the Bishop separated.'

'Surely you tried to persuade Aysgarth not to take part!'

'Of course, but as it was one of the biggest services of the year he absolutely refused to step down. He's a great one for keeping up appearances – only this time he was so drunk he could barely keep upright. In the end we entered the Cathedral with Tommy on one side of him and me on the other to ensure we'd steady him if he stumbled, although normally he'd have been on his own, walking ahead of the Bishop, while Tommy and I – or Paul – would have been walking together in front of him.'

'But surely the Bishop must have realised –'

'I don't think so. He probably thought our formation was odd but I suspect he'd have been too busy glancing around the congregation and mentally recapping his sermon to pay the oddity much attention.'

'So Aysgarth made it to the stall –'

'Yes, and once he was there he was out of sight of almost everyone except the extreme west wing of the choir. The Bishop was the celebrant and Tommy was reading the lessons, so Stephen didn't actually have to do anything until the administration of the sacrament.'

'What happened then?'

'Our worst dreams came true. Remember, this was the Midnight Eucharist, which is always like the feeding of the five thousand: a packed Cathedral, hordes of communicants and so much going on that a dean could go missing for a while without his absence being noticed. We had two tables in operation, one at the head of the nave, where the Bishop and Paul and half the clerical assistants were working, and one at the high altar where Tommy and I were labouring away with the other half of the helpers. Stephen was supposed to be at our table and of course we both noticed he wasn't. Tommy said: "Let him be – much better that he stays where he is," and I certainly wasn't going to argue with him, but after a while I said: "It's odd he hasn't at least attempted to join us." "Just what I was thinking," said Tommy, and using the excuse that he was going to get some more consecrated wine from the Bishop's table, he nipped away to investigate. However he never reached the Bishop's table. He was back in a flash, and the moment I saw his face I knew the worst had happened.

'Well, I palmed off my wafers on the nearest clerical assistant and followed Tommy to the Dean's stall. Stephen was out, absolutely unconscious, we couldn't rouse him. Tommy said: "We've got to get him away before Charles passes by," but of course that was easier said than done, even though, as you'll remember, there's an exit from the choir into the side-aisle by the vestry. So the route was obvious. What wasn't so obvious was how on earth we were going to get him out. Tommy and I are both around six feet tall and not exactly weaklings, but Stephen's heavy – or at least he was before he lost weight recently – and we feared he'd be difficult to manoeuvre. In the end Tommy just said: "It's speed that's important. We can't cover up the fact that he's being whisked out. All we can do is whisk him out in double-quick time." So I took his left side and Tommy took his right and then Tommy said: "All right, Eddie – say your prayers" – and I assure you that didn't seem in the least blasphemous because we were both sweating blood by that time, I can remember my heart banging away, I don't think I've been so consumed with horror since I was captured in Normandy in 'forty-four.

'Well, we did it, we draped his arms around our shoulders and we whipped him out with his feet two inches from the ground, and I don't think too many people noticed; all the attention was focused on the Bishop at the central table, and no one was anticipating any action in the choir. However Dido and the family saw us, of course; they'd noticed, even if no one else had, that he hadn't emerged from the stall earlier and they were wondering what was wrong. Dido came straight to the vestry with all four sons of the first marriage, and so fortunately there were plenty of strong helpers to smuggle him home. But none of the boys ever spoke of the incident afterwards, and Dido just treated it as an unfortunate case of food poisoning.'

'But what on earth did Aysgarth say the next day to you and Fitzgerald?'

'He claimed he'd had no sleep the night before and that the heavy Christmas Eve dinner had overpowered him.'

'But surely Fitzgerald made some sort of protest –'

'Of course – to me. Tommy's actually a little frightened of Stephen, and so's Paul. Stephen's a very strong personality. But both Tommy and Paul said after the catastrophe that I'd have to talk bluntly to Stephen – they knew he'd always listen to me even if he wouldn't listen to them – but as it turned out, nothing needed to be said. The disaster had given him the most colossal fright. He drank only soda-water after that for three weeks.'

There was a pause. Eddie refilled our glasses again before adding: 'Fortunately, as I mentioned earlier, he seems to be drinking less at present – in fact he's in amazingly high spirits, although considering the current batch of Cathedral crises I can't imagine why he should be so cheerful. He's almost treating the sculpture fiasco as a joke.'

'Well, I suppose it does have its funny side –'

'It doesn't, you know. There's nothing funny about increasing the Bishop's desire to pull out the long knife.'

'But Eddie –'

'A scandalous risk that doesn't come off – that's all Charles needs now to close in for the kill, and we're not home and dry on this sculpture yet, not by a long chalk. In fact I've even wondered – and now I'm really scraping the bottom of the barrel of horror – I've even wondered if Stephen's harmless penchant for young women has swung right out of control and he's indulging in some sort of crazy flirtation with Harriet March.'

'Oh, that's impossible.'

'Yes, I suppose it is. It would explain why he's in such high spirits, but . . . no, he couldn't, surely, be that much of a fool.'

'What on earth gave you the idea?'

'He was rather wild in one of our Chapter meetings not so long ago – I forget the exact context, but he described the Cathedral's spire as a phallic symbol. Afterwards I heard Tommy say to Paul: "I do hope this sculpture fiasco doesn't turn out to be a case of *cherchez la femme*," and as soon as he'd spoken I felt my blood run cold –'

'I think Fitzgerald's round the bend. I say, Eddie, while we're on the subject of sex . . . well, there's something I can't resist asking just out of sheer vulgar curiosity: what the hell do you think goes on between Aysgarth and Dido?'

'Anything from nightly copulation to absolutely nothing,' said Eddie gloomily, polishing off the hock, 'and with his history of heavy drinking I think the most likely answer is nothing. But who can tell? Only God can possibly know what goes on in that marriage. The whole thing's a complete mystery.'

But it no longer seemed such a mystery to me. Aysgarth's drinking could well have had a malign effect on his relationship with Dido, and even now that his alcohol intake had been reduced and his body had unmistakably recovered, he no longer needed to sleep with her because he had me; a psychological block prevented him from fully consummating our affair, but at least I was able to provide him with sexual satisfaction. The mystery had at last been unravelled and now I could relax – except that relaxation had simultaneously become impossible.

I started to torment myself with images of the Bishop, itching to pull out the long knife and close in for the kill.

XIV

'My darling,' wrote Aysgarth, 'I'm scribbling this in the weekly staff meeting which we always hold at eleven o'clock every Monday – the senior members of staff sit around a table in the sacristy (that's the large room where the ceremonial robes are kept). I'm at the top and my minions sit in no particular order on either side. Today I've got the Clerk of the Works on my left and the senior Verger on my right. The three residentiary Canons are here, of course (or, to give them their proper titles as canons of a cathedral of the Old Foundation: the Precentor, the Chancellor – to be distinguished from the Chancellor of the diocese who grants faculties – and the Treasurer). Then we have the Choirmaster, the Organist, the Master-Mason, the senior Cathedral Guide, the Manager of the Cathedral shop, the Architect, the Librarian and the Vicar of the Close (who does the day-to-day pastoral work for me among the people who live within the precincts). Neither the Accountant nor the Estate Agent nor the Investment Manager's present today because the agenda doesn't require their special skills. This is just going to be a cosy little chat, very Barchester, about various domestic matters such as how we pamper the tourists. (This is known as the Great Cafeteria Question.) However at the moment the senior Verger and the Organist are waffling about *The Archers*. I'll have to rein them in.

'(LATER) We embarked on our discussion of the proposed cafeteria, but we've somehow got back to *The Archers* and Gilbert the Librarian is saying it's not as good as *Mrs Dale's Diary*. Why we're so fixated on wireless serials this morning I can't imagine. I'll have to rein them in again.

'(LATER) HORRORS! The Vicar of the Close, who's finally been allowed to get a word in, has suggested that before we spend money building a cafeteria we'd better start glueing together the west front – apparently he was on the sward yesterday when an American tourist was grazed by a piece of falling masonry the size of a brick which dropped off one of the statues high up on the west wall. Runcival the Master-Mason says that's nothing new, the west front's been on the verge of disintegration for years, and didn't he say only six months ago ... etc., etc. The Clerk of the Works says we'd better shove up some scaffolding before an entire statue falls out of a niche with lethal results. That's all I need, of course: a dead tourist adorning the west front steps. Fitzgerald says to Runcival: "How much money are we talking about here?" and Runcival answers in his most sepulchral voice: "A thousand for a temporary safety measure and thousands for the full repairs." That means an appeal, which is always hell. The last one indirectly finished off Dean Carter. But before we can even launch an appeal I've got to raise a quick thousand to ensure a temporary safety. This is somewhat tricky because –

'(LATER) Had to stop because everyone was having hysterics at the thought of an appeal. However the Architect is now burbling on about quarrying the right kind of stone for the repairs. As I was saying, raising a quick thousand is going to be slightly tricky. The Cathedral finances are handled primarily by the Accountant and me. (Forget Eddie's formal title of Treasurer – he does liaise with the Accountant, but the title's a hang-over from the old days and means he has to keep an eye on the Cathedral treasures.) The Accountant deals with most of the money, but I have a private account, which I call the Dean's Fund, at the Cathedral's bank. I use it for what I call "glorifying the Cathedral" – buying miscellaneous articles of great artistic merit. Harriet's sculpture falls into this category, of course, but so also do small items such as the magnificent pair of cut-glass vases which we use for flowers.

'The money's raised mainly by staging concerts in the nave, but I made a packet when I got the Starbridge Playhouse to put on *Murder in the Cathedral* here a couple of years ago and I have various other fund-raising tricks up my sleeve. But these take time to pull off and time is just what I don't have at the moment as the thousand for the west front needs to be raised at once. It shouldn't actually come from the Dean's Fund at all, but the official funds are in low water at the moment, in fact they're in the red, and to tell the truth the Dean's Fund owes the main Cathedral account money which I've got to repay before the auditors move in for their next session. So what do I do? Heaven only knows, but the temptation to follow in Carter's footsteps and sell off burial plots in the cloisters is fast becoming irresistible!

'Must close, Fitzgerald's obviously wondering what I'm scribbling, desperate love, N.'

XV

'Dear Venetia,' wrote Eddie, 'I'm scrawling this at the weekly staff meeting where the possibility of killing off all the tiresome tourists is being discussed. Apparently we only have to let the west front disintegrate a little more and then all the statues will fall out of their niches with very effective results. Look, it was marvellous seeing you yesterday. Any chance of dinner at the Quill Pen this week? They have quite a dashing little Piesporter Goldtröpchen on the wine-list. Yours gratefully (for listening so sympathetically yesterday) EDDIE. PS. Stephen appears to be writing a three-volume novel. He shouldn't do it, people notice. Quick notes only!'

XVI

'Are you all right, Venetia?' said the Bishop suddenly after he had dictated his last sentence of the afternoon. 'You seem a little *distraite.*'

'Well, as a matter of fact I'm rather worried about a friend of mine who seems to be drifting deeper and deeper into a catastrophic mess. Sorry if I wasn't quite with it today.'

'Come and have some tea. My wife should be around somewhere —'

'How nice of you, Bishop, but I really have to dash back. So if you'll excuse me . . .'

I fled.

XVII

I was just pouring myself a stiff brandy and wondering what the legal definition of embezzlement was, when my brother Oliver telephoned about my mother's seventieth birthday.

'. . . and Sylvia's found a silver rose-bowl at Garrard's. The only difficulty is that everyone turns out to be absolutely bⴰoke and we were wondering, old girl, since you happen to be the only member of the family who has no worries or anxieties of any kind –'

'Look, pal,' I said, 'if everyone can't come up with their share you can count me out.'

'I say, Venetia, is anything the matter? You sound a bit –'

'Oh, run off and play at being an MP!' I hung up, then left the receiver off the hook.

The dim room darkened as night began to fall.

XVIII

'My darling, I thought we might go back to that nice little hollow at Castle Brigga –'

'I'm dreadfully sorry, Neville, but I've got to cancel – I'm feeling like death.'

He was painfully concerned. We had met in the car-park of the Crusader Hotel and I had just collapsed on the Humber's front seat.

'But how awful to think you had to drag yourself over here when you were unwell! Why didn't you phone the Deanery?'

'I did. Dido answered.'

'Damn. Darling, I'm so sorry . . . Are you registered with a doctor?'

'Don't need one. It's just a touch of food-poisoning.' It was a hang-over. I had drunk myself into a stupor the night before because I was so worried about him.

'If only I could look after you, make you tea –'

'No, don't worry, I just want to snooze.'

He drove me to the door of my flat and parted from me in an agony of anxiety. His last feverish words were: 'I'll write!'

Closing the front door I groped my way upstairs to bed and prayed he would somehow be saved from ruin.

FOUR

I

'Any news of Dinkie?' enquired Mrs Ashworth over coffee at the South Canonry the next morning.

'Yes, but it's suddenly become so ghastly that I'm not sure I can talk about it.'

'She's not suicidal, is she?'

'No, but it turns out her married man's on the brink of catastrophe, and she's so paralysed with horror that she can't work out what she should do next.'

'She should leave him.'

'Then he'll keel over into the abyss, she says.'

'On the contrary, the shock would probably prompt him to pull himself together.'

'That could be true, certainly. But in my view the most potent argument in favour of her leaving him is that Dinkie herself is a great danger to this man, possibly the greatest danger of all. If their affair's exposed he could wind up as ruined as Profumo.'

'The person who's in the greatest danger of all,' said Mrs Ashworth, 'is Dinkie. Tell her he's got a good chance of survival if she leaves him, but neither of them will survive if she stays.'

'Yes, I think I could coax Dinkie to believe that, but the trouble – the nightmare – the really spine-chilling truth is that he's now so heavily involved that I don't think he could bear to let her go. He'd never accept that the affair was over unless –' I stopped. Then I said: 'I'm sorry, Mrs Ashworth, I know I sound quite abnormally worried, but I really am very fond of Dinkie and one does get so fraught when one's friends are in a fix.'

'Of course,' said Mrs Ashworth. 'That's what friendship's all about, isn't it? I understand.'

Changing the subject abruptly I asked her for news of Charley.

II

'My darling, it was AGONY only being able to see you for such a short time this afternoon, I feel utterly stunned – and also, of course, demented to think of you suffering all alone in your flat with no one to look after you. I only wish I could send flowers and grapes by the ton, but I can only send you this letter – which comes as always with my very best love. I do hope you're now feeling better. I'd ring you but I do prefer to avoid the telephone, such a dangerous instrument, particularly since D's new hobby seems to be listening in on the extension.

'Can we meet on Friday afternoon instead? I've got an appointment but I can cancel it. It's only with the surveyors. Let the whole west front fall down! I just want to be with you in our dear little hollow. If you can make it but aren't well enough to reply to this letter by return, ring me at 7.00 a.m. on Friday. (D will never rouse herself at that hour, not even to listen in.) If I don't hear from you I'll know it's no good, but my darling, *please* drop everything, even the Bishop, because if I don't see you I'll go mad and drink a bottle of brandy and pass out before I can get to evensong. I feel absolutely DESPERATE. Deepest love, N.'

III

'I can't tell you how glad I am to see you,' said Eddie as we drank Piesporter Goldtröpchen and toyed with grilled trout at the Quill Pen on Thursday night. 'You're fast becoming a life-line! We've got a big crisis blowing up over the west front. Three years ago it could have been repaired with minimal expense, but Stephen shrugged off the warning reports by saying that surveyors were always over-pessimistic about old buildings. Now, of course, the repairs will cost a fortune and what's worse is that Stephen's being vague about money.'

'Vague about money?'

'The accounts are in a mess. Poor old Bob Carey, our account-ant, is practically gibbering with terror, but Stephen just says don't worry, he'll sort everything out.'

'But how on earth –'

'The whole trouble began three years ago when Stephen began to raise money for the Chagall window and opened a special account at the bank. It was all quite above board, but later he kept on the account while he continued his fund-raising for more works of art, and the net result was that this gave him a fatal leeway to take financial risks – he was able to write cheques without obtaining a counter-signature.'

'Don't tell me he –'

'He seems to have got careless and spent money before he'd actually raised it – Tommy's convinced Stephen lied to us about the cost of that sculpture. Anyway, what happened was that a few months ago Stephen borrowed some money for the Dean's Fund from the main Cathedral account. You may ask why Bob Carey didn't put his foot down, but he's such a nice old boy that I don't suppose he suspected anything was wrong – or perhaps he just didn't have the nerve to stand up to the Dean and say no. However, shortly after that the Cathedral dipped into the red when we had a problem with drainage under St Anselm's chapel. Bob asked for the repayment of the loan but Stephen put him off so the Cathedral's still in the red – although there's nothing particularly unusual about that, I hasten to add, because the Cathedral's often dipping into the red and out again as we struggle to keep up with the expenses. What's unusual about this particular sojourn in debt is that Stephen's directly to blame for it because he can't repay that loan.'

'But what on earth's he going to do?'

'Oh, he'll raise the money eventually by giving concerts, no doubt about that, but meanwhile we're in the soup because we need money immediately to shore up the west front. I suppose we'll have to mortgage one of our city properties, although that's not going to look good, and if the Bishop hears –'

'Oh, my God –'

'No, it's all right, he wouldn't make a visitation just because we'd been driven to mortgage property, but of course we all want to keep the accounts mess from him. My really big nightmare is that Harriet March will sue us for breach of contract if – when – we reject that sculpture. Heaven only knows what the legal position is –'

'But surely with her reputation she'll be able to sell the piece elsewhere!'

'I think she ought to bury it. And talking of burials we're knee-deep in another absolutely scandalous situation . . .' He told me about the Bone-Pelham fiasco. I gave up attempting to eat my trout and concentrated on trying not to drink my Piesporter Goldtröpchen as if it were lemonade.

'. . . and we simply can't start burying people again in the cloisters! The lawn's full up, chock-a-block with corpses going all the way back to the pre-Reformation canons –'

'But listen, Eddie, what do you think the real story is about this three thousand pounds that you say Sir George is reported to have paid to Dean Carter?'

'Tommy and Paul, who knew Carter very well, are quite sure he'd never have taken a bribe and I find it hard to believe too, but no matter what happened, the fact remains that Stephen's mishandled this business. He should never have got drawn into investigating the three thousand; it's essentially a red herring. He should have taken a very firm line with Lady Bone-Pelham right from the start and said sorry, I don't know what Dr

Carter arranged but it's impossible for us under public health regulations to bury anyone in the cloisters in 1963. Heaven only knows what the public health regulations are, of course, but that's a minor detail . . . I say, Venetia, is anything wrong with that trout?'

'No, it was divine but I'm just not particularly hungry. Marvellous wine, Eddie!'

'Very soothing, isn't it, and God knows I need soothing. The really important thing, as I see it, is to prevent word of this mess reaching the Bishop. If Lady Bone-Pelham blows her top –'

'She won't. Aysgarth will charm her somehow.'

'I think he's running out of charm. I think he's running out of luck. I think he's running out of everything –'

'Always the little ray of sunshine, aren't you, Eddie? I say, do you think I could possibly have a drop of Rémy Martin instead of pudding?'

IV

At seven o'clock on Friday morning I telephoned the Deanery. Aysgarth grabbed the receiver halfway through the first ring.

'It's me,' I said. 'I can come.'

'My darling, it's no good. I'm apoplectic with rage. Charles has summoned me to the South Canonry at three.'

'Oh, my God –'

'No, it's all right! It'll only be about the Bone-Pelham fiasco – Lady Bone-Pelham finally couldn't resist screeching to him that I was a blackguard who ought to be defrocked, but I've now got the mess under control. Yesterday I talked to Carter's son, who's a very respectable chartered accountant in London, and he says the three thousand was almost certainly a gift from Sir George to the Starbridge Sunlight Home for Handicapped Children – apparently Carter did a lot of work in his spare time for the Home and was treasurer of a fund-raising appeal a few years ago. The Widow Carter had obviously forgotten this and confused the donation with a sum of three thousand pounds which her husband raised (so his son tells me) from a building society to finance the purchase of the bungalow in Budleigh Salterton. So the situation's now crystal clear: Dean Carter is exonerated, the Widow Bone-Pelham is certifiable, off goes Sir George's corpse to the cemetery and off the hook drop the Dean and Chapter. Happy ending!'

'Thank God! So the Bishop has nothing to complain about?'

'Certainly not! Game, set and match to the Dean!'

'*Thank God*. Oh Neville –'

'My darling, I've got to see you – Lady Mary after evensong?'

'Can't wait . . .'

V

'My dear Venetia,' wrote Eddie in a note which was delivered by hand, 'I really enjoyed our dinner yesterday at the Quill Pen. Sorry I got a bit gloomy at the end. You were wonderful, so calm, so serene, so endlessly sympathetic and understanding. You couldn't possibly drop in for a drink some time over the weekend, could you? I promise to open the Château Lafite this time! I don't know why I got diverted by the hock the other day. Love, EDDIE.'

VI

'Venetia, it's Arabella. Look, sweetie, I've got the most ghastly crisis on at the moment, I'm simply knee-deep in divorce lawyers and everyone's threatening to sue everyone else and the bills keep mounting up and I'm so desperate I've even cancelled my weekly order from the florist. So could you be an absolute darling and pay my share of the rose-bowl for the time being? There's no *long-term* problem because Sebastian (my new dreamboat) is so rich he never even carries money, but I don't want to bother him when his divorce is at a slightly delicate stage, so –'

'I've opted out of the rose-bowl unless everyone pays their own way. Tell Dreamboat to get acquainted with a bunch of five-pound notes.'

'Venetia!' She was shattered.

I hung up.

VII

'Dear Eddie, Drooling at the thought of the Château Lafite. Do you have two bottles? Love, VENETIA.'

Having slipped this note through Eddie's letter-box I crossed the Cathedral sward to the north porch. The bell was tolling for evensong, and as the sidesman showed me to my usual place in the choir, the organ began to play. Five minutes later the procession emerged from the vestry, the congregation stood up –

But Aysgarth was nowhere to be seen.

After the service I did sit on Lady Mary for half an hour in the hope that he might still reach the cloisters, but no one came. I tried to work out what had happened. The appointment with the Bishop had been set for three o'clock. If Aysgarth was still at the South Canonry three and a half hours later, what on earth could be going on?

Returning home I poured myself a double brandy and prepared for a tense vigil by the phone.

VIII

He rang just before eight. 'Darling, I'm so sorry, I –' He stopped. Then he said to someone nearby: 'Just talking to Primrose – I won't be a moment.' Dido's voice droned in the background like a dentist's drill. Then he said to me: 'Listen, Primrose, I must go – I'd forgotten we were dining out. I'll talk to you tomorrow.' And the next moment I heard the click of the receiver being replaced and the buzz of the empty line.

IX

'My darling,' wrote Aysgarth, 'I had rather a rough ride at the South Canonry this afternoon, and when I got home Dido demanded a blow-by-blow description – which I didn't give her as she would have had hysterics, but nevertheless she suspected I wasn't being honest with her, and by the time I'd calmed her down and packed her off to her bedroom to nurse her headache it was nearly half-past five. I was just about to rush off to the Cathedral for evensong when disaster struck: the Architect turned up on my doorstep to discuss the west front, and by the time I'd got rid of him I knew I must have missed you, but I did dash to Lady Mary anyway, just to make sure. Gnashing my teeth at the thought that we'd probably only missed each other by seconds I raced back to phone you – only to find that some more visitors had arrived to see me, and although I did my best to liquidate them they lingered infuriatingly on. Then just as I finally got you on the line Dido surfaced to remind me that we were expected at the Chantry for dinner in five minutes! At that point, I can tell you, I was ready to climb every wall in sight and needed a very hefty scotch to help me keep both feet firmly on the ground. Darling, I'm sorry, sorry, sorry – what a disaster! I felt demented.

'Charles really wheeled on the big guns at the South Canonry. His power-mania is now running riot to such an extent that I feel his true home is in a City boardroom – he's the kind of potentate who would enjoy raising an eyebrow and seeing the Stock Market plunge in consequence. Thank God he's missed out on Canterbury! The Church of England's had a lucky escape.

'Of course I hardly expected the interview to be easy; he'd signalled the episcopal displeasure by summoning me not by phone ("Hullo, Stephen old boy – any chance of seeing you for a tot of Tio Pepe?") but by a letter, *typed*, if you please, by the hag Peabody and signed with the official episcopal signature – a cross (for bishop), then "Charles" and finally "Staro" (for Starbridge). The full text of this icy missive ran: "My dear Dean, I should be greatly obliged if you could come to the South Canonry at 3.00 p.m. to discuss a matter which requires an urgent resolution. Yours sincerely, ✠ CHARLES STARO."

'Very nasty. Well, I togged myself up in my best clerical suit and then I *drove* the three hundred yards to the South Canonry. (No turning up on foot like a suppliant.) The lay-chaplain admitted me in vilely aloof style and ushered me into the episcopal study with a sniff. (Why was I admitted by the *lay*-chaplain? Why not by the chaplain himself? That was a subtle piece of downgrading!) Charles, sitting behind his desk and exuding his very worst public-school/Cambridge snootiness, *didn't stand up*. Damn rude. He just looked at me as if I were some idle undergraduate who hadn't been studying for his exams and said: "Good afternoon, Stephen. Please sit down. I'm afraid we've reached the point where we must settle the fate of the Harriet March sculpture."

'I nearly passed out. I was all set to drag the rug from under his feet on the Bone-Pelham crisis. However, I pulled myself together, sat down and kept my mouth shut. Sometimes silence can be a disconcerting weapon, but Charles didn't turn a hair. He just said bluntly: "The diocesan committee's now been selected for the purpose of advising the Chancellor on this matter, but I see no point in them ever meeting. My mind's made up; I can no longer afford to procrastinate in the hope that you'll see reason. We just can't afford to air this case in the Consistory Court, and I must insist that you withdraw your application for a faculty."

'I said: "I dispute your decision, I dispute the wisdom of your attitude and I dispute your despotic attempt to deprive me of my rights under ecclesiastical law. I demand a hearing before the Chancellor." I thought that would stop him dead in his tracks, but he blasted back: "I deplore your hostility, I deplore your pigheadedness and above all I deplore your refusal to face reality. Do you seriously believe you'd ever be granted a faculty for that junk-heap?"

'I said: "Whether I'm granted a faculty or not is irrelevant. The fact remains that I'm entitled to a hearing in the Consistory Court, and no bishop is entitled to dispense with the law."

'"Don't flaunt that flabby liberal idealism at me!" exploded Charles. "You're just using it to cover up the fact that you're too proud to back down! You know as well as I do that all you'll achieve by a court hearing is nation-wide publicity in the gutter-press, and if you really think I'm going to stand by and let the unchurched masses split their sides laughing over the pornographic taste of the Dean of Starbridge, you'd better think again!"

'I shot back: "If you're so power-mad that you believe you're above the law, I'm complaining to the Archbishop of Canterbury!"

'"I'm the one who'll be complaining to the Archbishop of Canterbury!" shouts Charles. "Either you wash your hands of that sculpture or I'm making a visitation!"

'Silence. I'm winded. I feel as if I've wound up in a pool of blood on the floor, and for a moment I'm so shocked I can't speak. A visitation would be very nasty. In fact it would be very, very nasty indeed in my present circumstances. The last thing I want is the Bishop arriving on the doorstep like the wrath of God, particularly when I've got the west front falling down with the result that I'm obliged to do some juggling with the accounts. (If only I wasn't already juggling! It's true that commissioning the sculpture *was* a trifle more expensive than I'd anticipated, but I knew I could make up the deficit eventually. How was I to know I'd suddenly need a quick thousand to shore up the west front?)

'I see now what must have happened: Charles had the confidence to bludgeon me into a bloodstained heap because he knew I was vulnerable over the accounts. That *traitor* Fitzgerald! He'd tipped off the Archdeacon again.

'Well, I mopped up the blood (metaphorically) and I staggered to my feet (literally) and I said with dignity: "I'm sorry that you should find it necessary to threaten me in such an extremely unedifying manner, and even sorrier that your order puts me in a most awkward moral predicament. Perhaps, as my Bishop, you can advise me how I can face Mrs March with a clear conscience when I repudiate the contract for the sculpture."

'I thought that might make him give an embarrassed twitch, but no, he strokes his pectoral cross – I can't stand it when he does that, I'm sure he only does it to underline the fact that he's reached the episcopal bench in the House of Lords and I haven't – and he retorts: "If you can commission a sculpture on impulse, without consulting your Chapter, from an attractive young woman who batted her eyelashes at you over the dry-martini cocktails, I wouldn't have thought your conscience was too clear in the first place. Pay Mrs March in full so that she has no legal redress and then sever your connection with her. That, I think, will ensure your conscience is a little clearer in future than it is at present."

'I could have hit him.

'But I didn't. Successful clergymen don't go around hitting people and no clergyman in his right mind takes a swing at his bishop. I'm in my right mind. I didn't take a swing. But by heaven, I don't know how I restrained myself.

'When I trusted myself to speak I said: "I've already denied to you that my association with Mrs March is in any way improper. I must tell you that I strongly resent you raking up this slander a second time."

'"And I must tell you," said Charles, "that I've recently heard yet another rumour which implies your association with Mrs March is an improper one. I'm prepared to believe your denials, but I put it to you that the dean of a great cathedral is required to be as far above suspicion as Caesar's wife, and I must frankly declare that I don't wish to hear such scandalous gossip ever again."

'Well, of course, I knew I had to stand up to him, put up a tough front, so I said: "I'm much obliged to you for continuing to believe me innocent of adultery. In the circumstances I suppose I should regard that as an unprecedented favour."

'He just looked at me. I hoped he was going to give me details of this new rumour – naturally I wanted to demolish it – but to my disappointment he changed the subject and said: "Someone was asking about you the other day, someone who always takes an interest in you and wishes you well. Do you ever think of calling on Jon Darrow?"

'I was very surprised. However it was a relief to drop the subject of adultery, so I said amiably enough that I'd planned to look in at Starrington Manor next Christmas, and wasn't it marvellous that the old boy was still ticking over.

'Charles said: "Don't leave it till Christmas. Go soon – he'd really like to see you." And then having allowed himself this little piece of chit-chat in order to ease the truly appalling atmosphere between us, he said tersely: "But to return to the sculpture: I trust I can now rely on you to terminate the arrangement with Mrs March immediately and in a manner which generates no publicity of any kind."

'"As you wish," I said equally tersely, "but I'm sorry. The sculpture's a fine work of modern art – in the opinion of those who have the taste to appreciate it." Then I waited, but when he didn't offer me either his hand or a reply I walked out.

'Well, all I can say is that I've staved off a disastrous visitation. But what a scene! I feel as if he beat me up with that pectoral cross of his. I'd like to – but no, I must get a grip on myself. Violent feelings are utterly wrong for a clergyman. Perhaps I can work mine off by punching a pillow for ten minutes! No, on second thoughts I think it's time for a triple whisky. (The dinner-party tonight was an awful bore but at least the port flowed freely.)

'I haven't yet worked out what to say to Harriet, but I'm sure she'll be decent about the fiasco if I put all the blame squarely on Charles. The stupid part about the rumours is that I'm quite certain she's not interested in carrying on with any man at the moment because she's still wedded to the memory of her hero husband who was killed on Everest. That fact makes this new rumour all the more startling – and worrying too. Where did the story come from and how on earth did it get started? I don't think I can blame Fitzgerald for this one. Scandalous facts – yes. Romantic fiction – no. Not his line of country at all.

'But I must now leave the mystery unsolved and conclude this letter. I'll slip out early tomorrow morning, take the car to Butchers' Alley and pop the envelope through your door – I'll be tempted to ring the bell, I know, but you'd be in your nightdress and I might feel tempted to rip it off. I already feel like ripping everything in sight and giving primeval howls of rage. That **** of a Bishop! I can't *bear* being worsted in a power-struggle like that, I long to WIN! My darling, write *soon* – I feel so starved of your company that I can hardly endure it, vastest, devotedest love, N.'

X

'According to Stephen,' said Eddie as we sipped Château Lafite in his drawing-room and watched the Cathedral turn golden in the evening light, 'he and Charles had a stylish fencing match which Stephen eventually won by graciously withdrawing the sculpture in order to do the pathetically harassed Bishop a favour. I don't believe a word of it.'

'You don't?'

'No. I think Charles, as Dinkie would say, "took him to the cleaners". How *is* Dinkie, by the way?'

'Oh, she's in a ghastly state. She's having an affair with a married man who –' I stopped. I had only drunk half a glass of wine. I said: 'I think I'm going mad.'

'I thought Dinkie was carrying on with –'

'– with Simon, yes. Sorry. Mental aberration.'

'I say, Venetia, you wouldn't by any possible chance be free for the rest of the evening, would you? I've discovered this nice little restaurant where they have a most provocative Pouilly-Fuissé –'

I agreed to go out to dinner.

XI

'Well, thanks, Eddie – it's been fun –'

'Any chance of seeing you next week?'

'Why not? I might as well live it up a little before I have to face the ghastly family reunion at Lord North Street.'

'I'm glad your brother was finally able to buy the rose-bowl on credit.'

'God knows what he bought it on – I think he had to take someone to lunch at the Ritz in order to get the loan. The entire episode with all its shoddy scrounging and revolting extravagance makes me wonder why the British haven't long since guillotined their aristocracy.'

This amused Eddie. 'We seem to have reversed our roles!' he remarked. 'Now that the sculpture crisis is over I'm calm and cheerful, whereas now that you're facing the family reunion you're gloom personified!'

'Well, don't get too cheerful – there's still the problem of how you're going to raise the quick thousand to shore up the west front.'

Eddie said startled at once: 'How did you know about that?'

My stomach seemed to turn a full circle in a single second. My voice said: 'You told me.'

'I know I told you about the west front but I never mentioned any exact sum of money.'

'Then I must have got it from Primrose – you know how the Dean tells her everything.'

'I'm surprised he told her about the Chapter meeting yesterday morning. It developed into a real slanging match when Stephen had to reveal he'd led us astray about the cost of the sculpture.'

I said quickly: 'Primrose was talking about the staff meeting last Monday. Wasn't it Runcival who said the temporary repairs would cost a thousand?'

'Yes, it was, but that slang phrase you used, "a quick thousand", wasn't used by Runcival. As English isn't my native tongue I'm very sensitive to slang, and I know that particular colloquialism only surfaced at yesterday's Chapter meeting.'

'Well, now it's surfacing again,' I said. 'I don't see why the Dean and Chapter should have a monopoly on the well-worn phrase "a quick thousand". Heavens, look at the time, I mustn't keep you hanging around on the doorstep a second longer –'

'But we haven't yet made a date for –'

'Phone me,' I said, and escaped.

XII

'My dearest Venetia, last night was *tremendous*! I really enjoyed your dashing witticisms about Simone de Beauvoir and Jean-Paul Sartre. Listen, I've just seen in the *Starbridge Weekly News* that the latest Ingmar Bergman film is playing at the Rialto. Interested? Much love, EDDIE.'

XIII

'Dear Eddie, Glad you weren't appalled by my philosophical didacticism at dinner – I'm afraid I was tight as Old Harry after all the divine Château Lafite and the even diviner Pouilly-Fuissé. I really shouldn't have had that Rémy Martin afterwards, but never mind, we only live once (on earth, I mean) so one might as well forge ahead with élan. However I don't think I could quite forge ahead to Ingmar Bergman at present – I'm not in the mood for Scandinavian gloom and doom. Why don't I buy some fish and chips and a bottle of hooch so that we can indulge in the sin of gluttony at my flat? After demolishing Sartre's existentialism, I think it's time I behaved like a zombie. We might watch Martin Darrow on TV. Much love, VENETIA.'

XIV

'. . . and my darling, I couldn't help noticing at Castle Brigga this afternoon that you weren't quite yourself – although of course looking as beautiful as ever and being just as wonderfully sympathetic as always – and suddenly I had the dreadful thought that maybe you'd met the Great Paragon. Even though you were so generous to me in our dear little hollow I had the impression that you were somehow separated from me by something, and after we'd parted I felt in a cold panic for hours – although perhaps my imagination's running riot merely because I'm so dreading losing you. But my darling, if ever there *was* someone else, you would tell me, wouldn't you? I do like to think that we tell each other everything. Of course it would slaughter me to know that the Great Paragon had finally arrived, but I'd rather know than not know – even though I can't imagine how I'd ever survive without you, I love you so much and no words could ever express how grateful I am to you for so utterly restoring my self-esteem after my recent hellish confrontations with the Bishop and the Chapter. You've been so sweet, so understanding, so loving, so kind, so –'

XV

'This is very nice *vin ordinaire*, Venetia. A most interesting bouquet. It goes well with the fish and chips.'

'Shut up, Eddie, and let's enjoy Martin Darrow.'

'Will you kick me out if I hold your hand?'

'You sound as if you'd prefer to be kicked.'

'Oh Venetia, I –'

'*Shut up!* I want to have thirty minutes of absolute quiet while I goggle at the box.'

Eddie shut up.

We watched one of the summer repeats of *Down at the Surgery*. Martin Darrow, dark, debonair and richly amusing, lit up the screen with his presence. After a while Eddie reached out and encircled my fingers with his huge hot clammy paw.

I somehow managed to keep my fish and chips in my stomach.

XVI

'. . . and darling, *darling* Neville, I just don't know how you could have received such an utterly false impression – if I seemed *distraite* at Castle Brigga it was only because I was so worried about you. Of course there's no one else! I love you and no one but you, I'll love you for ever and ever – in fact, I love you so much that *I'd even lay down my life to save you*, so don't talk to me any more about loving someone else, never even think of it because *you're* the Great Paragon, *you*, my adored one, my dearest love, my *darling* Mr Dean –'

XVII

'Darling Venetia, I'm scribbling this in the Monday staff meeting because I've just had a tremendous idea and I can't wait to let you know about it: why don't I come up to town on the day after your mother's seventieth birthday and take you out to dinner at the Savoy? Say yes and I shall be in ecstasy. Passionate love, EDDIE.'

XVIII

'My darling, I'm scrawling this in the Monday staff meeting where Runcival the Master-Mason is going on and on and on about the blank-blank west front. My undying thanks for your magnificent and moving letter which made me want to sing the Hallelujah Chorus at the top of my voice on the Cathedral sward – only the thought of the sopranos' top notes deterred me! But thank God, darling, you're never likely to be in a position where you have to sacrifice your life to keep me safe.

'I think I'm recovering from THAT BISHOP. I've had a top-secret conference with the bank manager about raising the quick thousand and I'm now sure I can pull off a loan without mortgaging any property – I've promised him I'll stage a really gargantuan performance of "The Messiah" this Christmas to recoup my losses. Fitzgerald's bound to growl: "I thought we were running a cathedral, not a concert hall," but he can't raise any serious objection to "The Messiah", and I know I'll win through in the end.

'(LATER) The Clerk of the Works has just been reading us a doomsday script about the state of the fabric, and declares that in twenty years' time the spire will fall down. This gives a completely new twist, I must say, to the famous pronouncement: *"Après nous le déluge!"* Eddie's now scribbling furiously, probably eager to produce some earnest memorandum. Poor old Eddie, he's been a bit excitable lately – I think the sculpture crisis has told on him. When we met this morning he said he wanted to go up to London after Sunday evensong for a reunion with some old chums from the Anglo-German Churchmen's Fellowship, and could I stand in for him at the early services on Monday. Well, of course officially he's supposed to be tethered to the Cathedral this month as he's the canon-in-residence, but I think he deserves a short break and I'm very willing to help him out. What a tower of strength he's been to me recently! After Fitzgerald's betrayals I've got to the stage where I really appreciate loyalty, and as I told you once not so very long ago, at least I can always rely on Eddie never to stab me in the back. All my love, my darling, my angel, my –'

XIX

'Dear Eddie, Okay. Dinner at the Savoy on Sunday night. But I warn you, I'll be a basket-case after my mother's party and may well be unable to speak. You'd better come to Lord North Street at around six-thirty to have a drink and say "hiya" to the parents.

'Meanwhile there's something I want to ask you: when is a confession not a confession? An old school-friend of mine, Margaret Wharton, saw an Anglo-Catholic priest the other day and told him a lot of things about her married lover. Afterwards she found out to her horror that the priest counsels her lover's boss.

Margaret wasn't actually in the confessional with this priest, she was just chatting. Is there a remote possibility that the priest could pass on to the boss the fact that the married lover is up to his neck in adultery? Margaret can't sleep a wink at night for worrying about this. Please advise instantly. Lots of love, V.'

XX

'My darling Venetia, If the priest betrays a single syllable he should be reported to his bishop. Confidential conversations aren't confined to the confessional.

'Many thanks for the invitation to Lord North Street. I'll bring your mother a belated birthday present. She's very keen on plants, isn't she? In tremendous spirits, *much* love, EDDIE.'

XXI

'My darling Neville, I'm glad to report with enormous relief that the great family orgy is over and we now have ten years to recover before my mother reaches eighty. Everyone behaved well, although that idiot Harold made a revoltingly sentimental speech – my father and I looked at each other and knew instantly that we both wanted to throttle him – and Oliver arrived slightly tight from the Reform Club – and Henrietta would keep boring us with stories about her dogs – and Sylvia talked on and on about her pregnancy (if I were pregnant I hope I'd have the good taste to keep my mouth shut and not go so nauseously mumsy-wumsy) – and Absolutely-the-Bottom Arabella kept tossing her newly-blonded hair all over the place as she prattled about Sebastian, her current "dreamboat", who must be just about the most brainless hunk on earth to fall for all that rubbish.

'Mama was thrilled with the rose-bowl which Sylvia had tricked out with those ghastly scentless roses which always look like plastic. In fact Mama adored the whole circus and even shed a tear after Harold's frightful speech and said how lucky she was to have such a wonderful glorious family, and we all slobbered over her shamelessly and told her how lucky we were to have such a wonderful glorious mother. God knows how much champagne we all drank. Papa even started declaiming in classical Greek. The whole evening was a huge success.

'This morning I'm slightly hung-over but I did just want to dash off a letter so that you wouldn't feel "starved". Darling, I'm thinking of you constantly and counting the hours that separate us – in fact I hardly know how to wait until we're at Castle Brigga once more . . .'

XXII

'How very clever it was of you,' I said to Eddie as we dined at the Savoy, 'to give my mother that book. Victorian water-colours of plants! She'll be your friend for life now.'

'I hope so,' said Eddie blandly, sipping his champagne.

Silence fell. I toyed with my grilled sole and wished I felt hungry. Frantically I searched for a new topic of conversation. 'Well, don't keep me in suspense!' I said brightly, making an artistic mound of my spinach. 'I've been deprived of the Starbridge news for two whole days! What's the latest shattering development?'

'Dido came to see me.'

My knife clattered on my plate. I tried to grasp the handle again but something seemed to have happened to my fingers. Casually my voice said: 'Oh yes? What a bore! What did she want to talk about?'

'Stephen.'

'Well, that's hardly a new departure, I suppose.' I took a large gulp of champagne and managed to get my knife under control. 'But what did the old girl say?'

'She's terrified of the Bishop.'

'Oh God, don't tell me she had hysterics all over your drawing-room!'

'No, she was well in control of herself, although I wouldn't have been surprised to see a touch of hysteria. I think she's right to be terrified.'

'But why? The Bone-Pelham crisis was defused, the sculpture mess has now been swept under the rug and I'm sure the Dean will somehow raise the money to shore up the west front – why should Dido suddenly start twittering in terror?'

'Because my worst nightmare's come true and there's a rumour going around that Stephen's having an affair with Harriet March.'

I managed to say after only a fractional pause: 'You mean because he commissioned the sculpture on an impulse while she was simpering at him during a party?'

'No, there's a new rumour, and Dido says it's already reached the South Canonry. Apparently (and Stephen didn't tell me this) Charles indicated during their big showdown that the story was known to him. Of course Stephen must have denied everything, but I think this could finally be the point where the Bishop pulls out the long knife. We all know what he's like on the subject of sexual morality. He may overlook heavy drinking, commissioning pornographic sculpture and juggling with the accounts, but he's not going to turn a blind eye to a sexual indiscretion.'

I drained my glass. As a passing waiter immediately refilled it I said: 'What I'd like to know is how this bloody silly new rumour ever got off the ground.' Automatically I started drinking again.

'According to Dido, Stephen's been seen driving around with a glamorous, long-haired young woman on his day off – and of course that description does fit Harriet March.'

'Obviously someone's mistakenly identified the man as the Dean.'

'No, there's no question of mistaken identity. Apparently Stephen almost caused a traffic accident in Chasuble Lane a few weeks ago, and the policeman who happened to be passing by not only recognised him but spoke to him. Before joining the force this man had worked in the stonemasons' yard at the Cathedral, so –'

'But how did the story reach Dido if the policeman no longer has any connection with the Close?'

'Oh, a good story will always grow wings and fly! The policeman told his former work-mates in the pub that a young woman like a film star with long, wavy dark hair had jumped out of the Dean's car and vanished as if she was anxious to avoid publicity. The enthralled work-mates told Runcival who told the Clerk of the Works who told Tommy Fitzgerald who told Paul Dalton who told his sister who told Dido –'

'– who told you. I see. But then who told the Bishop?'

'It was almost certainly the Archdeacon. Tommy tipped him off about the sculpture, and the odds are he tipped him off again about the rumour. And of course once the Archdeacon knew –'

'But surely there could be a perfectly innocent explanation? For instance, two of the Archdeacon's daughters have long wavy hair, and Sally, if not Julie, could certainly be described as glamorous. Why shouldn't the Dean have been giving her a lift? And why, when he got stuck with the policeman in Chasuble Lane, shouldn't she have nipped out and popped home to the vicarage down Butchers' Alley?'

'Funnily enough I offered Dido the same explanation, but she just said that no matter how many innocent explanations were offered, the Bishop would continue to think the worst.'

'That sounds as if she's secretly suspecting the worst herself!'

'No, Dido seems absolutely convinced that Stephen would never have a fully consummated love affair with anyone. But of course a clergyman can get in a scandalous mess without committing an act which is legally defined as adultery, and what Dido's afraid of is that Stephen's dabbled in a flirtation that's somehow got out of control.'

'I just can't believe he'd be quite such a fool.' I drained my glass of champagne again. 'Dare I ask how this interview with Dido ended, or will that spoil the punchline of your story?'

'She asked me to intervene. She said none of the sons had ever been able to talk to him and I was the only man who could possibly help. That's true, of course. Funny how Dido always gets the personal relationships dead right –'

'But what on earth does she expect you to say?'

'She wants me to spell out the cold hard facts of life and bring him down to earth. She's convinced that having lost touch with reality by indulging in this heavy flirtation, he's now in the most frightful danger – and I'm bound to say,' said Eddie as he too finished his glass of champagne, 'I think she's absolutely right.'

'I think she's round the bend.'

'No, Venetia. You've got Dido dead wrong. I know she's tormented by a neurotic temperament, but she's honest, she's loyal and she's brave – brave enough to face this appalling crisis without flinching. She wants to save Stephen. And so do I. And so, I think, do you.'

'Well, of course I do! I'm just boggling at her melodramatic suggestion that you should stage some monstrous scene in which you spell out the cold hard facts of life like a teacher trying to educate a sub-normal pupil! You're not really going to do as she suggests, are you?'

'I've already done it,' said Eddie.

I nearly passed out. 'You mean you've seen him?'

'No. Not him. I came to the conclusion,' said Eddie, laying down his knife and fork, 'that it wasn't actually Stephen I had to see.'

And as I stared, too shocked to move or speak, he raised his head and looked me straight in the eyes.

FIVE

— ◆◆ —

'It is in his chapter on the "New Morality" that Catholics
would feel themselves unable to go far with Dr. Robinson.'

ANONYMOUS
The Honest to God Debate
ed. DAVID L. EDWARDS

I

I looked away.

I stared at my mangled fish. I stared at my sculpted spinach.
I stared at the shining cutlery and the snow-white table-cloth
and the champagne bottle in the ice-bucket and the carnation
in the vase.

There was a long, long silence.

Then Eddie spoke again. He spoke quietly, and as I listened
I noticed that a small potato remained on his plate. It's strange
what the mind registers in moments of overpowering horror
and fear.

Eddie said: 'Marry me.'

The outline of the dinner-plate began to blur.

He said: 'It's all right. I understand. It's all right.'

My hands were twisting my napkin into a lump in my lap. I
was unable to reply.

'We'll have fun,' he said. 'I know we would. We'd be good
friends. It would work. And we'd live in London, not just
because you wouldn't want to live permanently in the provinces,
but because ... well, I could no longer work in Starbridge,
and London's the place where I'd be most likely to land a
good job. I've worked there before and my curriculum vitae's
excellent.'

I managed to nod but still I could not speak.

'You could share in my career or you could be quite independent. I'm used to coping with the work on my own so I wouldn't insist that you converted yourself into a clerical wife.'

My voice said with difficulty: 'Sounds reasonable.'

'Think it over,' said Eddie as the waiter removed our plates. 'Of course I hardly need add that you have the complete freedom to say no – this isn't a bizarre attempt to blackmail you into marriage – but I honestly do think that you and I –'

'Quite.' I reached for my glass but it was empty. 'The trouble is,' I said, 'I can't imagine ever leaving Starbridge.'

'It'll be horrifically difficult for both of us. But even if you don't marry me, something's got to be done, Venetia. Things can't go on as they are.'

'Oh, I quite see that.' I fidgeted with my glass before adding: 'I don't love you.'

'I think you could. I'll take the risk.'

'All these scandalous risks –'

'There's nothing scandalous about marrying a girl one's loved for a long time, and I think it's a gamble that'll come off. We like each other, we get on –'

'Yes,' I said. 'Happy ending. Soaring violins. Golden sunset.' I started to cry.

'Darling Venetia – my dear, I'm so sorry, don't cry – please – everything's going to be all right –'

'Not for him. That Bishop –'

'The Bishop as yet has no proof. No witness has identified you as the girl in the Dean's car, and as you pointed out a moment ago, that girl could have been one of Malcolm Lindsay's daughters. The Bishop may suspect you – although in fact I can't think why he should – but if you now leave Starbridge he'll never know for certain.'

I tried to wipe away my tears with my napkin. At last I said: 'Does Dido suspect, do you think?'

'I'm sure of it. She never mentioned your name but I'm convinced she must know.'

'But how could she?' I was appalled. 'He was always so careful!'

'Yes, but Dido's so shrewd about personal relationships, and there was a lot of evidence lying around.'

'What evidence?'

'The sort of evidence which I can now clearly see with the wisdom of hindsight but which Dido would have picked up much earlier. I'd guess she suspected as soon as you stayed on in Starbridge but severed yourself from Primrose. It was all so odd, so mysterious . . . and you looked so stunning, so radiant, yet there was apparently no man in your life. I myself had no trouble swallowing the theory that you'd undergone a religious conversion – it's a well-known phenomenon and it does result in both radical change and enhanced vitality – but I doubt if Dido would have swallowed it so easily. Then there was the fact that Stephen was so buoyant at a time when he should have been bowed down by the Cathedral crises. This would have been glaringly obvious to Dido – it was glaringly obvious to me, but because I was wrapped up in the wrong theory I never actually connected you with Stephen until –'

'The quick thousand for the west front.' I dragged my napkin across my aching eyes.

'It just seemed such a coincidence that you should have used that same raffish phrase. And then as soon as the truth occurred to me everything seemed blindingly obvious.'

I realised I had ruined my make-up as usual. Black streaks marred the white napkin.

Mumbling an excuse I groped my way to my feet and stumbled to the cloakroom.

II

After I had finished vomiting I cleaned up my face, but my hands were trembling so much that I was unable to reapply my eye make-up.

'I'll take you home,' said Eddie as soon as he saw my haggard appearance.

'I'm terribly sorry –'

'No need to apologise.'

Halfway down Whitehall I said: 'I don't know what you think he and I got up to, but –'

'It doesn't matter.'

'– we didn't –'

'I don't want to know.'

I started to cry again. 'It'll kill him if I break it off.'

'No, it'll save him. It'll wake him from the dream.'

'He'll die of grief.'

'No, that only happens in books. He'll live. He'll only be destroyed if you stay and wreck his career.'

'But how terrible that it should be *you* – and *I* – who have to –'

'Sometimes you have to shed blood in order to save lives. Think of surgeons.'

But I could not think of surgeons. I could only think of my doomed Mr Dean. I began to weep uncontrollably.

'Lord North Street!' pronounced the taxi driver glumly after we had remained stationary for some time.

'Drive around Smith Square, please,' said Eddie, 'and drive slowly.'

As the car crawled on I succeeded in drying my eyes, but the realisation that I was almost home made me panic. 'My God, what can I look like? If my parents see me –'

'Shall I come in and create a diversion while you rush upstairs to bed?'

But I knew I could bear his company no longer. I told him I would manage.

'Travel back with me tomorrow,' he said. 'I'm getting the ten-fifteen.'

'No, I've got to be alone, I've got to think.'

'All right, but phone me if you change your mind. I'm staying at the Stafford.'

Having circled Smith Square at a funereal pace we wound up back in Lord North Street.

'Darling . . .' He gave me such a brief kiss that I barely noticed it. 'Remember: I love you. We'll have fun. It'll work.'

We parted. The taxi disappeared. Turning the key in the lock with shaking fingers I crept into the hall. Raucous laughter from the drawing-room upstairs indicated that a social gathering was in progress, but as I tiptoed past, praying that my presence in the house would not be immediately discovered, the door opened and my mother appeared. She exclaimed: 'Ah, Venetia!' But then her expression changed and she said no more.

I muttered: 'Rather tired. Long day. 'Night.' And fled to my room.

Later my mother tapped on my locked door and said: 'Anything I can do, darling?' but I pretended to be asleep and she went away.

III

'Darling Eddie, I've thought it over and concluded that you're right. We'd have fun. It'd work. But don't rush me. I've got to figure out how to tell him. That may take a little time and meanwhile please tell *no one* how things stand between us. Thanks for being so nice when I wrecked dinner. Lots of love, VENETIA.'

IV

'My darling Neville, I can't wait to see you – staying on an extra day in London was a big mistake. A party of us went to dine at the Savoy but I hated every moment and when I got home I lay awake all night longing for you. In fact I've missed you so much that I've felt quite ill, but at least these two days in London have proved to me beyond any doubt that I love you more than anyone else in the world, and I'm now utterly convinced that so long as you're drawing breath on this earth I could never be happy with anyone else. My darling Mr Dean, I hardly know how to wait for Wednesday but meanwhile this comes to you with undying – yes, *undying* – love from your adoring and devoted V.'

V

I sent both letters from the post office in Tufton Street, and as soon as Eddie's envelope slipped from my fingers I wanted to claw it back.

Yet even if I had been able to retrieve the letter I would have had no choice but to post it again. Unless I converted myself into a lost prize, Aysgarth would never let go of me and then without doubt he would be destroyed.

On my way home I reached the church in the centre of Smith Square. Round and round the church I walked, the church of St John the Evangelist. '"In the beginning was the Word,"' Father Darrow had said, quoting St John's Gospel, but it was a word I could no longer hear.

My head was throbbing. I could barely see. I hardly knew what I was doing.

'Darling Eddie . . . We'd have fun. It'd work . . .'

'My darling Neville, I can't wait to see you . . .'

Two people, I was being divided between two people, but no, I was dividing *into* two people, it was as if someone was hacking away with a meat cleaver and splitting my personality from top to bottom. I saw clearly then not only that I was mad but that we were all three of us mad, Aysgarth, Eddie and I – all mad and all in hell! – and all the time the Great Pollutant was spewing its filth across our lives.

VI

As I prepared to leave, my mother said again: 'Is there anything I can do, darling?' but I answered kindly: 'No, you run along and attend to your plants.' No point in bothering the old girl, particularly when she had just enjoyed such a splendid birthday with all her wonderful, glorious children.

My father said: 'Goodbye, Venetia. I enjoyed meeting Hoffenberg again. A thoroughly nice chap,' and patted me encouragingly on the shoulder, but of course he was always hopeless with women.

I caught the eleven-fifteen train and arrived in Starbridge ninety minutes later. At the flat I found a shoal of letters from Aysgarth. He was writing morning, noon and night, and suddenly the colossal weight of his love seemed suffocating; I felt as if not only all the breath but all the blood was being squeezed from my body. I couldn't even open the letters. I could only sit on the edge of the sofa and clutch the envelopes.

Eventually I managed to phone Eddie. 'Look,' I said, 'this morning I posted you a revoltingly graceless note saying I'd go ahead. I just want to say I'm sorry it was so revoltingly graceless. You deserve better.'

'Venetia!'

'I want very much to marry you and I'm quite sure it's the right thing to do.'

'But this is sensational! I –'

'I'm seeing him on Wednesday. I'll end it all then.'

'Darling, I'm so happy, so –'

I got rid of him but just as I was reaching for the gin bottle the phone rang. Wretched Eddie no doubt wanted to rush to the flat and slobber over me. Wanting only to be alone I grabbed the receiver in a rage. 'Yes?'

'My darling.'

My rage was wiped out. All memory of Eddie was wiped out. Everything was wiped out except the sound of that voice. Blindly I sank down on the sofa.

'I had to phone,' he said. 'Couldn't stop myself. Had to hear your voice.'

'Darling – oh Neville –'

'I can't wait till Wednesday, I've got to see you. Lady Mary after evensong?'

I agreed to meet him in the cloisters that evening.

VII

Well, of course, I couldn't do it, could I? I couldn't end the affair. I couldn't end it in the cloisters that evening, I couldn't end it on Wednesday at Castle Brigga, I couldn't end it when I wrote to him every day. I couldn't end it, and all the time Eddie was hovering in an agony of anxiety as I repeatedly promised him: 'I'll do it. I really will.'

At Castle Brigga I said idly to Aysgarth when he mentioned the subject of Primrose's limp friendship with Tait: 'Do you think Maurice has ever proposed?' and when to my surprise I received an affirmative answer, I asked: 'But do you think she's right to turn him down?'

'Of course!' He was shocked. 'No girl should ever marry a man she doesn't love.'

'But Maurice would nonetheless be a husband, wouldn't he? He'd give her status and self-respect and a real life at last.'

'Without love all that would be meaningless.'

'But she'd probably come to love him later.'

'That doesn't necessarily follow at all. I told Primrose: "Never marry a man you don't care for with passion," and she promised me she never would.'

'But darling, Prim doesn't exactly have the suitors queuing up, does she, and time's ticking on —'

'I'd rather she stayed a spinster than married without love.'

'Isn't that much too idealistic? Have you, a very masculine man, any real grasp of what spinsterhood actually means?'

But he only said stubbornly: 'One must have one's ideals; that's what separates us from the animals. To marry without love is a crime.'

That was the moment when I should have said: 'It's a crime I'm about to commit,' but I could only exclaim warmly: 'Darling Neville, what a romantic you are!' – and yet again poor Eddie slipped far to the back of my mind.

VIII

'You've got to tell him, Venetia,' said Eddie. 'I'm sorry, I know you don't want to be pushed but the time's come when I don't just have to push – I have to give you the biggest possible shove. He's in greater danger with every day that passes. Tommy Fitzgerald said to me today: "I think the Dean writes letters to a lady-love during the staff meetings. When I put on my distance glasses I could see the words 'My darling' at the top of the page."'

'Oh my God –'

'And if Tommy chooses to pass on *that* piece of information to the Archdeacon –'

'I'll end it tomorrow at Castle Brigga,' I said.

But I didn't see how I ever could.

I drank myself senseless with gin and passed out some time before dawn.

IX

'Neville! Thank God I've managed to get you on the phone. Look, I can't make it this afternoon, I feel appalling – no, don't panic, it's nothing for you to worry about, just menstruation de luxe – really, I can't think why God couldn't have made female organs more cleverly, they're nothing but trouble, even worse than teeth.'

'My poor darling, I'm so sorry – but I've got to see you soon or I'll go mad. What about tomorrow? I'll cancel everything –'

'No, tomorrow's no good. I've got to work for the Bishop. How about Friday?'

We agreed to meet in the car-park of the Rialto cinema on Friday afternoon. That gave me two days to decide how I was going to do the impossible, and for the first time in my life I began to understand why people committed suicide. But of course I wasn't the suicidal type.

Or was I?

Taking two aspirins to kill my hang-over I reached again for the gin bottle.

It was five minutes past seven in the morning.

X

'And now,' said the Bishop, smooth, powerful and dangerous in a pitch-black suit, 'having completed all the chapters except the one on ethics, I think it's finally time to demolish the New Morality.'

The sweat prickled on my forehead.

'We'll start,' said Dr Ashworth after a pause to survey the battlefield, 'with some random observations as usual. Are you ready?'

'Yes, Bishop.' My mouth was bone-dry.

'Number one: Dr Robinson is attempting to apply the principle of *Situationethik* –' He spelled the word before interpolating: '– better to use the German designation, I think, as that calls attention to the original writing on the subject – a theory of morals according to which there is no human action which would be morally wrong in every circumstance. This theory parts company with the traditional teaching of the Catholic Church which, while acknowledging that vast numbers of moral decisions are determined by the "situation" – that is, the circumstances of each particular case – nonetheless holds that some actions are intrinsically wrong and can never under any circumstances be justified.

'Dr Robinson contends that when attempting to resolve a moral dilemma nothing is prescribed – except love. The Catholic Church would agree with this, *but* – underline the "but", please – it would say that this prescription must take into account certain absolute limits to conduct; the maintaining of such absolute limits is a safeguard against the sinfulness and fallibility of man. Dr Robinson, however, rejecting objective standards in advocating a subjective approach, declares that a solution to each moral dilemma can be discovered merely by surveying all the facts with loving compassion.

'This is, of course, impossible.

'Human beings are not omniscient, and only God can ever know all the facts in any given case. For example, a well-meaning counsellor may approach a case with enormous loving compassion yet because of either ignorance or wishful thinking or misunderstanding or just plain stupidity come to a conclusion which is entirely wrong. Love is not enough. We must have objective standards which provide the poor, faltering, limited human race with at least some indication of how we should conduct ourselves in order to avoid misery and destruction. The Bishop, I fear, has far too high an opinion of modern man's ability to soar above his sinful, fallible nature and play God in ethical matters with impunity.

'Number two: the Bishop writes as if Christianity were no more than a weak love ethic. Christianity is indeed about love but it is also about salvation and redemption. It is directed not towards a so-called modern man who lives some idyllic existence in which every problem can be solved with a kiss and a cuddle. It deals with people as they are – and very often they're suffering, floundering amidst tragedy, perhaps even screaming in agony as the result of their wrong actions and the wrong actions of others. What has Dr Robinson to say to these people? Absolutely nothing. You must say rather more than: "All you need is love!" to someone who is tortured by guilt, racked with grief or overpowered by despair. When a man is being crucified during his personal Good Friday, he needs someone who symbolises Easter Sunday and the redemptive love of Christ, not some sunny-natured fool who bounces around at the foot of the cross and showers him with sentimental good will.

'Number three: the Bishop theorises a great deal about human relationships but seems to have only the sketchiest idea about how his theories would work in practice. If a young man and a young woman are in love, he suggests, the young man will ask himself not: do I sleep with her? But: do I love her? According to Dr Robinson, if the answer is yes, then the young man, glorified by his passion, will abstain from sexual intercourse in order not to take advantage of his girl-friend. However, I put it to Dr Robinson that this is sheer romantic idealism which has no relation to reality. The young man, in reality, will ask himself: do I sleep with her? And immediately he'll answer: you bet – if I can! He may be full of good intentions; he may sincerely believe he loves the girl; he may even wish to marry her eventually, but if a sexual attraction exists he'll want to take the young lady to bed. And perhaps he will marry her. And perhaps they will indeed live happily ever after. One must always allow for cases where both parties are blessed by extraordinary good luck. But perhaps, alternatively, he'll tire of her; perhaps he'll abuse her love; perhaps she'll abuse his; perhaps there'll be an abortion, a breakdown, even suicide. There are any number of possibilities inherent in this situation, but two things at least are certain: first, sex is the most powerful drive known to man and any ethical theory that fails to take this into account must be seriously deficient. And second, such a powerful force can lay waste, maim and kill as efficiently as a powerful force such as a hurricane or an earthquake. Bearing this fact of life in mind, it would seem prudent to devise rules and safeguards which will help to minimise the potential damage. Dr Robinson has very much more confidence than I have in both the wisdom of inexperienced young people and their ability to protect themselves from serious harm.

'Number four: the Bishop tells us we find God in loving relationships. Certainly we do. But supposing someone, through no fault of his own, has no loving relationships in his life; are we to say that in his loneliness he has no access to God? Or supposing a loving relationship comes to an end; are we to say that the parties concerned must part from God as well as each other? God cannot, I suggest, be confined merely to loving relationships, and I would also suggest that it is not only God who can be found there. The Devil can infiltrate any situation, and it's quite possible to have an extremely loving relationship which is absolutely wrong and utterly destructive, not only for the parties themselves but for the innocent people who depend on them. The classic example of this, of course,' said Dr Ashworth, pausing in his peregrinations to hover at my side, 'is adultery. Have you got that, Venetia?'

'Yes, Bishop.'

'You don't seem to be writing.'

'I . . .'

'Never mind, these are only rough notes. I'll go more slowly. The classic example (as I was saying) is adultery. Number five: by adopting this subjective approach to ethics the Bishop seems to be aligning himself with those people who declare that the real obscenity in our society today is not sex but violence. Sex, I agree, is not an obscenity. But the abuse of sex, I would argue, is deeply obscene. I think it not surprising that at this stage of the century there should be a backlash against strict standards in sexual conduct, but I prophesy that the people who are now busy tearing up the old rules will reap rather more than they bargained for. I also venture to suggest that more harm, more grief and more soul-destroying misery are caused to more people by the abuse of the sexual rules than by the use of violence. For example, anyone who has ever witnessed the carnage wrought by a devastating adulterous liaison could never forget the horror of seeing people slowly driven mad by their – Venetia! My dear girl, what's the matter?'

I finally broke down.

XI

'Right,' said the Bishop swiftly, 'don't move. Take this –' A handkerchief was stuffed into my shaking hand '– and hold on. Help's coming.' And sweeping to the door he flung it open and shouted: 'Darling!' just as he did when he returned home from an outing.

I sat glued to my chair and clutched his handkerchief and shuddered with dry, hoarse, racking sobs. Clear-eyed I stared at my open notebook and the shorthand which I knew I could never read back.

Voices sounded in the hall. I heard the Bishop say urgently: 'It's Venetia,' and I also heard Mrs Ashworth's lightning response: 'Leave this to me.'

Hurrying into the room she stooped over me and put an arm around my shoulders. 'You're exhausted, aren't you?' she said briskly. 'You must have a complete rest. I'll tell everyone you've got flu.'

Tears finally streamed down my cheeks. I clutched her. But I was unable to speak.

'Come along,' said Mrs Ashworth, mercifully unemotional. 'I'll put you to bed and give you a couple of sleeping pills so that you can switch off and pass out. Much the best thing to do.'

She helped me to my feet and steered me upstairs. No one was in the hall. The telephone started to ring but someone answered it. The stairs seemed to go on for ever. 'You can have the best spare-room,' said Mrs Ashworth. 'It's got a beautiful view of the meadows, very soothing and restful. I'll just get you a pair of Charley's pyjamas. I'm afraid my nightdresses wouldn't fit you.'

I sat down on the spare-room bed. The view was indeed very beautiful, and I thought how tactful it was of her not to give me a room which faced the Cathedral. But then I remembered she had no idea why I should now find any view of the Cathedral unbearable. The lapse frightened me. I had to remember I was among the enemy; I had to take fanatical care to make no mistakes.

Still shivering from head to toe I began to plot a plausible excuse for my collapse.

XII

'So sorry to be such a bore,' I said to Mrs Ashworth unsteadily when she brought me the sleeping tablets, 'but the truth is I didn't level with you earlier about Perry Palmer. I'm madly in love with him but he gave me a terrible time when I went up to London for my mother's birthday and I've done nothing but drink gin ever since. All rather a nightmare. But I'm sure I'll sort myself out eventually.'

'Poor Venetia,' said Mrs Ashworth, sounding sincerely sympathetic but remaining expressionless. 'I'm so very sorry. Now do please take these tablets and pass out.'

Downing the pills I keeled over out of torment into oblivion.

XIII

'Can I make any phone calls for you?' offered Mrs Ashworth as she brought me tea that evening. 'Is there anyone who might ring your flat and be concerned when there was no reply?'

I had to struggle to think. My brain was still sluggish from the pills but I thought of Aysgarth, receiving no letter from me at seven o'clock on the following morning and unable to contact me by phone. Then with horror I remembered that I was due to meet him in the afternoon for our postponed outing. If I failed to appear he would be demented.

'What's the matter?' said Mrs Ashworth sharply.

'Nothing.' My panic was so great I could hardly breathe.

'Now Venetia, that's quite obviously not true. You're white as a ghost and you look terrified –'

'Mrs Ashworth, I've got to talk to Eddie Hoffenberg.'

'I'll ring him for you.'

'No, no – I've got to speak to him myself, I must, I shan't sleep a wink unless I speak to him!'

'Very well.' Mrs Ashworth said no more but led me into a light airy bedroom where a white telephone sat on a table by a large double bed.

Having collapsed on the counterpane I waited till she had left the room and then feverishly started to dial.

'Eddie,' I said as he answered, 'listen carefully. This is an emergency. I collapsed at the South Canonry this afternoon – exhaustion, nothing more – and I'm staying here for a couple of days while Mrs Ashworth announces to everyone that I have flu. I told her –' I hesitated, acutely aware that my words could be falling among eavesdroppers '– I told her about my awful love affair with Perry,' I said. 'I had to explain why I was in such a state.'

'I understand,' said Eddie without hesitation. 'Would you like me to tell him you're temporarily out of circulation?'

'Could you? I'm meeting him tomorrow afternoon, and if I don't turn up –'

'Leave it to me. But Venetia, you'll really have to end this affair with Perry, you know.'

'Yes, but –'

'You must write to him. I was a fool to think you could break it off in any other way.'

'I'll write later, I promise –'

'No,' said Eddie, 'you'll write now. I'm not standing any more of this procrastination.'

'But Eddie, I'm ill, I –'

'Once the letter's written you'll feel better.'

'No, I can't do it now, I can't –'

'I tell you, YOU MUST! You'll ruin him, you'll ruin yourself, you'll ruin everyone if you go on like this one day longer!'

I started to sob.

'I'll be at the South Canonry at eleven o'clock tomorrow morning,' said Eddie, 'and if that letter's not written, I'll break the news to him myself.'

'No!' I screamed but he had hung up.

I sobbed and sobbed.

Eventually Mrs Ashworth appeared and without a word led me back to bed. I got rid of her by pretending to be asleep. Then I lay awake in agony until dawn.

XIV

'My darling Neville, There's no kind, gentle way to say this, but . . .'

'Dear Neville, How I hate to write this, but . . .'

'Darling Neville, I can hardly bring myself to tell you this, but . . .'

'Dearest Neville, You'll never forgive me, but . . .'

I paused to burn all these attempts at confession in the ashtray and tried yet again to find the words to express the unspeakable. It was now the morning after my collapse and I was still lying in bed. I had brushed my hair but made no attempt to apply make-up. Intermittently I wept. Charley's pyjamas, pale green cotton adorned with dark green piping, provided a touch of chic which was bizarrely at odds with my shadowed, drawn face. I looked like the worst kind of heroin addict, someone who could barely survive from one fix to the next. No wonder Mrs Ashworth had instantly diagnosed me as exhausted, and no wonder she had instinctively decided that such a seamy disintegration had to be passed off as a socially acceptable bout of flu.

With terror I realised it was almost eleven o'clock and the letter was still unwritten. Picking up my pen I wrote in a mindless daze of panic and pain: 'Neville, forgive me but I can't go on, I'm marrying Eddie, I don't want to hurt you but I can't go on, sorry, sorry, sorry but I can't go on, there are no more words, V.'

There was a knock on the door, and as I started violently my hostess looked in. 'Are you sure you feel up to seeing anyone?' she asked. 'If I rang Eddie now I could probably catch him before —' She broke off as the doorbell rang downstairs. 'That must be him,' she said. 'He's early. But Venetia, if you want to change your mind —'

'No.' I was stuffing the letter into an envelope, sealing the flap. 'I must see him.' My fingers were very stiff and I hardly knew what I was doing but I laid the unaddressed envelope on the bedside table beside the ashtray overflowing with cigarette butts. In the distance I was aware of voices followed by footsteps but I paid them no attention. I could only concentrate on straightening the bedclothes as if I thought that by smoothing the sheet I could smooth away my turmoil.

The next moment I had a shock: the door swung wide and the Bishop walked in. I had not seen him since my collapse, but no doubt that was because his wife had advised him to keep away. He was dressed formally in gaiters for some approaching official engagement, but by speaking in his kindest voice he avoided being intimidating.

'Well, Venetia,' he said lightly, 'it seems the clerical celebrities of Starbridge are all rushing to offer you sympathy!'

And as I looked past him I saw to my indescribable terror that not merely Eddie but Aysgarth had followed him up to my room.

XV

It was the most scandalous risk but he was faultlessly debonair, sauntering along with his hands in his pockets while his expression conveyed just the right amount of affectionate paternal concern, and beside him Eddie too was acting as if his life depended on it; he was exuding a sociable manner which flawlessly concealed what must have been an unadulterated horror and fear. Everyone was immaculately casual. The Bishop, who showed no inclination to leave, drifted to the window as if to check that the view was still there; Mrs Ashworth, also unable to tear herself away, began to readjust a flower in the vase which she had brought to the room earlier; Eddie wandered to the bedside until he stood within inches of the unaddressed envelope, and Aysgarth, keeping a relentlessly chaste distance from me, lounged against the tall chest of drawers. The conversation, insofar as I could register it, seemed to be light and inconsequential, like the opening phase of a drawing-room comedy. I almost felt we were waiting for the audience to settle in their seats so that Martin Darrow could make his big entrance.

I struggled to concentrate on the dialogue.

'. . . and when I happened to mention to Stephen that I was visiting you —' That was Eddie.

'— I decided it was time to pay a pastoral call!' That, of course, was Aysgarth.

'Quite right!' said the Bishop, very charming. 'Why should the Vicar of the Close have all the fun?'

'My sentiments exactly!' said Aysgarth.

They beamed at each other, a model of Christian amiability. No other dean and no other bishop could possibly have been on better terms.

'It's sweet of you to come,' I said, finally finding my place in the script. 'I'm terribly honoured.'

'How are you feeling?' enquired Eddie, looking straight at the envelope on the bedside table.

'Oh, just a trifle fragile.'

'She has a temperature of a hundred and one,' said Mrs

Ashworth, lying with effortless skill as she continued to remodel the flower arrangement.

'There's a lot of this flu about,' said Aysgarth. 'I hear the Archdeacon's daughters are going down like ninepins.'

'What a curious vision that conjures up!' said Eddie.

There was much casual laughter in which I managed to join. Everyone was having a splendid time.

'This is all rather Victorian, isn't it?' I heard the Bishop remark after an interval during which I lost the thread of the conversation. I was trying to work out how I could slip the envelope to Eddie without Aysgarth noticing. 'Wasn't there a novel by Trollope in which the heroine received a couple of clergymen when she was lying on her sick-bed?'

'The mother, I assume, was in attendance,' said Mrs Ashworth, finally abandoning the flowers and deciding for some reason to pick up the wastepaper basket.

'Was that *Orley Farm*, Charles?' asked Eddie with interest. 'I seem to recall the hero and heroine being drawn together over a sick-bed, but the hero wasn't a clergyman, and –'

'Surely it must have been one of the Barchester novels!' said Aysgarth.

'It could have been *The Vicar of Bullhampton*,' said the Bishop, 'but to be quite honest, I don't remember. Lyle, why are you wandering around with that wastepaper basket?'

'Just being a good housewife.' She emptied my overflowing ashtray.

'Very smart pyjamas, Venetia!'

'Thank you, Mr Dean! They're Charley's.'

'I seem to have seen them before somewhere –'

'Marks and Spencer's,' said Mrs Ashworth, looking around to see what she could tidy up next.

'Ah yes! Good old Marks –'

'How did we all live,' mused the Bishop rhetorically, 'before the advent of Marks and Spencer?'

'One of my daughters-in-law gave me a Marks and Spencer's string vest last Christmas,' said Aysgarth. 'I always feel very dashing when I'm wearing it.'

'I'm rather keen on their shirts,' said Eddie.

'They say the royal family shop there incognito,' I said, finding my place in the script again. I suddenly noticed my hands. They were gripping the edge of the sheet so hard that my knuckles ached. I tried to relax my fingers one by one but by the time I had finished I realised I had once more lost the thread of the conversation.

'– Jermyn Street,' said the Bishop, concluding a sentence. Recalling the conversation about clothes I made the brilliant deduction that he had been referring to the tailors who made his shirts.

'My father's been to the same tailor in Savile Row for fifty years,' I said. 'So unadventurous.'

There was a pause. To my horror I realised that my deduction had been wrong and that the conversation had moved on from clothes. What else happened in Jermyn Street apart from the tailoring of expensive shirts? I racked my brains in panic but could only recall the back entrance of Fortnum's.

'Talking of your father, Venetia,' said Eddie, rushing to the rescue, 'how did that family dinner-party of yours go? I completely forgot to ask.'

'Oh, it was fabulous!' I said, now feeling ill with the strain of keeping up with the conversation. 'We were all awash with champagne and sentimentality!'

'Eddie paid a quick visit to London that weekend,' said Aysgarth, 'but he won't say much about it. I can't think why he should be so secretive.'

I commented brightly: 'We all have our secrets!' before it struck me that this was quite the wrong thing to say. Or did I merely think it was wrong because my secrets were so all-consuming? 'I mean – what I'm trying to say is –'

'We ought to pay a quick visit to London ourselves, Lyle,' said the Bishop as I floundered to a halt. 'I want to see Thornton Wilder's play *The Ides of March*. Have you seen it, Venetia?'

'I think Venetia's flaking out,' said Mrs Ashworth, suddenly taking control of the scene, 'and after receiving a bishop, a dean and a canon simultaneously, I'm not one bit surprised. Charles would you like to lead the retreat?'

'I'll post this for you, Venetia,' said Eddie, picking up the envelope on the bedside table.

'It's not addressed,' said Aysgarth, who had also been watching the letter like a hawk.

'It's okay,' I said much too loudly. 'I –' But I had to stop. I was so terrified of saying the wrong thing. My mind went blank. Panic began to interfere with my breathing.

'It's a note for Lady Flaxton,' said Eddie, pocketing the envelope. 'Venetia told me about it on the phone last night. Don't worry, Venetia, I'll write the address and provide the stamp.'

'Well!' said the Bishop, moving to the door. 'Come along, gentlemen – the audience is at an end!'

I thought: I'm nearly there. I've only got to hold myself together for a few more seconds. We're all nearly there. No one's made any ghastly mistakes. We're going to survive.

'. . . so get well soon, Venetia –' That was Aysgarth.

'Yes, get well soon –' That was Eddie.

Nearly there. Nearly home.

'Would you like Primrose to look in with some magazines?'

I found my voice. 'Well, if she has five minutes to spare . . .'

I was going to make it. Only seconds to go.

'I'll ring her at the office when I get home –'

'Lovely – thanks so much –'

The countdown to safety had now begun. Ten – nine – eight –

'I'll be in touch, Venetia,' said Eddie. 'Let me know if there's anything you need.'

'Oh, I'll be all right now –'

Seven – six – five – four –

'Well, take care of yourself –'

'Yes, take care of yourself –'

Three – two –

''Bye, Venetia –'

''Bye, Venetia –'

One – ZERO! I'd done it. I'd survived. Thank God.

''Bye, Eddie,' I said, almost fainting with relief. ''Bye, Neville.'

The world at once stopped turning as everyone froze in their tracks.

PART FOUR

———◆———

THE LIGHT OF
THE WORLD

'Here was more than just a man: here was a window into God at work. For "God was in Christ reconciling the world to himself".'

JOHN A. T. ROBINSON
Suffragan Bishop of Woolwich 1959–1969
Honest to God

ONE

'It is this union-in-estrangement with the Ground of our
being . . . that we mean by hell.'

JOHN A. T. ROBINSON
Suffragan Bishop of Woolwich 1959–1969
Honest to God

I

Someone was screaming.

I couldn't think who it was.

It wasn't the Bishop, motionless in the doorway. It wasn't
Eddie, paralysed at the foot of the bed. It wasn't Aysgarth,
carved in stone in the middle of the carpet. It wasn't Mrs
Ashworth, transfixed by the dressing-table.

But someone was screaming. Someone was shouting: 'No,
no, NO!' over and over again in a rising crescendo of hysteria.

Then I realised the voice was connected with me. It belonged
to a fragment of my personality. I had begun to disintegrate
and now I was splitting into a thousand pieces . . .

I screamed and screamed, but Mrs Ashworth was coming to
the rescue; I saw her move, saw her swing round on the three
men and shout: 'OUT!' in a voice which made them jump. The
curious part was that they all obeyed her instantly. Afterwards
I never forgot that at the most crucial moment of my spiritual
sickness the Church of England, that ancient bastion of male
privilege, turned tail and fled *en masse*.

Mrs Ashworth flung her arms around me. She cried in agony:
'It's all right – don't reproach yourself –' but I could only weep:
'I've ruined him – I've given it all away.' Then huge sobs tore
at my throat, but she only held me closer and as I clung to her
in a frenzy of terror I heard her whisper: 'Oh my darling child,

do you think we hadn't guessed? I always knew you were Dinkie. I've suffered with you every inch of the way . . .'

II

After a long while when I was calmer and we had used up the box of Kleenex wiping away our tears, we sat in silence, holding hands. I felt safer now that I knew I was no longer alone. I was still unable to think clearly but I could breathe in a normal manner and know that only one person was doing the breathing. Mrs Ashworth had apparently glued together my fragmented self by enfolding me in a loving silence. Without words we were able to share the pain and thus, mysteriously, reduce it.

At last, after what seemed a great interval, I whispered five words. They were: 'What will the Bishop do?'

'Enlist Jon Darrow's help.'

'I know the Bishop dropped a hint earlier about Father Darrow, but Neville didn't seem to realise –'

'It's no good dropping delicate little hints to someone like Stephen. You have to slam him against a wall and shake him till his teeth rattle before he takes any notice. I told Charles that, but poor Charles! He does so hate taking a tough line!'

'Does he? But during that final row they had over the sculpture –'

'My dear, I was livid – *livid*! Charles was up all night afterwards, pacing the floor in a frenzy, and that sort of stress is extremely bad for him. He's got a very sensitive nature,' said Mrs Ashworth, exuding the fiery concern of a protective tigress, 'and he can't bear fights.'

'But he seems to be so good at them! I thought he was capable of pulling out a long knife at any moment and –'

'No, luckily for Stephen long knives aren't included in the regulation kit issued to bishops at their consecration.'

'But surely *now* –'

'Oh, it'll be ultimatum time of course – "Rehabilitate yourself with the aid of a skilled director or else I'll go straight to the

Archbishop" – but don't worry. Those old public schoolboys who run the Church of England always prefer to bury a mess six feet deep and then play cricket on top of it. Charles will press for rehabilitation, and Stephen – who's quite the most relentless survivor I've ever met – will fall into line.'

'So –'

'So assuming the affair's over, you shouldn't waste any more energy worrying about him.' She reached for the cigarettes on my bedside table but the packet was empty. 'Shall we smoke?' she said. 'There's a packet in my bedroom – just a minute.'

By the time she returned I had phrased my next question. 'Mrs Ashworth,' I said, 'when did you first realise what was going on?'

'Last May.' She paused to light our cigarettes. 'Charles told me he'd looked out of the window of the Cathedral library and seen the two of you holding hands in the cloisters. His comment was: "I do wish Stephen would stop this idiotic flirting with young women. I've no doubt it's all quite harmless but it's definitely not appropriate behaviour for a senior cleric." Then suddenly I had a twinge of feminine intuition. Of course I had no idea – how could I have had? – that Stephen might ever be capable of such serious clerical misconduct as adultery, but nevertheless I thought: supposing it's *not* harmless? And I suggested to Charles that we kept an eye on you. He hit on the idea of employing you as a secretary, and gradually as time passed –'

'It all became obvious.'

'To me, yes. But Charles kept saying: "We've no proof," and trying not to believe the worst. Poor Charles – such a very Christian nature! However in my experience,' said Mrs Ashworth, blowing smoke casually at the ceiling, 'the worst is usually true.'

'Neville and I . . . we never actually . . . we didn't quite . . .'

'No? I wonder why he held back. I suppose it was just his way of fooling himself that he wasn't committing adultery.'

'It seemed to be more complicated than that. He saw me as a great prize and he seemed to be frightened that if he won me he wouldn't want me any more.'

'How bizarre! But no doubt his capture of Dido taught him how unpleasant winning a great prize could be.'

'Oh, he never saw Dido as a prize! He married her out of compassion.'

Mrs Ashworth gave an incredulous laugh. 'My dear, his *amour fou* for a society girl was the talk of the Church! He was mad about her.'

There was a silence. Then slowly I said: 'Perhaps he still is. After all, I know he didn't abstain from going all the way with me just because he was afraid of winning a great prize and finding it unsatisfactory; he also abstained because he believed it would save Dido from destruction.'

'Well, of course I've long suspected that there's far more to that marriage than meets the eye. People are usually so busy noticing how obsessed she is with him that they overlook how utterly he's bound up with her.'

'But in that case why did he –'

' – fall for you? Oh, for all the usual reasons, I'm sure, but also, I suspect, because you represented an escape from the Dido obsession and he'd reached the stage where he needed a holiday. After all, what's the most satisfactory way of escaping from an obsession? You escape into another obsession and run the two of them in tandem.'

'So you think he didn't really love me at all?'

'On the contrary I'm sure he was mad about you, and that's why one should stress the peculiarity of his psychology. If he didn't consummate the affair there must have been very powerful mental forces holding him back.'

'It seems so stupid,' I said, 'to have gone through all this without ever –'

'It could be important for your recovery. Human beings are really very fragile, emotionally and spiritually, and need to keep a certain private space around their deepest selves where they feel they can be in control against any invading force. If you can feel later that there was at least one part of your deepest self which was untouched by this destruction, you'll find the healing will take place more easily.'

I said simply: 'I don't think I'll ever be healed.'

'My dearest Venetia –'

'I can't stop thinking about him. What on earth could have been said after they'd left the room?'

'Probably very little. They'd pretend your fatal slip never happened because they'd all need time to work out what they were going to do next.'

'Neville must be in the most frightful panic –'

'I doubt it. He'll have knocked back the whisky by this time.'

'My God, you mean you know about the drink?'

'Oh, we all know about that. The great thing is to hush it up, but fortunately those canons practise loyalty on a heroic scale . . . And talking of canons, Eddie's still very keen, isn't he?'

'I've actually agreed to marry him. I've just made the break with Neville. That letter Eddie took away –'

'Good heavens, now I see it all!'

I started to cry. 'He'll get the letter tomorrow – I can't bear to think of it – he'll be so hurt, so shattered, so crushed –'

'For a little while, perhaps.'

'But Mrs Ashworth –'

'My dear, that one's tough as old boots. They simply don't make them any tougher up in Yorkshire.'

'But if he loses me and loses his job –'

'He won't lose it. I've told you: he'll fall into line and trot off to Jon Darrow's spiritual workshop for a compulsory overhaul and comprehensive repairs. Of course if Stephen were a gentleman he'd do the decent thing and resign, but he'll never voluntarily give up that Deanery. It's much too big a prize to kiss goodbye.'

'But he doesn't approve of spiritual directors and he calls Father Darrow an ecclesiastical pirate!'

'It's really amazing what one can learn to like,' said Mrs Ashworth, 'when one's professional life is on the line. No, my dear, the big question here is not what's going to happen to Neville-Stephen; his future's clearly mapped out. The really big question is what's going to happen to you.'

I wiped my tears from my swollen eyes and whispered: 'What do you think I should do?' as if I now had a choice. But of course no new choice existed. I still had to end the affair to ensure Aysgarth's survival, and I knew there was only one way of making him let go.

'You really want to know what I think?' said Mrs Ashworth. 'I think you should marry the good, decent man who loves you.'

I started weeping again. 'But I don't love him.'

'So long as you like him and respect him, I don't think the absence of romantic love is important. And as for the real love, that can come later.'

'Can it?'

'Why not? When one's emerged from a disastrous affair, goodness and decency begin to seem immensely attractive.'

I was reassured by her confidence, and suddenly the future seemed less chilling. 'Mrs Ashworth,' I said, speaking reluctantly but driven on by a craving for further reassurance, 'am I right in thinking you speak from personal experience? You seem so very certain . . . I'm sorry, I don't want to pry, but –'

Mrs Ashworth said obliquely: 'I never cease to thank God that Charles wanted to marry me even though I was then too battered to love him as he deserved.'

'So before you met him –'

There was a knock at the door.

'Who is it?' called Mrs Ashworth sharply, and the Bishop answered: 'Me.'

'Just a moment.' She stubbed out her cigarette and left the room. I heard their voices murmur in the distance for some time but at last Mrs Ashworth returned to say briskly: 'Charles would very much like to see you on your own. It might be a good thing. He could convince you that the Christian response to Stephen's behaviour isn't to disembowel him with a long knife.'

After a pause I said: 'Okay.'

'I'll wait in the corridor. If you want to turf him out, all you have to do is yell.'

She slipped out and the Bishop slipped in. He was very quiet, very calm, very gentle. 'This won't take long,' he said, pulling up a chair and sitting down by the bed. 'Sometimes in a crisis it's best if no words are spoken but I think if I were silent now I would only add to your very great anxiety, so I want to say this: I know the Church must often seem to a layman to be just another worldly corporation staffed by ambitious executives, but in our own inadequate, imperfect way the churchmen in authority do try, by remembering God every day and praying to Him for the grace to serve Him as He desires, to live according to Christian precepts. My job is to be a shepherd. That's why I carry the crozier, the shepherd's crook, in the Cathedral. I have to care for the sheep, all of them, not just the sheep who stay bunched together and never put a foot wrong, but the sheep who stray out of sight and can't find their way home. My duty in caring for the flock is not to run around with a whip and a knife, flogging the strays into line and cutting the throats of the ones who cause trouble. My duty is to go after the strays and find them and carry them back one by one to safety. So you see, although bishops may seem very grand people, particularly when they're dressed up in their uniform, and although their job may seem rooted in a complex web of power, yet at the heart of their lives lies this great simplicity, the simplicity of the shepherd who serves God by caring for others and helping them when they're in distress.'

He paused as if to consider whether he should say more but then rose to his feet and silently replaced the chair. It was only when he reached the door that he spoke again. He said: 'I expect it's too difficult for you to talk to me, but if you should wish later when you're better to talk to a clergyman, I can easily arrange a meeting. Meanwhile I'm sure my wife is far more able to help you than I am.' And he slipped out again into the corridor.

Feeling that no man could possibly be of any use to me at that moment I reflected vaguely that it was a pity there were no women priests. But of course those old public schoolboys who ran the Church of England would never permit a woman to play cricket on their hallowed turf.

'Still conscious?' said Mrs Ashworth, returning to the room.

'Yes. He was rather sweet,' I said vaguely in a hopeless attempt to express my gratitude for the Bishop's kindness, and then overcome by my exhaustion I again started to cry.

III

When the tears finally stopped I felt as a patient must feel when he has been prepared for an operation and knows that he is powerless to do anything except wait for the ordeal to be over. I lay lifelessly in bed. Mrs Ashworth offered me a selection of novels but I was unable to read them. I could only listen to her transistor radio and thumb through some magazines.

In the afternoon a letter arrived, delivered by hand. The address on the envelope had been typed in order to preserve the author's anonymity among the prying eyes at the South Canonry. I could hardly bear to break the seal but I had to know what he had written.

'My darling,' I read, 'just a brief note which you can burn immediately in the ashtray. *Don't worry* about the slip. I said afterwards: "Venetia's obviously very ill and confused – why should she call me Neville when I specifically told her on holiday in the Hebrides that she could call me Stephen?" Eddie at once said: "Obviously she was almost delirious," and Charles said: "She's certainly most unwell." So that's all right. I thought it was rather clever of me to rake up the Hebrides – everyone always sinks into Christian names on holiday, and just because Eddie never actually heard you call me Stephen up there he can't prove I didn't invite you to dispense with formality. So my darling, *don't worry* and *get well soon*. Nobody suspects anything. Much, much, *much* love, N.'

Mrs Ashworth burnt the letter in the ashtray and produced a new box of Kleenex. Time dragged on and at intervals she would sit with me and knit. I wanted to ask her more about the man who had wrecked her life before the young Dr Ashworth had arrived on the scene like a white knight, but I was unable to frame any question beyond a preliminary enquiry. I did say: 'That story you told me about the young woman who was almost destroyed by a romance that went wrong – you were the young woman, weren't you, just as I was Dinkie,' but when she answered: 'It's best to draw a veil over that now,' I realised that the subject was one which she had no wish to discuss. Yet because I knew she had been through an experience similar to mine I was able to say to her: 'One of the most baffling aspects of the whole affair is that I feel I never really knew him. I just knew a "persona", a mask. He claimed it was the real him, but I suspect there were acres and acres of the real him that I never traversed at all; I suspect I just saw one corner of a vast field.'

'Oh, that's a very common feature of love affairs. Romance and fantasy fence off the cosy corner and leave reality out in the cold beyond the pale.'

'But what *was* reality here? How do I come to terms with it? How do I sort it all out in my mind when so much is either unknown or a mystery? You talked of twin obsessions running in tandem, but –'

'– but I was speculating. Yes, I do understand what you mean, but all you can do is concentrate on the facts which are beyond dispute: he was married; the two of you became emotionally involved with each other; he brought you to breakdown. Then you can expand a little on those basic facts with some degree of certainty: he was probably under stress for various reasons – and perhaps you too were under stress in some way, with the result that you each found an escape from your problems in the other; then during this great escape he displayed a passion which could well have been genuine but could also have been part of an elaborate fantasy generated by the journey away from reality. That all sounds very stark, I know, but that's really all it's possible to say.'

'I just feel that if only I knew the whole truth –'

'My dear, we never know the whole truth about anyone. Only God can ever know the whole truth. All we can do is struggle to grasp that part of the truth which God has made accessible to us and accept that not all mysteries are solvable.'

'But surely you know the whole truth about the Bishop?'

Mrs Ashworth smiled. Then she said: 'When I first met Charles long ago in 1937 he seemed very straightforward, a successful young clergyman from a comfortable middle-class home. But the reality behind the glittering image was far more complex, I assure you, than I could ever have imagined, and even now I daresay there are still mysteries in his past which I shall never unravel.' She hesitated but added: 'He was a widower when I met him. He's talked to me about that first marriage, but not in a way that has ever encouraged me to dig deep into what actually happened. I'd like to know more, of course, but I've accepted that there's nothing more he has to say; I've accepted that there's a limit on our knowledge of even those who are closest to us. The older one gets the more one realises how saturated life is in mystery, and the biggest mystery of all, it often seems to me, is the mystery of the human personality.'

I meditated on this conversation for some time while the sunshine dwindled into twilight and darkness began to fall. Later the Bishop looked in to see how I was. Later still Mrs Ashworth brought me a mug of cocoa and some more pills. Once again I sank thankfully into oblivion, but the next morning at seven o'clock I was awake, every muscle in my body aching with tension as I pictured the postman walking up to the front door of the Deanery with my letter in his hand.

IV

At eight o'clock Mrs Ashworth came to my room with Aysgarth's reply. All she said was: 'He's just delivered this. I heard the car in the drive and thought it might be him. He looked much as usual.'

My fingers were trembling so much that I was unable to open the envelope. Without a word she took it from my hands, ripped open the flap and handed me the folded sheet of paper within.

He had written: 'This breaks my heart. I'm now standing in

the worst wasteland I've ever known. I can only pray that God will bless you and keep you safe and ultimately grant you the happiness you deserve.' There was no opening 'my darling', no signature, no love sent, only the three bleak sentences which, carefully written in his clear handwriting, suggested a survivor in ruthless control of himself.

I wept with relief.

It was finally over.

Or was it?

V

'My darling, I feel I'm going stark staring mad. Can you not write *just one word*? Please, please, if you've ever loved me at all – which now seems doubtful – send me JUST ONE WORD. N.'

VI

'Darling Neville, You know how much I love you, but I'm ending our affair because there's no alternative; if I don't end it you'll be ruined. Please try to understand. I'm doing this – *all of it* – so that you can be saved. V.'

VII

'My darling, I was so utterly appalled by your letter that I nearly passed out. Listen, you *mustn't marry him*, you absolutely mustn't – the very idea that you could be marrying Eddie in order to save me is so horrific that I can't maintain a noble silence on the subject a second longer, I just can't, I'd wind up in a lunatic asylum.

'Darling, Eddie's dead wrong for you. God knows, no one's fonder of Eddie than I am – oh, the nightmare of it, the sheer unadulterated *hell* that I should be betrayed by the two people who are closest to me, I feel as if I've been disembowelled and abandoned to bleed to death, but never mind that now, I don't count, what's it matter if I bleed to death, what have I got to live for, but *you* count, *you* matter, you have *everything* to live for, and I can't bear that you should throw yourself away like this, CAN'T BEAR IT.

'The truth is poor Eddie's a very damaged sort of fellow – it's the result of his war experiences and losing all his family – and he's so neurotic, so enslaved by hypochondria and introspection, that he could only wear you down in no time if you married him. HE'S NOT GOOD ENOUGH FOR YOU. I've always tried to resign myself to the fact that you would marry one day but I wanted you to marry someone who was worthy of you, and he's not worthy, he'll never be worthy, and besides – I hate to say this because the images it conjures up are so revolting, but nevertheless it has to be said – how can you conceivably marry a man whom you find physically repulsive? It's all the most ghastly mistake and it'll wreck your life. Even if you go into the marriage with the idea of divorcing him eventually, you'll still have to live through an experience which could scar you for ever.

'Darling, I'll give you up, I'll never see you again, I'll never even write one letter, but please, *please*, PLEASE swear to me by return of post that you'll break off this absolutely *disastrous* engagement. Always your most devoted and loving N.'

VIII

'Dear Mr Dean,' dictated Mrs Ashworth as the tears streamed down my face and the pen shook in my hand, 'I'm afraid you must take it as settled that Eddie and I will be marrying shortly. I know this is very difficult for you and I'm sorry. But the sooner you accept the situation the sooner all three of us will begin to recover from this horrific ordeal. Yours sincerely, VENETIA.'

IX

'My darling, I can't believe you could have written that letter, and I refuse to take ANYTHING as settled. I'm going to fight to save you from tragedy. Eternal love from your devoted N.'

X

'My dear Stephen, Venetia has asked me to reply to your last letter. I assure you that it is indeed settled that she is to marry Eddie, and Charles and I both think that your correspondence with her should now cease. Yours sincerely, LYLE.'

XI

'. . . so unable to stand the suspense any longer I turned up at the Deanery,' wrote Eddie. 'Dido showed me straight into his study. It was a shock for him but he recovered quickly and was perfectly civil. He looked tired but sober. Certainly there was no whisky in sight. I told him of my intention to work in London and said I planned to marry you next month at St Margaret's Westminster. He nodded and said would I like him to write to the Bishop of London, but I said no, that was all right, Charles had already offered to pull strings on my behalf. That reply produced a deafening silence but I raced on and asked if he wanted me to resign the canonry straight away or whether he was content for me to stay on until the wedding.

'Then he became very proud, very grand, and said that was nothing to do with him, that was something I should discuss with the Bishop, he had no strong feelings on the subject, as far as he was concerned I could do exactly as I liked. So I said I didn't want to leave the Cathedral in the lurch by a sudden resignation and it might also be a good thing, from the point of view of avoiding gossip, if I stayed on until my marriage. Then I added that after the wedding we'd be renting a flat in

London until I got the house which will go with my new job. I thought perhaps I should make it clear that we shan't be returning to the Starbridge diocese, even temporarily.

'He said politely: "Quite. I wish you every happiness," and suddenly I couldn't bear it, I just had to say: "Stephen I'm so very sorry, but believe me, whatever happens either now or in the future, you'll always be the hero who saved me from despair in that POW camp and looked after me later as if I were your own son."

'He just sighed. Then he said in an exasperated voice: "You'll never be an Englishman, will you, Eddie? Englishmen just don't make that kind of remark," and I laughed – I think he did mean me to laugh, don't you? – and thanked him for seeing me and that was the end of the conversation. But he seemed well in control of himself and I think he's going to be all right . . .'

XII

'My dear Venetia, Eddie has just been here and, as you would say, "slobbered all over me". Why can't foreigners behave properly? However, I accept that he meant well. I also accept that I've lost my Great Prize and that our correspondence must inevitably end.

'I won't ask you to thank Lyle for her letter. What an old battle-axe that woman's turned into! She has a real talent for wielding what Eddie, with his Nazi memories, would call "the long knife". I could tell you a thing or two about her. But I won't. I may be just a Yorkshire draper's son but I trust I know when and how to behave like a gentleman.

'I went to see that old pirate Jon Darrow today. Thought I really ought to look in on the old boy as he was asking after me so persistently. I must say, old age has improved him; he's quieter now, more sedate. We had a little chat about this and that, talked about the past, just as one inevitably does with the elderly. By the way, I think he secretly took a fancy to you at the Starbridge Playhouse! "A most interesting girl!" he said, eyes gleaming. Funny old pirate. I promised I'd drop in on him again soon – and in fact I think I might drop in on him regularly for a while. He seemed so pathetically glad to receive a visitor, and one really does have a Christian duty to be kind to old people.

'I hope you're now completely recovered from the flu. Primrose has just succumbed – there's certainly a lot of it about – and has returned from her flat to her old room at the Deanery in order to be properly cosseted. Perhaps you might look in on her before you leave for London to make the wedding arrangements. It would be prudent, I think, if you made some small gesture towards renewing that friendship, because Primrose continues to wonder why you dropped her so abruptly and she needs the chance to write off your withdrawal as a mere temporary aberration resulting from Eddie's courtship.

'In sending you my best regards I hope I may sign myself your well-wisher, STEPHEN AYSGARTH.'

XIII

Arriving at the Deanery clutching a box of chocolates and the latest edition of *Punch*, I was admitted by Dido's companion-housekeeper Miss Carp and ushered upstairs to Primrose's room. Lying wanly in bed Primrose opened her eyes as I put my head around the door.

'Receiving callers, Prim?'

'Venetia! Good heavens, I *am* honoured.' She hauled herself up on the pillows and gave me a chilly smile. Her lank brown hair, frizzy at the ends, fell in strands towards her shoulders and her pink nightdress, possibly one of Dorothy Perkins' more unfortunate products, clung limply to her flat chest.

Leaving my offerings on the bed I enquired: 'Feeling ghastly?'

'Yes, but better than yesterday. Oh, *Punch*! How nice – thanks . . . Well, I suppose I ought to congratulate you, oughtn't I? We've all seen the announcement in today's *Times*.'

'Please don't feel obliged to congratulate me if you don't want to, Primrose.'

'Well, to be quite frank, Father and I think it's a very big mistake. We think you could do better for yourself.'

I was just wondering whether I should give up and walk out when the door behind me was swept wide open and Dido streamed into the room. It at once occurred to me that she had crept along the corridor to eavesdrop as soon as Miss Carp had informed her of my arrival.

'What utter nonsense, Primrose!' she exclaimed. 'You should be ashamed of yourself, sulking away so ungraciously in bed just because Venetia's getting married and you're still lying on the shelf!' And before this brutal remark could draw forth a stinging retort she added crisply: 'Venetia, how very kind of you to call on poor Primrose – I always did say you were a nice girl *au fond*, even though the *fond* was so seldom on display – and my dear! Too, too lovely about your engagement, I'm thrilled for you both! Take no notice of Primrose's sour grapes, because I assure you, my dear, that far from disapproving of your engagement Stephen told me last night – and of course he always tells me everything – that in his opinion marriage would be the making of both you *and* dear Eddie!'

'He doesn't tell you a damn thing!' said Primrose incensed. '*I'm* the one he confides in, and he told me this morning –'

'Well, obviously when he saw you were so *devoured* by jealousy he pretended to disapprove of the engagement so that you wouldn't feel quite such a failure!'

My voice said politely: 'I think I ought to be going now,' but when I turned towards the door I found that Aysgarth himself was standing on the threshold.

'Oh, there you are, darling!' cried Dido radiantly as I flinched and stopped dead in my tracks. 'Come on in and join the party! Primrose, silly girl, is refusing to believe you're in favour of Venetia's marriage – do tell her you're all for it!'

'I certainly wish Venetia every happiness.' He gave me a smile which was no more than a subtle upturning of his thin mouth. His blue eyes were expressionless.

'Father,' said Primrose, now pale with rage, 'you distinctly said to me –'

'Oh, dear, *dear* child,' said Dido in a voice which vibrated with exasperation, 'when are you ever going to abandon this pathetic illusion that you're in your father's confidence?'

'Darling,' said Aysgarth quietly to her. 'Please.'

'Father never lies to me, and he said –'

'Never lies to you? My God, that's a laugh! If you only knew the half of what's been going on in his life lately –'

Aysgarth and I spoke at the same moment. He said strongly: 'Dido, that's enough!' while I exclaimed with a dreadful false brightness: 'Well, I simply *must* be going!'

'Your trouble, Dido,' cried Primrose, outshouting us both, 'is that you're the one who's "devoured" by jealousy because I'm in his confidence and you're not! Why, he said to me only the other day: "Primrose," he said, "of course I know you'll marry eventually, but how am I going to bear it when you go away and I have no one to talk to?" And that's why you're quite wrong in thinking I'm jealous of Venetia – I don't want to get married, I'm never going to get married, I've made up my mind that I'm going to stay with Father and be a comfort to him in his marital hell!'

'Primrose, be quiet!' said Aysgarth violently, but the scene was now quite out of control and as I stood paralysed with horror Dido, throwing all self-restraint to the winds, tossed the lighted match into the keg of dynamite which we had all been circling for so long.

'My poor pet!' she said to Primrose in her most withering voice. 'You've been grossly deceived! He's just been playing a rôle for you, the rôle of the doting father, but in fact he's long past caring what you do with yourself. He's too busy doting elsewhere – as Venetia will be the first to testify!'

Primrose said blankly: 'Venetia?' at the exact same moment as Aysgarth whispered: 'That's enough – that's enough, I tell you –'

'You see?' said Dido to Primrose. 'You know nothing – nothing, nothing, nothing! But Venetia could tell you things you could never in your wildest dreams imagine, Venetia could tell you –'

I said in a loud voice: 'I'm going!' but quick as a flash Dido barred my path to the door.

'Oh no, you're not!' she said. 'I've *had* it with this girl, mooning over her father as if he were her lover and making my life hell for year after year, and this is it, this is where I refuse to tolerate her behaviour a second longer, this is where I draw the line.' She spun to face Primrose. 'Venetia's your father's little piece of nonsense. Not his mistress – she's still *virgo intacta* – but his trivial little plaything which he uses for relaxation during his leisure hours. It's been going on for some months. He takes her out on his afternoon off and they drive to some deserted spot – Castle Brigga, isn't it, Venetia dear? – and there they indulge in their amusing little sex-games –'

'I don't believe it,' said Primrose. She was now ashen. 'That's the foulest lie I've ever heard.' She looked at her father. 'Why don't you deny it?' she said in a shaking voice. 'Why are you just standing there? Why don't you say it's a lie?'

'Because it's the truth,' said Dido. She jerked my arm. 'It's all true, isn't it, Venetia? My God, look at you! I suppose you thought I didn't know anything about it! I suppose you thought I'd never heard of Castle Brigga! Who told her, you're thinking, who told her – and how does she know I'm still a virgin? Well, my dear, this is where you get your big surprise, the surprise you'll remember all your life, because *STEPHEN TELLS ME EVERYTHING*. He always has and he always will – and do you you know where he tells me everything, Venetia? In bed! And after sex! I suppose you thought, silly, ignorant girl, that you had him all to yourself; I suppose you thought you knew him through and through – but you were wrong. You never knew *Stephen* at all. You just knew a masked actor who indulged in some shallow play-acting, but I know *Stephen* and *Stephen* makes love only to *me*. He's always promised that there was one act he'd never do with anyone else, and that promise was given because he's dedicated his whole life to making me feel cherished and fulfilled. So what do I care about his little weaknesses?

What do I care about all the drink and the masked actor who amuses himself with young girls? All that matters is that *he's mine* and *he loves me* and I love him a thousand times better than *any other woman ever could*!' And turning her back on me abruptly she marched out with her head held high.

The door banged.

There was a silence.

I remember Primrose, blue eyes huge in her white shocked face. I remember Aysgarth, grey and drawn, the suffering etched deep in the heavy lines about his mouth. I remember the copy of *Punch* on the bed and the unopened box of chocolates and the curtains fluttering lightly in the breeze from the open window.

At last Aysgarth said unevenly to Primrose – not to me, but to Primrose, it was Primrose he turned to first: 'It's not true, I give you my word.'

'Of course it couldn't possibly be true,' said Primrose stiff-lipped. 'Not possibly.' She was unable to look at either of us.

Then Aysgarth turned to me and said: 'I apologise, Venetia, for all her lies. She's had a fixation about Castle Brigga ever since she discovered that I'd circled it on the Ordnance Survey map. I'd planned to take Pip there one day for an outing.'

'I see,' I said. 'Yes.'

The silence closed in on us again, and suddenly I saw the full dimensions of the destruction that had been wrought. Neither Primrose nor I could know for certain whether or not he spoke the truth. We would want to believe him, but the more we tried the more clearly we would remember Dido, fearlessly outspoken, shrewd about personal relationships, passionately devoted to her husband, voicing the horrors which we could never be sure were false. She had told the truth to Primrose about my affair with Aysgarth. How could I ever convince myself beyond doubt that she had lied to me about her marriage? I knew that logically it was possible that she had told the truth to Primrose and lied to me, but it was equally possible that she had told the truth to both of us. Faith had been wrecked, trust destroyed, love annihilated. Now indeed we all stood in a wasteland which stretched as far as the eye could see.

'My darling –'

I gave a start, but he was talking to Primrose – not to me but to Primrose – and as I glimpsed some seamy psychological shadow fall backwards across the past I felt my blood run cold with repulsion.

'– my darling, you must believe me, you must –'

'But of course I believe you!' said Primrose, somehow managing to look at him at last, but as soon as I saw the expression on her face I knew he had lost her for ever.

He knew it too. He had been moving towards her but now he swung back to face me. 'Venetia, tell her,' he said stricken, stammering in his agony. 'Tell her it's not true!'

'It's not true,' I said to Primrose in my politest voice, and walked away without looking back.

XIV

'My dear Venetia, I'm sorry to trouble you when you must be so busy with your wedding preparations, but I really felt I couldn't let that appalling scene at the Deanery pass without comment. Dido seems to have jumped to conclusions on the minimum of evidence. Of course I never told her anything about us. But she did find out I'd circled Castle Brigga on the map, she did find out that I was disappearing with the car on my afternoon off, and when she heard the rumour that I'd been seen in Chasuble Lane (at the end of my ill-fated attempt to play Juan Fangio) with a young woman, she realised it was you and not, as was popularly supposed, Harriet March.

'Her disclosure that I had promised never to consummate an extra-marital affair is true (and explains why she was confident you were still *virgo intacta*) but her allegation that I have a habit of gossiping garrulously in bed after sexual intercourse is, I assure you, a fable. In such circumstances I prefer to smoke a cigarette and pass out. No doubt there's more you'd like me to say on that particular subject, but I believe I've now implied all that requires to be said: namely that Dido's not above mixing truth with lies when she's ruthlessly pursuing her own ends. Yours sincerely, STEPHEN.'

XV

I never replied to that letter because I was too busy in London assembling my trousseau. Later he wrote to my sister Sylvia and asked for news of me. Sylvia was rather touched by this avuncular interest and struck up a correspondence with him; it helped pass the time as she waited for the baby to arrive. She showed me a couple of his letters. They were very amusing and charming, but I doubted that Sylvia could match this sparkling style in her replies.

He did write me one more letter. It read: 'My dearest Venetia, The time has come when I must wish you well in your new life and assure you that I shall be praying hard for your happiness. I suspect you no longer believe this, but you really were the very greatest prize I ever encountered, the love of my life, and now that I look back from a grey cold present into that brilliant past we shared together, I realise how very privileged I was to experience, no matter how fleetingly, such absolute perfection. I shall always cherish the memory of those walks through the woods and those kisses in the hollow – and even those prosaic journeys in the car when we merely laughed and gossiped together. What glorious times we had! I shall never forget them, never, I swear it – till my dying day I'll always dream of those shining hours when I loved the best girl in all the world and travelled with her through paradise. May God bless you, my darling, and in sending you all my love as always, I remain, now and forever, your most devoted MR DEAN.'

The letter arrived on my wedding-day.

It wrecked my eye make-up and nearly ruined my white gown.

God knows how I ever made it to the church.

TWO

---◆◆◆---

'But equally it is the union-in-love with the Ground of our being such as we see in Jesus Christ, that is the meaning of heaven. And it is the offer of that life, in all its divine depth, to overcome the estrangement and alienation of existence as we know it that the New Testament speaks of as the "new creation".'

JOHN A. T. ROBINSON
Suffragan Bishop of Woolwich 1959–1969
Honest to God

I

Eddie landed a very acceptable job as the rector of a smart Kensington parish, and the rectory was acceptable too, a cream-coloured, early Victorian, double-fronted town-house with plenty of space for entertaining. I bought my heart's desire in the country later. It was in Norfolk, a little out of the way perhaps, but the fine, austere, classical mansion had a lake at the bottom of the back lawn, and the members of the Coterie adored streaming down there from London at weekends. I never bothered with parish life, but I was always careful to keep up appearances by behaving properly in London – or if I did misbehave I made damned sure I was discreet.

The marriage, of course, was a disaster.

The 1960s were a disaster too, as those who were lucky enough to survive knew all too well. 'All you need is love!' sang the Beatles, as the Great Pollutant, seeping into the gap created by the absence of a strong religion, began systematically to poison our lives. Pascal wrote: 'It is natural for the mind to believe and for the will to love; so that for want of true objects they must attach themselves to false.' The true objects all went under in that part of the 1960s where I wasted what remained of my youth, and only the false gods survived to ensure our ruin.

The ranks of the Coterie were decimated. Dinkie overdosed on heroin, Emma-Louise crashed through three marriages, that nice Holly Carr committed suicide, Norman Aysgarth took to drink, man-eating Cynthia had a nervous breakdown, Robert Welbeck was crippled in a motorway smash-up, Simon drowned in a swimming-pool after freaking out on LSD, Don Latham dropped out of the BBC in order to meditate in India, Katie Aysgarth took to spiritualism and went peculiar, Christian –

Now, that was a great mystery. They say Nick Darrow unravelled that one in the end, Nick Darrow treading his mystical paths with his crystal ball in one hand and his crucifix in the other. He survived, of course. So, more surprisingly, did Michael Ashworth and Marina who married each other and lived (so far as I could tell) happily ever after. Michael still pounced around occasionally but Marina always became a devoted friend of any mistress who lasted longer than six months. Some people really are extraordinary.

Primrose's wedding took place a month after mine, and with an ambitious wife egging him on, Maurice Tait wound up running the Choir School. They had four children and Primrose was always reported to be radiant – as was Dido once she had finally got rid of her step-daughter. It was nice to know that the appalling scene at the Deanery eventually made Dido, Primrose and, presumably, Maurice ecstatically happy.

Eddie died young, just as he had so often threatened he would, but before the end came I tried to make amends to him for my shortcomings by having a baby. God knows who the father was but all that mattered was that Eddie thought the child was his. It turned out to be a girl, rather a bright little bit of fluff, but I never had much gift for being a mother.

The Bishop published his book *A Modern Heresy for Modern Man* to critical acclaim but minimal sales. However, later his distinguished good-looks were discovered by television and he used to appear, gorgeous in purple, pectoral cross flashing, on various discussion programmes. Unlike other eminent prelates who flirted with the medium he always took a very firm line with hedonistic pop stars.

I found I could never bear to watch him for more than a few seconds, but I was glad that in the Church of England, then enduring one of its most demoralised phases, there was at least someone who had the guts to speak up for the unfashionable views which he believed to be right.

I eventually severed all my Starbridge connections. Once I met Mrs Ashworth for lunch in London but that was a mistake and afterwards she said: 'I'm sorry, I remind you of it all, don't I? Don't worry, I understand.'

I liked that woman. I could never hold it against her that she had given me the wrong advice. How could she have known that what had been right for her and the Bishop would be wrong for Eddie and me? At least she had cared deeply about my welfare and I knew she saw me as the daughter she had never had. At that lunch in London she told me that in 1945 when her husband had returned from the war she had tried to have another baby but without success. That had obviously been a sadness to her, but at least both her sons did well.

Charley, surprisingly, turned out to be almost as sexy as his brother in the end – those golden eyes were really very compelling – and he married one of those ghastly wonderwomen spawned by the Women's Movement, someone who was capable of tossing off a master's thesis, bringing up a shoal of successful children and producing a gourmet dinner for eight – all with one hand tied behind her back while she continued to look like a film star. I loathe women like that, but perhaps I'm jealous because they made the most of their opportunities while I threw all mine away. And perhaps I'm jealous too of Charley's wonderwoman because I sometimes think I might have found Charley an entertaining husband. If only I could have hung on and waited while he completed his transformation from ugly duckling to sexy swan! But I couldn't have waited, could I? I had to save my Mr Dean.

I never recovered from him, of course. No man I met ever measured up to him. I often wondered if I would have been less enslaved by his memory if our love-affair had been fully consummated; naturally no real-life consummation could ever match the glittering dream which existed for all time in my imagination, but perhaps even if the affair had been completed in a conventional manner I would still have been unable to forget the memory of those 'shining hours' which Aysgarth had described in his final letter.

He ruined me, that was the truth of it. He ruined me, he ruined my marriage, he ruined every attempt I made to find happiness elsewhere. Religion? Oh, he ruined that for me too; I turned away from theology and I turned away from the Church. He and his New Reformation! I wanted no part of it, not after all I'd been through in Starbridge. The last thing I did before I left my home in Lord North Street for my wedding at St Margaret's was to tear up *Honest to God* and chuck the pieces in the wastepaper basket.

So the 'sixties came to an end and the 'seventies began for those who had survived. I certainly thought of myself as surviving; I hadn't OD'd on heroin or freaked out on LSD or died of cirrhosis of the liver. But as I see so clearly now, my survival was an illusion. The Great Pollutant had claimed another victim, and from my spiritual grave I could only look back in rage at the man whom I held responsible for my death.

Then one day in 1975 when I was in Norfolk, one day when the summer sun was shining on the lake, one day when I was a widow of thirty-eight, a letter arrived out of the blue.

II

'My dear Venetia, I have now reached the advanced age of seventy-three and look at least a hundred, even though in my head I feel no more than forty-five! What a curious phenomenon growing old is. I'm not able to go out and about much nowadays, but I've made a good recovery from my stroke – still *compos mentis* (or am I deluding myself?!) – and I can walk with the aid of two sticks. It was wonderful to wave the wheelchair goodbye. I was goaded into staging this spectacular recovery by the formidable alliance of Dido (still going strong, needless to say) and my new lady-friend, Mrs Jenny Hayman, a charming young widow who lives near us in Surrey and who drops in almost every day to chat with me and occasionally (if I'm very good) to hold my hand. Dido is devoted to Jenny, whose visits give her (D) the chance to escape from the useless old hulk (me) and roar round the village infuriating everyone in sight, so I have now followed the example of my mentor Alex Jardine (Bishop of Starbridge 1932–1937) and wound up in an irreproachably seemly *ménage à trois*.

'Anyway, when I was in the wheelchair and feeling a trifle glum, Dido and Jenny hatched a scheme to lure me off my bottom: Jenny offered to take me on an excursion to Norwich to see the Cotman exhibition. As you know, I've always been interested in art (I'm sure you've never forgotten that fatally ambivalent box of cigars!) and I particularly liked the thought of a little holiday in Norwich, such a beautiful city with such a magnificent cathedral. So to cut a long story short I shall merely add that the carrot dangled before the donkey proved too luscious to resist, and the donkey will soon be doddering through Norfolk.

'My darling, if you can't face me I shall understand, but I have only one desire at the moment and that's to see you again – just once more – before I die. Of course I may live for years (poor old Dido!) but if I'm called to meet my Maker before I've had the chance to fulfil this last alluring whim, I shall without doubt stage a tantrum in heaven. (Hell is out of the question, of course, since no good Liberal Protestant Modernist believes in it – although on reflection I recall there *are* no good Liberal Protestant Modernists nowadays, only a bunch of boring radical theologians who don't believe in anything – and I'm certainly not one of those!)

'Let me know what you think. Whatever your decision nothing can change the fact that I shall love you till the day I die. I remain – still – after all these many years – your most loyal and devoted MR DEAN.'

III

He was very stout and very old. His face had a high colour, possibly as the result of heart disease, and his white hair was thinner and wispier. He moved very slowly with his two sticks. His eyes were now only a faded blue, but his mouth still turned downwards in a sultry curve when his face was in repose.

As soon as I saw how impaired he was I knew beyond doubt that this visit was no mere exercise in nostalgia, no bizarre extension of the fantasy and illusion of 1963. He had struggled to see me at the very end of his life because his love was genuine, and once this truth had dawned all my anger vanished as if it had never existed. I ran out to meet him, and although he merely held out his hand I flung wide my arms and we hugged each other.

'Well!' he said afterwards. For a moment no other words were possible. 'Well!' He beamed at me.

I said only: 'My darling Mr Dean.'

The new lady-friend was a pleasant woman, very middle class, but then not everyone can be born with silver spoons in their mouths, and anyway every time I looked in the glass I despised the aristocracy. I think she was nervous of me. God knows what he had told her. I had invited another old friend to stay (homosexual, so restful) in case the going proved sticky, but there were no problems and we all chattered away happily throughout dinner. We had arranged that they should stay the night before travelling on to Norwich.

The only difficult moment came when Nanny brought in Vanessa, then aged four. Aysgarth said: 'So this is the child,' and when his faded eyes filled with tears I knew he was looking at the world of might-have-been, the world we would have inhabited if Dido had conveniently died and left him a widower. I had often thought of this world and had concluded in my anger that he would have made me very miserable once victory had finally dulled his appetite for his great prize, but now I knew I was looking, just as he was, at the lasting happiness we had been denied.

The next morning after breakfast he said to me: 'I'd so much like to walk to that seat overlooking the lake,' so we set off at a snail's pace across the lawn. Little Mrs Hayman stayed tactfully in the house, but no doubt he had given her orders beforehand about making herself scarce at the right moment.

When we were finally settled on the seat by the lake we held hands and waited in silence until he had recovered his breath. It was a clear, warm morning. The water was as still as glass. Birds skimmed over the surface and vanished in the reeds. Everywhere was very quiet.

At last he said with a smile: 'You've been very kind to me, haven't you?'

'For heaven's sake! What else did you expect?'

'Perhaps formal politeness masking a bitter resentment.'

I said at once with an incredulous laugh: 'You silly man, what on earth are you talking about?'

'My darling Venetia,' he said, 'do you think I never realised, as I listened to the gossip on the grapevine, that I ruined you? And do you really think that I – with my deep horror of destroying women – could ever die in peace unless I had made some attempt, no matter how feeble, to put right the great wrong that I've done?'

Tears sprang to my eyes. Then pressing his gnarled old hand against my cheek I passionately denied my own destruction.

IV

There was so much I had planned to discuss with him. I wanted to examine all the dark corners of our affair so that the mysteries were finally clarified. I wanted him to tell me truthfully, without prevarication, in words of one syllable, exactly what his relationship with Dido had been not only in 1963 but from the day he married her. I wanted to discover why he had been so 'bound up', as Mrs Ashworth had put it, with such an impossible woman who was so absolutely wrong for him. That was the real mystery, of course. In 1963 I had been so young and inexperienced that I had gone off at a tangent chasing a solution to the wrong problem. The mystery had not been whether he had slept with Dido while chasing me. Obviously he had. (Or had he?) At the age of twenty-six I would have found it a massive betrayal if he had been sleeping with another woman, but now I could see that any sex he might have had with her could have been of no more emotional significance than one of his 'triple whiskies', a mere tranquilliser which helped keep him calm in stressful times. No, the real mystery was not whether he had slept with Dido but how he had come to be so incurably entangled with her, and it was this question which I was determined he should now answer.

But once again he eluded me. He always did, I realise that now. And Mrs Ashworth was right. We're not meant to know everything about other people, even those who are closest to us, and we have to accept at the end of the day that not all mysteries are solvable.

Meanwhile he was busy saying he had destroyed me.

'Darling . . .' I suddenly realised the tears were streaming down my face. He was displaying all his old talent for wrecking my make-up. 'It wasn't your fault,' I said. 'You mustn't reproach yourself. And I'm not ruined, I did survive, I'm fine.' Finding a handkerchief I started mopping my cheeks. Fortunately I now used a waterproof mascara.

'Promiscuity is so often a mark of dislocation,' he said, 'of boredom, alienation and despair. One very seldom realises that when one's young, of course, because the transient pleasure's so overwhelming. But later the pleasure no longer heals, and then, as in all cases of alienation, one yearns for the putting-right, the making-whole, the unification of the fragmented self.'

Trying to speak lightly I said: 'This sounds like the theology of atonement!'

'That's right. At-one-ment. Do you ever go to church?'

I shook my head. No point in saying anything. Nothing worthwhile to say.

'God's not there any more?'

I made a big effort. All hostesses have a duty to be sociable, even with retired clergymen who are so *louche* as to talk about God at the wrong moment. 'Oh, God's there!' I said brightly, as if we were discussing some eccentric mutual friend, 'but He's not interested in me and I'm not interested in Him. We're irrelevant to each other nowadays.'

'If you love someone they never become irrelevant.'

'Well, obviously He and I don't love each other.' I did hope the old pet wasn't going to become tiresome and spoil our very successful reunion. I tried to work out how I could tell him tactfully that I hated discussing religion because it always reminded me of Starbridge, but then I realised that any such admission would only confirm his belief that he was responsible for my spiritual destruction. I was still floundering for the words which would direct the conversation away from God when he said with strength: 'You're saying you're estranged from God. You're saying you're alienated in the wasteland. But that's the tragedy of mankind which lies at the heart not only of the doctrine of atonement but the doctrine of the Incarnation. We may be estranged from God, but God's never estranged from us. He came into the world to be at one with us and share our suffering so that mankind may be raised up, reconciled and redeemed. "God was in Christ," as the famous quotation goes, "reconciling the world to himself."'

'Yes, I know all that, darling, and of course it's lovely, so idealistic, but what relation does it have to real life as we live it today in 1975?'

'I'll tell you exactly.' He was getting stronger and stronger. The years were falling away, the clock was being put back, and for a moment I could almost believe we were sitting together again on Lady Mary. 'I'll give you an example,' he said, 'an example of the principle of atonement in action, of the spirit of the Incarnation still ceaselessly on the move, of how pain and alienation and estrangement, no matter how deep, can be transmuted and healed by the power of love – which is the power of God. I wanted to put things right between us. I came here out of love, and when you saw me you knew that. Then you didn't just open the door and say hullo. You opened the door and you smiled and you ran down the steps and you took me in your arms and you hugged me – and the demons of alienation and estrangement were vanquished at last because my love and your response had cast them out. That old pirate Jon Darrow would have said: "No demon can withstand the power of Christ!" but as a Modernist I prefer to say: "This is the Christian principle in action!" In the end Love – Love with a capital L – is the only thing that matters. I was very wrong about many things back in 1963, but at least I was right about that.'

'You're saying Charles Ashworth won the battle but John Robinson won the war?' I said, again struggling to keep my emotions at bay by adopting a light, amused tone, but he only said urgently: 'The real truth lies far beyond Ashworth and Robinson – the real truth lies with God Himself. The power of His love is such that although you may consider yourself estranged from Him, He could never consider Himself estranged from you. He's always longing for the reconciliation – the moment when you turn back to Him, as you turned back to me, and fling wide your arms and vanquish the demon of alienation.'

'Quite. Well, this theological talk is just like the old days, but –'

He refused to give up. Stubborn, pig-headed old Yorkshireman. I might have known he'd battle on. Abruptly he said: 'You remember Holman Hunt's painting, *The Light of the World*?'

'Oh darling, such an awful old piece of Victorian tat!'

'The style may be dated, but the *kerygma*, the message, is eternal. Christ stands outside the closed door, the door with no handle, and waits with his lamp for admittance to the human heart beyond –'

'All right, it's *not* just an awful old piece of Victorian tat – I was being revoltingly over-sophisticated. But again, what does all this mean in practical terms today in 1975? I know I've made a complete and utter mess of my life, but it's far too late now to start all over again!'

'It's never too late. That's the point. It's always possible to rise from the grave of pain, alienation and despair.'

'Even when one's buried beneath a concrete slab?'

'Yes! Certainly! Even then!'

'But how do I achieve this resurrection? Go back to the Church?'

At once he became sombre. 'I know the Church failed you. The Church is as fallible and imperfect as the men who run it, and I could never blame you, after all your experiences, if you hold the Church in contempt. But if you could look past the Church now to the eternal truths which lie beyond –'

'Yes, they're still there, I realise that, but how do I connect with them, how do I tune in, how do I dial their number?'

'They're not at the end of a telephone line. They're waiting on your doorstep, and all you have to do is open the great closed door, the door that Holman Hunt painted, the door that has to be opened from within.'

There was a pause. Then I astonished myself by saying: 'I can picture Christ standing at the great closed door. But I can't see myself on the inside. I think I'm on the outside, watching him, and beyond the door is my new resurrected life, but I can't figure out how to get there. So it's no good Christ just standing by the door with his lamp. That's too passive. He's got to act – he's got to stretch out his hand and grab me so that he can heave me over the threshold.'

'Then that's what will happen. One day – and I shall pray it's one day soon – you'll see him standing at the great closed door and then as you watch he'll turn and stretch out his hand.'

'Darling!' I had to give him a kiss. He was trying so hard and I loved him so much. 'All right,' I said, wanting to make him feel he had succeeded, 'I'll pray for that too – we'll both pray for my much-needed resurrection, but darling, I can't have you blaming yourself any more for my futile existence. And for God's sake, don't think I'm secretly seething with anger towards you. I've been angry in the past, I admit, but I promise you I blame you for nothing now.'

It was true. I had forgiven him. But I had to blame someone

468

for my wasted life so all the anger which I had directed outward I now turned in upon myself. With a new ferocity I continued the all-consuming task of blotting out the pain of alienation, and although occasionally I remembered that image of the outstretched hand by the great closed door, no light pierced the darkness of the wasteland where the Great Pollutant still oozed its filth across my soul.

V

Then in 1988, thirteen years after my last meeting with Aysgarth and twenty-five years after the publication of *Honest to God*, I took that wrong turning on the motorway and saw once again as if in a dream the spire of Starbridge Cathedral soaring towards the sky to lure me back to my lost paradise of long ago. And it was there in the cloisters, where Lady Mary's seat was no longer to be found, that I saw among the milling crowds the man whom I still called my Talisman, the man who then led me into the deserted garden of the Choir School, and it was there, as we sat overlooking the river, that I wept yet again for the life that had been destroyed.

VI

'Well, the trouble was,' I said in a voice devoid of emotion as I confessed the emotion I could never forget, 'I became so very, very fond of my darling Mr Dean.' Then I broke down, quietly, with the minimum of fuss, and shed two or three discreet tears into a tastefully embroidered handkerchief. In my opinion middle-aged women, who will always look revolting in distress, have absolutely no excuse for bawling away like young girls who will inevitably wind up looking dewy-eyed and lovely.

Nick was very still. He was forty-five now; I was fifty-one. The gap in our ages which had seemed such an abyss quarter of a century ago had been wiped out. We were merely middle-aged contemporaries who had shared fragments of the past. Without the owlish spectacles which had given him such a serious air in his youth, his face had an angular individuality which was striking, and as always, he was intensely watchable. He was wearing off-white slacks, a casually-styled black jacket and one of those modern clerical shirts, pale grey with a thin strip of plastic woven around the neck to symbolise the stiff collar. The informality of his appearance conveyed the impression of a clergyman on the fringes of the Church, someone unconventional, daring, possibly a trifle unorthodox. I wondered vaguely how his life had turned out but I knew little about him beyond the fact that he worked at one of the Guild churches in the City of London. Somebody had told me he counselled AIDS cases, but that rumour was hardly surprising. Everyone counselled AIDS cases nowadays. It was the fashion.

'Sorry,' I said, giving my eyes one last dab with the tasteful handkerchief. 'Silly of me. Take no notice.'

He said again as he had said a few moments before: 'Forgive.'

'I did forgive him. Long ago.'

'But have you forgiven the most important person of all?'

'Who's that?'

'Yourself.'

I was transfixed. Then I scrabbled for my powder compact and tried to hide my confusion by giving my nose a quick pat with the puff. Despite the fact that my tears had been shed so discreetly, I had still wound up looking revolting. Poor Nick, landed with a middle-aged fright! I resolved to adopt a bright new sociable manner to extricate us both from embarrassment.

'What are you doing down here?' I enquired agreeably, dropping the powder compact back in my bag.

'I'm a consultant to the diocese of Starbridge. The Bishop calls me in sometimes.'

'Oh yes? What's your special expertise?'

'The paranormal.'

I boggled but made a quick recovery. 'Still treading your mystical paths?'

He smiled but said nothing.

'Laid any good ghosts lately?' I said gaily as if I were chatting to a difficult guest at a cocktail party.

'I'm beginning to think you yourself are a ghost,' he said, 'a spirit crying out to be laid to rest.'

'Well, darling, you can lay me any time you please! My pleasure.' I stood up, intent on giving the impression that I was well in command of myself again, and added briskly: 'Were you on your way to the South Canonry to see the Bishop when you rescued me?'

'No, I'd already been to the South Canonry and I'd decided to kill time in the cloisters while I waited for evensong . . . Will you stroll back with me to the north porch?'

We began to walk up the path away from the river to the door in the wall which separated us from the stonemasons' yard. After a long silence in which I was wholly absorbed in remembering the evensongs of 1963, he said: 'Why did you yourself come to Starbridge today?'

'God knows. But my dear, never mind about me – I'm just languishing on my own private scrap-heap! Tell me all about the Church of England in 1988 – does anyone still remember *Honest to God*?'

'Some books have just been published to mark the twenty-fifth anniversary. A few middle-aged churchmen are getting nostalgic, but I suspect the younger generation are largely indifferent to the dated theology of the 'sixties.'

'So all that starry-eyed radicalism which was going to create the New Reformation –'

'– expired. The New Reformation ran aground on the rocks of apathy, the Radicals are now thrashing about in a dead end and the Liberals are being knocked so hard that they can only reel punch-drunk from one crisis to the next. This is the day of the conservatives, and the Evangelicals are finally on the march.'

'My God, that's exactly what Charley Ashworth prophesied in 1963!'

'Ah well,' said Nick dryly, opening the door in the wall, 'it would be hard to find someone more conservative than Charley.'

'And where do you stand amidst all these warring factions?'

'Beyond them.'

We moved into the stonemasons' yard and as Nick closed the door behind us I said: 'I remember your father talking of the religion that was beyond fashion. But if you represent timeless mysticism and Charley represents the Evangelicals, who among our former acquaintances now stands for the Liberal-Radical wing?'

'Ah, that would be Primrose Tait,' said Nick. 'She's a great power nowadays in the Movement for the Ordination of Women.'

'Oh God!' I rolled my eyes heavenwards in mock horror, just as I always did whenever a successful woman appeared on the horizon to make me despise myself for my lost opportunities. 'Thank heavens I'm right outside it all! What a circus!'

Nick said swiftly: 'So you're happy on your scrap-heap, are you?' but pride made me retort: 'In total bliss, darling! It's the only place where a worthless old hag of a failure like me could ever feel thoroughly at home!'

'So that's how you see yourself, is it? Worthless? A failure? Unforgivable?'

'Well, be frank, Nick! How do you see me?'

'I follow a man,' said my Talisman, 'who believed that each one of us has worth, and that no one is unforgivable.'

To my horror I found I was unable to deliver a glib reply — or indeed any reply at all.

We re-entered the Close by the main entrance of the stone-masons' yard, and as we began to move around the vast west front of the Cathedral towards the north porch, I became painfully aware that although I was near enough to touch the walls I was utterly severed from the great mystery beyond them. Then at last the alienation and estrangement, that famous *angst* of twentieth-century man, seemed unbearable. My soul ached. I longed to shed the pollution which poisoned it, but I was so weak. I could only say mildly, absurdly, to Nick: 'Did you ever see *Ben Hur*?' No cry for help could ever have been more obscure.

'The Charlton Heston version?'

472

'Yes, there was one part I always remember and it wasn't that bloody chariot race. It was when Christ was preaching to the crowd – although one never saw the face of Christ, only his back, and one never heard him, they merely played a special kind of music –'

'I remember.'

'– and Ben Hur appeared on the edge of the crowd. He was right in the background and one saw him move around the outer fringes – just as we're doing now, moving around the edge of the Cathedral – and as Ben Hur moved, Christ moved too and one realised that Christ was watching him –'

'Yes, that was a very dramatic moment.'

'– but I can't quite remember what happened next.'

'Ben Hur was drawn in from the fringes.'

'He was? But not in that scene, surely.'

'Then it was later.'

We turned the corner and saw the north porch. Above us, somewhere in the tower below the spire, the bell was tolling for evensong.

'Well!' I said brightly, pausing by the porch and wondering what on earth had driven me to ramble on so disjointedly about an ancient Hollywood epic. 'It's been heavenly to see you again – keep treading those mystical paths! I suppose you'll eventually waft back into my orbit some day, just as you always do.'

In reply he took out his wallet, produced a card and handed it to me. The card read: 'The Reverend Nicholas Darrow, St Benet's-by-the-Wall, Egg Street, London E.C.2.' 'Give me a call,' he said, 'when you get back to town.'

'My dear, what fun! But I mustn't distract you from all your paranormal phenomena!' I was acutely aware that he had asked for neither my phone number nor my address. The card was a mere gesture of politeness, nothing more, a move which could be labelled 'concerned' and 'caring', a minor spiritual charade which would salve his Christian conscience.

'So long, Venetia,' he was saying with a smile as he turned away into the north porch. He even added that most meaningless of all Americanisms: 'Take care.'

'Goodbye, Nick.' I remained outside, staring after him, his card already screwed up in my hand for deposit in the nearest litter-bin.

Then he stopped. He had reached the huge oak door which led into the Cathedral, and for one long moment he stood there – he stood there as if waiting by the great closed door, and suddenly I thought: Holman Hunt. *The Light of the World.*

I knew then what was going to happen next, but I didn't dare believe it. My voice cried in my head: he won't, he can't, he couldn't –

But he did. And as I stared through my tears in wonder, unable to move or speak, he turned back to me and he stretched out his hand.

AUTHOR'S NOTE

Scandalous Risks is the fourth in a series of six novels about the Church of England in the twentieth century; each book is designed to be read independently of the others, but the more books are read the wider will be the view of the multi-sided reality which is being presented.

The first novel, *Glittering Images*, narrated by Charles Ashworth, was set in 1937. *Glamorous Powers*, narrated by Jon Darrow, opened in 1940, and *Ultimate Prizes* was narrated by Neville Aysgarth after the war. The fifth novel, *Mystical Paths*, will examine the Church in 1968 from the point of view of Nicholas Darrow.

*   *   *

Aysgarth's thought (though not his private life) derives from the writings of John Arthur Thomas Robinson (1919–1983) in the 1960s. Robinson was born in the shadow of Canterbury Cathedral where his father was a canon, and educated at Marlborough and at Jesus College, Cambridge; he gained a degree in classics, a first in theology and a doctorate in philosophy. After he was ordained in 1945 he was a curate at Bristol and a chaplain at Wells Theological College before he became Dean of Clare College, Cambridge and Lecturer in New Testament in the University Faculty of Divinity in 1951. He was still under forty when he was asked by Dr Mervyn Stockwood, then Bishop of Southwark, to be his suffragan (assistant) bishop at Woolwich. The Archbishop of Canterbury, Dr Geoffrey Fisher, was opposed to this appointment, mainly on the ground that Robinson was too young for episcopal rank, but Stockwood persisted and Robinson became Bishop of Woolwich in 1959. By this time he had been married for some years and had four children.

In 1960 he gained nationwide notoriety during the Crown's prosecution of Penguin Books for publishing an alleged obscene novel, the unexpurgated edition of *Lady Chatterley's Lover* by D. H. Lawrence. Robinson agreed to be a witness for the defence, but some of his opinions, taken out of context, provided sensational headlines for the press; his remark that sex was an act of holy communion (widely misinterpreted as Holy Communion) dates from this time. Archbishop Fisher commented: 'In my judgement the Bishop was mistaken to think that he could take part in the trial without becoming a stumbling-block to many ordinary Christians.'

Less than three years later, in March 1963, Robinson was hitting the national headlines again when the SCM Press published his most famous work, *Honest to God*. In the seven months following publication, 350,000 copies were sold and seven translations were about to be published. It was, so its publisher David L. Edwards claimed, the fastest-selling book of serious theology in the history of the world, and clearly by trying to restate Christianity in an up-to-date form and by introducing the general public to the writings of modern theologians Robinson connected with a vast religious interest buried deep in what was too often assumed to be a largely Godless and secular society. Dr Michael Ramsey, who had succeeded Dr Fisher as Archbishop of Canterbury, was at first hostile to the book but later revised this initial reaction and admitted: 'I was soon to grasp how many were the contemporary gropings and quests which lay behind *Honest to God*.' Robinson received over four thousand letters, some of which were published in *The Honest to God Debate*, edited by David L. Edwards, in October 1963. This book also contained, in addition to favourable reviews, strong criticism of the book from professional theologians.

After ten years as Bishop of Woolwich Robinson returned to Cambridge as Dean of Chapel at Trinity. This appointment was not altogether a success and Robinson did not become the prophetic voice of the 1970s as many in the Church had hoped that he would. It was noticeable that his New Testament scholarship became increasingly conservative. In 1983 he was diagnosed as suffering from cancer and he died in the December of that year. His last book, *The Priority of John*, was published posthumously, and in reviewing it Canon Leslie Houlden wrote: 'The public reputation of John Robinson . . . was at its height in the sixties. On the theological scene he seemed to epitomise the spirit of that period as well as anyone . . . yet to see him as a thrillingly shocking radical was a misconception . . . He hunted with no pack for long but went his own way . . . Those who have seen him as a late Victorian radical born out of due time are perhaps the most discerning.'

Honest to God is still in print, and in 1988 the SCM Press published *God's Truth*, a collection of essays to celebrate the twenty-fifth anniversary of this landmark in the history of the twentieth-century Church of England.